Ocular Treatment: Evidence Based

Ocular Treatment: Evidence Based

Frederick Hampton Roy MD FACS
Hampton Roy Eyecare
Little Rock, Arkansas, USA

Co-author

Renee Tindall RN
Director
Hampton Roy Eyecare
Little Rock, Arkansas, USA

JAYPEE The Health Sciences Publisher
New Delhi | London | Panama | Philadelphia

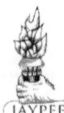 **Jaypee Brothers Medical Publishers (P) Ltd**

Headquarters

Jaypee Brothers Medical Publishers (P) Ltd.
4838/24, Ansari Road, Daryaganj
New Delhi 110 002, India
Phone: +91-11-43574357
Fax: +91-11-43574314
E-mail: jaypee@jaypeebrothers.com

Overseas Offices

J.P. Medical Ltd.
83, Victoria Street, London
SW1H 0HW (UK)
Phone: +44-20 3170 8910
Fax: +44(0)20 3008 6180
E-mail: info@jpmedpub.com

Jaypee Medical Inc.
The Bourse
111, South Independence Mall East
Suite 835, Philadelphia, PA 19106, USA
Phone: +1 267-519-9789
E-mail: jpmed.us@gmail.com

Jaypee Brothers Medical Publishers (P) Ltd.
Bhotahity, Kathmandu, Nepal
Phone: +977-9741283608
E-mail: kathmandu@jaypeebrothers.com

Jaypee-Highlights Medical Publishers Inc.
City of Knowledge, Bld. 237, Clayton
Panama City, Panama
Phone: +1 507-301-0496
Fax: +1 507-301-0499
E-mail: cservice@jphmedical.com

Jaypee Brothers Medical Publishers (P) Ltd.
17/1-B, Babar Road, Block-B, Shaymali
Mohammadpur, Dhaka-1207
Bangladesh
Mobile: +08801912003485
E-mail: jaypeedhaka@gmail.com

Website: www.jaypeebrothers.com
Website: www.jaypeedigital.com

Inquiries for bulk sales may be solicited at: jaypee@jaypeebrothers.com

Ocular Treatment: Evidence Based

First Edition: **2015**

ISBN 978-93-5152-246-1

Printed at Rajkamal Electric Press, Plot No. 2, Phase-IV, Kundli, Haryana.

Dedicated to

Kay, Charles, Frederick, Kimberly,
Robert, Hampton Nichols and Constance
Helena, Neeli, Blake, Tyler, Trey,
Cooper, Keetin and Cross

Preface

This text is the first edition. It is a combination of Ocular Differential Diagnosis and Ocular Syndrome and Systemic Diseases (Both published by Jaypee Brothers Medical Publishers (P) Ltd., New Delhi, India).

My approach is to take selected differential diagnosis from Ocular Differential Diagnosis (ODDX) and combine with Ocular Syndromes and Systemic Disease. This provides evidence-based differential diagnosis with listings with each item.

The book allows access to the disorder either anatomically or by classification of the disorder. Once the reader is in the proper section, a list of the more common entities is available with a concise description, diagnostic laboratory, and treatment. Some ophthalmologic disorders can only be diagnosed by clinical observation. In these cases a detailed physical description of the entity is listed.

Ptosis, for example, has large categories of congenital and adult-onset ptosis. These disease entities are divided into age of onset and then a descriptive list of possible causes are listed under each category.

Although drug dosages and methods of administration have been scrutinized, it is important that each physician exercise his or her own judgment in the choice or use of a drug. The physician is advised to check the product information included in the drug's package insert before drug administration. New data and individual clinical situations can change the drug regimen.

Frederick Hampton Roy

Contents

1. Infectious Diseases   **1**

- Acinetobacter (Mima Polymorpha; Acinetobacter Iwoffi)   1
- Acquired Immunodeficiency Syndrome (AIDS; Acquired Cellular Immunodeficiency; Acquired Immunodeficiency)   1
- Acute Hemorrhagic Conjunctivitis (AHC; Epidemic Hemorrhagic Keratoconjunctivitis, Apollo 11 Disease)   2
- Aspergillosis   3
- Bacillus Species Infections   3
- Blastomycosis   4
- Brucellosis (Bang Disease; Malta Fever; Mediterranean Fever; Pig Breeder Disease; Gibraltar Fever; Undulant Fever)   4
- Candidiasis   5
- Catscratch Oculoglandular Syndrome (Parinaud Conjunctiva-Adenitis Syndrome; Parinaud Oculoglandular Syndrome; Catscratch Disease; Bartonella Henselae)   5
- Coccidioidomycosis (Valley Fever, San Joaquin Fever)   6
- Deerfly Fever (Francis Disease; Rabbit Fever; Tularemia; Deerfly Tularemia)   6
- Dengue Fever   6
- Dermatophytosis (Epidermophytosis; Epidcrmomycosis; Rubrophytia; Tinea; Trichophytosis)   7
- Diphtheria   7
- Epidemic Keratoconjunctivitis   8
- Erysipelas (Saint Anthony Fire)   8
- Escherichia Coli   9
- Gonorrhea   9
- Haemophilus Aegyptius (Koch-Weeks Bacillus)   10
- Haemophilus Influenzae   10
- Hansen Disease (Leprosy)   10
- Herpes Simplex   11
- Herpes Simplex Masquerade Syndrome   11
- Inclusion Conjunctivitis (Chlamydia; Paratrachoma)   12

- Infectious Mononucleosis (Mononucleosis; Epstein-Barr Virus, Acute; Acute Epstein-Barr Virus, Glandular Fever)   12
- Influenza   13
- Leptospirosis (Weil Disease)   13
- Lyme Disease   14
- Marseilles Fever (Boutonneuse Fever)   14
- Microsporidial Infection   14
- Molluscum Contagiosum   15
- Moraxella Lacunata   15
- Mucormycosis (Phycomycosis)   16
- Mumps   16
- Newcastle Disease (Fowlpox)   16
- Nocardiosis   17
- Pappataci Fever (Phlebotomus Fever; Sandfly Fever)   17
- Pharyngoconjunctival Fever (Acute Follicular Conjunctivitis; Adenoviral Conjunctivitis; Syndrome of Beal)   18
- Pneumococcal Infections (Streptococcus Pneumoniae Infections)   18
- Presumed Ocular Histoplasmosis (Histoplasmosis Choroiditis; Histoplasmosis Maculopathy; Histoplasmosis Syndrome)   19
- Propionibacterium Acnes   19
- Proteus Infections   19
- Proteus Syndrome   20
- Pseudomonas Aeruginosa Infections   20
- Q Fever (Coxiella Burnetii)   21
- Rabies (Hydrophobia; Lyssa)   21
- Rhinosporidiosis   22
- Rocky Mountain Spotted Fever   22
- Rubella Syndrome (Congenital Rubella Syndrome; German Measles; Gregg Syndrome)   22
- Rubeola (Measles; Morbilli)   23
- Sporotrichosis   23
- Staphylococcus   24
- Streptococcus (Scarlet Fever)   24
- Syphilis (Acquired Lues; Acquired Syphilis; Lues Venerea; Malum Venereum)   25

- Syphilis, Congenital (Congenital Lues) 25
- Tetanus (Lockjaw) 26
- Trachoma 26
- Tuberculosis 27
- Typhoid Fever (Abdominal Typhus; Enteric Fever) 27
- Varicella (Chickenpox) 28
- Varicella Syndrome, Congenital 28
- Yersiniosis 28

2. **Parasitic Diseases** **29**

- Acanthamoeba 29
- Baylisascaris (Unilateral Subacute Neuroretinitis; Ocular Larva Migrans) 29
- Coenurosis (Tapeworm) 30
- Demodicosis 30
- Hydatid Cyst (Echinococcosis) 31
- Nematode Ophthalmia Syndrome (Visceral Larva Migrans Syndrome; Toxocariasis) 31
- Pediculosis and Phthiriasis 32
- Toxoplasmosis (Toxoplasmic Retinochoroiditis; Ocular Toxoplasmosis) 32
- Trichinellosis (Trichinosis) 33

3. **Nutritional Disorders** **34**

- Crohn Disease (Granulomatous Ileocolitis) 34
- Hypovitaminosis A (Xerophthalmia) 35
- Inflammatory Bowel Disease (Ulcerative Colitis; Regional Enteritis) 35

4. **Disorders of Protein Metabolism** **36**

- Lowe Syndrome (Oculo-Cerebro-Renal Syndrome) 36
- ML I (Mucolipidosis I; Lipomucopoly-saccharidosis; Dysmorphic Sialidosis; Spranger Syndrome) 36
- Tyrosinosis (Hanhart Syndrome; Richner Syndrome; Recessive Keratosis Palmoplantaris; Pseudoherpetic Keratitis; Richner-Hanhart Syndrome; Tyrosinemia II; Pseudodendritic Keratitis) 37

5. **Disorders of Carbohydrate Metabolism** **38**

- Diabetes Mellitus 38
- Fanconi Syndrome (Toni-Fanconi Syndrome; Amino Diabetes; Hypochloremic-Glycosuric Osteonephropathy Syndrome; De Toni-Fanconi Syndrome) 39

- Hunter Syndrome (MPS II Syndrome; Mucopolysaccharidosis II; Systemic Mucopolysaccharidosis Type II) 39
- Hurler Syndrome (Pfaundler-Hurler Syndrome; Gargoylism; Dysostosis Multiplex; MPS IH Syndrome; Systemic Mucopolysaccharidosis Type IH; Mucopolysaccharidosis IH) 40
- Juvenile Diabetes-Dwarfism-Obesity Syndrome (Mauriac Syndrome; Dwarfism-Hepatomegaly-Obesity-Juvenile Diabetes Syndrome) 40
- Kimmelstiel-Wilson Syndrome (Diabetes Mellitus-Hypertension-Nephrosis Syndrome; Diabetes-Nephrosis Syndrome; Diabetic Glomerulosclerosis; Intercapillary Glomerulosclerosis;Renal Glomerulohyalinosis-Diabetic Syndrome) 41
- Marquardt-Loriaux Syndrome (Wolfram Syndrome; Diabetes Insipidus-Diabetes Mellitus-OpticAtrophy-Deafness Syndrome; DIDMOAD Syndrome) 41
- Mucopolysaccharidosis VII (Beta-Glucuronidase Deficiency; MPS VII) 42
- Sanfilippo-Good Syndrome (Heparitinuria; Mucopolysaccharidosis III; MPS III) 42
- Scheie Syndrome (Mucopolysaccharidosis IS; MPS IS; MPS V; Mucopolysaccharidosis V) 43
- Spondyloepiphyseal Dysplasia (Morquio Syndrome; Morquio-Brailsford Syndrome; Brailsford-Morquio Dystrophy; Familial Osseous Dystrophy; Keratosulfaturia; MPS IV; Mucopolysaccharidosis IV; Osteochondrodystrophia Deformans; Infantile Hereditary Chondrodysplasia; Hereditary Polytopic Enchondral Dysostosis; Hereditary Osteochondro-dystrophy; Eccentro-Osteochondrodysplasia; Dysostosis Enchondralis Meta-Epiphysaria; Morquio-Ullrich Syndrome; Atypical Chondrodystrophy; Chondrodystrophia Tarda; Chondro-Osteodystrophy) 43
- Systemic Mucopolysaccharidosis Type VI (Mucopolysaccharidosis VI; Maroteaux-Lamy Syndrome; MPS VI Syndrome) 44
- Tropical Pancreatic Diabetes (TPD) (Background Retinopathy) 45
- Von Reuss Syndrome (Galactosemic Syndrome; Galactokinase Deficiency; Galactosemia), Nystagmus 45

6. Disorders of Lipid Metabolism   **46**

- Fabry Disease (Angiokeratoma Corporis
  Diffusum Syndrome; Diffuse Angiokeratosis;
  Fabry-Anderson Syndrome; Glycosphingolipid
  Lipidosis; Glycosphingolipidosis)   46
- Hyperlipoproteinemia   47

7. Hematologic and Cardiovascular Disorders   **48**

- Carotid Artery Syndrome
  (Cavernous Sinus Fistula Syndrome;
  Red-Eyed Shunt Syndrome)   48
- Carotid Artery Syndrome
  (Carotid Vascular Insufficiency Syndrome;
  Ocular Ischemic Syndrome)   49
- Foramen Lacerum Syndrome (Aneurysm of
  Internal Carotid Artery Syndrome)   49
- Herrick Syndrome (Dresbach Syndrome;
  Sickle Cell Disease; Drepanocytic Anemia)   50
- Scheie Syndrome (Mucopolysaccharidosis IS;
  MPS IS; MPS V; Mucopolysaccharidosis V)   50
- Thalassemia (Cooley Anemia;
  Thalassemia Major; Thalassemia Minor)   51
- Vaquez Disease (Polycythemia Vera;
  Erythema; Erythrocytosis Megalosplenica;
  Myelopathic Polycythemia; Vaquez-Osler
  Syndrome; Cryptogenic Polycythemia;
  Polycythemia Rubra; Splenomegalic
  Polycythemia)   51

8. Dermatologic Disorders   **52**

- Atopic Dermatitis (Atopic Eczema;
  Besnier Prurigo)   52
- Bullous Ichthyosiform Erythroderma
  (Collodion Baby; Congenital Ichthyosis;
  Epidermolytic Hyperkeratosis; Ichthyosis;
  Ichthyosis Vulgaris; Lamellar Ichthyosis;
  Nonbullous Ichthyosiform Erythroderma;
  Xeroderma; X-Linked Ichthyosis)   52
- Contact Dermatitis (Dermatitis Venenata)   53
- Dermatostomatitis [Stevens-Johnson
  Syndrome; Erythema Multiforme Exudativum;
  Syndroma Mucocutaneo-Oculare; Baader
  Dermatostomatitis Syndrome; Mucosal-
  Respiratory Syndrome; Fuchs (2) Syndrome;
  Mucocutaneous Ocular Syndrome]   53
- Disseminated Lupus Erythematosus (Systemic
  Lupus Erythematosus; Lupus Erythematosus;
  Kaposi-Libman-Sack Syndrome, SLE)   54
- Erythema Nodosum
  (Dermatitis Contusiformis)   54

- Mastocytosis (Urticaria; Mast Cell Leukemia)   55
- Acne Rosacea
  (Acne Erythematosa; Ocular Rosacea)   55
- Psoriasis (Psoriasis Vulgaris)   56
- Quincke Disease (Giant Edema;
  Giant Urticaria; Hives; Nettle Rash;
  Angioneurotic Edema)   56

9. Connective Tissue Disorders   **57**

- Amyloidosis (Primary Amyloidosis; Lubarsch-
  Pick Syndrome; Idiopathic Amyloidosis)   57
- Amyloidosis of Gingiva and Conjunctiva,
  with Mental Retardation
  (Primary Systemic Amyloidosis)   58
- Behçet Syndrome (Dermato-Stomato-
  Ophthalmic Syndrome; Oculobuccogenital
  Syndrome; Gilbert Syndrome)   58
- Cogan (2) Syndrome (Oculomotor Apraxia
  Syndrome; Wieacker Syndrome)   59
- Felty Syndrome (Chauffard-Still Syndrome;
  Primary Splenic Neutropenia with Arthritis;
  Rheumatoid Arthritis with Hypersplenism;
  Still-Chauffard Syndrome;
  Uveitis-Rheumatoid Arthritis Syndrome)   59
- Grönblad-Strandberg Syndrome
  (Systemic Elastodystrophy; Pseudoxanthoma
  Elasticum; Elastorrhexis; Darier-Grönblad-
  Strandberg Syndrome)   60
- Hamman-Rich Syndrome (Alveolar Capillary
  Block Syndrome; Diffuse Pulmonary Fibrosis
  Syndrome; Rheumatoid Lung Syndrome)   60
- Juvenile Rheumatoid Arthritis
  (JRA; Still Disease)   61
- Marfan Syndrome (Dolichostenomelia;
  Arachnodactyly; Hyperchondroplasia;
  Dystrophia; Mesodermalis Congenita)   61
- Morphea (Localized Scleroderma;
  Circumscribed Scleroderma)   62
- Relapsing Polychondritis (Jaksch-Wartenhost
  Syndrome; Meyenburg-Altherz-Vehlinger
  Syndrome; von Meyenberg II Syndrome)   62
- Rheumatoid Arthritis (Adult)   63
- Schaumann Syndrome (Besnier-Boeck-Schau-
  mann Syndrome; Boeck Sarcoid; Sarcoidosis)   63
- Scleroderma (Progressive Systemic Sclerosis;
  Systemic Scleroderma)   64
- Systemic Lupus Erythematosus (Disseminated
  Lupus Erythematosus; Lupus Erythematosus;
  Kaposi-Libman-Sack Syndrome, SLE)   64

- Temporal Arteritis Syndrome (Cranial Arteritis Syndrome; Giant Cell Arteritis; Hutchinson-Horton-Magath-Brown Syndrome) 65
- Uveitis, Juvenile Idiopathic Arthritis 65
- von Bekhterev-Strümpell Syndrome (Marie-Strümpell Spondylitis; Ankylosing Spondylitis; Pierre-Marie Syndrome; Bekhterev Disease; Rheumatoid Spondylitis), Optic Atrophy 66
- Wegener Syndrome (Wegener Granulomatosis) 66
- Weill-Marchesani Syndrome (Marchesani Syndrome; Inverted Marfan Syndrome; Brachymorphy with Spherophakia; Dystrophia Mesodermalis Congenita Hyperplastica) 67

10. Skeletal Disorders **68**

- Down Syndrome (Mongolism; Trisomy G; Trisomy 21 Syndrome; Mongoloid Idiocy) 68

11. Phakomatoses **69**

- Angiomatosis Retinae (von Hippel-Lindau Syndrome; Retinocerebral Angiomatosis; Cerebelloretinal Hemangioblastomatosis; Lindau Syndrome; Retinal Capillary Hamartoma) 69
- Neurofibromatosis Type I (von Recklinghausen Syndrome; Neurinomatosis) 69
- Sturge-Weber Syndrome (Meningocutaneous Syndrome; Vascular Encephalotrigeminal Syndrome; Neuro-Oculocutaneous Angiomatosis; Encephalofacial Angiomatosis; Encephalotrigeminal Syndrome) 70

12. Neurologic Disorders **71**

- Amblyopia (Functional Amblyopia, Lazy Eye) 71
- Aniridia, Cerebellar Ataxia, and Mental Deficiency (Gillespie Syndrome) 71
- Arnold-Chiari Syndrome (Platybasia Syndrome; Cerebellomedullary Malformation Syndrome; Basilar Impressions) 72
- Andersen-Warburg Syndrome (Whitnall-Norman Syndrome; Oligophrenia Microphthalmos Syndrome; Norrie Disease; Atrophia Oculi Congenital Fetal Iritis Syndrome; Congenital Progressive Oculo-Acoustico-Cerebral Dysplasia) 72
- Batten-Mayou Syndrome (Spielmeyer-Vogt Syndrome; Mayou-Batten Disease; Stock-Spielmeyer-Vogt Syndrome; Cerebroretinal Degeneration; Pigmentary Retinal Lipoid Neuronal Heredodegeneration; Vogt-Spielmeyer Syndrome; Juvenile Ganglioside Lipidosis; Neuronal Ceroid Lipofuscinosis; Myoclonic Variant of Cerebral Lipidosis; Batten Disease; Cerebromacular Dystrophy; Juvenile Amaurotic Family Idiocy; Spielmeyer-Sjögren Syndrome) 73
- Bell's Palsy (Idiopathic Facial Paralysis) 74
- Bielschowsky-Lutz-Cogan Syndrome (Internuclear Ophthalmoplegia) 74
- Bonnet-Dechaume-Blanc Syndrome (Cerebroretinal Arteriovenous Aneurysm Syndrome; Neuroretinoangiomatosis Syndrome; Wyburn-Mason Syndrome) 75
- Cerebellar Ataxia, Infantile, with Progressive External Ophthalmoplegia 75
- Cerebellar Ataxia, Cataract, Deafness and Dementia or Psychosis (Heredopathia Ophthalmo-Oto-Encephalica) 76
- Cerebellar Degeneration with Slow Movements 76
- Cerebral Autosomal Dominant Arteriopathy 76
- Cerebral Cholesterolosis (Cerebrotendinous Xanthomatosis; CTX) 77
- Cerebral Palsy 77
- Chronic Progressive External Ophthalmoplegia (CPEO; Ophthalmoplegia Plus) 78
- Claude Syndrome (Inferior Nucleus Ruber Syndrome; Rubrospinal-Cerebellar-Peduncle Syndrome) 78
- Congenital Dyslexia Syndrome (Developmental Dyslexia of Critchley; Congenital Word Blindness of Hermann; Primary Dyslexia; Dyslexia Syndrome; Minimal Brain Dysfunction Syndrome; Attention Deficit Disorder; Congenital Word Blindness) 79
- Creutzfeldt-Jakob Syndrome (Spastic Pseudosclerosis; Corticostriatospinal Degeneration; Disseminated Encephalopathy; Heidenhain Syndrome; Presenile Dementia with Spastic Paralysis; Presenile Dementia-Cortical Degeneration Syndrome) 79

- Cushing (2) Syndrome (Angle Tumor Syndrome; Cerebellopontine Angle Syndrome; Pontocerebellar Angle Tumor Syndrome; Acoustic Neuroma Syndrome)   80
- De Lange Syndrome (I) (Congenital Muscular Hypertrophy Cerebral Syndrome; Brachmann-De Lange Syndrome)   80
- Disseminated Sclerosis (Multiple Sclerosis)   81
- Friedreich Ataxia (Spinocerebellar Ataxia)   81
- Hartnup Syndrome (Pellagra-Cerebellar Ataxia-Renal Aminoaciduria Syndrome; H Disease; Niacin Deficiency)   82
- Hysteria (Malingering; Ophthalmic Flake Syndrome)   82
- Joubert Syndrome (Familial Cerebellar Vermis Agenesis)   83
- Marinesco-Sjögren Syndrome (Congenital Spinocerebellar Ataxia-Congenital Cataract-Oligophrenia Syndrome)   83
- Neuroparalytic Keratitis (Neurotropic Keratitis, Trigeminal Neuropathic Keratopathy)   84
- Nothnagel Syndrome (Ophthalmoplegia-Cerebellar Ataxia Syndrome)   84
- Obesity-Cerebral-Ocular-Skeletal Anomalies Syndrome   84
- Oculocerebellar Tegmental Syndrome   85
- Oculocerebral Syndrome with Hypopigmentation (Amish Oculocerebral Syndrome; Cross Syndrome)   85
- Oculopalatocerebral Dwarfism (OPC Dwarfism)   86
- Oculorenocerebellar Syndrome (ORC Syndrome)   86
- Olivopontocerebellar Atrophy III (OPCA III; OPCA with Retinal Degeneration)   87
- Optic Atrophy with Demyelinating Disease of CNS   87
- Parkinson Syndrome (Paralysis Agitans; Shaking Palsy)   87
- Raeder Syndrome (Paratrigeminal Paralysis; Horton Headache; Histamine Cephalalgia; Ciliary Neuralgia; Cluster Headache; Periodic Migrainous Neuralgia)   88
- Sotos Syndrome (Cerebral Gigantism)   88
- Spinocerebellar Atrophy with Pupillary Paralysis   89
- Stannus Cerebellar Syndrome   89
- Symonds Syndrome (Otitic Hydrocephalus Syndrome; Serous Meningitis Syndrome; Benign Intracranial Hypertension; Pseudotumor Cerebri)   90
- Thyrocerebroretinal Syndrome (Familial Thyrocerebral-Retinal Syndrome)   90
- Tolosa-Hunt Syndrome (Painful Ophthalmoplegia)   91
- Traumatic Encephalopathy Syndrome (Posttraumatic General Cerebral Syndrome; Postconcussion Syndrome; Punch-Drunk Syndrome), Nystagmus   91
- Weber Syndrome (Weber-Dubler Syndrome; Cerebellar Peduncle Syndrome; Alternating Oculomotor Paralysis; Ventral Medial Midbrain Syndrome), Ptosis   92

13. **Neoplasms**   **93**
- Actinic and Seborrheic Keratosis   93
- Basal Cell Carcinoma   93
- Basal Cell Nevus Syndrome (Nevoid Basal Cell Carcinoma Syndrome; Nevoid Basalioma Syndrome; Gorlin Syndrome; Gorlin-Goltz Syndrome; Multiple Basal Cell Nevi Syndrome)   94
- Squamous Cell Carcinoma, Conjunctival   94
- Squamous Cell Carcinoma of Eyelid   95
- Corneal Dermoids   95
  - Bloch-Sulzberger Syndrome (Incontinentia Pigmenti; Siemens-Bloch-Sulzberger Syndrome)   95
  - Cri-du-Chat Syndrome [Cat-Cry (5p-) Syndrome; Crying Cat Syndrome; BI Deletion Syndrome; Lejeune Syndrome]   96
  - Duane Syndrome   96
  - Coats Disease (Leber Miliary Aneurysm; Retinal Telangiectasia)   97
  - Neurocutaneous Syndrome   97
  - Linear Nevus Sebaceus of Jadassohn (Nevus Sebaceus of Jadassohn; Jadassohn-Type Anetoderma; Organoid Nevus Syndrome; Sebaceus Nevus Syndrome)   98
  - Goldenhar Syndrome (Oculo-Auriculo-Vertebral Dysplasia; Goldenhar-Gorlin Syndrome)   98
  - Ring Dermoid Syndrome (Amblyopia)   99

- Craniopharyngioma 99
- Dermoid (Dermoid Choristoma; Dermoid Cyst; Dermolipoma; Lipodermoid) 99
- Dermoid, Orbital 100
- Ring Dermoid Syndrome (Amblyopia) 100
- Ewing Sarcoma (Ewing Syndrome) 101
- Fibrosarcoma 101
- Hemangioma, Capillary 101
- Hodgkin Disease 102
- Hutchinson Syndrome (Adrenal Cortex Neuroblastoma with Orbital Metastasis; Pepper Syndrome) 102
- Juvenile Xanthogranuloma (JXG; Nevoxanthoendothelioma) 103
- Kaposi Disease (Kaposi Sarcoma; Kaposi Hemorrhagic Sarcoma; Multiple Idiopathic Hemorrhagic Sarcoma; Kaposi Varicelliform Eruption) 103
- Kasabach-Merritt Syndrome (CapillaryAngioma-Thrombocytopenia; Hemangioma-Thrombocytopenia; Thrombocytopenia Purpura-Hemangioma) 104
- Keratoacanthoma 104
- Leiomyoma 105
- Liposarcoma 105
- Lymphangioma 105
- Lymphoid Hyperplasia (Reactive Lymphoid Hyperplasia; Lymphoid Tumors; Malignant Lymphoma; Pseudolymphoma; Pseudotumor; Burkitt Lymphoma; Neoplastic Angioendotheliomatosis) 106
- Medulloepithelioma (Diktyoma) 106
- Meningioma 107
- Meningioma, Optic Nerve Sheath 107
- Meningioma, Sphenoid Wing 108
- Mucocele (Pyocele) 108
- Neurilemmoma (Schwannoma; Neurinoma, PTEN Hamartoma Tumor Syndrome) 108
- Neuroblastoma 109
- Optic Gliomas 109
- Orbital Lymphoma 110
- Orbital Rhabdomyosarcoma 110
- Papilloma (Wart; Verruca) 110
- Periocular Merkel Cell Carcinoma 111
- Periocular Metastatic Tumors (Ocular Metastatic Tumors) 111
- Reticulum Cell Sarcoma (Non-Hodgkin Lymphoma) 112
- Retinoblastoma 112
- Rhabdomyosarcoma (Corneal Edema) 113
- Sebaceous Gland Carcinoma 113

14. Mechanical and Non-Mechanical Injuries 114
- Acid Burns 114
- Alkaline Injury of the Eye 114
- Ciliary Body Concussions and Lacerations 115
- Conjunctival Lacerations 115
- Corneal Foreign Body 115
- Electrical Injury 116
- Extraocular Muscle Lacerations 116
- Eyelid Contusions, Lacerations and Avulsions 117
- Hypothermal Injury (Cryoinjury; Frostbite) 117
- Intraocular Foreign Body: Copper 117
- Intraocular Foreign Body: Nonmagnetic Chemically Inert 118
- Intraocular Foreign Body: Steel or Iron 118
- Lacrimal System Contusions and Lacerations 118
- Orbital Cellulitis and Abscess 119
- Orbital Compartment Syndrome, Acute 119
- Orbital Fracture, Apex 120
- Orbital Hemorrhages 120
- Orbital Implant Extrusion 120
- Orbital Infarction Syndrome 121
- Scleral Ruptures and Lacerations 121
- Shaken Baby Syndrome (Battered-Baby Syndrome; Battered-Child Syndrome; Child Abuse Syndrome; Silverman Syndrome) 122
- Thermal Burns 122

15. Unclassified Disease or Conditions 123
- Kimmelstiel-Wilson Syndrome (Diabetes Mellitus-Hypertension-Nephrosis Syndrome; Diabetes-Nephrosis Syndrome; Diabetic Glomerulosclerosis; Intercapillary Glomerulosclerosis; Renal Glomerulohyalinosis-Diabetic Syndrome) 123
- Papillorenal Syndrome (Renal-Coloboma Syndrome) 123
- Vogt-Koyanagi-Harada Disease (Harada Disease; Uveitis-Vitiligo-Alopecia-Poliosis Syndrome) 124

16. Anterior Chamber   **125**

- Anterior Chamber Cleavage Syndrome (Reese-Ellsworth Syndrome; Peters-Plus Syndrome)   125
- Anterior Segment Ischemia Syndrome   126
- Cholesterolosis of the Anterior Chamber   126
  - Chronic Uveitis, Anterior Granulomatous (Iritis)   126
  - Eales Disease (Periphlebitis)   127
  - Subluxation, Dislocation of the Lens   127
  - Microcephaly, Microphthalmia, Cataracts, and Joint Contractures   128
  - Phthisis Bulbi   128
  - Retinal Detachment/Giant Retinal Tears   128
  - Traumatic Cataract   129
  - Vitreous Hemorrhage   129
- Epithelial Ingrowth (Epithelial Downgrowth)   129
- Frenkel Syndrome (Ocular Contusion Syndrome; Anterior Segment Traumatic Syndrome)   130
- Gas Bubbles in the Anterior Chamber   130
  - Clostridium Perfringens   130
  - Escherichia Coli   131
- Glaucoma, Hyphema   131
- Hyphema (Bleeding into the Anterior Chamber)   132
  - Fuchs (1) Syndrome (Heterochromic Cyclitis Syndrome)   132
  - Gonorrhea   133
  - Herpes Zoster   133
  - Juvenile Rheumatoid Arthritis (JRA; Still Disease)   134
  - Von Bekhterev-Strumpell Syndrome (Marie-Strumpell Spondylitis; Ankylosing Spondylitis; Pierre-Marie Syndrome; Bekhterev Disease; Rheumatoid Spondylitis) Optic atrophy   134
  - Werlhof Disease (Hemophilia and Thrombocytopenic Purpura)   135
  - Leukemia   135
  - Henoch-Schönlein Purpura (Purpura; Anaphylactoid Purpura)   135
  - Herrick Syndrome (Dresbach Syndrome; Sickle Cell Disease; Drepanocytic Anemia)   136
  - Avitaminosis C (Scurvy; Vitamin C Deficiency)   136
  - Iris Neovascularization with Pseudoexfoliation Syndrome   137
  - Juvenile Xanthogranuloma (JXG; Nevoxanthoendothelioma)   137
  - Retinoblastoma   138
  - Pupillary Membrane, Persistent   138
- Hyphema (Traumatic Hyphema)   139
- UGH Syndrome (Uveitis-Glaucoma-Hyphema Syndrome) Glaucoma   139
- Hypopyon (Pus in Anterior Chamber)   139
  - Acanthamoeba   141
  - Acquired Immunodeficiency Syndrome (AIDS; Acquired Cellular Immunodeficiency; Acquired Immunodeficiency)   141
  - Aspergillosis   142
  - Candidiasis   142
  - Alkaline Injury of the Eye   143
  - Escherichia Coli   143
  - Fusobacterium   144
  - Herpes Simplex   144
  - Herpes Zoster   144
  - Measles (Morbilli; Rubeola)   145
  - Moraxella Lacunata   145
  - Gonorrhea   146
  - Proteus Infections   146
  - Pseudomonas Aeruginosa   147
  - Smallpox (Variola)   147
  - Staphylococcus   147
  - Streptococcus (Scarlet Fever)   148
  - Behçet Syndrome (Dermato-Stomato-Ophthalmic Syndrome; Oculobuccogenital Syndrome; Gilbert Syndrome)   148
  - Toxic Lens Syndrome (Toxic Anterior Segment Syndrome; TASS)   149
  - Acanthamoeba   149
  - Actinomycosis   150
  - Amebiasis (Amebic Dysentery, Entamoeba Histolytica)   150
  - Aspergillosis   151
  - Bacillus Cereus   151
  - Behçet Syndrome (Dermato-Stomato-Ophthalmic Syndrome; Oculobuccogenital Syndrome; Gilbert Syndrome)   151

– Candidiasis 152
– Coccidioidomycosis
 (Valley Fever, San Joaquin Fever) 152
– Coenurosis (Tapeworm) 153
– Cysticercosis 153
– Fusobacterium 154
– Hydatid Cyst (Echinococcosis) 154
– Influenza 155
– Listerellosis (Listeriosis) 155
– Lockjaw (Tetanus) 156
– Metastatic Bacterial Endophthalmitis 156
– Moraxella Lacunata 156
– Mucormycosis (Phycomycosis) 157
– Pseudomonas Aeruginosa Infections 157
– Relapsing Fever (Recurrent Fever) 158
– Staphylococcus 158
– Streptococcus (Scarlet Fever) 159
– Behçet Syndrome (Dermato-Stomato-
 Ophthalmic Syndrome;
 Oculobuccogenital Syndrome;
 Gilbert Syndrome) 159
– Histiocytosis X (Hand-Schuller-Christian
 Syndrome; Lipoid Granuloma;
 Xanthomatous Granuloma Syndrome;
 Schuller-Christian-Hand Syndrome;
 Letterer-Siwe Syndrome; Acute
 Histiocytosis X; Eosinophilic Granuloma;
 Reticuloendotheliosis Syndrome) 160
– Juvenile Rheumatoid Arthritis
 (JRA; Still Disease) 160
– Leukemia 161
– Von Bekhterev-Strumpell Syndrome
 (Marie-Strumpell Spondylitis;
 Ankylosing Spondylitis;
 Pierre-Marie Syndrome; Bekhterev
 Disease; Rheumatoid Spondylitis)
 Optic atrophy 161
– Stevens-Johnson Syndrome
 [Dermatostomatitis; Erythema
 Multiforme Exudativum; Syndroma
 Mucocutaneo-Oculare; Baader
 Dermatostomatitis Syndrome; Mucosal-
 Respiratory Syndrome; Fuchs (2)
 Syndrome; Mucocutaneous
 Ocular Syndrome] 162
– Neovascularization, Corneal Contact
 Lens Related 162

– Tuberculosis 163
– Weil Disease (Leptospirosis) 163
– Yersiniosis 164
– Ghost Cell Glaucoma 164
– Primary Angle-Closure Glaucoma
 (Primary Closed Angle Glaucoma) 164
– Reticulum Cell Sarcoma (Non-Hodgkin
 Lymphoma) 165
• Intraocular Epithelial Cysts 165
• Mesodermal Dysgenesis (Anterior Chamber
 Dysgenesis; Dysembryogenesis; Anterior
 Segment Ocular Dysgenesis Syndrome) 166
• Neovascularization of Anterior Chamber
 Angle (Newly Formed Vessels Extend
 into the Trabecular Meshwork) 166
– Hemangioma 167
– Iris Melanoma 167
– Retinal Venous Obstruction 168
– Fungal Enophthalmitis 168
– Retinal Detachment, Rhegmatogenous 168
– Uveitis, Anterior Nongranulomatous
 (Iritis, Chronic) 169
– Takayasu Syndrome (Martorell Syndrome;
 Aortic Arch Syndrome; Pulseless Disease;
 Reversed Coarctation Syndrome) 169
– Carotid Artery Syndrome (Cavernous
 Sinus Fistula Syndrome; Red-Eyed
 Shunt Syndrome) 170
– Temporal Arteritis Syndrome
 (Cranial Arteritis Syndrome;
 Giant Cell Arteritis; Hutchinson-
 Horton-Magath-Brown Syndrome) 170
– Coats Disease (Leber Miliary Aneurysm;
 Retinal Telangiectasia) 171
– Eales Disease (Periphlebitis) 171
– Malignant Melanoma of the Posterior
 Uvea (Choroidal Melanoma, Ciliary
 Body Melanoma, Uveal Melanoma,
 Intraocular Melanoma) 171
– Andersen-Warburg Syndrome
 (Whitnall-Norman Syndrome;
 Oligophrenia Microphthalmos
 Syndrome; Norrie Disease; Atrophia
 Oculi Congenital Fetal Iritis Syndrome;
 Congenital Progressive Oculo-
 Acoustico-Cerebral Dysplasia) 172
– Retinal Detachment, Rhegmatogenous 172
– Hemangioma 173

– Retinal Artery Occlusion 173
– Retinoblastoma 174
– Retrolental Fibroplasia (RLF; Retinopathy of Prematurity) 174
– Herrick Syndrome (Dresbach Syndrome; Sickle Cell Disease; Drepanocytic Anemia) 175
• Synechiae, Peripheral Anterior 175
• Peters Anomaly 176
• Postoperative Flat Anterior Chamber 176
• Recurrent Hyphema 177
• Shaken Baby Syndrome (Battered-Baby Syndrome; Battered-Child Syndrome; Child Abuse Syndrome; Silverman Syndrome) 177
• Spontaneous Hyphema 178
– Werlhof Disease (Hemophilia and Thrombocytopenic Purpura) 178
– Leukemia 179
– Lymphoid Hyperplasia (Reactive Lymphoid Hyperplasia; Lymphoid Tumors; Malignant Lymphoma; Pseudolymphoma; Pseudotumor; Burkitt Lymphoma; Neoplastic Angioendotheliomatosis) 179
– Henoch-Schönlein Purpura (Purpura; Anaphylactoid Purpura) 180
– Avitaminosis C (Scurvy; Vitamin C Deficiency) 180
– Retinoschisis (RS) 180
– Retrolental Fibroplasia (RLF; Retinopathy of Prematurity) 181
– Hypertension 181
– Juvenile Xanthogranuloma (JXG; Nevoxanthoendothelioma) 182
– Exophthalmos (Proptosis) 182
– Moraxella Lacunata 182
– Rubeosis Iridis 183
– Behçet Syndrome (Dermato-Stomato-Ophthalmic Syndrome; Oculobuccogenital Syndrome; Gilbert Syndrome) 184
– Diabetes Mellitus 184
– Gonorrhea 185
– Herpes Zoster 185
– Herpes Simplex 186
• Spontaneous Hyphema in Infants 186
– Juvenile Rheumatoid Arthritis (JRA; Still Disease) 186

– Anemia 187
– Leukemia 187
– Andersen-Warburg Syndrome (Whitnall-Norman Syndrome; Oligophrenia Microphthalmos Syndrome; Norrie Disease; Atrophia Oculi Congenital Fetal Iritis Syndrome; Congenital Progressive Oculo-Acoustico-Cerebral Dysplasia) 188
– Juvenile Xanthogranuloma (JXG; Nevoxanthoendothelioma) 188
– Persistent Hyperplastic Primary Vitreous (PHPV, Persistent Fetal Vasculature) 189
– Retinoblastoma 189
– Retinoschisis (RS) 190
– Retrolental Fibroplasia (RLF; Retinopathy of Prematurity) 190
• Toxic Lens Syndrome (Toxic Anterior Segment Syndrome; TASS) 191
• White Mass in Anterior Chamber 191
– Bacterial Endophthalmitis 191
– Aspergillosis 192

17. Choroid **193**
• Angioid Streaks 193
– Bassen-Kornzweig Syndrome (Abetalipoproteinemia; Acanthocytosis; Familial Hypolipoproteinemia) 194
– Cooley Anemia (Thalassemia; Thalassemia Major; Thalassemia Minor) 194
– Paget Disease (Osteitis Deformans; Congenital Hyperphosphatemia; Hyperostosis Corticalis Deformans; Pozzi Syndrome; Chronic Congenital Idiopathic Hyperphosphatemia; Osteochalasis Desmalis Familiaris; Familial Osteoectasia) 195
– Ehlers-Danlos Syndrome (Fibrodysplasia Elastica Generalisata; Cutis Hyperelastica; Meekeren-Ehlers-Danlos Syndrome; Indian Rubber Man Syndrome; Cutis Laxa) 195
– Hallermann-Streiff Syndrome [Dyscephalic-Mandibulo-Oculo-Facial Syndrome; Oculo-Mandibulo-Dyscephaly; Ullrich-Fremery-Dohna Syndrome; Francois Dyscephalic Syndrome; Mandibulo-Oculo-Facial Dyscephaly Syndrome; Francois-Hallermann-Streiff Syndrome; Hallermann-Streiff-Francois Syndrome;

Audry I Syndrome; Dohna Syndrome; Francois Syndrome (1); Dyscephaly-Teeth Abnormality-Dwarfism; Dyscephalia Oculomandibularis-Hypotrichosis; Mandibulo-Ocular Dyscephalia Hypotrichosis; Fremery-Dohna Syndrome; Oculo-Mandibulo-Facial Dyscephaly]   196

– Hemochromatosis   197

– Congenital Spherocytic Anemia (Congenital Hemolytic Jaundice; Hereditary Spherocytosis)   197

– Kasabach-Merritt Syndrome (Capillary Angioma-Thrombocytopenia; Hemangioma-Thrombocytopenia; Thrombocytopenia Purpura-Hemangioma)   197

– Lead Poisoning   198

– Von Recklinghausen Syndrome (Neurofibromatosis Type I; Neurinomatosis)   198

– Conjunctival Melanotic Lesions (Conjunctival Nevus, Conjunctival Juncional Nevus, Subepithelial Nevus, Compound Nevus, Blue Nevus, Melanosis Oculi, Conjunctival Melanosis, Epithelial Nelanosis, Racial Melanosis, Sub-Epithelial Melanocytosis, Congenital Melanocytosis, Primary Acquired Melanosis, Malignant Melanoma, Conjunctival Melanoma, Conjunctival Malignant Melanoma)   199

– Pseudopapilledema (Optic Nerve Head Drusen)   199

– Paget Disease (Osteitis Deformans; Congenital Hyperphosphatemia; Hyperostosis Corticalis Deformans; Pozzi Syndrome; Chronic Congenital Idiopathic Hyperphosphatemia; Osteochalasis Desmalis Familiaris; Familial Osteoectasia)   200

– Choroidal Detachment (Ciliochoroidal Detachment)   200

– Grönblad-Strandberg Syndrome (Systemic Elastodystrophy; Pseudoxanthoma Elasticum; Elastorrhexis; Darier-Grönblad-Strandberg Syndrome)   201

– Herrick Syndrome (Dresbach Syndrome; Sickle Cell Disease; Drepanocytic Anemia)   201

– Sturge-Weber Syndrome (Meningocutaneous Syndrome; Vascular Encephalotrigeminal Syndrome; Neuro-Oculocutaneous Angiomatosis; Encephalofacial Angiomatosis; Encephalotrigeminal Syndrome)   202

– Bourneville Syndrome (Bourneville-Pringle Syndrome; Tuberous Sclerosis; Epiloia)   202

• Central Serous Chorioretinopathy   203

• Choroid Coloboma   203

– Aicardi Syndrome   204

– Basal Cell Nevus Syndrome (Nevoid Basal Cell Carcinoma Syndrome; Nevoid Basalioma Syndrome; Gorlin Syndrome; Gorlin-Goltz Syndrome; Multiple Basal Cell Nevi Syndrome)   204

– Cat's-Eye Syndrome (Schachenmann Syndrome; Schmid-Fraccaro Syndrome; Partial Trisomy G Syndrome)   205

– Charge Association (Multiple Congenital Anomalies Syndrome; Coloboma, Heart Disease, Atresia, Retarded Growth, Genital Hypoplasia, Ear Malformation Association)   206

– Crouzon Syndrome (Dysostosis Craniofacialis; Oxycephaly; Craniofacial Dysostosis; Parrot-Head Syndrome; Möbius-Crouzon Syndrome; Hereditary Craniofacial Dysostosis)   206

– Zollinger-Ellison Syndrome (Polyglandular Adenomatosis Syndrome; Multiple Endocrine Adenomatosis Partial Syndrome) Optic atrophy   207

– Hallermann-Streiff Syndrome (Dyscephalic-Mandibulo-Oculo-Facial Syndrome; Oculo-Mandibulo-Dyscephaly; Ullrich-Fremery-Dohna Syndrome; Francois Dyscephalic Syndrome; Mandibulo-Oculo-Facial Dyscephaly Syndrome; Francois-Hallermann-Streiff Syndrome; Hallermann-Streiff-Francois Syndrome; Audry I Syndrome; Dohna Syndrome; Francois Syndrome (1); Dyscephaly-Teeth Abnormality-Dwarfism; Dyscephalia Oculomandibularis-Hypotrichosis; Mandibulo-Ocular Dyscephalia Hypotrichosis; Fremery-Dohna Syndrome; Oculo-Mandibulo-Facial Dyscephaly)   207

– Bloch-Sulzberger Syndrome
(Incontinentia Pigmenti; Siemens-
Bloch-Sulzberger Syndrome) 208

– Kartagener Syndrome (Sinusitis-
Bronchiectasis-Situs Inversus Syndrome;
Bronchiectasis-Dextrocardia-Sinusitis;
Kartagener Triad) 208

– Laurence-Moon-Bardet-Biedl Syndrome
(Bardet-Biedl Syndrome; Retinitis
Pigmentosa-Polydactyly-Adiposogenital
Syndrome) 209

– Pierre-Robin Syndrome
(Robin Syndrome; Micrognathia-
Glossoptosis Syndrome) 209

– Stickler Syndrome (Hereditary
Progressive Arthroophthalmopathy) 210

– Bourneville Syndrome
(Bourneville-Pringle Syndrome;
Tuberous Sclerosis; Epiloia) 210

– Goldenhar Syndrome
(Oculo-Auriculo-Vertebral Dysplasia;
Goldenhar-Gorlin Syndrome) 211

– Goltz Syndrome (Focal Dermal
Hypoplasia Syndrome) 211

– Joubert Syndrome (Familial Cerebellar
Vermis Agenesis) 212

– Klinefelter Syndrome (Gynecomastia-
Aspermatogenesis Syndrome;
XXY Syndrome; XXXY Syndrome;
XXYY Syndrome; Reifenstein-Albright
Syndrome) 212

– Lenz Microphthalmia Syndrome 213

– Linear Nevus Sebaceus of Jadassohn
(Nevus Sebaceus of Jadassohn;
Jadassohn-Type Anetoderma;
Organoid Nevus syndrome;
Sebaceus nevus syndrome) 213

– Frontonasal Dysplasia Syndrome
(Median Cleft Face Syndrome) 214

– Meckel Syndrome (Dysencephalia
Splanchnocystic Syndrome;
Gruber Syndrome) 214

– Retinoblastoma 214

– Rubinstein-Taybi Syndrome
(Broad-thumbs Syndrome) 215

– Triploidy Syndrome (Iris Coloboma) 215

– Trisomy 18 Syndrome (E Syndrome;
Edwards Syndrome), Congenital
Glaucoma 216

– Trisomy 13 Syndrome (Trisomy D1
Syndrome, Patau Syndrome,
Reese Syndrome) Iris Coloboma 216

– Turner Syndrome (Turner-Albright
Syndrome; Gonadal Dysgenesis;
Genital Dwarfism Syndrome;
Ullrich-Turner Syndrome;
Bonnevie-Ullrich Syndrome;
Pterygolymphangiectasia Syndrome;
Ullrich-Bonnevie Syndrome)
Cataract, Posterior 217

– Walker-Warburg Syndrome
(Cerebro-ocular Dysplasia-Muscular
Dystrophy; Warburg Syndrome;
COD-MD Syndrome; Fukuyama
Congenital Muscular Dystrophy;
Hard + or – E Syndrome) Cataract 217

• Choroidal Detachment
(Ciliochoroidal Detachment) 218

• Choroidal Folds 218

– Malignant Melanoma of the Posterior
Uvea (Choroidal Melanoma,
Ciliary Body Melanoma, Uveal
Melanoma, Intraocular Melanoma) 219

– Junius-Kuhnt Syndrome [Kuhnt-Junius
Disease; Macular Senile Disciform
Degeneration (I); Macula Lutea
Juvenile Degeneration (2)] 219

– Exophthalmos (Proptosis) 220

– Basedow Syndrome (Graves Disease;
Hyperthyroidism; Thyrotoxicosis;
Exophthalmic Goiter; Parry Disease) 220

– Hyperopia, High 221

– Ocular Hypotony 221

– Papilledema 221

– Choroidal Detachment
(Ciliochoroidal Detachment) 222

– Retinal Detachment, Rhegmatogenous 222

– Uveitis, Anterior Nongranulomatous
(Iritis, Chronic) 222

• Choroidal Hemorrhage 223

– Doyne Honeycomb Choroiditis
(Dominant Orbruch Membrane Drusen;
Hutchinson-Tays Central Guttate
Choroiditis; Holthouse-Batten
Superficial Choroiditis;
Malattia-Leventinese Syndrome) 223

– Sturge-Weber Syndrome
(Meningocutaneous Syndrome;

Vascular Encephalotrigeminal Syndrome; Neuro-Oculocutaneous Angiomatosis; Encephalofacial Angiomatosis; Encephalotrigeminal Syndrome) 224

– Arteriosclerosis 224

– Leukemia 225

– Addison Pernicious Anemia Syndrome (Pernicious Anemia Syndrome; Vitamin B12 Deficiency Anemia; Macrocytic Anemia; Biermer Syndrome) 225

– Kasabach-Merritt Syndrome (Capillary Angioma-Thrombocytopenia; Hemangioma-Thrombocytopenia; Thrombocytopenia Purpura-Hemangioma) 226

– Diabetes Mellitus 226

– Ehlers-Danlos Syndrome (Fibrodysplasia Elastica Generalisata; Cutis Hyperelastica; Meekeren-Ehlers-Danlos Syndrome; Indian Rubber Man Syndrome; Cutis Laxa) 227

– Paget Disease (Osteitis Deformans; Congenital Hyperphosphatemia; Hyperostosis Corticalis Deformans; Pozzi Syndrome; Chronic Congenital Idiopathic Hyperphosphatemia; Osteochalasis Desmalis Familiaris; Familial Osteoectasia) 227

– Purtscher Syndrome (Fat Embolism Syndrome; Traumatic Retinal Angiopathy; Traumatic Liporrhagia; Valsalva Retinopathy of Duane; Duane Retinopathy) 228

• Purtscher Syndrome (Fat Embolism Syndrome; Traumatic Retinal Angiopathy; Traumatic Liporrhagia; Valsalva Retinopathy of Duane; Duane Retinopathy) 228

• Choroidal Ruptures 229

• Choroideremia (Tapetochoroidal Dystrophy, Progressive; Choroidal Sclerosis) 229

• Choroiditis (Posterior Uveitis) 230

– Herpes Simplex 230

– Herpes Zoster 231

– Pars Planitis (Angiohyalitis, Chronic Cyclitis, Cyclitis Perpheral Uveitis, Peripheral Uveoretinitis Vitritis) 231

– Schaumann Syndrome (Besnier-Boeck-Schaumann Syndrome; Boeck Sarcoid; Sarcoidosis) 232

– Acquired Lues (Syphilis; Acquired Syphilis; Lues Venerea; Malum Venereum) 232

– Ocular Toxoplasmosis (Toxoplasmic Retinochoroiditis; Toxoplasmosis) 233

– Tuberculosis 233

– Vogt-Koyanagi-Harada Disease (Harada Disease; Uveitis-Vitiligo-Alopecia-Poliosis Syndrome) 234

– Acquired Immunodeficiency Syndrome (AIDS; Acquired Cellular Immunodeficiency; Acquired Immunodeficiency) 234

– Behçet Syndrome (Dermato-Stomato-Ophthalmic Syndrome; Oculobuccogenital Syndrome; Gilbert Syndrome) 235

– Birdshot Retinopathy (Vitiliginous Chorioretinitis) 235

– Candidiasis 236

– Parinaud Oculoglandular Syndrome (Parinaud Conjunctiva-Adenitis Syndrome; Catscratch Oculoglandular Syndrome; Catscratch Disease; Bartonella henselae) 236

– Cryptococcosis (Torulosis) 237

– Cytomegalic Inclusion Disease (Cytomegalovirus; Congenital Cytomegalic Inclusion Disease) 237

– Coccidioidomycosis (Valley Fever, San Joaquin Fever) 238

– Infectious Mononucleosis (Mononucleosis; Epstein-Barr Virus, Acute; Acute Epstein-Barr Virus, Glandular Fever) 238

– Lyme Disease 238

– Histoplasmosis (Histoplasmosis Choroiditis; Histoplasmosis Maculopathy; Presumed Ocular Histoplasmosis Syndrome) 239

– Disseminated Sclerosis (Multiple Sclerosis) 239

– Schaumann Syndrome (Besnier-Boeck-Schaumann Syndrome; Boeck Sarcoid; Sarcoidosis) 240

– Serpiginous Choroidopathy 240

– Acquired Lues (Syphilis; Acquired Syphilis; Lues Venerea; Malum Venereum) 241

- Disseminated Lupus Erythematosus (Systemic Lupus Erythematosus; Lupus Erythematosus; Kaposi-Libman-Sack Syndrome, SLE)   241
- Nematode Ophthalmia Syndrome (Visceral Larva Migrans Syndrome; Toxocariasis)   242
- Ocular Toxoplasmosis (Toxoplasmic Retinochoroiditis; Toxoplasmosis)   242
- Chickenpox (Varicella)   243
• Choroiditis (Posterior Uveitis) in Children   243
- Von Bekhterev-Strumpell Syndrome (Marie-Strumpell Spondylitis; Ankylosing Spondylitis; Pierre-Marie Syndrome; Bekhterev Disease; Rheumatoid Spondylitis) Optic atrophy   244
- Schaumann Syndrome (Besnier-Boeck-Schaumann Syndrome; Boeck Sarcoid; Sarcoidosis)   244
- Sympathetic Ophthalmia   245
- Vogt-Koyanagi-Harada Disease (Harada Disease; Uveitis-Vitiligo-Alopecia-Poliosis Syndrome)   245
- Behçet Syndrome (Dermato-Stomato-Ophthalmic Syndrome; Oculobuccogenital Syndrome; Gilbert Syndrome)   246
- Jensen Disease (Juxtapapillary Retinopathy)   246
- Cytomegalic Inclusion Disease (Cytomegalovirus; Congenital Cytomegalic Inclusion Disease)   247
- Diffuse Unilateral Subacute Neuroretinitis Syndrome (DUSN; Unilateral Wipeout Syndrome; Wipeout Syndrome)   247
- Herpes Simplex   248
- Acquired Immunodeficiency Syndrome (AIDS; Acquired Cellular Immunodeficiency; Acquired Immunodeficiency)   248
- Uveitis (Iritis, Iridocystitis, Intermediate and Posterior Uveitis, Noninfectious Chorioretinitis)   249
- Psoriatic Arthritis   249
- Juvenile Rheumatoid Arthritis (JRA; Still Disease)   250
- Nematode Ophthalmia Syndrome (Visceral Larva Migrans Syndrome; Toxocariasis)   250
- Reiter Syndrome (Fiessinger-Leroy Syndrome; Conjunctivo-Urethro-Synovial Syndrome; Idiopathic Blennorrheal Arthritis Syndrome; Polyarthritis Enterica)   251
- Reticulum Cell Sarcoma (Non-Hodgkin Lymphoma)   251
- Rubella Syndrome (Congenital Rubella Syndrome; German Measles; Gregg Syndrome)   252
- Dawson Disease (Dawson Encephalitis; Subacute Sclerosing Panencephalitis; Inclusion-Body Encephalitis)   252
- Acquired Lues (Syphilis; Acquired Syphilis; Lues Venerea; Malum Venereum)   253
- Ocular Toxoplasmosis (Toxoplasmic Retinochoroiditis; Toxoplasmosis)   254
- Tuberculosis   254
• Choroidoretinal Degeneration with Retinal Reflex in Heterozygous Women   255
• Choroidoretinal Dystrophy   255
• Crowded Disk Syndrome (Bilateral Choroidal Folds and Optic Neuropathy)   256
• Cytomegalic Inclusion Disease (Cytomegalovirus; Congenital Cytomegalic Inclusion Disease)   256
• Doyne Honeycomb Choroiditis (Dominant Orbruch Membrane Drusen; Hutchinson-Tays Central Guttate Choroiditis; Holthouse-Batten Superficial Choroiditis; Malattia-Leventinese Syndrome)   256
• Expulsive Choroidal Hemorrhage   257
• Histoplasmosis (Histoplasmosis Choroiditis; Histoplasmosis Maculopathy; Presumed Ocular Histoplasmosis Syndrome)   257
• Malignant Melanoma of the Posterior Uvea (Choroidal Melanoma, Ciliary Body Melanoma, Uveal Melanoma, Intraocular Melanoma)   258
• Ocular Toxoplasmosis (Toxoplasmic Retinochoroiditis; Toxoplasmosis)   258
• Pars Planitis (Angiohyalitis, Chronic Cyclitis, Cyclitis Peripheral Uveitis, Peripheral Uveoretinitis Vitritis)   259
• Serpiginous Choroidopathy   259
• Sympathetic Ophthalmia   259

- Giant Cell Arteritis (Temporal Arteritis Syndrome; Cranial Arteritis Syndrome; Hutchinson-Horton-Magath-Brown Syndrome) 260
- Disseminated Lupus Erythematosus (Systemic Lupus Erythematosus; Lupus Erythematosus; Kaposi-Libman-Sack Syndrome, SLE) 260
- Kussmaul Disease (Kussmaul-Maier Disease; Necrotizing Angiitis; PAN; Polyarteritis Nodosa) 261
- Rheumatoid Arthritis (Adult) 262
- Wegener Syndrome (Wegener Granulomatosis) 262
- Uveal Effusion 263
  - Arteriovenous Fistula (Arteriovenous Aneurysm; Arteriovenous Angioma; Arteriovenous Malformation; Cirsoid Aneurysm; Racemose Hemangioma; Varicose Aneurysm) 263
  - Disseminated Lupus Erythematosus (Systemic Lupus Erythematosus; Lupus Erythematosus; Kaposi-Libman-Sack Syndrome, SLE) 263
  - Uveitis, Anterior Nongranulomatous (Iritis, Chronic) 264
  - Sympathetic Ophthalmia 264
  - Vogt-Koyanagi-Harada Disease (Harada Disease; Uveitis-Vitiligo-Alopecia-Poliosis Syndrome) 265
- Coccidioidomycosis (Valley Fever, San Joaquin Fever) 265
- Vitreoretinochoroidopathy (VRCP; Autosomal Dominant Vitreoretinochoroidopathy; ADVIRC) Choroidal atrophy 266

18. Ciliary Body **267**

- Accommodative Spasm 267
- Ciliary Body Concussions and Lacerations 267
- Ciliary Body Detachment (*See* Hypotony) 268
- Long Ciliary Processes Extending to Dilated Pupillary Space 268
  - Aniridia (Congenital Aniridia, Hereditary Aniridia) 268
  - Chronic Angle Closure Glaucoma 269
  - Iris Cysts 269
  - Dislocation of the Lens 269
  - Plateau Iris Syndrome 270

  - Falciform Detachment 270
  - Bloch-Sulzberger Syndrome (Incontinentia Pigmenti; Siemens-Bloch-Sulzberger Syndrome) 270
  - Andersen-Warburg Syndrome (Whitnall-Norman Syndrome; Oligophrenia Microphthalmos Syndrome; Norrie Disease; Atrophia Oculi Congenital Fetal Iritis Syndrome; Congenital Progressive Oculo-Acoustico-Cerebral Dysplasia) 271
  - Persistent Hyperplastic Primary Vitreous (PHPV, Persistent Fetal Vasculature) 272
  - Retrolental Fibroplasia (RLF; Retinopathy of Prematurity) 272
  - Trisomy 13 Syndrome (Trisomy Dl Syndrome, Patau Syndrome, Reese Syndrome) Iris Coloboma 272
- Malignant Melanoma of the Posterior Uvea (Choroidal Melanoma, Ciliary Body Melanoma, Uveal Melanoma, Intraocular Melanoma) 273
- Pars Planitis (Peripheral Uveitis) 273
  - Disseminated Sclerosis (Multiple Sclerosis) 274
  - Rheumatoid Arthritis (Adult) 274
  - Schaumann Syndrome (Besnier-Boeck-Schaumann Syndrome; Boeck Sarcoid; Sarcoidosis) 275
  - Acquired Lues (Syphilis; Acquired Syphilis; Lues Venerea; Malum Venereum) 275
  - Ocular Toxoplasmosis (Toxoplasmic Retinochoroiditis; Toxoplasmosis) 276
  - Ulcerative Colitis (Regional Enteritis; Inflammatory Bowel Disease) 276
- Pigmented Ciliary Body Lesions 277
  - Malignant Melanoma of the Posterior Uvea (Choroidal Melanoma, Ciliary Body Melanoma, Uveal Melanoma, Intraocular Melanoma) 277

19. Conjunctiva **278**

- Acute Follicular Conjunctivitis (Adenoviral Conjunctivitis; Pharyngoconjunctival Fever; Syndrome of Beal) 278
- Acute Hemorrhagic Conjunctivitis (AHC; Epidemic Hemorrhagic Keratoconjunctivitis, Apollo 11 Disease) 278

- Acute Mucopurulent Conjunctivitis — 279
  - Pneumococcal Infections (Streptococcus Pneumoniae Infections) — 279
  - Staphylococcus — 280
  - Haemophilus Aegyptius (Koch-Weeks Bacillus) — 280
  - Rubella Syndrome (Congenital Rubella Syndrome; German Measles; Gregg Syndrome) — 281
  - Measles (Morbilli; Rubeola) — 281
  - Mumps — 282
  - Reiter Syndrome (Fiessinger-Leroy Syndrome; Conjunctivo-Urethro-Synovial Syndrome; Idiopathic Blennorrheal Arthritis Syndrome; Polyarthritis Enterica) — 282
  - Streptococcus (Scarlet Fever) — 283
  - Candidiasis — 283
  - Fuchs-Lyell Syndrome (Debré-Lamy-Lyell Syndrome; Toxic Epidermal Necrolysis) — 284
  - Relapsing Polychondritis (Jaksch Wartenhost Syndrome; Meyenburg-Altherz-Vehlinger Syndrome; Von Meyenberg II Syndrome) — 284
  - Sjögren Syndrome (Gougerot-Sjögren Syndrome; Secretoinhibitor Syndrome; Sicca Syndrome) — 285
- Allergic Conjunctivitis (Allergic Rhinoconjunctivitis, Hay Fever Conjunctivitis, Atopic Keratoconjunctivitis, Allergic Conjunctivitis, Giant Papillary Conjunctivitis) — 285
- Amyloidosis of Gingiva and Conjunctiva, with Mental Retardation (Primary Systemic Amyloidosis) — 286
- Angelucci Syndrome (Critical Allergic Conjunctivitis Syndrome) — 286
- Angular Conjunctivitis (Morax-Axenfeld Bacillus) — 287
- Bacterial Conjunctivitis (Infective Conjunctivitis, Mucopurulent Conjunctivitis) — 287
- Benign Mucosal Pemphigoid (Chronic Cicatricial Conjunctivitis; Cicatricial Pemphigoid; Essential Shrinkage of the Conjunctiva; Membrane Pemphigus; Ocular pemphigoid) — 288
- Bitot Spots — 288
  - Eyelid Coloboma — 288
  - Nystagmus — 289
  - Rieger Syndrome (Axenfeld-Rieger Syndrome; Dysgenesis Mesodermalis Corneae et Irides; Dysgenesis Mesostromalis; Axenfeld Posterior Embryotoxon-Juvenile Glaucoma) — 289
  - Corneal Snowflake Dystrophy — 290
  - Darier-White Syndrome (Keratosis Follicularis; Dyskeratosis Follicularis Syndrome; Psorospermosis) — 290
  - Vitamin A Deficiency — 291
- Blepharoconjunctivitis — 291
- Lesions of Caruncle — 292
  - Basal Cell Carcinoma — 292
  - Hemangioma, Capillary — 292
  - Dermoid (Dermoid Choristoma; Dermoid Cyst; Dermolipoma; Lipodermoid) — 293
  - Malignant Melanoma of the Posterior Uvea (Choroidal Melanoma, Ciliary Body Melanoma, Uveal Melanoma, Intraocular Melanoma) — 293
  - Papilloma (Wart; Verruca) — 294
  - Lymphoid Hyperplasia (Reactive Lymphoid Hyperplasia; Lymphoid Tumors; Malignant Lymphoma; Pseudolymphoma; Pseudotumor; Burkitt Lymphoma; Neoplastic Angioendotheliomatosis) — 294
  - Actinic and Seborrheic Keratosis — 295
  - Squamous Cell Carcinoma, Conjunctival — 295
- Chronic Follicular Conjunctivits (Conjunctivitis Giant Papillary) Lymphoid Follicles Cobblestoning of Conjunctiva with Long-Term Course — 295
  - Rothmund Syndrome (Rothmund-Thomson Syndrome; Telangiectasia-Pigmentation-Cataract Syndrome; Ectodermal Syndrome; Congenital Poikiloderma with Juvenile Cataract) Keratoconus — 296
  - Lymphoid Hyperplasia (Reactive Lymphoid Hyperplasia; Lymphoid Tumors; Malignant Lymphoma; Pseudolymphoma; Pseudotumor; Burkitt Lymphoma; Neoplastic Angioendotheliomatosis) — 297

- Chronic Mucopurulent Conjunctivitis (Mucopurulent Discharge, Moderate Hyperemia with a Chronic Course) 297
  - Angular Conjunctivitis (Morax-Axenfeld Bacillus) 298
  - Pediculosis and Phthiriasis 298
  - Staphylococcus 299
  - Ectropion 299
- Cicatricial Conjunctivitis (Cicatricial Pemphigoid) Scarring of Conjunctiva 299
  - Diphtheria 301
  - Streptococcus (Scarlet Fever) 301
  - Schaumann Syndrome (Besnier-Boeck-Schaumann Syndrome; Boeck Sarcoid; Sarcoidosis) 302
  - Progressive Systemic Sclerosis (Scleroderma; Systemic Scleroderma) 302
  - Benign Mucosal Pemphigoid (Chronic Cicatricial Conjunctivitis; Cicatricial Pemphigoid; Essential Shrinkage of the Conjunctiva; Membrane Pemphigus; Ocular Pemphigoid) 303
  - Lichen Planus 303
  - Blepharoconjunctivitis 304
  - Linear IgA Disease 304
  - Trachoma 304
  - Acne Rosacea (Acne Erythematosa; Ocular Rosacea) 305
  - Alkaline Injury of the Eye 305
  - Chlamydia (Inclusion Conjunctivitis; Paratrachoma) 306
  - Congenital Lues (Congenital Syphilis) 306
  - Dermatitis Herpetiformis (Duhring-Brocq Disease) 307
  - Epidemic Keratoconjunctivitis 307
  - Scalded Skin Syndrome (Toxic Epidermal Necrolysis; Ritter Disease; Toxic Epidermal Necrolysis of Lyell; Staphylococcal Scalded Skin Syndrome; Lyell Syndrome; Epidermolysis Acuta Toxica; Toxic Epidermal Necrolysis) Symblepharon 308
  - Goldscheider Syndrome (Weber-Cockayne Syndrome; Epidermolysis Bullosa; Dominant Epidermolysis Bullosa Dystrophiea Albopapuloidea) 308
  - Stevens-Johnson Syndrome [Dermatostomatitis; Erythema Multiforme Exudativum; Syndroma Mucocutaneo-Oculare; Baader Dermatostomatitis Syndrome; Mucosal-Respiratory Syndrome; Fuchs (2) Syndrome; Mucocutaneous Ocular Syndrome] 309
  - Bullous Ichthyosiform Erythroderma (Collodion Baby; Congenital Ichthyosis; Epidermolytic Hyperkeratosis; Ichthyosis; Ichthyosis Vulgaris; Lamellar Ichthyosis; Nonbullous Ichthyosiform Erythroderma; Xeroderma; X-Linked Ichthyosis) 310
  - Contact Dermatitis (Dermatitis Venenata) 310
  - Fuchs-Lyell Syndrome (Debré-Lamy-Lyell Syndrome; Toxic Epidermal Necrolysis) 311
  - Hydroa Vacciniforme 311
  - Impetigo 311
  - Bullous Ichthyosiform Erythroderma (Collodion Baby; Congenital Ichthyosis; Epidermolytic Hyperkeratosis; Ichthyosis; Ichthyosis Vulgaris; Lamellar Ichthyosis; Nonbullous Ichthyosiform Erythroderma; Xeroderma; X-Linked Ichthyosis) 312
  - Benign Mucosal Pemphigoid (Chronic Cicatricial Conjunctivitis; Cicatricial Pemphigoid; Essential Shrinkage of the Conjunctiva; Membrane Pemphigus; Ocular pemphigoid) 312
  - Lichen Planus 313
  - Reiter Syndrome (Fiessinger-Leroy Syndrome; Conjunctivo-Urethro-Synovial Syndrome; Idiopathic Blennorrheal Arthritis Syndrome; Polyarthritis Enterica) 313
  - Sjögren Syndrome (Gougerot-Sjögren Syndrome; Secretoinhibitor Syndrome; Sicca Syndrome) 314
  - Staphylococcus 314
  - Acquired Lues (Syphilis; Acquired Syphilis; Lues Venerea; Malum Venereum) 315
  - Progressive Systemic Sclerosis (Scleroderma; Systemic Scleroderma) 315
  - Vaccinia (Keratitis) 316

- Conjunctival Melanotic Lesions
  (Conjunctival Nevus, Conjunctival
  Juncional Nevus, Subepithelial Nevus,
  Compound Nevus, Blue Nevus,
  Melanosis Oculi, Conjunctival Melanosis,
  Epithelial Nelanosis, Racial Melanosis,
  Sub-Epithelial Melanocytosis, Congenital
  Melanocytosis, Primary Acquired
  Melanosis, Malignant Melanoma,
  Conjunctival Melanoma, Conjunctival
  Malignant Melanoma) 316
- Conjunctival Xerosis
  (Dryness of Conjunctiva) 317
  – Benign Mucosal Pemphigoid
    (Chronic Cicatricial Conjunctivitis;
    Cicatricial Pemphigoid; Essential
    Shrinkage of the Conjunctiva;
    Membrane Pemphigus;
    Ocular pemphigoid) 318
  – Exophthalmos (Proptosis) 318
  – Vitamin A Deficiency 319
  – Cystic Fibrosis Syndrome
    (Fibrocystic Disease of Pancreas) 319
  – Anorexia Nervosa (Apepsia Hystericci) 320
  – Crohn Disease
    (Granulomatous Ileocolitis) 320
  – Ulcerative Colitis (Regional Enteritis;
    Inflammatory Bowel Disease) 321
  – Pancreatitis 321
  – Ankylostomiasis (Hookworm Disease) 322
  – Mosse Syndrome (Polycythemia-
    Hepatic Cirrhosis Syndrome) 322
  – Malaria 322
  – Pregnancy 323
  – Tuberculosis 323
  – Pityriasis Rubra Pilaris
    [Kaposi Disease (2); Devergie Disease;
    Hebra Disease; Tarral-Besnier Disease;
    Lichen Ruber; Lichen Ruber
    Acuminatus; Pityriasis Pilaris] 324
  – Basedow Syndrome (Graves Disease;
    Hyperthyroidism; Thyrotoxicosis;
    Exophthalmic Goiter; Parry Disease) 324
  – Uyemura Syndrome
    (Fundus Albipunctatus with Hemeralopia
    and Xerosis) Night blindness 325
  – Alacrima 325
  – Keratoconjunctivitis Sicca and
    Sjögren's Syndrome 326
  – Riley-Day Syndrome
    (Congenital Familial Dysautonomia) 326
  – Sjögren Syndrome (Gougerot-Sjögren
    Syndrome; Secretoinhibitor Syndrome;
    Sicca Syndrome) 327
- Conjunctivitis, Ligneous 327
- Corneal and Conjunctival Calcifications 328
- Chlamydia (Inclusion Conjunctivitis;
  Paratrachoma) 328
- Conjunctivitis, Viral 328
- Conjunctivochalasis (CCH) 329
- Dry Eye Syndrome 329
- Elschnig Syndrome I
  (Meibomian Conjunctivitis) 330
- Epidemic Keratoconjunctivitis 330
- Filtering Blebs and Associated Problems 331
- Herpes Simplex 331
- Herpes Zoster 331
- Giant Papillary Conjunctivitis Syndrome 332
- Conjunctival Lacerations 332
- Ligneous Conjunctivitis 333
- Membranous Conjunctivitis 333
  – Acid Burns of the Eye 333
  – Alkaline Injury of the Eye 334
  – Diphtheria 334
  – Ligneous Conjunctivitis 335
  – Pneumococcal Infections
    (Streptococcus Pneumoniae Infections) 335
  – Streptococcus (Scarlet Fever) 336
  – Actinomycosis 336
  – Measles (Morbilli; Rubeola) 336
  – Smallpox (Variola) 337
  – Pseudomonas Aeruginosa 337
  – Herpes Simplex 338
  – Epidemic Keratoconjunctivitis 338
- Meningococcemia
  (Neisseria Meningitides; Meningitis) 338
- Mucous Membrane Pemphigoid 339
- Ophthalmia Neonatorum
  (Conjunctivitis Occurring in Newborns) 339
  – Diphtheria 340
  – Staphylococcus 340
  – Streptococcus (Scarlet Fever) 341
  – Pneumococcal Infections
    (Streptococcus Pneumoniae Infections) 341

- Escherichia Coli 342
- Haemophilus Influenzae 342
- Acinetobacter (Mima Polymorpha; Acinetobacter Iwoffi) 342
- Gonorrhea 343
- Meningococcemia (Neisseria Meningitides; Meningitis) 343
- Proteus Infections 344
- Pseudomonas Aeruginosa 344
- Herpes Simplex 344
- Acinetobacter 345
- Clostridium Perfringens 345
- Listerellosis (Listeriosis) 346
- Moraxella Lacunata 346
- Propionibacterium Acnes 346
• Parinaud Oculoglandular Syndrome (Parinaud Conjunctiva-Adenitis Syndrome; Catscratch Oculoglandular Syndrome; Catscratch Disease; Bartonella henselae) 347
• Petzetakis-Takos Syndrome (Phlyctenular Keratoconjunctivitis) 347
• Pseudomembranous Conjunctivitis 348
- Diphtheria 352
- Gonorrhea 353
- Meningococcemia (Neisseria Meningitides; Meningitis) 353
- Pneumococcal Infections (Streptococcus Pneumoniae Infections) 353
- Staphylococcus 354
- Streptococcus (Scarlet Fever) 354
- Haemophilus Aegyptius (Koch-Weeks Bacillus) 355
- Haemophilus Influenzae 355
- Pseudomonas Aeruginosa 356
- Escherichia Coli 356
- Bacillus Subtilis (Hay Bacillus) 356
- Shigellosis (Bacillary Dysentery) 357
- Tuberculosis 357
- Epidemic Keratoconjunctivitis 358
- Herpes Simplex 358
- Herpes Zoster 358
- Reiter Syndrome (Fiessinger-Leroy Syndrome; Conjunctivo-Urethro-Synovial Syndrome; Idiopathic Blennorrheal Arthritis Syndrome; Polyarthritis Enterica) 359

- Vaccinia (Keratitis) 359
- Candidiasis 360
- Stevens-Johnson Syndrome [Dermatostomatitis; Erythema Multiforme Exudativum; Syndroma Mucocutaneo-Oculare; Baader Dermatostomatitis Syndrome; Mucosal-Respiratory Syndrome; Fuchs (2) Syndrome; Mucocutaneous Ocular Syndrome] 360
- Scalded Skin Syndrome (Toxic Epidermal Necrolysis; Ritter Disease; Toxic Epidermal Necrolysis of Lyell; Staphylococcal Scalded Skin Syndrome; Lyell Syndrome; Epidermolysis Acuta Toxica; Toxic Epidermal Necrolysis) Symblepharon 361
- Pemphigus Vulgaris 361
- Acid Burns of the Eye 362
- Alkaline Injury of the Eye 362
- Graft Versus Host Disease 363
- Hoof and Mouth Disease 363
- Haemophilus Aegyptius (Koch-Weeks Bacillus) 363
- Ligneous Conjunctivitis 364
- Urbach-Wiethe Syndrome (Rossle-Urbach-Wiethe Syndrome; Lipoproteinosis; Hyalinosis Cutis et Mucosae; Lipoid Proteinosis; Proteinosis-Lipoidosis) Dry Eyes 364
- Superior Limbic Keratoconjunctivitis (Theodores Superior Limbic Keratoconjunctivitis, SLK) 365
- Wegener Syndrome (Wegener Granulomatosis) 365
• Pterygium of Conjunctiva and Cornea 366
• Purulent Conjunctivitis 366
- Pneumococcal Infections (Streptococcus Pneumoniae Infections) 367
- Staphylococcus 367
- Streptococcus (Scarlet Fever) 368
- Enterobiasis (Oxyuriasis; Pinworm; Seatworm) 368
- Escherichia Coli 368
- Haemophilus Influenzae 369
- Rhinoscleroma (Klebsiella Rhinoscleromatis) 369
- Moraxella Lacunata 370
- Gonorrhea 370

– Meningococcemia
  (Neisseria Meningitides; Meningitis)   370

– Proteus Infections   371

– Pseudomonas Aeruginosa   371

– Vaccinia (Keratitis)   372

– Actinomycosis   372

– Candidiasis   372

– Nocardiosis   373

– Wiskott-Aldrich Syndrome
  (Corneal Ulcer)   373

• Stevens-Johnson Syndrome
  [Dermatostomatitis; Erythema Multiforme
  Exudativum; Syndroma Mucocutaneo-
  Oculare; Baader Dermatostomatitis
  Syndrome; Mucosal-Respiratory
  Syndrome; Fuchs (2) Syndrome;
  Mucocutaneous Ocular Syndrome]   374

• Superior Limbic Keratoconjunctivitis
  (Theodores Superior Limbic
  Keratoconjunctivitis, SLK)   374

• Tumors of the Conjunctiva   375

  – Keratoacanthoma   376

  – Bowen Disease (Intraepithelial
    Epithelioma; Carcinoma in Situ;
    Dyskeratosis)   376

  – Bourneville Syndrome
    (Bourneville-Pringle Syndrome;
    Tuberous Sclerosis; Epiloia)   376

• Vernal Keratoconjunctivitis
  (Atopic Keratoconjunctivitis,
  Allergic Conjunctivitis, Giant
  Papillary Conjunctivitis)   377

20. Cornea   **378**

• Degeneration   378

  – Anterior Embryotoxon (Arcus)   378

  – Alagille Syndrome (AGS; Alagille-Watson
    Syndrome, AWS; Cholestasis with
    Peripheral Pulmonary Stenosis;
    Arteriohepatic Dysplasia, AHD; Hepatic
    Ductular Hypoplasia, Syndromatic)   379

  – Alport Syndrome (Hereditary Familial
    Congenital Hemorrhagic Nephritis;
    Hereditary Nephritis; Familial Nephritis)   379

  – Schnyder's Crystalline
    Corneal Dystrophy   380

  – Band-Shaped Keratopathy   380

  – Episkopi Blindness   381

– Mercury Poisoning
  (Minamata Syndrome)   382

– De Barsy Syndrome   382

– Disseminated Lupus Erythematosus
  (Systemic Lupus Erythematosus;
  Lupus Erythematosus; Kaposi-
  Libman-Sack Syndrome, SLE)   383

– Gout (Hyperuricemia)   383

– Williams-Beuren Syndrome
  (Supravalvular Aortic Stenosis;
  Beuren Elfin Face; Hypercalcemia
  Supravalvular Aortic Stenosis;
  Hypercalcemic Face) Hypertelorism   384

– Schaumann Syndrome
  (Besnier-Boeck-Schaumann Syndrome;
  Boeck Sarcoid; Sarcoidosis)   384

– Heerfordt Syndrome (Uveoparotid Fever;
  Uveoparotitis; Uveoparotitic Paralysis)   385

– Hyperparathyroidism   385

– Hypophosphatasia
  (Phosphoethanolaminuria)   386

– Drummond Syndrome (Idiopathic
  Hypercalcemia; Blue Diaper Syndrome)   386

– Burnett Syndrome (Milk Drinker
  Syndrome; Milk-Alkali Syndrome)   387

– Paget Disease (Osteitis Deformans;
  Congenital Hyperphosphatemia;
  Hyperostosis Corticalis Deformans;
  Pozzi Syndrome; Chronic Congenital
  Idiopathic Hyperphosphatemia;
  Osteochalasis Desmalis Familiaris;
  Familial Osteoectasia)   387

– Lignac-Fanconi Syndrome
  (Fanconi-Lignac Syndrome; Cystinosis
  Syndrome; Cystine Storage-
  Aminoaciduria-Dwarfism Syndrome;
  Renal Rickets; Nephropathic Cystinosis)   388

– Bullous Ichthyosiform Erythroderma
  (Collodion Baby; Congenital Ichthyosis;
  Epidermolytic Hyperkeratosis;
  Ichthyosis; Ichthyosis Vulgaris; Lamellar
  Ichthyosis; Nonbullous Ichthyosiform
  Erythroderma; Xeroderma; X-Linked
  Ichthyosis)   388

– Phthisis Bulbi   389

– Juvenile Rheumatoid Arthritis
  (JRA; Still Disease)   389

– Rheumatoid Arthritis (Adult)   389

– Interstitial Keratitis   390

– Felty Syndrome (Chauffard-Still Syndrome; Primary Splenic Neutropenia with Arthritis; Rheumatoid Arthritis with Hypersplenism; Still-Chauffard Syndrome; Uveitis-Rheumatoid Arthritis Syndrome) 390

– Romberg Syndrome (Parry-Romberg Syndrome; Progressive Hemifacial Atrophy; Progressive Facial Hemiatrophy; Facial Hemiatrophy) Enophthalmus 391

– Bourneville Syndrome (Bourneville-Pringle Syndrome; Tuberous Sclerosis; Epiloia) 391

– Wagner Syndrome (Hyaloideoretinal Degeneration; Hereditary Hyaloideoretinal Degeneration and Palatoschisis; Clefting Syndrome; Goldmann-Favre Syndrome; Favre Hyaloideoretinal Degeneration; Retinoschisis with Early Hemeralopia) Nystagmus 392

– Bietti Disease (Bietti Marginal Crystalline Dystrophy) 393

– Erosion Syndrome 393

– Pterygium of Conjunctiva and Cornea 394

– Fuchs-Salzmann-Terrien Syndrome 394

– Terrien Disease (Terrien Marginal Degeneration; Gutter Dystrophy; Peripheral Furrow Keratitis; Senile Marginal Atrophy) 394

• Dystrophy 395

– Cogan-Guerry Syndrome (Microcystic Corneal Dystrophy; Map-Dot Fingerprint Dystrophy) 395

– Corneal Dystrophy, Meesmann Epithelial (Meesmann Epithelial Dystrophy of Cornea) 395

– Thygeson Syndrome (Keratitis Superficialis Punctata) 396

– Reis-Bucklers Corneal Dystrophy (Corneal Dystrophy of Bowman's Layer, Superficial Variant of Granular Dystrophy, Granular Corneal Dystrophy Type III) 396

– Francois (1) Dystrophy (Francois-Neetens Syndrome; Central Cloudy Dystrophy; Cloudy Central Corneal Dystrophy) 397

– Granular Corneal Dystrophy 397

– Lattice Corneal Dystrophy (Lattice Dystrophy Type I, Lattice Dystrophy Type II, Lattice Dystrophy Type III, LCD-I, LCD-II, LCD-III, Meretoja's Syndrome, Biber-Haab-Dimmer Dystrophy, Familial Myloid Polyneuropathy Type IV, Avellino Dystrophy) 398

– Corneal Dystrophy, Macular Type (Groenouw Type II Corneal Dystrophy) 398

– Fuchs' Corneal Dystrophy (Fuchs' Endothelial Dystrophy of the Cornea, Combined Dystrophy of Fuchs', Endothelial Dystrophy of the Cornea, Epithelial Dystrophy of Fuchs', Fuchs' Epithelial-Endothelial Dystrophy) 399

– Posterior Polymorphous Dystrophy 399

– Corneal Snowflake Dystrophy 400

– Schnyder's Crystalline Corneal Dystrophy 400

• Keratoconus (Conical Cornea) 400

– Alagille Syndrome (AGS; Alagille-Watson Syndrome, AWS; Cholestasis with Peripheral Pulmonary Stenosis; Arteriohepatic Dysplasia, AHD; Hepatic Ductular Hypoplasia, Syndromatic) 401

– Aniridia (Congenital Aniridia, Hereditary Aniridia) 402

– Apert Syndrome (Acrocephalosyndactylism Syndrome; Acrocranio-dysphalangia; Acrodysplasia; Sphenoacrocranio-syndactyly; Absent-Digits-Cranial-Defects Syndrome) 402

– Asthma (Hayfever) 403

– Atopic Dermatitis (Atopic Eczema; Besnier Prurigo) 403

– Lattice Corneal Dystrophy (Lattice Dystrophy Type I, Lattice Dystrophy Type II, Lattice Dystrophy Type III, LCD-I, LCD-II, LCD-III, Meretoja's Syndrome, Biber-Haab-Dimmer Dystrophy, Familial Myloid Polyneuropathy Type IV, Avellino Dystrophy) 404

– Van Der Hoeve Syndrome (Osteogenesis Imperfecta; Osteopsathyrosis; Ekman Syndrome; Lobstein Syndrome; Spurway Syndrome; Vrolik Syndrome; Eddowes Syndrome; Brittle Bone Disease) Glaucoma 404

– Iris Nevus Syndrome (Cogan-Reese Syndrome; Chandler Syndrome; Iridocorneal Endothelial Syndrome; ICE Syndrome) — 405

– Neovascularization, Corneal Contact Lens Related — 405

– Crouzon Syndrome (Dysostosis Craniofacialis; Oxycephaly; Craniofacial Dysostosis; Parrot-Head Syndrome; Möbius-Crouzon Syndrome; Hereditary Craniofacial Dysostosis) — 406

– Ehlers-Danlos Syndrome (Fibrodysplasia Elastica Generalisata; Cutis Hyperelastica; Meekeren-Ehlers-Danlos Syndrome; Indian Rubber Man Syndrome; Cutis Laxa) — 406

– Floppy Eyelid Syndrome — 407

– Goltz Syndrome (Focal Dermal Hypoplasia Syndrome) — 407

– Fuchs' Corneal Dystrophy (Fuchs' Endothelial Dystrophy of the Cornea, Combined Dystrophy of Fuchs, Endothelial Dystrophy of the Cornea, Epithelial Dystrophy of Fuchs, Fuchs' Epithelial-Endothelial Dystrophy) — 408

– Grönblad-Strandberg Syndrome (Systemic Elastodystrophy; Pseudoxanthoma Elasticum; Elastorrhexis; Darier-Grönblad-Strandberg Syndrome) — 408

– Leber Tapetoretinal Dystrophy Syndrome (Amaurosis Congenita; Retinal Aplasia; Retinal Abiotrophy; Pigmentary Retinitis with Congenital Amaurosis; Dysgenesis Neuroepithelialis Retinae; Alstrom-Olsen Syndrome) — 409

– Kuru Syndrome (Laughing Death) — 410

– Laurence-Moon-Bardet-Biedl Syndrome (Bardet-Biedl Syndrome; Retinitis Pigmentosa-Polydactyly-Adiposogenital Syndrome) — 410

– Little Syndrome (Nail-Patella Syndrome; Hereditary Osteo-Onycho-Dysplasia; HOOD Syndrome) — 411

– Lymphogranuloma Venereum (Nicolas-Favre Disease; Tropical Bubo LGV; Lymphogranuloma Inguinale) — 411

– Marfan Syndrome (Dolichostenomelia; Arachnodactyly; Hyperchondroplasia; Dystrophia Mesodermalis Congenita) — 411

– Measles (Morbilli; Rubeola) — 412

– Down Syndrome (Mongolism) — 412

– Mulvihill-Smith Syndrome — 413

– Neurodermatitis (Lichen Simplex Chronicus) — 413

– Von Recklinghausen Syndrome (Neurofibromatosis Type I; Neurinomatosis) — 414

– Noonan Syndrome (Male Turner Syndrome) — 414

– Ocular Hypertension — 415

– Pellucid Marginal Degeneration — 415

– Lenticonus and Lentiglobus — 415

– Posterior Polymorphous Dystrophy — 416

– Retinal Disinsertion Syndrome (Keratoconus) — 416

– Retinitis Pigmentosa — 416

– Retrolental Fibroplasia (RLF; Retinopathy of Prematurity) — 417

– Rieger Syndrome (Axenfeld-Rieger Syndrome; Dysgenesis Mesodermalis Corneae et Irides; Dysgenesis Mesostromalis; Axenfeld Posterior Embryotoxon-Juvenile Glaucoma) — 418

– Tourette Syndrome (Gilles de la Tourette Syndrome; Brissaud II Syndrome; Caprolalia Generalized Tic; Guinon Myospasia Impulsiva) — 418

• Berardinelli-Seip Syndrome (Congenital Generalized Lipodystrophy) — 419

• Brittle Cornea Syndrome (Brittle Cornea, Blue Sclera and Red Hair Syndrome; Blue Sclera Syndrome) — 419

• Cataract, Microcornea Syndrome — 419

• Colobomatous, Microphthalmia and Microcornea Syndrome — 420

• Cataract, Congenital or Juvenile (Cataract, Juvenile, Hutterite Type) — 420

• Congenital Clouding of the Cornea — 421

• Spinocerebellar Degeneration and Corneal Dystrophy (Corneal Cerebellar Syndrome; Corneal Dystrophy with Spinocerebellar Degeneration) — 421

• Cornea Plana — 422

• Down Syndrome (Mongolism; Trisomy G; Trisomy 21 Syndrome; Mongoloid Idiocy) — 422

• Francois (2) Dystrophy (Francois-Evens Syndrome; Speckled Corneal Dystrophy) — 422

- Megalocornea (Cornea having a Horizontal Diameter of more than 14 mm) 423
  - Aarskog Syndrome (Facial-Digital-Genital Syndrome) 423
  - Congenital and Infantile Cataracts 424
  - Craniosynostosis-Mental Retardation-Clefting Syndrome 424
  - Down Syndrome (Mongolism; Trisomy G; Trisomy 21 Syndrome; Mongoloid Idiocy) 424
  - Marchesani Syndrome (Weill-Marchesani Syndrome; Inverted Marfan Syndrome; Brachymorphy with Spherophakia; Dystrophia Mesodermalis Congenita Hyperplastica) 425
  - Marfan Syndrome (Dolichostenomelia; Arachnodactyly; Hyperchondroplasia; Dystrophia Mesodermalis Congenita) 425
  - MMMM Syndrome (Neuhauser Syndrome; Megalocornea, Macrocephaly, Mental and Motor Retardation) 426
  - Scheie Syndrome (Mucopolysaccharidosis IS; MPS IS; MPS V; Mucopolysaccharidosis V) 426
  - Neuhauser Syndrome (Megalocornea, Macrocephaly, Mental and Motor Retardation) 427
  - Lowe Syndrome (Oculo-Cerebro-Renal Syndrome) 427
  - Oculodental Syndrome (Peters Syndrome; Rutherford Syndrome) 428
  - Van Der Hoeve Syndrome (Osteogenesis Imperfecta; Osteopsathyrosis; Ekman Syndrome; Lobstein Syndrome; Spurway Syndrome; Vrolik Syndrome; Eddowes Syndrome; Brittle Bone Disease) Glaucoma 428
  - Crouzon Syndrome (Dysostosis Craniofacialis; Oxycephaly; Craniofacial Dysostosis; Parrot-Head Syndrome; Möbius-Crouzon Syndrome; Hereditary Craniofacial Dysostosis) 429
  - Pierre-Robin Syndrome (Robin Syndrome; Micrognathia-Glossoptosis Syndrome) 429
  - Rieger Syndrome (Axenfeld-Rieger Syndrome; Dysgenesis Mesodermalis Corneae et Irides; Dysgenesis Mesostromalis; Axenfeld Posterior Embryotoxon-Juvenile Glaucoma) 430
  - Rubella Syndrome (Congenital Rubella Syndrome; German Measles; Gregg Syndrome) 430
  - Sturge-Weber Syndrome (Meningocutaneous Syndrome; Vascular Encephalotrigeminal Syndrome; Neuro-Oculocutaneous Angiomatosis; Encephalofacial Angiomatosis; Encephalotrigeminal Syndrome) 431
- Microcornea (Cornea with a Horizontal Diameter of less than 10 mm) 431
  - Aniridia (Congenital Aniridia, Hereditary Aniridia) 432
  - Dislocation of the Lens 433
  - Axenfeld-Rieger Syndrome (Posterior Embryotoxon; Axenfeld Syndrome) 433
  - Colobomatous, Microphthalmia and Microcornea Syndrome 434
  - Glaucoma, Congenital 434
  - Hyperopia, High 434
  - Meckel Syndrome (Dysencephalia Splanchnocystic Syndrome; Gruber Syndrome) 435
  - Primary Angle-Closure Glaucoma (Primary Closed Angle Glaucoma) 435
  - Sclerocornea 436
  - Aberfeld Syndrome (Schwartz-Jampel Syndrome; Congenital Blepharophimosis Associated with Generalized Myopathy Syndrome; Ocular and Facial Abnormalities Syndrome) 436
  - Carpenter Syndrome (Acrocephalopolysyndactyly Type II) 437
  - Cataract, Microcornea Syndrome 437
  - Chromosome 18 Partial Deletion (Long-Arm) Syndrome [Monosomy 18 Partial (Long-Arm) Syndrome; De Grouchy Syndrome] 437
  - Ehlers-Danlos Syndrome (Fibrodysplasia Elastica Generalisata; Cutis Hyperelastica; Meekeren-Ehlers-Danlos Syndrome; Indian Rubber Man Syndrome; Cutis Laxa) 438
  - Gansslen Syndrome (Familial Hemolytic Icterus; Hematologic-Metabolic Bone Disorder) 439
  - Hallermann-Streiff Syndrome [Dyscephalic-Mandibulo-Oculo-Facial Syndrome; Oculo-Mandibulo-Dyscephaly; Ullrich-Fremery-Dohna Syndrome; Francois Dyscephalic

Syndrome; Mandibulo-Oculo-Facial
Dyscephaly Syndrome; Francois-
Hallermann-Streiff Syndrome;
Hallermann-Streiff-Francois Syndrome;
Audry I Syndrome; Dohna Syndrome;
Francois Syndrome (1); Dyscephaly-Teeth
Abnormality-Dwarfism; Dyscephalia
Oculomandibularis-Hypotrichosis;
Mandibulo-Ocular Dyscephalia
Hypotrichosis; Fremery-Dohna Syndrome;
Oculo-Mandibulo-Facial Dyscephaly]   439

– Hemifacial Microsomia Syndrome
   (Unilateral Facial Agenesis;
   Otomandibular Dysostosis;
   Francois-Haustrate Syndrome)   440

– Hutchinson-Gilford Syndrome (Progeria)   441

– Laurence-Moon-Bardet-Biedl
   Syndrome (Bardet-Biedl Syndrome;
   Retinitis Pigmentosa-Polydactyly-
   Adiposogenital Syndrome)   441

– Lenz Microphthalmia Syndrome   442

– Little Syndrome (Nail-Patella Syndrome;
   Hereditary Osteo-Onycho-Dysplasia;
   HOOD Syndrome)   442

– Marchesani Syndrome (Weill-Marchesani
   Syndrome; Inverted Marfan Syndrome;
   Brachymorphy with Spherophakia;
   Dystrophia Mesodermalis
   Congenita Hyperplastica)   442

– Marfan Syndrome (Dolichostenomelia;
   Arachnodactyly; Hyperchondroplasia;
   Dystrophia Mesodermalis Congenita)   443

– Meckel Syndrome (Dysencephalia
   Splanchnocystic Syndrome;
   Gruber Syndrome)   444

– Meyer-Schwickerath-Weyers Syndrome
   (Microphthalmos Syndrome;
   Oculodentodigital Dysplasia)   444

– Morgagni Syndrome (Hyperostosis
   Frontalis Interna Syndrome;
   Intracranial Exostosis;
   Metabolic Craniopathy)   445

– Micro Syndrome   446

– Rieger Syndrome (Axenfeld-Rieger
   Syndrome; Dysgenesis Mesodermalis
   Corneae et Irides; Dysgenesis
   Mesostromalis; Axenfeld Posterior
   Embryotoxon-Juvenile Glaucoma)   446

– Ring Chromosome 6 (Aniridia, Congenital
   Glaucoma, and Hydrocephalus)   447

– Roberts Pseudothalidomide
   Syndrome (Glaucoma)   447

– Rubella Syndrome (Congenital Rubella
   Syndrome; German Measles;
   Gregg Syndrome)   448

– Sabin-Feldman Syndrome
   (Chorioretinitis)   448

– Schwartz Syndrome
   (Retinal Detachment)   449

– Smith-Magenis Syndrome   449

– Triploidy Syndrome (Iris Coloboma)   450

– Trisomy 13 Syndrome (Trisomy D1
   Syndrome, Patau Syndrome,
   Reese Syndrome) Iris Coloboma   450

– Waardenburg Syndrome (Van Der
   Hoeve-Halberstam-Waardenburg
   Syndrome; Waardenburg-Klein
   Syndrome; Embryonic Fixation
   Syndrome; Interoculo-
   Iridodermato-Auditive Dysplasia;
   Piebaldism) Hypertelorism   451

• MIDAS Syndrome (Microphthalmia,
   Dermal Aplasia and Sclerocornea)   451

• MMMM Syndrome (Neuhauser Syndrome;
   Megalocornea, Macrocephaly, Mental and
   Motor Retardation)   452

• Myotonic Dystrophy Syndrome (Myotonia
   Atrophica Syndrome; Dystrophia Myotonica;
   Curschmann-Steinert Syndrome)   452

• Multiple Endocrine Neoplasia
   2B or 3 (MEN 2B or 3)   453

• Ring Dermoid Syndrome (Amblyopia)   454

• Sclerocornea   454

• Senter Syndrome (Keratitis-Ichthyosis-
   Deafness Syndrome; KID Syndrome;
   Ichthyosiform Erythroderma, Corneal
   Involvement, and Deafness (Keratitis)   455

• Snail Tracks of Cornea   455

• Weyers Syndrome (2) (Weyers IV
   Syndrome; Iridodental Dysplasia;
   Dentoirideal Dysplasia; Dysgenesis
   Iridodentalis; Dysgenesis Mesodermalis
   Corneae et Irides with Digodontia)
   Corneal Opacity   455

• Whipple Disease
   (Intestinal Lipodystrophy) Papilledema   456

• Keratitis   456

   – Actinomycosis   456

   – Corneal Ulcer (Bacterial Corneal Ulcers,
      Bacterial Keratitis)   457

   – Central Sterile Corneal Ulceration   457

   – Corneal Opacity-Diffuse   457

– Cockayne Syndrome (Dwarfism with Retinal Atrophy and Deafness; Mickey Mouse Syndrome)   458

– Lignac-Fanconi Syndrome (Fanconi-Lignac Syndrome; Cystinosis Syndrome; Cystine Storage-Aminoaciduria-Dwarfism Syndrome; Renal Rickets; Nephropathic Cystinosis)   458

– Rubella Syndrome (Congenital Rubella Syndrome; German Measles; Gregg Syndrome)   459

– Gangliosidosis GMI Type 1 [Generalized Gangliosidosis (Infantile); Norman-Landing Syndrome; Pseudo-Hurler Lipoidosis]   459

– Hurler Syndrome (Pfaundler-Hurler Syndrome; Gargoylism; Dysostosis Multiplex; MPS IH Syndrome; Systemic Mucopolysaccharidosis Type IH; Mucopolysaccharidosis IH)   460

– Maroteaux-Lamy Syndrome (Systemic Mucopolysaccharidosis Type VI; MPS VI Syndrome; Mucopolysaccharidosis VI)   461

– Morquio Syndrome (Morquio-Brailsford Syndrome; Brailsford-Morquio Dystrophy; Familial Osseous Dystrophy; Keratosulfaturia; MPS IV; Mucopolysaccharidosis IV; Spondyloepiphyseal Dysplasia; Osteochondrodystrophia Deformans; Infantile Hereditary Chondrodysplasia; Hereditary Poly topic Enchondral Dysostosis; Hereditary Osteochondrodystrophy; Eccentro-Osteochondrodysplasia; Dysostosis Enchondralis Meta-Epiphysaria; Morquio-Ullrich Syndrome; Atypical Chondrodystrophy; Chondrodystrophia Tarda; Chondro-Osteodystrophy)   461

– ML III (Pseudo-Hurler Polydystrophy; Mucolipidosis III)   462

– ML IV (Mucolipidosis IV; Berman Syndrome)   462

– Arylsulfatase A Deficiency (Metachromatic Leukodystrophy; Sulfatide Lipoidosis Syndrome; Greenfield Disease; Scholz Syndrome; Scholz-Bielschowsky-Henneberg Syndrome; Van Bogaert-Nyssen Disease; Van Bogaert-Nyssen-Peiffer Disease; Familial Progressive Cerebral Sclerosis; Infantile Progressive Cerebral Sclerosis;

Infantile Metachromatic Leukodystrophy; Leukodystrophia Cerebri Progressiva Metachromatica Diffusa; Opticochleodentate Degeneration)   463

– Beta-Glucuronidase Deficiency (Mucopolysaccharidosis VII; MPS VII)   463

– Jadassohn-Lewandowsky Syndrome (Pachyonychia Congenita)   464

– Cerebro-Oculo-Facio-Skeletal Syndrome (COFS Syndrome)   464

– Oculodental Syndrome (Peters Syndrome; Rutherford Syndrome)   465

– Scheie Syndrome (Mucopolysaccharidosis IS; MPS IS; MPS V; Mucopolysaccharidosis V)   465

– Sclerocornea   466

– Berardinelli-Seip Syndrome (Congenital Generalized Lipodystrophy)   466

– Goldberg Disease   467

– Corneal Opacity-Localized, Congenital   467

– ACL Syndrome (Acromegaloid, Cutis Verticis Gyrata, Corneal Leukoma Syndrome)   467

– Cataract, Microcornea Syndrome   468

– Fetal Alcohol Syndrome   468

– Rubella Syndrome (Congenital Rubella Syndrome; German Measles; Gregg Syndrome)   469

– Keratoconus Posticus Circumscriptus (KPC; KPC with Associated Malformations)   469

– Corneal Dystrophy, Meesmann Epithelial (Meesmann Epithelial Dystrophy of Cornea)   470

– Peters Anomaly   470

– Pillay Syndrome (Ophthalmomandibulomelic Dysplasia)   471

– Anterior Chamber Cleavage Syndrome (Reese-Ellsworth Syndrome; Peters-Plus Syndrome)   471

– Hanhart Syndrome (Richner Syndrome; Recessive Keratosis Palmoplantaris; Pseudoherpetic Keratitis; Richner-Hanhart Syndrome; Tyrosinemia II; Tyrosinosis; Pseudodendritic Keratitis)   472

– Rieger Syndrome (Axenfeld-Rieger Syndrome; Dysgenesis Mesodermalis Corneae et Irides; Dysgenesis Mesostromalis; Axenfeld Posterior Embryotoxon-Juvenile Glaucoma)   472

– Waardenburg Syndrome (Van Der Hoeve-Halberstam-Waardenburg Syndrome; Waardenburg-Klein Syndrome; Embryonic Fixation Syndrome; Interoculo-Iridodermato-Auditive Dysplasia; Piebaldism) Hypertelorism ... 473

– 11q- Syndrome ... 473

– 18q- Syndrome (18q Deletion Syndrome) ... 474

– Sands of the Sahara Syndrome (Diffuse Lamellar Keratitis) ... 474

– Filamentary Keratitis ... 474

– Fungal Keratitis ... 475

– HLA-B27 Syndromes ... 475

– Interstitial Keratitis ... 476

– Keratitis Fugax Hereditaria ... 476

– Senter Syndrome (Keratitis-Ichthyosis-Deafness Syndrome; KID Syndrome; Ichthyosiform Erythroderma, Corneal Involvement, and Deafness (Keratitis) ... 476

– Dimmer Syndrome (Keratitis Nummularis) ... 477

– Epithelial Erosion Syndrome (Metaherpetic Keratitis; Kaufman Syndrome; Franceschetti Dystrophy; Posttraumatic Keratitis) ... 477

– Mooren's Ulcer (Chronic Serpiginous Ulcer of the Cornea, Ulcus) ... 478

– Neuroparalytic Keratitis (Neutropic Keratitis, Trigeminial Neuropathic Keratopathy) ... 478

– Cogan (1) Syndrome (Nonsyphilitic Interstitial Keratitis) ... 479

– Pannus (Superficial Vascular Invasion Confined to a Segment of the Cornea or Extending Around the Entire Limbus) ... 479

– Acne Rosacea (Acne Erythematosa; Ocular Rosacea) ... 480

– Anoxic Overwear Syndrome ... 480

– Avitaminosis B2 (Ariboflavinosis; Pellagra) ... 481

– Neovascularization, Corneal Contact Lens Related ... 481

– Deerfly Fever (Francis Disease; Rabbit Fever; Tularemia; Deerfly Tularemia) ... 482

– Corneal Edema (Bullous Keratopathy, Epithelial Edema, Stromal Edema) ... 482

– Dermatitis Herpetiformis (Duhring-Brocq Disease) ... 482

– Fuchs' Corneal Dystrophy (Fuchs' Endothelial Dystrophy of the Cornea, Combined Dystrophy of Fuchs', Endothelial Dystrophy of the Cornea, Epithelial Dystrophy of Fuchs', Fuchs' Epithelial-Endothelial Dystrophy) ... 483

– Haemophilus Influenzae ... 483

– Histiocytosis X (Hand-Schuller-Christian Syndrome; Lipoid Granuloma; Xanthomatous Granuloma Syndrome; Schuller-Christian-Hand Syndrome; Letterer-Siwe Syndrome; Acute Histiocytosis X; Eosinophilic Granuloma; Reticuloendotheliosis Syndrome) ... 484

– Hypoparathyroidism ... 485

– Chlamydia (Inclusion Conjunctivitis; Paratrachoma) ... 485

– Keratoconjunctivitis Sicca and Sjögren's Syndrome ... 486

– Leishmaniasis ... 486

– Terrien Disease (Terrien Marginal Degeneration; Gutter Dystrophy; Peripheral Furrow Keratitis; Senile Marginal Atrophy) ... 486

– Peripheral Ulcerative Keratitis ... 487

– PISK (Pressure Induced Intralamellar Stromal Keratitis) ... 487

– Hanhart Syndrome (Richner Syndrome; Recessive Keratosis Palmoplantaris; Pseudoherpetic Keratitis; Richner-Hanhart Syndrome; Tyrosinemia II; Tyrosinosis; Pseudodendritic Keratitis) ... 488

– Relapsing Fever (Recurrent Fever) ... 488

– Rocky Mountain Spotted Fever ... 489

– Sandwich Infectious Keratitis Syndrome (SIK Syndrome) ... 489

– Superior Limbic Keratoconjunctivitis (Theodores Superior Limbic Keratoconjunctivitis, SLK) ... 489

– Peripheral Ulcerative Keratitis ... 490

– Ultraviolet Keratitis ... 490

– Vernal Keratoconjunctivitis (Atopic Keratoconjunctivitis, Allergic Conjunctivitis, Giant Papillary Conjunctivitis) ... 491

• Trauma ... 491

– Corneal Abrasions, Contusions, Lacerations and Perforations ... 491

– Cogan (1) Syndrome (Nonsyphilitic Interstitial Keratitis) ... 491

– Corneal Edema (Bullous Keratopathy, Epithelial Edema, Stromal Edema) 492
– Corneal Edema, Postoperative 492
– Descemet Membrane Folds 493
– Corneal Foreign Body 493
– Corneal Graft Rejection or Failure 493
– Herpes Simplex 494
– Corneal Melt Postoperative 494
– Corneal Mucous Plaques 495
– Myopia, Intracorneal Rings 495
– Neovascularization, Corneal Contact Lens Related 495
– Mucous Membrane Pemphigoid 496
– Ultraviolet Keratitis 496

21. Extraocular Muscles 497

• Paralysis of Sixth Nerve (Abducens Palsy) 497
– Foville Syndrome (Foville Peduncular Syndrome) 499
– Gaucher Syndrome (Glucocerebroside Storage Disease; Glucosyl Ceramide Lipidosis; Cerebroside Lipidosis) 499
– Extreme Hydrocephalus Syndrome (Kleeblattschädel Syndrome; Cloverleaf Skull Syndrome; Hydrocephalus; Chondrodystrophicus Congenita) 500
– Leukemia 500
– Millard-Gubler Syndrome (Abducens-Facial Hemiplegia Alternans) 501
– Pneumococcal Infections (Streptococcus Pneumoniae Infections) 501
– Arnold-Chiari Syndrome (Platybasia Syndrome; Cerebellomedullary Malformation Syndrome; Basilar Impressions) 502
– Vertebral Basilar Artery Syndrome (Intranuclear Ophthalmoplegia) 502
– Craniopharyngioma 503
– Hemangioma 503
– Wernicke Syndrome I (Superior Hemorrhagic Polioencephalopathic Syndrome; Hemorrhagic Polioencephalitis Superior Syndrome; Encephalitis Hemorrhagica Superioris; Avitaminosis B; Thiamine Deficiency; Beriberi; Gayet-Wernicke Syndrome; Wernicke-Korsakoff Syndrome) Ptosis 504

– Foramen Lacerum Syndrome (Aneurysm of Internal Carotid Artery Syndrome) 504
– Cushing (2) Syndrome (Angle Tumor Syndrome; Cerebellopontine Angle Syndrome; Pontocerebellar Angle Tumor Syndrome; Acoustic Neuroma Syndrome) 505
– Chickenpox (Varicella) 505
– Coccidioidomycosis (Valley Fever, San Joaquin Fever) 506
– Dandy-Walker Syndrome (Atresia of the Foramen of Magendie) 506
– Diphtheria 506
– Gradenigo Syndrome (Temporal Syndrome; Lannois-Gradenigo Syndrome) 507
– Greig Syndrome (Ocular Hypertelorism Syndrome; Hypertelorism; Primary Embryonic Hypertelorism; Hypertelorism Ocularis) 507
– Hydrophobia (Lyssa; Rabies) 508
– Extreme Hydrocephalus Syndrome (Kleeblattschädel Syndrome; Cloverleaf Skull Syndrome; Hydrocephalus; Chondrodystrophicus Congenita) 508
– Malaria 509
– Measles (Morbilli; Rubeola) 509
– Meningococcemia (Neisseria Meningitides; Meningitis) 509
– Möbius II Syndrome (Congenital Facial Diplegia; Congenital Paralysis of the Sixth and Seventh Nerves; Congenital Oculofacial Paralysis; Von Graefes Syndrome) 510
– Diabetes Mellitus 510
– Herpes Zoster 511
– Poliomyelitis (Infantile Paralysis) 511
– Disseminated Sclerosis (Multiple Sclerosis) 512
– Acquired Lues (Syphilis; Acquired Syphilis; Lues Venerea; Malum Venereum) 512
– Bang Disease (Brucellosis; Malta Fever; Mediterranean Fever; Pig Breeder Disease; Gibraltar Fever; Undulant Fever) 513
– Ophthalmoplegic Migraine Syndrome 513
– Passow Syndrome (Bremer Status Dysraphicus; Status Dysraphicus Syndrome; Syringomyelia; Syringobulbia) 514

- Symonds Syndrome (Otitic Hydrocephalus Syndrome; Serous Meningitis Syndrome; Benign Intracranial Hypertension; Pseudotumor Cerebri) 515
- Raymond Syndrome [Raymond-Cestan Syndrome; Cestan (2) Syndrome; Pontine Syndrome; Disassociation of Lateral Gaze Syndrome] 515
- Relapsing Polychondritis (Jaksch Wartenhost Syndrome; Meyenburg-Altherz-Vehlinger Syndrome; Von Meyenberg II Syndrome) 516
- Trichinellosis (Trichinosis) 516
- Foix Syndrome (Cavernous Sinus Syndrome; Hypophyseal-Sphenoidal Syndrome; Cavernous Sinus Neuralgia Syndrome; Godtfredsen Syndrome; Cavernous Sinus-Nasopharyngeal Tumor Syndrome; Cavernous Sinus Thrombosis) 517
- Orbital Fracture, Apex 517
- Sphenocavernous Syndrome 518
- Sluder Syndrome (Sphenopalatine Ganglion Neuralgia Syndrome; Lower Facial Neuralgia Syndrome) 518
- Rochon-Duvigneaud Syndrome (Superior Orbital Fissure Syndrome) Optic Atrophy 519
- Tolosa-Hunt Syndrome (Painful Ophthalmoplegia) 519
- Raeder Syndrome (Paratrigeminal Paralysis; Horton Headache; Histamine Cephalalgia; Ciliary Neuralgia; Cluster Headache; Periodic Migrainous Neuralgia) 520
- Cretinism (Hypothyroid Goiter; Hypothyroidism; Juvenile Hypothyroidism; Myxedema) 520
- Duane Syndrome (Retraction Syndrome; Stilling Syndrome; Turk-Stilling Syndrome) 521
- Engelmann Syndrome [Osteopathia Hyperostotica (Scleroticans) Multiplex Infantilis; Diaphyseal Dysplasia; Camurati-Engelmann Disease; Hereditary Multiple Diaphyseal Sclerosis; Juvenile Paget Disease] 521
- Kahler Disease (Myelomatosis; Multiple Myeloma) 522
- Disseminated Lupus Erythematosus (Systemic Lupus Erythematosus; Lupus Erythematosus; Kaposi-Libman-Sack Syndrome, SLE) 522

- Erb-Goldflam Syndrome (Erb II Syndrome; Hoppe-Goldflam Disease; Pseudoparalytic Syndrome; Myasthenia Gravis) 523
- Eclampsia and Preeclampsia (Toxemia of Pregnancy; Preeclampsia) 524
- Schaumann Syndrome (Besnier-Boeck-Schaumann Syndrome; Boeck Sarcoid; Sarcoidosis) 524
- Millard-Gubler Syndrome (Abducens-Facial Hemiplegia Alternans) 525
- Accommodative Esotropia 525
- Acquired Nonaccommodative Esotropia 526
- A Esotropia Syndrome 526
- Axenfeld-Schurenberg Syndrome (Cyclic Oculomotor Paralysis) 526
- Cogan (2) Syndrome (Oculomotor Apraxia Syndrome; Wieacker Syndrome) 527
- Congenital Esotropia (Infantile Esotropia) 527
- Esotropia: High Accommodative Convergence to Accommodation Ratio 528
- Marcus Gunn Syndrome (Jaw-Winking Syndrome; Congenital Trigeminooculomotor Synkinesis) 528
- Paralysis of Third Nerve (Oculomotor Nerve) 528
  - Benedikt Syndrome (Tegmental Syndrome) 531
  - Erb-Goldflam Syndrome (Erb II Syndrome; Hoppe-Goldflam Disease; Pseudoparalytic Syndrome; Myasthenia Gravis) 531
  - Parinaud Oculoglandular Syndrome (Parinaud Conjunctiva-Adenitis Syndrome; Catscratch Oculoglandular Syndrome; Catscratch Disease; Bartonella henselae) 532
  - Koerber-Salus-Elschnig Syndrome (Sylvian Aqueduct Syndrome; Nystagmus Retractorius Syndrome) 532
  - Axenfeld-Schurenberg Syndrome (Cyclic Oculomotor Paralysis) 533
  - Bruns Syndrome (Postural Change Syndrome) 533
  - Claude Syndrome (Inferior Nucleus Ruber Syndrome; Rubro-Spinal-Cerebellar-Peduncle Syndrome) 533
  - Nothnagel Syndrome (Ophthalmoplegia-Cerebellar Ataxia Syndrome) 534
  - Vertebral Basilar Artery Syndrome (Intranuclear Ophthalmoplegia) 534

– Migraine (Vascular Headache) 535
– Weber Syndrome (Weber-Dubler Syndrome; Cerebellar Peduncle Syndrome; Alternating Oculomotor Paralysis; Ventral Medial Midbrain Syndrome) Ptosis 535
– Amebiasis (Amebic Dysentery, Entamoeba Histolytica) 536
– Botulism 536
– Chickenpox (Varicella) 537
– Craniopharyngioma 537
– Dengue Fever 538
– Devic Syndrome (Ophthalmoencephalomyelopathy; Optic Myelitis; Neuromyelitis Optica) 538
– Diphtheria 539
– Encephalitis, Acute 539
– Influenza 539
– Lockjaw (Tetanus) 540
– Malaria 540
– Measles (Morbilli; Rubeola) 541
– Meningococcemia (Neisseria Meningitides; Meningitis) 541
– Disseminated Sclerosis (Multiple Sclerosis) 541
– Ophthalmoplegic Migraine Syndrome 542
– Kussmaul Disease (Kussmaul-Maier Disease; Necrotizing Angiitis; PAN) 543
– Poliomyelitis (Infantile Paralysis) 543
– Alcoholism 544
– Herpes Zoster 544
– Mumps 545
– Hydrophobia (Lyssa; Rabies) 545
– Relapsing polychondritis (Jaksch Wartenhost Syndrome; MeyenbUrg-Altherz-Vehlinger Syndrome; Von MeyEnberg II Syndrome) 546
– Smallpox (Variola) 546
– Acquired Lues (Syphilis; Acquired Syphilis; Lues Venerea; Malum Venereum) 547
– Temporal Arteritis Syndrome (Cranial Arteritis Syndrome; Giant Cell Arteritis; Hutchinson-Horton-Magath-Brown Syndrome) 547
– Tuberculosis 548
– Carotid Artery Syndrome (Cavernous Sinus Fistula Syndrome; Red-Eyed Shunt Syndrome) 548

– Arteriovenous Fistula (Arteriovenous Aneurysm; Arteriovenous Angioma; Arteriovenous Malformation; Cirsoid Aneurysm; Racemose Hemangioma; Varicose Aneurysm) 549
– Carotid Artery Syndrome (Cavernous Sinus Fistula Syndrome; Red-Eyed Shunt Syndrome) 549
– Tolosa-Hunt Syndrome (Painful Ophthalmoplegia) 550
– Rochon-Duvigneaud Syndrome (Superior Orbital Fissure Syndrome) Optic Atrophy 550
– Foramen Lacerum Syndrome (Aneurysm of Internal Carotid Artery Syndrome) 551
– Sphenocavernous Syndrome 551
– Gradenigo Syndrome (Temporal Syndrome; Lannois-Gradenigo Syndrome) 552
– Rochon-Duvigneaud Syndrome (Superior Orbital Fissure Syndrome) Optic Atrophy 552
– Albers-Schonberg Disease (Marble Bone Disease; Osteosclerosis Fragilis Generalisata; Osteopetrosis; Osteopoikilosis; Osteosclerosis Congenita Diffusa) 553
– Hodgkin Disease 553
– Disseminated Lupus Erythematosus (Systemic Lupus Erythematosus; Lupus Erythematosus; Kaposi-Libman-Sack Syndrome, SLE) 554
– Erb-Goldflam Syndrome (Erb II Syndrome; Hoppe-Goldflam Disease; Pseudoparalytic Syndrome; Myasthenia Gravis) 554
– Passow Syndrome (Bremer Status Dysraphicus; Status Dysraphicus Syndrome; Syringomyelia; Syringobulbia) 555
– Porphyria Cutanea Tarda 555
– Schaumann Syndrome (Besnier-Boeck-Schaumann Syndrome; Boeck Sarcoid; Sarcoidosis) 556
• V Esotropia Syndrome 556
• Weber Syndrome (Weber-Dubler Syndrome; Cerebellar Peduncle Syndrome; Alternating Oculomotor Paralysis; Ventral Medial Midbrain Syndrome) Ptosis 557

- Sixth Nerve 557
  - Acquired Exotropia 557
  - A Exotropia Syndrome 558
  - Basic and Intermittent Exotropia 558
  - V Exotropia Syndrome 558
- Fourth Nerve 559
  - Brown Syndrome (Superior Oblique Tendon Sheath Syndrome) 559
  - Canine Tooth Syndrome (Class VII Superior Oblique Palsy) 559
  - Congenital Epiblepharon Inferior Oblique Insufficiency Syndrome 560
  - Proximal and Distal Click Syndrome of the Superior Oblique Tendon (Simulated Superior Oblique Tendon Syndrome) 560
  - Superior Oblique Myokymia 561
  - Trochlear Nerve Palsy (Fourth Nerve Palsy) 561
- Nystagmus 561
  - Blocked Nystagmus Syndrome (Nystagmus Blockage Syndrome; Nystagmus Compensation Syndrome) 561
  - Cataract, Microphthalmia and Nystagmus 562
  - Epiphyseal Dysplasia, Microcephaly, and Nystagmus 562
  - Hennebert Syndrome (Luetic-Otitic-Nystagmus Syndrome) 563
  - Karsch-Neugebauer Syndrome (Nystagmus-Split Hand Syndrome) 563
  - Koerber-Salus-Elschnig Syndrome (Sylvian Aqueduct Syndrome; Nystagmus Retractorius Syndrome) 564
  - Lenoble-Aubineau Syndrome (Nystagmus-Myoclonia Syndrome) 564
  - Nystagmus 565
  - Nystagmus Compensation Syndrome 565
  - Nystagmus, Congenital (Congenital Idiopathic Nystagmus) 565
  - Nystagmus, Primary Hereditary (Congenital Nystagmus) 566
  - Nystagmus, Voluntary 566
- Ophthalmoplegia 567
  - Acute Ophthalmoplegia (Acute Onset of Extraocular Muscle Palsy) 567
  - Internal Orbital Fractures (Blowout Fracture) 570
  - Orbital Cellulitis and Abscess 570
  - Ophthalmoplegic Migraine Syndrome 571
  - Erb-Goldflam Syndrome (Erb II Syndrome; Hoppe-Goldflam Disease; Pseudoparalytic Syndrome; Myasthenia Gravis) 571
  - Rhabdomyosarcoma (Corneal Edema) 572
  - Retinal Artery Occlusion 572
  - Fisher Syndrome (Ophthalmoplegia Ataxia Areflexia Syndrome; Miller-Fisher Syndrome) 573
  - Hydrophobia (Lyssa; Rabies) 573
  - Chickenpox (Varicella) 574
  - Smallpox (Variola) 574
  - Measles (Morbilli; Rubeola) 574
  - Mumps 575
  - Influenza 575
  - Herpes Zoster 576
  - Abdominal Typhus (Enteric Fever; Typhoid Fever) 576
  - Streptococcus (Scarlet Fever) 577
  - Pertussis (Whooping Cough) 577
  - Pneumococcal Infections (Streptococcus Pneumoniae Infections) 578
  - Japanese River Fever (Mite-Borne Typhus; Rural Typhus; Scrub Typhus; Tropical Typhus; Tsutsugamushi Disease; Typhus) 578
  - Malaria 579
  - Guillain-Barré Syndrome (Landry Paralysis; Acute Infectious Neuritis; Acute Polyradiculitis; Acute Febrile Polyneuritis; Acute Idiopathic Polyneuritis; Inflammatory Polyradiculoneuropathy; Landry-Guillain-Barré-Strohl Syndrome; Postinfectious Polyneuritis) 579
  - Acquired Immunodeficiency Syndrome (AIDS; Acquired Cellular Immunodeficiency; Acquired Immunodeficiency) 580
  - Tuberculosis 580
  - Cryptococcosis (Torulosis) 581
  - Diphtheria 581
  - Lockjaw (Tetanus) 582
  - Botulism 582
  - Schaumann Syndrome (Besnier-Boeck-Schaumann Syndrome; Boeck Sarcoid; Sarcoidosis) 582

- Wernicke Syndrome I (Superior Hemorrhagic Polioencephalopathic Syndrome; Hemorrhagic Polioencephalitis Superior Syndrome; Encephalitis Hemorrhagica Superioris; Avitaminosis B; Thiamine Deficiency; Beriberi; Gayet-Wernicke Syndrome; Wernicke-Korsakoff Syndrome) Ptosis   583
- Diabetes Mellitus   583
- Leukemia   584
- Porphyria Cutanea Tarda   584
- Temporal Arteritis Syndrome (Cranial Arteritis Syndrome; Giant Cell Arteritis; Hutchinson-Horton-Magath-Brown Syndrome)   585
- Bielschowsky-Lutz-Cogan Syndrome (Internuclear Ophthalmoplegia)   585
- Bilateral Complete Ophthalmoplegia (Bilateral Palsy of Ocular Muscles, Ptosis, with Pupil and Accommodation Involvement)   586
- Cushing (2) Syndrome (Angle Tumor Syndrome; Cerebellopontine Angle Syndrome; Pontocerebellar Angle Tumor Syndrome; Acoustic Neuroma Syndrome)   586
- Encephalitis, Acute   587
- Fisher Syndrome (Ophthalmoplegia Ataxia Areflexia Syndrome; Miller-Fisher Syndrome)   587
- Temporal Arteritis Syndrome (Cranial Arteritis Syndrome; Giant Cell Arteritis; Hutchinson-Horton-Magath-Brown Syndrome)   588
- Kiloh-Nevin Syndrome (Muscular Dystrophy of External Ocular Muscles; Ocular Myopathy)   588
- Disseminated Sclerosis (Multiple Sclerosis)   589
- Mucormycosis (Phycomycosis)   589
- OHAHA Syndrome (Ophthalmoplegia, Hypotonia, Ataxia, Hypoacusis, Athetosis)   590
- Parinaud Oculoglandular Syndrome (Parinaud Conjunctiva-Adenitis Syndrome; Catscratch Oculoglandular Syndrome; Catscratch Disease; Bartonella Henselae)   590
- Rochon-Duvigneaud Syndrome (Superior Orbital Fissure Syndrome) Optic Atrophy   591
- Rollet Syndrome (Orbital Apex-Sphenoidal Syndrome) Optic Neuritis   591
- Acquired Lues (Syphilis; Acquired Syphilis; Lues Venerea; Malum Venereum)   592
- Wernicke Syndrome I (Superior Hemorrhagic Polioencephalopathic Syndrome; Hemorrhagic Polioencephalitis Superior Syndrome; Encephalitis Hemorrhagica Superioris; Avitaminosis B; Thiamine Deficiency; Beriberi; Gayet-Wernicke Syndrome; Wernicke-Korsakoff Syndrome) Ptosis   592
- Whipple Disease (Intestinal Lipodystrophy) Papilledema   593
- Internal Orbital Fractures (Blowout Fracture)   593
- Cerebellar Ataxia, Infantile, with Progressive External Ophthalmoplegia   593
- Chronic Ophthalmoplegia (CPEO) Slow Onset of Extraocular Muscle Palsy   594
- Ophthalmoplegia, Progressive External   594
- Friedreich Ataxia (Spinocerebellar Ataxia)   595
- Brown-Marie Syndrome (Brown-Marie Ataxic Syndrome; Sanger Brown Syndrome; Hereditary Ataxia Syndrome; Marie Hereditary Ataxia)   595
- Steele-Richardson-Olszewski Syndrome (Progressive Supranuclear Palsy)   596
- Passow Syndrome (Bremer Status Dysraphicus; Status Dysraphicus Syndrome; Syringomyelia; Syringobulbia)   596
- Basedow Syndrome (Graves Disease; Hyperthyroidism; Thyrotoxicosis; Exophthalmic Goiter; Parry Disease)   597
- Disseminated Sclerosis (Multiple Sclerosis)   597
- Acquired Lues (Syphilis; Acquired Syphilis; Lues Venerea; Malum Venereum)   598
- Chronic Progressive External Ophthalmoplegia (CPEO; Ophthalmoplegia Plus)   598
- Dominant Optic Atrophy Syndrome (Dominant Optic Atrophy, Deafness, Ptosis, Ophthalmoplegia, Dystaxia, and Myopathy)   599
- External Ophthalmoplegia (Paralysis of Ocular Muscles Including Ptosis with Sparing of Pupil and Accommodation)   599

- Lubarsch-Pick Syndrome
  (Primary Amyloidosis;
  Idiopathic Amyloidosis; Amyloidosis) 600
- Foramen Lacerum Syndrome
  (Aneurysm of Internal Carotid
  Artery Syndrome) 601
- Bassen-Kornzweig Syndrome
  (Abetalipoproteinemia; Acanthocytosis;
  Familial Hypolipoproteinemia) 601
- Bee Sting of the Eye
  (Bee Sting of the Cornea) 602
- Chronic Progressive External
  Ophthalmoplegia
  (CPEO; Ophthalmoplegia Plus) 602
- Diabetes Mellitus 602
- Diphtheria 603
- Encephalitis, Acute 603
- Friedreich Ataxia
  (Spinocerebellar Ataxia) 604
- Garcin Syndrome (Half-Base Syndrome;
  Schmincke Tumor-Unilateral
  Cranial Paralysis) 604
- Basedow Syndrome (Graves Disease;
  Hyperthyroidism; Thyrotoxicosis;
  Exophthalmic Goiter; Parry Disease) 605
- Jacod Syndrome (Negri-Jacod Syndrome;
  Petrosphenoidal Space Syndrome) 605
- Kearns-Sayre Syndrome
  (Ophthalmoplegia Plus Syndrome;
  Kearns-Shy Syndrome; Kearns Disease) 606
- Mumps 606
- Erb-Goldflam Syndrome
  (Erb II Syndrome; Hoppe-Goldflam
  Disease; Pseudoparalytic Syndrome;
  Myasthenia Gravis) 606
- Myotonic Dystrophy Syndrome
  (Myotonia Atrophica Syndrome;
  Dystrophia Myotonica;
  Curschmann-Steinert Syndrome) 607
- Linear Nevus Sebaceus of Jadassohn
  (Nevus Sebaceus of Jadassohn;
  Jadassohn-Type Anetoderma;
  Organoid Nevus syndrome;
  Sebaceus Nevus Syndrome) 608
- Nothnagel Syndrome
  (Ophthalmoplegia-Cerebellar
  Ataxia Syndrome) 608
- Oculopharyngeal Syndrome
  (Progressive Muscular Dystrophy with
  Ptosis and Dysphagia; Oculopharyngeal
  Muscular Dystrophy) 609

- Olivopontocerebellar Atrophy III
  (OPCA III; OPCA with
  Retinal Degeneration) 609
- Progressive External Ophthalmoplegia
  and Scoliosis 610
- Addison Pernicious Anemia Syndrome
  (Pernicious Anemia Syndrome;
  Vitamin B12 Deficiency Anemia;
  Macrocytic Anemia; Biermer Syndrome) 610
- Guillain-Barré Syndrome
  (Landry Paralysis; Acute Infectious
  Neuritis; Acute Polyradiculitis; Acute
  Febrile Polyneuritis; Acute Idiopathic
  Polyneuritis; Inflammatory
  Polyradiculoneuropathy;
  Landry-Guillain-Barré-Strohl
  Syndrome; Postinfectious Polyneuritis) 611
- Fisher Syndrome (Ophthalmoplegia
  Ataxia Areflexia Syndrome;
  Miller-Fisher Syndrome) 611
- Romberg Syndrome (Parry-Romberg
  Syndrome; Progressive Hemifacial
  Atrophy; Progressive Facial Hemiatrophy;
  Facial Hemiatrophy) Enophthalmus 612
- Refsum Syndrome (Heredopathia Atactica
  Polyneuritiformis Syndrome; Phytanic
  Acid Oxidase Deficiency; Phytanic Acid
  Storage Disease; Refsum-Thiebaut
  Syndrome) 612
- Progressive Systemic Sclerosis
  (Scleroderma; Systemic Scleroderma) 613
- Shy-Drager Syndrome
  (Orthostatic Hypotension Syndrome;
  Shy-MeGee-Drager Syndrome) 613
- Shy-Gonatas Syndrome 614
- Lyme Disease 614
- Rocky Mountain Spotted Fever 615
- Wernicke Syndrome I (Superior
  Hemorrhagic Polioencephalopathic
  Syndrome; Hemorrhagic Polioencephalitis
  Superior Syndrome; Encephalitis
  Hemorrhagica Superioris;
  Avitaminosis B; Thiamine Deficiency;
  Beriberi; Gayet-Wernicke Syndrome;
  Wernicke-Korsakoff Syndrome) Ptosis 615
- Fisher Syndrome (Ophthalmoplegia
  Ataxia Areflexia Syndrome;
  Miller-Fisher Syndrome) 616
- Internuclear Ophthalmoplegia 616
- Arnold-Chiari Syndrome
  (Platybasia Syndrome;
  Cerebellomedullary Malformation
  Syndrome; Basilar Impressions) 617

– Fabry Disease (Angiokeratoma Corporis Diffusum Syndrome; Diffuse Angiokeratosis; Fabry-Anderson Syndrome; Glycosphingolipid Lipidosis; Glycosphingolipidosis)   617

– Disseminated Sclerosis (Multiple Sclerosis)   618

– Erb-Goldflam Syndrome (Erb II Syndrome; Hoppe-Goldflam Disease; Pseudoparalytic Syndrome; Myasthenia Gravis)   618

– Oculocerebellar Tegmental Syndrome   619

– Acquired Lues (Syphilis; Acquired Syphilis; Lues Venerea; Malum Venereum)   619

– Temporal Arteritis Syndrome (Cranial Arteritis Syndrome; Giant Cell Arteritis; Hutchinson-Horton-Magath-Brown Syndrome)   620

– Craniocervical Syndrome (Whiplash Injury)   620

– WEBINO Syndrome (Wall-Eyed Bilateral Internuclear Ophthalmoplegia)   621

– Wernicke Syndrome I (Superior Hemorrhagic Polioencephalopathic Syndrome; Hemorrhagic Polioencephalitis Superior Syndrome; Encephalitis Hemorrhagica Superioris; Avitaminosis B; Thiamine Deficiency; Beriberi; Gayet-Wernicke Syndrome; Wernicke-Korsakoff Syndrome) Ptosis   621

– Bielschowsky-Lutz-Cogan Syndrome (Internuclear Ophthalmoplegia)   622

– Cryptococcosis (Torulosis)   622

– Disseminated Sclerosis (Multiple Sclerosis)   623

– Erb-Goldflam Syndrome (Erb II Syndrome; Hoppe-Goldflam Disease; Pseudoparalytic Syndrome; Myasthenia Gravis)   623

– Behçet Syndrome (Dermato-Stomato-Ophthalmic Syndrome; Oculobuccogenital Syndrome; Gilbert Syndrome)   624

– IVIC Syndrome (Radial Ray Defects, Hearing Impairment, Internal Ophthalmoplegia, Thrombocytopenia)   624

– Kearns-Sayre Syndrome (Ophthalmoplegia Plus Syndrome; Kearns-Shy Syndrome; Kearns Disease)   625

– Myopia-Ophthalmoplegia Syndrome   625

– Nothnagel Syndrome (Ophthalmoplegia-Cerebellar Ataxia Syndrome)   626

– OHAHA Syndrome (Ophthalmoplegia, Hypotonia, Ataxia, Hypoacusis, Athetosis)   626

– Ophthalmoplegia, Familial Static   627

– Painful Ophthalmoplegia (Palsy of Ocular Muscles with Pain)   627

– Foix Syndrome (Cavernous Sinus Syndrome; Hypophyseal-Sphenoidal Syndrome; Cavernous Sinus Neuralgia Syndrome; Godtfredsen Syndrome; Cavernous Sinus-Nasopharyngeal Tumor Syndrome; Cavernous Sinus Thrombosis)   627

– Ophthalmoplegic Migraine Syndrome   628

– Mucormycosis (Phycomycosis)   628

– Acquired Immunodeficiency Syndrome (AIDS; Acquired Cellular Immunodeficiency; Acquired Immunodeficiency)   629

– Rollet Syndrome (Orbital Apex-Sphenoidal Syndrome) Optic Neuritis   629

– Hunt Syndrome (Ramsay-Hunt Syndrome; Geniculate Neuralgia; Herpes Zoster Auricularis)   630

– Rochon-Duvigneaud Syndrome (Superior Orbital Fissure Syndrome) Optic Atrophy   631

– Temporal Arteritis Syndrome (Cranial Arteritis Syndrome; Giant Cell Arteritis; Hutchinson-Horton-Magath-Brown Syndrome)   631

– Tic Douloureux (Trigeminal Neuralgia)   632

– Tolosa-Hunt Syndrome (Painful Ophthalmoplegia)   632

– Ophthalmoplegia, Progressive External   632

– Ophthalmoplegia, Progressive External, with Ragged Red Fibers   633

– Ophthalmoplegia, Progressive External, with Scrotal Tongue and Mental Deficiency   633

– Progressive External Ophthalmoplegia and Scoliosis   634

– Pseudoophthalmoplegia Syndrome (Roth-Bielschowsky Syndrome)   634

– Tolosa-Hunt Syndrome (Painful Ophthalmoplegia)   635

– WEBINO Syndrome (Wall-Eyed Bilateral Internuclear Ophthalmoplegia)   635

- Congenital Vertical Retraction Syndrome 635
- Duane Syndrome (Retraction Syndrome; Stilling Syndrome; Turk-Stilling Syndrome) 636
- General Fibrosis Syndrome (Congenital Enophthalmos with Ocular Muscle Fibrosis and Ptosis; Congenital Fibrosis of the Inferior Rectus with Ptosis; Strabismus Fixus; Vertical Retraction Syndrome (Congenital Fibrosis Syndrome) 636

22. Eyelids **638**

- Disorders 638
  - Aberfeld Syndrome (Schwartz-Jampel Syndrome; Congenital Blepharophimosis Associated with Generalized Myopathy Syndrome; Ocular and Facial Abnormalities Syndrome) 638
  - Bell's Palsy (Idiopathic Facial Paralysis) 638
  - Blepharochalasis 639
  - Blepharophimosis Syndrome (Simosa Syndrome) 639
  - Blepharoptosis, Myopia, Ectopia Lentis 640
  - Charge Association (Multiple Congenital Anomalies Syndrome; Coloboma, Heart Disease, Atresia, Retarded Growth, Genital Hypoplasia, Ear Malformation Association) 640
  - Lid Coloboma 641
  - Amniogenic Band Syndrome (Ring Constriction; Streeter Dysplasia) 641
  - Epidermal Nevus Syndrome (Ichthyosis Hystrix) 641
  - Cryptophthalmia Syndrome (Cryptophthalmos Syndactyly Syndrome; Fraser Syndrome) 642
  - Frontonasal Dysplasia Syndrome (Median Cleft Face Syndrome) 642
  - Goldenhar Syndrome (Oculo-Auriculo-Vertebral Dysplasia; Goldenhar-Gorlin Syndrome) 643
  - Miller Syndrome (Postaxial Acrofacial Dysostosis; Genee-Wiedemann Syndrome) 643
  - Nager Syndrome (Nager Acrofacial Dyostosis) 644
  - Linear Nevus Sebaceus of Jadassohn (Nevus Sebaceus of Jadassohn; Jadassohn-Type Anetoderma; Organoid Nevus Syndrome; Sebaceus Nevus Syndrome) 644
  - Palpebral Coloboma-Lipoma Syndrome (Nasopalpebral Lipoma-Coloboma) 645
  - Franceschetti Syndrome (Franceschetti-Zwahlen-Klein Syndrome; Treacher Collins Syndrome; Mandibulofacial Dysostosis; Mandibulofacial Syndrome; Eyelid-Malar-Mandible Syndrome; Oculovertebral Syndrome; Berry Syndrome; Franceschetti-Zwahlen Syndrome; Zwahlen Syndrome; Bilateral Facial Agenesis; Berry-Franceschetti-Klein Syndrome; Franceschetti-Klein Syndrome; Franceschetti Syndrome (II); Treacher Collins-Franceschetti Syndrome; Weyers-Thier Syndrome) 645
  - Eyelid Contusions, Lacerations, and Avulsions 646
  - Dermatochalasis 646
  - Dominant Optic Atrophy Syndrome (Dominant Optic Atrophy, Deafness, Ptosis, Ophthalmoplegia, Dystaxia, and Myopathy) 646
  - Duck-Bill Lips and Ptosis 647
  - Ectropion (Lid Margin Turned Outward from the Eyeball) 647
  - Distichiasis (Distichiasis with Congenital Anomalies of the Heart and Peripheral Vasculature) 648
  - Eyelid Coloboma 649
  - Franceschetti Syndrome (Franceschetti-Zwahlen-Klein Syndrome; Treacher Collins Syndrome; Mandibulofacial Dysostosis; Mandibulofacial Syndrome; Eyelid-Malar-Mandible Syndrome; Oculovertebral Syndrome; Berry Syndrome; Franceschetti-Zwahlen Syndrome; Zwahlen Syndrome; Bilateral Facial Agenesis; Berry-Franceschetti-Klein Syndrome; Franceschetti-Klein Syndrome; Franceschetti Syndrome (II); Treacher Collins-Franceschetti Syndrome; Weyers-Thier Syndrome) 649
  - Pediatric Congenital Glaucoma (Primary Infantile Glaucoma, Buphthalmos) 650
  - Cerebro-Oculo-Facio-Skeletal Syndrome (COFS Syndrome) 650
  - Down Syndrome (Mongolism; Trisomy G; Trisomy 21 Syndrome; Mongoloid Idiocy) 651

- Hartnup Syndrome (Pellagra-Cerebellar Ataxia-Renal Aminoaciduria Syndrome; H Disease; Niacin Deficiency)   651
- Lowe Syndrome (Oculo-Cerebro-Renal Syndrome)   652
- Miller Syndrome (Postaxial Acrofacial Dysostosis; Genee-Wiedemann Syndrome)   652
- Nonne-Milroy-Meige Disease (Chronic Hereditary Lymphedema; Milroy Disease; Meige Disease; Meige-Milroy Syndrome; Nonne-Milroy Syndrome; Chronic Hereditary Edema; Chronic Hereditary Trophedema; Chronic Trophedema; Elephantiasis Congenita Hereditaria; Familial Hereditary Edema; Hereditary Edema; Idiopathic Hereditary Lymphedema; Pseudoedematous Hypodermal Hypertrophy; Pseudoelephantiasis Neuroarthritica; Oromandibular Dystonia; Blepharospasm-Oromandibular Dystonia; Congenital Trophedema; Tropholymphedema; Trophoneurosis; Elephantiasis Arabum Congenita)   653
- Robinow-Silverman-Smith Syndrome (Achondroplastic Dwarfism; Mesomelic Dwarfism; Robinow Dwarfism)   653
- Sjögren-Larsson Syndrome (Oligophrenia Ichthyosis Spastic Diplegia Syndrome)   654
- Ectropion   654
- Blepharophimosis Syndrome (Simosa Syndrome)   655
- Erb-Goldflam Syndrome (Erb II Syndrome; Hoppe-Goldflam Disease; Pseudoparalytic Syndrome; Myasthenia Gravis)   655
- Hereditary Ectodermal Dysplasia Syndrome (Siemens Syndrome; Keratosis Follicularis Spinulosa Syndrome; Hypohidrotic Ectodermal Dysplasia; Christ-Siemens-Touraine Syndrome; Weech Syndrome; Anhidrotic Ectodermal Dysplasia; Ichthyosis Follicularis)   656
- Bell's Palsy (Idiopathic Facial Paralysis)   656
- Guillain-Barré Syndrome (Landry Paralysis; Acute Infectious Neuritis; Acute Polyradiculitis; Acute Febrile Polyneuritis; Acute Idiopathic Polyneuritis; Inflammatory Polyradiculoneuropathy; Landry-Guillain-Barré-Strohl Syndrome; Postinfectious Polyneuritis)   657
- Lagophthalmos   657
- Ectropion   658
- Amendola Syndrome   658
- Blastomycosis   659
- Harlequin Syndrome (Bullous Ichthyosiform Erythroderma; Collodion Baby; Congenital Ichthyosis; Epidermolytic Hyperkeratosis; Ichthyosis; Ichthyosis Vulgaris; Lamellar Ichthyosis; Nonbullous Ichthyosiform Erythroderma; Xeroderma; X-Linked Ichthyosis)   659
- Kabuki Makeup Syndrome (Niikawa-Kuroki Syndrome)   660
- Hansen Disease (Leprosy)   660
- Orbital Fracture, Apex   661
- Keratodermia Palmaris ET Plantaris (Palmoplantar Keratodermia; Keratosis Palmoplantaris)   661
- Psoriasis (Psoriasis Vulgaris)   661
- Mycosis Fungoides Syndrome (Sézary Syndrome; Malignant Cutaneous Reticulosis Syndrome)   662
- Zinsser-Engman-Cole Syndrome (Dyskeratosis Congenita with Pigmentation; Cole-Rauschkolb-Toomey Syndrome) Ectropion   663
- Danbolt-Closs Syndrome (Acrodermatitis Enteropathica; Brandt Syndrome)   663
- Elschnig Syndrome I (Meibomian Conjunctivitis)   664
- Kaposi Disease (Kaposi Sarcoma; Kaposi Hemorrhagic Sarcoma; Multiple Idiopathic Hemorrhagic Sarcoma; Kaposi Varicelliform Eruption)   664
- Leiomyoma   664
- Ehlers-Danlos Syndrome (Fibrodysplasia Elastica Generalisata; Cutis Hyperelastica; Meekeren-Ehlers-Danlos Syndrome; Indian Rubber Man Syndrome; Cutis Laxa)   665
- Entropion (Inversion of Lid Margin)   665
- Dental-Ocular-Cutaneous Syndrome   666
- Hereditary Ectodermal Dysplasia Syndrome (Siemens Syndrome; Keratosis Follicularis Spinulosa Syndrome; Hypohidrotic Ectodermal Dysplasia; Christ-Siemens-Touraine Syndrome; Weech Syndrome; Anhidrotic Ectodermal Dysplasia; Ichthyosis Follicularis)   666

– Anophthalmos 667
– General Fibrosis Syndrome (Congenital Enophthalmos with Ocular Muscle Fibrosis and Ptosis; Congenital Fibrosis of the Inferior Rectus with Ptosis; Strabismus Fixus; Vertical Retraction Syndrome (Congenital Fibrosis Syndrome) 667
– Lymphedema 668
– Hansen Disease (Leprosy) 668
– Trachoma 669
– Amendola Syndrome 669
– Smallpox (Variola) 670
– Epicanthus (Fold of Skin over Inner Canthus of Eye) 670
– Aminopterin-induced Syndrome 671
– Basal Cell Nevus Syndrome (Nevoid Basal Cell Carcinoma Syndrome; Nevoid Basalioma Syndrome; Gorlin Syndrome; Gorlin-Goltz Syndrome; Multiple Basal Cell Nevi Syndrome) 672
– Bassen-Kornzweig Syndrome (Abetalipoproteinemia; Acanthocytosis; Familial Hypolipoproteinemia) 672
– Blepharophimosis Syndrome (Simosa Syndrome) 673
– Turner Syndrome (Turner-Albright Syndrome; Gonadal Dysgenesis; Genital Dwarfism Syndrome; Ullrich-Turner Syndrome; Bonnevie-Ullrich Syndrome; Pterygolymphangiectasia Syndrome; Ullrich-Bonnevie Syndrome) Cataract, Posterior 673
– Carpenter Syndrome (Acrocephalopolysyndactyly Type II) 674
– Cat's-Eye Syndrome (Schachenmann Syndrome; Schmid-Fraccaro Syndrome; Partial Trisomy G Syndrome) 674
– Smith-Lemli-Opitz Syndrome (Cerebrohepatorenal Syndrome) 675
– Conradi Syndrome (Multiple Epiphyseal Dysplasia Congenita; Dysplasia Epiphysealis Congenita; Chondrodystrophia Foetalis Hypoplastica; Calcinosis Universalis; Congenital Calcifying Chondrodystrophy; Stippled Epiphyses Syndrome; Conradi-Hünermann Syndrome; Chondrodysplasia Punctata) 675

– Chromosome 18 Partial Deletion (Long-Arm) Syndrome [Monosomy 18 Partial (Long-Arm) Syndrome; De Grouchy Syndrome] 676
– Freeman-Sheldon Syndrome (Cranio-Carpo-Tarsal Dysplasia; Whistling Face Syndrome) 676
– Wolf Syndrome (Monosomy 4 Partial Syndrome; Chromosome 4 Partial Deletion Syndrome; Hirschhorn-Cooper Syndrome) Ptosis 677
– Chromosome 13q Partial Deletion (Long-Arm Syndrome; 13q Syndrome) 677
– Möbius II Syndrome (Congenital Facial Diplegia; Congenital Paralysis of the Sixth and Seventh Nerves; Congenital Oculo facial Paralysis; Von Graefes Syndrome) 678
– Baller-Gerold Syndrome (Craniosynostosis Radial Aplasia) 678
– Cri-du-Chat Syndrome [Cat-Cry (5p-) Syndrome; Crying Cat Syndrome; BI Deletion Syndrome; Lejeune Syndrome] 679
– Dubowitz Syndrome (Dwarfism-Eczema-Peculiar Facies) 679
– Down Syndrome (Mongolism; Trisomy G; Trisomy 21 Syndrome; Mongoloid Idiocy) 679
– Drummond Syndrome (Idiopathic Hypercalcemia; Blue Diaper Syndrome) 680
– Ehlers-Danlos Syndrome (Fibrodysplasia Elastica Generalisata; Cutis Hyperelastica; Meekeren-Ehlers-Danlos Syndrome; Indian Rubber Man Syndrome; Cutis Laxa) 680
– 18q- Syndrome (18q Deletion Syndrome) 681
– Aberfeld Syndrome (Schwartz-Jampel Syndrome; Congenital Blepharophimosis Associated with Generalized Myopathy Syndrome; Ocular and Facial Abnormalities Syndrome) 681
– Fetal Alcohol Syndrome 682
– Freeman-Sheldon Syndrome (Cranio-Carpo-Tarsal Dysplasia; Whistling Face Syndrome) 682
– 4q- Syndrome (4q Deletion Syndrome) 683
– Gansslen Syndrome (Familial Hemolytic Icterus; Hematologic-Metabolic Bone Disorder) 683

- Greig Syndrome (Ocular Hypertelorism Syndrome; Hypertelorism; Primary Embryonic Hypertelorism; Hypertelorism Ocularis) 683
- Hurler Syndrome (Pfaundler-Hurler Syndrome; Gargoylism; Dysostosis Multiplex; MPS IH Syndrome; Systemic Mucopolysaccharidosis Type IH; Mucopolysaccharidosis IH) 684
- Jacobs Syndrome (Triple X Syndrome; XXX Syndrome; Super Female Syndrome) 685
- Klinefelter Syndrome (Gynecomastia-Aspermatogenesis Syndrome; XXY Syndrome; XXXY Syndrome; XXYY Syndrome; Reifenstein-Albright Syndrome) 685
- Kohn-Romano Syndrome (BPES Syndrome) 685
- Komoto Syndrome (Congenital Eyelid Tetrad; CET) 686
- Laurence-Moon-Bardet-Biedl Syndrome (Bardet-Biedl Syndrome; Retinitis Pigmentosa-Polydactyly-Adiposogenital Syndrome) 686
- Multiple Lentigines Syndrome (LEOPARD Syndrome) 687
- Leroy Syndrome 687
- Little Syndrome (Nail-Patella Syndrome; Hereditary Osteo-Onycho-Dysplasia; HOOD Syndrome) 688
- Michel Syndrome 688
- Mohr-Claussen Syndrome (Oral-Facial-Digital Syndrome Type II; OFD Syndrome; Orofaciodigital Syndrome II) 688
- Noonan Syndrome (Male Turner Syndrome) 689
- Lowe Syndrome (Oculo-Cerebro-Renal Syndrome) 689
- Meyer-Schwickerath-Weyers Syndrome (Microphthalmos Syndrome; Oculodentodigital Dysplasia) 690
- Potter Syndrome (Renal Agenesis Syndrome; Renofacial Syndrome) 690
- Ring Chromosome 6 (Aniridia, Congenital Glaucoma, and Hydrocephalus) 691
- Robinow-Silverman-Smith Syndrome (Achondroplastic Dwarfism; Mesomelic Dwarfism; Robinow Dwarfism) 691
- Rubinstein-Taybi Syndrome (Optic Atrophy) 692
- Schonenberg Syndrome (Dwarf-Cardiopathy Syndrome) Blepharophymosis 692
- Smith Syndrome (Facio-Skeleto-Genital Dysplasia) 692
- TAR Syndrome (Thrombocytopenia-Absent Radius Syndrome) 693
- Cooley Anemia (Thalassemia; Thalassemia Major; Thalassemia Minor) 693
- Trisomy 18 Syndrome (E Syndrome; Edwards Syndrome) Congenital Glaucoma 694
- Turner Syndrome (Turner-Albright Syndrome; Gonadal Dysgenesis; Genital Dwarfism Syndrome; Ullrich-Turner Syndrome; Bonnevie-Ullrich Syndrome; Pterygolymphangiectasia Syndrome; Ullrich-Bonnevie Syndrome) Cataract, Posterior 694
- Waardenburg Syndrome (Van Der Hoeve-Halberstam-Waardenburg Syndrome; Waardenburg-Klein Syndrome; Embryonic Fixation Syndrome; Interoculo-Iridodermato-Auditive Dysplasia; Piebaldism) Hypertelorism 695
- X-Linked Mental Retardation Syndrome (XLMR) Glaucoma 695
- XXXXX Syndrome (Penta X Syndrome, Tetra X Syndrome) Hypertelorism 696
- Facial Palsy (Bell's Palsy) 696
- Erb-Goldflam Syndrome (Erb II Syndrome; Hoppe-Goldflam Disease; Pseudoparalytic Syndrome; Myasthenia Gravis) 698
- Botulism 699
- Möbius II Syndrome (Congenital Facial Diplegia; Congenital Paralysis of the Sixth and Seventh Nerves; Congenital Oculofacial Paralysis; Von Graefes Syndrome) 699
- Kugelberg-Welander Syndrome (Juvenile Muscular Atrophy) 700
- Weber Syndrome (Weber-Dubler Syndrome; Cerebellar Peduncle Syndrome; Alternating Oculomotor Paralysis; Ventral Medial Midbrain Syndrome) Ptosis 700

– Guillain-Barré Syndrome (Landry Paralysis; Acute Infectious Neuritis; Acute Polyradiculitis; Acute Febrile Polyneuritis; Acute Idiopathic Polyneuritis; Inflammatory Polyradiculoneuropathy; Landry-Guillain-Barré-Strohl Syndrome; Postinfectious Polyneuritis)   701

– Foville Syndrome (Foville Peduncular Syndrome)   701

– Millard-Gubler Syndrome (Abducens-Facial Hemiplegia Alternans)   702

– Passow Syndrome (Bremer Status Dysraphicus; Status Dysraphicus Syndrome; Syringomyelia; Syringobulbia)   702

– Charge Association (Multiple Congenital Anomalies Syndrome; Coloboma, Heart Disease, Atresia, Retarded Growth, Genital Hypoplasia, Ear Malformation Association)   703

– Wernicke Syndrome I (Superior Hemorrhagic Polio-encephalopathic Syndrome; Hemorrhagic Polioencephalitisz Superior Syndrome; Encephalitis Hemorrhagica Superioris; Avitaminosis B; Thiamine Deficiency; Beriberi; Gayet-Wernicke Syndrome; Wernicke-Korsakoff Syndrome) Ptosis   703

– Acquired Lues (Syphilis; Acquired Syphilis; Lues Venerea; Malum Venereum)   704

– Tuberculosis   704

– Arteriosclerosis   705

– Bell's Palsy (Idiopathic Facial Paralysis)   705

– Herpes Zoster   706

– Hypertension   706

– Hansen Disease (Leprosy)   707

– Acquired Lues (Syphilis; Acquired Syphilis; Lues Venerea; Malum Venereum)   707

– Melkersson-Rosenthal Syndrome (Melkersson Idiopathic Fibroedema; Miescher Cheilitis Granulomatosis)   708

– Heerfordt Syndrome (Uveoparotid Fever; Uveoparotitis; Uveoparotitic Paralysis)   708

– Mikulicz-Radecki Syndrome (Mikulicz Syndrome; Dacryosialoadenopathy; Mikulicz-Sjögren Syndrome)   709

– Floppy Eyelid Syndrome   709

– Granuloma Faciale   710

– Horner Syndrome   710

– Arnold-Chiari Syndrome (Platybasia Syndrome; Cerebellomedullary Malformation Syndrome; Basilar Impressions)   712

– Acquired Lues (Syphilis; Acquired Syphilis; Lues Venerea; Malum Venereum)   713

– Iris Melanoma   713

– Disseminated Sclerosis (Multiple Sclerosis)   714

– Wallenberg Syndrome (Dorsolateral Medullary Syndrome; Lateral Bulbar Syndrome) Ptosis   714

– Passow Syndrome (Bremer Status Dysraphicus; Status Dysraphicus Syndrome; Syringomyelia; Syringobulbia)   715

– Acquired Lues (Syphilis; Acquired Syphilis; Lues Venerea; Malum Venereum)   715

– Poliomyelitis (Infantile Paralysis)   716

– Meningococcemia (Neisseria Meningitides; Meningitis)   716

– Progressive Systemic Sclerosis (Scleroderma; Systemic Scleroderma)   716

– Dejerine-Klumpke Syndrome (Lower Radicular Syndrome; Klumpke Syndrome; Klumpke Paralysis)   717

– Pancoast Syndrome (Hare Syndrome; Superior Pulmonary Sulcus Syndrome)   717

– Hodgkin Disease   718

– Leukemia   718

– Tuberculosis   719

– Raeder Syndrome (Paratrigeminal Paralysis; Horton Headache; Histamine Cephalalgia; Ciliary Neuralgia; Cluster Headache; Periodic Migrainous Neuralgia)   719

– Foix Syndrome (Cavernous Sinus Syndrome; Hypophyseal-Sphenoidal Syndrome; Cavernous Sinus Neuralgia Syndrome; Godtfredsen Syndrome; Cavernous Sinus-Nasopharyngeal Tumor Syndrome; Cavernous Sinus Thrombosis)   720

– Raeder Syndrome (Paratrigeminal Paralysis; Horton Headache; Histamine Cephalalgia; Ciliary Neuralgia; Cluster Headache; Periodic Migrainous Neuralgia)   720

- Herpes Zoster — 721
- Migraine (Vascular Headache) — 721
- Congenital Varicella Syndrome — 722
- Hypomelanosis of Ito Syndrome (Incontinentia Pigmenti Achromians; Systematized Achromic Nevus) — 722
- Lagophthalmos — 723
- Lid Myokymia — 723
- Madarosis (Loss of Lashes) — 723
- Marcus Gunn Syndrome (Jaw-Winking Syndrome; Congenital Trigeminooculomotor Synkinesis) — 724
- Marin Amat Syndrome (Inverted Marcus Gunn Phenomenon) — 724
- Melkersson-Rosenthal Syndrome (Melkersson Idiopathic Fibroedema; Miescher Cheilitis Granulomatosis) — 725
- Erb-Goldflam Syndrome (Erb II Syndrome; Hoppe-Goldflam Disease; Pseudoparalytic Syndrome; Myasthenia Gravis) — 725
- Oculopharyngeal Syndrome (Progressive Muscular Dystrophy with Ptosis and Dysphagia; Oculopharyngeal Muscular Dystrophy) — 726
- Palpebral Coloboma-Lipoma Syndrome (Nasopalpebral Lipoma-Coloboma) — 726
- Pierre-Robin Syndrome (Robin Syndrome; Micrognathia-Glossoptosis Syndrome) — 727
- Comprehensive Ptosis Classification — 727
- Aarskog-Scott Syndrome (Faciogenital Dysplasia) — 739
- Acrorenoocular Syndrome — 739
- Alacrima — 740
- Albers-Schonberg Disease (Marble Bone Disease; Osteosclerosis Fragilis Generalisata; Osteopetrosis; Osteopoikilosis; Osteosclerosis Congenita Diffusa) — 740
- Lubarsch-Pick Syndrome (Primary Amyloidosis; Idiopathic Amyloidosis; Amyloidosis) — 741
- Apert Syndrome (Acrocephalosyndactylism Syndrome; Acrocranio-dysphalangia; Acrodysplasia; Sphenoacrocranio-syndactyly; Absent-Digits-Cranial-Defects Syndrome) — 741
- Retinitis Pigmentosa — 742
- Axenfeld-Schurenberg Syndrome (Cyclic Oculomotor Paralysis) — 742
- Baraitser-Winter Syndrome — 743
- Bassen-Kornzweig Syndrome (Abetalipoproteinemia; Acanthocytosis; Familial Hypolipoproteinemia) — 743
- Blepharophimosis Syndrome (Simosa Syndrome) — 744
- Bonnet-Dechaume-Blanc Syndrome (Cerebroretinal Arteriovenous Aneurysm Syndrome; Neuroretinoangiomatosis Syndrome; Wyburn-Mason Syndrome) — 744
- Turner Syndrome (Turner-Albright Syndrome; Gonadal Dysgenesis; Genital Dwarfism Syndrome; Ullrich-Turner Syndrome; Bonnevie-Ullrich Syndrome; Pterygolymphangiectasia Syndrome; Ullrich-Bonnevie Syndrome) Cataract, Posterior — 745
- Brown Syndrome (Superior Oblique Tendon Sheath Syndrome) — 745
- Carpenter Syndrome (Acrocephalopolysyndactyly Type II) — 746
- Cerebral Palsy — 746
- Chromosome 11 Long-Arm Deletion Syndrome — 747
- Chromosome 18 Partial Deletion (Long-Arm) Syndrome [Monosomy 18 Partial (Long-Arm) Syndrome; De Grouchy Syndrome] — 747
- Chromosome 18 Partial Deletion (Short-Arm) Syndrome [Monosomy 18 Partial (Short-Arm) Syndrome] — 748
- General Fibrosis Syndrome [Congenital Enophthalmos with Ocular Muscle Fibrosis and Ptosis; Congenital Fibrosis of the Inferior Rectus with Ptosis; Strabismus Fixus; Vertical Retraction Syndrome (Congenital Fibrosis Syndrome)] — 748
- Ophthalmoplegia, Progressive External — 749
- Freeman-Sheldon Syndrome (Cranio-Carpo-Tarsal Dysplasia; Whistling Face Syndrome) — 749
- Cretinism (Hypothyroid Goiter; Hypothyroidism; Juvenile Hypothyroidism; Myxedema) — 750

– Cri-du-Chat Syndrome
[Cat-Cry (5p-) Syndrome; Crying Cat
Syndrome; BI Deletion Syndrome;
Lejeune Syndrome]   750
– Crouzon Syndrome (Dysostosis
Craniofacialis; Oxycephaly; Craniofacial
Dysostosis; Parrot-Head Syndrome;
Möbius-Crouzon Syndrome; Hereditary
Craniofacial Dysostosis)   751
– Dandy-Walker Syndrome
(Atresia of the Foramen of Magendie)   751
– De Lange Syndrome (I) (Congenital
Muscular Hypertrophy Cerebral
Syndrome; Brachmann-De
Lange Syndrome)   752
– Dubowitz Syndrome
(Dwarfism-Eczema-Peculiar Facies)   752
– Duck-Bill Lips and Ptosis   752
– Ehlers-Danlos Syndrome
(Fibrodysplasia Elastica Generalisata;
Cutis Hyperelastica; Meekeren-Ehlers-
Danlos Syndrome; Indian Rubber Man
Syndrome; Cutis Laxa)   753
– Engelmann Syndrome [Osteopathia
Hyperostotica (Scleroticans) Multiplex
Infantilis; Diaphyseal Dysplasia;
Camurati-Engelmann Disease;
Hereditary Multiple Diaphyseal
Sclerosis; Juvenile Paget Disease]   753
– Arthrogryposis Multiplex Congenita   754
– Cockayne Syndrome (Dwarfism
with Retinal Atrophy and Deafness;
Mickey Mouse Syndrome)   755
– Cryptophthalmia Syndrome
(Cryptophthalmos Syndactyly
Syndrome; Fraser Syndrome)   755
– Duane Syndrome (Retraction
Syndrome; Stilling Syndrome;
Turk-Stilling Syndrome)   756
– Freeman-Sheldon Syndrome
(Cranio-Carpo-Tarsal Dysplasia;
Whistling Face Syndrome)   756
– General Fibrosis Syndrome
(Congenital Enophthalmos with
Ocular Muscle Fibrosis and Ptosis;
Congenital Fibrosis of the Inferior
Rectus with Ptosis; Strabismus Fixus;
Vertical Retraction Syndrome
(Congenital Fibrosis Syndrome)   757

– Greig Syndrome (Ocular Hypertelorism
Syndrome; Hypertelorism; Primary
Embryonic Hypertelorism;
Hypertelorism Ocularis)   757
– Hemifacial Microsomia Syndrome
(Unilateral Facial Agenesis;
Otomandibular Dysostosis;
Francois-Haustrate Syndrome)   758
– Klippel-Trenaunay-Weber Syndrome
(Parkes-Weber Syndrome; Angio-Osteo-
Hypertrophy Syndrome)   758
– Krause Syndrome (Congenital
Encephalo-Ophthalmic Dysplasia;
Encephalo-Ophthalmic Syndrome)   759
– Branched-Chain Ketoaciduria
(Maple Syrup Urine Disease)   759
– Morquio Syndrome (Morquio-Brailsford
Syndrome; Brailsford-Morquio Dystrophy;
Familial Osseous Dystrophy;
Keratosulfaturia; MPS IV;
Mucopolysaccharidosis IV;
Spondyloepiphyseal Dysplasia;
Osteochondrodystrophia Deformans;
Infantile Hereditary Chondrodysplasia;
Hereditary Poly topic Enchondral
Dysostosis; Hereditary
Osteochondrodystrophy; Eccentro-
Osteochondrodysplasia; Dysostosis
Enchondralis Meta-Epiphysaria;
Morquio-Ullrich Syndrome; Atypical
Chondrodystrophy; Chondrodystrophia
Tarda; Chondro-Osteodystrophy)   760
– Von Recklinghausen Syndrome
(Neurofibromatosis Type I;
Neurinomatosis)   760
– Romberg Syndrome (Parry-Romberg
Syndrome; Progressive Hemifacial Atrophy;
Progressive Facial Hemiatrophy; Facial
Hemiatrophy) Enophthalmus   761
– Passow Syndrome (Bremer Status
Dysraphicus; Status Dysraphicus
Syndrome; Syringomyelia; Syringobulbia)   761
– Epidermal Nevus Syndrome
(Ichthyosis Hystrix)   762
– Fabry Disease (Angiokeratoma
Corporis Diffusum Syndrome;
Diffuse Angiokeratosis; Fabry-Anderson
Syndrome; Glycosphingolipid Lipidosis;
Glycosphingolipidosis)   762
– Gillum-Anderson Syndrome   763

- Hemangioma   763
- Von Bekhterev-Strumpell Syndrome (Marie-Strumpell Spondylitis; Ankylosing Spondylitis; Pierre-Marie Syndrome; Bekhterev Disease; Rheumatoid Spondylitis) Optic Atrophy   764
- Hunter Syndrome (MPS II Syndrome; Mucopolysaccharidosis II; Systemic Mucopolysaccharidosis Type II)   764
- Hurler Syndrome (Pfaundler-Hurler Syndrome; Gargoylism; Dysostosis Multiplex; MPS IH Syndrome; Systemic Mucopolysaccharidosis Type IH; Mucopolysaccharidosis IH)   765
- Hyperammonemia I (Carbamyl Phosphate Synthetase Deficiency; Hyperammonemia II; Ornithine Transcarbamylase Deficiency; Hyperammonemia-Hyperornithinemia-Homocitrullinuria Syndrome)   766
- Kiloh-Nevin Syndrome (Muscular Dystrophy of External Ocular Muscles; Ocular Myopathy)   766
- Kohn-Romano Syndrome (BPES Syndrome)   767
- Komoto Syndrome (Congenital Eyelid Tetrad; CET)   767
- Kugelberg-Welander Syndrome (Juvenile Muscular Atrophy)   767
- Laurence-Moon-Bardet-Biedl Syndrome (Bardet-Biedl Syndrome; Retinitis Pigmentosa-Polydactyly-Adiposogenital Syndrome)   768
- Leigh Syndrome (Subacute Necrotizing Encephalomyelopathy; Infantile Subacute Necrotizing Encephalomyelopathy; Hyperpyruvicemia with Hyper-Alpha-Alaninemia; Gangliosidosis G_{M_2} Type 3)   768
- Little Syndrome (Nail-Patella Syndrome; Hereditary Osteo-Onycho-Dysplasia; HOOD Syndrome)   769
- MERRF Syndrome   769
- Colobomatous, Microphthalmia and Microcornea Syndrome   770
- Sjögren-Larsson Syndrome (Oligophrenia Ichthyosis Spastic Diplegia Syndrome)   770
- Retinitis Pigmentosa   771
- Aicardi Syndrome   771
- Bloch-Sulzberger Syndrome (Incontinentia Pigmenti; Siemens-Bloch-Sulzberger Syndrome)   772
- Goltz Syndrome (Focal Dermal Hypoplasia Syndrome)   772
- Lenz Microphthalmia Syndrome   773
- Ellis-Van Creveld Syndrome (Chondroectodermal Dysplasia)   773
- Joubert Syndrome (Familial Cerebellar Vermis Agenesis)   774
- Kartagener Syndrome (Sinusitis-Bronchiectasis-Situs Inversus Syndrome; Bronchiectasis-Dextrocardia-Sinusitis; Kartagener Triad)   774
- Laurence-Moon-Bardet-Biedl Syndrome (Bardet-Biedl Syndrome; Retinitis Pigmentosa-Polydactyly-Adiposogenital Syndrome)   775
- Marinesco-Sjögren Syndrome (Congenital Spinocerebellar Ataxia-Congenital Cataract-Oligophrenia Syndrome)   775
- Meckel Syndrome (Dysencephalia Splanchnocystic Syndrome; Gruber Syndrome)   776
- Micro Syndrome   776
- Sjögren-Larsson Syndrome (Oligophrenia Ichthyosis Spastic Diplegia Syndrome)   777
- Walker-Warburg Syndrome (Cerebroocular Dysplasia-Muscular Dystrophy; Warburg Syndrome; COD-MD Syndrome; Fukuyama Congenital Muscular Dystrophy; Hard + or - E Syndrome) Cataract   777
- Marfan Syndrome (Dolichostenomelia; Arachnodactyly; Hyperchondroplasia; Dystrophia Mesodermalis Congenita)   778
- Crouzon Syndrome (Dysostosis Craniofacialis; Oxycephaly; Craniofacial Dysostosis; Parrot-Head Syndrome; Möbius-Crouzon Syndrome; Hereditary Craniofacial Dysostosis)   778
- Stickler Syndrome (Hereditary Progressive Arthro-ophthalmopathy)   779
- Franceschetti Syndrome (Franceschetti-Zwahlen-Klein Syndrome; Treacher Collins Syndrome; Mandibulofacial Dysostosis; Mandibulofacial Syndrome; Eyelid-Malar-Mandible Syndrome; Oculovertebral Syndrome;

Berry Syndrome; Franceschetti-Zwahlen Syndrome; Zwahlen Syndrome; Bilateral Facial Agenesis; Berry-Franceschetti-Klein Syndrome; Franceschetti-Klein Syndrome; Franceschetti Syndrome (II); Treacher Collins-Franceschetti Syndrome; Weyers-Thier Syndrome) 779

– Bourneville Syndrome (Bourneville-Pringle Syndrome; Tuberous Sclerosis; Epiloia) 780

– Zellweger Syndrome (Cerebrohepatorenal Syndrome of Zellweger) 780

– 4q Syndrome 781

– 11q- Syndrome 781

– 13q-Syndrome (13q Deletion Syndrome) 782

– 18q- Syndrome (18q Deletion Syndrome) 782

– Triploidy Syndrome (Iris Coloboma) 783

– Trisomy 8 Mosaicism Syndrome (Exotropia) 783

– Trisomy 9q Syndrome (Hypertelorism) 784

– Trisomy 13 Syndrome (Trisomy DL Syndrome, Patau Syndrome, Reese Syndrome) Iris Coloboma 785

– Trisomy 18 Syndrome (E Syndrome; Edwards Syndrome) Congenital Glaucoma 785

– XXXXY Syndrome (Hypertelorism) 785

– Amniogenic Band Syndrome (Ring Constriction; Streeter Dysplasia) 786

– Cat's-Eye Syndrome (Schachenmann Syndrome; Schmid-Fraccaro Syndrome; Partial Trisomy G Syndrome) 786

– CHARGE Association (Multiple Congenital Anomalies Syndrome; Coloboma, Heart Disease, Atresia, Retarded Growth, Genital Hypoplasia, Ear Malformation Association) 787

– Ullrich Syndrome (Ullrich-Feichtiger Syndrome; Dyscraniopylophalangy) Corneal Ulcer 787

– Frontonasal Dysplasia Syndrome (Median Cleft Face Syndrome) 788

– Goldenhar Syndrome (Oculo-Auriculo-Vertebral Dysplasia; Goldenhar-Gorlin Syndrome) 788

– Hemifacial Microsomia Syndrome (Unilateral Facial Agenesis; Otomandibular Dysostosis; Francois-Haustrate Syndrome) 789

– Linear Nevus Sebaceus of Jadassohn (Nevus Sebaceus of Jadassohn; Jadassohn-Type Anetoderma; Organoid Nevus Syndrome; Sebaceus Nevus Syndrome) 789

– Rubinstein-Taybi Syndrome (Optic Atrophy) 790

– Andersen-Warburg Syndrome (Whitnall-Norman Syndrome; Oligophrenia Microphthalmos Syndrome; Norrie Disease; Atrophia Oculi Congenital Fetal Iritis Syndrome; Congenital Progressive Oculo-Acoustico-Cerebral Dysplasia) 790

– Forsius-Eriksson Syndrome (Aland Disease) 791

– Lowe Syndrome (Oculo-Cerebro-Renal Syndrome) 791

– Cerebro-Oculo-Facio-Skeletal Syndrome (COFS Syndrome) 792

– Conradi Syndrome (Multiple Epiphyseal Dysplasia Congenita; Dysplasia Epiphysealis Congenita; Chondrodystrophia Foetalis Hypoplastica; Calcinosis Universalis; Congenital Calcifying Chondrodystrophy; Stippled Epiphyses Syndrome; Conradi-Hünermann Syndrome; Chondrodysplasia Punctata) 792

– Oculocerebral Syndrome with Hypopigmentation (Amish Oculocerebral Syndrome; Cross Syndrome) 793

– Diamond Blackfan Syndrome 793

– Fanconi Syndrome (Toni-Fanconi Syndrome; Amino Diabetes; Hypochloremic-Glycosuric Osteonephropathy Syndrome; De Toni-Fanconi Syndrome) 794

– Obesity-Cerebral-Ocular-Skeletal Anomalies Syndrome 794

– Blatt Syndrome (Cranio-Orbito-Ocular Dysraphia) 795

– Gansslen Syndrome (Familial Hemolytic Icterus; Hematologic-Metabolic Bone Disorder) 795

– Hypomelanosis of Ito Syndrome (Incontinentia Pigmenti Achromians; Systematized Achromic Nevus) 796

– Leri Syndrome (Pleonosteosis Syndrome; Carpal Tunnel Syndrome) 796

– Myotonic Dystrophy Syndrome
(Myotonia Atrophica Syndrome;
Dystrophia Myotonica;
Curschmann-Steinert Syndrome)   797

– Rieger Syndrome (Axenfeld-Rieger
Syndrome; Dysgenesis Mesodermalis
Corneae et Irides; Dysgenesis
Mesostromalis; Axenfeld Posterior
Embryotoxon-Juvenile Glaucoma)   798

– Trisomy 10q Syndrome
(10q+ Syndrome) Optic Disk   798

– Trisomy 21q- Syndrome
(21q Deletion Syndrome)   799

– X Chromosomal Deletion (Optic Atrophy)   799

– Beal Syndrome   800

– Gorlin-Chaudhry-Moss Syndrome   800

– Hallermann-Streiff Syndrome
(Dyscephalic-Mandibulo-Oculo-Facial
Syndrome; Oculo-Mandibulo-Dyscephaly;
Ullrich-Fremery-Dohna Syndrome;
Francois Dyscephalic Syndrome;
Mandibulo-Oculo-Facial Dyscephaly
Syndrome; Francois-Hallermann-Streiff
Syndrome; Hallermann-Streiff-Francois
Syndrome; Audry I Syndrome; Dohna
Syndrome; Francois Syndrome (1);
Dyscephaly-Teeth Abnormality-Dwarfism;
Dyscephalia Oculomandibularis-
Hypotrichosis; Mandibulo-Ocular
Dyscephalia Hypotrichosis; Fremery-
Dohna Syndrome; Oculo-
Mandibulo-Facial Dyscephaly)   801

– Hutchinson-Gilford Syndrome (Progeria)   802

– Krause Syndrome (Congenital
Encephalo-Ophthalmic Dysplasia;
Encephalo-Ophthalmic Syndrome)   802

– Meyer-Schwickerath-Weyers Syndrome
(Microphthalmos Syndrome;
Oculodentodigital Dysplasia)   803

– Pierre-Robin Syndrome (Robin Syndrome;
Micrognathia-Glossoptosis Syndrome)   803

– Retinal Disinsertion Syndrome
(Keratoconus)   804

– Sabin-Feldman Syndrome
(Chorioretinitis)   804

– Weyers Syndrome (2) (Weyers IV
Syndrome; Iridodental Dysplasia;
Dentoirideal Dysplasia; Dysgenesis
Iridodentalis; Dysgenesis Mesodermalis
Corneae et Irides with Digodontia)
Corneal Opacity   805

– Rubella Syndrome (Congenital Rubella
Syndrome; German Measles;
Gregg Syndrome)   805

– Congenital Spherocytic Anemia
(Congenital Hemolytic Jaundice;
Hereditary Spherocytosis)   806

– Ocular Toxoplasmosis (Toxoplasmic
Retinochoroiditis; Toxoplasmosis)   806

– Cytomegalovirus Retinitis   807

– Infectious Mononucleosis
(Mononucleosis; Epstein-Barr Virus,
Acute; Acute Epstein-Barr Virus,
Glandular Fever)   807

– Chickenpox (Varicella)   807

– Fetal Alcohol Syndrome   808

– Folling Syndrome (Phenylketonuria;
Phenylpyruvic Oligophrenia; Ikiotia
Phenylketonuria Syndrome)   808

– Möbius II Syndrome (Congenital Facial
Diplegia; Congenital Paralysis of the
Sixth and Seventh Nerves; Congenital
Oculofacial Paralysis;
Von Graefes Syndrome)   809

– Morquio Syndrome (Morquio-
Brailsford Syndrome; Brailsford-
Morquio Dystrophy; Familial Osseous
Dystrophy; Keratosulfaturia; MPS IV;
Mucopolysaccharidosis IV;
Spondyloepiphyseal Dysplasia;
Osteochondrodystrophia Deformans;
Infantile Hereditary Chondrodysplasia;
Hereditary Poly topic Enchondral
Dysostosis; Hereditary
Osteochondrodystrophy; Eccentro-
Osteochondrodysplasia; Dysostosis
Enchondralis Meta-Epiphysaria;
Morquio-Ullrich Syndrome; Atypical
Chondrodystrophy; Chondrodystrophia
Tarda; Chondro-Osteodystrophy)   809

– Myotonic Dystrophy Syndrome
(Myotonia Atrophica Syndrome;
Dystrophia Myotonica;
Curschmann-Steinert Syndrome)   810

– Von Recklinghausen Syndrome
(Neurofibromatosis Type I;
Neurinomatosis)   811

– Nonne-Milroy-Meige Disease
(Chronic Hereditary Lymphedema;
Milroy Disease; Meige Disease;
Meige-Milroy Syndrome; Nonne-Milroy
Syndrome; Chronic Hereditary Edema;

Chronic Hereditary Trophedema;
Chronic Trophedema; Elephantiasis
Congenita Hereditaria; Familial
Hereditary Edema; Hereditary Edema;
Idiopathic Hereditary Lymphedema;
Pseudoedematous Hypodermal
Hypertrophy; Pseudoelephantiasis
Neuroarthritica; Oromandibular
Dystonia; Blepharospasm-Oromandibular
Dystonia; Congenital Trophedema;
Tropholymphedema; Trophoneurosis;
Elephantiasis Arabum Congenita) 811

– Noonan Syndrome
(Male Turner Syndrome) 812

– Oculopharyngeal Syndrome
(progressive Muscular Dystrophy with
Ptosis and Dysphagia; Oculopharyngeal
Muscular Dystrophy) 812

– Papillon-Leage-Psaume Syndrome
(Oro-Digital-Facial Syndrome;
Linguofacial Dysplasia of Grob;
Gorlin Syndrome; Dysplasia
Linguofacialis; OFD Syndrome;
Oro-Digital-Facial Dysostosis;
Grob Linguofacial Dysplasia) 813

– Touraine-Solente-Gole Syndrome
(Pachydermoperiostosis; Acropachyderma;
Audry II Syndrome; Brugsch Syndrome;
Friedrich-Erb-Arnold Syndrome;
Hehlinger Syndrome) 813

– Romberg Syndrome (Parry-Romberg
Syndrome; Progressive Hemifacial
Atrophy; Progressive Facial Hemiatrophy;
Facial Hemiatrophy) Enophthalmus 814

– Shy-Gonatas Syndrome 814

– Smith-Lemli-Opitz Syndrome
(Cerebrohepatorenal Syndrome) 815

– Smith Syndrome (Facio-Skeleto-
Genital Dysplasia) 815

– Ectopia Lentis with Ectopia of Pupil
(Ectopia Lentis et Pupillae) 816

– Passow Syndrome (Bremer Status
Dysraphicus; Status Dysraphicus
Syndrome; Syringomyelia; Syringobulbia) 816

– Treft Syndrome (Optic Atrophy) 817

– Tunbridge-Paley Disease (Optic Atrophy) 817

– Van Bogaert-Hozay Syndrome (Esotropia) 818

– Waardenburg Syndrome (Van Der
Hoeve-Halberstam-Waardenburg
Syndrome; Waardenburg-Klein

Syndrome; Embryonic Fixation
Syndrome; Interoculo-Iridodermato-
Auditive Dysplasia; Piebaldism)
Hypertelorism 818

– Arteriovenous Fistula (Arteriovenous
Aneurysm; Arteriovenous Angioma;
Arteriovenous Malformation; Cirsoid
Aneurysm; Racemose Hemangioma;
Varicose Aneurysm) 819

– Horner Syndrome (Bernard-Horner
Syndrome; Cervical Sympathetic
Paralysis Syndrome; Claude-Bernard-
Horner Syndrome; Horner
Oculopupillary Syndrome) 819

– Marcus Gunn Syndrome
(Jaw-Winking Syndrome; Congenital
Trigeminooculomotor Synkinesis) 820

– Marin Amat Syndrome
(Inverted Marcus Gunn Phenomenon) 820

– Misdirected Third Nerve Syndrome 821

– Riley-Day Syndrome
(Congenital Familial Dysautonomia) 821

– Von Herrenschwand Syndrome
(Sympathetic Heterochromia) Ptosis 822

– Blepharochalasis 822

– Lubarsch-Pick Syndrome (Primary
Amyloidosis; Idiopathic Amyloidosis;
Amyloidosis) 822

– Botulism 823

– Brown Syndrome (Superior Oblique
Tendon Sheath Syndrome) 823

– Cestan-Chenais Syndrome
[Cestan (1) Syndrome] 824

– Craniocervical Syndrome
(Whiplash Injury) 824

– Cretinism (Hypothyroid Goiter;
Hypothyroidism; Juvenile
Hypothyroidism; Myxedema) 825

– Dejean Syndrome
(Orbital Floor Syndrome) 825

– Dejerine-Klumpke Syndrome
(Lower Radicular Syndrome;
Klumpke Syndrome; Klumpke Paralysis) 826

– Horner Syndrome (Bernard-Horner
Syndrome; Cervical Sympathetic
Paralysis Syndrome; Claude-Bernard-
Horner Syndrome; Horner
Oculopupillary Syndrome) 826

- Krause Syndrome (Congenital Encephalo-Ophthalmic Dysplasia; Encephalo-Ophthalmic Syndrome)   827
- Naffziger Syndrome (Scalenus Anticus Syndrome)   827
- Pancoast Syndrome (Hare Syndrome; Superior Pulmonary Sulcus Syndrome)   828
- Raeder Syndrome (Paratrigeminal Paralysis; Horton Headache; Histamine Cephalalgia; Ciliary Neuralgia; Cluster Headache; Periodic Migrainous Neuralgia)   828
- Retroparotid Space Syndrome (Villaret Syndrome; Posterior Retroparotid Space Syndrome) Enophthalmos   829
- Silent Sinus Syndrome   829
- Jugular Foramen Syndrome (Vernet Syndrome)   830
- Wallenberg Syndrome (Dorsolateral Medullary Syndrome; Lateral Bulbar Syndrome) Ptosis   830
- Abdominal Typhus (Enteric Fever; Typhoid Fever)   831
- Basedow Syndrome (Graves Disease; Hyperthyroidism; Thyrotoxicosis; Exophthalmic Goiter; Parry Disease)   831
- Erb-Goldflam Syndrome (Erb II Syndrome; Hoppe-Goldflam Disease; Pseudoparalytic Syndrome; Myasthenia Gravis)   832
- Pregnancy   833
- Guillain-Barré Syndrome (Landry Paralysis; Acute Infectious Neuritis; Acute Polyradiculitis; Acute Febrile Polyneuritis; Acute Idiopathic Polyneuritis; Inflammatory Polyradiculoneuropathy; Landry-Guillain-Barré-Strohl Syndrome; Postinfectious Polyneuritis)   833
- Horner Syndrome (Bernard-Horner Syndrome; Cervical Sympathetic Paralysis Syndrome; Claude-Bernard-Horner Syndrome; Horner Oculopupillary Syndrome)   834
- Laurence-Moon-Bardet-Biedl Syndrome (Bardet-Biedl Syndrome; Retinitis Pigmentosa-Polydactyly-Adiposogenital Syndrome)   834
- Diencephalic Syndrome (Diencephalic Epilepsy Syndrome; Autonomic Epilepsy Syndrome; Penfield Syndrome; Anterior Diencephalic Autonomic Epilepsy Syndrome)   835
- Arnold-Chiari Syndrome (Platybasia Syndrome; Cerebellomedullary Malformation Syndrome; Basilar Impressions)   835
- Acquired Lues (Syphilis; Acquired Syphilis; Lues Venerea; Malum Venereum)   836
- Wallenberg Syndrome (Dorsolateral Medullary Syndrome; Lateral Bulbar Syndrome) Ptosis   836
- Passow Syndrome (Bremer Status Dysraphicus; Status Dysraphicus Syndrome; Syringomyelia; Syringobulbia)   837
- Acquired Lues (Syphilis; Acquired Syphilis; Lues Venerea; Malum Venereum)   837
- Poliomyelitis (Infantile Paralysis)   838
- Meningococcemia (Neisseria Meningitides; Meningitis)   838
- Progressive Systemic Sclerosis (Scleroderma; Systemic Scleroderma)   839
- Dejerine-Klumpke Syndrome (Lower Radicular Syndrome; Klumpke Syndrome; Klumpke Paralysis)   839
- Pancoast Syndrome (Hare Syndrome; Superior Pulmonary Sulcus Syndrome)   840
- Hodgkin Disease   840
- Leukemia   841
- Foix Syndrome (Cavernous Sinus Syndrome; Hypophyseal-Sphenoidal Syndrome; Cavernous Sinus Neuralgia Syndrome; Godtfredsen Syndrome; Cavernous Sinus-Nasopharyngeal Tumor Syndrome; Cavernous Sinus Thrombosis)   841
- Raeder Syndrome (Paratrigeminal Paralysis; Horton Headache; Histamine Cephalalgia; Ciliary Neuralgia; Cluster Headache; Periodic Migrainous Neuralgia)   842
- Herpes Zoster   842
- Migraine (Vascular Headache)   843
- Chickenpox (Varicella)   843
- Oculomotor Paralysis (III Nerve Palsy)   843
- Benedikt Syndrome (Tegmental Syndrome)   844

- Erb-Goldflam Syndrome (Erb II Syndrome; Hoppe-Goldflam Disease; Pseudoparalytic Syndrome; Myasthenia Gravis)   844
- Parinaud Syndrome (Divergence Paralysis; Subthalamic Syndrome; Paralysis of Vertical Movements; Pretectal Syndrome)   845
- Axenfeld-Schurenberg Syndrome (Cyclic Oculomotor Paralysis)   846
- Bruns Syndrome (Postural Change Syndrome)   846
- Claude Syndrome (Inferior Nucleus Ruber Syndrome; Rubrospinal-Cerebellar-Peduncle Syndrome)   847
- Congenital Vertical Retraction Syndrome   847
- Nothnagel Syndrome (Ophthalmoplegia-Cerebellar Ataxia Syndrome)   847
- Migraine (Vascular Headache)   848
- Weber Syndrome (Weber-Dubler Syndrome; Cerebellar Peduncle Syndrome; Alternating Oculomotor Paralysis; Ventral Medial Midbrain Syndrome) Ptosis   848
- Amebiasis (Amebic Dysentery, Entamoeba Histolytica)   849
- Oculomotor Paralysis (III Nerve Palsy)   849
- Botulism   850
- Chickenpox (Varicella)   850
- Craniopharyngioma   851
- Dengue Fever   851
- Devic Syndrome (Ophthalmoencephalomyelopathy; Optic Myelitis; Neuromyelitis Optica)   852
- Diphtheria   852
- Encephalitis, Acute   853
- Hepatic Failure   853
- Influenza   853
- Lockjaw (Tetanus)   854
- Reticulum Cell Sarcoma (Non-Hodgkin Lymphoma)   854
- Malaria   855
- Measles (Morbilli; Rubeola)   855
- Meningococcemia (Neisseria Meningitides; Meningitis)   855
- Disseminated Sclerosis (Multiple Sclerosis)   856

- Ophthalmoplegic Migraine Syndrome   856
- Kussmaul Disease (Kussmaul-Maier Disease; Necrotizing Angiitis; PAN; Polyarteritis Nodosa)   857
- Poliomyelitis (Infantile Paralysis)   858
- Herpes Zoster   858
- Mumps   859
- Hydrophobia (Lyssa; Rabies)   859
- Relapsing Polychondritis (Jaksch Wartenhost Syndrome; Meyenburg-Altherz-Vehlinger Syndrome; Von Meyenberg II Syndrome)   860
- Smallpox (Variola)   860
- Acquired Lues (Syphilis; Acquired Syphilis; Lues Venerea; Malum Venereum)   861
- Temporal Arteritis Syndrome (Cranial Arteritis Syndrome; Giant Cell Arteritis; Hutchinson-Horton-Magath-Brown Syndrome)   861
- Tuberculosis   862
- Foix Syndrome (Cavernous Sinus Syndrome; Hypophyseal-Sphenoidal Syndrome; Cavernous Sinus Neuralgia Syndrome; Godtfredsen Syndrome; Cavernous Sinus-Nasopharyngeal Tumor Syndrome; Cavernous Sinus Thrombosis)   862
- Arteriovenous Fistula (Arteriovenous Aneurysm; Arteriovenous Angioma; Arteriovenous Malformation; Cirsoid Aneurysm; Racemose Hemangioma; Varicose Aneurysm)   863
- Carotid Artery Syndrome (Cavernous Sinus Fistula Syndrome; Red-Eyed Shunt Syndrome)   863
- Tolosa-Hunt Syndrome (Painful Ophthalmoplegia)   864
- Foramen Lacerum Syndrome (Aneurysm of Internal Carotid Artery Syndrome)   864
- Foix Syndrome (Cavernous Sinus Syndrome; Hypophyseal-Sphenoidal Syndrome; Cavernous Sinus Neuralgia Syndrome; Godtfredsen Syndrome; Cavernous Sinus-Nasopharyngeal Tumor Syndrome; Cavernous Sinus Thrombosis)   865
- Gradenigo Syndrome (Temporal Syndrome; Lannois-Gradenigo Syndrome)   865

- Rochon-Duvigneaud Syndrome (Superior Orbital Fissure Syndrome) Optic Atrophy — 866
- Albers-Schonberg Disease (Marble Bone Disease; Osteosclerosis Fragilis Generalisata; Osteopetrosis; Osteopoikilosis; Osteosclerosis Congenita Diffusa) — 866
- Hodgkin Disease — 867
- Disseminated Lupus Erythematosus (Systemic Lupus Erythematosus; Lupus Erythematosus; Kaposi-Libman-Sack Syndrome, SLE) — 867
- Erb-Goldflam Syndrome (Erb II Syndrome; Hoppe-Goldflam Disease; Pseudoparalytic Syndrome; Myasthenia Gravis) — 868
- Passow Syndrome (Bremer Status Dysraphicus; Status Dysraphicus Syndrome; Syringomyelia; Syringobulbia) — 869
- Porphyria Cutanea Tarda — 869
- Schaumann Syndrome (Besnier-Boeck-Schaumann Syndrome; Boeck Sarcoid; Sarcoidosis) — 870
- Botulism — 870
- Blepharochalasis — 871
- Pneumococcal Infections (Streptococcus Pneumoniae Infections) — 871
- Staphylococcus — 872
- Haemophilus Aegyptius (Koch-Weeks Bacillus) — 872
- Influenza — 873
- Rubella Syndrome (Congenital Rubella Syndrome; German Measles; Gregg Syndrome) — 873
- Measles (Morbilli; Rubeola) — 873
- Mumps — 874
- Reiter Syndrome (Fiessinger-Leroy Syndrome; Conjunctivo-Urethro-Synovial Syndrome; Idiopathic Blennorrheal Arthritis Syndrome; Polyarthritis Enterica) — 874
- Candidiasis — 875
- Scalded Skin Syndrome (Toxic Epidermal Necrolysis; Ritter Disease; Toxic Epidermal Necrolysis of Lyell; Staphylococcal Scalded Skin Syndrome; Lyell Syndrome; Epidermolysis Acuta Toxica; Toxic Epidermal Necrolysis) Symblepharon — 875
- Relapsing Polychondritis (Jaksch Wartenhost Syndrome; Meyenburg-Altherz-Vehlinger Syndrome; Von Meyenberg II Syndrome) — 876
- Sjögren Syndrome (Gougerot-Sjögren Syndrome; Secretoinhibitor Syndrome; Sicca Syndrome) — 877
- Angular Conjunctivitis (Morax-Axenfeld Bacillus) — 877
- Pediculosis and Phthiriasis — 878
- Staphylococcus — 878
- Actinomycosis — 879
- Epidemic Keratoconjunctivitis — 879
- Glander Syndrome — 880
- Meningococcemia (Neisseria Meningitides; Meningitis) — 880
- Pseudomonas Aeruginosa Infections — 881
- Herpes Simplex — 881
- Smallpox (Variola) — 881
- Acute Follicular Conjunctivitis (Adenoviral Conjunctivitis; Pharyngoconjunctival Fever; Syndrome of Beal) — 882
- Epidemic Keratoconjunctivitis — 882
- Chlamydia (Inclusion Conjunctivitis; Paratrachoma) — 883
- Herpes Zoster — 883
- Newcastle Disease (Fowlpox) — 884
- Influenza — 884
- Herpes Zoster — 885
- Parinaud Oculoglandular Syndrome (Parinaud Conjunctiva-Adenitis Syndrome; Catscratch Oculoglandular Syndrome; Catscratch Disease; Bartonella henselae) — 885
- Trachoma — 886
- Moraxella Lacunata — 886
- Streptococcus — 887
- Pinta (Nonvenereal Treponematosis) — 887
- Chlamydia (Inclusion Conjunctivitis; Paratrachoma) — 887
- Ophthalmia Neonatorum (Neonatal Conjunctivitis) — 888
- Angelucci Syndrome (Critical Allergic Conjunctivitis Syndrome) — 888
- Anoxic Overwear Syndrome — 889
- Benjamin-Allen Syndrome — 889

- Floppy Eyelid Syndrome — 889
- Giant Papillary Conjunctivitis Syndrome — 890
- Beal Syndrome — 890
- Angular Conjunctivitis (Morax-Axenfeld Bacillus) — 891
- Rothmund Syndrome (Rothmund-Thomson Syndrome; Telangiectasia-Pigmentation-Cataract Syndrome; Ectodermal Syndrome; Congenital Poikiloderma with Juvenile Cataract) Keratoconus — 891
- Molluscum Contagiosum — 892
- Neurocutaneous Syndrome — 892
- Parinaud Syndrome (Divergence Paralysis; Subthalamic Syndrome; Paralysis of Vertical Movements; Pretectal Syndrome) — 892
- Trachoma — 893
- Neovascularization, Corneal Contact Lens Related — 893
- Benign Mucosal Pemphigoid (Chronic Cicatricial Conjunctivitis; Cicatricial Pemphigoid; Essential Shrinkage of the Conjunctiva; Membrane Pemphigus; Ocularpemphigoid) — 894
- Diphtheria — 894
- Streptococcus (Scarlet Fever) — 895
- Schaumann Syndrome (Besnier-Boeck-Schaumann Syndrome; Boeck Sarcoid; Sarcoidosis) — 895
- Progressive Systemic Sclerosis (Scleroderma; Systemic Scleroderma) — 896
- Lichen Planus — 896
- Blepharoconjunctivitis — 897
- Linear IgA Disease — 897
- Trachoma — 897
- Acne Rosacea (Acne Erythematosa; Ocular Rosacea) — 898
- Alkaline Injury of the Eye — 898
- Chlamydia (Inclusion Conjunctivitis; Paratrachoma) — 899
- Benign Mucosal Pemphigoid (Chronic Cicatricial Conjunctivitis; Cicatricial Pemphigoid; Essential Shrinkage of the Conjunctiva; Membrane Pemphigus; Ocularpemphigoid) — 899
- Congenital Lues (Congenital Syphilis) — 900
- Dermatitis Herpetiformis (Duhring-Brocq Disease) — 900
- Epidemic Keratoconjunctivitis — 901
- Scalded Skin Syndrome (Toxic Epidermal Necrolysis; Ritter Disease; Toxic Epidermal Necrolysis of Lyell; Staphylococcal Scalded Skin Syndrome; Lyell Syndrome; Epidermolysis Acuta Toxica; Toxic Epidermal Necrolysis) Symblepharon — 901
- Goldscheider Syndrome (Weber-Cockayne Syndrome; Epidermolysis Bullosa; Dominant Epidermolysis Bullosa Dystrophiea Albopapuloidea) — 902
- Stevens-Johnson Syndrome [Dermatostomatitis; Erythema Multiforme Exudativum; Syndroma Mucocutaneo-Oculare; Baader Dermatostomatitis Syndrome; Mucosal-Respiratory Syndrome; Fuchs (2) Syndrome; Mucocutaneous Ocular Syndrome] — 902
- Bullous Ichthyosiform Erythroderma (Collodion Baby; Congenital Ichthyosis; Epidermolytic Hyperkeratosis; Ichthyosis; Ichthyosis Vulgaris; Lamellar Ichthyosis; Nonbullous Ichthyosiform Erythroderma; Xeroderma; X-Linked Ichthyosis) — 903
- Contact Dermatitis (Dermatitis Venenata) — 904
- Fuchs-Lyell Syndrome (Debré-Lamy-Lyell Syndrome; Toxic Epidermal Necrolysis) — 904
- Hydroa Vacciniforme — 905
- Impetigo — 905
- Bullous Ichthyosiform Erythroderma (Collodion Baby; Congenital Ichthyosis; Epidermolytic Hyperkeratosis; Ichthyosis; Ichthyosis Vulgaris; Lamellar Ichthyosis; Nonbullous Ichthyosiform Erythroderma; Xeroderma; X-Linked Ichthyosis) — 905
- Benign Mucosal Pemphigoid (Chronic Cicatricial Conjunctivitis; Cicatricial Pemphigoid; Essential Shrinkage of the Conjunctiva; Membrane Pemphigus; Ocularpemphigoid) — 906
- Lichen Planus — 906
- Reiter Syndrome (Fiessinger-Leroy Syndrome; Conjunctivo-Urethro-Synovial Syndrome; Idiopathic Blennorrheal Arthritis Syndrome; Polyarthritis Enterica) — 907

- Keratoconjunctivitis Sicca and Sjögren's Syndrome 907
- Staphylococcus 908
- Acquired Lues (Syphilis; Acquired Syphilis; Lues Venerea; Malum Venereum) 908
- Progressive Systemic Sclerosis (Scleroderma; Systemic Scleroderma) 909
- Vaccinia (Keratitis) 909
- Listerellosis (Listeriosis) 910
- Pneumococcal Infections (Streptococcus Pneumoniae Infections) 910
- Staphylococcus 911
- Escherichia Coli 911
- Haemophilus Influenzae 911
- Rhinoscleroma (Klebsiella Rhinoscleromatis) 912
- Moraxella Lacunata 912
- Gonorrhea 913
- Meningococcemia (Neisseria Meningitidis; Meningitis) 913
- Proteus Syndrome 913
- Pseudomonas Aeruginosa 914
- Vaccinia (Keratitis) 914
- Actinomycosis 915
- Candidiasis 915
- Nocardiosis 916
- Wiskott-Aldrich Syndrome (Corneal Ulcer) 916
- Floppy Eyelid Syndrome 917
- Molluscum Contagiosum 917
- Basal Cell Carcinoma 918
- Squamous Cell Carcinoma of Eyelid 918
- Hemangioma 918
- Lymphangioma 919
- Juvenile Xanthogranuloma (JXG; Nevoxanthoendothelioma) 919
- Malignant Melanoma of the Posterior Uvea (Choroidal Melanoma, Ciliary Body Melanoma, Uveal Melanoma, Intraocular Melanoma) 920
- Rhabdomyosarcoma (Corneal Edema) 920
- Passow Syndrome (Bremer Status Dysraphicus; Status Dysraphicus Syndrome; Syringomyelia; Syringobulbia) 921
- Papilloma (Wart; Verruca) 921
- Basal Cell Nevus Syndrome (Nevoid Basal Cell Carcinoma Syndrome;
- Nevoid Basalioma Syndrome; Gorlin Syndrome; Gorlin-Goltz Syndrome; Multiple Basal Cell Nevi Syndrome) 922
- Melanocytic Lesions of the Eyelids (Ephelis, Lentigo, Neovascular Nevus, Dermal Melanocytosis, Malignant Melanoma) 922
- Mucocele (Pyocele) 923
- Sebaceous Gland Carcinoma 923
- Urbach-Wiethe Syndrome (Rossle-Urbach-Wiethe Syndrome; Lipoproteinosis; Hyalinosis Cutis et Mucosae; Lipoid Proteinosis; Proteinosis-Lipoidosis) Dry Eyes 924
- Lubarsch-Pick Syndrome (Primary Amyloidosis; Idiopathic Amyloidosis; Amyloidosis) 924
- Corneal Abrasions, Contusions, Lacerations and Perforations 925
- Lower Lid Ptosis 925
- Lid Retraction 925
- Pseudo-Graefe Syndrome (Fuchs Sign) 927
- Brown Syndrome (Superior Oblique Tendon Sheath Syndrome) 927
- Parkinson Syndrome (Paralysis Agitans; Shaking Palsy) 928
- Steele-Richardson-Olszewski Syndrome (Progressive Supranuclear Palsy) 928
- Duane Syndrome (Retraction Syndrome; Stilling Syndrome; Turk-Stilling Syndrome) 929
- Poliomyelitis (Infantile Paralysis) 929
- Chorea (Acute Chorea; Sydenham Chorea; St Vitus Dance; Huntington Hereditary Chorea) 930
- Craniostenosis 930
- Encephalitis, Acute 930
- Hydrophobia (Lyssa; Rabies) 931
- Hysteria (Malingering; Ophthalmic Flake Syndrome) 931
- Meningococcemia (Neisseria MeningitidIs; Meningitis) 932
- Disseminated Sclerosis (Multiple Sclerosis) 932
- Parinaud Syndrome (Divergence Paralysis; Subthalamic Syndrome; Paralysis of Vertical Movements; Pretectal Syndrome) 933

– Parkinson Syndrome
(Paralysis Agitans; Shaking Palsy) 933

– Russell Syndrome (Nystagmus) 934

– Koerber-Salus-Elschnig Syndrome
(Sylvian Aqueduct Syndrome;
Nystagmus Retractorius Syndrome) 934

– Acquired Lues (Syphilis;
Acquired Syphilis; Lues Venerea;
Malum Venereum) 935

– Von Economo Syndrome
(Encephalitis Lethargica; Sleeping
Sickness; Iceland Disease) Nystagmus 935

– Basedow Syndrome (Graves Disease;
Hyperthyroidism; Thyrotoxicosis;
Exophthalmic Goiter; Parry Disease) 936

– Horner Syndrome (Bernard-Horner
Syndrome; Cervical Sympathetic
Paralysis Syndrome; Claude-Bernard-
Horner Syndrome; Horner
Oculopupillary Syndrome) 937

– Mosse Syndrome (Polycythemia-
Hepatic Cirrhosis Syndrome) 937

– Basedow Syndrome (Graves Disease;
Hyperthyroidism; Thyrotoxicosis;
Exophthalmic Goiter; Parry Disease) 938

– Marcus Gunn Syndrome (Jaw-Winking
Syndrome; Congenital
Trigeminooculomotor Synkinesis) 938

– Trichiasis 939

– Xanthelasma
(Xanthelasma Palpebrarum) 939

– Xeroderma Pigmentosum
(Symblepharon) 940

• Acquired Immunodeficiency
Syndrome (AIDS; Acquired Cellular
Immunodeficiency; Acquired
Immunodeficiency) 940

• Blepharitis (Seborrheic Blepharitis,
Adult Blepharitis, Meibomian
Gland Dysfunction) 941

• Chalazion 941

• Temporal Arteritis Syndrome
(Cranial Arteritis Syndrome;
Giant Cell Arteritis;
Hutchinson-Horton-Magath-
Brown Syndrome) 942

• Granuloma Venereum 942

• Hordeolum (Internal Hordeolum, Acute
Meibonitis, External Hordeolum, Stye) 943

• Orbital Cellulitis and Abscess 943

• Streptococcus (Scarlet Fever) 943

• Basedow Syndrome (Graves Disease;
Hyperthyroidism; Thyrotoxicosis;
Exophthalmic Goiter;
Parry Disease) 944

• Trachoma 944

• Wegener Syndrome
(Wegener Granulomatosis) 945

• Yellow Fever 945

• Basal Cell Carcinoma 946

• Actinic and Seborrheic Keratosis 946

• Lymphangioma 946

• Melanocytic Lesions of the Eyelids
(Ephelis, Lentigo, Neovascular Nevus,
Dermal Melanocytosis,
Malignant Melanoma) 947

• Malignant Melanoma of the Posterior
Uvea (Choroidal Melanoma, Ciliary Body
Melanoma, Uveal Melanoma,
Intraocular Melanoma) 947

• Sebaceous Gland Carcinoma 948

23. Glaucoma **949**

• Open Angle Glaucoma 949

– Normal-Tension Glaucoma
(Low Tension Glaucoma) 949

– Angle Recession Glaucoma 950

– Aphakic and Pseudophakic Glaucoma 950

– UGH Syndrome (Uveitis-Glaucoma-
Hyphema Syndrome) Glaucoma 950

– Corticosteroid-Induced Glaucoma 951

– Glaucoma Associated with Elevated
Venous Pressure 951

– Ghost Cell Glaucoma 952

– Iris Nevus Syndrome (Cogan-Reese
Syndrome; Chandler Syndrome;
Iridocorneal Endothelial
Syndrome; ICE Syndrome) 952

– Lens-Induced Glaucoma (Phacolytic,
Lens Particle and Phacoantigenic) 953

– Malignant Glaucoma (Ciliary Block
Glaucoma, Aqueous Misdirection,
Cilolenticular/Ciliovitreal Block) 953

– Glaucoma Following Penetrating
Keratoplasty 954

– Pigmentary Dispersion Syndrome and
Pigmentary Glaucoma 954

– Posner-Schlossman Syndrome
(Glaucomatocyclitic Crisis) 954

– Pseudoexfoliation Syndrome 955

– Pupillary Block Glaucoma 955

– Primary Angle-Closure Glaucoma
(Primary Closed Angle Glaucoma) 956

– Chronic Angle Closure Glaucoma 956

– Glaucoma Associated with Intraocular
Tumors (Tumor Related Glaucoma,
Melanomalytic Glaucoma, Neovascular
Glaucoma, Angle Closure Glaucoma) 957

– Iridal Adhesion Syndrome
(Iris Adhesion Syndrome,
Iridocorneal Endothelial Syndrome) 957

– Malignant Glaucoma (Ciliary Block
Glaucoma, Aqueous Misdirection,
Cilolenticular/Ciliovitreal Block) 958

– Phacomorphic Glaucoma 958

– Plateau Iris Syndrome 958

– Rubeosis Iridis Neovascular Glaucoma 959

• Aniridia (Congenital Aniridia,
Hereditary Aniridia) 959

• Congenital Cataract, Microcornea,
Abnormal Irides, Nystagmus, and
Congenital Glaucoma Syndrome 960

• Glaucoma, Congenital 960

• Juvenile Glaucoma 961

• Glaucoma, Hereditary Juvenile 961

• Glaucoma, Recessive Juvenile 961

• Microphthalmos, Pigmentary
Retinopathy, Glaucoma 962

• Axenfeld-Rieger Syndrome (Posterior
Embryotoxon; Axenfeld Syndrome) 962

• Rieger Syndrome (Axenfeld-Rieger
Syndrome; Dysgenesis Mesodermalis
Corneae et Irides; Dysgenesis
Mesostromalis; Axenfeld Posterior
Embryotoxon-Juvenile Glaucoma) 963

• Ring Chromosome 6 (Aniridia,
Congenital Glaucoma, and Hydrocephalus) 963

• Ocular Hypotony 964

24. Globe **965**

• Clinical Anophthalmos
(Apparent Absence of Globe) 965

– Anencephaly 965

– Frontonasal Dysplasia Syndrome
(Median Cleft Face Syndrome) 966

– Ullrich Syndrome (Ullrich-Feichtiger
Syndrome; Dyscraniopylophalangy)
Corneal Ulcer 966

– Goldenhar Syndrome (Oculo-
Auriculo-Vertebral Dysplasia;
Goldenhar-Gorlin Syndrome) 966

– Goltz Syndrome
(Focal Dermal Hypoplasia Syndrome) 967

– Hallermann-Streiff Syndrome
[Dyscephalic-Mandibulo-Oculo-Facial
Syndrome; Oculo-Mandibulo-Dyscephaly;
Ullrich-Fremery-Dohna Syndrome;
Francois Dyscephalic Syndrome;
Mandibulo-Oculo-Facial Dyscephaly
Syndrome; Francois-Hallermann-Streiff
Syndrome; Hallermann-Streiff-Francois
Syndrome; Audry I Syndrome; Dohna
Syndrome; Francois Syndrome (1);
Dyscephaly-Teeth Abnormality-Dwarfism;
Dyscephalia Oculomandibularis-
Hypotrichosis; Mandibulo-Ocular
Dyscephalia Hypotrichosis; Fremery-
Dohna Syndrome; Oculo-Mandibulo-
Facial Dyscephaly] 967

– Hypervitaminosis A 968

– Klinefelter Syndrome (Gynecomastia-
Aspermatogenesis Syndrome;
XXY Syndrome; XXXY Syndrome;
XXYY Syndrome; Reifenstein-Albright
Syndrome) 969

– Lanzieri Syndrome 969

– Leri Syndrome (Pleonosteosis
Syndrome; Carpal Tunnel Syndrome) 970

– Meckel Syndrome
(Dysencephalia Splanchnocystic
Syndrome; Gruber Syndrome) 970

– Franceschetti Syndrome [Franceschetti-
Zwahlen-Klein Syndrome; Treacher
Collins Syndrome; Mandibulofacial
Dysostosis; Mandibulofacial Syndrome;
Eyelid-Malar-Mandible Syndrome;
Oculovertebral Syndrome;
Berry Syndrome; Franceschetti-Zwahlen
Syndrome; Zwahlen Syndrome;
Bilateral Facial Agenesis; Berry-
Franceschetti-Klein Syndrome;
Franceschetti-
Klein Syndrome;
Franceschetti Syndrome (II); Treacher
Collins-Franceschetti Syndrome;
Weyers-Thier Syndrome] 971

– Otocephaly 971

- Trisomy 13 Syndrome (Trisomy D1 Syndrome, Patau Syndrome, Reese Syndrome) Iris Coloboma 972
- Waardenburg Syndrome (Van Der Hoeve-Halberstam-Waardenburg Syndrome; Waardenburg-Klein Syndrome; Embryonic Fixation Syndrome; Interoculo-Iridodermato-Auditive Dysplasia; Piebaldism) Hypertelorism 972
- Bacterial Endophthalmitis 973
- Escherichia Coli 973
- Fungal Endophthalmitis 973
- Metastatic Bacterial Endophthalmitis 974
- Metastatic Fungal Endophthalmitis 974
- Phacoanaphylactic Endophthalmitis (Endophthalmitis Phacoanaphylactica, Phacoanaphylactic Uveitis, Phacoantigenic Uveitis) 974
- MIDAS Syndrome (Microphthalmia, Dermal Aplasia and Sclerocornea) 975
- Behçet Syndrome (Dermato-Stomato-Ophthalmic Syndrome; Oculobuccogenital Syndrome; Gilbert Syndrome) 975
- Filtering Blebs and Associated Problems 976
- Schaumann Syndrome (Besnier-Boeck-Schaumann Syndrome; Boeck Sarcoid; Sarcoidosis) 976
- Sympathetic Ophthalmia 977
- Acquired Lues (Syphilis; Acquired Syphilis; Lues Venerea; Malum Venereum) 977
- Vogt-Koyanagi-Harada Disease (Harada Disease; Uveitis-Vitiligo-Alopecia-Poliosis Syndrome) 978
- Retraction of the Globe (on Horizontal Conjugate Gaze) 978
  - Duane Syndrome (Retraction Syndrome; Stilling Syndrome; Turk-Stilling Syndrome) 979
  - Acrorenoocular Syndrome 979
  - Goldenhar Syndrome (Oculo-Auriculo-Vertebral Dysplasia; Goldenhar-Gorlin Syndrome) 980
  - Hanhart Syndrome (Richner Syndrome; Recessive Keratosis Palmoplantaris; Pseudoherpetic Keratitis; Richner-Hanhart Syndrome; Tyrosinemia II; Tyrosinosis; Pseudodendritic Keratitis) 980

- Okihiro Syndrome 981
- Wildervanck Syndrome (Cervicooculoacousticus Syndrome; Franceschetti-Klein-Wildervanck Syndrome; Wildervanck-Waardenburg Syndrome; Cervicooculofacial Dysmorphia; Cervicooculofacial Syndrome) Nystagmus 981
- Dermoid (Dermoid Choristoma; Dermoid Cyst; Dermolipoma; Lipodermoid) 982
- Hemangioma 982
- Lymphangioma 982
- Basedow Syndrome (Graves Disease; Hyperthyroidism; Thyrotoxicosis; Exophthalmic Goiter; Parry Disease) 983

25. Headache **984**

- Raeder Syndrome (Paratrigeminal Paralysis; Horton Headache; Histamine Cephalalgia; Ciliary Neuralgia; Cluster Headache; Periodic Migrainous Neuralgia) 984
- Temporal Arteritis Syndrome (Cranial Arteritis Syndrome; Giant Cell Arteritis; Hutchinson-Horton-Magath-Brown Syndrome) 984
- Hypertension 985
- Migraine (Vascular Headache) 985
- Muscle Contraction Headache 986
- Pseudotumor 986

26. Iris **987**

- Aniridia and Absent Patella 987
- Aniridia (Absence of Iris, Partial or Complete) 987
  - Aniridia, Cerebellar Ataxia, and Mental Deficiency (Gillespie Syndrome) 988
  - Homocystinuria Syndrome 988
  - Marinesco-Sjögren Syndrome (Congenital Spinocerebellar Ataxia-Congenital Cataract-Oligophrenia Syndrome) 989
  - Miller Syndrome (Wilms Aniridia Syndrome; WAGR Syndrome; Wilms Tumor-Aniridia-Genitourinary Abnormalities-Mental Retardation Syndrome) 989
  - Oculodental Syndrome (Peters Syndrome; Rutherford Syndrome) 990

– Rieger Syndrome (Axenfeld-Rieger Syndrome; Dysgenesis Mesodermalis Corneae et Irides; Dysgenesis Mesostromalis; Axenfeld Posterior Embryotoxon-Juvenile Glaucoma) 991

– Ring Chromosome 6 (Aniridia, Congenital Glaucoma, and Hydrocephalus) 991

– Scaphocephaly Syndrome (Papilledema) 992

– Hereditary Ectodermal Dysplasia Syndrome (Siemens Syndrome; Keratosis Follicularis Spinulosa Syndrome; Hypohidrotic Ectodermal Dysplasia; Christ-Siemens-Touraine Syndrome; Weech Syndrome; Anhidrotic Ectodermal Dysplasia; Ichthyosis Follicularis) 992

– Ullrich Syndrome (Ullrich-Feichtiger Syndrome; Dyscraniopylophalangy) Corneal Ulcer 993

• Aniridia, Partial with Unilateral Renal Agenesis and Psychomotor Retardation 993

• Uveitis, Anterior Nongranulomatous (Iritis, Chronic) 994

• Uveitis, Anterior Granulomatous (Iritis) 994

• Fuchs (1) Syndrome (Heterochromic Cyclitis Syndrome) 995

• Juvenile Rheumatoid Arthritis (JRA; Still Disease) 995

• Charlin Syndrome (Nasal Nerve Syndrome; Nasociliaris Nerve Syndrome; Nasociliary Syndrome) 996

• Chikungunya Fever 996

• Coloboma of Iris 997

– Acrorenoocular Syndrome 998

– Aicardi Syndrome 998

– Aniridia (Congenital aniridia, Hereditary Aniridia) 999

– Biemond Syndrome 999

– Cat's-Eye Syndrome (Schachenmann Syndrome; Schmid-Fraccaro Syndrome; Partial Trisomy G Syndrome) 1000

– CHARGE Association (Multiple Congenital Anomalies Syndrome; Coloboma, Heart Disease, Atresia, Retarded Growth, Genital Hypoplasia, Ear Malformation Association) 1000

– Chromosome 18 Partial Deletion (Short-Arm) Syndrome [Monosomy 18 Partial (Short-Arm) Syndrome] 1001

– Ellis-Van Creveld Syndrome (Chondroectodermal Dysplasia) 1001

– Epidermal Nevus Syndrome (Ichthyosis Hystrix) 1002

– Goltz Syndrome (Focal Dermal Hypoplasia Syndrome) 1002

– Hallermann-Streiff Syndrome (Dyscephalic-Mandibulo-Oculo-Facial Syndrome; Oculo-Mandibulo-Dyscephaly; Ullrich-Fremery-Dohna Syndrome; Francois Dyscephalic Syndrome; Mandibulo-Oculo-Facial Dyscephaly Syndrome; Francois-Hallermann-Streiff Syndrome; Hallermann-Streiff-Francois Syndrome; Audry I Syndrome; Dohna Syndrome; Francois Syndrome (1); Dyscephaly-Teeth Abnormality-Dwarfism; Dyscephalia Oculomandibularis-Hypotrichosis; Mandibulo-Ocular Dyscephalia Hypotrichosis; Fremery-Dohna Syndrome; Oculo-Mandibulo-Facial Dyscephaly) 1003

– Hemifacial Microsomia Syndrome (Unilateral Facial Agenesis; Otomandibular Dysostosis; Francois-Haustrate Syndrome) 1004

– Hurler Syndrome (Pfaundler-Hurler Syndrome; Gargoylism; Dysostosis Multiplex; MPS IH Syndrome; Systemic Mucopolysaccharidosis Type IH; Mucopolysaccharidosis IH) 1004

– Heterochromia Iridis 1005

– Jeune Disease (Asphyxiating Thoracic Dystrophy; Thoracic-Pelvic-Phalangeal Dystrophy) 1005

– Joubert Syndrome (Familial Cerebellar Vermis Agenesis) 1006

– Kartagener Syndrome (Sinusitis-Bronchiectasis-Situs Inversus Syndrome; Bronchiectasis-Dextrocardia-Sinusitis; Kartagener Triad) 1006

– Klinefelter Syndrome (Gynecomastia-Aspermatogenesis Syndrome; XXY Syndrome; XXXY Syndrome; XXYY Syndrome; Reifenstein-Albright Syndrome) 1007

– Klippel-Trenaunay-Weber Syndrome (Parkes-Weber Syndrome; Angio-Osteo-Hypertrophy Syndrome) 1007

– Langer-Giedion Syndrome (Trichorhinophalangeal Syndrome, Type II) 1008

– Lanzieri Syndrome 1008

– Laurence-Moon-Bardet-Biedl Syndrome (Bardet-Biedl Syndrome; Retinitis Pigmentosa-Polydactyly-Adiposogenital Syndrome) 1008

– Marfan Syndrome (Dolichostenomelia; Arachnodactyly; Hyperchondroplasia; Dystrophia Mesodermalis Congenita) 1009

– Vitamin A Deficiency 1010

– Meckel Syndrome (Dysencephalia Splanchnocystic Syndrome; Gruber Syndrome) 1010

– Frontonasal Dysplasia Syndrome (Median Cleft Face Syndrome) 1011

– Meyer-Schwickerath-Weyers Syndrome (Microphthalmos Syndrome; Oculodentodigital Dysplasia) 1011

– Basal Cell Nevus Syndrome (Nevoid Basal Cell Carcinoma Syndrome; Nevoid Basalioma Syndrome; Gorlin Syndrome; Gorlin-Goltz Syndrome; Multiple Basal Cell Nevi Syndrome) 1012

– Linear Nevus Sebaceus of Jadassohn (Nevus Sebaceus of Jadassohn; Jadassohn-Type Anetoderma; Organoid Nevus syndrome; Sebaceus nevus syndrome) 1012

– Obesity-Cerebral-Ocular-Skeletal Anomalies Syndrome 1013

– Hemifacial Microsomia Syndrome (Unilateral Facial Agenesis; Otomandibular Dysostosis; Francois-Haustrate Syndrome) 1013

– Rieger Syndrome (Axenfeld-Rieger Syndrome; Dysgenesis Mesodermalis Corneae et Irides;Dysgenesis Mesostromalis; Axenfeld Posterior Embryotoxon-Juvenile Glaucoma) 1014

– Rubinstein-Taybi Syndrome (Optic Atrophy) 1014

– Franceschetti Syndrome (Franceschetti-Zwahlen-Klein Syndrome; Treacher Collins Syndrome; Mandibulofacial Dysostosis; Mandibulofacial Syndrome; Eyelid-Malar-Mandible Syndrome; Oculovertebral Syndrome; Berry Syndrome; Franceschetti-Zwahlen Syndrome; Zwahlen Syndrome; Bilateral Facial Agenesis; Berry-Franceschetti-Klein Syndrome; Franceschetti-Klein Syndrome; Franceschetti Syndrome (II); Treacher Collins-Franceschetti Syndrome; Weyers-Thier Syndrome) 1015

– Trisomy 13 Syndrome (Trisomy D1 Syndrome, Patau Syndrome, Reese Syndrome) Iris Coloboma 1015

– Trisomy 18 Syndrome (E Syndrome; Edwards Syndrome) Congenital Glaucoma 1016

– Turner Syndrome (Turner-Albright Syndrome; Gonadal Dysgenesis; Genital Dwarfism Syndrome; Ullrich-Turner Syndrome; Bonnevie-Ullrich Syndrome; Pterygolymphangiectasia Syndrome; Ullrich-Bonnevie Syndrome) Cataract, Posterior 1016

– Walker-Warburg Syndrome (Cerebroocular Dysplasia-Muscular Dystrophy; Warburg Syndrome; COD-MD Syndrome; Fukuyama Congenital Muscular Dystrophy; Hard + or – E Syndrome) Cataract 1017

– Wolf Syndrome (Monosomy 4 Partial Syndrome; Chromosome 4 Partial Deletion Syndrome; Hirschhorn-Cooper Syndrome) Ptosis 1017

– 11q- Syndrome 1018

– Chromosome 13q Partial Deletion (Long-Arm Syndrome; 13q Syndrome) 1018

– 18q- Syndrome (18q Deletion Syndrome) 1018

– XYY Syndrome 1019

• Concave Peripheral Iris 1019

– Pigmentary Dispersion Syndrome and Pigmentary Glaucoma 1019

– Pseudoexfoliation Syndrome 1020

• Floppy Iris Syndrome 1020

• Fuchs (1) Syndrome (Heterochromic Cyclitis Syndrome) 1021

• Gray Iris Syndrome 1021

• Heterochromia Iridis 1021

- Iridal Adhesion Syndrome
  (Iris Adhesion Syndrome,
  Iridocorneal Endothelial Syndrome) ... 1022
- Iris Bombe ... 1022
- Iris Cysts ... 1022
- Iris Dysplasia Hypertelorism-
  Psychomotor Retardation Syndrome ... 1023
- Iris Melanoma ... 1023
- Iris Pigment Layer Cleavage ... 1024
- Iris Prolapse ... 1024
- Iris Retraction Syndrome (Posterior
  Synechiae and Iris Retraction Syndrome) ... 1024
- Jabs Syndrome (Synovitis, Granulomatous
  Uveitis, and Cranial Neuropathies) ... 1025
- Juvenile Xanthogranuloma
  (JXG; Nevoxanthoendothelioma) ... 1025
- Iris Laceration and Iris Holes, and
  Iridodialysis ... 1026
- Lens-Iris Diaphram Retropulsion
  Syndrome ... 1026
- Iris Melanoma ... 1026
- Miller Syndrome (Wilms' Aniridia
  Syndrome; WAGR Syndrome;
  Wilms' Tumor-Aniridia-Genitourinary
  Abnormalities-Mental Retardation
  Syndrome) ... 1027
- Iris Neovascularization with
  Pseudoexfoliation Syndrome ... 1027
- Albinism (Brown Oculocutaneous
  Albinism; Nettleship Falls Syndrome) ... 1028
- Iris Pigment Layer Cleavage ... 1028
- Plateau Iris Syndrome ... 1029
- Posterior Iris Chafing Syndrome ... 1029
- Ring Chromosome 6 (Aniridia,
  Congenital Glaucoma, and Hydrocephalus) ... 1029
- Rubeosis Iridis [Neovacularization
  (Newly Formed Blood Vessels) on the Iris] ... 1030
  - Takayasu Syndrome (Martorell
    Syndrome; Aortic Arch Syndrome;
    Pulseless Disease; Reversed
    Coarctation Syndrome) ... 1031
  - Carotid Artery Syndrome (Cavernous
    Sinus Fistula Syndrome; Red-Eyed
    Shunt Syndrome) ... 1032
  - Temporal Arteritis Syndrome
    (Cranial Arteritis Syndrome;
    Giant Cell Arteritis; Hutchinson-
    Horton-Magath-Brown Syndrome) ... 1032

- Central or Branch Retinal
  Artery Occlusion ... 1033
- Diabetes Mellitus ... 1033
- Eales Disease (Periphlebitis) ... 1034
- Andersen-Warburg Syndrome
  (Whitnall-Norman Syndrome;
  Oligophrenia Microphthalmos
  Syndrome; Norrie Disease;
  Atrophia Oculi Congenital Fetal Iritis
  Syndrome; Congenital Progressive
  Oculo-Acoustico-Cerebral Dysplasia) ... 1034
- Persistent Hyperplastic Primary Vitreous
  (PHPV, Persistent Fetal Vasculature) ... 1035
- Retinal Detachment, Rhegmatogenous ... 1035
- Hemangioma ... 1035
- Retinoblastoma ... 1036
- Retrolental Fibroplasia
  (RLF; Retinopathy of Prematurity) ... 1036
- Herrick Syndrome (Dresbach
  Syndrome; Sickle Cell Disease;
  Drepanocytic Anemia) ... 1037
- Hemangioma ... 1037
- Exfoliation Syndrome
  (Capsular Exfoliation Syndrome) ... 1038
- Fibrinoid Syndrome ... 1038
- Fungal Enophthalmitis ... 1039
- Iris Neovascularization with
  Pseudoexfoliation Syndrome ... 1039
- Uveitis, Anterior Granulomatous (Iritis) ... 1039
- Adult Cataracts ... 1040
- Diabetes Mellitus ... 1040
- Myotonic Dystrophy Syndrome
  (Myotonia Atrophica Syndrome;
  Dystrophia Myotonica;
  Curschmann-Steinert Syndrome) ... 1041
- Ocular Hypotony ... 1042
- Uveitis, Anterior Granulomatous (Iritis) ... 1042
  - Uveitis, Anterior Nongranulomatous
    (Iritis, Chronic) ... 1042
  - Uveitis (Iritis, Iridocystitis,
    Intermediate and Posterior Uveitis,
    Noninfectious Chorioretinitis) ... 1043
- Uveitis Masquerade Syndrome(s)
  (VMS) Uveitis 1286 ... 1043
- UGH Syndrome (Uveitis-Glaucoma-
  Hyphema Syndrome) Glaucoma ... 1044

27. Lacrimal System **1045**

- Alacrima 1045
- Branchial Clefts with Characteristic Facies, Growth Retardation, Imperforate Nasolacrimal Duct, and Premature Aging 1045
- Congenital Anomalies of the Lacrimal System (Congenital Nasolacrimal Duct Obstruction, Dacryocystitis, Dacryocystocele, ACCESSORY Punctum, Punctal Stenosis, Canalicular Stenosis) 1046
- Dacryoadenitis 1046
- Autoimmunologically Mediated Syndrome (Lymphocytic Hypophysitis Associated with Dacryoadenitis Syndrome) 1047
- Dry Eye Syndrome 1047
- Epiphoria 1048
- Heerfordt Syndrome (Uveoparotid Fever; Uveoparotitis; Uveoparotitic Paralysis) 1048
- Lacrimal Duct Defect 1048
- Lacrimal Gland Tumors 1049
- Lacrimal Hypersecretion 1049
- Lacrimal System Contusions and Lacerations 1049
- Parinaud Oculoglandular Syndrome (Parinaud Conjunctiva-Adenitis Syndrome; Catscratch Oculoglandular Syndrome; Catscratch Disease; Bartonella henselae) 1050
- Parotid Aplasia or Hypoplasia (Salivary Gland Absence; Lacrimal Puncta Absence) 1050
- Riley-Day Syndrome (Congenital Familial Dysautonomia) 1051
- Keratoconjunctivitis Sicca and Sjögren's Syndrome 1051
- Werner Syndrome (Progeria of Adults) Blue Sclera 1051
- Congenital Anomalies of the Lacrimal System (Congenital Nasolacrimal Duct Obstruction, Dacryocystitis, Dacryocystocele, Accessory Punctum, Punctal Stenosis, Canalicular Stenosis) 1052
- Stasis 1052
- Epiphoria 1053
- Branchial Clefts with Characteristic Facies, Growth Retardation, Imperforate Nasolacrimal Duct, and Premature Aging 1053

- Walker-Clodius Syndrome (Lobster Claw Deformity with Nasolacrimal Obstruction; EEC; Ectrodactyly, Ectodermal Dysplasia, and Cleft Lip/Palate) 1053

28. Lens **1055**

- Adult Cataracts 1055
- After Cataracts 1055
- Alström Disease (Cataract and Retinitis Pigmentosa) 1056
- Andogsky Syndrome (Atopic Cataract Syndrome; Dermatogenous Cataract) 1056
- Cataract, Anterior Polar 1057
- Cataract and Congenital Ichthyosis 1057
- Cataract, Congenital or Juvenile (Cataract, Juvenile, Hutterite Type) 1058
- Cataract, Congenital Total with Posterior Sutural Opacities 1058
- Cataract, Crystalline Aculeiform or Frosted 1059
- Cataract, Crystalline Coralliform 1059
- Cataract, Floriform 1059
- Cataract, Membranous 1060
- Cataract, Microcornea Syndrome 1060
- Cataract, Microphthalmia and Nystagmus 1060
- Cataract, Nuclear (Coppock Cataract; Cataract, Discoid) 1061
- Cataract, Nuclear Diffuse Nonprogressive 1061
- Cataract, Posterior Polar 1062
- Cerebellar Ataxia, Cataract, Deafness, and Dementia or Psychosis (Heredopathia Ophthalmo-Oto-Encephalica) 1062
- Cerebellar Ataxia, Infantile, with Progressive External Ophthalmoplegia 1062
- Congenital Cataracts Facial Dysmorphism Neuropathy Syndrome 1063
- Congenital Cataract, Microcornea, Abnormal Irides, Nystagmus and Congenital Glaucoma Syndrome 1063
- Congenital Cataract with Oxycephaly (Tower Skull Syndrome) 1064
- Desert Lung and Cataract Syndrome 1064
- Dislocation of Intraocular Lens 1064
- Dislocation of the Lens 1065
- Foveal Hypoplasia and Presenile Cataract Syndrome (O'Donnell-Pappas Syndrome) 1065
- Hypogonadism-Cataract Syndrome 1066

- Iridescent Crystalline Deposits in Lens 1066
- Cretinism (Hypothyroid Goiter; Hypothyroidism; Juvenile Hypothyroidism; Myxedema) 1067
- Hypocalcemia 1067
  - Cretinism (Hypothyroid Goiter; Hypothyroidism; Juvenile Hypothyroidism; Myxedema) 1068
  - Hypoparathyroidism 1068
  - Pseudohypoparathyroidism Syndrome (Chronic Renal Tubular Insufficiency Syndrome; Seabright-Bantam Syndrome; Albright Hereditary Osteodystrophy) 1069
  - Myotonic Dystrophy Syndrome (Myotonia Atrophica Syndrome; Dystrophia Myotonica; Curschmann-Steinert Syndrome) 1069
  - Cataract, Crystalline Coralliform 1070
  - Cataract, Crystalline Aculeiform or Frosted 1070
- Koby Syndrome (Floriform Cataract) 1071
- Lens Induced Glaucoma (Phacolytic, Lens Particle and Phacoantigenic) 1071
- Lens-Iris Diaphragm Retropulsion Syndrome 1072
- Lenticonus and Lentiglobus 1072
- Lost Lens Syndrome 1072
- Malignant Hyperpyrexia Syndrome (Postcataract Hyperpyrexia Syndrome; Postinduction Hyperpyrexia Syndrome) 1073
- Marinesco-Sjögren Syndrome (Congenital Spinocerebellar Ataxia-Congenital Cataract-Oligophrenia Syndrome) 1073
- Microcephaly, Microphthalmia, Cataracts, and Joint Contractures 1074
- Microspherophakia 1074
- Microspherophakia with Hernia 1074
- Myopathy, Mitochondrial, with Cataract 1075
- Nieden Syndrome (Telangiectasia-Cataract Syndrome) 1075
- Osteogenesis Imperfecta Congenita, Microcephaly and Cataracts 1076
- Pseudoexfoliation Syndrome 1076
- Rubella Syndrome (Congenital Rubella Syndrome; German Measles; Gregg Syndrome) 1077

- Toxic Lens Syndrome (Toxic Anterior Segment Syndrome; TASS) 1077
- Traumatic Cataract 1078
- Z Syndrome 1078

29. Macula **1079**

- Age-Related Macular Degeneration 1079
- Batten-Mayou Syndrome (Spielmeyer-Vogt Syndrome; Mayou-Batten Disease; Stock-Spielmeyer-Vogt Syndrome; Cerebroretinal Degeneration; Pigmentary Retinal Lipoid Neuronal Heredodegeneration; Vogt-Spielmeyer Syndrome; Juvenile Ganglioside Lipidosis; Neuronal Ceroid Lipofuscinosis; Myoclonic Variant of Cerebral Lipidosis; Batten Disease; Cerebromacular Dystrophy; Juvenile Amaurotic Family Idiocy; Spielmeyer-Sjögren Syndrome) 1080
- Central Serous Chorioretinopathy 1080
- Choroidoretinal Degeneration with Retinal Reflex in Heterozygous Women 1081
- Coloboma of Macula (Agenesis of Macula) 1081
- Coloboma of Macula with Type B Brachydactyly (Apical Dystrophy) 1082
- Diabetic Macular Edema 1082
- Dialinas-Amalric Syndrome (Amalric-Dialinas Syndrome; Deaf Mutism-Retinal Degeneration Syndrome) 1083
- Epimacular Proliferation (Macular Pucker) 1083
- Franceschetti Disease (Fundus Flavimaculatus) 1083
- Grouped Pigmentation of the Macula 1084
- Histoplasmosis (Histoplasmosis Choroiditis; Histoplasmosis Maculopathy; Presumed Ocular Histoplasmosis Syndrome) 1084
- Jensen Disease (Juxtapapillary Retinopathy) 1085
- Junius-Kuhnt Syndrome [Kuhnt-Junius Disease; Macular Senile Disciform Degeneration (1); Macula Lutea Juvenile Degeneration (2)] 1085
- Macular Edema, Pseudophakic (Irvine-Gass) 1086
- Macular Hole 1086
  - Papilledema 1087
  - Retinal Detachment, Rhegmatogenous 1087

– Retinoschisis 1087

– Electrical Injury 1088

– Central Serous Chorioretinopathy 1088

– Coloboma of Macula
(Agenesis of Macula) 1088

– Dawson Disease (Dawson Encephalitis;
Subacute Sclerosing Panencephalitis;
Inclusion-Body) 1089

– Herrick Syndrome (Dresbach Syndrome;
Sickle Cell Disease;
Drepanocytic Anemia) 1090

• Marseilles Fever (Boutonneuse Fever) 1090

• Progressive Foveal Dystrophy
(Central Retinal Pigment
Epithelial Dystrophy) 1091

• Solar Retinopathy 1091

• Sorsby I Syndrome
(Hereditary Macular Coloboma Syndrome) 1091

• Stargardt Disease
(Juvenile Macular Degeneration) 1092

30. Optic Nerve **1093**

• Crowded Disk Syndrome (Bilateral
Choroidal Folds and Optic Neuropathy) 1093

• Meningioma, Optic Nerve Sheath 1093

• Nasal Retinal Nerve Fiber
Layer Attenuation 1094

• Optic Atrophy 1094

– GAPO Syndrome (Growth Retardation,
Alopecia, Pseudoanodontia, Optic
Atrophy Syndrome) 1095

– Leber Hereditary Optic Neuropathy
(Optic Atrophy Amaurosis;
Pituitary Syndrome; Leber Syndrome) 1095

– Marquardt-Loriaux Syndrome
(Wolfram Syndrome; Diabetes
Insipidus-Diabetes Mellitus-Optic
Atrophy-Deafness Syndrome;
DIDMOAD Syndrome) 1096

– Optic Atrophy, Nerve Deafness 1096

– Optic Atrophy, Non-Leber-Type,
with Early Onset 1097

– Spastic Paraplegia, Optic Atrophy,
Dementia 1097

– Toxic/Nutritional Optic Neuropathy 1097

– X-Chromosomal Deletion
(Optic Atrophy) 1098

– Yellow Fever 1098

• Optic Neuritis 1098

– Optic Neuropathy, Anterior Ischemic 1099

– Botulism 1099

– Optic Neuritis, Childhood 1100

– Optic Neuropathy, Compressive 1100

– Optic Nerve Decompression for
Traumatic Neuropathy 1100

– Lyme Disease 1101

– Rocky Mountain Spotted Fever 1101

• Pseudopapilledema
(Optic Nerve Head Drusen) 1102

• Optic Nerve Hypoplasia, Familial
(Bilateral, Unilateral) 1102

• Optic Pit Syndrome 1102

• Papilledema 1103

• Symonds Syndrome (Otitic Hydrocephalus
Syndrome; Serous Meningitis Syndrome;
Benign Intracranial Hypertension;
Pseudotumor Cerebri) 1103

31. Orbit **1104**

• Acute Orbital Compartment Syndrome 1104

• Foramen Lacerum Syndrome
(Aneurysm of Internal Carotid Artery
Syndrome) 1104

• Blatt Syndrome (Cranio-Orbito-
Ocular Dysraphia) 1105

• Carotid Artery Syndrome (Cavernous
Sinus Fistula Syndrome; Red-Eyed
Shunt Syndrome) 1105

• Foix Syndrome (Cavernous Sinus
Syndrome; Hypophyseal-Sphenoidal
Syndrome; Cavernous Sinus Neuralgia
Syndrome; Godtfredsen Syndrome;
Cavernous Sinus-Nasopharyngeal Tumor
Syndrome; Cavernous Sinus Thrombosis) 1106

• Orbital Cellulitis and Abscess 1106

• Exophthalmos (Proptosis) 1107

• General Fibrosis Syndrome [Congenital
Enophthalmos with Ocular Muscle
Fibrosis and Ptosis; Congenital Fibrosis
of the Inferior Rectus with Ptosis;
Strabismus Fixus; Vertical Retraction
Syndrome (Congenital Fibrosis Syndrome)] 1107

• Orbital Infarction Syndrome 1108

• Sphenocavernous Syndrome 1108

• Yellow Fever 1109

- Carotid Artery Syndrome
  (Cavernous Sinus Fistula Syndrome;
  Red-Eyed Shunt Syndrome)   1109
- Foix Syndrome (Cavernous Sinus
  Syndrome; Hypophyseal-Sphenoidal
  Syndrome; Cavernous Sinus Neuralgia
  Syndrome; Godtfredsen Syndrome;
  Cavernous Sinus-Nasopharyngeal Tumor
  Syndrome; Cavernous Sinus Thrombosis)   1110
- External Orbital Fractures   1110
- Internal Orbital Fractures
  (Blowout Fracture)   1110
- Orbital Fracture, Apex   1111
- Optic Foramen Fractures   1111
- Orbital Hemorrhages   1112
- Dermoid, Orbital   1112
- Basedow Syndrome (Graves Disease;
  Hyperthyroidism; Thyrotoxicosis;
  Exophthalmic Goiter; Parry Disease)   1112
- Hemangioma   1113
- Hemangioma, Capillary   1113
- Hemangioma, Cavernous   1114
- Lacrimal Gland Tumors   1114
- Leukemia   1115
- Lymphoid Hyperplasia (Reactive
  Lymphoid Hyperplasia; Lymphoid
  Tumors; Malignant Lymphoma;
  Pseudolymphoma; Pseudotumor;
  Burkitt Lymphoma; Neoplastic
  Angioendotheliomatosis)   1115
- Meningioma, Optic Nerve Sheath   1116
- Meningioma, Sphenoid Wing   1116
- Neuroblastoma   1117
- Von Recklinghausen Syndrome
  (Neurofibromatosis Type I;
  Neurinomatosis)   1117
- Orbital Lymphoma   1118
- Rhabdomyosarcoma (Corneal Edema)   1118

32. Pupil   **1119**

- Horner Syndrome (Bernard-Horner
  Syndrome; Cervical Sympathetic
  Paralysis Syndrome; Claude-Bernard-
  Horner Syndrome; Horner
  Oculopupillary Syndrome)   1119
- Pupillary Membrane, Persistent   1120

33. Retina   **1121**

- Acute Posterior Multifocal Placoid Pigment
  Epitheliopathy (White Dot Syndrome)   1121
- Acute Retinal Necrosis Syndrome
  (ARN Syndrome; Bilateral Acute
  Retinal Necrosis; Barn Syndrome)   1121
- Albinism (Brown Oculocutaneous Albinism;
  Nettleship Falls Syndrome)   1122
- Best Disease (Best Macular Degeneration;
  Vitelliruptive Macular Dystrophy;
  Polymorphic Macular Degeneration
  of Braley; Vitelliform Dystrophy)   1122
- Birdshot Retinopathy
  (Vitiliginous Chorioretinitis)   1123
- Blackwater Fever   1123
- CAR Syndrome (Cancer-Associated
  Retinopathy Syndrome)   1124
- Ceroid Lipofuscinosis   1124
- Chloroquine/Hydroxychloroquine Toxicity
  (Bull's Eye Maculopathy)   1125
- Choroidoretinal Dystrophy   1125
- Coats Disease (Leber Miliary Aneurysm;
  Retinal Telangiectasia)   1126
- Congenital Hereditary Retinoschisis
  (CHRS; Juvenile X-Linked Retinoschisis)   1126
- Central Serous Chorioretinopathy   1126
- Cytomegalovirus Retinitis   1127
- Diffuse Unilateral Subacute Neuroretinitis
  Syndrome (DUSN; Unilateral Wipeout
  Syndrome; Wipeout Syndrome)   1127
- Eales Disease (Periphlebitis)   1128
- Fleck Retina of Kandori Syndrome
  (Kandori Syndrome)   1128
- Giant Retinal Tears   1128
- Gyrate Atrophy (Ornithine Ketoacid
  Aminotransferase Deficiency)   1129
- Jensen Disease
  (Juxtapapillary Retinopathy)   1129
- Lattice Degeneration and
  Retinal Detachment   1129
- Metaphyseal Chondrodysplasia with
  Retinitis Pigmentosa   1130
- Microcephaly with Chorioretinopathy   1130
- Peripheral Retinal Breaks and
  Degeneration   1130
- Proliferative Vitreoretinopathy (PVR)   1131

- Refsum Syndrome (Heredopathia Atactica Polyneuritiformis Syndrome; Phytanic Acid Oxidase Deficiency; Phytanic Acid Storage Disease; Refsum-Thiebaut Syndrome) 1131
- Retinal Capillaritis 1132
- Retinoblastoma 1132
- Retrolental Fibroplasia (RLF; Retinopathy of Prematurity) 1133
- Diverticulosis of Bowel, Hernia, Retinal Detachment 1133
- Retinal Detachment, Exudative 1134
- Retinal Detachment, Proliferative 1134
- Retinal Detachment, Rhegmatogenous 1134
- Schwartz Syndrome (Retinal Detachment) 1135
- Retinal Detachment, Tractional 1135
- Alstrom Disease (Cataract and Retinitis Pigmentosa) 1136
- Laurence-Moon-Bardet-Biedl Syndrome (Bardet-Biedl Syndrome; Retinitis Pigmentosa-Polydactyly-Adiposogenital Syndrome) 1136
- Usher Syndrome (Hereditary Retinitis Pigmentosa-Deafness Syndrome) Retinitis Pigmentosa 1137
- Hallgren Syndrome (Retinitis Pigmentosa-Deafness-Ataxia Syndrome; Usher Syndrome Type I) 1137
- Retinopathy, Pigmentary, and Mental Retardation (Mirhosseini-Holmes-Walton Syndrome) 1138
- Pallidal Degeneration, Progressive, with Retinitis Pigmentosa (Hypoprebetalipoproteinemia, Acanthocytosis, Retinitis Pigmentosa, and Pallidal Degeneration; HARP Syndrome) 1138
- Spastic Quadriplegia, Retinitis Pigmentosa, Mental Retardation 1139
- Retinoschisis, Acquired [Acquired Retinoschisis (RS)] 1139
- Retinoschisis, Autosomal Dominant 1139
- Retinoschisis, Congenital 1140
- Retinoschisis of Fovea 1140
- Terson Syndrome (Subarachnoid Hemorrhage Syndrome) 1140
- Abdominal Typhus (Enteric Fever; Typhoid Fever) 1141
- Ocular Toxoplasmosis (Toxoplasmic Retinochoroiditis; Toxoplasmosis) 1141
- Oliver-McFarlane Syndrome (Trichomegaly Syndrome) 1142
- Usher Syndrome (Hereditary Retinitis Pigmentosa-Deafness Syndrome) Retinitis Pigmentosa 1142
- Von Hippel-Lindau Syndrome (Retinocerebral Angiomatosis; Angiomatosis Retinae; Cerebelloretinal Hemangioblastomatosis; Lindau Syndrome; Retinal Capillary Hamartoma) Glaucoma 1143
- Wagner Syndrome (Hyaloideoretinal Degeneration; Hereditary Hyaloideoretinal Degeneration and Palatoschisis; Clefting Syndrome; Goldmann-Favre Syndrome; Favre Hyaloideoretinal Degeneration; Retinoschisis with Early Hemeralopia) Nystagmus 1143
- Central or Branch Retinal Artery Occlusion 1144
- Carotid Artery Syndrome (Carotid Vascular Insufficiency Syndrome; Ocular Ischemic Syndrome) 1144
- Diabetes Mellitus 1145
  - Diabetic Retinopathy, Background 1145
  - Diabetic Retinopathy, Proliferative 1146
- Hypertension 1146
- Jensen Disease (Juxtapapillary Retinopathy) 1147
- Macroaneurysm 1147
- Herrick Syndrome (Dresbach Syndrome; Sickle Cell Disease; Drepanocytic Anemia) 1148
- Rendu-Osler Syndrome [Rendu-Osler-Weber Syndrome; Hereditary Hemorrhagic Telangiectasis; Babington Disease; Goldstein Hematemesis; Osler Syndrome (2)] 1148
- Retinal Venous Obstruction 1149

34. Sclera **1150**

- Episcleritis 1150
- Blue Sclera 1150
  - Folling Syndrome (Phenylketonuria; Phenylpyruvic Oligophrenia; Ikiotia Phenylketonuria Syndrome) 1151
  - Hypophosphatasia (Phosphoethanolaminuria) 1152
  - Lowe Syndrome (Oculo-Cerebro-Renal Syndrome) 1152

- De Lange Syndrome (I) (Congenital Muscular Hypertrophy Cerebral Syndrome; Brachmann-De Lange Syndrome)   1153
- Brittle Cornea Syndrome (Brittle Cornea, Blue Sclera and Red Hair Syndrome; Blue Sclera Syndrome)   1153
- Crouzon Syndrome (Dysostosis Craniofacialis; Oxycephaly; Craniofacial Dysostosis; Parrot-Head Syndrome; Möbius-Crouzon Syndrome; Hereditary Craniofacial Dysostosis)   1154
- Hallermann-Streiff Syndrome [Dyscephalic-Mandibulo-Oculo-Facial Syndrome; Oculo-Mandibulo-Dyscephaly; Ullrich-Fremery-Dohna Syndrome; Francois Dyscephalic Syndrome; Mandibulo-Oculo-Facial Dyscephaly Syndrome; Francois-Hallermann-Streiff Syndrome; Hallermann-Streiff-Francois Syndrome; Audrey I Syndrome; Dohna Syndrome; Francois Syndrome (1); Dyscephaly- Teeth Abnormality-Dwarfism; Dyscephalia Oculomandibularis-Hypotrichosis; Mandibulo-Ocular Dyscephalia Hypotrichosis; Fremery-Dohna Syndrome; Oculo-Mandibulo-Facial Dyscephaly]   1154
- Marfan Syndrome (Dolichostenomelia; Arachnodactyly; Hyperchondroplasia; Dystrophia Mesodermalis Congenita)   1155
- Marshall-Smith Syndrome   1156
- Maroteaux-Lamy Syndrome (Systemic Mucopolysaccharidosis Type VI; MPS VI Syndrome; Mucopolysaccharidosis VI)   1156
- Osteogenesis Imperfecta Congenita, Microcephaly and Cataracts   1157
- Paget Disease (Osteitis Deformans; Congenital Hyperphosphatemia; Hyperostosis Corticalis Deformans; Pozzi Syndrome; Chronic Congenital Idiopathic Hyperphosphatemia; Osteochalasis Desmalis Familiaris; Familial Osteoectasia)   1157
- Pierre-Robin Syndrome (Robin Syndrome; Micrognathia-Glossoptosis Syndrome)   1158
- Roberts Pseudothalidomide Syndrome (Glaucoma)   1158
- Werner Syndrome (Progeria of Adults) Blue Sclera   1159

- Turner Syndrome (Turner-Albright Syndrome; Gonadal Dysgenesis; Genital Dwarfism Syndrome; Ullrich-Turner Syndrome; Bonnevie-Ullrich Syndrome; Pterygolymphangiectasia Syndrome; Ullrich-Bonnevie Syndrome) Cataract, Posterior   1159
- Scleral Staphylomas and Dehiscences   1160
- Ehlers-Danlos Syndrome (Fibrodysplasia Elastica Generalisata; Cutis Hyperelastica; Meekeren-Ehlers-Danlos Syndrome; Indian Rubber Man Syndrome; Cutis Laxa)   1160
- Goltz Syndrome (Focal Dermal Hypoplasia Syndrome)   1161
- Bloch-Sulzberger Syndrome (Incontinentia Pigmenti; Siemens-Bloch-Sulzberger Syndrome)   1161
- OTA Syndrome (Nevus of Ota; Oculodermal Melanocytosis; Nevus Fuscoceruleus Ophthalmomaxillaris Syndrome)   1162
- Grönblad-Strandberg Syndrome (Systemic Elastodystrophy; Pseudoxanthoma Elasticum; Elastorrhexis; Darier-Grönblad-Strandberg Syndrome)   1162
- Relapsing Polychondritis (Jaksch-Wartenhost Syndrome; Meyenburg-Altherz-Vehlinger Syndrome; Von Meyenberg II Syndrome)   1163
- Aspergillosis   1163
- Candidiasis   1164
- Cytomegalovirus Retinitis   1164
- Diffuse Unilateral Subacute Neuroretinitis Syndrome (DUSN; Unilateral Wipeout Syndrome; Wipeout Syndrome)   1165
- Histoplasmosis (Histoplasmosis Choroiditis; Histoplasmosis Maculopathy; Presumed Ocular Histoplasmosis Syndrome)   1165
- Propionibacterium Acnes   1166
- Ocular Toxoplasmosis (Toxoplasmic Retinochoroiditis; Toxoplasmosis)   1166
- Behçet Syndrome (Dermato-Stomato-Ophthalmic Syndrome; Oculobuccogenital Syndrome; Gilbert Syndrome)   1167
- Blackwater Fever   1167
- Familial Mediterranean Fever   1168

- Kussmaul Disease (Kussmaul-Maier Disease; Necrotizing Angiitis; PAN; Polyarteritis Nodosa) 1168
- Porphyria Cutanea Tarda 1169
- Relapsing Polychondritis (Jaksch Wartenhost Syndrome; Meyenburg-Altherz-Vehlinger Syndrome; Von Meyenberg II Syndrome) 1169
- Rheumatoid Arthritis (Adult) 1170
- Schaumann Syndrome (Besnier-Boeck-Schaumann Syndrome; Boeck Sarcoid; Sarcoidosis) 1170
- Disseminated Lupus Erythematosus (Systemic Lupus Erythematosus; Lupus Erythematosus; Kaposi-Libman-Sack Syndrome, SLE) 1171
- Takayasu Syndrome (Martorell Syndrome; Aortic Arch Syndrome; Pulseless Disease; Reversed Coarctation Syndrome) 1171
- Temporal Arteritis Syndrome (Cranial Arteritis Syndrome; Giant Cell Arteritis; Hutchinson-Horton-Magath-Brown Syndrome) 1172
- Wegener Syndrome (Wegener Granulomatosis) 1172

35. Vitreous **1173**
- Anterior Vitreous Detachment 1173
- Familial Exudative Vitreoretinopathy 1173
- Vitreous Hemorrhage 1174
- Hydatid Cyst (Echinococcosis) 1174
- Intraocular Foreign Body: Copper 1174
- Intraocular Foreign Body: Nonmagnetic Chemically Inert 1175
- Intraocular Foreign Body: Steel or Iron 1175
- Persistent Fetal Vasculature 1176
- Persistent Hyperplastic Primary Vitreous (PHPV, Persistent Fetal Vasculature) 1176
- Proliferative Vitreoretinopathy (PVR) 1176
- Retinal Vascular Hypoplasia with Persistence of Primary Vitreous 1177
- Vitreous Wick Syndrome 1177

Index *1179*

CHAPTER

1

Infectious Diseases

🗗 1. ACINETOBACTER (MIMA POLYMORPHA; ACINETOBACTER IWOFFI)

General

Gram-negative pleomorphic bacillus *Mima*; generally occurs in patient with lowered resistance.

Ocular

Conjunctivitis and chemosis; corneal ulcer; blepharitis; iris prolapse; endophthalmitis.

Clinical

Meningitis; pneumonitis; endocarditis; urethritis; vaginitis; arthritis; dermatitis; intracranial abscess; subdural empyema.

Laboratory

Culture of the appropriate body fluid that is properly transported, plated, and incubated grows *Acinetobacter baumannii*.

Treatment

An infectious disease specialist should be consulted to differentiate colonization from infection and for antibiotic recommendations.

🗗 BIBLIOGRAPHY

1. Cunha BA. (2011). Acinetobacter. [online] Available from www.emedicine.com/med/TOPIC3456.HTM. [Accessed July, 2013].

🗗 2. ACQUIRED IMMUNODEFICIENCY SYNDROME (AIDS; ACQUIRED CELLULAR IMMUNODEFICIENCY; ACQUIRED IMMUNODEFICIENCY)

General

Acquired breakdown of the immune system followed by disease that takes advantage of the body's collapsed defenses; acquired by shared drug needles or sexual intercourse; occurs most frequently in homosexually active men (75%), intravenous drug abusers (13%), and Haitian immigrants (6%).

Ocular

Retinal cotton-wool spots; cytomegalovirus (CMV) retinitis; retinal periphlebitis; conjunctival Kaposi sarcoma; necrotizing retinitis; retinal hemorrhages; conjunctivitis sicca; orbital Burkitt lymphoma; peripheral retinochoroiditis; vitreitis; fungal corneal ulcer; hypopyon; acute glaucoma; third nerve palsy; anterior uveitis; atypical retinitis; orbital pseudotumor; herpes zoster ophthalmicus; herpes simplex keratitis; bacterial keratitis; molluscum contagiosum; toxoplasma retinitis; acute retinal necrosis; HIV retinitis; syphilitic retinitis; *Pneumocystis carinii* choroiditis; fungal and bacterial endophthalmitis; fungal choroiditis; conjunctival microvasculopathy; keratitis sicca; subconjunctival hemorrhage.

Clinical

Because of lowered immunity, one third develops Kaposi sarcoma; pneumonia caused by *P. carinii*; death.

Laboratory

Enzyme-linked immunosorbent assay (ELISA) test is used. For screening, other tests are used to evaluate false-positive and false-negative test results.

Treatment

Medical consultations are required for systemic treatment. The treatment of CMV retinitis can include drugs such as ganciclovir, valganciclovir, fomivirsen, foscarnet and cidofovir. All of these drugs have specific adverse effects and complicate the decision to use for treatment.

BIBLIOGRAPHY

1. Copeland RA. (2011). Ocular Manifestations of HIV Infection. [online] Available from www.emedicine.com/oph/TOPIC417.HTM. [Accessed July, 2013].
2. Dubin J. (2011). Rapid Testing for HIV. [online] Available from www.emedicine.com/emerg/TOPIC253.HTM. [Accessed July, 2013].

3. ACUTE HEMORRHAGIC CONJUNCTIVITIS (AHC; EPIDEMIC HEMORRHAGIC KERATOCONJUNCTIVITIS, APOLLO 11 DISEASE)

General

First reported in 1969, first epidemic in United States in 1981; enterovirus; explosive onset; usually bilateral; coxsackie virus A24 and enterovirus 70 have been implicated in the most recent outbreaks.

Ocular

Chemosis; follicular conjunctivitis; petechial bulbar hemorrhages; seromucous discharge; keratitis; lacrimation; lid edema; photophobia; preauricular lymphadenopathy.

Clinical

Systemic symptoms are rare, although several cases of lumbosacral radiculomyelitis have occurred late in the course of the disease; polio-like paralysis (associated with enterovirus 70).

Laboratory

Antisera have been used with good results. These are being supplanted by polymerase chain reaction (PCR) methods, which reduce the time needed for viral typing.

Treatment

Very contagious with transmitted eye to hand to eye contact. Self-limited course; generally no treatment is necessary.

BIBLIOGRAPHY

1. Plechaty G. (2011). Acute Hemorrhagic Conjunctivitis. [online] Available from www.emedicine.com/oph/TOPIC492.HTM. [Accessed July, 2013].

4. ASPERGILLOSIS

General

Systemic infection common in poultry farmers, feeders or breeders of pigeons, and persons who work with grains; should be considered in immunocompromised patients.

Ocular

Corneal ulcer; blepharitis; keratitis; scleritis; endophthalmitis; exophthalmos; retinal hemorrhages; retinal detachment; vitreitis; cataract; conjunctivitis; orbital cellulitis; paresis of extraocular muscles; secondary glaucoma; scleromalacia perforans; endogenous endophthalmitis; anterior chamber mass; invasion of choroid and anterior optic nerve.

Clinical

Pulmonary infections; invasive fungal disease.

Laboratory

Culture from superficial scrapings from bed of infection.

Treatment

Voriconazole is the drug of choice. Although disease outcomes substantially improve with antifungal treatment, patient survival and infection resolution depend on improved immunosuppression.

BIBLIOGRAPHY

1. Batra V. (2011). Pediatric Aspergillosis. [online] Available from www.emedicine.com/ped/TOPIC148.HTM. [Accessed July, 2013].

5. BACILLUS SPECIES INFECTIONS

General

Aerobic, Gram-positive spore-forming rods which are the cause of many ocular infections; most common cause of post-traumatic endophthalmitis in rural settings. Most commonly enters the eye as a result of penetrating trauma with a contaminated foreign body but can be related to intravenous drug use. Extremely poor visual outcome is associated with this infection.

Clinical

Fever, leukocytosis.

Ocular

Corneal ring infiltrate, diffuse subepithelial infiltrates, hypopyon, vitritis.

Laboratory

Gram stain reveals a Gram-positive rod.

Treatment

Antibiotic (generally vancomycin) should be given intravitreal, topical and systemic. Due to the aggressive nature of *Bacillus cereus*, a vitreous tap with antibiotic injection alone is not recommended. Pars plana vitrectomy with intravitreal injection of vancomycin is the treatment of choice.

BIBLIOGRAPHY

1. Egan DJ. (2011). Endophthalmitis. [online] Available from www.emedicine.com/emerg/TOPIC880.HTM. [Accessed July, 2013].

⊟ 6. BLASTOMYCOSIS

General

Chronic fungal disease caused by *Blastomyces dermatitidis*.

Ocular

Hypopyon; mycotic keratitis; corneal ulcer; choroidal granuloma; nodules of iris; cicatrization of eyelid; ectropion; descemetocele; panophthalmitis; recurrent papillomatous lesion upper lid; granulomatous conjunctivitis.

Clinical

Granulomatous lesions of skin, lung, bone, or any part of the body.

Laboratory

Periodic acid-Schiff and Gomori methenamine-silver stains.

Treatment

Therapeutic approaches involve the use of oral azoles, primarily itraconazole. Ocular treatment may include surgical draining of the lid in addition to antifungal therapy.

⊟ BIBLIOGRAPHY

1. Steele RW. (2011). Pediatric blastomycosis. [online] Available from www.emedicine.com/ped/TOPIC254.HTM. [Accessed July, 2013].

⊟ 7. BRUCELLOSIS (BANG DISEASE; MALTA FEVER; MEDITERRANEAN FEVER; PIG BREEDER DISEASE; GIBRALTAR FEVER; UNDULANT FEVER)

General

Transmitted to man from animals or animal products containing bacteria of the genus *Brucella*; human infection results from ingestion of infected animal tissue and milk products or through skin wounds directly bathed in freshly killed animal tissues.

Ocular

Conjunctivitis; punctate keratitis; optic neuritis; swollen optic nerves; chorioretinitis; extraocular muscle palsies; phlyctenules; dacryoadenitis; papilledema; episcleritis; macular edema; phthisis bulbi; uveitis; vitreous opacities; changes in intraocular pressure (early decrease or late increase).

Clinical

Fever; icterus; weakness; sweats; general malaise; mammary abscess.

Laboratory

Increasing serum agglutination test.

Treatment

The goal of medical therapy is to prevent complications and relapses. Multidrug antimicrobial regimens are the mainstay of therapy. Ocular treatment includes topical steroids and cycloplegics for uveitis.

⊟ BIBLIOGRAPHY

1. Al-Nassir W. (2011). Brucellosis. [online] Available from www.emedicine.com/med/TOPIC248.HTM. [Accessed July, 2013].

🗗 8. CANDIDIASIS

General

Yeast-like opportunistic fungal infection caused by *Candida albicans*.

Ocular

Uveitis; hypopyon; conjunctivitis; keratitis; corneal ulcer; blepharitis; endophthalmitis; dacryocystitis; papillitis; retinal atrophy; Roth spot; vitreous abscess; retrobulbar abscess; retinal detachment; panophthalmitis; chorioretinitis; infectious crystalline keratopathy.

Clinical

C. albicans normally is present as an intestinal saprophyte in 35–75% of the human population; in situations of internal environmental change, however, *Candida* can become pathogenic (e.g. obesity, diabetes mellitus, malignancy, and other debilitating conditions).

Laboratory

Common yeast from up to 50% of healthy individuals isolate directly from the eye should be attempted to confirm the presence of organism. Blood agar and Sabouraud's dextrose agar may be used; PCR for species identification.

Treatment

Mucocutaneous infection typically responds to topical therapy. Antifungal therapy should be started immediately after necessary cultures have been obtained from all suspected sites of infection. Infectious disease specialists are typically involved in cases of invasive candidiasis.

🗗 BIBLIOGRAPHY

1. Hedayati T. (2012). Candidiasis in Emergency Medicine. [online] Available from www.emedicine.com/emerg/TOPIC76.HTM. [Accessed July, 2013].

🗗 9. CATSCRATCH OCULOGLANDULAR SYNDROME (PARINAUD CONJUNCTIVA-ADENITIS SYNDROME; PARINAUD OCULOGLANDULAR SYNDROME; CATSCRATCH DISEASE; BARTONELLA HENSELAE)

General

Most frequently seen in children; incubation time 7-10 days; caused by small pleomorphic Gram-negative bacillus; good prognosis; affects both sexes; about 90% of patients with this condition have serologic evidence of infection by *Rochalimaea henselae*.

Ocular

Conjunctivitis; retrotarsal conjunctival granulations; formation of granulomata in anterior segment about 3 mm high and 2-6 mm in diameter; inferior fornix usually affected; ulceration common; neuroretinitis; optic neuritis.

Clinical

Tender, red papule at the site of a cat scratch; regional preauricular and cervical lymphadenitis (often only one gland involved); irregular fever for 4–5 days and malaise; fever; parotid gland swelling.

Laboratory

Histopathology of biopsied lymph node of Warthin-Starry silver stain.

Treatment

Symptomatic treatment includes warm compresses, analgesics and antipyretics. Aspiration of lymph node if distention causes pain. Antibiotics may be necessary in severe cases.

🗗 BIBLIOGRAPHY

1. Nervi SJ. (2011). Catscratch Disease. [online]. Available from www.emedicine.com/med/TOPIC304.HTM. [Accessed July, 2013].
2. Chi SL, Stinnett S, Eggenberger E, et al. Clinical characteristics in 53 patients with cat scratch optic neuropathy. Ophthalmology. 2012;119:183–7.

🗗 10. COCCIDIOIDOMYCOSIS (VALLEY FEVER, SAN JOAQUIN FEVER)

General

Caused by fungus *Coccidioides immitis*.

Ocular

Conjunctivitis; choroiditis; uveitis; retinal hemorrhages; vitreal opacity; vitreal floaters; episcleritis; hypopyon; granulomatous lesion of optic nerve head; paralysis of sixth cranial nerve; secondary glaucoma; papilledema; mutton fat keratitic precipitates; necrotizing granulomatous conjunctivitis; iridocyclitis.

Clinical

Mild respiratory illness; cavity lung lesion.

Laboratory

Routine culture media, IgM antibody of acute, IgG antibody for present or past infection.

Treatment

Systemic fluconazole or amphotericin B is the treatment of choice. Ocular treatment includes topical amphotericin B and use of steroids sparingly.

🗗 BIBLIOGRAPHY

1. Hospenthal DR. (2011) Coccidioidomycosis. [online] Available from www.emedicine.com/ped/TOPIC423.HTM. [Accessed July, 2013].

🗗 11. DEERFLY FEVER (FRANCIS DISEASE; RABBIT FEVER; TULAREMIA; DEERFLY TULAREMIA)

General

Acute infectious disease caused by *Francisella (Pasteurella) tularensis*.

Ocular

Chemosis; conjunctivitis; corneal ulcer; endophthalmitis; dacryocystitis; optic atrophy; iris prolapse; chalazion; corneal opacity; pannus.

Clinical

Local ulcerative lesion; suppuration of regional lymph nodes; fever; prostration; myalgia; severe headache; pneumonia.

Laboratory

Diagnosis is usually based on serology results. Tularemia tube agglutination testing is the most commonly used serological test.

Treatment

Systemic antibiotics

🗗 BIBLIOGRAPHY

1. Cleveland KO, Gelfand M, Raugi GJ. (2013). Tularemia. [online]. Available from www.emedicine.com/med/TOPIC2326.HTM. [Accessed July, 2013].

🗗 12. DENGUE FEVER

General

Endemic over the tropics and subtropics; caused by four distinct serogroups of dengue viruses: types 1, 2, 3 and 4, group B arboviruses; transmitted solely by mosquitoes of the genus *Aedes*.

Ocular

Lid edema; conjunctivitis; ocular and retrobulbar pain accentuated by ocular movement; dacryoadenitis; keratitis; corneal ulcer; iritis; retinal or vitreous hemorrhages; ocular motor paresis; optic atrophy.

Clinical

Hemorrhagic fever, severe headache; backache; joint pain; rigors; insomnia; anorexia; loss of taste; epistaxis; rashes; maculopapular rash; myalgia; human infection with of four serotypes of dengue virus causing two diseases: classic dengue fever and dengue hemorrhagic fever (50% mortality).

Laboratory

Basic metabolic panel, liver function test, coagulation studies, chest X-ray, serial ultrasonography.

Treatment

A self-limited illness, and only supportive care is required. Acetaminophen may be used to treat patients with symptomatic fever. Dengue hemorrhagic fever warrant closer observation. Rehydration with intravenous fluids, plasma expander, transfusion and shock therapy may be necessary.

BIBLIOGRAPHY

1. Shepherd SM, Hinfey PB, Shoff WH. (2013). Dengue. [online] Available from www.emedicine.com/med/TOPIC528.HTM. [Accessed July, 2013].

13. DERMATOPHYTOSIS (EPIDERMOPHYTOSIS; EPIDERMOMYCOSIS; RUBROPHYTIA; TINEA; TRICHOPHYTOSIS)

General

Superficial infection of the skin; ringworm fungi; most frequently seen in children during hot, humid weather.

Ocular

Conjunctivitis; corneal ulcer; madarosis; scaly rash; folliculitis; blepharitis; lid edema.

Clinical

Scalp, facial, and lid ringworm lesions.

Laboratory

Rapid identification on PCR. Septate hyphae branches on 20% potassium hydroxide stain.

Treatment

Topical treatment involves antifungal cream. Systemic treatment involves use of ketoconazole for 2–4 weeks.

BIBLIOGRAPHY

1. Kao GF. (2011). Tinea Capitis. [online] Available from www.emedicine.com/derm/TOPIC420.HTM. [Accessed July, 2013].

14. DIPHTHERIA

General

Acute infectious disease caused by *Corynebacterium diphtheriae*; severity is dependent upon the amount of exotoxin absorbed prior to initiation of specific therapy.

Ocular

Conjunctivitis; xerophthalmia; keratitis; corneal ulcer; blepharitis; cellulitis of lid; meibomianitis; ptosis; dacryocystitis; cataract; central retinal artery occlusion; optic neuritis; accommodative spasm or paralysis; convergence paralysis; divergence paralysis; paralysis of third, fourth, or sixth nerve; paralysis of accommodation (in children); ocular motor nerve paresis; choroiditis; cranial neuropathies involving the trigeminal, vagus, and hypoglossal cranial nerves; myocarditis.

Clinical

Local inflammatory lesion, with effect on heart, kidneys, and nervous system.

Laboratory

Gram-positive rods commonly affect children younger than 10 years.

Treatment

Systemic treatment involves use of diphtheria antitoxin and antibiotics. Ocular treatment includes diphtheria antitoxin and high titer y-globulin preparation. Topical penicillin-G ointment helps to eradicate the bacilli.

BIBLIOGRAPHY

1. Demirci CS. (2011). Pediatric Diphtheria. [online] Available from www.emedicine.com/ped/TOPIC596.HTM. [Accessed July, 2013].

15. EPIDEMIC KERATOCONJUNCTIVITIS

General

Highly communicable; adenovirus types 8 and 19; usually bilateral; epidemic keratoconjunctivitis has been reported worldwide associated with 11 virus serotypes, with serotypes 8, 11, and 19 being the most common responsible ones.

Ocular

Follicular or membranous conjunctivitis; chemosis; subconjunctival hemorrhages; corneal opacity; punctate epithelial keratitis; corneal ulcer; blepharospasm; lid edema; serous discharge; uveitis; epiphora.

Clinical

Submaxillary and cervical lymphadenopathy.

Laboratory

Viral isolation on cell culture from conjunctival scrapings.

Treatment

No effective topical or systemic treatment available. Topical steroids may be used if epithelial keratitis occurs.

BIBLIOGRAPHY

1. Bawazeer A. (2011). Epidemic Keratoconjunctivitis. [online] Available from www.emedicine.com/oph/TOPIC677.HTM. [Accessed July, 2013].

16. ERYSIPELAS (SAINT ANTHONY FIRE)

General

Acute localized inflammation of the skin and subcutaneous tissue; erysipelas is a febrile infection of the skin and subcutaneous tissue, most commonly caused by *Streptococcus*, characterized by the acute onset of a red, indurated expanding plaque that nearly disappears with the use of antibiotics; sometimes caused by *Staphylococcus*.

Ocular

Conjunctivitis; blepharitis; elephantiasis and gangrene of lid; ptosis; dacryocystitis; cellulitis of orbit; keratitis; panophthalmitis; uveitis; eyelid involvement.

Clinical

Edema; fever; rigor; vesicles; tenderness; headache; vomiting; localized pain.

Laboratory

Blood cultures, needle aspirates or biopsy yields less than 10% positive cultures; direct immunofluorescence is useful to detect *Streptococcus* in skin specimens.

Treatment

Systemic treatment is penicillin G. Ocular treatment is to clean and debridement of wound and use of a broad-spectrum antibiotic ointment.

BIBLIOGRAPHY

1. Binford RT, Lindo SD. Dermatologic conditions affecting the eye. In: Dunlap EA (Ed). Gordon's Medical Management of Ocular Disease, 2nd edition. New York: Harper & Row; 1976. pp. 91–110.
2. Bratton RL, Nesse RE. St. Anthony's fire: diagnosis and management of erysipelas. Am Fam Physician. 1995;51:401–4.
3. Duane TD. Clinical Ophthalmology. Philadelphia: JB Lippincott; 1987.
4. Roy FH, Fraunfelder FH, Fraunfelder FT. Roy and Fraunfelders's Current Ocular Therapy, 6th edition. Philadelphia: WB Saunders; 2008.
5. McHugh D, Fison PN. Ocular erysipelas. Arch Ophthalmol. 1992;110:1315.

17. ESCHERICHIA COLI

General

Gram-negative rod found in the gastrointestinal tract; urinary tract is the usual portal of entry.

Ocular

Uveitis; hyphema; hypopyon; gas bubbles in anterior chamber; purulent conjunctivitis; keratitis; corneal edema; panophthalmitis; endophthalmitis; glaucoma.

Clinical

Diarrhea; gastroenteritis; dehydration.

Laboratory

Anaerobic Gram-negative rod.

Treatment

Antibiotic therapy should start with ampicillin until sensitivity reports return.

BIBLIOGRAPHY

1. Suh DW. (2011). Ophthalmologic Manifestations of Escherichia Coli. [online] Available from www.emedicine.com/oph/TOPIC496.HTM. [Accessed July, 2013].

18. GONORRHEA

General

Caused by *Neisseria gonorrhoeae*, which is transmitted sexually.

Ocular

Conjunctivitis; eyelid edema; keratitis; uveitis.

Clinical

Pelvic inflammatory disease; arthritis; dermatitis; carditis; meningitis.

Laboratory

Gram stain smear demonstrates Gram-negative diplococci with polymorphonuclear leukocytes in conjunctival exudates.

Treatment

Therapy consists of systemic antibiotics; topical antibiotics are relatively ineffective in the treatment of eye disease. It is important to treat all sexual partners simultaneously to prevent reinfection.

BIBLIOGRAPHY

1. Wong B. (2012). Gonorrhea. [online] Available from www.emedicine.com/oph/TOPIC497.HTM. [Accessed July, 2013].

🗗 19. HAEMOPHILUS AEGYPTIUS (KOCH-WEEKS BACILLUS)

General

Caused by Gram-negative Koch-Weeks bacillus in warm climate regions; characterized by a 24- to 48-hour incubation period; now classified as *Haemophilus influenzae* biotype III; *H. influenzae* is divided into biotypes based on biochemical reactions (indole production, urease activity, ornithine decarboxylase activity) and into serotypes based on their capsular polysaccharides; common cause of purulent conjunctivitis and preseptal cellulitis in children.

Ocular

Conjunctivitis; corneal opacity; corneal ulcer; phlyctenular keratoconjunctivitis; keratitis; cellulitis oflid; pseudoptosis; uveitis; petechial subconjunctival hemorrhages.

Clinical

Coryza; systemic symptoms are rare.

Laboratory

Poorly staining Gram-negative bacilli or coccobacilli. Culture on chocolate agar.

Treatment

Antibiotics are the mainstay of treatment. Invasive and serious infections are best treated with an intravenous third-generation cephalosporin until antibiotic sensitivities are available.

🗗 BIBLIOGRAPHY

1. Devarajan VR. (2012) Haemophilus Influenzae Infections. [online]. Available from. www.emedicine.com/med/TOPIC936.HTM. [Accessed July, 2013].

🗗 20. HAEMOPHILUS INFLUENZAE

General

Gram-negative rod.

Ocular

Conjunctivitis; cellulitis; tenonitis; uveitis; vitreous opacity; pannus; corneal opacity.

Clinical

Pharyngitis; epiglottitis; laryngotracheitis; pneumonia; bronchitis; otitis media; meningitis; cellulitis; septic arthritis; sinusitis.

Laboratory

Gram-negative coccobacillus with eight biotypes and six serotypes. Gram stain and culture.

Treatment

Antibiotics are the mainstay of treatment. Invasive and serious infections are best treated with an intravenous third-generation cephalosporin until antibiotic sensitivities are available.

🗗 BIBLIOGRAPHY

1. Devarajan VR. (2012). Haemophilus Influenzae Infections. [online] Available from www.emedicine.com/med/TOPIC936.HTM. [Accessed July, 2013].

🗗 21. HANSEN DISEASE (LEPROSY)

General

Communicable disease caused by *Mycobacterium leprae*.

Ocular

Keratitis; leukoma; pannus; corneal ulcer; uveitis; iris atrophy; dacryocystitis; anisocoria; multiple pupils; decreased or absent pupillary reaction to light; paralysis of seventh nerve; episcleritis; blepharospasm; lagophthalmos; madarosis; secondary glaucoma; decreased intraocular pressure; subconjunctival fibrosis; punctate epithelial keratopathy; posterior subcapsular cataract; corneal hypesthesia; prominent corneal nerves; iridocyclitis; foveal avascular keratitis; scleritis; interstitial keratitis; iris pearls; dry eye.

Clinical

Disease affects primarily the skin, mucous membrane, and peripheral nerves.

Laboratory

Skin biopsy specimens contain vacuolated macrophages, few lymphocytes, and numerous acid-fast bacilli often in clumps or globi.

Treatment

The World Health Organization (WHO) recommends multiple drug therapy (MDT) for all forms of leprosy. MDT 14 consists of rifampin, ofloxacin, and minocycline.

BIBLIOGRAPHY

1. Kim EC. (2011) Ocular Manifestations of Leprosy. [online] Available from www.emedicine.com/oph/TOPIC743.HTM. [Accessed July, 2013].

22. HERPES SIMPLEX

General

Large, complex deoxyribonucleic acid (DNA) virus.

Ocular

Conjunctivitis; keratitis; iridocyclitis; corneal ulcer; uveitis; hyphema; hypopyon; iris atrophy; cataract; scleritis; dacryoadenitis; blepharitis; acute retinal necrosis.

Clinical

Recurrent skin vesicles on lids, perioral area, nose and genitalia; meningitis, encephalitis.

Laboratory

Viral cultures.

Treatment

Antiviral therapy, topical or oral, is an effective treatment of epithelial herpes infection.

BIBLIOGRAPHY

1. Shaohui L, Pavan-Langston D, Colby KA. Pediatric herpes simplex of the anterior segment: characteristics, treatment, and outcomes. Ophthalmology. 2012;119:2003–8.
2. Wang JC. (2010). Ophthalmologic Manifestations of Herpes Simplex Keratitis. [online] Available from www.emedicine.com/oph/TOPIC100.HTM. [Accessed July, 2013].

23. HERPES SIMPLEX MASQUERADE SYNDROME

General

Acanthamoeba keratitis occurs in those who wear soft contact lenses daily; confused with herpes simplex; Acanthamoeba culbertsoni, Acanthamoeba castellanii and Acanthamoeba polyphaga are causative agents; agents found in distilled water, hot tubs, and swimming pools (*see* Acanthamoeba).

Ocular

Keratitis; corneal ulcer; corneal cysts; stromal infiltrates and necrosis; scleritis; uveitis; epiphora; pseudodendrites.

Clinical

None.

Laboratory

Corneal smears and cultures.

Treatment

Antibiotics are used to treat the ulcer, lubrication, oral tetracycline, proper wear of contact lens.

BIBLIOGRAPHY

1. Hoft RH, Mondino BJ. The diagnosis and clinical management of acanthamoeba keratitis. Semin Ophthalmol. 1991;6:106.
2. Johns KJ, O'Day DM, Head WS, et al. Herpes simplex masquerade syndrome: acanthamoeba keratitis. Curr Eye Res. 1987;6:207-212.
3. Moore MB, McCulley JP, Luckenbach M, et al. Acanthamoeba keratitis associated with soft contact lenses. Am J Ophthalmol. 1985;100:396-403.
4. Samples JR, Binder PS, Luibel FJ, et al. Acanthamoeba keratitis possibly acquired from a hot tub. Arch Ophthalmol. 1984;102:707-10.
5. Wilhelmus KR. Parasitic keratitis and conjunctivitis. In: Smolin G, Thoft RA (Eds). The Cornea, 3rd edition. Boston: Little, Brown and Company; 1994. pp. 262-6.

24. INCLUSION CONJUNCTIVITIS (CHLAMYDIA; PARATRACHOMA)

General

Organism that infects the epithelium of mucoid surfaces; sexually transmitted; major cause of non-gonococcal urethritis in men and cervicitis in women; major cause of neonatal ophthalmia; *Chlamydia trachomatis* is an intracellular bacterium lacking respiratory enzymes that has an affinity for mucosal epithelium; serotypes A through C have been epidemiologically associated with trachoma; serotypes E through K have been associated with genital infection and keratoconjunctivitis in sexually active adults and neonates; other serotypes have been associated with lymphogranuloma venereum and Reiter syndrome.

Ocular

Follicular conjunctivitis; corneal opacities; keratitis; corneal ulcer; lid edema; uveitis.

Clinical

Pneumonia; gastrointestinal disturbances; genital discharge.

Laboratory

Giemsa stain, cell culture—time intensive, direct fluorescent monoclonal antibiotics to stain smears.

Treatment

Three to six weeks of oral tetracycline (500 mg qid), oral doxycycline (100 mg bid), or oral erythromycin stearate (500 mg qid). Simultaneous treatment of all sexual partners is important to prevent reinfection.

BIBLIOGRAPHY

1. Bashour M. (2012). Ophthalmologic Manifestations of Chlamydia. [online] Available from www.emedicine.com/oph/TOPIC494.HTM. [Accessed July, 2013].

25. INFECTIOUS MONONUCLEOSIS (MONONUCLEOSIS; EPSTEIN-BARR VIRUS, ACUTE; ACUTE EPSTEIN-BARR VIRUS, GLANDULAR FEVER)

General

Asymptomatic in childhood; manifested in late adolescence of early adulthood; associated with Burkitt lymphoma and nasopharyngeal carcinoma.

Ocular

Conjunctivitis; ptosis; hippus; dacryocystitis; episcleritis; hemianopsia; nystagmus; retinal and subconjunctival hemorrhages; optic neuritis; orbital edema; scotoma; paralysis of extraocular muscles; uveitis; peripheral choroiditis; keratitis; papilledema; scleritis; retrobulbar neuritis, Sjögren syndrome; retinitis, choroiditis.

Clinical

Fever; widespread lymphadenopathy; pharyngitis; hepatic involvement; presence of atypical lymphocytes and heterophile antibodies in the blood; fatigue.

Treatment

A self-limited illness that does not usually require specific therapy. Splenic rupture is an acute abdominal emergency that usually requires surgical intervention.

BIBLIOGRAPHY

1. Cunha BA. (2011). Infectious Mononucleosis. [online]. Available from www.emedicine.com/med/TOPIC1499. HTM. [Accessed July, 2013].

26. INFLUENZA

General

Acute respiratory infection of specific viral etiology which includes H1N1.

Ocular

Conjunctivitis; subconjunctival hemorrhages; keratitis; tenonitis; ptosis; cellulitis of orbit and lid; dacryocystitis; retinal hemorrhage; cataract; episcleritis; hypopyon; optic neuritis; uveitis; panophthalmitis; vitreal hemorrhage; paralysis of third or fourth nerve; uveitis following vaccination for influenza.

Clinical

Headache; fever; malaise; muscular aching; substernal soreness; nasal stuffiness; nausea.

Laboratory

The criterion standard for diagnosing influenza A and B is a viral culture of nasal-pharyngeal samples, throat samples, or both.

Treatment

Prevention is the most effective therapy. Two new drugs have been marketed recently for treatment of influenza A and B. These are the neuraminidase inhibitors, oseltamivir and zanamivir.

BIBLIOGRAPHY

1. Derlet RW. (2012). Influenza. [online] Available from www.emedicine.com/med/TOPIC1170.HTM. [Accessed July, 2013].

27. LEPTOSPIROSIS (WEIL DISEASE)

General

Acute severe infection caused by *Leptospira* transmitted by ingestion of food contaminated by the reservoir bacterium.

Ocular

Acute conjunctivitis; episcleritis; fibrinous iridocyclitis with vitreal haze; hypopyon; keratitis; pain on ocular movement; uveitis; optic neuritis; cataract; hemorrhagic retinitis; ptosis.

Clinical

Jaundice; fever; headaches; chills; vomiting; anemia; psychologic disturbances.

Laboratory

Complete blood count (CBC), urinalysis and isolation of organism in blood, urine or cerebrospinal fluid.

Treatment

Intravenous penicillin G for a week. Ceftriaxone can also be used.

BIBLIOGRAPHY

1. Hickey PW. (2012). Pediatric Leptospirosis. [online] Available from www.emedicine.com/ped/TOPIC1298.HTM. [Accessed July, 2013].

28. LYME DISEASE

General

Caused by tick bite; symptoms resolve after treatment.

Ocular

Keratitis may occur up to 5 years after the first episode; diplopia; photophobia; ischemic optic neuropathy; iritis; panophthalmitis; conjunctivitis; exudative retinal detachment; choroiditis; vitreitis; multiple cranial nerve palsies; association with acute, posterior, multifocal, placoid, pigment epitheliopathy; branch retinal artery occlusion.

Clinical

Arthritis; increased intracranial pressure; effusion of knees; swelling of wrists.

Laboratory

Immunofluorescent assay (IFA) and ELISA.

Treatment

Oral antibiotics for 2–3 weeks: tetracycline 500 mg four times a day, doxycycline 100 mg two times a day, phenoxymethyl penicillin 500 mg four times a day, or amoxicillin 500 mg three to four times a day.

BIBLIOGRAPHY

1. Zaidman GW. (2011). Ophthalmic Aspects of Lyme Disease Overview of Lyme Disease. [online] Available from www.emedicine.com/oph/TOPIC262.HTM. [Accessed July, 2013].

29. MARSEILLES FEVER (BOUTONNEUSE FEVER)

General

Caused by *Rickettsia conorii* and transmitted by ticks.

Ocular

Conjunctivitis; central serous retinopathy; retinal detachment; perivasculitis; uveitis; papillitis; keratitis.

Clinical

Fever; lymph node enlargement; papular rash.

Laboratory

Serology is usually a confirmatory method; however, these tests are useful only after an acute infection. Culture of the organism may be used for diagnosis early in the course of the disease.

Treatment

Tetracyclines with chloramphenicol and quinolones may be considered first-line antibiotics. Patients with the benign form are usually treated with antibiotics for 7 days. Patients with the malignant form are usually treated with antibiotics for 2 weeks.

BIBLIOGRAPHY

1. Zalewska A, Schwartz RA. (2011). Boutonneuse Fever. [online] Available from www.emedicine.com/derm/TOPIC759.HTM. [Accessed July, 2013].

30. MICROSPORIDIAL INFECTION

General

Obligate intracellular, spore-forming, mitochondrial-lacking eukaryotic protozoan parasites.

Clinical

None.

Ocular

Photophobia, blepharospasm, nonspecific or papillary conjunctival hyperemia.

Laboratory

Gram stain smear show Gram-positive, void spores in the cytoplasm of epithelial cells.

Treatment

Topical fumagillin which can be prepared from fumagillin bicylohexylammonium salt (Fumadil B).

⊟ BIBLIOGRAPHY

1. Roy FH, Fraunfelder FW, Fraunfelder FT. Roy and Fraunfelder's Current Ocular Therapy, 6th edition. London: Elsevier; 2008.

⊟ 31. MOLLUSCUM CONTAGIOSUM

General

Etiologic agent of this disease is a poxvirus that can cause proliferative skin lesions anywhere on the body; commonly found in patients who are immunosuppressed.

Ocular

Lesions of lid, lid margin, conjunctiva, and cornea; conjunctivitis; keratitis; corneal ulcer.

Clinical

Well-defined, pearly appearing papules with umbilicated centers of varying size (3–10 mm); eczematization of the surrounding skin.

Laboratory

Craters have epithelial cells with large eosinophilic intra-cytoplasmic inclusion bodies (molluscum or Henderson Patterson bodies) when virus particles migrate to the granular layer of the epidermis, the inclusion bodies become basophilic.

Treatment

Topical agents cantharidin, tretinoin, podophllin, trichloroacetic acid, tincture of iodine, silver nitrate or phenol, potassium hydroxide. Systemic agents include griseofulvin, methisazone and cimetidine.

⊟ BIBLIOGRAPHY

1. Bhatia AC. (2012). Molluscum Contagiosum. [online] Available from www.emedicine.com/oph/TOPIC500.HTM. [Accessed July, 2013].

⊟ 32. MORAXELLA LACUNATA

General

Gram-negative rod; causes chronic angular blepharoconjunctivitis; without treatment, may persist for months or years; normally found in flora of respiratory tract; seen more frequently in alcoholics and those with poor sanitary habits; *Moraxella* organisms produce proteases, although those are not related directly to their pathogenetic mechanism.

Ocular

Catarrhal angular conjunctivitis; corneal ulcer; hypopyon, chronic blepharitis; eczema; lateral canthal skin erythema; iridocyclitis.

Clinical

Alcoholism; impaired nutrition; dermatitis.

Laboratory

Aerobic, oxidasc positive, Gram-negative diplococcus or coccobacilli morphologically indistinguishable from *Neisseria*.

Treatment

Artificial tears, cold compresses, antibiotics.

⊟ BIBLIOGRAPHY

1. Baum J, Fedukowicz HB, Jordan A. A survey of Moraxella corneal ulcers in a derelict population. Am J Ophthalmol. 1980;90:476–80.
2. Burd EM. Bacterial keratitis and conjunctivitis. In: Smolin G, Thoft RA (Eds). The Cornea. Boston: Little, Brown and Company; 1994. pp. 20–1.
3. Roy FH, Fraunfelder FW. Current Ocular Therapy, 6th edition. Philadelphia: WB Saunders; 2008.
4. van Bijsterveld OP. The incidence of Moraxella on mucous membranes and the skin. Am J Ophthalmol. 1972;74:72–6.

🗗 33. MUCORMYCOSIS (PHYCOMYCOSIS)

General

Acute, often fatal infection caused by saprophytic fungi; associated with diabetes mellitus and ketoacidosis.

Ocular

Corneal ulcer; striate keratopathy; ptosis; panophthalmitis; proptosis; cellulitis of orbit; immobile pupil; retinitis; optic neuritis; paralysis of extraocular muscles; central retinal artery thrombosis.

Clinical

Epistaxis; nasal discharge; facial pain; facial palsies; anhidrosis; cranial nerve or peripheral motor and sensory nerve deficits may occur.

Laboratory

Tissue biopsy and culture of paranasal sinuses demonstrate the presence of the fungi, which appear as broad, irregular, nonseptate, branching hyphae on Hematoxylin and Eosin (H & E) stain.

Treatment

Amphotericin B.

🗗 BIBLIOGRAPHY

1. Crum-Cianflone NF. (2011). Mucormycosis. [online] Available from www.emedicine.com/oph/TOPIC225.HTM. [Accessed July, 2013].

🗗 34. MUMPS

General

Viral infection.

Ocular

Conjunctivitis; keratitis; corneal ulcer; tenonitis; exophthalmos; microphthalmos; optic atrophy; optic neuritis; papillitis; scleritis; uveitis; cortical blindness; congenital punctal occlusion; paralysis of extraocular muscles; dacryoadenitis; iritis; paralysis of accommodation; internal and external ophthalmoparesis.

Clinical

Affects the parotid glands, but infection of other glandular tissue occurs, including the lacrimal gland and testicles; encephalitis; meningitis.

Laboratory

Mumps virus by acute serologic studies.

Treatment

Generous hydration and alimentation, analgesics for headaches. No antiviral agent is available.

🗗 BIBLIOGRAPHY

1. Defendi GL. (2012). Mumps. [online] Available from www.emedicine.com/ped/TOPIC1503.HTM. [Accessed July, 2013].

🗗 35. NEWCASTLE DISEASE (FOWLPOX)

General

Acquired directly by people handling chickens (*see* Parinaud Oculoglandular Syndrome); self-limiting conjunctivitis caused by a paramyxovirus.

Ocular

Acute follicular conjunctivitis, unilateral; keratitic precipitates; lid edema; decreased accommodation and visual acuity.

Clinical

Fatigue; fever; headache; pulmonary complications; preauricular lymphadenopathy.

Laboratory/conjunctivitis

Diagnosis is made by clinical findings.

Treatment

Topical antibiotics, cold compresses, artificial tears.

🗗 BIBLIOGRAPHY

1. Gordon S. Viral keratitis and conjunctivitis. Adenovirus and other nonherpetic viral diseases. In: Smolin G, Thoft RA (Eds). The Cornea. Boston: Little, Brown and Company; 1994.
2. Pau H. Differential diagnosis of eye diseases. New York: Thieme; 1987.
3. Roy FH, Fraunfelder FW, Fraunfelder FT. Roy and Fraunfelder's Current Ocular Therapy, 6th edition. London: Elsevier; 2008.

🗗 36. NOCARDIOSIS

General

Aerobic Actinomycetaceae that may cause a chronic suppurative process; aerobic Gram-positive filamentous bacteria with branching pattern which resemble fungi.

Ocular

Conjunctivitis; keratitis; corneal ulcer; uveitis; lid involvement; orbital cellulitis; endophthalmitis; glaucoma; external ophthalmoplegia; scleritis; canaliculitis; preseptal cellulitis.

Clinical

Granuloma; draining sinuses; brain abscess; meningitis.

Laboratory

Gram-positive filamentous structures with an intermittent or a beaded staining pattern, weakly acid-fast. Organism culture from the infection (i.e. respiratory secretion, skin biopsies, or aspirates from abscesses).

Treatment

Antimicrobial therapy is the treatment of choice.

🗗 BIBLIOGRAPHY

1. DeCroos FC, Garg P, Reddy AK, et al. Optimizing diagnosis and management of nocardia keratitis, scleritis, and endophthalmitis: 11 year microbial and clinical overview. Ophthalmology. 2011;118:1193–200.
2. Greenfield RA. (2011). Nocardiosis. [online] Available from www.emedicine.com/med/TOPIC1644.HTM. [Accessed July, 2013].

🗗 37. PAPPATACI FEVER (PHLEBOTOMUS FEVER; SANDFLY FEVER)

General

Viral etiology; transmitted by the sandfly *Phlebotomus papatasii.*

Ocular

Pick sign of conjunctiva (conjunctival injection limited to the exposed portion of the conjunctiva); uveitis; optic neuritis; papilledema; papillitis; blepharospasm; retinal venous engorgement; vitreal exudates.

Clinical

Fever; headaches; myalgia; pain; stiffness of the neck and back.

Laboratory

Parasite can be detected through direct evidence from peripheral blood, bone marrow, or splenic aspirates.

Treatment

Sodium stibogluconate, a pentavalent antimonial compound (SbV), is the drug of choice.

🗗 BIBLIOGRAPHY

1. Vidyashankar C, Agrawal R. (2011). Pediatric Leishmaniasis. [online] Available from www.emedicine.com/ped/TOPIC1292.HTM. [Accessed July, 2013].

38. PHARYNGOCONJUNCTIVAL FEVER (ACUTE FOLLICULAR CONJUNCTIVITIS; ADENOVIRAL CONJUNCTIVITIS; SYNDROME OF BEAL)

General

Infectious disease produced by adenovirus; serotypes 3, 4, 7, 8, 19, 37, and several others may cause acute conjunctivitis with or without upper respiratory tract involvement; epidemic keratoconjunctivitis has been reported worldwide associated with 11 virus serotypes, with serotypes 8, 11, and 19 being the most commonly responsible.

Ocular

Conjunctivitis; chemosis; keratitis; blepharitis; blepharospasm.

Clinical

Fever; pharyngitis; lymph node enlargement; malaise; myalgia; headache; diarrhea.

Laboratory

Laboratory tests generally are not useful. Cell cultures from infected areas and adenoviral antibody titer allows for precise identification of serotype.

Treatment

Symptomatic control may include cold compresses, artificial tears; nonsteroidal and occasionally steroidal drops to relieve itching.

BIBLIOGRAPHY

1. Scott IU. (2012). Pharyngoconjunctival Fever. [online] Available from www.emedicine.com/oph/TOPIC501.HTM. [Accessed July, 2013].

39. PNEUMOCOCCAL INFECTIONS (STREPTOCOCCUS PNEUMONIAE INFECTIONS)

General

Gram-positive diplococcus *Streptococcus pneumoniae*; some strains are encapsulated while others are not; ocular infections usually are caused by the encapsulated strains; conjunctivitis and corneal scarring produced in an animal model have been attributed to a hemolytic cytolytic exopeptidase.

Ocular

Hypopyon; conjunctivitis; keratitis; corneal ulcer; endophthalmitis; dacryocystitis; uveitis; orbital cellulitis; secondary glaucoma; ophthalmia neonatorum.

Clinical

Upper respiratory infection; chills; sharp pain in hemithorax; cough with sputum production; fever; headache; gastrointestinal symptoms.

Laboratory

Gram stain demonstrates Gram-positive cocci in pairs. The unattached end of each cocci is slightly pointed outward.

Treatment

Impetigo, oral antibiotics and topical antibiotic ointment; preseptal cellulitis, oral antibiotics; orbital celluliti, need team of infectious diseases, otolaryngology and ophthalmology to develop plan of therapy; dacryocystitis, oral and topical antibiotics, dacryocystorhinostomy may be necessary; conjunctivitis, topical antibiotic; keratitis, topical antibiotics; poststreptococcal reactive arthritis can occur with uveitis, topical steroids and cycloplegics; endophthalmitis, prompt and aggressive therapy with topical, intravitreal and sometimes systemic antibiotics and pars plana vitrectomy; post-refractive surgery keratitis, flap raised, cultured and treated. Occasionally the flap should be amputated.

BIBLIOGRAPHY

1. Muench DF. (2012). Pneumococcal Infections. [online] Available from www.emedicine.com/med/TOPIC1848.HTM. [Accessed July, 2013].

⊟ 40. PRESUMED OCULAR HISTOPLASMOSIS (HISTOPLASMOSIS CHOROIDITIS; HISTOPLASMOSIS MACULOPATHY; HISTOPLASMOSIS SYNDROME)

General

Fungal infection caused by *Histoplasma capsulatum.*

Ocular

Circumpapillary atrophy; maculopathy; scattered yellow "histo" spots; optic disk edema; disseminated choroiditis (immunocompromised patients); vitreous hemorrhage; punched-out chorioretinal lesions; choroidal neovascular membrane; exogenous endophthalmitis (isolated report).

Clinical

Pulmonary infection; fever; malaise.

Laboratory

Sixty percent of the adult population from the Ohio and Mississippi river valleys have a positive histoplasmin skin test; therefore clinic course is most helpful.

Treatment

Although the diagnosis is clinical, certain ancillary tests help in confirming it. Fluorescein angiography, human leukocyte antigen (HLA) typing B7 and DRw2 may be indicated.

⊟ BIBLIOGRAPHY

1. Wu L. (2012). Presumed Ocular Histoplasmosis Syndrome. [online] Available from www.emedicine.com/oph/TOP-IC406.HTM. [Accessed July, 2013].

⊟ 41. PROPIONIBACTERIUM ACNES

General

Gram-positive, pleomorphic, non-spore forming bacillus that is considered part of the normal eyelid and conjunctival anaerobic flora. Pathogenic if introduced intraocular.

Clinical

None

Ocular

Chronic keratitis, endophthalmitis, vitritis.

Laboratory

Aerobic and anaerobic cultures must be incubated for 14 days. Capsular biopsy may demonstrate Gram-positive, pleomorphic, non-spore forming bacillus or Gram stain.

Treatment

Vancomycin, intravitreal or systemic

⊟ BIBLIOGRAPHY

1. Roy FH, Fraunfelder FW, Fraunfelder FT. Roy and Fraunfelder's Current Ocular Therapy, 6th edition. London: Elsevier; 2008.

⊟ 42. PROTEUS INFECTIONS

General

Gram-negative bacilli found in water, soil and decaying organic substances.

Ocular

Conjunctivitis; keratitis; corneal ulcers; endophthalmitis; panophthalmitis; dacryocystitis; gangrene of eyelid; uveitis; hypopyon; paralysis of seventh nerve.

Clinical

Cutaneous infection after surgery; usually occurs as a secondary infection of the skin, ears, mastoid sinuses, eyes, peritoneal cavity, bone, urinary tract, meninges, lung, or bloodstream; meningitis; intracranial subdural and epidural empyema; brain abscess; intracranial septic thrombophlebitis affecting cavernous/lateral sinuses.

Laboratory

Proteus organisms are easily recovered through routine laboratory cultures. An ultrasound of the kidneys or a CT scan should be considered as part of a workup.

Treatment

Traditional treatment includes oral quinolone for 3 days or trimethoprim/sulfamethoxazole.

BIBLIOGRAPHY

1. Struble K. (2011). Proteus Infections. [online] Available from www.emedicine.com/med/TOPIC1929.HTM. [Accessed July, 2013].

43. PROTEUS SYNDROME

General

A harmarteo neoplastic disorder with variable clinical manifestations.

Ocular

Myopia; band keratopathy; cataract; vitreous hemorrhage; chorioretinal mass; serous retinal detachment.

Clinical

Thickening of the bones of the external auditory meatus and cranial fossa; enlargement of the left internal auditory meatus; deformities of the feet and toes.

Laboratory

Proteus organisms are easily recovered through routine laboratory cultures. An ultrasound of the kidneys or a CT scan should be considered as part of a workup.

Treatment

Traditional treatment includes oral quinolone for 3 days or trimethoprim/sulfamethoxazole.

BIBLIOGRAPHY

1. Struble K. (2011). Proteus Infections. [online] Available from www.emedicine.com/med/TOPIC1929.HTM. [Accessed July, 2013].

44. PSEUDOMONAS AERUGINOSA INFECTIONS

General

Gram-negative rod with secondary contaminant of superficial wounds; *Pseudomonas* organisms produce a variety of enzymes that cause pathologic changes, including hemolysins and exotoxins as well as a glycocalyx that increases adherence.

Ocular

Hypopyon; conjunctivitis; keratitis; ulcerative abscess of cornea; endophthalmitis; panophthalmitis.

Clinical

Local tissue damage and diminished host resistance, which may occur in ear, lung, skin, and urinary tract.

Laboratory

Complete blood count may reveal leukocytosis with a left shift and bandemia. Positive results on blood culture in the absence of extracardiac sites of infection may indicate pseudomonal endocarditis.

Treatment

Antimicrobials are the mainstay of therapy. Two-drug combination therapy such as an antipseudomonal beta-lactam antibiotic with an aminoglycoside.

BIBLIOGRAPHY

1. Klaus-Dieter L. (2012). Pseudomonas aeruginosa Infections. [online] Available from www.emedicine.com/med/TOPIC1943.HTM. [Accessed July, 2013].

45. Q FEVER (COXIELLA BURNETII)

General

Acute rickettsial infection caused by *Coxiella burnetii*; at least eleven serotypes of this organism are capable of causing human infection; elevated inflammatory response results in granulomatous formation.

Ocular

Conjunctivitis; gangrene of eyelids; retinal hemorrhages; perivasculitis; episcleritis; optic neuritis; uveitis; papilledema; nystagmus; ocular motor nerve pareses; Miller-Fisher syndrome.

Clinical

Fever; severe headache; tissue necrosis; pneumonia; self-limited fever; endocarditis; hepatitis.

Laboratory

Small Gram-negative rod which grows inside eukaryotic cells. Diagnosis is made based on detection of phase I and II antibodies a four fold rise in complement-fixing antibody titer against phase II antigen occurs and yields the highest specificity.

Serologic test

Compliment fixation is specific but lacks sensitivity and indirect immunofluorescence is Q fever highly specific and sensitive.

Treatment

Adequate antibiotic therapy initiated early in the first week of illness is highly effective and is associated with the best outcome. Doxycycline is the drug of choice.

BIBLIOGRAPHY

1. Rathore MH. (2011). Rickettsial Infection. [online] Available from www.emedicine.com/ped/TOPIC2015.HTM. [Accessed July, 2013].

46. RABIES (HYDROPHOBIA; LYSSA)

General

Acute viral zoonosis of the central nervous system.

Ocular

Lid retraction; widening of palpebral fissure; retinal hemorrhages; mydriasis; paralysis of third, fourth, fifth, or seventh nerve; bilateral optic neuritis; branch retinal artery occlusion; vaccine-induced autoimmune demyelinative optic neuritis.

Clinical

Fever; headache; nausea; numbness; tingling; acute sensitiveness to sound and light; laryngeal and pharyngeal spasms; increased muscle tonus; convulsions; delirium; coma; death.

Laboratory

Saliva can be tested by virus isolation or reverse transcription followed by PCR. Suspected infectious animal should be quarantined for 10 days.

Treatment

Before the onset of symptoms, both passive and active immunizations are effective for preventing progression to full-blown rabies. In exposures to high-risk species, initiate treatment immediately pending laboratory examination of the animal, if it is caught.

BIBLIOGRAPHY

1. Gompf SG. (2011). Rabies. [online] Available from www.emedicine.com/med/TOPIC1374.HTM. [Accessed July, 2013].

⬄ 47. RHINOSPORIDIOSIS

General

Rare fungal infection, primarily affecting the mucous membranes of the nose and eye. Causative agent is *Rhinosporidium seeberi.*

Clinical

Respiratory mucosa, vaginal mucosa, skin and metastatic-like involvement of the internal organs.

Ocular

Conjunctival lesions, photophobia and conjunctival infection.

Treatment

Complete surgical excision remains the most effective treatment. Cautery or cryopexy to the base of the excised lesion may be beneficial to prevent recurrence.

⬄ BIBLIOGRAPHY

1. Roy FH, Fraunfelder FW, Fraunfelder FT. Roy and Fraunfelder's Current Ocular Therapy, 6th edition. London: Elsevier; 2008.

⬄ 48. ROCKY MOUNTAIN SPOTTED FEVER

General

Acute systemic disease caused by *Rickettsia rickettsii* transmitted by a wood tick or dog tick.

Ocular

Conjunctivitis; optic atrophy; cotton-wool spots; scotoma; uveitis; optic neuritis; paralysis of accommodation; paralysis of extraocular muscles; retinal vascular occlusion; vitreal opacity; hypopyon; anterior uveitis with fibrin clots.

Clinical

Fever; chills; headache; muscle aches; rash.

Laboratory

Early diagnosis depends on clinical and epidemiologic grounds. Polymerase chain reaction has high sensitivity and specificity.

Treatment

Intravenous tetracycline and chloramphenicol should be started as soon as possible. Oral doxycycline, tetracycline and chloramphenicol may be considered but only if patient is not acutely ill.

⬄ BIBLIOGRAPHY

1. Cunha BA. (2011). Rocky Mountain Spotted Fever. [online] Available from www.emedicine.com/oph/TOPIC503.HTM. [Accessed July, 2013].

⬄ 49. RUBELLA SYNDROME (CONGENITAL RUBELLA SYNDROME; GERMAN MEASLES; GREGG SYNDROME)

General

Rubella infection of the mother during first trimester of pregnancy; ocular disease is the most commonly found abnormality in patients with congenital rubella syndrome (75%), multiorgan disease is common (> 75%); no significant association has been found between gestational age and time of maternal infection and incidence of individual ocular conditions.

Ocular

Nystagmus; glaucoma; corneal haziness; cataracts; retinal pigmentary changes; appearance and central distribution of lesions are quite distinguishable from retinitis pigmentosa; retinopathy is not progressive and has little, if any, effect on vision; waxy atrophy of optic disk; conjunctivitis; megalocornea or microcornea; buphthalmos; microphthalmos; uveitis; iris atrophy; spherophakia; strabismus.

Clinical

Low-birth weight; diarrhea; pneumonia; urinary infection; hearing loss; heart disease; hepatosplenomegaly; mental retardation; inguinal hernias; ataxia; cardiac abnormalities.

Laboratory

Diagnosis is made by clinical findings. If in doubt, a rising titer of immunoglobulin M will indicate a recent infection.

Treatment

Treatment for rubella of the eye centers on glaucoma and cataract.

🗗 BIBLIOGRAPHY

1. Lombardo PC. (2011). Dermatologic Manifestations of Rubella. [online] Available from www.emedicine.com/derm/TOPIC380.HTM. [Accessed July, 2013].

🗗 50. RUBEOLA (MEASLES; MORBILLI)

General

Acute, extremely communicable disease that affects young school-aged children; caused by paramyxovirus.

Ocular

Hypopyon; uveitis; conjunctivitis; Koplik (Hirschberg) spots of conjunctiva; keratitis; corneal ulcer; cellulitis of lid; dacryocystitis; congenital cataract; optic atrophy; optic neuritis; strabismus; pigmentary retinopathy; iris prolapse; hemianopsia; secondary glaucoma; central retinal artery occlusion; orbital cellulitis; accommodative spasm; paralysis of sixth nerve; keratoconus.

Clinical

Maculopapular rash; fever.

Laboratory

Diagnosis made by clinical findings.

Treatment

Good hydration.

🗗 BIBLIOGRAPHY

1. Chen SSP. (2011). Measles. [online] Available from www.emedicine.com/derm/TOPIC259.HTM. [Accessed July, 2013].

🗗 51. SPOROTRICHOSIS

General

Chronic fungal infection caused by *Sporothrix schenckii*; lesion usually occurs on exposed skin and is characterized by nodules or pustules that may develop into small ulcers; infectious agent usually gains entrance into the skin by traumatic implantation of soil or plant materials; disseminated sporotrichosis is uncommon, usually occurring in alcoholics or immunosuppressed patients.

Ocular

Conjunctivitis; keratitis; corneal ulcer; blepharitis; endophthalmitis; iris atrophy; dacryocystitis; osteitis; periosteitis; scleritis; erosion of bony walls of the orbit.

Clinical

Enlargement of regional lymph nodes; pulmonary lesions; granulomas in the joints and genitourinary system.

Laboratory

Cultured on Sebouraud dextrose agar, cream-colored to black, folded, leathery.

Treatment

Potassium iodide drops as a saturated solution is the treatment of choice. Amphotericin B may be necessary in more severe forms with visceral and intraocular or orbital involvement.

🗗 BIBLIOGRAPHY

1. Greenfield RA. (2012). Sporotrichosis. [online] Available from www.emedicine.com/med/TOPIC2161.HTM. [Accessed July, 2013].

52. STAPHYLOCOCCUS

General

Gram-positive coccus *Staphylococcus aureus*; most common cause of suppurative infection in humans; more common in patients with a previous disorders, such as diabetes, thyroid disease, renal failure, or malnutrition; although most *S. aureus* isolates from other sources are encapsulated, capsules have not been noted in ocular isolates.

Ocular

Uveitis; hypopyon; conjunctivitis; keratitis; cellulitis of lid; meibomianitis; ptosis; blepharitis; endophthalmitis; dacryocystitis; increased intraocular pressure; orbital periosteitis.

Clinical

Tissues hypertonic, edematous, and painful; lesion liquefies, forming creamy yellow pus; fever; nausea; vomiting; cough; dyspnea; abdominal pain; diarrhea; bloody stools; dehydration; shock.

Laboratory

Aerobic Gram-positive cocci bacteria grow in grape-like clusters. Coagulase positive indicates pathogenicity.

Treatment

Specific antimicrobial therapy is chosen based on the site and severity of the infection and the antimicrobial sensitivities of the organism involved.

BIBLIOGRAPHY

1. Tolan RW. (2012). Staphylococcus Aureus Infection. [online] Available from www.emedicine.com/ped/TOPIC2704.HTM. [Accessed July, 2013].

53. STREPTOCOCCUS (SCARLET FEVER)

General

Gram-positive bacteria that can invade any tissue.

Ocular

Conjunctivitis; corneal ulcer; blepharitis; scarlatinal rash of lid; erysipelas dermatitis of lid; gangrene of lid; endophthalmitis; proptosis; dacryocystitis; optic neuritis; orbital cellulitis; uveitis; hypopyon; secondary glaucoma; paralysis of extraocular muscles; infectious crystalline keratopathy; scleritis.

Clinical

Pharyngitis; impetigo; scarlet fever; pneumonia; bacteremia; rheumatic fever; glomerulonephritis.

Laboratory

Gram-positive cocci growing in pairs or chains. Throat culture and sensitivity are useful.

Treatment

Penicillin is the drug of choice.

BIBLIOGRAPHY

1. Zabawski EJ. (2011). Scarlet Fever. [online] Available from www.emedicine.com/emerg/TOPIC518.HTM. [Accessed July, 2013].

54. SYPHILIS (ACQUIRED LUES; ACQUIRED SYPHILIS; LUES VENEREA; MALUM VENEREUM)

General

Causative agent, *Treponema pallidum*, usually transmitted sexually.

Ocular

Conjunctival chancroid; conjunctivitis; keratitis; blepharitis; ptosis; iris atrophy; hippus; dacryocystitis; optic nerve atrophy; optic neuritis; periostitis; episcleritis; scleritis; nystagmus; uveitis; vitreous hemorrhages; paralysis of sixth nerve; papilledema; retinal hemorrhages; retinitis proliferans; oculogyric crisis; neuroretinitis; papilledema (associated with aseptic meningitis); diffuse or multifocal chorioretinitis; vertical supranuclear gaze palsy; Benedikt syndrome.

Clinical

Primary lesion associated with regional lymphadenopathy; secondary bacteremic stage associated with generalized mucocutaneous lesions; tertiary stage characterized by destructive mucocutaneous, musculoskeletal, or parenchymal lesions, aortitis, or central nervous system disease; syphilis and human immunodeficiency virus (HIV) infection often coexist in the same patient who experiences a higher incidence and greater severity of neurologic and ocular manifestations; a significant percentage of patients infected with HIV-I and *T. pallidum* become seronegative to syphilis testing.

Laboratory

Serologic nontreponemal tests include Venereal Disease Research Laboratory (VDRL) and rapid plasma reagin (RPR).

Treatment

The goals are to reduce morbidity and to prevent complications. Penicillin is the antibiotic of choice for treating syphilis. Ocular syphilis should be treated the same as patients with neurosyphilis.

BIBLIOGRAPHY

1. Majmudar PA. (2011). Interstitial Keratitis Overview of Interstitial Keratitis. [online]. Available from www.emedicine.com/oph/TOPIC453.HTM. [Accessed July, 2013].
2. Euerle B. (2012). Syphilis. [online] Available from www.emedicine.com/med/TOPIC2224.HTM. [Accessed July, 2013].

55. SYPHILIS, CONGENITAL (CONGENITAL LUES)

General

Caused by intrauterine transplacental infection of fetus by *T. pallidum* (*see* Syphilis).

Ocular

Conjunctivitis; keratitis; dacryocystitis; optic nerve atrophy; periostitis; anisocoria; Argyll Robertson pupil; retinal degeneration; nystagmus; gumma of conjunctiva, eyelids, and orbit; paresis of extraocular muscles; secondary glaucoma; uveitis; iridoschisis.

Clinical

Cutaneous and mucous membrane lesions; periostitis; anemia; hepatosplenomegaly; ectodermal defects; central nervous system involvement; gummatous lesions.

Laboratory

Fluorescent treponemal antibody-absorption (FTA-ABS) and microhemagglutination assay for *Treponema pallidum* (MHA-TP) are the standard test. All patients with syphilis should also be tested for HIV.

Treatment

Parenteral penicillin is the preferred treatment for all stages of syphilis. The treatment varies from primary and secondary syphilis, late latent syphilis, tertiary syphilis and neurosyphilis. Ocular treatment includes topical steroids and cycloplegics and it can relieve the symptoms of anterior uveitis and interstitial keratitis. Subconjunctival steroids have been used to relieve recurrent anterior segment inflammation. Severe corneal opacification may require keratoplasty; however, with recurrent inflammation and graft rejection.

BIBLIOGRAPHY

1. Waseem M. (2011). Pediatric Syphilis. [online] Available from www.emedicine.com/ped/TOPIC2193.HTM. [Accessed July, 2013].

56. TETANUS (LOCKJAW)

General

Acute infectious disease affecting nervous system; causative agent is *Clostridium tetani*; bacteria enters body through a puncture wound, abrasion, cut, or burn.

Ocular

Chemosis; keratitis; nystagmus; uveitis; corneal ulcer; cellulitis of orbit; hypopyon; panophthalmitis; pupil paralysis; pseudoptosis; blepharospasm; paralysis of third or seventh nerve; may occur following perforating ocular injuries.

Clinical

Severe muscle spasms; dysphagia; trismus; facial palsy; muscle stiffness; irritability.

Laboratory

Gram-positive spore-forming bacteria; laboratory studies are of little value.

Treatment

Passive immunization with human tetanus immune globulin shortens the course of tetanus and may lessen its severity. Benzodiazepines have emerged as the mainstay of symptomatic therapy for tetanus.

BIBLIOGRAPHY

1. Hinfey PB. (2012). Tetanus. [online] Available from www.emedicine.com/med/TOPIC2254.HTM. [Accessed July, 2013].

57. TRACHOMA

General

Most common in rural communities of the Middle East, Africa, Asia, and South and Central America; caused by *C. trachomatis*; associated with poor sanitation and medical care.

Ocular

Chronic keratoconjunctivitis; papillae follicles; keratitis; opacities of cornea; scars of palpebral conjunctiva; ptosis; tearing; entropion.

Clinical

Rhinitis; otitis media; upper respiratory tract infection.

Laboratory

Most endemic areas, lab tests are unavailable. Commercial PCR based assay has high sensitivity and specificity.

Treatment

Tetracycline eye ointment for 6 weeks or a single dose azithromycin systemically.

BIBLIOGRAPHY

1. Solomon AW. (2011). Trachoma. [online] Available from www.emedicine.com/oph/TOPIC118.HTM. [Accessed July, 2013].

🔖 58. TUBERCULOSIS

General

Communicable disease caused by the acid-fast bacillus *Mycobacterium tuberculosis*.

Ocular

Conjunctivitis; subconjunctival nodules (tuberculomas); keratitis; pannus; corneal ulcer; blepharitis; cellulitis; meibomianitis; uveitis; dacryocystitis; chronic orbital cellulitis; retinitis; scleritis; scleral perforation; hypopyon; vitreous hemorrhages; optic neuritis; optic atrophy; tuberculous panophthalmitis; choroidal tubercles; intraorbital extraocular lesions.

Clinical

Pulmonary infection; pyuria; hematuria; epididymitis; dysuria; flank pain; distorted calyces; productive cough.

Laboratory

Acid-fast bacillus culture of body fluids including vitreous and aqueous. Polymerase chain reaction is 89% positive for pulmonary infection.

Treatment

A course of chemotherapy (isoniazid, rifampin, pyrazinamide and ethambutol or streptomycin) for a period of 6 months is the recommended therapy.

🔖 BIBLIOGRAPHY

1. Collins JK. Handbook of Clinical Ophthalmology. New York: Masson; 1982.
2. DeVoe AG, Locatcher-Khorazo D. The external manifestations of ocular tuberculosis. Trans Am Ophthalmol Soc. 1964;62:203–12.
3. D'Souza P, Garg R, Dhaliwal RS, et al. Orbital tuberculosis. Int Ophthalmol. 1994;18:149–52.
4. Gupta V, Gupta A, Arora S, et al. Presumed tubercular serpiginous like choroiditis. Ophthalmology. 2003;110: 1744–9.
5. Patkar S, Singhania BK, Agrawal A. Intraorbital extraocular tuberculosis: a report of three cases. Surg Neurol. 1994; 42:320–1.
6. Roy FH, Fraunfelder FW, Fraunfelder FT. Roy and Fraunfelder's Current Ocular Therapy, 6th edition. London: Elsevier; 2008.
7. Tejada P, Mendez MJ, Negreira S. Choroidal tubercles with tuberculous meningitis. Int Ophthalmol. 1994;18:115–8.

🔖 59. TYPHOID FEVER (ABDOMINAL TYPHUS; ENTERIC FEVER)

General

Causative agent, *Salmonella typhi*.

Ocular

Conjunctivitis; chemosis; corneal ulcer; tenonitis; paralysis of extraocular muscles; endophthalmitis; panophthalmitis; optic neuritis; retinal detachment; central scotoma; central retinal artery emboli; iritis with or without hypopyon; choroiditis; retinal hemorrhages; bilateral optic neuritis; abnormal ocular motility (likely secondary to thrombotic infarcts affecting the ocular motor nerve nuclei, fascicles, brainstem, or cerebral hemispheres).

Clinical

Fever; headache; bradycardia; splenomegaly; maculopapular rash; leukopenia; encephalitis. Salmonella may produce an illness characterized by fever and bacteremia without any other manifestations of enterocolitis or enteric fever, which is particularly common in patients with acquired immunodeficiency syndrome (AIDS).

Laboratory

Gram-negative bacillus isolation from blood culture (50–70% of cases). Positive stool culture is less frequent.

Treatment

Early detection, antibiotic therapy and adequate fluids, electrolytes, and nutrition reduce the rate of complications and reduce the case-fatality rate.

🔖 BIBLIOGRAPHY

1. Brusch JL. (2011). Typhoid Fever. [online] Available from www.emedicine.com/med/TOPIC2331.HTM. [Accessed July, 2013].

60. VARICELLA (CHICKENPOX)

General

Acute exanthematous disease; highly contagious; children ages between 2 and 8 years.

Ocular

Conjunctival ulcer; corneal ulcer; descemetocele; corneal opacity; keratitis; paresis of third, fourth, and sixth nerves; optic neuritis; papilledema; retinitis; hemorrhagic retinopathy; uveitis; cataract; paralytic mydriasis; phthisis bulbi; unifocal choroiditis; dendritic keratitis; acute retinal necrosis (in a patient with AIDS); disciform keratitis.

Clinical

Fever; malaise; rash; pruritus.

Laboratory

Diagnosis is made by clinical findings.

Treatment

Isolation oral antihistamines, such as diphenhydramine and hydroxyzine, are used for severe pruritus and acetaminophen is recommended for use for the reduction of fever.

BIBLIOGRAPHY

1. Bechtel KA. (2011). Pediatric Chickenpox. [online] Available from www.emedicine.com/emerg/TOPIC367.HTM. [Accessed July, 2013].

61. VARICELLA SYNDROME, CONGENITAL

General

Varicella passed in utero from mother to fetus.

Ocular

Microphthalmia; microcornea; persistent hyperplastic primary vitreous.

Clinical

Urinary tract infection; neurogenic bladder.

Laboratory

Clinical.

Treatment

See persistent hyperplastic primary vitreous.

BIBLIOGRAPHY

1. Anderson WE. (2011). Varicella-Zoster Virus. [online] Available from www.emedicine.com/med/TOPIC2361.HTM. [Accessed July, 2013].

62. YERSINIOSIS

General

Infection with one of the invasive rod-shaped *Yersinia* bacteria.

Clinical

Gastroenteritis, high fever, acute terminal ileitis.

Ocular

Corneal perforation, panophthalmitis, anterior uveitis, photophobia, lacrimation, pericorneal ciliary injection, aqueous flare and cell, keratic precipitates and macular edema.

Laboratory

Small, non-motile, Gram-negative coccobacilli found in stool samples and conjunctiva.

Treatment

Tetracycline or chloramphenicol is drug of choice.

BIBLIOGRAPHY

1. Roy FH, Fraunfelder FW, Fraunfelder FT. Roy and Fraunfelder's Current Ocular Therapy, 6th edition. London: Elsevier; 2008.

CHAPTER
2

Parasitic Diseases

⊟ 1. ACANTHAMOEBA

General

It is caused by *Acanthamoeba polyphaga* and *Acanthamoeba cartel* (*see* Herpes simplex masquerade syndrome); all types of contact lenses have been associated with *Acanthamoeba* keratitis, particularly daily-wear soft contact lenses.

Ocular

Hypopyon; uveitis; conjunctivitis and chemosis; keratitis; pannus; corneal ring abscess; papillitis; vitreitis; retinal perivasculitis; secondary glaucoma; post-keratoplasty *Acanthamoeba* keratitis may present as an infectious crystalline keratopathy in the periphery of the graft.

Clinical

Meningoencephalitis; meningitis; hemorrhagic encephalitis.

Laboratory

Polygonal double-walled cysts, under bright-field or phase-contrast microscopy or stained with hematoxylin and eosin, Gram stain, Giemsa stain or celluflor white.

Treatment

Medical therapy for *Acanthamoeba* infection is not well established. Topical antimicrobial agents that achieve high concentrations at the site of the infection can be considered. Treatment of keratitis consists of early diagnosis and aggressive surgical and medical therapies.

⊟ BIBLIOGRAPHY

1. Crum-Cianflone NF. (2011). Acanthamoeba. [online] Available from www.emedicine.com/med/TOPIC10.HTM. [Accessed July, 2013].
2. Wang JC. (2010). Ophthalmologic Manifestations of Herpes Simplex Keratitis. [online] Available from www.emedicine.com/oph/TOPIC100.HTM. [Accessed July, 2013].

⊟ 2. BAYLISASCARIS (UNILATERAL SUBACUTE NEURORETINITIS, OCULAR LARVA MIGRANS)

General

A diffuse unilateral subacute neuroretinitis caused by *Baylisascaris procyonis* which is the common raccoon roundworm or *Ancylostoma caninum*.

Clinical

Eosinophilic meningoencephalitis.

Ocular

Retinal or subretinal tracks, optic disk edema, pallor, vitritis, snowbanking in pars plana and iritis.

Laboratory

Baylisascaris tests can be performed using serum and CSF. ELISA and Western blot are available from the Department of Veterinary Pathobiology at Purdue University.

Treatment

Prompt laser photocoagulation of the motile worm in the retina is the preferred and most effective treatment.

BIBLIOGRAPHY

1. Roy FH, Fraunfelder FW, Fraunfelder FT. Roy and Fraunfelder's Current Ocular Therapy, 6th edition. London: Elsevier; 2008.

3. COENUROSIS (TAPEWORM)

General

Rare human infestation of the cystic larval stage of the dog tapeworm; usually infestation in the muscle, subcutaneous tissue, eye, nervous system, or brain; three species may be involved: (1) *Multiceps taenia*,(2) *Multiceps serialis* and (3) *Multiceps glomeratus.*

Ocular

Hypopyon; retinal detachment; retinal edema; anterior uveitis; conjunctivitis; proptosis; miosis; vitreal haze; increased intraocular pressure; coenurus cysts of the conjunctiva and iris.

Clinical

Ataxia; headache; loss of weight; somnolence; stiffness of neck and shoulders.

Laboratory

Perianal and stool examinations are useful.

Treatment

Anthelmintic drugs are used to rid the gastrointestinal (GI) tract of worms or systemically to rid the body of the helminth forms that invade organs and tissues.

BIBLIOGRAPHY

1. Irizarry L. (2011). Tapeworm Infestation. [online] Available from www.emedicine.com/emerg/TOPIC567.HTM. [Accessed July, 2013].

4. DEMODICOSIS

General

Demodex folliculorum and *Demodex brevis* infestation; exact role in causing blepharitis is unclear; most patients are asymptomatic.

Ocular

Blepharitis; follicular distention and hyperplasia; lid hyperemia; lid hyperkeratinization; madarosis; Meibomian gland destruction; mite colonies of eyelashes and eyebrows.

Clinical

Pruritus.

Laboratory

Presence of parasites on epilated eyelashes.

Treatment

Brushed vigorously across the external lid margin, following 0.5% proparacaine instillation. Five minutes later, a solution of 70% alcohol is applied in a similar manner.

This regimen is reported to successfully reduce both the symptoms and the observed number of mites by the end of 3 weekly visits. Ether and alcohol should be used with caution, and corneal contact should be prevented. Home regimen includes scrubbing the eyelids twice daily with baby shampoo diluted with water to yield a 50% dilution and applying an antibiotic ointment at night until resolution of symptoms. Discard makeup, clean sheets, check household members and pets.

⊟ BIBLIOGRAPHY

1. Li J, O'Reilly N, Sheha H, et al. Correlation between ocular demodex infestation and serum immunoreactivity to bacillus proteins in patients with facial rosacea. Ophthalmology. 2010;117:870–7.
2. Roque MR. (2011). Demodicosis. [online] Available from www.emedicine.com/oph/TOPIC517.HTM. [Accessed July, 2013].

⊟ 5. HYDATID CYST (ECHINOCOCCOSIS)

General

Caused by *Echinococcus granulosus* acquired by contact with a dog host.

Ocular

Conjunctivitis; keratitis; exophthalmos; phthisis bulbi; optic atrophy; optic neuritis; papilledema; abscesses of orbit and cornea; retinal detachment; retinal hemorrhages; cataract; hypopyon; secondary glaucoma; hydatid cysts of the conjunctiva, eyelid, orbit, and lacrimal system; acute visual loss; vitreous mass.

Clinical

Pruritus; urticaria; pulmonary cysts; brain cysts; anaphylactic shock; death.

Laboratory

Plain orbital radiographs may show enlarged orbital diameters and increased soft-tissue density. Ultrasonography demonstrates a cystic lesion without internal reflectivity; computed tomography discloses a well-defined cystic mass.

Treatment

Echinococcosis is rare and can be severe. Refer patients to reference centers to confirm their diagnosis and to obtain advice on therapeutic strategy.

⊟ BIBLIOGRAPHY

1. Vuitton DA. (2011). Echinococcosis. [online] Available from www.emedicine.com/med/TOPIC326.HTM. [Accessed July, 2013].

⊟ 6. NEMATODE OPHTHALMIA SYNDROME (VISCERAL LARVA MIGRANS SYNDROME; TOXOCARIASIS)

General

Usually found in children; invasion by larvae of *Toxocara canis* and *Toxocara cati* of viscera and eyes; pronounced eosinophilia; as many as 30% of asymptomatic children demonstrate serologic evidence of prior *Toxocara* infestations.

Ocular

Leukocoria; uveitis; cataract; marked vitreous reaction with large floaters; choroiditis; large, cyst-like white masses extending into vitreous; optic neuritis; papillitis; strabismus; hemorrhagic, exudative, or granulomatous retinitis; retinal detachment; endophthalmitis; larvae present in the cornea.

Clinical

Hepatosplenomegaly; pulmonary infiltration; fever; cough; lack of appetite.

Laboratory

Eosinophilia in patients with visceral disease. ELISA test is best to document systemic or ocular infection with *T. canis*.

Treatment

Treatment is by case-by-case basis; in most cases no treatment is needed; systemic anthelmintic agents; vitrectomy may be necessary.

⊟ BIBLIOGRAPHY

1. Biglan AW, Glickman LT, Lobes LA. Serum and vitreous Toxocara antibody in nematode endophthalmitis. Am J Ophthalmol. 1979;88:898–901.

2. Roy FH, Fraunfelder FW, Fraunfelder FT. Roy and Fraunfelder's Current Ocular Therapy, 6th edition. London: Elsevier; 2008.

3. Maguire AM, Green WR, Michels RG, et al. Recovery of intraocular Toxocara Canis by pars plana vitrectomy. Ophthalmology. 1990;97:675–80.

4. Raistrick ER, Hart JC. Ocular toxocariasis in adults. Br J Ophthalmol. 1976;60:365–70.

5. Wilder HC. Nematode endophthalmitis. Trans Am Acad Ophthalmol Otolaryngol. 1950;55:99.

6. Wilkinson C. Ocular toxocariasis. In: Ryan SJ (Ed). Retina, 2nd edition. St. Louis: Mosby; 1994. pp. 1545–52.

⊟ 7. PEDICULOSIS AND PHTHIRIASIS

General

Infestation of lice on head, body, or pubic area.

Ocular

Conjunctivitis; keratitis; infestation of lice or nits glued to shafts of eyelashes and eyebrow.

Clinical

Pruritus; skin excoriation; impetigo; pyoderma with lymphadenitis and febrile episodes.

Laboratory

Removal from hair shaft and examination under microscope.

Treatment

Treatments involve spreading an ointment at the base of the eyelashes at night to trap mites as they emerge from their burrow and/or move from one follicle to another.

⊟ BIBLIOGRAPHY

1. Guenther L. (2013). Pediculosis (Lice). [online] Available from www.emedicine.com/med/TOPIC1769.HTM. [Accessed July, 2013].

⊟ 8. TOXOPLASMOSIS (TOXOPLASMIC RETINOCHOROIDITIS; OCULAR TOXOPLASMOSIS)

General

Parasite infestation caused by *Toxoplasma gondii;* cell-mediated immunity is believed to be the major defence mechanism against *Toxoplasma* infection; ocular toxoplasmosis occurs in approximately 1% of patients with acquired immunodeficiency syndrome (AIDS); AIDS-related toxoplasma retinochoroiditis may have several atypical clinical manifestations.

Ocular

Keratitis; uveitis; optic atrophy; papillitis; anisocoria; persistent pupillary membrane; focal retinochoroiditis; scleritis; cataract; microphthalmos; myopia; nystagmus; esotropia.

Clinical

Cysts are seen in many organs, including brain and muscle; hydrocephalus; intracerebral calcification; various CNS complaints.

Laboratory

Serologic tests for anti-*T. gondii.* Antibodies are common.

Treatment

Triple drug therapy pyrimethamine, sulfadiazine and prednisone. Pyrimethamine should be combined with folinic acid. Surgical care includes photocoagulation, cryotherapy or vitrectomy.

⊟ BIBLIOGRAPHY

1. Lasave AF, Llopis MD, Muccioli C, et al. Intravitreal clindamycin and dexamethasone for zone 1 toxoplasmic retinochoroiditis at twenty-four months. Ophthalmology. 2010;1831–8.
2. Soheilian M, Ramezani A, Azimzadeh A, et al. Randomized trial of intravitreal clindamycin and dexamethasone versus pyrimethamine, sulfadiazine and prednisolone in treatment of ocular toxoplasmosis. Ophthalmology. 2011;118:134–41.
3. Wuh L. (2011). Ophthalmologic Manifestations of Toxoplasmosis. [online] Available from www.emedicine.com/oph/TOPIC707.HTM. [Accessed July, 2013].

⊟ 9. TRICHINELLOSIS (TRICHINOSIS)

General

Parasite *Trichinella* enters the body by ingestion of infected meat (usually poorly cooked pork).

Ocular

Conjunctivitis; splinter hemorrhages of conjunctiva; paralysis of sixth nerve; exophthalmos; proptosis; uveitis; optic neuritis; papilledema; retinal hemorrhages; dyschromatopsia; scotoma; secondary glaucoma; encysted parasites in the extraocular muscles.

Clinical

Fever; urticaria; respiratory symptoms; muscle pain; myalgias and severe proximal muscle weakness; impaired coordination.

Laboratory

Leukocytosis and eosinophilia elevated serum levels of lactic dehydrogenase, aldolase and creatine phosphokinase (50% cases).

Treatment

Mebendazole orally is the treatment of choice. In severe cases, prednisone may be used in conjunction with anthelmintic agent.

⊟ BIBLIOGRAPHY

1. Arnold LK. (2013). Trichinellosis/Trichinosis. [online] Available from www.emedicine.com/emerg/TOPIC612.HTM. [Accessed July, 2013].

CHAPTER
3

Nutritional Disorders

1. CROHN DISEASE (GRANULOMATOUS ILEOCOLITIS)

General

Autoimmune or hypersensitivity inflammatory change; slight prevalence in males; Jewish people most frequently affected; onset at any age; more severe in young people; remission; relapses.

Ocular

Recurrent conjunctivitis; marginal corneal ulcers; keratitis; blepharitis; dry eye; scleritis; episcleritis; iris atrophy; uveitis; pupil immobility and dilatation; macular edema; macular hemorrhages; extraocular muscles palsy; vitreal haze; retinal vasculitis; subconjunctival nodules; conjunctival ulcer; pannus; acute dacryoadenitis; orbital pseudotumor.

Clinical

Inflammatory bowel disease; abdominal distention; tenderness of abdomen; mass in right lower quadrant of abdomen; diarrhea; abdominal cramps; bloating; flatulence; weight loss; nervousness; tension; depression; pyoderma gangrenosum.

Laboratory

Test result positive for anti-*Saccharomyces cerevisiae* antibodies (ASCA) and negative for perinuclear anti-neutrophil cytoplasmic antibody (p-ANCA) antigen suggests the presence of Crohn's disease. Computed tomography (CT), magnetic resonance imaging (MRI), barium contrast studies, colonoscopy and upper endoscopy may also be useful.

Treatment

Treat diarrhea; antibiotic and anti-inflammatory drugs, antimetabolites, anti-tumor necrosis factor antibody, immunosuppressive agents; surgical correction for fibrostenotic obstruction may be necessary.

BIBLIOGRAPHY

1. Rangasamy P, Yung-Hsin C, Coash ML, et al. (2011). Crohn Disease. [online] Available from www.emedicine.com/med/TOPIC477.HTM. [Accessed July, 2013].

⊟ 2. HYPOVITAMINOSIS A (XEROPHTHALMIA)

General

Deficient serum levels of vitamin A; principal cause of infantile blindness in the world; it is due to insufficient intake of vitamin A or interference with its absorption from the intestinal tract; transport or storage in the liver; obstruction of biliary tract or pancreatic ducts.

Ocular

Bitot's spot; xerosis; keratomalacia; keratitis; corneal perforation and ulcer; corneal opacity; hyperkeratosis; retinal degeneration; scotoma.

Clinical

Inadequate dietary intake or interference with absorptive storage or transport capacities, as occurs in liver disease, sprue, regional enteritis, gastic bypass and chronic gastroenteritis; respiratory infection; diarrhea; reduced childhood mortality.

Laboratory

Serum vitamin A levels.

Treatment

Oral administration of vitamin A 200,000 IU at presentation, the following day, and a third dose a week later is recommended. Infants should receive half doses.

⊟ BIBLIOGRAPHY

1. Schwartz RA, Centurion SA, Gascon P. (2012). Dermatologic Manifestations of Vitamin A Deficiency. [online] Available from www.emedicine.com/derm/TOPIC794.HTM. [Accessed July, 2013].

⊟ 3. INFLAMMATORY BOWEL DISEASE (ULCERATIVE COLITIS; REGIONAL ENTERITIS)

General

Chronic inflammatory disease of unknown etiology; both sexes affected; onset at all ages, most frequently between ages of 20 and 40 years; usually abrupt onset; psychosomatic pathogenesis possible.

Ocular

Iritis; uveitis; episcleritis; papillomatous changes of palpebral conjunctiva; scleritis; serous retinal detachment; choroidal infiltrates; retrobulbar neuritis; papillitis; retinal pigment epithelium disturbance; choroidal folds.

Clinical

Abdominal pain; cramps; diarrhea; arthritis; weight loss; erythema nodosum; aphthous stomatitis; pallor; tenderness over colon; nutritional deficiency; carcinoma; associations with Sjögren syndrome and Takayasu disease have been reported.

Laboratory

Elevated white blood count and erythrocyte sedimentation rate. Radiography demonstrates the "sting sign" of narrowed lumen in the terminal ileum.

Treatment

Systemic corticosteroids, metronidazole, pain medication and antispasmodic drugs give relief.

⊟ BIBLIOGRAPHY

1. Khan AN, Sheen AJ, Varia H. (2011). Ulcerative Colitis Imaging. [online] Available from www.emedicine.com/radio/TOPIC785.HTM. [Accessed July, 2013].

CHAPTER
4

Disorders of Protein Metabolism

1. LOWE SYNDROME (OCULO-CEREBRO-RENAL SYNDROME)

General

Essential enzyme or protein abnormality is unknown; sex-linked recessive trait (male incidence only); onset in early infancy.

Ocular

Nystagmus; congenital glaucoma; miotic pupils; no pupillary reaction; ectropion uveae; malformation of the anterior chamber angle and of the iris; Schlemm's canal may be absent with imperfect angle cleavage; blue sclera; cloudy cornea; cataracts; megalocornea; corneal dystrophy; buphthalmos; microphthalmos; microphakia; mydriasis; strabismus; lens punctate cortical opacities.

Clinical

Mental, psychomotor, and growth retardation; aminoaciduria; albuminuria; glycosuria; renal tubular acidosis; rickets; osteomalacia; muscular hypotony; hyporeflexia; hyperactivity with bizarre choreoathetoid movements and screaming.

Laboratory

Urine—aminoaciduria, proteinuria, calciuria, phosphaturia; serum-elevated acid phosphate; imaging studies—brain magnetic resonance imaging (MRI)—mild ventriculomegaly (one-third cases); ocular ultrasound—if dense cataract, rule out mass or retinal detachment posterior.

Treatment

Monitor and treat for glaucoma. If glaucoma develops, intraocular pressure lowering agents must be used. Often, these patients require surgical intervention with goniotomy, trabeculotomy, or a drainage filtration device. Congenital cataracts should be removed, ideally in the first 6 weeks of life, to optimize the visual potential.

BIBLIOGRAPHY

1. Alcorn DM. (2012). Oculocerebrorenal syndrome. [online] Available from www.emedicine.com/oph/TOPIC516.HTM. [Accessed July, 2013].

2. ML I (MUCOLIPIDOSIS I; LIPOMUCOPOLYSACCHARIDOSIS; DYSMORPHIC SIALIDOSIS; SPRANGER SYNDROME)

General

Rare storage disease; autosomal recessive; increased sialic acid and deficiency of the enzyme alpha-N-acetyl-neuraminidase in cultured mucolipidosis I fibroblasts.

Ocular

Variable corneal clouding; macular cherry-red spot; optic atrophy; lens opacity; pupillary reflexes anomaly; grayish area around cherry-red spot.

Clinical

Moderate progressive mental retardation; skeletal changes of dysostosis multiplex; peripheral neuropathy; myoclonic jerks; tremor; cerebellar signs; gait abnormalities.

Laboratory

Detecting deficiency of alpha-N-acetylneuraminidase activity.

Treatment

Limited only to supportive care and symptomatic relief.

⊟ BIBLIOGRAPHY

1. Roth KS, Rizzo WB, McGovern MM. (2012). Sialidosis (Mucolipidosis I). Available from www.emedicine.com/ped/TOPIC2093.HTM. [Accessed July, 2013].

⊟ 3. TYROSINOSIS (HANHART SYNDROME; RICHNER SYNDROME; RECESSIVE KERATOSIS PALMOPLANTARIS; PSEUDOHERPETIC KERATITIS; RICHNER-HANHART SYNDROME; TYROSINEMIA II; PSEUDODENDRITIC KERATITIS)

General

Autosomal recessive; consanguinity.

Ocular

Excess tearing; photophobia; dendritic lesions of the cornea with corneal sensitivity not affected; keratitis; papillary hypertrophy of conjunctiva; corneal haze; neovascularization of cornea; cataract; nystagmus.

Clinical

Dyskeratosis palmoplantaris; diffuse keratosis; dystrophy of nails; hypotrichosis; mental retardation (usually pronounced); sensorineural hearing loss.

Laboratory

Serum-plasma tyrosine 16–62 mg/dL; urine-tyrosinuria and tyrosyluria; liver biopsy—decreased cytoplasmic tyrosine aminotransferase (cTAT) activity.

Treatment

Topical keratolytics, topical retinoids, potent topical steroids with or without keratolytics in dermatoses with an inflammatory component.

⊟ BIBLIOGRAPHY

1. Lee RA, Yassaee M, Bowe WP, et al. (2011). Keratosis Palmaris et Plantaris. [online] www.emedicine.com/derm/TOPIC589.HTM. [Accessed July, 2013].

CHAPTER
5

Disorders of Carbohydrate Metabolism

1. DIABETES MELLITUS

General

Complex disorder of carbohydrate, lipid and protein metabolism characterized by hyperglycemia and a relative or total lack of insulin. Development is influenced by both genetic and environmental factors. Most commonly occurs in middle or late life (type II) and is seen most commonly in the obese. Diabetes can occur in the first or second decade of life (type I) and usually involves the lack of insulin production by the pancreas and the need for insulin therapy.

Clinical

Atherosclerosis; nephropathy; neuropathy; polyuria; polydipsia; polyphagia; obesity; elevated plasma glucose and elevated glycated hemoglobin (A1C).

Ocular

Diabetic retinopathy; vitreous hemorrhage; macular edema; cataract; glaucoma; asteroid hyalosis; extraocular muscle paralysis; rubeosis iridis; corneal hypesthesia; optic nerve atrophy; papillopathy.

Laboratory

Diagnosis made by fasting plasma glucose of greater than 126 mg/dL and 2 hours post glucose load (75 g) plasma glucose of greater than 200 mg/dL and confirmed by repeat test.

Treatment

Goals include elimination of symptoms, by reduction of blood sugar and blood pressure. Smoking cessation, aspirin therapy, weight loss, exercise, diabetic diet as well as oral medication and/or insulin are all used in the treatment of diabetes. Diabetic retinopathy is most successfully treated with retinal photocoagulation. Pars plana vitrectomy is sometimes necessary to remove vitreous hemorrhage. Other ocular problems caused by diabetes such as cataracts and glaucoma are treated in traditional methods.

BIBLIOGRAPHY

1. Khardori R. (2012). Type 2 diabetes mellitus. [online] Available from emedicine.medscape.com/article/117853-overview. [Accessed July, 2013].

2. FANCONI SYNDROME (TONI-FANCONI SYNDROME; AMINO DIABETES; HYPOCHLOREMIC-GLYCOSURIC OSTEONEPHROPATHY SYNDROME; DE TONI-FANCONI SYNDROME)

General

Autosomal recessive inheritance; hematologic manifestations mainly in young patients; in adults the syndrome resembles milkman syndrome with disorder of calcium and phosphorus metabolism; chronic organic acidosis in Fanconi syndrome due to an inborn error of protein metabolism.

Ocular

Massive retinal hemorrhage may be present secondary to blood dyscrasia; bilateral anterior uveitis.

Clinical

Ecchymoses and mucous membrane hemorrhages; skin hyperpigmentation; osteomalacia; pseudofractures; deformities of radius and absence of thumbs; hypophosphatemia.

Laboratory

Diagnosis is made by clinical findings.

Treatment

Treat the underlying cause as quickly as possible; vitrectomy.

BIBLIOGRAPHY

1. Fanconi G, Turler U. Kogenitale Kleinhirnatrophie mit Supranuklearen Storungen der Motilitat der Augenmuskein. Helv Paediatr Acta. 1951;6:475–83.
2. Geeraets WJ. Ocular Syndromes, 3rd edition. Philadelphia: Lea & Febiger; 1976.
3. Tsilou ET, Giri N, Weinstein S, et al. Ocular and orbital manifestations of the inherited bone marrow failure syndromes: Fanconi anemia and dyskeratosis congenita. Ophthalmology. 2010;117:615–22.

3. HUNTER SYNDROME (MPS II SYNDROME; MUCOPOLYSACCHARIDOSIS II; SYSTEMIC MUCOPOLYSACCHARIDOSIS TYPE II)

General

Sex-linked recessive inheritance; clinically less severe than Hurler syndrome (MPS I) with a longer life span (into adulthood); similar to MPS I (Hurler syndrome), with chondroitin sulfate B and heparitin sulfate excreted in excess in the urine (*see* Sanfilippo-Good Syndrome; Morquio-Brailsford Syndrome; Scheie Syndrome; Maroteaux-Lamy Syndrome); X-linked recessive inheritance; decreased iduronate sulfatase.

Ocular

Visual fields may be constricted; splitting or absence of Bowman membrane in the periphery; stromal haze may be present; pigmentary degeneration of the retina; night blindness; narrowed retinal vessels and central choroidal sclerosis; bushy eyebrows; coarse eyelashes; ptosis; optic atrophy; papilledema; proptosis; angle-closure glaucoma; corneal clouding; scleral thickening; uveal effusion.

Clinical

Dwarfism; stiff joints; hepatosplenomegaly; gargoyle-like facies.

Laboratory

Urine-dermatan and heparin sulfate; serum-assay of iduronate 2-sulfatase (IDS) activity; assay for activity of sulfoiduronate sulfatase in fibroblasts.

Treatment

The relevant enzyme (IDS in the case of MPS type II) can be given in the form of enzyme replacement therapy (ERT) or by bone marrow transplantation (BMT); surgical intervention for chronic hydrocephalus, nerve entrapment (carpal tunnel syndrome), abdominal wall hernias, tracheostomy, and joint contractures.

BIBLIOGRAPHY

1. Braverman NE, Fenton CL, Conover-Walker MK. (2011). Genetics of Mucopolysaccharidosis Type II. Available from www.emedicine.com/ped/TOPIC1029.HTM. [Accessed July, 2013].

4. HURLER SYNDROME (PFAUNDLER-HURLER SYNDROME; GARGOYLISM; DYSOSTOSIS MULTIPLEX; MPS IH SYNDROME; SYSTEMIC MUCOPOLYSACCHARIDOSIS TYPE IH; MUCOPOLYSACCHARIDOSIS IH)

General

Autosomal recessive inheritance; in addition to corneal opacities and enlargement of the head at birth, other symptoms become apparent at the end of the first year; death occurs usually before 20 years; gross excess of chondroitin sulfate band, heparitin sulfate in the urine (*see* Hunter Syndrome; Sanfilippo-Good Syndrome; Morquio-Brailsford Syndrome; Scheie Syndrome; Maroteaux-Lamy Syndrome). Jensen suggested that the pathogenesis of the various mucopolysaccharidoses is the same but that the variations in the defective enzymes cause the different types; most common mucopolysaccharidosis (MPS), decreased iduronidase.

Ocular

Proptosis; hypertelorism; thick, enlarged lids; esotropia; diffuse haziness of the cornea at birth progressive to milky opacity; retinal pigmentary changes may exist; macular edema and absence of foveal reflex; optic atrophy; megalocornea; bushy eyebrows; coarse eyelashes; mucopolysaccharide deposits of iris, lens, and sclera; enlarged optic foramen; retinal detachment; anisocoria; buphthalmos; nystagmus; secondary open-angle glaucoma; progressive retinopathy with vascular narrowing; hyperpigmentation of the fundus; bone spicule; papilledema.

Clinical

Dorsolumbar kyphosis; head deformities with depressed nose bridge; short cervical spine; short limbs; macroglossia; enlarged liver and spleen; short stature; facial dysmorphism; progressive psychomotor retardation.

Laboratory

Blood smears-abnormal cytoplasmic inclusions in lymphocytes; urine: increased excretion of dermatan sulfate and heparin sulfate.

Treatment

- *Macular edema*: Use of corticosteroids, carbonic anhydrase inhibitors and nonsteroidal anti-inflammatory drugs (NSAIDs) are the mainstay of treatment. If traditional therapy is not effective, intraocular injections of Avastin® may be helpful. In cases that have vitreous strand tugging against the macula, pars plana vitrectomy may be necessary.
- *Retinal detachment*: Scleral buckle, pneumatic retinopexy and vitrectomy may be used to close all the breaks.
- *Glaucoma*: Glaucoma medication should be the first plan of action. If medication is unsuccessful, a filtering surgical procedure with or without antimetabolites may be beneficial.
- *Papilledema*: Underlying cause should be determined and treated. Systemic acetazolamide is the medical therapy of choice.

BIBLIOGRAPHY

1. Banikazemi M. (2012). Genetics of Mucopolysaccharidosis Type I. [online] Available from www.emedicine.com/ped/TOPIC1031.HTM. [Accessed July, 2013].

5. JUVENILE DIABETES-DWARFISM-OBESITY SYNDROME (MAURIAC SYNDROME; DWARFISM-HEPATOMEGALY-OBESITY-JUVENILE DIABETES SYNDROME)

General

Etiology is obscure, although nutritional deficiencies, metabolic disorders and deficiency of insulin have been considered; develops slowly, with slow growth and difficulties in management of diabetic condition.

Ocular

Cataract; diabetic retinopathy with retinal hemorrhages, exudates, microaneurysms, neovascularization, vaso-glial proliferation (grades I to IV diabetic retinopathy; hypertensive retinopathy); occasional optic neuritis.

Clinical

Hepatomegaly; diminished growth; osteoporosis; hypertension; arteriosclerosis; obesity (with moon face); juvenile diabetes; abdominal colic.

Laboratory

Random plasma glucose level of greater than 200 mg/dL is adequate to establish the diagnosis of diabetes.

Treatment

Insulin therapy, self-monitor blood glucose levels, diabetic diet and education.

⬚ BIBLIOGRAPHY

1. Khardori R. (2012). Type 1 Diabetes Mellitus. [online] Available from www.emedicine.com/emerg/TOPIC133.HTM. [Accessed July, 2013].

⬚ 6. KIMMELSTIEL-WILSON SYNDROME (DIABETES MELLITUS-HYPERTENSION-NEPHROSIS SYNDROME; DIABETES-NEPHROSIS SYNDROME; DIABETIC GLOMERULOSCLEROSIS; INTERCAPILLARY GLOMERULOSCLEROSIS; RENAL GLOMERULOHYALINOSIS-DIABETIC SYNDROME)

General

Occurs in patients with diabetes mellitus of several years' duration.

Ocular

Retinal lesions, including hemorrhages, exudates, and neovascularization.

Clinical

Hypertension; proteinuria; edema; glomerulonephrosis; arteriosclerosis; capillary or intercapillary glomerulosclerosis; eosinophilic nodules; hyaline degeneration of the renal arterioles.

Laboratory

Serum—hyperglycemia; urine—glycosuria

Treatment

Pharmacologic therapy allowing glycemic control, diet modification and weight loss are the main therapies for diabetes.

⬚ BIBLIOGRAPHY

1. Khardori R. (2012). Type 2 diabetes mellitus. [online]. Available from www.emedicine.com/med/TOPIC547.HTM. [Accessed July, 2013].

⬚ 7. MARQUARDT-LORIAUX SYNDROME (WOLFRAM SYNDROME; DIABETES INSIPIDUS-DIABETES MELLITUS-OPTIC ATROPHY-DEAFNESS SYNDROME; DIDMOAD SYNDROME)

General

Autosomal recessive; present from childhood; age of onset varies.

Ocular

Optic nerve atrophy; color blindness; visual field defects; anisocoria; diabetic retinopathy; nystagmus; cataract; pigmentation of retina.

Clinical

Juvenile diabetes mellitus; diabetes insipidus; neurosensory hearing loss; hypertension; cerebellar dysfunction; vertigo; atony of urinary tract; anosmia; peripheral neuropathy; mitochondrial abnormalities; moderate hearing loss.

Laboratory

Diagnosis is made by clinical findings.

Treatment

Optic nerve atrophy: Intravenous steroids may be used with optic neuritis or ischemic neuropathy. Stem cell treatment may be the future treatment of choice.

🖶 BIBLIOGRAPHY

1. Bundey S, Poulton K, Whitwell H, et al. Mitochondrial abnormalities in the DIDMOAD syndrome. J Inherit Metab Dis. 1992;15:315–9.

2. Higashi K. Otologic findings of DIDMOAD syndrome. Am J Otol. 1991;12:57–60.
3. Mtanda AT, Cruysberg JR, Pinckers AJ. Optic atrophy in Wolfram syndrome. Ophthalmol Paediatr Genet. 1986;7:159–65.
4. Niemeyer G, Marquardt JL. Retinal function in an unique syndrome of optic atrophy, juvenile diabetes mellitus, diabetes insipidus, neurosensory hearing loss, autonomic dysfunction, and hyperalanineuria. Invest Ophthalmol. 1972;11:617–24.
5. Wolfram DJ. Diabetes mellitus and simple optic atrophy among siblings: report of four cases. Mayo Clin Proc. 1938;13:715.

🖶 8. MUCOPOLYSACCHARIDOSIS VII (BETA-GLUCURONIDASE DEFICIENCY; MPS VII)

General

Autosomal recessive disorder associated with enzyme deficiency of β-glucuronidase; disorder combines clinical and biochemical features of the Morquio and Sanfilippo syndromes.

Ocular

Clouding of the cornea.

Clinical

Dwarfism; hepatosplenomegaly; skeletal deformity; mental retardation; hernias; unusual facies; delayed psychomotor development; frequent symptomatic pulmonary infections.

Laboratory

Urine—elevated glycosaminoglycans and oligosaccharides; blood—vacuoles in lymphocytes and fibroblasts. Metachromatic granular inclusions (Alder bodies) in leukocytes.

Treatment

No treatment is available for the underlying disorder, and care must be supportive.

🖶 BIBLIOGRAPHY

1. Banikazemi M, Varma S. (2011). Genetics of Mucopolysaccharidosis Type VII. [online] Available from www.emedicine.com/ped/TOPIC858.HTM. [Accessed July, 2013].

🖶 9. SANFILIPPO-GOOD SYNDROME (HEPARITINURIA; MUCOPOLYSACCHARIDOSIS III; MPS III)

General

Autosomal recessive; excess urinary excretion of heparitin sulfate (*see* Hunter Syndrome; Hurler Syndrome; Maroteaux-Lamy Syndrome; Morquio Syndrome; Scheie Syndrome). Lack of a β-galactosaminidase-like enzyme causing accumulation of glycolipids, acid mucopolysaccharides, and their precursors; both sexes affected; death occurs by second decade in the majority of cases; autosomal recessive; divided into type A (with decreased levels of heparan sulfatase) and type B (with decreased levels of N-acetyl-a-D-glucosaminidase).

Ocular

Night blindness; slight narrowing of retinal vessels; pigment deposits in the fundi; bushy eyebrows; coarse eyelashes; acid mucopolysaccharide deposits in cornea, iris, lens, and sclera; retinal degeneration; optic nerve atrophy.

Clinical

Mental deficiency progressing to severe degrees within a few years; seizures; gargoyle features very mild; dwarfism; stiff joints; hepatosplenomegaly; hirsutism; mitral valve insufficiency.

Laboratory

Urine—excessive heparin sulfate MPS urine spot test is positive.

Treatment

Bone marrow transplant improves systemic health but there is no therapy to prevent long-term function.

BIBLIOGRAPHY

1. Bittar T, Washington ER. (2012). Mucopolysaccharidosis. [online] Available from www.emedicine.com/orthoped/TOPIC203.HTM. [Accessed July, 2013].

10. SCHEIE SYNDROME (MUCOPOLYSACCHARIDOSIS IS; MPS IS;MPS V; MUCOPOLYSACCHARIDOSIS V)

General

Autosomal recessive; chondroitin sulfate B excreted in excess in the urine; formerly MPS V (*see* Hurler Syndrome; Hunter Syndrome; Sanfilippo-Good Syndrome; Morquio Syndrome; Maroteaux-Lamy Syndrome). Both sexes affected; deficiency of a-L-iduronidase; increased urinary dermatan and heparan sulfate; fibrous long-spacing collagen on histopathologic examination; least severe form of MPS.

Ocular

Night blindness; fields may show general constriction; ring scotoma; diffuse corneal haze to marked corneal clouding (progressive); bushy eyebrows; coarse eyelashes; optic atrophy; anisocoria; cataracts; proptosis; acid mucopolysaccharide deposits in the iris and sclera; tapetoretinal degeneration; glaucoma.

Clinical

Normal intelligence; broad facies; thickened joints; aortic valvular disease; psychosis; claw hand; carpal tunnel syndrome; excessive body hair; progressive juxta-articular cystic lesions.

Laboratory

Thin layer chromatography and radiography.

Treatment

Enzyme replacement therapy—patients with joint contractures may need surgery. Corneal transplant may be necessary if vision problems are severe.

BIBLIOGRAPHY

1. Banikazemi M. (2012). Genetics of Mucopolysaccharidosis Type I. [online] Available from www.emedicine.com/ped/TOPIC2052.HTM. [Accessed July, 2013].

11. SPONDYLOEPIPHYSEAL DYSPLASIA (MORQUIO SYNDROME; MORQUIO-BRAILSFORD SYNDROME; BRAILSFORD-MORQUIO DYSTROPHY; FAMILIAL OSSEOUS DYSTROPHY; KERATOSULFATURIA; MPS IV; MUCOPOLYSACCHARIDOSIS IV; OSTEOCHONDRODYSTROPHIA DEFORMANS; INFANTILE HEREDITARY CHONDRODYSPLASIA; HEREDITARY POLYTOPIC ENCHONDRAL DYSOSTOSIS; HEREDITARY OSTEOCHONDRODYSTROPHY; ECCENTRO-OSTEOCHONDRODYSPLASIA; DYSOSTOSIS ENCHONDRALIS META-EPIPHYSARIA; MORQUIO-ULLRICH SYNDROME; ATYPICAL CHONDRODYSTROPHY; CHONDRODYSTROPHIA TARDA; CHONDRO-OSTEODYSTROPHY)

General

Autosomal recessive dystrophy of cartilage and bone; slight predilection for males; apparent between ages 4 and 10 years; excess production of keratosulfate (*see* Hurler Syndrome; Hunter Syndrome; Sanfilippo-Good Syndrome; Scheie Syndrome; Maroteaux-Lamy Syndrome); autosomal recessive; abnormal N-acetylgalactosamine-G-sulfate sulfatase.

Ocular

Enophthalmos; ptosis; excessive tear secretion; ocular hypotony; miosis; occasionally hazy cornea; bushy eyebrows; optic nerve atrophy; moderate-to-late corneal clouding.

Clinical

Dwarfism; skeletal deformities (progressive); delayed ossification of epiphyses; decreased muscle tone; deafness; weak extremities; waddling gait; coarse broad mouth; spaced teeth; aortic regurgitation; normal intelligence.

Laboratory

Blood-Reilly's granules in leukocytes; X-ray—flat vertebrae and odontoid hypoplasia.

Treatment

Treatment is limited to supportive care.

BIBLIOGRAPHY

1. Bittar T, Washington ER. (2012). Mucopolysaccharidosis. [online] Available from www.emedicine.com/orthoped/TOPIC203.HTM. [Accessed July, 2013].

12. SYSTEMIC MUCOPOLYSACCHARIDOSIS TYPE VI (MUCOPOLYSACCHARIDOSIS VI; MAROTEAUX-LAMY SYNDROME; MPS VI SYNDROME)

General

Onset in infancy; etiology unknown; autosomal recessive; excessive urinary excretion of chondroitin sulfate B; lysosomal storage disease; deficiency of the enzyme arylsulfatase B; multiple clinical phenotypes.

Ocular

Corneal haziness and opacities; pupillary membrane remnants.

Clinical

Skeleton deformities; restriction of articular movements; dyspnea; heart murmur; hearing impairment.

Laboratory

Urine—excessive glycosaminoglycan dermatan sulfate or chondroitin sulfate B.

Treatment

Enzyme replacement, bone marrow transplant and stem cell therapy is in the experimental.

BIBLIOGRAPHY

1. Roy FH, Fraunfelder FT, Fraunfelder FW. Current Ocular Therapy, 6th edition. Philadelphia: WB Saunders; 2008.
2. Kenyon KR, Topping TM, Green WR, et al. Ocular pathology of the Maroteaux-Lamy syndrome (systemic mucopolysaccharidosis type VI). Histologic and ultrastructural report of two cases. Am J Ophthalmol. 1972;73:718–41.
3. Matalon R, Arbogast B, Dorfman A, et al. Deficiency of chondroitin sulfate N-acetylgalactosamine 4-sulfate sulfatase in Maroteaux-Lamy syndrome. Biochem Biophys Res Commun. 1974;61:1450–7.
4. Quigley HA, Kenyon KR. Ultrastructural and histochemical studies of a newly recognized form of systemic mucopolysaccharidosis (Maroteaux-Lamy syndrome, mild phenotype). Am J Ophthalmol. 1974;77:809–18.
5. Voskoboeva E, Isbrandt D, von Figura K, et al. Four novel mutant alleles of the arylsulfatase B gene in two patients with intermediate form of mucopolysaccharidosis VI (Maroteaux-Lamy syndrome). Hum Genet. 1994;93:259–64.

☐ 13. TROPICAL PANCREATIC DIABETES (TPD) (BACKGROUND RETINOPATHY)

General

Secondary diabetes as a result of chronic calcific pancreatitis; limited geographically to a few tropical countries; highest prevalence in southern India; male predominance; onset at young age; associated with protein calorie malnutrition; possible cause is cassava ingestion; malnutrition has been postulated as a possible etiology.

Ocular

Background retinopathy; proliferative retinopathy; fibrous retinitis proliferans; microaneurysms; macular edema; hemorrhages; exudates; decreased visual acuity.

Clinical

Chronic pancreatitis; recurrent abdominal pain; steatorrhea.

Laboratory/ocular

Fasting glucose and hemoglobin A1C.

Treatment/ocular

Laser photocoagulation.

☐ BIBLIOGRAPHY

1. Bhavsar AR, Atebara NH, Drouilhet JH. (2012). Diabetic retinopathy. [online] www.emedicine.com/oph/TOPIC414.HTM. [Accessed July, 2013].

☐ 14. VON REUSS SYNDROME (GALACTOSEMIC SYNDROME; GALACTOKINASE DEFICIENCY; GALACTOSEMIA), NYSTAGMUS

General

Autosomal recessive; consanguinity; conversion of galactose into glucose is blocked, leading to galactosemia; onset after a few days or weeks of milk ingestion; deficiency of galactose-1-phosphate uridyltransferase.

Ocular

Searching-type nystagmus; bilateral nuclear or cortical cataracts appear clinically as oil droplets; bilateral zonular cataracts with fine punctate opacities in the lens periphery.

Clinical

Vomiting; refusal of food; diarrhea; weight loss; hepatomegaly with ascites; jaundice; galactosuria; aminoaciduria; dehydration; hypoglycemic crisis; failure to thrive; hypotonia; lethargy; severe mental and neurologic manifestations.

Laboratory

Test for galactosuria and aminoaciduria.

Treatment

Dietary and cataract treatment as needed.

☐ BIBLIOGRAPHY

1. Cordes FC. Galactosemia cataract: a review. Am J Ophthalmol. 1960;50:1151.
2. Fraunfelder FT, Roy FH. Current Ocular Therapy, 6th edition. Philadelphia: WB Saunders; 2008.
3. Lerman S. The lens in congenital galactosemia. Arch Ophthalmol. 1959;61:88–92.
4. Okajima K, Yazaki M, Wada Y. Thymidase-kinase activity in individuals with galactokinase deficiency. Am J Hum Genet. 1987;41:503–4.

CHAPTER
6

Disorders of Lipid Metabolism

⊟ 1. FABRY DISEASE (ANGIOKERATOMA CORPORIS DIFFUSUM SYNDROME; DIFFUSE ANGIOKERATOSIS; FABRY-ANDERSON SYNDROME; GLYCOSPHINGOLIPID LIPIDOSIS; GLYCOSPHINGOLIPIDOSIS)

General

Lipoid storage disorder; X-linked recessive inheritance; lack of α-galactosidase A enzyme.

Ocular

Swelling of eyelids; varicosities of palpebral and bulbar conjunctiva; corneal dystrophy; corneal opacities; increased tortuosity of retinal vessels and aneurysmal dilatations; cornea verticillata; cataract; central retinal artery occlusion; internuclear paralysis of extraocular muscles; papilledema; tortuosity and caliber irregularity of conjunctival vessels; characteristic cream-colored whorl-like opacity in deep part of corneal epithelium; posterior cataract; occasional edema of optic disk and retina.

Clinical

Angiokeratoma of the skin with small, grouped papular lesions mainly over the scrotum, thighs, buttocks, sacral area, umbilical area, and lips; elevated blood pressure; disturbance in sweat secretion; pain in arms and legs; enlarged heart; albuminuria.

Laboratory

Reduced α-galactosidase A level in plasma; elevated trihexosyl ceramide levels in urine and plasma.

Treatment

Primarily surgical and is usually a corneal transplant. After surgery, treatment of amblyopia and optical therapy can be helpful.

⊟ BIBLIOGRAPHY

1. Banikazemi M, Desnick RJ, Astrin KH. (2012). Genetics of Fabry disease. [online] Available from www.emedicine.com/ped/TOPIC2888.HTM. [Accessed July, 2013].

⊟ 2. HYPERLIPOPROTEINEMIA

General

Metabolic disorder characterized by abnormally elevated concentrations of specific lipoprotein particles in the plasma.

Ocular

Arcus; lipid keratopathy; xanthelasma; lipemia retinalis; lipemia of limbal vessels; xanthomata of choroid, conjunctiva, eyelids, iris, and retina; central retinal vein occlusion; Schnyder crystalline corneal dystrophy (association).

Clinical

Deposition of lipids at various sites throughout the body, such as skin, tendons, and vascular system.

Laboratory

Serum-lipid profile consists of total cholesterol, triglycerides and high-density lipoprotein (HDL)-cholesterol to detect hyperlipoproteinemia; measure plasma lipid and lipoprotein levels while the patient is on a regular diet after an overnight fast of 12–16 hours.

Treatment

Drugs are used to lower cholesterol and triglyceride levels.

⊟ BIBLIOGRAPHY

1. Roy H. (2011). Hyperlipoproteinemia. [online] Available from www.emedicine.com/oph/TOPIC505.HTM. [Accessed July, 2013].

CHAPTER 7

Hematologic and Cardiovascular Disorders

⊟ 1. CAROTID ARTERY SYNDROME (CAVERNOUS SINUS FISTULA SYNDROME; RED-EYED SHUNT SYNDROME)

General

Seventy-five percent of cases caused by trauma; others occur spontaneously or are congenital; fistula from carotid artery to cavernous sinus.

Ocular

Progressive, pulsating exophthalmos; distended pulsating superior orbital vein; venous congestion of lids; variable ophthalmoplegia, depending on involvement of cranial nerves III to VI; secondary glaucoma; congestion of conjunctiva with chemosis; corneal ulcerations; eversion of the lower lid; loss of corneal sensation; retinal edema; engorgement of retinal veins; papilledema; optic atrophy; ocular bruit that may be subjective and/or objective; diplopia; visual decrease; choroidal folds; dilated superior ophthalmic vein.

Clinical

Severe unilateral headache; buzzing noise.

Laboratory

Orbital ultrasonography, CT, six-vessel cranial digital subtraction angiography—characterization of the arterial supply and venous drainage of fistula.

Treatment

Use of intraocular pressure lowering agent and topical lubrication is the ocular treatment of choice.

⊟ BIBLIOGRAPHY

1. Dailey EJ, Holloway JA, Murto RE, et al. Evaluation of ocular signs and symptoms in cerebral aneurysms. Arch Ophthalmol. 1964;71:463-74.
2. Duane TD. Clinical Ophthalmology. Philadelphia: JB Lippincott; 1987.
3. Flaharty PM, Lieb WE, Sergott RC, et al. Color Doppler imaging. A new noninvasive technique to diagnose and monitor carotid cavernous sinus fistulas. Arch Ophthalmol. 1991;109:522-6.
4. Gonshor LG, Kline LB. Choroidal folds and dural cavernous sinus fistula. Arch Ophthalmol. 1991;109:1065-6.
5. Phelps CD, Thompson HS, Ossoinig KC. The diagnosis and prognosis of atypical carotid cavernous fistula. Am J Ophthalmol. 1982;93:423-36.
6. Roy FH, Fraunfelder FW, Fraunfelder FT. Current Ocular Therapy, 6th edition. Philadelphia: WB Saunders; 2008.
7. Travers B. A case of aneurysm by anastomosis in the orbit, cured by ligation of common carotid artery. Med Chir Trans. 1917;2:1-420.

⧉ 2. CAROTID ARTERY SYNDROME (CAROTID VASCULAR INSUFFICIENCY SYNDROME; OCULAR ISCHEMIC SYNDROME)

General

Causes include microemboli, atherosclerotic plaques, arteritis, arterial compression by cicatricial tissue surrounding the vessel, and tumors; male preponderance; onset between ages 50 and 70 years.

Ocular

Lacrimation; homolateral transient, painless visual loss; photopsia; hemianopsia; retinal infarcts; cholesterol plaques may be seen in retinal arteries on funduscopic examination; optic atrophy; hypoxic retinopathy; low-tension glaucoma; anterior uveitis; cataract; visual acuity 20/400 or less; iris neovascularization; angle neovascularization; optic disk pale; retinal hemorrhages; Homer syndrome; amaurosis fugax; retinal artery occlusion; ophthalmoparesis; proptosis; chemosis; conjunctival hyperemia; acute orbital infarction.

Clinical

Transient cerebral ischemia with contralateral weakness of arm and leg; hemisensory disturbances; mental confusion and dysphasia; headache; dizziness; epileptiform seizures; carotid dissection.

Laboratory

Erythrocyte sedimentation rate and C-reactive protein levels in patients with suspected giant cell arteritis (GCA); fluorescein angiography.

Treatment

Panretinal photocoagulation to treat neovascularization of the iris, optic nerve, or retina. It was reported to cause regression of neovascularization. Antiplatelet therapy may be useful. Carotid endarterectomy has shown to benefit symptomatic patients.

⧉ BIBLIOGRAPHY

1. Leibovitch I, Calonje D, El-Harazi SM. (2011). Ocular ischemic syndrome. [online] Available from www.emedicine.com/oph/TOPIC487.HTM. [Accessed July, 2013].

⧉ 3. FORAMEN LACERUM SYNDROME (ANEURYSM OF INTERNAL CAROTID ARTERY SYNDROME)

General

Most commonly caused by congenital aneurysm involving the intradural portion of the carotid artery.

Ocular

Periorbital pain; ptosis; oculomotor paralysis with ptosis, diplopia, and internal ophthalmoplegia; cranial nerves IV and VI may be involved; homonymous hemianopia (occasionally); loss of pupillary reflexes for light and accommodation; papilledema; optic atrophy.

Clinical

Meningism; mental disturbances; unilateral frontal or orbital headache; migraine attacks.

Laboratory

Computed tomography (CT); magnetic resonance imaging (MRI); angiography; magnetic resonance angiography (MRA).

Treatment

Endovascular balloon occlusion.

⧉ BIBLIOGRAPHY

1. Dailey EJ, Holloway JA, Murto RE, et al. Evaluation of ocular signs and symptoms in cerebral aneurysms. Arch Ophthalmol. 1964;71:463-74.
2. Geeraets WJ. Ocular Syndromes. 3rd edition. Philadelphia: Lea & Febiger; 1976.
3. Misra M, Mohanty AB, Rath S. et al. Giant aneurysm of internal carotid artery presenting features of retrobulbar neuritis. Indian J Ophthalmol. 1991;39:28-9.

4. HERRICK SYNDROME (DRESBACH SYNDROME; SICKLE CELL DISEASE; DREPANOCYTIC ANEMIA)

General

Usually occurs in members of the black race; poor prognosis.

Ocular

Secondary glaucoma; telangiectasia of conjunctival vessels; scleral icterus; vitreous hemorrhages; cataract; retinal hemorrhages; exudates, and neovascularization; retinitis proliferans; microaneurysms; thrombosis of retinal venules; retinal vascular sheathing; central vein occlusion; angioid streaks; retinopathy with "black sunburst sign" in patients with SS hemoglobin; "sea-fan sign" in patients with SC hemoglobin; comma signs of conjunctiva; fan-shaped neovascularization of iris; sector ischemic atrophy of iris; optic atrophy; white cotton mass of vitreous; retinal holes; color vision defects; central retinal artery obstruction; branch retinal artery obstruction; white without pressure; venous tortuosity; sickling maculopathy.

Clinical

Severe anemia with hemolytic crises; bone and joint aches; hemarthrosis; jaundice; hepatosplenomegaly.

Laboratory

Blood-sickling of red blood cells, newborn screening for hemoglobin disorders.

Treatment

Transfusion is required in an aplastic crisis; erythrocytapheresis is an automated red-cell exchange and bone marrow transplantation may be useful. Pain is the hallmark of sickle cell disease. While frequency and severity vary greatly, most patients have interval symptoms. Once pain has begun, no therapy reverses the process. Analgesics may provide a reasonable degree of comfort. While certain dosing guidelines are available, the amount of drug given should be titrated to the degree of pain experienced. Vitrectomy may be necessary.

BIBLIOGRAPHY

1. Maakaron JE, Taher A, Woermann UJ. (2012). Sickle cell anemia. [online] Available from www.emedicine.com/ped/TOPIC2096.HTM. [Accessed July, 2013].

5. SCHEIE SYNDROME (MUCOPOLYSACCHARIDOSIS IS; MPS IS; MPS V; MUCOPOLYSACCHARIDOSIS V)

General

Autosomal recessive; chondroitin sulfate B excreted in excess in the urine; formerly MPS V (*see* Hurler Syndrome; Hunter Syndrome; Sanfilippo-Good Syndrome; Morquio Syndrome; Maroteaux-Lamy Syndrome). Both sexes affected; deficiency of a-L-iduronidase; increased urinary dermatan and heparan sulfate; fibrous long-spacing collagen on histopathologic examination; least severe form of MPS.

Ocular

Night blindness; fields may show general constriction; ring scotoma; diffuse corneal haze to marked corneal clouding (progressive); bushy eyebrows; coarse eyelashes; optic atrophy; anisocoria; cataracts; proptosis; acid mucopolysaccharide deposits in the iris and sclera; tapetoretinal degeneration; glaucoma.

Clinical

Normal intelligence; broad facies; thickened joints; aortic valvular disease; psychosis; claw hand; carpal tunnel syndrome; excessive body hair; progressive juxta-articular cystic lesions.

Laboratory

Thin layer chromatography and radiography.

Treatment

Enzyme replacement therapy—patients with joint contractures may need surgery. Corneal transplant may be necessary if vision problems are severe.

BIBLIOGRAPHY

1. Banikazemi M. (2012). Genetics of Mucopolysaccharidosis Type I. [online] Available from www.emedicine.com/ped/TOPIC2052.HTM. [Accessed July, 2013].

6. THALASSEMIA (COOLEY ANEMIA; THALASSEMIA MAJOR; THALASSEMIA MINOR)

General

Autosomal dominant in synthesis of α or β chain of hemoglobin; most prevalent in Mediterranean and Oriental populations.

Ocular

Retinal hemorrhages; angioid streaks; macular vascular abnormalities; pigmented chorioretinal scars (black sunbursts); occlusion of peripheral retinal arteries; vitreous hemorrhages.

Clinical

Hemolytic anemia; hypochromic anemia.

Laboratory

Blood—hypochromic, microcystic anemia.

Treatment

Goals of medical therapy are correction of anemia, suppression of erythropoiesis, and inhibition of increased gastrointestinal (GI) iron.

BIBLIOGRAPHY

1. Takeshita K. (2012). Beta thalassemia. [online]. Available from www.emedicine.com/med/TOPIC438.HTM. [Accessed July, 2013].

7. VAQUEZ DISEASE (POLYCYTHEMIA VERA; ERYTHEMA; ERYTHROCYTOSIS MEGALOSPLENICA; MYELOPATHIC POLYCYTHEMIA; VAQUEZ-OSLER SYNDROME; CRYPTOGENIC POLYCYTHEMIA; POLYCYTHEMIA RUBRA; SPLENOMEGALIC POLYCYTHEMIA)

General

Increased number of red blood cells; myeloproliferative disorder.

Ocular

Conjunctival vascular engorgement; dilated tortuous retinal veins; retinal hemorrhages; optic disk edema; central retinal vein occlusion; visual field defects; visual hallucinations; diplopia.

Clinical

Elevated red blood cells; systemic vascular congestion; leukocytosis; thrombocytosis; central nervous system involvement; splenomegaly; hepatomegaly; bleeding diathesis; gingival/mucosal bleeding; ecchymosis; epistaxis; neurologic abnormal dizziness; vertigo; ataxia.

Laboratory

The serum erythropoietin (Epo) level should be decreased in nearly all patients with polycythemia vera (PV) and no recent hemorrhage.

Treatment

Phlebotomy or bloodletting has been the mainstay of therapy.

BIBLIOGRAPHY

1. Besa EC, Woermann UJ. (2012). Polycythemia vera. [online] Available from www.emedicine.com/med/TOPIC1864.HTM. [Accessed July, 2013].

CHAPTER

8

Dermatologic Disorders

⊟ 1. ATOPIC DERMATITIS (ATOPIC ECZEMA; BESNIER PRURIGO)

General

Highly specific disease resulting from heredity determined lowered cutaneous threshold to pruritus and characterized by intense itching; elevated total and specific immunoglobulin E.

Ocular

Keratoconjunctivitis; keratoconus; cataract; atopic dermatitis of lid; secondary glaucoma; uveitis; possible association with retinal detachment; pannus; blepharo-conjunctivitis; corneal scarring; suppurative keratitis.

Clinical

In infants, it involves the face with dry or oozing erythematous patches; in children and adolescents, itching localized in the neck, antecubital spaces, popliteal folds, and ears; seborrheic changes.

Laboratory

Diagnosis is made by clinical findings.

Treatment

Topical corticosteroids are the mainstay of treatment. Adequate rehydration will minimize the direct effects of irritants and allergens on the skin and maximize the effect of topically applied therapies, thus decreasing the need for topical steroids.

⊟ BIBLIOGRAPHY

1. Schwartz AR. (2011). Pediatric atopic dermatitis. [online] Available from www.emedicine.com/ped/TOPIC2567.HTM. [Accessed July, 2013].

⊟ 2. BULLOUS ICHTHYOSIFORM ERYTHRODERMA (COLLODION BABY; CONGENITAL ICHTHYOSIS; EPIDERMOLYTIC HYPERKERATOSIS; ICHTHYOSIS; ICHTHYOSIS VULGARIS; LAMELLAR ICHTHYOSIS; NONBULLOUS ICHTHYOSIFORM ERYTHRODERMA; XERODERMA; X-LINKED ICHTHYOSIS)

General

Autosomal inherited disorder; affects both sexes; normal at birth; onset within first 7 days; X-linked; pathogenesis may be secondary to physicochemical changes of corneal tissues including accumulation of cholesterol sulfate.

Ocular

Keratopathy; corneal scarring; keratitis; conjunctivitis; lagophthalmos; photophobia; ectropion; lid erythema; lacrimation; keratoconus; deep corneal punctate/filiform lesions.

Clinical

At birth, the skin surface is moist, red and tender; within several days, thick scales form.

Laboratory

Diagnosis is made by clinical findings.

Treatment

Genetic counseling and prenatal diagnosis also can be offered. Newborns with denuded skin are at increased risk for infection, secondary sepsis, and electrolyte imbalance and should be transferred to the neonatal intensive care unit (NICU) for monitoring and treatment as needed.

⊟ BIBLIOGRAPHY

1. Chen TS, Metz BJ. (2012). Epidermolytic Hyperkeratosis (Bullous Congenital Ichthyosiform Erythroderma). [online] www.emedicine.com/derm/TOPIC590.HTM. [Accessed July, 2013].

⊟ 3. CONTACT DERMATITIS (DERMATITIS VENENATA)

General

Reaction of skin due to contact with foreign material; inflammatory disorder of the skin that may result from immunologic hypersensitivity (allergic contact dermatitis) or cutaneous injury not involving immunologic mechanisms (irritant contact dermatitis) from offending topical agents.

Ocular

Keratoconjunctivitis; chemosis; leukoma; corneal ulcer; pruritus of lids.

Clinical

Dermatitis; itching, erythema; vesiculation; edema with weeping and crusting.

Laboratory

Diagnosis is made by clinical findings.

Treatment

Adequate hygiene and avoidance of the contactant may be helpful. Many cases of localized mild contact dermatitis respond well to cool compresses and adequate wound care. Antibiotic therapy may be necessary for secondary infection. Low-strength topical steroids, such as hydrocortisone; may be effective in decreasing inflammation and symptoms associated with very mild contact dermatitis. Systemic steroids are the mainstay of therapy in acute episodes of severe extensive allergic contact dermatitis.

⊟ BIBLIOGRAPHY

1. Crowe MA. (2011). Pediatric Contact Dermatitis. [online] Available from www.emedicine.com/ped/TOPIC2569. HTM. [Accessed July, 2013].

⊟ 4. DERMATOSTOMATITIS [STEVENS-JOHNSON SYNDROME; ERYTHEMA MULTIFORME EXUDATIVUM; SYNDROMA MUCOCUTANEO-OCULARE; BAADER DERMATOSTOMATITIS SYNDROME; MUCOSAL-RESPIRATORY SYNDROME; FUCHS (2) SYNDROME; MUCOCUTANEOUS OCULAR SYNDROME]

General

Etiology unknown; affects all ages; most frequently seen between 1st decade and 3rd decades of life; prevalent in males; drugs are the most commonly identified etiologic factor in this condition.

Ocular

Hypopyon; iritis; keratitis; corneal ulcers; keratoconjunctivitis sicca; chemosis; conjunctivitis; widespread fibrinoid necrosis of conjunctival vessels; blepharitis; endophthalmitis; phthisis bulbi; uveitis; cataracts; pannus; optic neuritis; keratoconus; adenoviral conjunctivitis has been reported to have precipitated Stevens-Johnson syndrome; orbital cyst may be a complication.

Clinical

General malaise, headaches, chills and fever; severe skin and mucous membrane eruptions (erythema multiforme); dorsa of hands and feet are most frequently affected; rhinitis; balanitis; vulvovaginitis; urethritis (nonspecific); cystitis; patients with acquired immunodeficiency syndrome (AIDS) are at higher risk of developing Stevens-Johnson syndrome.

Laboratory

No laboratory tests are specific to Stevens-Johnson syndrome. Diagnosis is made from clinical findings.

Treatment

Systemic treatment with steroids is controversial. Antibiotics are used based on clinical course. Eyelid hygiene performed as needed.

BIBLIOGRAPHY

1. Plaza JA, Dronen SC, Foster J, et al. (2011). Erythema multiforme. [online] Available from www.emedicine.com/med/TOPIC727.HTM. [Accessed July, 2013].

5. DISSEMINATED LUPUS ERYTHEMATOSUS (SYSTEMIC LUPUS ERYTHEMATOSUS; LUPUS ERYTHEMATOSUS; KAPOSI-LIBMAN-SACK SYNDROME, SLE)

General

Possible etiology includes viral infections and genetic predisposition; immunologic abnormalities.

Ocular

Keratitis; keratoconjunctivitis sicca; corneal ulcer; optic nerve atrophy; optic neuritis; papilledema; arteritis; central retinal vein occlusion; retinal detachment; microaneurysm; scleritis; uveitis; ptosis; conjunctivitis; paralysis of third nerve; homonymous hemianopsia; multifocal microinfarcts; mydriasis; nystagmus; proptosis; orbital myositis; pseudoretinitis pigmentosa; photophobia.

Clinical

Polyarthritis; morning stiffness; fever; malaise; fatigue; polyserositis; renal disease; central nervous system disease; anemia; leukopenia; maculopapular rash in a "butterfly" distribution over malar region; alopecia.

Laboratory

Antibodies to double-stranded DNA or the Smith (Sm) antigen or a false-positive serology test for syphilis; positive antinuclear antibody test that is caused by a medication.

Treatment

Fever, rash, musculoskeletal and serositis manifestations respond to hydroxychloroquine and nonsteroidal anti-inflammatory drugs (NSAIDs). Low-to-moderate dose steroids are necessary for acute flares. Central nervous system (CNS) involvement and renal disease constitute more serious disease and often require high-dose steroids and other immunosuppression agents. Diffuse proliferative lupus nephritis has been treated with cyclophosphamide induction therapy.

BIBLIOGRAPHY

1. Bartles CM, Muller D. (2012). Systemic erythematosus lupus. [online] Available from www.emedicine.com/med/TOPIC2228.HTM. [Accessed July, 2013].

6. ERYTHEMA NODOSUM (DERMATITIS CONTUSIFORMIS)

General

Young females; hypersensitive reaction secondary to viral, bacterial and fungal infections; duration 2–4 weeks; recurrences possible.

Ocular

Subcutaneous nodules involving lids; keratitis; uveitis.

Clinical

Painful nodules on surface of thighs, arms and face; fever; malaise; red lesions that progress to bruise like and disappear in a few days to 3 weeks; cervical lymphadenopathy; exquisitely tender, erythematous nodules distributed symmetrically on the extensor surfaces of the lower extremities.

Laboratory

Throat culture as part of the initial workup to exclude group A β-hemolytic streptococcal infection erythrocyte sedimentation rates are often very high. Antistreptolysin titer is elevated in some patients with streptococcal disease, but normal values do not exclude streptococcal infection. Evaluate titer levels during the initial workup, since streptococcal disease is a common cause of erythema nodosum (EN). Order stool examination, since along with the appropriate history of gastrointestinal complaints, a stool examination can exclude infection by *Yersinia*, *Salmonella*, and *Campylobacter* organisms.

Order blood cultures according to preliminary indications and findings.

Treatment

Self-limited disease and requires only symptomatic relief using NSAIDs, cool wet compresses, elevation, and bed rest.

BIBLIOGRAPHY

1. Hebel JL, Habif T. (2012). Erythema nodosum. [online] Available from www.emedicine.com/derm/TOPIC138.HTM. [Accessed July, 2013].

7. MASTOCYTOSIS (URTICARIA; MAST CELL LEUKEMIA)

General

Increased mast cells found in tissues and organs; range from cutaneous to systemic condition.

Ocular

Conjunctival pigmentation; keratitis; pingueculae.

Clinical

Urticarial wheals; mast cells infiltrate into liver, spleen, gastrointestinal system and bones.

Laboratory

Complete blood count (CBC), plasma or urinary histamine, total tryptase levels, bone marrow biopsy.

Treatment

H1 and H2 antihistamines, oral disodium cromoglycate.

BIBLIOGRAPHY

1. Hogan DJ, Mastrodomenico CM. (2012). Mastocytosis. [online] www.emedicine.com/derm/TOPIC258.HTM. [Accessed July, 2013].

8. ACNE ROSACEA (ACNE ERYTHEMATOSA; OCULAR ROSACEA)

General

Etiology unknown; usually occurs in women 30–50 years of age; pathogenetic mechanism remains unclear.

Ocular

Conjunctivitis; corneal neovascularization (wedge-shaped); keratitis; meibomianitis; blepharitis; recurrent chalazion; conjunctival hyperemia; superficial punctate keratopathy; corneal vascularization, thinning, perforation, and scarring; episcleritis; scleritis; iritis; nodular conjunctivitis.

Clinical

Symmetrical erythema; papules; pustules; telangiectasia; sebaceous gland hypertrophy of the forehead, malar eminences, and nose.

Laboratory

Diagnosis is made from clinical findings.

Treatment

Systemic antibiotics are useful in most cases.

BIBLIOGRAPHY

1. Banasikowaska AK, Singh S. (2012). Rosacea. [online] Available from www.emedicine.com/derm/TOPIC377.HTM. [Accessed July, 2013].

9. PSORIASIS (PSORIASIS VULGARIS)

General

Chronic skin disease of unknown etiology; both sexes affected; onset at any age; disease peaks at puberty; strong human leukocyte antigen (HLA) association resulting in heritable disease susceptibility.

Ocular

Desquamative psoriatic plaques of lids resulting in madarosis, trichiasis, or ectropion; corneal plaques; xerosis, symblepharon; keratitis; chronic corneal ulceration; phthisis bulbi; iritis.

Clinical

Thick, dry, elevated red patches of skin covered with coarse silvery scales that usually affect areas of skin not exposed to sun, such as scalp, sacrum, elbows, and knees; positive association with Sjögren syndrome and keratitis sicca.

Laboratory

Diagnosis is made by clinical findings.

Treatment

The simplest treatment of psoriasis is daily sun exposure, sea bathing, topical moisturizers and relaxation. Moisturizers, such as petrolatum jelly, are helpful. Anthralin, coal or wood tar, corticosteroids, salicylic acid, phenolic compounds, and calcipotriene (a vitamin D analog) also may be effective. Ocular lubricants and punctal occlusion, oral and topical corticosteroids are sometimes beneficial.

BIBLIOGRAPHY

1. Meffert J, Arffa R, Gordon R, et al. (2012). Psoriasis. [online]. Available from www.emedicine.com/oph/TOPIC483.HTM. [Accessed July, 2013].

10. QUINCKE DISEASE (GIANT EDEMA; GIANT URTICARIA; HIVES; NETTLE RASH; ANGIONEUROTIC EDEMA)

General

Vascular reaction involving subcutaneous tissues or submucosa; both sexes affected; allergy to various agents, including medications; emotional factor may be involved; recurrent.

Ocular

Optic neuritis; papilledema; central serous retinopathy; corneal edema; exophthalmos; nystagmus; secondary glaucoma; uveitis; periorbital and lid edema.

Clinical

Transient erythema; angioneurotic edema of loose subcutaneous tissue; sporadic urticaria; nausea; vomiting; diarrhea; cephalalgia; severe respiratory distress; polyuria.

Laboratory

Plasma levels for the diagnosis include the following: C4 level less than 104 mg/L (diagnostic).

Treatment

The goal is to prevent episodes of swelling. Minor episodes of subepithelial swelling need no treatment, but the patient with edema of the face and neck should be closely observed for spread of edema and signs of airway involvement. When hoarseness or other signs of a compromised airway occur, an otolaryngologist should be consulted for possible tracheostomy.

BIBLIOGRAPHY

1. Huang SW. (2012). Pediatric angioedema. [online] Available from www.emedicine.com/ped/TOPIC101.HTM. [Accessed July, 2013].

CHAPTER
9

Connective Tissue Disorders

⊟ 1. AMYLOIDOSIS (PRIMARY AMYLOIDOSIS; LUBARSCH-PICK SYNDROME; IDIOPATHIC AMYLOIDOSIS)

General

Rare condition of unknown etiology; inherited as a dominant trait, with male preponderance; characterized by amyloid accumulation in muscles and in gastrointestinal and genitourinary tracts.

Ocular

Internal and external ophthalmoplegia; diminished lacrimation; amyloid deposits in conjunctival, episcleral and ciliary vessels; vitreous opacities; amyloid deposits in the corneal stroma; retinal hemorrhages and perivascular exudates; paralysis of extraocular muscles; pseudopodia lentis; strabismus fixus convergens; keratoconus.

Clinical

Peripheral neuropathy (extremities); heart failure; defective hepatic and renal functions with hepatosplenomegaly; waxy skin lesions; muscular weakness (progressive); multiple myeloma; hoarseness; chronic gastrointestinal symptoms.

Laboratory

Biopsy staining with Congo red demonstrates apple-green birefringence under polarized light; distinctive fibrillar ultrastructure.

Treatment

Deoxydoxorubicin had demonstrated some clinical benefits.

⊟ BIBLIOGRAPHY

1. Biswas J, Badrinath SS, Rao NA. Primary nonfamilial amyloidosis of the vitreous. A light microscopic and ultrastructural study. Retina. 1992;12(3):251-3.
2. Goebel HH, Friedman AH. Extraocular muscle involvement in idiopathic primary amyloidosis. Am J Ophthalmol. 1971;71(5):1121-7.
3. Lubarsch O. Zur Kenntnis Ungewohnlicher Amyloidablagerungen. Virchows Arch Pathol Anat. 1929;271:867-89.
4. Magalini SI, Scrascia E. Dictionary of Medical Syndromes, 2nd edition. Philadelphia: Lippincott Williams & Wilkins; 1981.
5. Sharma P, Gupta NK, Arora R, et al. Strabismus fixus convergens secondary to amyloidosis. J Pediatr Ophthalmol Strabismus. 1991;28(4):236-7.
6. Wong VG, McFarlin DE. Primary familial amyloidosis. Arch Ophthalmol. 1967;78(2):208-13.

2. AMYLOIDOSIS OF GINGIVA AND CONJUNCTIVA, WITH MENTAL RETARDATION (PRIMARY SYSTEMIC AMYLOIDOSIS)

General

Autosomal recessive; primary amyloidosis differs from secondary by the mesodermal tissues being affected and nodular form of deposits; no pre-existing medical condition; preferential involvement of mesenchymal tissues; variable staining of deposits.

Ocular

Conjunctivitis with deposits; corneal leukoma; waxy eyelid papules with purpura; proptosis; diplopia; decreased vision; ptosis; keratitis sicca; upper lid mass; tonic pupil; accommodative paresis; diffuse yellow conjunctival mass.

Clinical

Hyperplastic gingivitis, tongue, skin and muscles; lungs with icing-like coating; mental retardation; peripheral neuropathy; congestive heart failure; polyarthropathy; spontaneous, incidental purpura; macroglossia; bleeding diathesis; idiopathic carpal tunnel syndrome.

Laboratory

Echocardiography is valuable in the evaluation of amyloid heart disease. Doppler studies are useful and may show abnormal relaxation early in the course of disease. Advanced involvement is characterized by restrictive hemodynamics.

Treatment

The treatment is often unsatisfactory. No reliable method for the accurate assessment of the total amount of amyloid in the body exists. The similarity with multiple myeloma suggests that chemotherapy may be useful. Using different regimens of intermittent oral melphalan and prednisone may also be useful.

BIBLIOGRAPHY

1. Nyirady J, Schwartz RA. (2012). Primary systemic amyloidosis. [online] Available from www.emedicine.com/derm/TOPIC19.HTM. [Accessed August, 2013].

3. BEHÇET SYNDROME (DERMATO-STOMATO-OPHTHALMIC SYNDROME; OCULOBUCCOGENITAL SYNDROME; GILBERT SYNDROME)

General

Virus infection; occurs in adults; chronic disease; complete remission is rare; etiology is unknown.

Ocular

Muscle palsies (occasional); nystagmus (occasional); conjunctivitis; hypopyon; iritis; recurrent uveitis; keratoconjunctivitis sicca; keratitis; vitreous hemorrhages; thrombophlebitis retinal veins (occasional); retinal hemorrhages; optic neuritis (occasional); macular edema; optic nerve atrophy; retinitis; secondary glaucoma; retinal vasculitis; disk edema; panophthalmitis; optic neuropathy; skin lesions, posterior uveitis and systemic complications have been associated with loss of vision with this disorder; corneal immune ring opacity.

Clinical

Aphthous lesions of mucous membranes of the mouth and genitalia; cerebellar signs; convulsions; paraplegia; skin erythema (multiforme, bullosum); arthritis; urethritis; glossitis; recurrent fever.

Laboratory

Nonspecific human leukocyte antigen (HLA) B51 positive may help to support diagnosis.

Treatment

The goals of therapy are to suppress inflammation, to reduce the frequency and severity of recurrences, and to minimize involvement of the retina. To be effective, treatment must be started early. Extent of involvement and severity of disease determine the choice of medication. Treatment options include corticosteroids, cytotoxic agents, cyclosporine and colchicine.

BIBLIOGRAPHY

1. Bashour M. (2012). Ophthalmologic manifestations of Behcet disease. [online] Available from www.emedicine.com/oph/TOPIC425.HTM. [Accessed August, 2013].

⊟ 4. COGAN (2) SYNDROME (OCULOMOTOR APRAXIA SYNDROME; WIEACKER SYNDROME)

General

X-linked; oculomotor apraxia and muscle atrophy; prevalent in males; corpus callosum can be hypoplastic.

Ocular

Rapid and frequent blinking; conjugate palsy; congenital oculomotor apraxia with patient unable to move eyes voluntarily to one side but with otherwise normal ocular movements; patient fixes objects by head tilt and turning, which causes further ocular deviation via the vestibular reflex; compensation for this overshoot is accomplished by some jerky eye movements with final fixation possible and gradual return of the head to the primary position; may be associated with abnormal electroretinographic responses.

Clinical

Slow progression, predominantly distal muscle atrophy; congenital contracture of feet; dyspraxia of face and tongue muscles; mild mental retardation.

Laboratory

Clinical.

Treatment

None.

⊟ BIBLIOGRAPHY

1. Borchert MS, Sadun AA, Sommers JD, et al. Congenital ocular motor apraxia in twins. Findings with magnetic resonance imaging. J Clin Neuroophthalmol. 1987;7(2):104-7.
2. Cogan DG. A type of congenital ocular motor apraxia presenting jerky head movements. Trans Am Acad Ophthalmol Otolaryngol. 1952;56(6):853-62.
3. Magni R, Spadea L, Pece A, et al. Electroretinographic findings in congenital oculomotor apraxia (Cogan's syndrome). Doc Ophthalmol. 1994;86(3):259-66.
4. Vassella F, Lütschg J, Mumenthaler M. Cogan's congenital ocular motor apraxia in two successive generations. Dev Med Child Neurol. 1972;14(6):788-96.

⊟ 5. FELTY SYNDROME (CHAUFFARD-STILL SYNDROME; PRIMARY SPLENIC NEUTROPENIA WITH ARTHRITIS; RHEUMATOID ARTHRITIS WITH HYPERSPLENISM; STILL-CHAUFFARD SYNDROME; UVEITIS-RHEUMATOID ARTHRITIS SYNDROME)

General

Etiology not fully understood, possibly infection or allergy; onset in middle-aged patients or children; prognosis poor; collagen disorder; occasionally can occur without articular disease.

Ocular

Decreased tear formation; scleromalacia perforans; keratoconjunctivitis; chronic anterior uveitis; scleritis; vitreous opacities; macular edema; choroidal inflammation; papillitis; keratic precipitates; band-shaped keratopathy.

Clinical

Rheumatoid arthritis (RA); splenomegaly; leukopenia; anemia (mild); oral lesion with ulcers and atrophy.

Laboratory

Complete blood count (CBC) with differential, computed tomography (CT), erythrocyte sedimentation rate (ESR) and serum immunoglobulin (Ig) levels invariably are elevated.

Treatment

Control the underlying RA with immunosuppressive therapy for RA often improves granulocytopenia and splenomegaly.

⊟ BIBLIOGRAPHY

1. Keating RM. (2012). Felty Syndrome. [online] Available from www.emedicine.com/med/TOPIC782.HTM. [Accessed August, 2013].

6. GRÖNBLAD-STRANDBERG SYNDROME (SYSTEMIC ELASTODYSTROPHY; PSEUDOXANTHOMA ELASTICUM; ELASTORRHEXIS; DARIER-GRÖNBLAD-STRANDBERG SYNDROME)

General

Autosomal recessive; female-to-male ratio of 2:1; in-heritance is usually autosomal recessive, but it also has reported as autosomal dominant.

Ocular

"Angioid streaks" of the retina; macular hemorrhages and transudates not infrequent; choroidal sclerosis; retinal detachment; keratoconus; cataract; paralysis of extraocular muscles [secondary to vascular lesions of central nervous system (CNS)]; subluxation of lens; exophthalmos; optic atrophy; vitreous hemorrhages; Salmon spot multiple atrophic peripheral retinal pigment epithelium (RPE) lesions; reticular pigment dystrophy of the macula; optic disk drusen; multiple small crystalline bodies associated with atrophic RPE changes.

Clinical

Pseudoxanthoma elasticum with thickening, softening and relaxation of the skin; skin changes are symmetrical in skin folds near large joints (axilla, elbow, inguinal region, lower abdomen, neck); flattening of the pulse curve and peripheral vascular disturbances; gastrointestinal hemorrhages.

Laboratory

Characteristic skin and retinal findings. Fluorescein angiography is done to detect angioid streaks and choroidal neovascular membranes.

Treatment

Dietary calcium and phosphorus restriction to minimum daily requirement levels has shown arrest in progression of the disease.

BIBLIOGRAPHY

1. Dahl AA, Calonje D, El-Harazi SM. (2012). Ophthalmologic manifestations of pseudoxanthoma elasticum. [online] Available from www.emedicine.com/oph/TOPIC475.HTM. [Accessed August, 2013].

7. HAMMAN-RICH SYNDROME (ALVEOLAR CAPILLARY BLOCK SYNDROME; DIFFUSE PULMONARY FIBROSIS SYNDROME; RHEUMATOID LUNG SYNDROME)

General

Etiology unknown; insidious onset with progressive exertional dyspnea; association with RA or scleroderma; autosomal recessive; occurs between 40 and 50 years.

Ocular

Xerophthalmia; keratomalacia; retinal venous congestion and engorgement; ischemic retinopathy; cystic macular changes.

Clinical

Cyanosis; dyspnea; cough; weight loss; clubbing of fingers; high sodium and chloride concentrations in sweat; heart failure.

Laboratory

Most patients have abnormal chest radiography findings. Bilateral diffuse reticular or reticulonodular infiltrates are observed.

Treatment

Oxygen therapy should be prescribed for patients with documented hypoxemia. Pulmonary specialist should be involved.

BIBLIOGRAPHY

1. Godfrey A, Ouellette DR. (2012). Idiopathic pulmonary fibrosis. [online] Available from www.emedicine.com/med/TOPIC1960.HTM. [Accessed August, 2013].

🗗 8. JUVENILE RHEUMATOID ARTHRITIS (JRA; STILL DISEASE)

General

Onset before age of 16 years; greater occurrence of systemic manifestations, monoarticular and oligoarticular joint involvement, and iridocyclitis.

Ocular

Hypopyon; band keratopathy; uveitis; cataract; papillitis; glaucoma; macular edema; ocular pain; vitreous cells; synechiae; scleritis; presumed to have an autoimmune etiology; antiocular antibodies, including iris protein antibodies, have been found in the sera of patients.

Clinical

Salmon pink macular rash; arthritis; hepatosplenomegaly; leukocytosis; chronic pain; joint swelling; low-grade fever; anemia; rheumatoid nodules.

Laboratory

Antinuclear antibody (ANA), rheumatoid factor, HLA-B27, X-ray imaging of joints.

Treatment

Uveitis is treated initially with topical corticosteroids. Systemic immunomodulatory agents may be useful for patients with limited or no response to topical or systemic corticosteroids.

🗗 BIBLIOGRAPHY

1. Roque MR, Roque BL, Miserocchi E, et al. (2012). Juvenile idiopathic arthritis uveitis. [online] Available from www.emedicine.com/oph/TOPIC675.HTM. [Accessed August, 2013].

🗗 9. MARFAN SYNDROME (DOLICHOSTENOMELIA; ARACHNODACTYLY; HYPERCHONDROPLASIA; DYSTROPHIA; MESODERMALIS CONGENITA)

General

Hypoplastic form of dystrophia mesodermalis congenita; autosomal dominant; affects both sexes. It has been demonstrated that an abnormality of the gene coding for the connective tissue protein fibrillin is responsible for chronic Marfan syndrome.

Ocular

Exotropia; nystagmus; paralysis of accommodation; myopia (axial or lenticular); iridodonesis; miosis; persistent pupillary membrane; blue sclera; spherophakia; lens dislocation; cataract; megalocornea; retinal detachment (less frequently); pigmentary retinopathy; colobomata of macula, iris, optic nerve and uveal tract (less frequently); keratoconus; central retinal artery occlusion; rhegmatogenous retinal detachment; syringoma.

Clinical

Arachnodactyly; skeletal anomalies; asymmetric thorax; dolichocephaly and high-arched palate; dissecting aneurysm; mitral valve prolapse; prominent ears; kyphoscoliosis; pectus excavatum; flat feet; hammer toes; pulmonary and kidney defects.

Laboratory

Genetic testing, molecular studies.

Treatment

- *Keratoconus*: Spectacle correction, hard contacts, avoid eye rubbing. If hydrops occur, discontinue contact lens, use sodium chloride (NaCl) drops and ointment, patching, and short course of steroids. As disease advances, penetrating keratoplasty, deep anterior lamellar keratoplasty intacs with laser grooves or collagen stabilization of cornea.
- *Cataract*: Change in glasses can sometimes improve a patient's visual function temporarily; however the most common treatment is cataract surgery.
- *Glaucoma*: Glaucoma medication should be the first plan of action. If medication is unsuccessful, a filtering surgical procedure with or without antimetabolites may be beneficial.
- *Strabismus*: Equalized vision with correct refractive error; surgery may be helpful in patient with diplopia.

🗗 BIBLIOGRAPHY

1. Chen H. (2011). Genetics of Marfan syndrome. [online] Available from www.emedicine.com/ped/TOPIC1372.HTM. [Accessed August, 2013].

10. MORPHEA (LOCALIZED SCLERODERMA; CIRCUMSCRIBED SCLERODERMA)

General

Localized chronic connective tissue disease of unknown etiology; etiology remains unknown, although there is a possible association with *Borrelia burgdorferi* infection.

Ocular

Circumscribed plaque-like lesions of the eyelid; prevalent in females; onset usually in second to fourth decades of life; onset occasionally associated with trauma, pregnancy, or menopause.

Clinical

Firm skin plaques over entire body, but most frequently on trunk, lower extremities, upper extremities, face and genitalia; abdominal pain; migraine; generalized joint pain; renal crisis; Raynaud's phenomenon; systemic sclerosis; eosinophilia; positive antinuclear factor; increased IgG; seizures; skin sclerosis; alterations in tryptophan metabolism.

Laboratory

Tests are limited and are on a case-by-case basis.

Treatment

No definite treatment is available.

BIBLIOGRAPHY

1. Nguyen JV, Werth VP, Fett N. (2012). Morphea. [online] Available from www.emedicine.com/derm/TOPIC272. HTM. [Accessed August, 2013].

11. RELAPSING POLYCHONDRITIS (JAKSCH-WARTENHOST SYNDROME; MEYENBURG-ALTHERZ-VEHLINGER SYNDROME; VON MEYENBERG II SYNDROME)

General

Episodic, yet generally progressive; onset usually in middle life; possibly caused by lysosomal labilizing factor of endogenous or exogenous toxic nature or immunologic reactions; possible association with Reiter's syndrome.

Ocular

Conjunctivitis; corneal ulcer; exophthalmos; pan-ophthalmitis; phthisis bulbi; proptosis; optic neuritis; papilledema; retinal detachment; blue sclera; episcleritis; scleromalacia; vitreous opacity; cataracts; nystagmus; retinal artery thrombosis; keratoconjunctivitis sicca; secondary glaucoma; scotoma; uveitis; paresis of third or sixth nerve; conjunctival mass (salmon patch); chorioretinitis.

Clinical

Destruction of cartilage and eventual replacement with connective tissue; polyarthritis; chondritis; tracheal collapse; bronchial collapse; anemia; liver dysfunction; death; malaise; fever; dyspnea; changes in pitch of voice; hearing impairment; vertigo; deformed ears; aortic valve insufficiency.

Laboratory

No specific serologic markers.

Treatment

No therapy.

BIBLIOGRAPHY

1. Compton N, Buckner JH, Harp KI, et al. (2012). Polychondritis. [online] Available from emedicine.medscape.com/article/331475-overview. [Accessed January, 2013].

🔲 12. RHEUMATOID ARTHRITIS (ADULT)

General

Systemic disease of unknown cause; more common in women (3:1); thought to have a strong autoimmune pathogenesis with positive IgM, IgG and IgA directed against the fragment crystallizable (Fc) portion of IgG.

Ocular

Sjögren syndrome; episcleritis; scleritis; keratitis; corneal ulcers; corneal perforation; uveitis; motility disorders; dry eyes; posterior scleritis (rare).

Clinical

Synovitis; stiffness; swelling; cartilaginous hypertrophy; joint pain; fibrous ankylosis; malaise; weight loss; vas-omotor disturbance.

Laboratory

About 80% are positive for rheumatoid factor but it is also found in systemic lupus erythematosus (SLE), Sjögren syndrome, sarcoidosis, hepatitis B and tuberculosis.

Treatment

Nonsteroidal anti-inflammatory drugs (NSAIDs), disease-modifying antirheumatic drugs (DMARDs), corticosteroids and immunosuppressant can be used.

🔲 BIBLIOGRAPHY

1. Temprano KK, Smith HR. (2012). Rheumatoid arthritis. [online] Available from www.emedicine.com/emerg/TOPIC48.HTM. [Accessed August, 2013].

🔲 13. SCHAUMANN SYNDROME (BESNIER-BOECK-SCHAUMANN SYNDROME; BOECK SARCOID; SARCOIDOSIS)

General

Etiology unknown; theories include tuberculosis, hypersensitivity to pine pollen, virus infection; affects blacks most often; chronic course with spontaneous remissions (*see* Heerfordt's syndrome); hilar or paratracheal nodes with erythema nodosum; onset most often in middle and old age; ocular involvement in 20–25% of all cases.

Ocular

Orbital granulomatous mass; bony defects; cutaneous and subcutaneous nodules; myogenic palsy; lacrimal gland adenopathy; decreased tear formation; secondary glaucoma; granulomatous uveitis with iris nodules, cells and flare; mutton fat keratic precipitates; keratitis sicca; vitreous floaters; band-shaped keratitis; complicated cataract; inflammatory retinal exudates; "candle wax drippings"; optic nerve atrophy; neuritis; eyelid nodules; ocular nerve enlargement (granuloma).

Clinical

Lymphadenopathy; hilar nodes; fatigue; cystic, punched-out or reticulated changes in small bones (mainly, hands and feet); muscle wasting; contractures; weakness in legs and arms.

Laboratory

Chest X-ray, CT scan and magnetic resonance imaging (MRI) of the brain.

Treatment

Glucocorticoids are the treatment of choice.

🔲 BIBLIOGRAPHY

1. Sharma GD. (2011). Pediatric sarcoidosis. [online] Available from www.emedicine.com/ped/TOPIC2043.HTM. [Accessed August, 2013].

14. SCLERODERMA (PROGRESSIVE SYSTEMIC SCLEROSIS; SYSTEMIC SCLERODERMA)

General

Chronic connective tissue disease of unknown etiology; chronic and usually progressive disorder; typical onset is in 3rd to 5th decade; ratio of women to men is 4:1; primary sites of pathology are the arterioles and capillaries of affected organs.

Ocular

Marginal corneal ulcers; shortened fornices of the conjunctiva; ptosis; cotton-wool patches of retina; papilledema; retinal hemorrhages; cicatrization of conjunctiva and cornea; blepharitis; blepharospasm; thready, tenacious yellow-white conjunctival discharge; hypertrophy of lacrimal gland; episcleritis; ocular myositis; Sjögren syndrome; uveitis; vitreous haze; keratitis sicca; decreased corneal sensation; iritis; ischemic choroidopathy; iris sectorial atrophy; blepharophimosis; heterochromia; keratoconus; central retinal vein occlusion; branch retinal vein occlusion.

Clinical

Vascular insufficiency; Raynaud's phenomenon; malaise; weight loss; stiffness; fever; polyarticular arthritis; diffuse edema of the hands; calcinosis; esophageal involvement; sclerodactyly; telangiectasis; esophageal stricture; renal failure; diffuse interstitial fibrosis.

Laboratory

No specific test establishes diagnosis. Hypergammaglobulinemia—50% of cases ANA increased in 40–70% cases.

Treatment

Skin thickening can be treated with D-penicillamine and other experimental drugs. Pruritus can be treated with moisturizers and histamine. Raynaud's phenomenon can be treated with calcium channel blockers. Renal crisis episodes are best prevented and treated with the aggressive use of angiotensin-converting enzyme (ACE) inhibitors. Myositis may be treated cautiously with steroids.

BIBLIOGRAPHY

1. Jimenez SA, Cronin PM, Koenig AS, et al. (2012). Scleroderma. [online] Available from www.emedicine.com/med/TOPIC2076.HTM. [Accessed August, 2013].

15. SYSTEMIC LUPUS ERYTHEMATOSUS (DISSEMINATED LUPUS ERYTHEMATOSUS; LUPUS ERYTHEMATOSUS; KAPOSI-LIBMAN-SACK SYNDROME, SLE)

General

Possible etiology includes viral infections and genetic predisposition; immunologic abnormalities.

Ocular

Keratitis; keratoconjunctivitis sicca; corneal ulcer; optic nerve atrophy; optic neuritis; papilledema; arteritis; central retinal vein occlusion; retinal detachment; microaneurysm; scleritis; uveitis; ptosis; conjunctivitis; paralysis of third nerve; homonymous hemianopsia; multifocal microinfarcts; mydriasis; nystagmus; proptosis; orbital myositis; pseudoretinitis pigmentosa; photophobia.

Clinical

Polyarthritis; morning stiffness; fever; malaise; fatigue; polyserositis; renal disease; CNS disease; anemia; leukopenia; maculopapular rash in a "butterfly" distribution over malar region; alopecia.

Laboratory

Antibodies to double-stranded deoxyribonucleic acid (DNA) or the Smith (Sm) antigen or a false-positive serology test for syphilis; positive ANA test that is caused by a medication.

Treatment

Fever, rash, musculoskeletal and serositis manifestations respond to hydroxychloroquine and NSAIDs. Low-to-moderate-dose steroids are necessary for acute flares. Central nervous system involvement and renal disease constitute more serious disease and often require high-dose steroids and other immunosuppression agents. Diffuse proliferative lupus nephritis has been treated with cyclophosphamide induction therapy.

🖶 BIBLIOGRAPHY

1. Bartels CM, Muller D. (2012). Systemic lupus erythematosus (SLE). [online] Available from www.emedicine.com/med/TOPIC2228.HTM. [Accessed August, 2013].

🖶 16. TEMPORAL ARTERITIS SYNDROME (CRANIAL ARTERITIS SYNDROME; GIANT CELL ARTERITIS; HUTCHINSON-HORTON-MAGATH-BROWN SYNDROME)

General

Etiology unknown; mainly females; mainly Whites; ages 55–80 years; temporal artery shows inflammatory thickening; arteritis of the vessels supplying the optic nerve.

Ocular

Transient ptosis; partial or complete loss of vision on the affected side; retinal detachment; exudates and hemorrhages; narrowing of retinal vessels; obstruction of the central retinal artery; optic atrophy; ischemic optic neuropathy; acute decreased intraocular pressure (IOP); corneal hypesthesia; palsies of extraocular muscles; hemorrhagic glaucoma; diplopia; hemorrhages on or around the disk.

Clinical

Throbbing headache; hyperalgesia of the scalp; malaise; anorexia; weakness; weight loss; fever; nodular pulmonary nodules; cough; otitis with deafness.

Laboratory

Elevated ESR greater than 50 mm/hour, positive temporal artery biopsy.

Treatment

Systemic corticosteroids are the therapy of choice.

🖶 BIBLIOGRAPHY

1. Allen AW, Biega T, Varma MK. (2012). Temporal arteritis imaging. [online] Available from www.emedicine.com/radio/TOPIC675.HTM. [Accessed August, 2013].
2. Walvick MD, Walvick MP. Giant cell arteritis: laboratory predictors of a positive temporal artery biopsy. Ophthalmology. 2011;118(6):1201-4.

🖶 17. UVEITIS, JUVENILE IDIOPATHIC ARTHRITIS

General

Uveitis in children is approximately 6% of all cases. The most frequent cause of juvenile uveitis is juvenile idiopathic arthritis (JIA).

Ocular

The affected eye is often healthy in appearance, yet 30–40% of patients with JIA uveitis have demonstrated severe loss of vision due to the condition.

Clinical

Past medical and ocular history; chief complaint and history of illnesses; other manifestations such as anemia, fever, rash, back pain, diarrhea, weight loss and fatigue.

Treatment

Initial treatment should begin with topical corticosteroids. If vitreous cells are present, the risk of cystoid macular edema (CME) increases, continuing corticosteroids and additional NSAIDs may be helpful.

Laboratory

Antinuclear antibody, rheumatoid factor, HLA-B27. X-ray of joint. Additional serologic test may include: syphilis serologies, Lyme titers, serum lysozyme, ACE.

BIBLIOGRAPHY

1. Roque MR, Roque BL, Miserocchi E, et al. (2012). Juvenile idiopathic arthritis uveitis. [online] Available from emedicine.medscape.com/article/1209891-overview. [Accessed August, 2013].

18. VON BEKHTEREV-STRÜMPELL SYNDROME (MARIE-STRÜMPELL SPONDYLITIS; ANKYLOSING SPONDYLITIS; PIERRE-MARIE SYNDROME; BEKHTEREV DISEASE; RHEUMATOID SPONDYLITIS), OPTIC ATROPHY

General

Variant of RA; etiology unknown; autosomal dominant; male preponderance; onset at age 20–40 years; although genetic background determines susceptibility to uveitis, the disease pattern suggests the possibility of random environmental triggers unrelated to the course of the underlying rheumatologic disorder.

Ocular

Nongranulomatous anterior uveitis; optic nerve atrophy (occasionally); hypopyon; band keratopathy; spontaneous hyphema.

Clinical

Spondylitis of vertebra and sacroiliac joints; ankylosis; general arthralgia; kyphosis; scoliosis; displaced head and total rigidity of spine.

Laboratory

Histocompatibility antigen HLA-B27 and a negative rheumatoid factor and ANA; X-ray evidence of narrowing of sacroiliac joint space and sclerosis.

Treatment

Oral NSAIDs, urethritis in Reiter's disease should be treated with tetracycline, topical steroids and cycloplegic agents.

BIBLIOGRAPHY

1. Vives MJ, Garfin SR. (2011). Rheumatoid arthritis of the cervical spine overview of rheumatoid spondylitis. [online] Available from www.emedicine.com/orthoped/TOPIC551.HTM. [Accessed August, 2013].

19. WEGENER SYNDROME (WEGENER GRANULOMATOSIS)

General

Etiology unknown; occurs in fourth and fifth decades of life; persistent rhinitis or sinusitis; three characteristic features are: (1) necrotizing granulomatous lesions in the respiratory tract, (2) generalized focal arthritis, and (3) necrotizing thrombotic glomerulitis.

Ocular

Exophthalmos; lid and conjunctival chemosis; papillitis; conjunctivitis; corneal ulcer; corneal abscess; optic atrophy; optic neuritis; orbital cellulitis; episcleritis; sclerokeratitis; cataract; peripheral ring corneal ulcers; ptosis; dacryocystitis; retinal periphlebitis; cotton-wool spots; retinal and vitreous hemorrhages; rubeosis iridis; neovascular glaucoma.

Clinical

Severe sinusitis; pulmonary inflammation; arteritis; weakness; fever; weight loss; bony destruction; granulomatous vasculitis of the upper and lower respiratory tracts; glomerulonephritis; diffuse pulmonary infiltrates; lymphadenopathy; diffuse pulmonary hemorrhage; overlap with giant cell arteritis.

Laboratory

Histopathology: Necrotizing, granulomatous vasculitis with infiltrating neutrophils, lymphocytes and giant cells; urine—proteinuria, hematuria and urinary casts.

Treatment

Topical eye lubricants, ophthalmic antibiotic solution or ointments and corticosteroid drops may prove to be beneficial. Orbital decompression is needed when medical treatment is unresponsive to treat optic nerve compression.

⊟ BIBLIOGRAPHY

1. Collins JF. Handbook of Clinical Ophthalmology. New York Chicago: Year Book Medical PublicationMasson; 1982.
2. Flach AJ. Ocular manifestations of Wegener's Wegener's granulomatosis [Letter]. JAMA. 1995; 274(15):1199–200.
3. Haynes BF, Fishman ML, Fauci AS, et al. The ocular manifestations of Wegener's Wegener's granulomatosis. Fifteen years' years' experience and review of the literature. Am J Med. 1977; 63(1):131–41.
4. Leavitt RY, Fauci AS. Less common manifestations and presentations of Wegener's Wegener's granulomatosis. Curr Opin Rheumatol. 1992; 4(1):16–22.
5. Robinson MR, Lee SS, Sneller MC, et al. Tarsal-conjunctival disease associated with Wegener's granulomatosis. Ophthalmology. 2003; 110(9): 1770–80.
6. Roy FH, Fraunfelder FW, Fraunfelder FT. Roy and Fraunfelder's Current Ocular Therapy, 6th edition. London: Elsevier; 2008.
7. Straatsma BR. Ocular manifestations of Wegener's Wegener's granulomatosis. Am J Ophthalmol. 1957;44(6):789-99.

⊟ 20. WEILL-MARCHESANI SYNDROME (MARCHESANI SYNDROME; INVERTED MARFAN SYNDROME; BRACHYMORPHY WITH SPHEROPHAKIA; DYSTROPHIA MESODERMALIS CONGENITA HYPERPLASTICA)

General

Pattern of inheritance uncertain; manifest at age of 9 months to 13 years.

Ocular

Lenticular myopia; secondary glaucoma (rare), caused by luxation of the lens; iridodonesis; ectopia lentis; spherophakia; optic atrophy; megalocornea; corneal opacity; acute pupillary block glaucoma.

Clinical

Brachydactyly; reduced growth; athletic build with abundant subcutaneous tissue; short neck and large thorax; short and clumsy hands and feet; decreased joint flexibility; hearing defects; inheritable connective tissue disorder, usually inherited as an autosomal recessive.

Laboratory

X-ray detects delayed carpal ossification.

Treatment/Glaucoma

Beta-blockers, carbonic anhydrase inhibitors and prostaglandin analogs. Surgery may be needed if IOP is uncontrolled.

⊟ BIBLIOGRAPHY

1. Hamosh A, Scott AF, Amberger J, et al. Online Mendelian Inheritance in Man, (OMIM),. a knowledgebase of human genes and genetic disorders. Nucleic Acids Res. 2002;30(1):52–5 McKusick-Nathans Institute for Genetic Medicine, Johns Hopkins University and National Center for Biotechnology Information, National Library of Medicine, February 12, 2007. World Wide Web URL: http://.
2. Jensen AD, Cross HE, Paton D, et al. Ocular complications in the Weill-Marchesani syndrome. Am J Ophthalmol. 1974; 77(2):261 9.
3. Marchesani O. Brachydactylie und Angeborene Kugellinse als Systemerkrankung. Klin Monatsbl Augenheilkd. 1939; 103:392.
4. McKusick VA. Mendelian Inheritance in Man; A Catalog of Human Genes and Genetic Disorders, 12th edition. Baltimore: The Johns Hopkins University Press; 1998.
5. Roy FH, Fraunfelder FW, Fraunfelder FT. Roy and Fraunfelder's Current Ocular Therapy, 6th edition. London: Elsevier; 2008.
6. Willi M, Kut L, Cotlier E, et al. Pupillary-block glaucoma in the Marchesani syndrome. Arch Ophthalmol. 1973;90(6):504-8.
7. Young ID, Fielder AR, Casey TA, et al. Weill-Marchesani syndrome in mother and son. Clin Genet. 1986;30(6):475-80.

CHAPTER
10

Skeletal Disorders

1. DOWN SYNDROME (MONGOLISM; TRISOMY G; TRISOMY 21 SYNDROME; MONGOLOID IDIOCY)

General

Trisomy of chromosome 21.

Ocular

Hypertelorism; epicanthus; blepharitis; ectropion; nystagmus; esotropia; high myopia (30%); hyperopia; color blindness; yellow spots on the iris; hypoplasia of the iris; blepharoconjunctivitis; lens opacities (50%); keratoconus (may be acute); corneal hydrops; corneal ectasia; corneal edema; leukoma; lateral displacement of canaliculi and puncta; megaloblepharon; euryblepharon; decreased accommodation; Lebes congenital amaurosis.

Clinical

Mental retardation; skeletal abnormalities; overextension of joints; deformed and low-set ears; short fifth finger; transverse palmar crease; fissured tongue; heart anomalies.

Laboratory

Amniocentesis during second trimester to check mothers who have low alpha-fetoprotein serum values, prenatal echography, craniofacial X-ray to check features and echocardiography.

Treatment

Primary care provider should coordinate the multisystemic evaluation. Awareness of systemic and ocular findings is essential for managing patients.

BIBLIOGRAPHY

1. Izquierdo NJ, Townsend W. (2011). Ophthalmologic manifestations of down syndrome. [online] Available from/www.emedicine.com/oph/TOPIC522.HTM. [Accessed August, 2013].

CHAPTER
11

Phakomatoses

1. ANGIOMATOSIS RETINAE (VON HIPPEL-LINDAU SYNDROME; RETINOCERE-BRAL ANGIOMATOSIS; CEREBELLORETINAL HEMANGIOBLASTOMATOSIS; LINDAU SYNDROME; RETINAL CAPILLARY HAMARTOMA)

General

Dominant inheritance; angiomata in the cerebellum and the walls of the fourth ventricle; young adults.

Ocular

Secondary glaucoma; angiomatosis of the iris; vitreous hemorrhages; tortuosity of dilated retinal artery and vein (feeder vessels); retinal exudates and hemorrhages; retinitis proliferans; angiomata of optic nerve and retina; papilledema; retinal detachment; lipid accumulation in macula; keratoconus; bilateral macular holes; choroid plexus papilloma; bilateral optic nerve hemangioblastomas.

Clinical

Cerebellar angiomatosis; epilepsy; psychic disturbances to dementia.

Laboratory

Diagnosis is made from clinical findings.

Treatment

Smaller tumors can be treated with argon laser photocoagulation. Cryotherapy is used to treat larger posterior angiomas. Vitreoretinal surgery is effective for the treatment of severe von Hippel-Lindau (VHL) retinal hemangiomas.

BIBLIOGRAPHY

1. Gaudric A, Krivosic V, Duguid G, et al. Vitreoretinal surgery for severe retinal capillary hemangiomas in von Hippel-Lindau disease. Ophthalmology. 2011;118(1):142-9.
2. Khan AN, Turnbull I, Al-Okaili R. (2011). Imaging in von Hippel-Lindau syndrome. [online] Available from www.emedicine.com/radio/TOPIC742.HTM. [Accessed August, 2013].

2. NEUROFIBROMATOSIS TYPE I (VON RECKLINGHAUSEN SYNDROME; NEURINOMATOSIS)

General

Dominant inheritance activated at puberty, during pregnancy and at menopause; strong evidence supports the existence of neurofibromatosis type I (NF-I) as a tumor suppressor gene.

Ocular

Proptosis; displacement of the globe; pulsation of the globe; ptosis; elephantiasis of the lids; pigment spots on lids; hydrophthalmos; nodular swelling of corneal nerves; cataracts; optic atrophy; choroidal melanoma; neurofibroma of the choroid, iris, eyelid and ciliary body; enlarged optic foramen; underdevelopment of orbital bones; café-au-lait spots on fundus; hamartoma of retina; congenital glaucoma; focal iris nodules; choroidal nevi; optic nerve gliomas; orbital neurofibroma; keratoconus.

Clinical

Café-au-lait skin pigmentations; fibroma molluscum; lipomas and sebaceous adenomas; schwannomas; growth abnormalities; spontaneous fractures; facial hemihypertrophy.

Laboratory

T2-weighted magnetic resonance images demonstrate multiple bright lesions in the basal ganglia, cerebellum, and brain in 80% optic nerve gliomas often develop perineural arachnoidal hyperplasia, which appears as an expanded cerebrospinal fluid (CSF) space around the nerve.

Treatment

Oral ketotifen may reduce the pain, tenderness and itchiness associated with neurofibromas.

BIBLIOGRAPHY

1. Dahl AA. (2011). Ophthalmologic manifestations of neurofibromatosis type. [online] Available from www.emedicine.com/oph/TOPIC338.HTM. [Accessed August, 2013].

3. STURGE-WEBER SYNDROME (MENINGOCUTANEOUS SYNDROME; VASCULAR ENCEPHALOTRIGEMINAL SYNDROME; NEURO-OCULOCUTANEOUS ANGIOMATOSIS; ENCEPHALOFACIAL ANGIOMATOSIS; ENCEPHALOTRIGEMINAL SYNDROME)

General

Trisomy 22 or partial trisomy inheritance. Variations include Jahnke syndrome (neuro-oculocutaneous angiomatosis without glaucoma), Schirmer syndrome (oculocutaneous angiomatosis with early glaucoma), Lawford syndrome (oculocutaneous angiomatosis with late glaucoma and no increase in volume of globe) and Mille syndrome (oculocutaneous syndrome with choroidal angioma but no glaucoma).

Ocular

Unilateral hydrophthalmos; secondary glaucoma (late) conjunctival angiomata (telangiectases); iris decoloration; nevoid marks or vascular dilation of the episclera; glioma; serous retinal detachment; choroidal angiomata; deep anterior chamber angle; port-wine stain of eyelids; buphthalmos; optic nerve cupping; anisometropia; hemianopsia; increased corneal diameter; enophthalmos; exophthalmos; optic atrophy; choroidal hemangioma; anterior chamber angle vascularization.

Clinical

Vascular port-Wine nevus (face, scalp, limbs, trunk, leptomeninges); acromegaly; facial hemihypertrophy; intracranial angiomas; convulsion; mental retardation; obesity; limb atrophy.

Laboratory

Neuroimaging studies and the clinical examination have been the procedures of choice to establish the diagnosis.

Treatment

Anticonvulsants for seizure control, symptomatic and prophylactic therapy for headache and glaucoma treatment to reduce the intraocular pressure (IOP).

BIBLIOGRAPHY

1. Del Monte MA, Taravella M. (2012). Sturge-Weber syndrome. [online] Available from www.emedicine.com/oph/TOPIC348.HTM. [Accessed August, 2013].
2. Takeoka M, Riviello JJ. (2010). Pediatric Sturge-Weber syndrome. [online] Available from www.emedicine.com/neuro/TOPIC356.HTM. [Accessed August, 2013].

CHAPTER
12

Neurologic Disorders

1. AMBLYOPIA (FUNCTIONAL AMBLYOPIA, LAZY EYE)

General

Reduction of best-corrected visual acuity that cannot be explained by structural abnormalities. It is usually associated with strabismus or anisometropia. Onset in childhood.

Clinical

None.

Ocular

Decreased central visual acuity; decreased contrast sensitivity; strabismus; anisometropia.

Laboratory

Diagnosis is made by clinical findings.

Treatment

If there is an obstacle to vision such as cataract, corneal opacity, ptosis or refractive error, this must be treated first. Occlusion of the sound eye is the mainstay of treatment and the success depends on the compliance. Atropine ophthalmic drops can be used in the sound eye in mild or moderate cases of amblyopia. Early diagnosis and treatment provide the best chance of regaining useful vision.

BIBLIOGRAPHY

1. Yen KG. (2012). Amblyopia. [online] Available from www.emedicine.com/oph/TOPIC316.HTM. [Accessed August, 2013].

2. ANIRIDIA, CEREBELLAR ATAXIA, AND MENTAL DEFICIENCY (GILLESPIE SYNDROME)

General

Autosomal recessive; onset at birth.

Ocular

Congenital cataracts; incomplete formation of iris; bilateral congenital mydriasis.

Clinical

Cerebellar ataxia; mental deficiency; delayed developmental milestones; persistent hypotonia of muscles; gross incoordination; attention tremor; scanning speech.

Laboratory

Chromosomal deletion is detected by cytogenetic testing with the use of high-resolution banding.

Treatment

The goal is directed towards the control of intraocular pressure with use of topical drops. Frequently, this goal is not met. Photophobia can be treated with tinted glasses. Strabismus, amblyopia, refractive errors and nystagmus may also require treatment with traditional methods.

⊟ BIBLIOGRAPHY

1. Singh D, Verma A. (2012). Aniridia. [online] Available from www.emedicine.com/oph/TOPIC43.HTM. [Accessed August, 2013].

⊟ 3. ARNOLD-CHIARI SYNDROME (PLATYBASIA SYNDROME; CEREBELLOMEDULLARY MALFORMATION SYNDROME; BASILAR IMPRESSIONS)

General

Malformation of the hindbrain; developmental deformity of the occipital bone and upper cervical spine; recognized in children or adults; clinical picture may be indistinguishable from that of Dandy-Walker syndrome in infants.

Ocular

Horizontal, vertical and rotary forms of nystagmus; vertical nystagmus in both up gaze and down gaze is most common; papilledema; esotropia; Duane retraction syndrome (association); oscillopsia.

Clinical

Hydrocephalus; cerebellar ataxia; bilateral pyramidal tract signs.

Laboratory

Computed tomography (CT) scans are used most commonly for the diagnosis of hydrocephalus and for the evaluation of suspected shunt malfunction.

Treatment

Early recognition and treatment is important because of the potential life-threatening symptoms. Early surgical intervention, especially in infants may prevent irreversible changes and death.

⊟ BIBLIOGRAPHY

1. Incesu L, Khosla A, Aiello MR. (2011). Imaging in Chiari II malformation. [online] Available from www.emedicine.com/radio/TOPIC150.HTM. [Accessed August, 2013].

⊟ 4. ANDERSEN-WARBURG SYNDROME (WHITNALL-NORMAN SYNDROME; OLIGOPHRENIA MICROPHTHALMOS SYNDROME; NORRIE DISEASE; ATROPHIA OCULI CONGENITAL FETAL IRITIS SYNDROME; CONGENITAL PROGRESSIVE OCULO-ACOUSTICO-CEREBRAL DYSPLASIA)

General

Sex-linked inheritance; gross deformation of both eyes; only males affected; onset at birth; putative gene for Norrie disease has been isolated and mapped to Xp11.3.

Ocular

Bilateral microphthalmos with extensive destruction of all ocular structures often resembling a pseudotumor; blindness at birth; iris atrophy; iritis; corneal opacification and lenticular destruction with a mass visible behind the lens as long as the lens is still clear; malformed retina and choroid with retinal pseudotumors; retinal detachment; retrolental vascular mass.

Clinical

Mental retardation ranging from imbecility to idiocy (may begin at any age) in about two-thirds of the cases; deafness of differing severity with onset between ages 9 and 45 years.

Laboratory

Diagnosis is made by clinical findings.

Treatment

Topical treatment for iritis; retinal detachment surgery and vitrectomy may be necessary. Immediate laser treatment is recommended following birth.

🖻 BIBLIOGRAPHY

1. Andersen SR, Warburg M. Norrie's disease: congenital bilateral pseudotumor of the retina with recessive X-chromosomal inheritance; Preliminary Report. Arch Ophthalmol. 1961;66(5):614-8.
2. Black G, Redmond RM. The molecular biology of Norrie's disease. Eye (Lond). 1994;8(5):491-6.
3. Chow CC, Kiernam DF, Chau FY, et al. Laser photocoagulation at birth prevents blindness in Norrie's disease diagnosed using amniocentesis. Ophthalmology. 2010;117(12):2402-6.
4. Enyedi LB, de Juan E, Gaitan A. Ultrastructural study of Norrie's disease. Am J Ophthalmol. l991;111(4):439-45.
5. Liberfarb RM, Eavey RD, De Long GR, et al. Norrie's disease: a study of two families. Ophthalmology. 1985;92(10):1445-51.
6. Norrie G. Causes of blindness in children; Twenty-five years' experience of Danish institutes for the blind. Acta Ophthalmologica. 1927;5(1-3):357-86.
7. Warburg M. Norrie's disease: differential diagnosis and treatment. Acta Ophthalmologica. 1975;53(2):217-36.
8. Wong F, Goldberg MF, Hao Y. Identification of a nonsense mutation at codon 128 of the Norrie's disease gene in a male infant. Arch Ophthalmol. 1993;111(11):1553-7.

🖻 5. BATTEN-MAYOU SYNDROME (SPIELMEYER-VOGT SYNDROME; MAYOU-BATTEN DISEASE; STOCK-SPIELMEYER-VOGT SYNDROME; CEREBRORETINAL DEGENERATION; PIGMENTARY RETINAL LIPOID NEURONAL HEREDODEGENERATION; VOGT-SPIELMEYER SYNDROME; JUVENILE GANGLIOSIDE LIPIDOSIS; NEURONAL CEROID LIPOFUSCINOSIS; MYOCLONIC VARIANT OF CEREBRAL LIPIDOSIS; BATTEN DISEASE; CEREBROMACULAR DYSTROPHY; JUVENILE AMAUROTIC FAMILY IDIOCY; SPIELMEYER-SJÖGREN SYNDROME)

General

Autosomal recessive; some cases of autosomal dominant; possible disturbance in lipid metabolism; most common in Jewish families; onset between ages 5–8 years; mean age at death is 17 years; poor prognosis (*see* Tay-Sachs disease; Dollinger-Bielschowsky syndrome). The lipopigment storage diseases are divided into four types based on clinical and electron microscopic features: (1) infantile (Hagberg-Santavuori syndrome), (2) late infantile (Jansky-Bielschowsky disease), (3) juvenile (Spielmeyer-Vogt disease) and (4) adult (Kufs disease).

Ocular

Vision initially reduced, progressing to total blindness; fat deposition in the retina with gradual development of pigment disturbances resembling retinitis pigmentosa; progressive primary optic atrophy; granular pigmentary change of macula; there is clinical evidence supporting the idea that the primary lesion of the retina is in the inner layers.

Clinical

Mental disturbances; convulsions (later); apathy; irritability; ataxia; upper and lower motor neuron palsies; rigidity; complete paralysis and dementia in terminal stage; hypertonus; death from intercurrent infection.

Laboratory

Palmitoyl-protein thioesterase (PPT) levels can be measured in leukocytes, cultured fibroblasts, dried blood spots, and saliva. Tripeptidyl peptidase 1 (TTP1) levels can be measured in leukocytes, cultured fibroblasts, dried blood spots, and saliva. Fibroblast TTP1 activity is approximately 17,000 μM of amino acids produced per hour per mg of protein. The TTP1 activity in CLN2 is less than 4% of normal.

Treatment

No specific treatment is available for these diseases.

🗗 BIBLIOGRAPHY

1. Chang CH. (2009). Neuronal ceroid lipofuscinoses. [online] Available from www.emedicine.com/neuro/TOPIC498. HTM. [Accessed August, 2013].

🗗 6. BELL'S PALSY (IDIOPATHIC FACIAL PARALYSIS)

General

Unilateral facial nerve paralysis of sudden onset and gradual recovery involving the nerve as it runs through the fallopian canal; etiology unknown; more common in adults.

Ocular

Corneal ulcer; paralysis of seventh nerve; ectropion; lagophthalmos; ptosis; epiphora; decreased visual acuity; diplopia; ocular irritation; exposure keratitis.

Clinical

Aching in the ear or mastoid; tingling or numbness of cheek or mouth; alteration of taste; hyperacusis; epiphora; facial weakness; most commonly and frequently affected cranial nerve with herpes zoster is the facial nerve.

Laboratory

Diagnosed by clinical findings.

Treatment

Most patients recover without treatment. If spontaneous recovery does not occur, the most widely accepted treatment is corticosteroids.

🗗 BIBLIOGRAPHY

1. Taylor DC, Khoromi S, Zachariah SB. (2012). Bell palsy. [online] Available from www.emedicine.com/neuro/TOPIC413.HTM. [Accessed August, 2013].

🗗 7. BIELSCHOWSKY-LUTZ-COGAN SYNDROME (INTERNUCLEAR OPHTHALMOPLEGIA)

General

Lesion in the medial longitudinal fasciculus; anterior internuclear ophthalmoplegia consists of paresis of convergence with paresis of homolateral medial rectus muscle during lateral gaze toward opposite side of the lesion; in the posterior internuclear ophthalmoplegia, convergence is not affected, while the homolateral medial rectus muscle is paralytic on lateral gaze; the most common cause in young patients include a demyelinating process such as multiple sclerosis (MS), whereas an ischemic process is more common in the elderly; other reported causes of brainstem infarction associated with internuclear ophthalmoplegia include sickle cell trait, periarteritis nodosa, Wernicke encephalopathy, "crack" cocaine smoking.

Ocular

Unilateral or bilateral palsy of the medial rectus muscle during conjugate lateral gaze but with or without normal function of this muscle during convergence, depending on the type of internuclear ophthalmoplegia; dissociated nystagmus in the maximal abducted contralateral eye.

Laboratory

Computed tomography and magnetic resonance imaging (MRI).

Treatment

Intravenous (IV) and oral steroids may be beneficial.

🗗 BIBLIOGRAPHY

1. Lee AG, Berlie CL, Costello F. (2012). Ophthalmologic manifestations of multiple sclerosis. [online] Available fromwww.emedicine.com/oph/TOPIC179.HTM.[Accessed August, 2013].
2. Luzzio C, Dangond F. (2012). Multiple sclerosis. [online] Available from www.emedicine.com/emerg/TOPIC321. HTM. [Accessed August, 2013].

8. BONNET-DECHAUME-BLANC SYNDROME (CEREBRORETINAL ARTERIOVENOUS ANEURYSM SYNDROME; NEURORETINOANGIOMATOSIS SYNDROME; WYBURN-MASON SYNDROME)

General

Dominant inheritance; unilateral or bilateral arteriovenous aneurysm of the midbrain with ipsilateral retinal angioma and skin nevi; severity and extent of symptoms depend on location of cerebral aneurysm and structures it may involve; not regarded as hereditary; incidence is equal in men and women; usually becomes symptomatic at the age of 30 years.

Ocular

Exophthalmos; ptosis; strabismus; nystagmus; hemianopsia due to lesion in optic tract or pulvinar; sluggish pupils; anisocoria; retinal arteriovenous aneurysm; varicosity of retinal veins; arteriovenous angiomas; papilledema; optic atrophy of fellow eye; vitreous hemorrhage; rubeosis iridis; optic neuropathy secondary to compression by vascular malformation; proptosis; partial ophthalmoplegia.

Clinical

Arteriovenous angiomas of the thalamus and mesencephalon; facial vascular and pigmented nevi, usually in the trigeminal distribution; psychic disturbances; slow and scanning speech; hydrocephalus; headache; dizziness; hemiplegia; congenital defects of bone, muscle, kidneys and gastrointestinal tract.

Laboratory

MRI, magnetic resonance angiography (MRA), fluorescein angiography.

Treatment

Referral for neurologic evaluation is indicated since intracranial vascular malformations are associated more commonly with larger retinal vascular lesions. Stability of the retinal lesions limits the need for ocular treatment.

BIBLIOGRAPHY

1. Bidwell AE. (2012). Wyburn-Mason syndrome. [online] Available from www.emedicine.com/oph/TOPIC357.HTM. [Accessed August, 2013].

9. CEREBELLAR ATAXIA, INFANTILE, WITH PROGRESSIVE EXTERNAL OPHTHALMOPLEGIA

General

Autosomal recessive; neurologic lesion.

Ocular

Paralysis of all extraocular muscles; ptosis; retinal degeneration; blindness.

Clinical

Spinocerebellar degeneration; ataxia.

Laboratory

None.

Treatment

None.

BIBLIOGRAPHY

1. Hamosh A, Scott AF, Amberger J, et al. Online Mendelian Inheritance in Man (OMIM), a knowledge base of human genes and genetic disorders. Nucleic Acids Res. 2002;30(1):52-5.
2. Jampel RS, Okazaki H, Bernstein H. Ophthalmoplegia and retinal degeneration associated with spinocerebellar ataxia. Arch Ophthalmol. 1961;66(2):247-59.
3. McKusick VA. Mendelian Inheritance in Man; A Catalog of Human Genes and Genetic Disorders, 12th edition. Baltimore, USA: The Johns Hopkins University Press; 1998.

10. CEREBELLAR ATAXIA, CATARACT, DEAFNESS AND DEMENTIA OR PSYCHOSIS (HEREDOPATHIA OPHTHALMO-OTO-ENCEPHALICA)

General

Autosomal dominant.

Ocular

Posterior polar cataracts.

Clinical

Tremor, paranoid psychosis; dementia; deafness.

Laboratory

None.

Treatment

Cataract surgery if vision decreases.

BIBLIOGRAPHY

1. Hamosh A, Scott AF, Amberger J, et al. Online Mendelian Inheritance in Man, (OMIM), a knowledgebase of human genes and genetic disorders. Nucleic Acids Res. 2002; 30(1):52-5.
2. McKusick VA. Mendelian Inheritance in Man; A Catalog of Human Genes and Genetic Disorders, 12th edition. Baltimore, USA: The Johns Hopkins University Press; 1998.
3. Stromgren E. Heredopathia ophthalmo-oto-encephalica. Neurogenetic directory, part 1. Handbook Clin Neurol. 1981;42:150-2.

11. CEREBELLAR DEGENERATION WITH SLOW MOVEMENTS

General

Autosomal dominant; described only in Indian families; associated with spinocerebellar degeneration and abnormal eye movements.

Ocular

Paramedian pontine reticular formation (horizontal gaze center); absent rapid movements of both eyes and abnormally slow movements.

Clinical

Brainstem lesion of paramedian pontine reticular formation; progressive mental deterioration.

Laboratory

Computed tomography and MRI.

Treatment

None.

BIBLIOGRAPHY

1. Dalvi AI, Rauschkolb PK, Berman SA. (2012). Striatonigral degeneration. [online] Available from www.emedicine.com/neuro/TOPIC354.HTM. [Accessed August, 2013].

12. CEREBRAL AUTOSOMAL DOMINANT ARTERIOPATHY

General

Autosomal dominant, generalized nonatherosclerotic nonamyloid arteriopathy.

Ocular

Scotoma with migraine, cataract, iris atrophy, retinal microinfarction.

Clinical

Recurrent stroke, cognitive decline, subcortical vascular dementia.

Laboratory

It is diagnosed by clinical findings.

Treatment

Change in glasses can sometimes improve patient's visual function temporarily; however, the most common treatment is cataract surgery.

🗗 BIBLIOGRAPHY

1. Alagiakrishnan K, Masaki K. (2012). Vascular dementia. [online] Available from www.emedicine.com/med/TOPIC3150.HTM. [Accessed August, 2013].

🗗 13. CEREBRAL CHOLESTEROLOSIS (CEREBROTENDINOUS XANTHOMATOSIS; CTX)

General

Autosomal recessive; lipid storage is characterized by progressive neurologic dysfunction; large amounts of cholestanol and cholesterol in every tissue in the body, particularly in brain and lungs.

Ocular

Cataracts; juvenile cataracts.

Clinical

Cerebellar ataxia; systemic spinal cord involvement; atherosclerosis; mental retardation; unsteady gait; liver damage; jaundice; chronic diarrhea.

Laboratory

Lipid levels.

Treatment

Change in glasses can sometimes improve a patient's visual function temporarily; however, the most common treatment is cataract surgery.

🗗 BIBLIOGRAPHY

1. Berginer VM, Salen G, Shefer S. Long-term treatment of cerebrotendinous xanthomatosis with chenodeoxycholic acid. N Engl J Med. 1984;311(26):1649-52.
2. Cruysberg JR, Wevers RA, Tolboom JJ. Juvenile cataract associated with chronic diarrhea in pediatric cerebrotendinous xanthomatosis. Am J Ophthalmol. 1991;112(5):606-7.
3. Katz DA, Scheinberg L, Horoupian DS, et al. Peripheral neuropathy in cerebrotendinous xanthomatosis. Arch Neurol. 1985;42(10):1008-10.

🗗 14. CEREBRAL PALSY

General

Group of diverse nonprogressive syndromes resulting from injury to the motor centers of the brain; lesions may occur prenatally, in infancy or in childhood up to age of 5 years or more; constitutes the most common cause of permanent physical handicap in children.

Ocular

Strabismus; ptosis; congenital cataract; optic nerve atrophy; papilledema; iris coloboma; nystagmus; uveitis; paresis of extraocular muscles; blepharospasm; leukoma.

Clinical

Systemic abnormalities such as mental retardation, seizures, microcephalus, hydrocephalus, speech delays, and behavioral or emotional disturbances; motor defect; central visual impairment due to cerebral cortex and white matter malformation.

Laboratory

No diagnosis is made by clinical findings.

Treatment

Multiple medical complications require orthopedics, neurologists and rehabilitation medicine specialists.

🗗 BIBLIOGRAPHY

1. Abdel-Hamid HZ, Zeldin AS, Bazzano AT, et al. (2011). Cerebral palsy. [online] Available from www.emedicine.com/neuro/TOPIC533.HTM. [Accessed August, 2013].

15. CHRONIC PROGRESSIVE EXTERNAL OPHTHALMOPLEGIA (CPEO; OPHTHALMOPLEGIA PLUS)

General

A general term covering many conditions; onset at any age; familial history; conditions associated with chronic progressive external ophthalmoplegia (CPEO) include myotonic dystrophy, Kearns-Sayre syndrome and oculopharyngeal dystrophy; disorders that rarely cause external ophthalmoplegia include congenital disorders (abetalipoproteinemia, Refsum disease, extraocular fibrosis syndrome, Möbius syndrome), progressive supranuclear palsy, endocrine exophthalmos, myasthenia gravis and MS; now considered to be a mitochondrial cytopathy with varied clinical presentation; four distinct disorders of ophthalmic importance are: (1) CPEO or Kearns-Sayre syndrome, (2) myoclonus epilepsy with ragged-red fibers (MERRF), (3) mitochondrial encephalopathy, lactic acidosis and stroke-like episodes (MELAS) and (4) Leber optic neuropathy.

Ocular

Exposure keratopathy; filamentary keratitis; keratoconjunctivitis sicca; corneal scarring; esotropia; exotropia; gaze paralysis; ptosis; levator paralysis; cataract; optic atrophy; diplopia; tapetoretinal degeneration; constriction of visual field; retinitis pigmentosa.

Clinical

Weakness; weight loss; myopathic or Hutchinson facies; cardiac abnormalities; central nervous system (CNS) abnormalities.

Laboratory

No specific test; diagnosis is based on the clinical evidence.

Treatment

A complex disorder requiring the involvement of physicians from various specialties, including neurology, cardiology, ophthalmology and endocrinology.

BIBLIOGRAPHY

1. Roy H. (2011). Chronic progressive external ophthalmoplegia. [online] Available from www.emedicine.com/oph/TOPIC510.HTM. [Accessed August, 2013].

16. CLAUDE SYNDROME (INFERIOR NUCLEUS RUBER SYNDROME; RUBROSPINAL-CEREBELLAR-PEDUNCLE SYNDROME)

General

Paramedian mesencephalic lesion starting in midbrain; often occlusion of terminal branches of the paramedian arteries supplying the inferior portion of the nucleus ruber.

Ocular

Paralysis of ipsilateral oculomotor and trochlear nerves (III, IV).

Clinical

It may be associated with motor hemiplegia.

Laboratory

Diagnosis is made by clinical findings.

Treatment

Prisms may be useful for small deviations. Botulinum toxin may also be useful. For deviation greater than 15 prism diopters, strabismus surgery may be required.

BIBLIOGRAPHY

1. Claude H. Inferior nucleus ruber syndrome. Rev Neurol. 1912;1:311.
2. Cremieux G, Serratrice G. A case of retraction nystagmus associated with Claude's syndrome. Mars Med (Fre). 1972;109:635.
3. Gaymard B, Saudeau D, de Toffol B, et al. Two mesencephalic lacunar infarcts presenting as Claude's syndrome and pure motor hemiparesis. Eur Neurol. 1991;31:152-5.
4. Geeraets WJ. Ocular Syndromes, 3rd edition. Philadelphia, PA: Lea & Febiger; 1976.

🗇 17. CONGENITAL DYSLEXIA SYNDROME (DEVELOPMENTAL DYSLEXIA OF CRITCHLEY; CONGENITAL WORD BLINDNESS OF HERMANN; PRIMARY DYSLEXIA; DYSLEXIA SYNDROME; MINIMAL BRAIN DYSFUNCTION SYNDROME; ATTENTION DEFICIT DISORDER; CONGENITAL WORD BLINDNESS)

General

Primary reading disability in children with an average or above average intelligence; male preponderance; dysfunction of the dominating parietotemporal lobe; Levinson postulates a primary cerebellar-vestibular (inner ear) dysfunction underlying this syndrome resulting in a secondary scrambled sensory input and motor output.

Ocular

No obvious connection seems to exist between coordination of ocular functions and dyslexia, although associated ocular findings may exist in reading problems (e.g. abnormal optokinetic nystagmus, metamorphopsia, defective color vision, convergence insufficiency, muscle imbalance, refractive errors); low accommodative converge/accommodation associated with decreased visual acuity and contrast sensitivity.

Clinical

General clumsiness; disorientation (time-space, right-left); behavioral changes; lack of integration of visual and auditory stimuli.

Laboratory

An educational diagnostician, an educator trained as a reading specialist, and a school psychologist are the professionals charged with evaluation.

Treatment

No medical care is indicated. Appropriate referrals to a special education (SPED) setting, specialized tutoring setting, or both can prove important for long-term progress.

🗇 BIBLIOGRAPHY

1. Crouch ER, Dozier PM. (2011). Reading learning disorder. [online] Available from www.emedicine.com/ped/TOPIC2792.HTM. [Accessed August, 2013].

🗇 18. CREUTZFELDT-JAKOB SYNDROME (SPASTIC PSEUDOSCLEROSIS; CORTICOSTRIATOSPINAL DEGENERATION; DISSEMINATED ENCEPHALOPATHY; HEIDENHAIN SYNDROME; PRESENILE DEMENTIA WITH SPASTIC PARALYSIS; PRESENILE DEMENTIA-CORTICAL DEGENERATION SYNDROME)

General

Heredofamilial occurrence; caused by degenerative changes in cerebral cortex, basal ganglion, and spinal cord; disease is progressive; begins in middle or later age; occurs in both sexes.

Ocular

Cortical blindness; myoclonic conjugate eye movements; paralysis of seventh nerve; ptosis; dyschromatopsia; homonymous hemianopsia; nystagmus; slow vertical saccades; mild demyelination of the optic nerve.

Clinical

Mental deterioration; psychosis; stupor; weakness and stiffness of extremities; slow development of pyramidal signs; loss of reflexes; tremor, rigidity; dysarthria; aphasia; ataxia; myoclonus; convulsive seizures; cerebellar ataxia decerebrate posture.

Laboratory

Diagnosis is based on the clinical and biological tests.

Treatment

There is no effective therapy but discontinuing medications that cause confusion and possibly psychiatric care may be beneficial.

🗇 BIBLIOGRAPHY

1. Thomas FP. (2012). Variant Creutzfeldt-Jakob disease and Bovine spongiform encephalopathy. [online] Available from www.emedicine.com/neuro/TOPIC725.HTM. [Accessed August, 2013].

🗗 19. CUSHING (2) SYNDROME (ANGLE TUMOR SYNDROME; CEREBELLOPONTINE ANGLE SYNDROME; PONTOCEREBELLAR ANGLE TUMOR SYNDROME; ACOUSTIC NEUROMA SYNDROME)

General

Tumor involving cranial nerves V, VI, VII, and VIII and brainstem; occurs between ages 30 and 45 years.

Ocular

Paresis orbicularis muscle (VII); paresis external rectus muscle (VI); mixed nystagmus with head tilt; palsies of extraocular muscles are accounted for by increased intracranial pressure if the aqueduct of Sylvius is closed by the growing tumor; decreased corneal reflex V (homolateral and early sign); bilateral papilledema (increased intracranial pressure).

Clinical

Deafness (homolateral); labyrinth function disturbed or lost; tinnitus; hyperesthesia of the face; homolateral facial nerve paresis (total paralysis rare); hoarseness; difficulties in swallowing; unilateral limb ataxia; gait ataxia; nuchal headache; emesis; facial pain, numbness and paresis; progressive unilateral hearing loss.

Laboratory

The diagnostic test for acoustic tumors is gadolinium-enhanced MRI.

Treatment

Surgical excision of the tumor; arresting tumor growth using stereotactic radiation therapy; careful serial observation.

🗗 BIBLIOGRAPHY

1. Kutz JW, Roland PS, Isaacson B. (2012). Acoustic neuroma. [online] Available from www.emedicine.com/ent/TOPIC239.HTM. [Accessed August, 2013].

🗗 20. DE LANGE SYNDROME (I) (CONGENITAL MUSCULAR HYPERTROPHY CEREBRAL SYNDROME; BRACHMANN-DE LANGE SYNDROME)

General

Etiology not known; autosomal recessive inheritance.

Ocular

Antimongoloid slant of palpebral fissures; mild exophthalmos; hypertrichosis of eyebrows; long eyelashes; telecanthus; ptosis; blepharophimosis; nystagmus on lateral gaze; constant coarse nystagmus; strabismus; alternating exotropia; high myopia; anisocoria; chronic conjunctivitis; blue sclera; pallor of optic disk.

Clinical

Mental retardation; growth retardation; extrapyramidal motor disturbances; multiple skeletal abnormalities with congenital muscular hypertrophy; long philtrum; thin lips; crescent-shaped mouth.

Laboratory

Molecular diagnosis with screening of the nipped-B-like (NIPBL) gene, X-ray, ultrasonography, echocardiography.

Treatment

Early intervention for feeding problems, hearing and visual impairment, congenital heart disease, and urinary system abnormalities and psychomotor delay.

🗗 BIBLIOGRAPHY

1. Tekin M, Bodurtha J. (2011). Cornelia De Lange syndrome. [online] Available from www.emedicine.com/ped/TOPIC482.HTM. [Accessed August, 2013].

🗗 21. DISSEMINATED SCLEROSIS (MULTIPLE SCLEROSIS)

General

Disseminated demyelination affecting white matter of the brain, spinal cord and optic nerves; etiology is unknown.

Ocular

Nystagmus; ptosis; myokymia; optic atrophy; papillitis; optic neuritis; anisocoria; Argyll Robertson pupil; Marcus Gunn pupil; hippus, decreased or absent papillary reaction to light; periphlebitis; visual field defects; gaze palsy; paralysis of third or sixth nerve; uveitis; oscillopsia; Uhthoff symptom (reduction of visual acuity with exercise or ocular hyperthermia); pars planitis; retinal venous sheathing; retinitis; granulomatous uveitis.

Clinical

Incoordination; paresthesia; spasticity; tic douloureux; urinary frequency and infections; progressive disability; paralysis; death.

Laboratory

MRI, cerebrospinal fluid positive for oligoclonal band, albumin and immunoglobulin G (IgG) index; brainstem auditory-evoked response (BAER) and somatosensory-evoked potentials (SEP).

Treatment

Patients with MS may require multiple consultations to rule out other causes for their symptoms. Drugs such as immunomodulators, immunosuppressors, antiparkinson agents, CNS stimulants are all used in the management of the disease.

🗗 BIBLIOGRAPHY

1. Luzzio C, Dangond F. (2012). Multiple sclerosis. [online] Available from www.emedicine.com/neuro/topic228.htm. [Accessed August, 2013].

🗗 22. FRIEDREICH ATAXIA (SPINOCEREBELLAR ATAXIA)

General

Etiology unknown, either autosomal recessive or dominant; progressive; incapacitating by the age of 20 years; death from secondary diseases or cardiac failure; prevalent in males.

Ocular

Nystagmus; optic atrophy; there is a form of Friedreich ataxia (FA) associated with congenital glaucoma.

Clinical

Kyphoscoliosis; tremor; dysmetria; asynergia; slow ataxic speech; paresthesias; Babinski sign; headache; retarded growth; mental retardation; polyuria; polydipsia; deformity of feet (onset in first year of life); clumsy gait and difficult to turn arms, head and trunk; deafness.

Laboratory

MRI is the study of choice in the evaluation of the atrophic changes.

Treatment

Results of treating ataxia in FA have generally been disappointing. No therapeutic measures are known to alter the natural history of the neurological disease.

🗗 BIBLIOGRAPHY

1. Chawla J. (2012). Friedreich ataxia. [online] Available from www.emedicine.com/neuro/TOPIC139.HTM. [Accessed August, 2013].

⊟ 23. HARTNUP SYNDROME (PELLAGRA-CEREBELLAR ATAXIA-RENAL AMINOACIDURIA SYNDROME; H DISEASE; NIACIN DEFICIENCY)

General

Recessive; inborn error in amino acid metabolism with abnormal metabolism of tryptophan; both sexes affected; presents from infancy.

Ocular

Ectropion; symblepharon; nystagmus; scleral ulcers; corneal leukoma; photophobia; diplopia during attacks.

Clinical

Dermatitis (similar to pellagra) with skin eruptions; progressive mental retardation; cerebellar ataxia.

Laboratory

Therapeutic response to niacin in a patient with the typical symptoms and signs establishes the diagnosis.

Treatment

Oral therapy with nicotinamide or niacin usually is effective in reversing the clinical manifestations.

⊟ BIBLIOGRAPHY

1. Hegyi V, Schwartz RA. (2012). Dermatologic manifestations of pellagra. [online] Available from www.emedicine.com/derm/TOPIC621.HTM. [Accessed August, 2013].

⊟ 24. HYSTERIA (MALINGERING; OPHTHALMIC FLAKE SYNDROME)

General

Willful or unwillful exaggeration or simulation of symptoms of an illness without physiologic cause; frequently secondary to a state of anxiety; may be seen more in children; physical or sexual abuse may be a predisposing factor.

Ocular

Anxiety-induced angiospastic or central serous retinopathy; self-induced conjunctivitis; traumatic epithelial erosions; herpetic keratitis; angioneurotic edema; contact dermatitis; ptosis; recurrent herpetic vesicles; anisocoria; peculiar pupillary reflexes; accommodative spasm; amaurosis fugax; anxiety-induced optic neuritis; disturbance of conjugate movement; dyschromatopsia; facial tic; hypersecretion glaucoma; increased or decreased tear secretion; night blindness; nystagmus; photophobia; strabismus; visual loss; psychogenic amaurosis with headaches.

Clinical

Aphonia; deafness; paralysis of limb; hemiplegia; dissociative state; anxiety; insomnia; tachycardia; shortness of breath; fatigue; vertigo, chest pains.

Laboratory

Eye examination to rule out pathology. Visual-evoked responses, electroretinopathy and electrooculography all should be normal.

Treatment

Psychiatric intervention is required in severe cases.

⊟ BIBLIOGRAPHY

1. Barris MC, Kaufman DI, Barberio D. Visual impairment in hysteria. Documenta Ophthalmologica. 1992;82:369-82.
2. Catalono RA, Simon JW, Krohel GB, et al. Functional visual loss in children. Ophthalmology. 1986;93(3):385-90.
3. Kramer KK, La Piana FG, Appleton B. Ocular malingering and hysteria: diagnosis and management. Surv Ophthalmol. 1979;24(2):89-96.
4. Miller BW. A review of practical tests for ocular malingering and hysteria. Surv Ophthalmol. 1973;17(4):241-6.
5. Roy FH, Fraunfelder FW, Fraunfelder FT. Roy and Fraunfelder's Current Ocular Therapy, 6th edition. Philadelphia, PA: WB Saunders; 2008.
6. Ziegler DK, Schlemmer RB. Familial psychogenic blindness and headache: a case study. J Clin Psychiatry. 1994;55(3):114-7.

25. JOUBERT SYNDROME (FAMILIAL CEREBELLAR VERMIS AGENESIS)

General

Autosomal recessive; both sexes affected; onset in early infancy.

Ocular

Choroidal coloboma; nystagmus; ocular fibrosis, telecanthus.

Clinical

Episodic hyperpnea; apnea; ataxia; psychomotor retardation; rhythmic protrusion of tongue; mental retardation; micrognathia; complex cardiac malformation; cutaneous dimples over wrists and elbows.

Laboratory

Urine culture, renal ultrasonography, dimercaptosuccinic acid (DMSA) renal scanning.

Treatment

Lifetime follow-up is required whether or not involution has occurred or a nephrectomy.

BIBLIOGRAPHY

1. Swiatecka-Urban A. (2011). Multicystic renal dysplasia. [online] Available from www.emedicine.com/ped/TOPIC1493.HTM. [Accessed August, 2013].

26. MARINESCO-SJÖGREN SYNDROME (CONGENITAL SPINOCEREBELLAR ATAXIA-CONGENITAL CATARACT-OLIGOPHRENIA SYNDROME)

General

Autosomal recessive trait; onset when child learns to walk; mitochondrial disease.

Ocular

Cataracts; aniridia; rotary and horizontal nystagmus; nystagmus; strabismus; optic atrophy.

Clinical

Cerebellar ataxia; oligophrenia; small stature; scoliosis; genu valgum; restricted extensibility of the knee; defects of fingers and toes; mental retardation; hair sparse; hypersalivation; sensorineural hearing loss.

Laboratory

Diagnosis is made by clinical findings.

Treatment

Cataracts: Change in glasses can sometimes improve a patient's visual function temporarily; however, the most common treatment is cataract surgery.

BIBLIOGRAPHY

1. Dotti MT, Bardelli AM, De Stefano N, et al. Optic atrophy in Marinesco-Sjögren syndrome: an additional ocular feature: Report of three cases in two families. Ophthalmic Genet. 1993;14(1):5-7.
2. Gillespie FD. Aniridia, cerebellar ataxia, and oligophrenia in siblings. Arch Ophthalmol. 1965;73(3):338-41.
3. Linda S, Lund I, Torbergsen T, et al. Mitochondrial diseases and myopathies: a series of muscle biopsy specimens with ultrastructural changes in the mitochondria. Ultrastruct Pathol. 1992;16(3):263-75.
4. Marinesco G, Draganesco S, Vasiliu. Nouvelle maladie familiale caractérisée par une tcataracte congénitale et un arrêt du developpement somatoneuropsychique. L'Encephale. 1931;26:97.
5. Sjögren T. Hereditary congenital spinocerebellar ataxia combined with congenital cataracts and oligophrenia. Acta Psychiatrica Scandinavica. 1947;22(S46):286-9.

27. NEUROPARALYTIC KERATITIS (NEUROTROPIC KERATITIS, TRIGEMINAL NEUROPATHIC KERATOPATHY)

General

Numbness of the cornea from injury of trigeminal nerve. Causes include surgery of trigeminal neuralgias, surgery of acoustic neuroma and herpes zoster ophthalmicus and Riley-Day syndrome.

Clinical

None.

Ocular

Abnormalities of the tear film and cornea, punctate keratopathy, epithelial detachment, stromal lysis.

Laboratory

Diagnosis is made by clinical findings.

Treatment

- *Stage 1:* Punctate keratopathy treated with intermittent patching. Oral tetracyclines and discontinuing contact lens may be helpful.
- *Stage 2:* Epithelial detachment—atropine, Blenderm or temporary tarsorrhaphy. Botulinum toxin into levator palpebral superioris.
- *Stage 3:* Closure of lid—atropine and botulinum toxin and antibiotics and systemic antibiotic. Permanent tarsorrhaphy.

BIBLIOGRAPHY

1. Graham RH, Hendrix MA. (2012). Neurotrophic keratopathy. [online] Available from www.emedicine.com/oph/TOPIC106.HTM. [Accessed August, 2013].

28. NOTHNAGEL SYNDROME (OPHTHALMOPLEGIA-CEREBELLAR ATAXIA SYNDROME)

General

Lesion of superior cerebellar peduncle, red nucleus and emerging oculomotor fibers such as pineal tumor, or tumor or vascular disturbance in corpora quadrigemina or vermis cerebelli (*see* Bruns syndrome).

Ocular

Oculomotor paresis; gaze paralysis most frequently upward, combined with some degree of internal or external ophthalmoplegia.

Clinical

Cerebellar ataxia; poor upper extremity movements; neoplasia; infarction; midbrain lesion.

Laboratory

Computed tomography and MRI of brain.

Treatment

See neurologist.

BIBLIOGRAPHY

1. Magalini SI, Scrascia E. Dictionary of Medical Syndromes, 2nd edition. Philadelphia, PA: Lippincott Williams and Wilkins; 1981.
2. Nothnagel H. Topische Diagnostik Der Gehirnkrankheiten. Berlin: Nabu Press; 2010. p. 220.

29. OBESITY-CEREBRAL-OCULAR-SKELETAL ANOMALIES SYNDROME

General

Rare, autosomal recessive disease; similar to Prader-Willi and Laurence-Moon-Bardet-Biedl syndromes.

Ocular

Microphthalmia; antimongoloid slant of lid fissure; asymmetrical size of fissure; strabismus; myopia; iris and chorioretinal colobomata; mottled retina; prominent choroidal vessels.

Clinical

Obesity (mid-childhood onset); hypotonia; mental retardation; craniofacial anomalies with microcephaly; tapering extremities; hyperextensibility at elbows and proximal interphalangeal joints; cubitus valgus; genu valgum; Simian creases; syndactyly.

Laboratory

Diagnosis is made by clinical findings.

Treatment

Strabismus: Equalized vision with correct refractive error; surgery may be helpful in patient with diplopia.

BIBLIOGRAPHY

1. Cohen MM, Hall BD, Smith DW, et al. A new syndrome with hypotonia, obesity, mental deficiency, and facial, oral, ocular, and limb anomalies. J Pediatr. 1973;83(2):280-4.
2. Hall BD, Smith DW. Prader-Willi syndrome: A resumé of 32 cases including an instance of affected first cousins, one of whom is of normal stature and intelligence. J Pediatr. 1972;81(2):286-93.

30. OCULOCEREBELLAR TEGMENTAL SYNDROME

General

Vascular lesion of mesencephalon with softening in peduncular area.

Ocular

Paralysis of associated ocular movements (internuclear anterior ophthalmoplegia).

Clinical

Sudden onset of hemiplegia with rapid recovery; bilateral cerebellar syndrome.

Laboratory

Diagnosis is made by clinical findings.

Treatment

Treat vascular lesion.

BIBLIOGRAPHY

1. Fournier A, Ducoulombier H, Cousin J, et al. [Oculo-cerebello-myoclonic syndrome and neuroblastoma]. J Sci Med Lille. 1972;90(5):189-97.
2. Rodriquez B, et al. A new type of peduncular syndrome: internuclear ophthalmoplegia and bilateral cerebellar syndrome from a tegmental lesion. Arch Urug Med. 1945;10:353; Am J Ophthalmol. 1946;29:511.

31. OCULOCEREBRAL SYNDROME WITH HYPOPIGMENTATION (AMISH OCULOCEREBRAL SYNDROME; CROSS SYNDROME)

General

Autosomal recessive.

Ocular

Spastic ectropion; microphthalmos; enophthalmos; microcornea; corneal opacification; corneal vascularization; palpebral conjunctival injection; narrow lid fissures; aniridia; nystagmus; bilateral optic atrophy.

Clinical

Spastic diplegia; cutaneous hypopigmentation; mental retardation; hypogonadism; growth retardation; developmental defects of the CNS such as cystic malformation of the posterior fossa of the Dandy-Walker type.

Laboratory

Diagnosis is made by clinical findings.

Treatment

See enophthalmos.

⊟ BIBLIOGRAPHY

1. Cross HE, McKusick VA, Breen W, et al. A new oculocerebral syndrome with hypopigmentation. J Pediatr. 1967;70(3): 398-406.
2. De Jong G, Fryns JP. Oculocerebral syndrome with hypopigmentation (Cross syndrome): the mixed pattern of hair pigmentation as an important diagnostic sign. Genet Couns. 1991;2(3):151-5.
3. Lerone M, Possagno A, Taccone A, et al. Oculocerebral syndrome with hypopigmentation (Cross syndrome): report of a new case. Clin Genet. 1992;41(2):87-9.
4. Pinsky L, DiGeorge AM, Harley RD, et al. Microphthalmos, corneal opacity, mental retardation, and spastic cerebral palsy: An oculocerebral syndrome. J Pediatr. 1965;67(3):387-98.

⊟ 32. OCULOPALATOCEREBRAL DWARFISM (OPC DWARFISM)

General

Autosomal recessive; persistent hyperplastic primary vitreous.

Ocular

Persistent hypertrophic primary vitreous; microphthalmos; leukocoria; retrolental fibrovascular membrane.

Clinical

Microcephaly; mental retardation; spasticity; cleft palate; short stature.

Laboratory

Diagnosis is made by clinical findings.

Treatment

Persistent hyperplastic primary vitreous—monocular congenital cataract surgery and amblyopia therapy. Posterior transciliary for pars plana vitrectomy and removal of tissue.

⊟ BIBLIOGRAPHY

1. Frydman M, Kauschansky A, Leshem I, et al. Oculo-palato-cerebral dwarfism: a new syndrome. Clin Genet. 1985; 27(4):414-419.
2. Hamosh A, Scott AF, Amberger J, et al. Online Mendelian Inheritance in Man, (OMIM), a knowledgebase of human genes and genetic disorders. Nucleic Acids Res. 2002;30(1):52-5.
3. McKusick VA. Mendelian Inheritance in Man; A Catalog of Human Genes and Genetic Disorders, 12th edition. Baltimore, USA: The Johns Hopkins University Press; 1998.

⊟ 33. OCULORENOCEREBELLAR SYNDROME (ORC SYNDROME)

General

Autosomal recessive.

Ocular

Progressive tapetoretinal degeneration with loss of retinal vessels.

Clinical

Mental retardation; continuous jerky movements; spastic diplegia; glomerulopathy with most renal glomeruli completely sclerosed.

Laboratory

Diagnosis is made by clinical findings.

Treatment

None—ocular.

⊟ BIBLIOGRAPHY

1. Hamosh A, Scott AF, Amberger J, et al. Online Mendelian Inheritance in Man, (OMIM), a knowledgebase of human genes and genetic disorders. Nucleic Acids Res. 2002;30(1): 52-5.
2. Hunter AGW, Jurenka S, Thompson D, et al. Absence of cerebellar granular layer, mental retardation, tapetoretinal degeneration and progressive glomerulopathy: An autosomal recessive oculo-renal-cerebellar syndrome. Am J Med Genet. 1982;11(4):383-95.
3. McKusick VA. Mendelian Inheritance in Man; A Catalog of Human Genes and Genetic Disorders, 12th edition. Baltimore, USA: The Johns Hopkins University Press; 1998.

34. OLIVOPONTOCEREBELLAR ATROPHY III (OPCA III; OPCA WITH RETINAL DEGENERATION)

General

Autosomal dominant; neurologic lesion; dominant with variable penetration.

Ocular

Retinopathy variable: peripheral, macular and circumpapillary; retinal degeneration; blindness; external ophthalmoplegia; variable electroretinogram function.

Clinical

Ataxia.

Laboratory

Anti-Purkinje cell antibodies, MRI.

Treatment

Treatment is directed to symptoms.

BIBLIOGRAPHY

1. Azevedo CJ, Berman SA. (2012). Olivopontocerebellar atrophy. [online] Available from www.emedicine.com/neuro/TOPIC282.HTM. [Accessed August, 2013].

35. OPTIC ATROPHY WITH DEMYELINATING DISEASE OF CNS

General

Autosomal dominant; demyelinated optic nerves appear smaller than normal and are pale white or gray in color; blood vessels may seem to be less prominent than normal.

Ocular

Optic neuritis; Leber optic atrophy.

Clinical

Ataxia; leg weakness; dysarthria; hemiparesis.

Laboratory/Ocular

Lumbar puncture, cerebrospinal fluid studies, MRI of brain and orbits.

Treatment/Ocular

Prednisolone, methylprednisolone.

BIBLIOGRAPHY

1. Gandhi R, Amula GM. (2012). Optic atrophy. [online] Available from www.emedicine.com/oph/TOPIC777.HTM. [Accessed August, 2013].

36. PARKINSON SYNDROME (PARALYSIS AGITANS; SHAKING PALSY)

General

Late stages of epidemic encephalitis; present with arteriosclerosis and with manganese and carbon monoxide poisoning; widespread destruction of pigmented cells in substantia nigra.

Ocular

Decreased blinking; lid fluttering; blepharospasm; oculogyric crises; ocular hypotony; blepharoplegia; ptosis; nystagmus; paralysis of convergence; paralysis of lateral rectus muscle; absent or sluggish pupillary reactions to light or convergence; mydriasis or anisocoria; optic neuritis; papilledema; abnormal saccades.

Clinical

Slowness of movements; loss of facial expression; "cogwheel" rigidity of the arms; rhythmical tremors; drooling; shuffling gait; stooping; monotonous voice.

Laboratory

MRI and CT scan reveal calcium and ceruloplasmin to exclude other conditions.

Treatment

The goal of medical management is to provide control of signs and symptoms for as long as possible while minimizing adverse effects. Medications usually provide good symptomatic control.

BIBLIOGRAPHY

1. Garcia-Martin E, Satue M, Fuertes I, et al. Ability and reproducibility of Fourier-domain optical coherence tomography to detect retinal nerve fiber layer atrophy in Parkinson's disease. Ophthalmology. 2012;119(10):2161-7.
2. Hauser RA, Lyons KE, McClain TA, et al. (2012). Parkinson disease. [online] Available from www.emedicine.com/neuro/TOPIC304.HTM. [Accessed August, 2013].

37. RAEDER SYNDROME (PARATRIGEMINAL PARALYSIS; HORTON HEADACHE; HISTAMINE CEPHALALGIA; CILIARY NEURALGIA; CLUSTER HEADACHE; PERIODIC MIGRAINOUS NEURALGIA)

General

Interruption of sympathetic fibers about the carotid artery and involvement of the fifth nerve; meningioma and aneurysm of the internal carotid artery are the most frequent causes; prominent in males; possible pathogenetic mechanism of this condition is an ischemic injury of the gasserian ganglion.

Ocular

Mild enophthalmos; mild ptosis (unilateral); epiphora; scotoma possible; hypotonia; unilateral miosis; increased tear secretion; periocular pain; Homer syndrome.

Clinical

Facial pain; occasionally weakness of the jaw muscles; headaches (V-region); hypertension; associated inflammatory processes are not infrequent.

Laboratory

Brain scan to rule out meningioma and basilar artery aneurysm.

Treatment

Oxygen inhalation and sumatriptan subcutaneous is useful in acute attacks.

BIBLIOGRAPHY

1. Bardorf CM, van Stavern G, Garcia-Valenzuela E. (2012). Horner syndrome. [online] Available from www.emedicine.com/oph/TOPIC336.HTM. [Accessed August, 2013].

38. SOTOS SYNDROME (CEREBRAL GIGANTISM)

General

Idiopathic disturbance of the diencephalon; etiology unknown; cerebral gigantism in childhood, Russell syndrome and total lipodystrophy are related forms of the same entity.

Ocular

Hypertelorism; antimongoloid lid aperture; high refractive error (hyperopia); nystagmus; strabismus.

Clinical

Acromegaly; large skull with frontal bossing; mental retardation; incoordination; abnormal excessive growth, mainly during the first 2 years of life.

Laboratory

Diagnosis is made by clinical findings.

Treatment

Strabismus: Equalized vision with correct refractive error; surgery may be helpful in patient with diplopia.

BIBLIOGRAPHY

1. Maino DM, Kofman J, Flynn MF, et al. Ocular manifestations of Sotos syndrome. J Am Optom Assoc. 1994;65(5):339-46.
2. Milunski A, Cowie VA, Donoghue EC. Cerebral gigantism in childhood: a report of two cases and a review of the literature. Pediatrics. 1967;40(3):395-402.
3. Sotos JF, Dodge PR, Muirhead D, et al. Cerebral gigantism in childhood. A syndrome of excessively rapid growth and acromegalic features and a nonprogressive neurologic disorder. N Engl J Med. 1964;271:109-16.
4. Yeh H, Price RL, Lonsdale D. Cerebral gigantism (Sotos' syndrome) and cataracts. J Pediatr Ophthalmol Strabismus. 1978;15(4):231-2.

39. SPINOCEREBELLAR ATROPHY WITH PUPILLARY PARALYSIS

General

Autosomal dominant; rare.

Ocular

Absence of pupillary reaction to light or convergence.

Clinical

Spinocerebellar atrophy.

Laboratory

Diagnosis is made by clinical findings.

Treatment

None.

BIBLIOGRAPHY

1. Hamosh A, Scott AF, Amberger J, et al. Online Mendelian Inheritance in Man (OMIM), a knowledgebase of human genes and genetic disorders. Nucleic Acids Res. 2002;30(1):52-5.
2. McKusick VA. Mendelian Inheritance in Man; A Catalog of Human Genes and Genetic Disorders, 12th edition. Baltimore, USA: The Johns Hopkins University Press; 1998.
3. Sutherland JM, Tyrer JH, Eadie MJ, et al. Atrophic spino-cerébelleuse familiale avec mydriase fixe. Rev Neurol. 1963;108:439-42.

40. STANNUS CEREBELLAR SYNDROME

General

Vitamin B (riboflavin) deficiency.

Ocular

Nystagmus; increased lacrimation; asthenopia; blepharitis; angular conjunctivitis; iris nodules; perilimbal vasodilation and pigmentation; corneal vascularization; superficial—diffuse keratitis; epithelial edema and corneal opacities; cataracts; brownish retinal patches.

Clinical

Muscular asthenia; hypotonia; ataxia; dysdiadochokinesia; mucocutaneous lesions resembling monilial intertrigo and glossitis.

Treatment

- Nystagmus
  - *Seesaw nystagmus:* Visual field to consider neoplastic or vascular etiologies.
  - *Upbeat nystagmus:* It may indicate MS, cerebellar degeneration, tumors or infarcts. Treatment is directed toward identification and resolution of underlying cause.
  - *Downbeat nystagmus:* It affects the cerebellum or craniocervical junction including Arnold-Chiari malformation, MS, trauma, tumor, infarction and many toxic metabolic entities. MRI may indicate a surgically correctable lesion. Periodic alternating nystagmus is continuous horizontal nystagmus from stroke, tumor, MS, trauma, infection, drug intoxication. It can occur from cataract, vitreous hemorrhage or optic atrophy.

- *Corneal vascularization:* Check for elevated intraocular pressure. Medical treatment includes the use of hyperosmotic drops, nonsteroidal and steroid eye drops. Corneal transplant may be necessary.
- *Cataract:* Change in glasses can sometimes improve a patient's visual function temporarily; however the most common treatment is cataract surgery.

BIBLIOGRAPHY

1. Osuntokun BO, Langman MJ, Wilson J, et al. Controlled trial of combinations of hydroxocobalamin-cysteine and riboflavin-cysteine, in Nigerian ataxic neuropathy. J Neurol Neurosurg Psychiatry. 1974;37:102-4.
2. Roe DA. Riboflavin deficiency: mucocutaneous signs of acute and chronic deficiency. Semin Dermatol. 1991;10(4):293-5.
3. Stannus HS. Some problems in riboflavin and allied deficiencies. Br Med J. 1944;2(4359):103-40.

41. SYMONDS SYNDROME (OTITIC HYDROCEPHALUS SYNDROME; SEROUS MENINGITIS SYNDROME; BENIGN INTRACRANIAL HYPERTENSION; PSEUDOTUMOR CEREBRI)

General

Children and adolescents; protracted course; increased cerebrospinal fluid, but without increase in protein or cells.

Ocular

Sixth nerve palsy, ipsilateral side with otitis media; retinal hemorrhages and exudates; moderate-to-marked papilledema followed by secondary optic atrophy; unilateral or bilateral swelling of the optic nerve head have been reported; cranial nerve third and fourth involvement; bilateral retinal vein occlusion.

Clinical

Greatly increased pressure of spinal fluid, often greater than 300 mm Hg, without increased cells or protein; intermittent headaches; otitis media; chronic renal failure; chronic myeloid leukemia.

Laboratory

Imaging studies such as MRI to rule out tumors of brain and spinal cord and lumbar puncture.

Treatment

Carbonic anhydrase inhibitors such as acetazolamide and furosemide are useful.

BIBLIOGRAPHY

1. Chang D, Nagamoto G, Smith WE. Benign intracranial hypertension and chronic renal failure. Cleve Clin J Med. 1992;59(4):419-22.
2. Chari C, Rao NS. Benign intracranial hypertension—its unusual manifestations. Headache. 1991;31(9):599-600.
3. Chern S, Magargal LE, Brav SS. Bilateral central retinal vein occlusion as an initial manifestation of pseudotumor cerebri. Ann Ophthalmol. 1991;23(2):54-7.
4. Roy FH, Fraunfelder FW, Fraunfelder FT. Roy and Fraunfelder's Current Ocular Therapy, 6th edition. Philadelphia, PA: WB Saunders; 2008.
5. Venable HP. Pseudo-tumor cerebri. J Natl Med Assoc. 1970;62(6):435-40.
6. Venable HP. Pseudo-tumor cerebri: further studies. J Natl Med Assoc. 1973;65(3):194-7.

42. THYROCEREBRORETINAL SYNDROME (FAMILIAL THYROCEREBRAL-RETINAL SYNDROME)

General

Autosomal recessive; renal, neurologic, and thyroid disease.

Ocular

Retinal hemorrhages; central vision defect; retinal edema; optic atrophy.

Clinical

Thrombocytopenia; chronic renal disease; colloid goiter.

Treatment/Ocular

Blood test, CT scans and MRI are essential in the evaluation and diagnosis. Corticosteroids are useful. Excision or decompression is needed when orbital tumors compress the optic nerve.

BIBLIOGRAPHY

1. McKusick VA. Mendelian Inheritance in Man, 12th edition. Baltimore, USA: The Johns Hopkins University Press; 1998.

43. TOLOSA-HUNT SYNDROME (PAINFUL OPHTHALMOPLEGIA)

General

Symptoms last from days to weeks; attacks recur at intervals of months or years; inflammatory lesion of cavernous sinus; onset most frequent in fifth decade of life; recurrent Tolosa-Hunt syndrome has been observed in some patients.

Ocular

Steadily "growing" retro-orbital pain; ptosis; involvement of cranial nerves III, IV, VI, and first division of V; scintillating scotomata; sluggish pupil reaction to light; corneal sensitivity diminished; optic neuritis.

Clinical

Inflammatory lesions of cavernous sinus.

Laboratory

MRI with axial and coronal views of brain, typically showing thickening and enhancement of involved cavernous sinus. Cerebral angiography is done to rule out aneurysm. Blood count, erythrocyte sedimentation rate, antinuclear antibody, antineutrophil cytoplasmic antibody and angiotensin-converting enzyme levels may be abnormal.

Treatment

Corticosteroids is often used to treat the chronic granulomatous inflammation of the cavernous sinus.

BIBLIOGRAPHY

1. Taylor DC. (2012). Tolosa-Hunt syndrome. [online] Available from www.emedicine.com/neuro/TOPIC373.HTM. [Accessed August, 2013].

44. TRAUMATIC ENCEPHALOPATHY SYNDROME (POSTTRAUMATIC GENERAL CEREBRAL SYNDROME; POSTCONCUSSION SYNDROME; PUNCH-DRUNK SYNDROME), NYSTAGMUS

General

Small focal hemorrhages within the cerebrum and/or cerebellum causing functional brain damage; minor traumatic brain injury is the most common type of traumatic encephalopathy.

Ocular

Nystagmus or nystagmoid ocular movements.

Clinical

Personality change; rigid face without expression; staggering gait; dysphonia.

Laboratory

Computed tomography and MRI can detect intracranial abnormalities.

Treatment

No specific treatment has been proven effective.

BIBLIOGRAPHY

1. Legome EL, Alt R, Wu T. (2011). Postconcussive syndrome in emergency medicine. [online] Available from www.emedicine.com/emerg/TOPIC865.HTM. [Accessed August, 2013].

45. WEBER SYNDROME (WEBER-DUBLER SYNDROME; CEREBELLAR PEDUNCLE SYNDROME; ALTERNATING OCULOMOTOR PARALYSIS; VENTRAL MEDIAL MIDBRAIN SYNDROME), PTOSIS

General

Lesion of the peduncle (crus), pons or medulla, which interrupts the third nerve before it emerges from the peduncle and interrupts fibers in the pyramidal tract above the level of the third nuclei; hemorrhage and thrombosis; tumor of the pituitary region, extending posteriorly; also may result in secondary to cerebrovascular disease.

Ocular

Ptosis; homolateral third nerve palsy (usually complete); fixed, dilated pupil.

Clinical

Contralateral hemiplegia; contralateral paralysis of face and tongue (supranuclear type).

Laboratory

Diagnosis is made by clinical findings.

Treatment

Ptosis: If visual acuity is affected, most cases require surgical correction and there are several procedures that may be used including levator resection, repair or advancement and Fasanella-Servat.

BIBLIOGRAPHY

1. Kistler JP, Ropper AH, Martin JB. Cerebrovascular diseases. In: Isselbacher KJ, Braunwald E, Wilson JD, Martin JB, Fauci A, Kasper DL (Eds). Harrison's Principles of Internal Medicine, 13th edition. New York: McGraw-Hill; 1994.
2. Miller NR (Ed). Walsh and Hoyt's Clinical Neuro-Ophthalmology, 44th edition. Baltimore, USA: Williams & Wilkins; 1995.
3. Newman NJ. Third, fourth and sixth-nerve lesions and the cavernous sinus. In: Albert DM, Jakobiec FA (Eds). Albert & Jakobiec's Principles and Practice of Ophthalmology: Clinical Practice, 5th edition. Philadelphia, PA: WB Saunders; 1994.
4. Weber H. A contribution to the pathology of the crura cerebri. Med Chir Trans. 1863;46:121-40.1.
5. Wolf BS, Newman CM, Khilnani MT. The posterior inferior cerebellar artery on vertebral angiography. Am J Roentgenol Radium Ther Nucl Med. 1962;87:322-37.

CHAPTER
13

Neoplasms

⊟ 1. ACTINIC AND SEBORRHEIC KERATOSIS

General

Actinic keratosis is a precancerous lesion that occurs most commonly on sunlight-exposed areas of the skin. Seborrheic keratosis is a benign epithelial tumor that appears predominantly on the trunk and head.

Clinical

Lupus.

Ocular

Eyebrow and eyelids lesions.

Laboratory

Diagnosis is made by clinical findings.

Treatment

Cryosurgery is the treatment of choice.

⊟ BIBLIOGRAPHY

1. Roy FH, Fraunfelder FW, Fraunfelder FT. Roy and Fraunfelder's Current Ocular Therapy, 6th edition. London: Elsevier, 2008.

⊟ 2. BASAL CELL CARCINOMA

General

Most common malignant neoplasm of lids; it can occasionally occur as a primary basal cell cancer of the conjunctiva and in the lacrimal canaliculus.

Ocular

Neoplasm most common on lower lid and medial canthus; lacrimation.

Clinical

Tumors of skin and other regions, including sinuses.

Laboratory

Typical histology findings. Imaging studies only for invading or deep tumor in the medial canthus.

Treatment

Surgery involves local excision, advanced and recurrent tumors are best managed by a multidisciplinary approach involving head and neck surgical oncologists. Photodynamic therapy and cryosurgery are also effective.

⊟ BIBLIOGRAPHY

1. Bader RS, Santacroce L, Diomede L, et al. (2012). Basal Cell Carcinoma. [online] Available from/www.emedicine.com/ent/TOPIC722.HTM. [Accessed August, 2013].

3. BASAL CELL NEVUS SYNDROME (NEVOID BASAL CELL CARCINOMA SYNDROME; NEVOID BASALIOMA SYNDROME; GORLIN SYNDROME; GORLIN-GOLTZ SYNDROME; MULTIPLE BASAL CELL NEVI SYNDROME)

General

Autosomal dominant; onset of skin lesions in childhood, usually at puberty.

Ocular

Basal cell carcinomas of eyelids; strabismus; hypertelorism; congenital cataracts; choroidal colobomas; glaucoma; medullated nerve fibers; prominence of supraorbital ridges; corneal leukoma; basalioma of the skin; coloboma of the choroid and optic nerve.

Clinical

Basal cell tumors with facial involvement; shallow pits of the skin of the hands and feet; jaw cysts; rib anomalies; kyphoscoliosis and fusion of vertebrae; medulloblastoma; frontal and temporoparietal bossing and broad nasal root.

Laboratory

Computed tomography (CT) scanning, ultrasonography, or magnetic resonance imaging (MRI) to evaluate neoplasms. Endoscopy to evaluate for the degree of polyposis and survey for malignant transformation is done.

Treatment

Patients may require medical attention for craniofacial, vertebral, dental, and ophthalmologic abnormalities, in addition to diagnosis and treatment of potential neoplasia.

BIBLIOGRAPHY

1. Hsu EK, Mamula P, Ruchelli ED. (2011). Intestinal polyposis syndromes. [online] Available from/www.emedicine.com/ped/TOPIC828.HTM [Accessed August, 2013].

4. SQUAMOUS CELL CARCINOMA, CONJUNCTIVAL

General

Malignant epithelial neoplasm characterized by basement membrane invasion or distant metastasis. Believed to arise from limbal stem cells and present as a mass in the interpalpebral fissure. Seen more frequently in Caucasians and individuals with exposure to sunlight but multiple infectious agents may play a role in the development. Human papillomavirus, human immunodeficiency virus (HIV), actinic exposure, the use of petroleum products and cigarette smoking may also be factors.

Clinical

Human papillomavirus, HIV, actinic exposure, the use of petroleum products, cigarette smokers.

Ocular

Gelatinous and velvety papilliform or leukoplakic mass on the nasal or temporal limbal area; irritation, chronic conjunctivitis.

Laboratory

Excisional biopsy is used to make positive diagnosis.

Treatment

Excisional biopsy is the treatment of choice. Careful monitoring is necessary to look for orbital invasion. Oncologist should be consulted if metastatic disease is suspected.

BIBLIOGRAPHY

1. Monroe M. (2012). Head and neck cutaneous squamous cell carcinoma. [online] Available from emedicine.medscape.com/article/1192041-overview. [Accessed August, 2013].

5. SQUAMOUS CELL CARCINOMA OF EYELID

General

Relatively rare periocular malignancy which usually occurs in the lower eyelid.

Clinical

None.

Ocular

Tumor of the eyelid.

Laboratory

Careful biopsy and histologic examination.

Treatment

Systemic or intralesional chemotherapy, or both has been effective when used in conjunction with surgery or radiation.

BIBLIOGRAPHY

1. Monroe M. (2012). Head and neck cutaneous squamous cell carcinoma. [online] Available from emedicine.medscape.com/article/1212601-overview. [Accessed August, 2013].

6. CORNEAL DERMOIDS

These congenital corneal limbal lesions grow slowly. Tumors are yellowish, elevated and variable in size; they consist of fibrofatty tissue covered by epidermal rather than by conjunctival epithelium and may contain ectodermal derivatives such as hair follicles, sebaceous glands and sweat glands. Trauma, irritation, and puberty hasten their growth.

1. Bloch-Sulzberger syndrome (incontinentia pigmenti)
2. Cri-du-chat syndrome (cat-cry syndrome)
3. Duane retraction syndrome
4. Multiple dermoids of the cornea associated with miliary aneurysms of the retina
5. Neurocutaneous syndrome (ectomesodermal dysgenesis)
6. Nevus sebaceous of Jadassohn (linear nevus sebaceous of Jadassohn)
7. Oculoauriculovertebral dysplasia (Goldenhar syndrome)
†8. Organoid nevus syndrome
9. Ring dermoid syndrome-autosomal dominant
†10. Sporadic
†11. Thalidomide teratogenicity.

BIBLIOGRAPHY

1. Arffa RC. Grayson's Diseases of the Cornea, 3rd edition. St. Louis: Mosby-Year Book; 1991.
2. Benjamin SN, Allen HF. Classification for limbal dermoid choristomas and brachial arch anomalies. Presentation of an unusual case. Arch Ophthalmol. 1972;87(3):305-14.
3. Brodsky MC, Kincannon JM, Nelson-Adesokan P, et al. Oculocerebral dysgenesis in the linear nevus sebaceous syndrome. Ophthalmology. 1997;104(3):497-503.
4. Roy FH. Ocular Syndromes and Systemic Diseases, 5th edition. New Delhi: Jaypee Brothers; 2013.

†Indicates a general entry and therefore has not been described in detail in the text

6.1 BLOCH-SULZBERGER SYNDROME (INCONTINENTIA PIGMENTI; SIEMENS-BLOCH-SULZBERGER SYNDROME)

General

Familial disorder affecting ectoderm; manifestations at birth; female predominance; X-linked dominant phenotype; disturbance of skin pigmentation.

Ocular

Orbital mass; retrolental fibroplasia; pseudoglioma; strabismus; blue sclera; cataract; optic nerve atrophy; papillitis; nystagmus; chorioretinitis; anomalies of chamber angle;

neovascularization of retina; retinal hemorrhages and edema; microphthalmia; tractional retinal detachment.

Clinical

Dental and skeletal anomalies common; neurologic abnormalities; recurrent inflammatory lesions; skin melanin pigmentation on the trunk: (marble cake); occipital lobe infarct; neonatal infarction of the macula.

Laboratory

CT scan or MRI of the brain should be performed.

Treatment

No specific treatment. Lesions should be left intact and kept clean and meticulous dental care is very important.

BIBLIOGRAPHY

1. Chang CH. (2012). Neurologic manifestations of incontinentia pigmenti. [online] Available from www.emedicine.com/neuro/TOPIC169.HTM. [Accessed August, 2013].

6.2. CRI-DU-CHAT SYNDROME [CAT-CRY (5P-) SYNDROME; CRYING CAT SYNDROME; BI DELETION SYNDROME; LEJEUNE SYNDROME]

General

Short arm deletion of a no. 5 chromosome (5p-); increased inheritance risk; 13% have one parent with balanced translocation; female preponderance 2:1 (*see* Wolf Syndrome).

Ocular

Hypertelorism; epicanthal folds; antimongoloid slanting of palpebral fissures; strabismus; increased tortuosity of retinal vessels.

Clinical

High-pitched, plaintive cry by an infant (reminiscent of a crying cat); mental retardation; broad nasal root; micrognathia or retrognathia; low-set ears; simian crease; congenital heart defect; small larynx and epiglottis.

Laboratory

Conventional cytogenetic studies, skeletal radiography, MRI, echocardiography.

Treatment

No treatment exists for the underlying disorder. Correction of congenital heart defects may be indicated.

BIBLIOGRAPHY

1. Chen H. (2013). Cri-du-Chat syndrome. [online] Available from www.emedicine.com/ped/TOPIC504.HTM. [Accessed August, 2013].

6.3. DUANE SYNDROME

Congenital ocular motility disorder is characterized by limited abduction or limited adduction. The palpebral fissure narrows on attempted adduction.

1. *Type 1 characteristics*
   a. A or V phenomena
   b. Defective abduction
   c. Palpebral fissure narrowing on adduction
   d. Retraction of the globe
   e. Updrift or downdrift of the affected eye on adduction or attempted abduction.
2. *Type 2 characteristics*
   a. Abduction appears to be normal or only slightly limited.
   b. Distinct narrowing of the palpebral fissure and retraction of the globe on attempted adduction.
   c. Limitation or complete palsy of adduction with exotropia of the paretic eye.
3. *Type 3 characteristics*
   a. Limitation or absence of both abduction and adduction of the affected eye.
   b. Globe retraction and narrowing of the palpebral fissure on attempted adduction.

Treatment

Surgery may be necessary to eliminate or improve head turn.

BIBLIOGRAPHY

1. Verma A. (2011). Duane syndrome. [online] Available from www.emedicine.com/oph/TOPIC326.HTM. [Accessed September, 2013].

6.4. COATS DISEASE (LEBER MILIARY ANEURYSM; RETINAL TELANGIECTASIA)

General

Exudative retinitis; rare; more common in males than females; 95% unilateral.

Ocular

Leukocoria; telangiectatic retinal vessels; solid gray-yellow retinal detachment; optic atrophy; vitreous hemorrhage; anterior uveitis; glaucoma; intraocular calcification (rare); fibro-osseous retinal nodules (atypical); hemorrhagic retinal macrocysts; cystoid macular edema.

Clinical

None.

Laboratory

Fluorescein angiography demonstrates large aneurysmal (light bulb) dilatation of the retinal vessels.

Treatment

Cryotherapy and vitrectomy can be used to obliterate the vascular abnormalities.

BIBLIOGRAPHY

1. Cameron JO. Coats' disease and Turner's syndrome. Am J Ophthalmol. 1974;78:852-4.
2. Senft SH, Hidayat AA, Cavender JC. Atypical presentation of Coats disease. Retina. 1994;14:36-8.

6.5. NEUROCUTANEOUS SYNDROME

General

Triad of linear nevus sebaceous; seizures; mental retardation.

Ocular

Colobomas of irides and choroid; nystagmus; keratoconus; corneal vascularization; optic glioma; epibulbar choristomas; connective tissue nevi of the eyelids.

Clinical

Multiple nevi; seizures; mental retardation; failure to thrive; hydrocephalus; deformities of skull; lipoma of the cranium; alopecia of the scalp.

Laboratory

Clinical.

Treatment

Spectacle correction, hard contacts, avoid eye rubbing. If hydrops occur, discontinue contact lens, use NaCl drops and ointment, patching, and short course of steroids. As disease advances penetrating keratoplasty, deep anterior lamellar keratoplasty intacs with laser grooves or collagen stabilization of cornea can be used.

BIBLIOGRAPHY

1. Kodsi SR, Bloom KE, Egbert JE, et al. Ocular and systemic manifestations of encephalocraniocutaneous lipomatosis. Am J Ophthalmol. 1994;118:77-82.

6.6. LINEAR NEVUS SEBACEUS OF JADASSOHN (NEVUS SEBACEUS OF JADASSOHN; JADASSOHN-TYPE ANETODERMA; ORGANOID NEVUS SYNDROME; SEBACEUS NEVUS SYNDROME)

General

Skin nevus caused by failure of separation of skin appendages from adjacent epithelium during the third month of gestation.

Ocular

Proptosis; epibulbar lipodermoids; colobomata of eyelids, iris, and choroid; antimongoloid fissures; ocular motor palsies; nystagmus; teratomas of orbit and aberrant lacrimal glands; corneal vascularization; vision defects; conjunctival dermolipomas; choristomas of conjunctiva, sclera; corneal vascularization/opacification; colobomas of uvea, retina, optic disk, and lids; optic nerve hypoplasia; microphthalmia; anophthalmia; hemangioma of the sclera/conjunctiva.

Clinical

Circumscribed lesions of the face and scalp with excessively large sebaceous glands; papillomatous epidermal hyperplasia; seizures; skeletal abnormalities, particularly in skull; failure to thrive; convulsion; mental retardation.

Laboratory

Epidermis shows papillomatous hyperplasia. In the dermis, the numbers of mature sebaceous glands are increased. Ectopic apocrine glands are often found in the deep dermis beneath sebaceous glands.

Treatment

Photodynamic therapy with topical aminolevulinic acid. Full-thickness skin excision is usually required, and topical destruction.

BIBLIOGRAPHY

1. Al Hammadi A, Lebwohl MG. (2012). Nevus Sebaceus. [online] Available from www.emedicine.com/derm/TOPIC296.HTM. [Accessed September, 2013].

6.7. GOLDENHAR SYNDROME (OCULO-AURICULO-VERTEBRAL DYSPLASIA; GOLDENHAR-GORLIN SYNDROME)

General

Most cases have been sporadic, but cases of autosomal dominant and recessive inheritance have been reported; male preponderance (60%); present at birth.

Ocular

Anophthalmia; colobomata of choroid, iris, and eyelid; antimongolian slant of lid fissure; epibulbar dermoid or lipodermoids of conjunctiva, cornea, and orbit; tilted optic disk; nerve hypoplasia; microphthalmia; macular heterotopia; tortuous retinal vessels.

Clinical

Frontal bulging of the skull; receding chin; malar hypoplasia; micrognathia and macrostomia; auricular appendices (single or multiple); multiple vertebral anomalies; preauricular fistulas; mental retardation.

Laboratory

Clinical.

Treatment

Dermoids: Surgery for function or cosmesis.

BIBLIOGRAPHY

1. Tewfik TL, Al-Noury KI. (2013). Manifestations of craniofacial syndromes. [online] Available from www.emedicine.com/ent/TOPIC319.HTM. [Accessed September, 2013].

6.9. RING DERMOID SYNDROME (AMBLYOPIA)

General

Autosomal dominant; usually bilateral.

Ocular

Dermoid choristoma; conjunctival plaques of keratinization; corneal lipid deposition; irregular corneal astigmatism; amblyopia; concomitant strabismus.

Laboratory

Clinical.

Treatment

Strabismus: Equalized vision with correct refractive error; surgery may be helpful in patient with diplopia.

BIBLIOGRAPHY

1. Henkind P, Marinoff G, Manas A, et al. Bilateral corneal dermoids. Am J Ophthalmol. 1973;76:972-7.
2. Mattos J, Contreras F, O'Donnell FE. Ring dermoid syndrome. Arch Ophthalmol. 1980;98:1059-61.
3. McKusick VA. Mendelian Inheritance in Man; A Catalog of Human Genes and Genetic Disorders, 12th edition. Baltimore: The Johns Hopkins University Press; 1998.

7. CRANIOPHARYNGIOMA

General

Benign congenital tumors arising from epithelial remnants of Rathke's pouch; most common non-glial intracranial tumors in childhood; second most common sellar-parasellar tumor primarily in children or young adults; 35% of cases occur in patients over age of 40 years.

Ocular

Paresis of third or sixth nerve; optic nerve atrophy; optic neuritis; papilledema; dilation of pupil; diplopia; hemianopia; nystagmus; scotoma; visual field defects; visual loss.

Clinical

Hydrocephalus; infantilism; diabetes insipidus; abnormal sexual development; headaches; acute aseptic meningitis.

Laboratory

Cranial CT and MRI are the current imaging standards.

Treatment

Although controversial, aggressive surgical treatment to attempt gross total resection is sometimes considered. Second option is planned limited surgery followed by radiotherapy.

BIBLIOGRAPHY

1. Bobustuc GC, Groves MD, Fuller GN, et al. (2012). Craniopharyngioma. [online] Available from www.emedicine.com/neuro/TOPIC584.HTM. [Accessed August, 2013].

8. DERMOID (DERMOID CHORISTOMA; DERMOID CYST; DERMOLIPOMA; LIPODERMOID)

General

Benign tumors composed of epidermal tissue, dermal adnexal structures, skin appendages, hair follicles, sebaceous gland and sweat glands; slowly growing.

Ocular

Dermoid of conjunctiva, cornea and lids; keratitis; extraocular muscle paralysis; exophthalmos; astigmatism; visual loss; orbital lesions causing diplopia and proptosis; may be connected with the lacrimal canaliculum.

Clinical

Subcutaneous dermoids of the skin; aplasia cutis congenita possibly associated with strabismus has been reported.

Laboratory

Radiographs of the orbit reveal the deeper orbital cysts; CT is commonly used to image orbital cysts; MRI of dermoid cyst is especially valuable in deeper orbital lesions.

Treatment

Surgery for function or cosmesis.

BIBLIOGRAPHY

1. Schwartz RA, Ruszczak Z. (2012). Dermoid cyst. [online] Available from www.emedicine.com/derm/TOPIC686. HTM. [Accessed August, 2013].

9. DERMOID, ORBITAL

General

Choristomas, tumors that originate from aberrant primordial tissue; may displace structures in the orbit, especially the globe. If the displacement is great, interference with vision by compression of the optic nerve.

Ocular

Mass in the orbital area; decreased visual acuity, color vision and brightness perception; afferent pupillary defect; optic nerve compression.

Laboratory

Radiography, CT, MRI and ultrasound can be used for diagnosis.

Treatment

No treatment is generally required unless there is optic nerve compression or for cosmetic problems. If surgery is required the location of the cyst helps to determine the appropriate type of orbitotomy.

BIBLIOGRAPHY

1. Cooper T (Ted), Nugent AK, (2012). Orbital dermoid. [online] Available from emedicine.medscape.com/article/1218740-overview. [Accessed August, 2013].

10. RING DERMOID SYNDROME (AMBLYOPIA)

General

Autosomal dominant; usually bilateral.

Ocular

Dermoid choristoma; conjunctival plaques of keratinization; corneal lipid deposition; irregular corneal astigmatism; amblyopia; concomitant strabismus.

Laboratory

Diagnosis is made by clinical findings.

Treatment

Strabismus—equalized vision with correct refractive error. Surgery may be helpful in patient with diplopia.

BIBLIOGRAPHY

1. Henkind P, Marinoff G, Manas A, et al. Bilateral corneal dermoids. Am J Ophthalmol. 1973;76(6):972-7.
2. Mattos J, Contreras F, O'Donnell FE JrMattos J, et al. Ring dermoid syndrome. A new syndrome of autosomal dominantly inherited, bilateral, annular limbal dermoids with corneal and conjunctival extension. Arch Ophthalmol. 1980;98(6):1059-61.
3. McKusick VA. Mendelian Inheritance in Man: A Catalog of Human Genes and Genetic Disorders, 12thth edition. Baltimore: The Johns Hopkins University Press; 1998.
4. McKusick-Nathans Institute for Genetic Medicine, Johns Hopkins University and National Center for Biotechnology Information, National Library of Medicine (2007). Online Mendelian Inheritance in Man®, (OMIM®). [online] Available from www.ncbi.nlm.nih.gov/omim. [Accessed August, 2013].
5. Oakman JH, Lambert SR, Grossniklaus HE, et al. Corneal dermoid: case report and review of classification. J Pediatr Ophthalmol Strabismus. 1993;30(6):388-91.

11. EWING SARCOMA (EWING SYNDROME)

General

Highly metastatic round cell tumor of bone; most commonly involves long or trunk bones; metastasizes at high rate; usually occurs between ages 10 and 25 years; seen more frequently in males than in females.

Ocular

Exophthalmos; orbital hemorrhages; orbital necrosis; commonly found as the second malignancy in patients with hereditary retinoblastoma.

Clinical

Lytic bone destruction; pain; edema; slight fever.

Laboratory

Histologic testing requires fresh tissue. Biopsy site to be in area of radiation.

Treatment

Tumor spread must be recognized, and methods such as positron emission tomography (PET) scanning with fluorodeoxyglucose (FDG) and/or bone scanning can help in detecting metastases.

BIBLIOGRAPHY

1. Strauss LG. (2011). Ewing sarcoma imaging. [online] Available from www.emedicine.com/radio/TOPIC275.HTM. [Accessed August, 2013].

12. FIBROSARCOMA

General

Malignant tumor of fibrous connective tissue; most commonly seen in persons 30–70 years old; frequent metastases to lung; true fibrosarcoma has a tendency to occur in children (better prognosis); most fibrosarcomas now would be classified as malignant fibrous histiocytomas.

Ocular

Paralysis of extraocular muscles; proptosis; orbital edema; erosion of orbital bony walls; increased intraorbital pressure; metastases to choroid/orbit.

Clinical

Tumors of mesenchymal soft tissues of the extremities, especially in the knee region; progressive pain; edema; tumors of the sinuses; tumors of the lungs.

Laboratory

Neuroimaging with CT and MRI are not used for diagnosis. Excisional or incisional biopsy is used for diagnosis.

Treatment

Surgical resection with a cuff of normal tissue and reconstruction of the subsequent defect are necessary. Radiation treatment and chemotherapy may also be necessary.

BIBLIOGRAPHY

1. Dickey ID, Floyd J. (2012). Fibrosarcoma. [online] Available from www.emedicine.com/orthoped/TOPIC599.HTM. [Accessed August, 2013].

13. HEMANGIOMA, CAPILLARY

General

Benign orbital tumors of infancy, rapid growth; thought to be of placental origin due to a unique microvascular phenotype shared by juvenile hemangiomas and human placenta.

Clinical

Kasabach-Merritt syndrome; congestive heart failure; nasopharyngeal obstruction; thrombocytopenia; hemolytic anemia.

Ocular

Red, thickened spot in the periorbital area, lid or brow; amblyopia; anisometropia.

Laboratory

Neuroimaging studies are useful to establish the diagnosis; CT, MRI and ultrasound may be beneficial.

Treatment

Corticosteroids topically, systemically and injected are the first line of treatment. Interferon may also be used in resistant cases. Laser and incisional surgical techniques hav had variable success.

BIBLIOGRAPHY

1. Al Dhaybi R, Superstein R, Milet A, et. al Treatment of periocular infantile hemangiomas with propranolol: case series of 18 children Ophthalmology. 2011;118(6):118488.
2. Seiff S, Zwick OM, DeAngelis DD, et al. (2011). Capillary Hemangioma. [online] Available from emedicine.medscape.com/article/1218805-overview. [Accessed August, 2013].

14. HODGKIN DISEASE

General

Hodgkin disease begins in the lymph nodes and usually spreads in a predictable fashion along contiguous chains of nodes; etiology may be viral; prevalent in males.

Ocular

Keratitis; uveitis; cataract; retinal hemorrhages; vasculitis; Horner syndrome; cortical blindness; papilledema; paralysis of oculomotor nerve; episcleritis; visual field defects; infiltration of choroid, conjunctiva, lacrimal gland, and orbit; papillitis; retrobulbar neuritis; opsoclonus-myoclonus; keratitis sicca; infiltrative optic neuropathy; association with Vogt-Koyanagi-Harada syndrome; bilateral serous detachments of the macula.

Clinical

Painless cervical, axillary, or inguinal lymph node swelling; fever; weight loss; anemia; generalized pruritus.

Laboratory

Biopsy of lymph glands is diagnostic.

Treatment

The goal of therapy is to induce a complete remission with radiation therapy, chemotherapy or bone marrow transplantation.

BIBLIOGRAPHY

1. Lash BW, Dessain SK, Argiris A. (2012). Hodgkin Lymphoma. [online] Available from www.emedicine.com/med/TOPIC1022.HTM. [Accessed August, 2013].

15. HUTCHINSON SYNDROME (ADRENAL CORTEX NEUROBLASTOMA WITH ORBITAL METASTASIS; PEPPER SYNDROME)

General

Metastatic infraorbital neuroblastoma after hematogenous dissemination of primary tumor; occurs in infants and children up to age of 6 years; poor prognosis; in children, neuroblastoma commonly involves the orbit; 15% of patients with neuroblastoma had proptosis and ecchymosis.

Ocular

Exophthalmos; lid hematoma; extraocular muscle palsy; subconjunctival hemorrhages; choroidal metastatic tumor; papilledema; optic atrophy.

Clinical

Severe anemia; increased sedimentation rate; urinary excretion of 3-methoxy-4-hydroxy mandelic acid.

Laboratory

Computed tomography and MRI are diagnostic.

Treatment

Chemotherapy and bone marrow or stem cell transplantation are used for therapy.

BIBLIOGRAPHY

1. Volpe NJ, Albert DM. Metastases to the uvea. In: Albert DM, Jakobiec FA (Eds). Principles and Practice of Ophthalmology, Philadelphia: WB Saunders; 1994. pp. 3260-70.

16. JUVENILE XANTHOGRANULOMA (JXG; NEVOXANTHOENDOTHELIOMA)

General

Childhood disease; unknown etiology.

Ocular

Uveal tract tumor presenting as spontaneous hyphema; secondary glaucoma; uveitis; corneal, lid and epibulbar tumors; proptosis; retinal and choroidal lesions (rare).

Clinical

Multiple benign tumors, primarily of the skin; usually appear in the first 3 years of life; lesions appear as yellow-to-brown papules or nodules.

Laboratory

Diagnostic techniques include biomicroscopy, high-frequency ultrasound and cytologic examination of anterior chamber paracentesis material.

Treatment

Topical, subconjunctival, intralesional and systemic corticosteroids are useful. Low-dose radiation may be the treatment of choice for diffuse uveal lesions. Glaucoma medications should be used in the setting of hyphema and increased intraocular pressure.

BIBLIOGRAPHY

1. Curtis T, Wheeler DT. (2012). Juvenile Xanthogranuloma. [online] Available from www.emedicine.com/oph/TOPIC588.HTM. [Accessed August, 2013].

17. KAPOSI DISEASE (KAPOSI SARCOMA; KAPOSI HEMORRHAGIC SARCOMA; MULTIPLE IDIOPATHIC HEMORRHAGIC SARCOMA; KAPOSI VARICELLIFORM ERUPTION)

General

Vascular tumor of unknown cause; seen most often in males, Jews, and those from eastern Europe, the southern Mediterranean, and Africa; HIV-related Kaposi syndrome is the most common type of cancer seen in acquired immunodeficiency syndrome patients.

Ocular

Ocular adnexa, varicelliform eruption, including lids, conjunctivae, lacrimal glands, and orbit, may be involved; hemorrhage; extensive injection and thickening of conjunctival tissues; conjunctival involvement more evident in bulbar conjunctiva.

Clinical

Vascular sarcomas usually occur on the legs, although widespread cutaneous and visceral tumors may develop; secondary malignancies are very common; lymphedema.

Laboratory

Diagnosis is histopathologic.

Treatment

Cutaneous or conjunctival biopsy of the lesion may be necessary for a definitive diagnosis.

BIBLIOGRAPHY

1. Freudenthal J, Yuhan KR, You TT. (2012). Ophthalmologic manifestations of Kaposi sarcoma. [online] Available from www.emedicine.com/oph/TOPIC481.HTM. [Accessed September, 2013].

18. KASABACH-MERRITT SYNDROME (CAPILLARY ANGIOMA-THROMBOCYTOPENIA; HEMANGIOMA-THROMBOCYTOPENIA; THROMBOCYTOPENIA PURPURA-HEMANGIOMA)

General

Angioma causing sequestration of platelets and platelet deficiency.

Ocular

Capillary hemangiomas of the orbit; retinal detachments.

Clinical

Extraorbital hemangiomas found on trunk, extremities and palate or in subglottic space; thrombocytopenia; found in infants; purpura and bleeding.

Laboratory

B-scan ultrasound, CT and MRI.

Treatment

Corticosteroids topical, injectable and systemic is the treatment of choice. Interferon alfa-2a has emerged as a new modality; laser surgery and incisional surgical techniques may be necessary.

BIBLIOGRAPHY

1. Seiff S, Zwick OM, DeAngelis DD, et al. (2011). Capillary Hemangioma. [online] Available from/www.emedicine.com/oph/TOPIC691.HTM [Accessed August, 2013].

19. KERATOACANTHOMA

General

Benign epithelial tumor that arises on hair follicles in exposed skin of Caucasians.

Clinical

Keratoacanthoma can occur in other parts of the body.

Ocular

Conjunctival nodules may result in foreign body sensation and tearing.

Laboratory

Biopsy of lesion can be diagnostic.

Treatment

Excisional biopsy, curettage, cryotherapy, radiation.

BIBLIOGRAPHY

1. Roy FH, Fraunfelder FW, Fraunfelder FT. Roy and Fraunfelder's Current Ocular Therapy, 6th edition. London: Elsevier; 2008.

🗗 20. LEIOMYOMA

General

Rare, benign tumor that arises from smooth muscle; usually well encapsulated.

Ocular

Pigmented tumor of ciliary body; proptosis; distorted pupil; ectropion; iris tumor; glaucoma; cataract; preferential location: ciliary body, peripheral choroid, supraciliary or suprachoroidal space; it has a predilection for younger patients and females.

Clinical

Metastases have not been described.

Laboratory

Diagnosis is made on histologic examination.

Treatment

Excise the leiomyoma from the iris and ciliary body if tumors increase in size.

🗗 BIBLIOGRAPHY

1. Roque MR, Roque BL. (2012). Iris leiomyoma. [online] Available from www.emedicine.com/oph/TOPIC589.HTM. [Accessed August, 2013].

🗗 21. LIPOSARCOMA

General

Aggressive malignant neoplasms of lipogenic cells; occurs at any age, but rarely before age of 30 years and most commonly in the 5th decade; occurs almost exclusively in adults and is found most often in the thigh or retroperitoneum.

Ocular

Paresis of extraocular muscle; proptosis; orbital liposarcoma; eyelid edema.

Clinical

Neoplasms of deeper soft tissues; metastasis to lungs, liver, lymph nodes, and periosteum.

Laboratory

Magnetic resonance imaging may be diagnostic, ultrasonography helps to separate true orbital cysts from liposarcoma and diagnosis is usually made only after biopsy.

Treatment

Consultation with oncologist as necessary.

🗗 BIBLIOGRAPHY

1. Khan AN, Chandramohan M, MacDonald S, et al. (2011). Liposarcoma imaging. [online] Available from www.emedicine.com/radio/TOPIC392.HTM. [Accessed August, 2013].

🗗 22. LYMPHANGIOMA

General

Poorly circumscribed infiltrating lesions consisting of lymphatic/dysplastic blood vessels; occurs predominantly in children and young adults.

Ocular

Conjunctival hemorrhages; cellulitis of lid; ptosis; exophthalmos; amblyopia; astigmatism; extraocular muscle imbalance; optic disk edema; retinal striae.

Clinical

Benign tumors of the lymph system.

Laboratory

Ultrasonography lacks specificity and soft-tissue detail; CT images bone deformity and MRI provides superior soft-tissue details.

Treatment

• *Ptosis*: Most cases require surgical correction if visual acuity is affected and there are several procedures that may be used including levator resection, repair or advancement and Fasanella-Servat procedure.

• *Exophthalmos*: Reversing the problem which is causing the exophthalmos is the treatment of choice and will minimize the ocular complications. Ocular lubricants are beneficial for control of the corneal exposure.

BIBLIOGRAPHY

1. Schwartz RA, Fernandez G. (2012). Lymphangioma. [online] Available from www.emedicine.com/derm/TOP-IC866.HTM. [Accessed August, 2013].

23. LYMPHOID HYPERPLASIA (REACTIVE LYMPHOID HYPERPLASIA; LYMPHOID TUMORS; MALIGNANT LYMPHOMA; PSEUDOLYMPHOMA; PSEUDOTUMOR; BURKITT LYMPHOMA; NEOPLASTIC ANGIOENDOTHELIOMATOSIS)

General

Occurs in tropical Africa; young children; idiopathic orbital inflammation; systemic disease is rarely associated but occasionally occurs with either vasculitis or lymphomas; etiology of Burkitt lymphoma currently includes three factors: (1) Epstein-Barr virus, (2) malaria and (3) chromosomal translocations activating the c-Myc oncogene, which induces uncontrolled B-cell proliferation.

Ocular

Proptosis; extraocular motility disturbances; lesions of orbit, lacrimal gland, conjunctiva, and uvea; cortical blindness; retinal artery occlusion; retinal vascular and pigment epithelial alterations; vitreitis.

Clinical

Maxillary tumor; Epstein-Barr virus; cranial neuropathy.

Laboratory

Generally diagnosed with a lymph node biopsy.

Treatment

Chemotherapy, monoclonal antibody therapy and bone marrow or stem cell infusions may be chosen as therapy.

BIBLIOGRAPHY

1. Brooks HL, Downing J, McClure JA, et al. Orbital Buritt's lymphoma in a homosexual man with acquired immune deficiency. Arch Ophthalmol. 1984;102(10):1533-7.
2. Cheung MK, Martin DF, Chan CC, et al. Diagnosis of reactive lymphoid hyperplasia by chorioretinal biopsy. Am J Ophthalmol. 1994;118(4):457-62.

24. MEDULLOEPITHELIOMA (DIKTYOMA)

General

Rare embryonic ocular tumor which usually arises from the primitive non-pigmented medullary epithelium of the ciliary body and less commonly affects the optic nerve, iris and retina.

Clinical

None.

Ocular

Decreased vision, leukocoria, rubeosis iridis, ectopia lentis, heterochromia, exophthalmos and hyphema.

Laboratory

Indirect ophthalmoscopy, slit-lamp examination and echography aid in diagnosis. CT and MRI may also be helpful. Diagnosis is confirmed on histological examination.

Treatment

Iridocyclectomy is useful for small tumors in the ciliary body. Enucleation is recommended for large tumors.

BIBLIOGRAPHY

1. Roy FH, Fraunfelder FW, Fraunfelder FT. Roy and Fraunfelder's Current Ocular Therapy, 6th edition. London: Elsevier, 2008.

25. MENINGIOMA

General

Benign, slow-growing tumors that arise from the arachnoid matter, the middle layer of meninges that lies inside the dura mater, and outside the pia mater; more common in females; peak incidence in the 7th decade of life.

Ocular

Exposure keratopathy; paralysis of extraocular muscles; proptosis; optic nerve atrophy; papilledema; choroidal folds; hyperopia; visual field defect; afferent pupil defect; optociliary shunt veins.

Clinical

Headache; intracranial pressure; vomiting.

Laboratory

Computed tomography or MRI will denote a well-circumscribed mass, extra-axial and adherent to dura. Due to location may compress brain, spinal cord or optic nerve.

Treatment

Total microsurgical intervention usually can be curative; radiation therapy after surgery.

BIBLIOGRAPHY

1. Zachariah SB, Khoromi S. (2012). Sphenoid wing meningioma. [online] Available from www.emedicine.com/oph/TOPIC670.HTM. [Accessed August, 2013].

26. MENINGIOMA, OPTIC NERVE SHEATH

General

Primary meningioma arises from the cap cells of the arachnoid surrounding the intraorbital or, less frequently, the intracanalicular optic nerve. Secondary meningioma are extensions of intracranial meningioma into the orbit. Secondary meningioma are much more common than primary, but the unqualified term "optic nerve sheath meningioma" ordinarily refers to primary. It may be caused by radiation, head trauma, hormonal factors and infectious agents.

Clinical

Headache, head trauma.

Ocular

Compressive optic neuropathy; transient visual obscurations; visual loss; proptosis; exophthalmos; ptosis; diplopia.

Laboratory

Computed tomography and MRI are the best imaging techniques.

Treatment

Radiotherapy following surgical removal. Chemotherapy is reserved for unresectable or recurrent meningioma.

BIBLIOGRAPHY

1. Gossman MV, Zachariah SB, Khoromi S. (2012). Optic nerve sheath meningioma. [online] Available from emedicine.medscape.com/article/1217466-overview. [Accessed August, 2013].

27. MENINGIOMA, SPHENOID WING

General

Arise from arachnoid cap cells which are attached to the dura at any location where meninges exist; may be associated with hyperostosis of the sphenoid ridge and be very invasive; may expand into the wall for the cavernous sinus and anteriorly into the orbit.

Clinical

Diffuse tumor infiltration; transient ischemic attack; anosmia; mental changes; increased intracranial pressure.

Ocular

Unilateral exophthalmos; proptosis; oculomotor palsy; painful ophthalmoplegia; blindness; papilledema.

Laboratory

Endocrine testing; CT and MRI allow definitive diagnosis.

Treatment

Tumor resection without injury to the optic nerve if the bone has not been invaded; if resection is not complete radiation therapy will be necessary; anti-hormonal agents may be useful in atypical and malignant meningioma as an adjunct to surgery.

BIBLIOGRAPHY

1. Zachariah SB, Khoromi S. (2012). Sphenoid Wing Meningioma. [online] Available from emedicine.medscape.com/article/1215752-overview. [Accessed August, 2013].

28. MUCOCELE (PYOCELE)

General

Accumulation and retention of mucoid material within the sinus as a result of continuous or periodic obstruction of the sinus ostium.

Ocular

Paralysis of extraocular muscles; exophthalmos; lacrimation; erosion of bony walls of orbit; decreased visual acuity; diplopia; elevation of lower lid; ptosis; compression optic neuropathy; globe distortion; enophthalmos; epiphora; scleral indentation; choroidal folds; discharging lesion of the upper lid; pseudotelecanthus; spontaneous non-traumatic enophthalmos; local anesthesia.

Clinical

Headaches; epidural abscess; subdural empyema; meningitis; brain abscess; occlusion of nasal passage; loosening of teeth.

Laboratory

Computed tomography scanning helps to outline bony changes; MRI helps to differentiate mucoceles from neoplasms in the paranasal sinuses.

Treatment

Gamma-linolenic acid.

BIBLIOGRAPHY

1. Flaitz CM, Hicks MJ. (2012). Mucocele and Ranula. [online] Available from www.emedicine.com/derm/TOPIC648.HTM. [Accessed August, 2013].

29. NEURILEMMOMA (SCHWANNOMA; NEURINOMA, PTEN HAMARTOMA TUMOR SYNDROME)

General

Slow-growing encapsulated neoplasm from the Schwann cells of nerves; seen most frequently with patients with von Recklinghausen disease.

Ocular

Ptosis; exophthalmos; visual loss; pupillary dilation; lacrimal sac mass.

Clinical

Facial numbness; retro-orbital headaches; intermittent pain radiating from the distribution of the appropriate sensory nerve branch.

Laboratory

Computed tomography scan can characterize the tumor's size and extent. MRI has high sensitivity to define nature and invasiveness of the tumor. Orbital and ocular echography shows sharply outlined capsule, a well-defined central cystic space, slight compressibility and blood flow.

Treatment

- *Ptosis*: Most cases require surgical correction if visual acuity is affected and there are several procedures that may be used including elevator resection, repair or advancement and Fasanella-Servat procedure.
- *Exophthalmos*: Reversing the problem, which is causing the exophthalmos, is the treatment of choice and will minimize the ocular complications. Ocular lubricants are beneficial for control of the corneal exposure.

⊟ BIBLIOGRAPHY

1. Kao GF. (2012). Dermatologic manifestations of neurilemmoma. [online] Available from www.emedicine.com/derm/TOPIC285.HTM. [Accessed August, 2013].

⊟ 30. NEUROBLASTOMA

General

Highly malignant solid tumor arising from undifferentiated sympathetic neuroblasts of the adrenal medulla, sympathetic ganglia, ectopic adrenal, and theoretically the ciliary ganglion; autosomal dominant.

Ocular

Ptosis; exophthalmos; optic atrophy; optic neuritis; papilledema; metastatic tumor of orbit; retinal hemorrhage; convergent strabismus; paralysis of sixth or seventh nerve; nonreactive pupil; primary differentiated neuroblastoma of the orbit also has been reported; tonic pupils; microphthalmia; choroidal metastases (rare); iris metastases (rare).

Clinical

Skeletal metastasis to the cranium.

Laboratory

Serum lactate dehydrogenase (LDH), ferritin, CBC count, serum creatinine, liver function test, CT and MRI test, echocardiogram.

Treatment

Treatment is provided by a multidisciplinary team.

⊟ BIBLIOGRAPHY

1. Lacayo NJ, Davis KA. (2012). Pediatric neuroblastoma. [online] Available from www.emedicine.com/ped/TOPIC1570.HTM. [Accessed August, 2013].

⊟ 31. OPTIC GLIOMAS

General

Juvenile pilocytic astrocytomas type I tumors intrinsic to the optic nerve, chiasm or tracts are termed optic gliomas.

Clinical

None.

Ocular

Proptosis, afferent pupil defect, hypotropia.

Laboratory

Magnetic resonance imaging with gadolinium contrast is essential.

Treatment

Observation—no proven efficacy has shown for excision of tumor to prevent contralateral eye involvement.

⊟ BIBLIOGRAPHY

1. Woodcock RJ. (2011). Optic nerve glioma imaging. [online] Available from www.emedicine.com/radio/TOPIC486. HTM. [Accessed August, 2013].

⊟ 32. ORBITAL LYMPHOMA

General

Localized form of systemic lymphoma affecting the orbit, lacrimal gland, lid and conjunctiva.

Clinical

Systemic lymphoma.

Ocular

Diplopia; exophthalmos; ocular pain; salmon-colored mass of the conjunctiva or eyelid.

Laboratory

Open biopsy and MRI or CT of the orbit.

Treatment

Radiation is the most frequently used treatment. Chemotherapy may be indicated for large diffuse B-cell lymphoma or with systemic treatment; excision of localized lesions; cryotherapy may be beneficial.

⊟ BIBLIOGRAPHY

1. EyeWiki™. Orbital lymphoma. [online] Available from eyewiki.aao.org/Orbital_Lymphoma. [Accessed August, 2013].

⊟ 33. ORBITAL RHABDOMYOSARCOMA

General

Embryonal or alveolar varieties of this tumor have a tendency to affect the orbit and adjacent structures.

Clinical

Skeletal, muscles and renal tumors.

Ocular

Rapid onset of painless proptosis, ptosis, ocular congestion, decreased extraocular motility.

Laboratory

Complete blood count, liver function test, renal function, and CT of lung and orbit.

Treatment

Local debulking of the orbital mass and adjunctive radiotherapy and chemotherapy.

⊟ BIBLIOGRAPHY

1. Roy FH, Fraunfelder FW, Fraunfelder FT. Roy and Fraunfelder's Current Ocular Therapy, 6th edition. London: Elsevier; 2008.

⊟ 34. PAPILLOMA (WART; VERRUCA)

General

Cutaneous or mucosal tumor of proliferating epithelial and fibrovascular tissues; viral etiology or noninfectious.

Ocular

Papillary conjunctivitis; pseudopterygium; corneal opacity; epithelial keratitis; corneal vascularization; lid ulcers; lacrimal system obstruction; hemorrhages of conjunctiva, lids and lacrimal system.

Clinical

Mulberry or cauliflower-like tumors that may occur on any cutaneous or mucosal surface.

Laboratory

Histologic evaluation is diagnostic.

Treatment

Salicylic acid is a first-line therapy used to treat warts, intralesional immunotherapy using injections, cryosurgery, carbon dioxide lasers, electrodesiccation and curettage or surgical excision.

⊟ BIBLIOGRAPHY

1. Shenefelt PD. (2012). Nongenital warts. [online] Available from www.emedicine.com/derm/TOPIC457.HTM. [Accessed August, 2013].

⊟ 35. PERIOCULAR MERKEL CELL CARCINOMA

General

Aggressive primary cutaneous neoplasm that frequently involves the eyelids and periocular region.

Clinical

Skin cancer.

Ocular

Uvea, eyelid tumors.

Laboratory

Histologic diagnosis.

Treatment

Chemotherapy, radiation, full-thickness resection of lid tumor.

⊟ BIBLIOGRAPHY

1. Roy FH, Fraunfelder FW, Fraunfelder FT. Roy and Fraunfelder's Current Ocular Therapy, 6th edition. London: Elsevier; 2008.

⊟ 36. PERIOCULAR METASTATIC TUMORS (OCULAR METASTATIC TUMORS)

General

Neoplasms that develop from malignant cells and are carried from a primary site of malignancy.

Ocular

Retinal detachment; retinal hemorrhages; enophthalmos; exophthalmos; proptosis; rubeosis iridis; uveitis; papilledema; orbital hemorrhages; hyphema; paralysis of extraocular muscles; secondary glaucoma.

Clinical

Metastasis in the bloodstream and lymphatic system is common; tumors of the lung or breast metastasize to globe; neoplasms that most commonly metastasize to orbit are neuroblastomas of suprarenal medulla and retroperitoneal ganglia; Wilms' tumor may involve the orbit.

Laboratory

Systemic studies include blood cell count, erythrocyte sedimentation rate and liver function tests. Ultrasound is useful with intraocular tumors.

Treatment

Chemotherapy or radiation with teletherapy if orbital tumor is nonresponsive to radiation; debulking is an option.

⊟ BIBLIOGRAPHY

1. Mercandetti M, Cohen AJ. (2011). Orbital tumors. [online] Available from www.emedicine.com/oph/TOPIC758.HTM. [Accessed August, 2013].

37. RETICULUM CELL SARCOMA (NON-HODGKIN LYMPHOMA)

General

Autosomal recessive; large-cell lymphoma with chronic inflammation with a predominance of cells in vitreous cavity; average age at time of diagnosis is 60 years; female to male ratio is approximately 2:1; 80% bilateral (frequently asymmetrical).

Ocular

Chronic uveitis; chorioretinal lesions; mycosis fungoides; necrosis of orbital tissues; phthisis bulbi; endophthalmos; exophthalmos; exudative retinal detachment; iris neovascularization; glaucoma; branch retinal vein occlusion; macular edema; optic neuropathy; vitreous hemorrhage; partial cranial nerve III palsy; multiple retinal pigment epithelium masses.

Clinical

Lymphocytic hyperplasia; fever; anemia; thrombocytopenia; liver and spleen enlargement; associated with immune dysfunction states, such as acquired immunodeficiency syndrome, or following transplantation.

Laboratory

Computed tomography/MRI scan, HIV evaluation, complete blood count (CBC), lumbar puncture.

Treatment

Radiation, chemotherapy.

BIBLIOGRAPHY

1. Vinjamaram S, Estrada-Garcia DA, Hernandez-Ilizaliturri FJ, et al. (2012). Non-Hodgkin lymphoma. [online] Available from emedicine.medscape.com/article/203399-overview. [Accessed August, 2013].

38. RETINOBLASTOMA

General

Malignant tumor arising in one or both retinas of young children, usually under the age of 2 years; usually unilateral; autosomal dominant; most common intraocular malignancy of childhood; incidence is 1 in 20,000 live births; origin is questionably neuroectodermal cells capable of multipotentiality; one-third of patients have heritable (bilateral or have a positive family history) autosomal dominant and two-thirds are sporadic; genetic transmission obeys two-mutation hypothesis of Knudson; trilateral retinoblastoma is bilateral retinoblastoma plus midline central nervous system tumor (most commonly pinealoma); most common second tumor is an osteogenic sarcoma (begins in second decade).

Ocular

Hyphema; hypopyon; corneal tumor; lid edema; endophthalmitis; exophthalmos; intraocular calcification of globe; heterochromia; neovascularization of iris or retina; papilledema; panophthalmitis; retinoblastoma extension into orbit and choroid; cat's-eye reflex; leukocoria; mydriasis; vitreous hemorrhage tumor seeding; esotropia; exotropia; glaucoma; visual loss.

Clinical

Metastasis into the lymph system, bone marrow and subarachnoid space; basal meningitis; death.

Laboratory

Computed tomography shows calcification of lesion which is a hallmark of disease; ultrasound-demonstrates calcification and MRI demonstrates presence and extent of extraocular disease.

Treatment

External beam radiation therapy is recommended on patients with significant vitreous seeding. Radioactive isotope plaques and chemotherapy are also an option. Removal of the tumor is the standard management for retinoblastoma.

BIBLIOGRAPHY

1. Abramson DH, Dunkel IJ, Brodie SE, et al. Superselective ophthalmic artery chemotherapy as primary treatment for retinoblastoma (chemosurgery). Ophthalmology. 2010;117(8):1623-9.
2. Isidro MA, Roque MR. (2012). Retinoblastoma. [online] Available from www.emedicine.com/oph/TOPIC346.HTM. [Accessed August, 2013].

⎂ 39. RHABDOMYOSARCOMA (CORNEAL EDEMA)

General

Most common malignant orbital neoplasm of childhood; usually occurs before the age of 10 years; more commonly seen in males; rarely may develop in adults; shows evidence of striated muscle differentiation; has been divided into three histopathologic types: (1) embryonal, (2) alveolar and (3) pleomorphic.

Ocular

Choroidal folds; corneal edema; exposure keratitis; rhabdomyosarcoma (RMS) of orbit or extraocular muscles; decreased motility; proptosis; papilledema; orbital edema; enlarged optic foramen; erosion of bony walls of orbit; pupil irregularity; epiphora; glaucoma; visual loss; nasolacrimal duct obstruction; conjunctival mass.

Clinical

Metastasis to the lymph system, bone marrow and lungs; headaches.

Laboratory

Liver, renal and cytogenetic testing; CT and bone scanning; MRI, ultrasonography and echocardiography.

Treatment

Chemotherapy radiation and surgically removing the tumor are used to treat patients with RMS.

⎂ BIBLIOGRAPHY

1. Cripe TP. (2011). Pediatric rhabdomyosarcoma. [online] Available from www.emedicine.com/ped/TOPIC2005. HTM. [Accessed August, 2013].

⎂ 40. SEBACEOUS GLAND CARCINOMA

General

Ocular adnexa contains various sebaceous glands from which carcinomas may arise; predilection for the upper lids but may involve both lids; usually in older age groups; slight female preponderance.

Ocular

Blepharitis; madarosis; meibomianitis; sebaceous carcinoma of lids or orbit; orbital edema; proptosis; conjunctivitis; superficial keratitis; lacrimal gland tumor.

Clinical

Metastasis to preauricular or cervical lymph nodes, or submandibular area.

Laboratory

Biopsy diagnosis in chronic non-healing chalazia or suspicious unresolved chronic blepharitis.

Treatment

Mohs' technique appears to have the highest success rate.

⎂ BIBLIOGRAPHY

1. Glassman ML, Bashour M. (2012). Sebaceous gland carcinoma. [online] Available from/www.emedicine.com/oph/ TOPIC716.HTM. [Accessed August, 2013].

CHAPTER 14

Mechanical and Non-Mechanical Injuries

⊟ 1. ACID BURNS

General

Acid injuries of the eyes are characterized by protein coagulation and precipitation with the anion. Direct tissue damage produced by the hydrogen ion.

Clinical

None.

Ocular

Chemosis, corneal epithelial defects, limbal blanching, corneal clouding, photophobia, corneal neovascularization, symblepharon formation.

Laboratory

Diagnosis is made from clinical history and findings.

Treatment

Immediate irrigation, topical antibiotics for bacterial infection if needed, contact lenses aid in re-epithelialization of the cornea.

⊟ BIBLIOGRAPHY

1. Roy FH, Fraunfelder FW, Fraunfelder FT. Roy and Fraunfelder's Current Ocular Therapy, 6th edition. London: Elsevier; 2008.

⊟ 2. ALKALINE INJURY OF THE EYE

General

A splash of alkaline solution causes the pH to rise and results in immediate damage to the external ocular tissues. These injuries are frequently seen from household chemicals or farming injuries from liquid ammonia used as fertilizer.

Ocular

Pain; lacrimation; blepharospasm; rise in intraocular pressure; rapid penetration of the cornea and sclera; chemical injury to iris, lens or ciliary body; symblepharon; phthisis bulbi; ankyloblepharon.

Laboratory

Diagnosis is made by clinical findings and history.

Treatment

Immediate copious irrigation, sticky paste of lime should be removed with a cotton-tipped applicator, mydriasis and topical antibiotics, pain medications, treatment of glaucoma with carbonic anhydrase inhibitors, patching and soft contact lenses may facilitate re-epithelialization, insertion of a methyl methacrylate ring may prevent fibrinous adhesions, lysis of adhesions with or without mucous membrane grafts, corneal stem cell transplantation, corneal transplantation, keratoprosthesis and conjunctival autographs.

BIBLIOGRAPHY

1. Roy FH, Fraunfelder FW, Fraunfelder FT. Roy and Fraunfelder's Current Ocular Therapy, 6th edition. London: Elsevier; 2008.

3. CILIARY BODY CONCUSSIONS AND LACERATIONS

General

Trauma which can frequently result in damage to other structures of the eye as well as the ciliary body. Choroid can be separated from the sclera and allow aqueous humor to drain into the suprachoroidal space.

Ocular

Hypotony, iris atrophy, angle-closure glaucoma, cataract, loss of retinal pigment epithelium, choroidal folds, cystoid macular edema, optic atrophy, phthisis bulbi.

Laboratory

Diagnosis is made by clinical findings.

Treatment

Topical steroids and cyclopentolate; surgery—sodium hyaluronate into the anterior chamber to close the cyclodialysis cleft, argon laser photocoagulation.

BIBLIOGRAPHY

1. Roy FH, Fraunfelder FW, Fraunfelder FT. Roy and Fraunfelder's Current Ocular Therapy, 6th edition. London: Elsevier; 2008.

4. CONJUNCTIVAL LACERATIONS

General

Usually not serious; however, they may mask an underlying ocular injury or retain foreign body.

Clinical

None.

Ocular

Subconjunctival hemorrhage, symblepharon.

Laboratory

Diagnosis is made by clinical findings.

Treatment

Surgery repair is rarely necessary. Packs may be used to minimize swelling.

BIBLIOGRAPHY

1. Roy FH, Fraunfelder FW, Fraunfelder FT. Roy and Fraunfelder's Current Ocular Therapy, 6th edition. London: Elsevier; 2008.

5. CORNEAL FOREIGN BODY

General

Foreign body lodged in the corneal epithelium; usually metal, glass or organic material; may be superficial or embedded. It is seen in males more frequently than females secondary to their activities.

Clinical

None.

Ocular

Pain, photophobia, tearing, conjunctival and ciliary injection; epithelial defect; corneal edema; rust ring with metallic injury.

Laboratory

Slit-lamp examination; Seidel test, and if intraocular involvement is suspected, B-scan, orbital CT scan and ultrasound biomicroscopy.

Treatment

Removal with a sterile spud or needle under topical anesthesia; if a rust ring remains a rust ring drill may be used. The patient is treated with antibiotics, cycloplegics and a pressure patch or bandage contact lens.

BIBLIOGRAPHY

1. Bashour M. (2012). Corneal Foreign Body Treatment & Management. [online] Available from emedicine.medscape.com/article/1195581-treatment. [Accessed August, 2013].

6. ELECTRICAL INJURY

General

Electric current passes through the body; voltage ranging from 100 million volts to 200 million volts may cause electrical burns.

Ocular

Choroidal atrophy; corneal perforation; necrosis of cornea or lids; blepharospasm; anterior or posterior subcapsular cataracts and vacuoles; optic neuritis; optic nerve atrophy; retinal edema; retinal hemorrhage; pigmentary degeneration; retinal holes; anterior uveitis; hyphema; hypotony; glaucoma; night blindness; nystagmus; paralysis of extraocular muscles; visual field defects; dilation of retinal veins.

Clinical

Skin burns; injury to cardiovascular, central nervous and musculoskeletal systems; tissue necrosis; vascular injury.

Laboratory

Diagnosis is made from clinical findings.

Treatment

Basics of supportive care, and appropriate advanced cardiac life support measures should be administered. Limb-saving measures, such as escharotomy and fasciotomy, may be needed to restore tissue perfusion.

BIBLIOGRAPHY

1. Cushing TA, Wright RK. (2010). Electrical Injuries in Emergency Medicine. [online] Available from www.emedicine.com/derm/TOPIC859.HTM. [Accessed August, 2013].

7. EXTRAOCULAR MUSCLE LACERATIONS

General

Rare without damage to globe, eyelid and adjacent structures.

Clinical

None.

Ocular

Laceration of extraocular muscles, most frequently the lateral or medial muscle.

Laboratory

Diagnosis is made by clinical findings and history.

Treatment

Reattachment of lacerated ends of muscle or tendon immediately after trauma.

BIBLIOGRAPHY

1. Roy FH, Fraunfelder FW, Fraunfelder FT. Roy and Fraunfelder's Current Ocular Therapy, 6th edition. London: Elsevier; 2008.

⊟ 8. EYELID CONTUSIONS, LACERATIONS AND AVULSIONS

General

Trauma to the eyelid, blowout fracture.

Clinical

None.

Ocular

Eyelid contusion, laceration or avulsion.

Laboratory

Computed tomography (CT) scan for orbital fracture, magnetic resonance imaging (MRI) for soft tissue contrast.

Treatment

Oral and topical antibiotics, debridement of wound, repair of laceration with sutures, repair of canalicular injury. Laceration of canthus may require an oculoplastic surgeon.

⊟ BIBLIOGRAPHY

1. Ing E. (2012). Eyelid Laceration. [online] Available from www.emedicine.com/oph/TOPIC219.HTM. [Accessed August, 2013].

⊟ 9. HYPOTHERMAL INJURY (CRYOINJURY; FROSTBITE)

General

Loss of body heat to the point of local cold injury or freezing of tissue.

Ocular

Localized cryoinjury that can cause choroidal atrophy, retinal hemorrhages, hyperpigmentation of retina, uveitis, corneal edema, neovascularization of cornea, ectropion, lid edema, madarosis, pseudoepitheliomatous hyperplasia, iris atrophy, and paresis of extraocular muscles.

Clinical

Vesicles and blebs of affected tissue, especially ears, fingers, toes and nose; contractures; dry gangrene of affected tissues.

Laboratory

Diagnosis is made by clinical findings.

Treatment

The management of frostbite may be divided into three phases: (1) field management, (2) rewarming, and (3) post-rewarming management. Rewarm the affected area in warm water at 40–42ºC (104–108ºF) for 15–30 minutes or until thawing is complete by clinical assessment. Debridement of white or clear blisters and topical treatment is necessary in the post-rewarming management.

⊟ BIBLIOGRAPHY

1. Mechem CC, Cheng D, Thompson TM, et al. (2011). Frostbite. [online] Available from www.emedicine.com/med/TOPIC2815.HTM. [Accessed August, 2013].

⊟ 10. INTRAOCULAR FOREIGN BODY: COPPER

General

Injury with copper foreign body. Ocular response results from the chemistry of the copper ion and the eye.

Clinical

None.

Ocular

Endophthalmitis, recurrent non-granulomatous inflammation, fibrous encapsulation.

Laboratory

Computed tomography to localize the foreign body, B-scan ultrasonography, radiographic spectrometry to define the presence of intraocular copper ions.

Treatment

Antibiotic to prevent endophthalmitis. Oral prednisone to reduce intraocular inflammation. Repair of laceration. Vitrectomy may be needed.

⊟ BIBLIOGRAPHY

1. Kuhn F, Wong DT, Giavedoni L. (2011). Intraocular Foreign Body. [online] Available from www.emedicine.com/oph/TOPIC648.HTM. [Accessed August, 2013].

⊟ 11. INTRAOCULAR FOREIGN BODY: NONMAGNETIC CHEMICALLY INERT

General

Intraocular foreign bodies that are nonmagnetic and chemically inert.

Clinical

None.

Ocular

Endopthalmitis, ocular laceration.

Laboratory

Computed tomography to localize foreign body and B-scan ultrasonography.

Treatment

Topical antibiotics are recommended. Topical steroid may be useful with traumatic uveitis. Repair of ocular laceration. Vitrectomy may be needed.

⊟ BIBLIOGRAPHY

1. Kuhn F, Wong DT, Giavedoni L. (2011). Intraocular Foreign Body. [online] Available from www.emedicine.com/oph/TOPIC648.HTM. [Accessed August, 2013].

⊟ 12. INTRAOCULAR FOREIGN BODY: STEEL OR IRON

General

Intraocular foreign body of either steel or iron. Foreign bodies are the major cause of ocular trauma legal blindness.

Clinical

None.

Ocular

Subconjunctival hemorrhage or edema, iris defect, lens disruption, retinal hemorrhage, inflammation or edema, endophthalmitis.

Laboratory

Computed tomography to define and localize the foreign body and B-scan ultrasonography. MRI is contraindicated because it may shift the position of the foreign body.

Treatment

Antibiotics via IV (intravenous) are recommended to prevent endophthalmitis; intravitreal antibiotics; repair of laceration and other ocular injury. Vitrectomy may be needed.

⊟ BIBLIOGRAPHY

1. Kuhn F. Wong DT, Giavedoni L. (2011). Intraocular Foreign Body. [online] Available from www.emedicine.com/oph/TOPIC648.HTM. [Accessed August, 2013].

⊟ 13. LACRIMAL SYSTEM CONTUSIONS AND LACERATIONS

General

Sharp and blunt trauma.

Clinical

None.

Ocular

Laceration of upper or lower eyelid medially.

Laboratory

Diagnosis is made by clinical findings.

Treatment

Repair canaliculus.

🗗 BIBLIOGRAPHY

1. Mawn LA. (2012). Canalicular Laceration. [online] Available from www.emedicine.com/oph/TOPIC218.HTM. [Accessed August, 2013].

🗗 14. ORBITAL CELLULITIS AND ABSCESS

General

Potentially life threatening; requires prompt evaluation and treatment.

Clinical

Sinusitis, ear infection, diabetes, dental disease.

Ocular

Orbital pain, proptosis, diplopia, decreased ocular motility, eyelid swelling and erythema, vision loss.

Laboratory

Diagnosis is made by clinical findings.

Treatment

Intravenous and oral antibiotic.

🗗 BIBLIOGRAPHY

1. Harrington JN. (2012). Orbital Cellulitis. [online] Available from www.emedicine.com/oph/TOPIC205.HTM. [Accessed August, 2013].

🗗 15. ORBITAL COMPARTMENT SYNDROME, ACUTE

General

Increased pressure within the confined orbital space generally secondary to facial trauma or surgery; blindness can occur without prompt treatment.

Clinical

Facial trauma; head trauma.

Ocular

Decreased visual acuity; ischemic optic neuropathy; retrobulbar hematoma; diplopia; proptosis; eye pain; reduction of ocular motility; papilledema; cherry-red macula; ecchymosis of lids; chemosis; increased intraocular pressure; afferent pupillary defect; ophthalmoplegia.

Laboratory

Computed tomography or MRI may be useful to identify the etiology of compression.

Treatment

Immediate osmotic agents and carbonic anhydrase inhibitors should be used; lateral orbital canthotomy should be used as soon as diagnosis is made and life-threatening injuries are stabilized to prevent permanent visual loss.

🗗 BIBLIOGRAPHY

1. Peak DA, Green TA. (2011). Acute Orbital Compartment Syndrome. [online] Available from emedicine.medscape.com/article/799528-overview. [Accessed August, 2013].

⊟ 16. ORBITAL FRACTURE, APEX

General

It affects the most posterior portion of the pyramidal-shaped orbit, positioned at the craniofacial junction. It is usually associated with blunt or penetrating trauma to the face or skull.

Clinical

Intracranial or facial trauma.

Ocular

Visual loss; optic neuropathy; optic nerve sheath hematoma; optic nerve impingement; optic nerve compression; retrobulbar hemorrhage; extraocular muscle nerve palsy; diplopia; afferent pupil defect; periocular ecchymosis; proptosis.

Laboratory

Computed tomography scan is the most appropriate to make diagnosis.

Treatment

In cases that involve decreased vision and optic nerve injury, medical or surgical nerve decompression should be considered. Corticosteroids should be the initial treatment and if it is not effective, surgical intervention is necessary.

⊟ BIBLIOGRAPHY

1. Patel B, Taylor SF. (2012). Apex Orbital Fracture. [online] Available from emedicine.medscape.com/article/1218196-overview. [Accessed August, 2013].

⊟ 17. ORBITAL HEMORRHAGES

General

Occurs acutely; substantial hemorrhage behind the orbit septum will raise intraorbital and intraocular pressure.

Clinical

None.

Ocular

Elevated intraocular pressure, orbital pain, diplopia, vision loss, ptosis, lid retraction, immobile globe, cloudy cornea, hemorrhagic conjunctiva, disk pallor, hyperemia of the disk, disk edema and choroidal folds.

Laboratory

Diagnosis is made by clinical findings.

Treatment

Topical medication to lower intraocular pressure, lateral canthotomy and inferior cantholysis.

⊟ BIBLIOGRAPHY

1. Roy FH, Fraunfelder FW, Fraunfelder FT. Roy and Fraunfelder's Current Ocular Therapy, 6th edition. London: Elsevier; 2008.

⊟ 18. ORBITAL IMPLANT EXTRUSION

General

Involves the displacement of implants' use in enucleations to replace volume loss.

Clinical

None.

Ocular

Superior tarsal sulcus deformity, defect in conjunctiva and Tenon's capsule.

Laboratory

Diagnosis is made by clinical findings.

Treatment

Immediate replacement with a fascia-enveloped sphere. If socket is infected, systemic and topical antibiotics are recommended.

BIBLIOGRAPHY

1. Roy FH, Fraunfelder FW, Fraunfelder FT. Roy and Fraunfelder's Current Ocular Therapy, 6th edition. London: Elsevier; 2008.

19. ORBITAL INFARCTION SYNDROME

General

Rare disorder secondary to ischemia of the intraorbital tissue due to occlusion of the ophthalmic artery and its branches.

Clinical

Occlusion of carotid artery; giant-cell arteritis; mucormycosis; systemic vasculitis; acute perfusion failure; sickle cell disease.

Ocular

Proptosis; ophthalmoplegia; lid edema; restricted motility; compressive optic neuropathy; reduced visual acuity; pain.

Laboratory

Magnetic resonance imaging is more specific than CT or nuclear scintigraphy in the evaluation of orbital changes.

Treatment

Orbital decompression.

BIBLIOGRAPHY

1. Maier P, Feltgen N, Lagrèze WA. Bilateral orbital infarction syndrome after bifrontal craniotomy. Arch Ophthalmol. 2007;125(3):422-3.

20. SCLERAL RUPTURES AND LACERATIONS

General

Ruptures caused by large, blunt objects that exert pressure on the eye. Lacerations are caused by sharp objects that enter the eye at the point of contact.

Clinical

None.

Ocular

Iris prolapse, endophthalmitis, cataract vitreous hemorrhage, hemorrhagic chemosis and decreased visual acuity.

Laboratory

Diagnosis is made on clinical findings.

Treatment

Complete vitrectomy, repair of laceration, systemic and local antibiotic therapy.

BIBLIOGRAPHY

1. Roy FH, Fraunfelder FW, Fraunfelder FT. Roy and Fraunfelder's Current Ocular Therapy, 6th edition. London: Elsevier; 2008.

21. SHAKEN BABY SYNDROME (BATTERED-BABY SYNDROME; BATTERED-CHILD SYNDROME; CHILD ABUSE SYNDROME; SILVERMAN SYNDROME)

General

Associated with parental abuse or accidents.

Ocular

Exophthalmos with orbital hemorrhages; lid hematoma; lid edema; secondary glaucoma; hyphema; vitreous hemorrhages; retinal exudates and hemorrhages (Berlin edema); choroidal atrophy; retinal detachment; papilledema; optic nerve sheath hemorrhage; preretinal, intraretinal, and subretinal hemorrhages; optic disk edema; choroidal hemorrhage.

Clinical

Soft tissue bruises; multiple fractures of long bones, ribs and skull; pharyngeal bruising, subdural hematoma; seizures; failure to thrive; vomiting associated with lethargy or drowsiness; respiratory irregularities; coma or death; intracranial hemorrhage.

Laboratory

Computed tomography of head to quantify degree of head trauma. MRI to define intraparenchymal brain lesions and subdural hematoma skeletal survey detects fractures of bones.

Treatment

Vitreous hemorrhage—if possible the source of the bleeding needs to be isolated and treated with laser. Vitrectomy may be necessary. Retinal detachment—scleral buckle, pneumatic retinopexy and vitrectomy may be used to close all the breaks. Orbital hemorrhage—topical medication to lower intraocular pressure, lateral canthotomy and inferior cantholysis.

BIBLIOGRAPHY

1. Budenz DL, Farber MG, Mirchandani HG, et al. Ocular and optic nerve hemorrhages in abused infants with intracranial injuries. Ophthalmology. 1994;101(3):559-65.
2. Coody D, Brown M, Montgomery D, et al. Shaken baby syndrome: identification and prevention for nurse practitioners. J Pediatr Health Care. 1994;8(2):50-6.
3. Lambert SR, Johnson TE, Hoyt CS. Optic nerve sheath and retinal hemorrhages associated with the shaken baby syndrome. Arch Ophthalmol. 1986;104(10):1509-12.
4. Munger CE, Peiffer RL, Bouldin TW, et al. Ocular and associated neuropathologic observations in suspected whiplash shaken infant syndrome. A retrospective study of 12 cases. Am J Forensic Med Pathol. 1993;14(3):193-200.

22. THERMAL BURNS

General

May occur to any body tissue.

Ocular

Conjunctival necrosis; corneal ulcer; exposure keratitis; ectropion; contracture deformity of lids; lid edema; entropion; endophthalmitis; proptosis; dacryocystitis; chronic epiphora; cellulitis; corneal perforation; symblepharon.

Clinical

Burns of any body tissue; edema; contractures; secondary infections.

Laboratory

Diagnosis is made by clinical findings.

Treatment

Pain management and topical medication are two therapeutic interventions.

BIBLIOGRAPHY

1. Jenkins JA, Schraga EG. (2011). Emergent Management of Thermal Burns. [online] Available from www.emedicine.com/emerg/TOPIC72.HTM. [Accessed August, 2013].

CHAPTER 15

Unclassified Disease or Conditions

1. KIMMELSTIEL-WILSON SYNDROME (DIABETES MELLITUS-HYPERTENSION-NEPHROSIS SYNDROME; DIABETES-NEPHROSIS SYNDROME; DIABETIC GLOMERULOSCLEROSIS; INTERCAPILLARY GLOMERULOSCLEROSIS; RENAL GLOMERULOHYALINOSIS-DIABETIC SYNDROME)

General

Occurs in patients with diabetes mellitus of several years duration.

Ocular

Retinal lesions, including hemorrhages, exudates, and neovascularization.

Clinical

Hypertension; proteinuria; edema; glomerulonephrosis; arteriosclerosis; capillary or intercapillary glomerulosclerosis; eosinophilic nodules; hyaline degeneration of the renal arterioles.

Laboratory

Serum—hyperglycemia; urine—glucosuria.

Treatment

Pharmacologic therapy allowing glycemic control, diet modification and weight loss are the main therapy for diabetes.

BIBLIOGRAPHY

1. Khardori R. (2013). Type 2 Diabetes Mellitus. [online] Available from www.emedicine.com/med/TOPIC547.HTM. [Accessed August, 2013].

2. PAPILLORENAL SYNDROME (RENAL-COLOBOMA SYNDROME)

General

Inherited condition often characterized by the association of bilateral centrally excavated optic disks with multiple cilioretinal vessels and dysplastic kidneys.

Clinical

Dysplastic kidneys, glomerulonephropathy and proteinuria.

Ocular

Retinal detachment, disk abnormalities.

Laboratory

Ultrasound of the kidneys, elevated blood urea nitrogen and creatinine levels, urinalysis to show proteinuria, and blood for PAZ2 mutation analysis.

BIBLIOGRAPHY

1. Roy FH, Fraunfelder FW, Fraunfelder FT. Roy and Fraunfelder's Current Ocular Therapy, 6th edition. London: Elsevier; 2008.

3. VOGT-KOYANAGI-HARADA DISEASE (HARADA DISEASE; UVEITIS-VITILIGO-ALOPECIA-POLIOSIS SYNDROME)

General

Viral infection; occurs predominantly among Italian and Japanese individuals; young adults; chronic.

Ocular

White lashes; secondary glaucoma; bilateral uveitis; sympathetic ophthalmitis; exudative iridocyclitis; vitreous opacities; bilateral serous retinal detachment and edema with spontaneous reattachment after weeks; depigmentation and patches of scattered pigment later; bilateral acute diffuse exudative choroiditis; papilledema; macular hemorrhage; cataracts; phthisis bulbi; poliosis; scleromalacia; intraocular lymphoma.

Clinical

Poliosis; vitiligo; hearing defect; headache; vomiting; meningeal irritation; reported to occur rarely in children.

Laboratory

Immunohistochemistry specimens demonstrate infiltration of CD4+ T-cells, epithelioid cells and multinucleated giant cells.

Treatment

Systemic therapy involves the use of high-dose corticosteroids. Topical steroids may be needed in conjunction with the use of systemic steroids.

BIBLIOGRAPHY

1. Walton RC, Choczaj-Kukula A, Janniger CK. (2012). Vogt-Koyanagi-Harada Disease. [online] Available from www.emedicine.com/oph/TOPIC459.HTM. [Accessed August, 2013].

CHAPTER
16

Anterior Chamber

🔲 1. ANTERIOR CHAMBER CLEAVAGE SYNDROME
(REESE-ELLSWORTH SYNDROME; PETERS-PLUS SYNDROME)

General

Abnormalities in the embryologic development of the anterior chamber due to failure of normal migration of mesodermal cells across the anterior segment of the eye or failure of later differentiation of the mesodermal elements; various conditions described as congenital: central anterior synechiae, persistent mesenchymal tissue in the chamber angle, posterior embryotoxon, congenital corneal hyaline membrane, posterior marginal dysplasia, prominent Schwalbe's line, mesodermal dysgenesis, and internal corneal ulcer seem all to fall in this same category of the anterior chamber cleavage syndrome; condition is present at birth; about 80% are bilateral; autosomal dominant inheritance; may be associated with congenital sensory neuropathy and ichthyosis.

Ocular

Increased intraocular pressure (IOP); adhesions between the iris and cornea; persistence of mesenchymal tissue in the chamber angle; usually shallow anterior chamber; iris coloboma and hypoplasia; prominent Schwalbe's ring; contiguous hyaloid membrane; corneal opacities of various density with or without edema, usually at the site of iris adhesion; anterior pole cataract; remains of hyaloid artery.

Clinical

Dental anomalies; mental retardation; cleft palate; syndactyly; craniofacial dysostosis; myotonic dystrophy.

Laboratory

Diagnosis is made by clinical findings.

Treatment

- *Glaucoma:* Glaucoma medication should be the first plan of action. If medication is unsuccessful, a filtering surgical procedure with or without antimetabolites may be beneficial.
- *Cataract:* Change in glasses can sometimes improve a patient's visual function temporarily; however, the most common treatment is cataract surgery.

🔲 BIBLIOGRAPHY

1. Giri G. (2012). Peters Anomaly. [online] Available from www.emedicine.com/oph/TOPIC112.HTM. [Accessed August, 2013].

2. ANTERIOR SEGMENT ISCHEMIA SYNDROME

General

Occasional complication of strabismus surgery; usually occurs in adult patients who have paretic strabismus after extensive transposition procedures; also may be secondary to giant cell arteritis or develop following trabeculectomy or strabismus surgery.

Ocular

Corneal edema; corneal ulceration; uveitis; iris atrophy; ectopic pupil; posterior synechiae; cataract; hypotony; phthisis bulbi.

Laboratory

Diagnosis is made by clinical findings.

Treatment

- *Uveitis:* Topical steroids and cycloplegic medication should be the initial treatment of choice. Oral steroids if not responsive to topical steroids, immunosuppressants if bilateral disease that does not respond to oral steroids, periocular steroids for unilateral or posterior uveitis. Vitrectomy can be used for severe vitreous opacification. Cryotherapy and laser photocoagulation may be used for localized pars plana exudates.
- *Cataract:* Change in glasses can sometimes improve a patient's visual function temporarily; however, the most common treatment is cataract surgery.

BIBLIOGRAPHY

1. Birt CM, Slomovic A, Motolko M, et al. Anterior segment ischemia in giant cell arteritis. Can J Ophthalmol. 1994; 29(2):93-4.
2. Hiatt RL. Production of anterior segment ischemia. J Pediatr Ophthalmol Strabismus. 1978;15(4):197-204.
3. Saunders RA, Sandall GS. Anterior segment ischemia syndrome following rectus muscle transposition. Am J Ophthalmol. 1982;93(1):34-8.
4. Saunders RA, Bluestein EC, Wilson ME, et al. Anterior segment ischemia after strabismus surgery. Surv Ophthalmol. 1994;38(5):456-66.
5. Watson NJ. Anterior segment ischemia. Ophthalmic Surg. 1992;23(6):429-31.

3. CHOLESTEROLOSIS OF THE ANTERIOR CHAMBER

In this condition, cholesterol crystals develop in the anterior chamber; usually in a blind eye following trauma, but can be associated with hyphema or secondary glaucoma. It is also associated with the following:
- Chronic uveitis
- Eales disease (periphlebitis)
- Lens subluxation
- †Mature or hypermature cataract
- Microphthalmia
- Phthisis bulbi
- Retinal detachment
- Traumatic cataract
- †Vascular disorders
- Vitreous hemorrhage

†Indicates a general entry and therefore has not been described in detail in the text

BIBLIOGRAPHY

1. Mishra RK, Ghosh M, Ghosh A. Cholesterol crystals in Eales disease. Indian J Ophthalmol. 1980;28:67-8.
2. Wand M, Garn RA. Cholesterolosis of the anterior chamber. Am J Ophthalmol. 1974;78:143-4.

3.1. CHRONIC UVEITIS, ANTERIOR GRANULOMATOUS (IRITIS)

General

Ocular inflammation of the iris and ciliary body. Etiology is idiopathic but certain systemic diseases may be the underlying cause.

Clinical

Herpes zoster, sarcoidosis, syphilis, Lyme disease, tuberculosis, multiple sclerosis, leprosy, toxoplasmosis, coccidiodomycosis, Vogt-Koyanagi-Harada disease, brucellosis.

Ocular

Photophobia, red eye, dull aching eye pain, perilimbal injection, keratic precipitates, flare and cell of anterior chamber, posterior synechiae, lenticular precipitates.

Laboratory

Diagnosis is made by clinical findings. If granulomatous iritisis recurrent, studies are necessary to determine the cause. Enzyme linked immunosorbent assay (ELISA), serologic testing for syphilis, sarcoidosis and Lyme may be indicated.

Treatment

Topical corticosteroids are the mainstay of therapy. Subconjunctival corticosteroids may be necessary in nonresponding cases. Cycloplegia is useful for control of pain and photophobia.

BIBLIOGRAPHY

1. Levinson RD. (2012). Uveitis, Anterior, Granulomatous. [online] Available from www.emedicine.com/oph/TOPIC586.HTM. [Accessed August, 2013].

3.2. EALES DISEASE (PERIPHLEBITIS)

General

Common; young adults.

Ocular

Sheathing of peripheral veins; hemorrhage in new vessels and later retinal detachment; retinal vascular tortuosity; microaneurysms of retina; post-neovascularization of vitreous; internuclear ophthalmoplegia.

Clinical

Epilepsy and hemiplegia have been reported; chronic encephalitis; ulcerative colitis; central nervous infarction.

Laboratory

Fluorescein angiography and tuberculosis screening test.

Treatment

Thyroid extract, osteogenic hormones, androgenic hormones, and systemic steroids. The antioxidant vitamins A, C, and E have been suggested as a possible therapy because antioxidizing enzymes are deficient in the vitreous samples.

BIBLIOGRAPHY

1. Roth DB, Fine HF. (2012). Eales Disease. [online] Available from www.emedicine.com/oph/TOPIC637.HTM. [Accessed August, 2013].

3.3. SUBLUXATION, DISLOCATION OF THE LENS

General

Ectopia lentis, occurs when the lens is not in its normal position.

Clinical

Marfan syndrome, Weill-Marchesani syndrome, sulfite oxidase deficiency.

Laboratory

Diagnosis is made by clinical findings.

Treatment

Careful phacoemulsification, topical steroids to control ocular inflammation.

BIBLIOGRAPHY

1. Eifrig CW. (2013). Ectopia Lentis. [online] Available from www.emedicine.com/oph/TOPIC55.HTM. [Accessed August, 2013].

3.5. MICROCEPHALY, MICROPHTHALMIA, CATARACTS, AND JOINT CONTRACTURES

General

Autosomal dominant; ocular features like Hagberg-Santavuori syndrome.

Ocular

Microphthalmia; cataracts; hypopigmented retinal degeneration.

Clinical

Microcephaly; shortening or wasting of muscle fibers, causing excess scar tissue over joints.

Laboratory

Clinical.

Treatment

Cataracts: Change in glasses can sometimes improve a patient's visual function temporarily, however the most common treatment is cataract surgery.

BIBLIOGRAPHY

1. Bateman JB, Philippart M. Ocular features of Hagberg-Santavuori syndrome. Am J Ophthalmol. 1986;102:262-71.
2. McKusick VA. Mendelian Inheritance in Man; A Catalog of Human Genes and Genetic Disorders, 12th edition. Baltimore: The Johns Hopkins University Press; 1998.
3. McKusick-Nathans Institute for Genetic Medicine, Johns Hopkins University and National Center for Biotechnology Information, National Library of Medicine. (2007). Online Mendelian Inheritance in Man, OMIM. [online] Available from www.ncbi.nlm.nih.gov/omim. [Accessed August, 2013].

3.6. PHTHISIS BULBI

General

Shrunken, not functional eye secondary to trauma, infection, radiation or other ocular abnormalities.

Clinical

None.

Ocular

Scarred swollen cornea; low IOP; distorted globe; cataract; ocular pain; blind.

Laboratory

Diagnosis is made by clinical observation.

Treatment

No treatment is available to improve. Alcohol injection can sometimes be used to reduce pain. Enucleation may also be necessary to eliminate the pain.

BIBLIOGRAPHY

1. Moran Eye Center. (2013). Phthisis bulbi. [online] Available from uuhsc.utah.edu/MoranEyeCenter/opatharch/uvea/phthisis_bulbi.htm. [Accessed August, 2013].

3.7. RETINAL DETACHMENT/GIANT RETINAL TEARS

General

Seen most commonly in the highly myopic; tear extends across at least 25% of the retina; tear commonly folds over itself.

Clinical

None.

Ocular

Lesions of the retina; loss of vision.

Laboratory

Diagnosis is made by clinical findings.

Treatment

Perfluoron can be used to unravel the retina and then laser is applied to reattach the retina.

BIBLIOGRAPHY

1. Retinal Consultants of San Antonio. (2010). Giant Retinal Tear Treatment. [online] Available from www.retinasanantonio.com/services/giant-retinal-tear-treatment. [Accessed August, 2013].

3.8. TRAUMATIC CATARACT

General

Injury resulting in lens opacification which can be diagnosed at the time of the trauma or years later.

Clinical

None.

Ocular

Visual loss, amblyopia, trauma to cornea, loose iris zonules.

Laboratory

Diagnosis is made by clinical findings.

Treatment

Extracapsular cataract extraction or phacoemulsification is the procedure of choice.

BIBLIOGRAPHY

1. Graham RH, Mulrooney BC. (2012). Traumatic cataract. [online] Available from www.emedicine.com/oph/TOPIC52.HTM. [Accessed August, 2013].

3.10. VITREOUS HEMORRHAGE

General

Hemorrhage into vitreous.

Clinical

Reduced vision secondary to bleeding in vitreous.

Ocular

Retinal vascular with proliferation or non-proliferation of retinal vessels, traction on retinal vessel, trauma, uveal tract.

Laboratory

Identify the cause with complete blood count (CBC), sickle cell prep, fetal bovine serum (FBS), clotting time, B-scan ultrasonography.

Treatment

Prophylaxis: Treat the underlying pathology; vitreous surgery—vitrectomy for non-clearing.

BIBLIOGRAPHY

1. Phillpotts BA, Blair NP, Gieser JP. (2013). Vitreous hemorrhage. [online] Available from www.emedicine.com/oph/TOPIC421.HTM. [Accessed August, 2013].

4. EPITHELIAL INGROWTH (EPITHELIAL DOWNGROWTH)

General

Epithelial ingrowth in a sheet-like fashion which is a rare complication of ocular trauma or anterior segment surgery.

Clinical

None.

Ocular

Hypotony, prolonged inflammation.

Laboratory

Diagnosis is made from clinical findings.

Treatment

Excision of epithelial sheets has been reported with variable success. A corneoscleral graft is necessary following this procedure.

⊟ BIBLIOGRAPHY

1. Roy FH, Fraunfelder FW, Fraunfelder FT. Roy and Fraunfelder's Current Ocular Therapy, 6th edition. London: Elsevier; 2008.

⊟ 5. FRENKEL SYNDROME (OCULAR CONTUSION SYNDROME; ANTERIOR SEGMENT TRAUMATIC SYNDROME)

General

Minor blunt trauma to the anterior segment of the globe.

Ocular

Sluggish pupil reaction; traumatic mydriasis; iris dialysis; heavy pigment deposits on the vitreous surface; subluxation of the lens; transient posterior cortical lens opacities; permanent anterior or posterior capsular opacities; coronary opacities; late anterior cortical rosette; late total traumatic cataract; Vossius ring following hyphema; peripheral pigment disturbance resembling atypical retinitis pigmentosa; macular edema; retinal detachment.

Clinical

None.

Laboratory

Diagnosis is made by clinical findings.

Treatment

Cataract surgery and retinal detachment surgery may be necessary.

⊟ BIBLIOGRAPHY

1. Frenkel H. Sur la Valeur Medico-Legale du Syndrome Traumatique du Segment Anterieur. Arch Ophthalmol. 1931;48:5.
2. Magalini SI, Scrascia E. Dictionary of Medical Syndromes, 2nd edition. Philadelphia: JB Lippincott; 1981.

⊟ 6. GAS BUBBLES IN THE ANTERIOR CHAMBER

- *Clostridium perfringens*
- *Escherichia coli*
- †Yttrium-aluminum-garnet (YAG) laser treatment to the anterior segment
- †Postoperative intraocular surgery

---

†Indicates a general entry and therefore has not been described in detail in the text

⊟ BIBLIOGRAPHY

1. Frantz JF, Lemp MA, Font RL, et al. Acute endogenous panophthalmitis caused by Clostridium perfringens. Am J Ophthalmol. 1974;78:295-303.
2. Obertymski H, Dyson C. Clostridium perfringens panophthalmitis. Can J Ophthalmol. 1974;9:258-9.

⊟ 6.1. CLOSTRIDIUM PERFRINGENS

General

Gram-positive rod; most important cause of gas gangrene infection.

Ocular

Hypopyon; gas bubbles in anterior chamber; endophthalmitis; proptosis; glaucoma; coffee-colored discharge; eyelid edema; severe ocular pain; endophthalmitis after penetrating trauma or metastatic.

Clinical

Traumatized ischemic skeletal muscle, abdominal wall, or uterus; hemolytic anemia; shock; death.

Laboratory

ELISA of the wound exudate, tissue samples, or serum can confirm diagnosis.

Treatment

Antibiotic therapy and hyperbaric oxygen may be useful. In more severe cases fasciotomy, debridement and amputation may be necessary.

BIBLIOGRAPHY

1. Ho H, Figueroa-Casas JB, Maxfield DG, et al. (2011). Gas gangrene. [online] Available from www.emedicine.com/med/TOPIC843.HTM. [Accessed August, 2013].

6.2. ESCHERICHIA COLI

General

Gram-negative rod found in the gastrointestinal tract; urinary tract is the usual portal of entry.

Ocular

Uveitis; hyphema; hypopyon; gas bubbles in anterior chamber; purulent conjunctivitis; keratitis; corneal edema; panophthalmitis; endophthalmitis; glaucoma.

Clinical

Diarrhea; gastroenteritis; dehydration.

Laboratory

Anaerobic Gram-negative rod.

Treatment

Antibiotic therapy should start with ampicillin until sensitivity reports return.

BIBLIOGRAPHY

1. Suh DW. (2012). Ophthalmologic manifestations of Escherichia coli. [online] Available from www.emedicine.com/oph/TOPIC496.HTM. [Accessed August, 2013].

7. GLAUCOMA, HYPHEMA

General

Collection of red blood cells in the anterior chamber.

Clinical

Most common following trauma; bleeding disorders; sickle cell disease.

Ocular

Blood in the anterior chamber, corneal bloodstaining; pupillary block; rubeosis iridis; intraocular tumors, older style intraocular lens (2L and 4L Binkhorst styles).

Laboratory

Slit-lamp examination; measurement of IOP; history of trauma, CT scan and ultrasonography to exclude orbital fracture and other associated eye injuries.

Treatment

Limiting activities that cause rapid movement of the globe; sleeping with head elevated; topical and oral ocular hypotensive medications; cycloplegics and topical steroids; avoiding medications such as aspirin that thin the blood.

BIBLIOGRAPHY

1. Dersu II. (2012). Hyphema Glaucoma. [online] Available from www.emedicine.medscape.com/article/1206635-overview [Accessed August, 2013].

8. HYPHEMA (BLEEDING INTO THE ANTERIOR CHAMBER)

- †*Trauma*
  - †Following laser iridectomy or strabismus surgery in aphakia
  - Honan balloon use in Fuchs heterochromic iridocyclitis
  - †Tear of ciliary body—post contusion deformity of anterior chamber
  - †To ciliary body, such as cyclodialysis
  - †To iris, such as in iridodialysis or intraocular lens irritation
  - †After airbag inflation
  - †Metallic intraocular foreign body during magnetic resonance imaging
- †*Overdistention of vessels*
  - Obstruction of central retinal vein
  - Sudden lowering of high IOP
- *Fragility of vessel walls*
  - Acute gonorrheal iridocyclitis
  - Acute herpes iridocyclitis
  - Acute rheumatoid iridocyclitis
  - Ankylosing spondylitis

---

†Indicates a general entry and therefore has not been described in detail in the text

- *Blood abnormality*
  - †Anemias
  - †Association with use of aspirin
  - Hemophilia
  - Leukemia
  - Purpura
  - Sickle cell disease
- *Metabolic disease*
  - †Diabetes mellitus (Willis disease)
  - Scurvy (avitaminosis C)
- *Neovascularization of iris*
- *Vascularized tumors of iris (see pigmented and nonpigmented iris lesions)*
  - †Angioma
  - †Iris vascular tufts
  - Juvenile xanthogranuloma (JXG)
  - †Lymphosarcoma
  - Retinoblastoma
- †Wound vascularization following cataract extraction
- *Persistent pupillary membrane hemorrhage*

BIBLIOGRAPHY

1. Sheppard JD, Crouch ER, Williams PB, et al. (2011). Hyphema. [online] Available from www.emedicine.com/oph/TOPIC 765.HTM. [Accessed August, 2013].

8.1B. FUCHS (1) SYNDROME (HETEROCHROMIC CYCLITIS SYNDROME)

General

Etiology unknown; mild infective cyclitis is the most likely cause; etiology remains unclear, although it is likely to be autoimmune; positive epidemiologic association with ocular toxoplasmosis has been investigated.

Ocular

Secondary glaucoma; unilateral hypochromic heterochromia; painless cyclitis with absence of synechiae and little or no ciliary injection; secondary cataract; vitreous opacities; small white discrete keratic precipitates with fine filaments between the precipitates; corneal epithelium may be slightly edematous; peripheral choroiditis occasionally; keratoconus.

Clinical

Occasional dysraphia of the cervical cord.

Laboratory

Diagnosis is made by clinical findings.

Treatment

Generally no treatment is necessary. Occasionally discomfort and ciliary injection is treated with topical steroids. With cataract surgery there is a higher rate of vitreous debri and hemorrhage. Glaucoma surgery may be indicated and rubeotic glaucoma may require enucleation.

BIBLIOGRAPHY

1. Arif M, Foster CS, Wong IG. (2011). Fuchs heterochromic uveitis. [online] Available from www.emedicine.com/oph/ TOPIC432.HTM. [Accessed August, 2013].

⊟ 8.3A. GONORRHEA

General

Caused by *Neisseria gonorrhoeae*, which is transmitted sexually.

Ocular

Conjunctivitis; eyelid edema; keratitis; uveitis.

Clinical

Pelvic inflammatory disease; arthritis; dermatitis; carditis; meningitis.

Laboratory

Gram stain smear demonstrates Gram-negative diplococci with polymorphonuclear leukocytes in conjunctival exudates.

Treatment

Therapy consists of systemic antibiotics; topical antibiotics are relatively ineffective in the treatment of eye disease. It is important to treat all sexual partners simultaneously to prevent reinfection.

⊟ BIBLIOGRAPHY

1. Wong B. (2013). Gonorrhea. [online] Available from www.emedicine.com/oph/TOPIC497.HTM. [Accessed August, 2013].

⊟ 8.3B. HERPES ZOSTER

General

It is caused by varicella zoster virus; about 75% of cases occur in persons over age 45 years; condition is more frequent with advancing age and in patients who are immunocompromised by drugs or disease; in particular, an increasing number of patients with herpes zoster ophthalmicus are immunosuppressed.

Ocular

Conjunctivitis; keratitis; recurrent corneal ulcer; neuralgia; zoster rash of eyelids; uveitis; iris atrophy; scleritis; cataract; optic neuritis; paralysis of third nerve; proptosis; paralysis of lids; orbital apex syndrome; retinitis; neurotrophic keratitis; acute retinal necrosis; progressive outer retinal necrosis; ocular motor nerve pareses; tonic pupil; encephalitis; vasculitis.

Clinical

Local lesions involving the posterior or root ganglia; nerve damage; tissue scarring.

Laboratory

Diagnosed mostly on the basis of the characteristic pain and appearance of the dermatomal rashes.

Treatment

Antiviral agents, systemic corticosteroids, antidepressants, and adequate pain control. Immunocompetent adults aged 60 years or older, benefit from receipt of the herpes zoster vaccine and have a lower incidence of herpes zoster.

⊟ BIBLIOGRAPHY

1. Ghaznawi N, Virdi A, Dayan A, et al. Herpes zoster ophthalmicus: comparison of disease in patients 60 years and older versus younger than 60 years. Ophthalmology. 2011;118: 2242-50.
2. Ho J, Xirasagar S, Lin H. Increased risk of a cancer diagnosis after herpes zoster ophthalmicus: a nationwide population-based study. Ophthalmology. 2011;118:1076-81.
3. Janniger CK, Eastern JS, Hospenthal DR, et al. (2013). Herpes zoster. [online]. Available from www.emedicine.com/oph/ TOPIC257.HTM. [Accessed August, 2013].
4. Tseng HF, Smith N, Harpaz R, et al. Herpes zoster vaccine in older adults and the risk of subsequent herpes zoster disease. JAMA. 2011;305:160-6.

8.3C. JUVENILE RHEUMATOID ARTHRITIS (JRA; STILL DISEASE)

General

Onset before age 16 years; greater occurrence of systemic manifestations, monarticular and oligoarticular joint involvement, and iridocyclitis.

Ocular

Hypopyon; band keratopathy; uveitis; cataract; papillitis; glaucoma; macular edema; ocular pain; vitreous cells; synechiae; scleritis; presumed to have an autoimmune etiology; antiocular antibodies, including iris protein antibodies, have been found in the sera of patients.

Clinical

Salmon pink macular rash; arthritis; hepatosplenomegaly; leukocytosis; chronic pain; joint swelling; low-grade fever; anemia; rheumatoid nodules.

Laboratory

Antinuclear antibody, rheumatoid factor, human leukocyte antigen B27, X-ray imaging of joints.

Treatment

Uveitis treated initially with topical corticosteroids. Systemic immunomodulatory agents may be useful for patients with limited or no response to topical or systemic corticosteroids.

BIBLIOGRAPHY

1. Roque MR, Roque BL, Miserocchi E, et al. (2012). Juvenile idiopathic arthritis uveitis. [online] Available from www.emedicine.com/oph/TOPIC675.HTM. [Accessed August, 2013].
2. Thorne JE, Woreta FA, Dunn JP, et al. Risk of cataract development amoung children with juvenile idiopathic arthritis-related uveitis treated with topical corticosteroids. Ophthalmology. 2010;117:1436-41.

8.3D. VON BEKHTEREV-STRUMPELL SYNDROME (MARIE-STRUMPELL SPONDYLITIS; ANKYLOSING SPONDYLITIS; PIERRE-MARIE SYNDROME; BEKHTEREV DISEASE; RHEUMATOID SPONDYLITIS) OPTIC ATROPHY

General

Variant of rheumatoid arthritis; etiology unknown; autosomal dominant; male preponderance; onset at age 20–40 years; although genetic background determines susceptibility to uveitis, the disease pattern suggests the possibility of random environmental triggers unrelated to the course of the underlying rheumatologic disorder.

Ocular

Non-granulomatous anterior uveitis; optic nerve atrophy (occasionally); hypopyon; band keratopathy; spontaneous hyphema.

Clinical

Spondylitis of vertebra and sacroiliac joints; ankylosis; general arthralgia; kyphosis; scoliosis; displaced head and total rigidity of spine.

Laboratory

Histocompatibility antigen HLA-B27 and a negative rheumatoid factor and antinuclear antibody; X-ray evidence of narrowing of sacroiliac joint space and sclerosis.

Treatment

Oral nonsteroidal anti-inflammatory drugs, urethritis in Reiter's disease should be treated with tetracycline, topical steroids and cycloplegic agents.

BIBLIOGRAPHY

1. Vives MJ, Garfin SR. (2011). Rheumatoid arthritis of the cervical spine overview of rheumatoid spondylitis. [online] Available from www.emedicine.com/orthoped/TOPIC551. HTM. [Accessed August, 2013].

8.4C. WERLHOF DISEASE (HEMOPHILIA AND THROMBOCYTOPENIC PURPURA)

General

Hemorrhagic disease of unknown etiology.

Ocular

Retinal hemorrhages; degeneration or severe intraocular hemorrhages with resultant retinitis proliferans.

Clinical

Petechiae and ecchymoses of skin and mucous membranes; tendency to bruise; decreased level of circulating platelets with a normal clotting time.

Laboratory

Diagnosis is made by clinical findings.

Treatment

See hemotologist.

BIBLIOGRAPHY

1. Kobayashi H, Honda Y. Intraocular hemorrhage in a patient with hemophilia. Metab Ophthalmol. 1985;8:27-30.
2. Pau H. Differential diagnosis of eye diseases. New York: Thieme; 1987.
3. Werlhof PG. Disquisitio Medica et Philogica de Variolis et Anthracibus. Brunswick: 1735.

8.4D. LEUKEMIA

General

Acute or chronic blood disorder.

Ocular

Engorgement of conjunctival vessels; papillary hypertrophy; aggregations of tumor cells in conjunctiva, choroid, and orbit; secondary glaucoma; retinal venous engorgement and tortuosity with pronounced constrictions; retinal hemorrhages; retinal detachment; cotton-wool spots; macular edema; papilledema; optic atrophy; optic neuritis; paralysis of extraocular muscles; hypopyon; vitreous opacities; retinal sea fans; perilimbal subconjunctival infiltrates; corneal leukemic infiltration (rare); shallow serous retinal detachments; hyphema; iris neovascularization; central retinal vein occlusion; vitreous infiltrates.

Clinical

Frequent involvement of central nervous system; intracranial hemorrhage; thrombocytopenia; rising white cell count.

Laboratory

CBC and differential, bone marrow aspiration, immunophenotyping, chromosomal analysis.

Treatment

Chemotherapy with or without radiotherapy.

BIBLIOGRAPHY

1. Wu L, Evans T, Martinez J. (2012). Leukemias. [online]. Available from www.emedicine.com/oph/TOPIC489.HTM. [Accessed August, 2013].

8.4E. HENOCH-SCHÖNLEIN PURPURA (PURPURA; ANAPHYLACTOID PURPURA)

General

Occurs chiefly in children, although it can affect persons of any age; frequently follows an upper respiratory tract infection within 3 weeks.

Ocular

Retinal hemorrhages; iritis; optic neuritis.

Clinical

Purpuric skin rash; concentrated on lower extremities; joint pain; abdominal pain; hematuria; central nervous system involvement.

Laboratory

Diagnosis is made by clinical findings.

Treatment

See hematologist.

⊟ BIBLIOGRAPHY

1. Harley RD (Ed). Pediatric Ophthalmology, 4th edition. Philadelphia: WB Saunders; 1998.

2. Lorentz WB, Weaver RG. Eye involvement in anaphylactoid purpura. Am J Dis Child. 1980;134:524-5.

3. Ryder HG, Marcus O. Henoch-Schonlein purpura: a case report. S Afr Med J. 1976;50:2005-6

⊟ 8.4F. HERRICK SYNDROME (DRESBACH SYNDROME; SICKLE CELL DISEASE; DREPANOCYTIC ANEMIA)

General

Usually occurs in members of the black race; poor prognosis.

Ocular

Secondary glaucoma; telangiectasia of conjunctival vessels; scleral icterus; vitreous hemorrhages; cataract; retinal hemorrhages, exudates, and neovascularization; retinitis proliferans; microaneurysms; thrombosis of retinal venules; retinal vascular sheathing; central vein occlusion; angioid streaks; retinopathy with "black sunburst sign" in patients with SS hemoglobin; "sea fan sign" in patients with SC hemoglobin; comma signs of conjunctiva; fan-shaped neovascularization of iris; sector ischemic atrophy of iris; optic atrophy; white cotton mass of vitreous; retinal holes; color vision defects; central retinal artery obstruction; branch retinal artery obstruction; white without pressure; venous tortuosity; sickling maculopathy.

Clinical

Severe anemia with hemolytic crises; bone and joint aches; hemarthrosis; jaundice; hepatosplenomegaly.

Laboratory

Blood-sickling of red blood cells, newborn screening for hemoglobin disorders.

Treatment

Transfusion is required in an aplastic crisis; erythrocytapheresis is an automated red-cell exchange and bone marrow transplantation may be useful. Pain is the hallmark of sickle cell disease. While frequency and severity vary greatly, most patients have interval symptoms. Once pain has begun, no therapy reverses the process. Analgesics may provide a reasonable degree of comfort. While certain dosing guidelines are available, the amount of drug given should be titrated to the degree of pain experienced. Vitrectomy may be necessary.

⊟ BIBLIOGRAPHY

1. Maakaron JE, Taher AT. (2013). Sickle cell anemia. [online] Available from www.emedicine.com/ped/TOPIC2096.HTM. [Accessed August, 2013].

⊟ 8.5B. AVITAMINOSIS C (SCURVY; VITAMIN C DEFICIENCY)

General

Vitamin C deficiency.

Ocular

Hemorrhages of lids, anterior chamber, vitreous cavity, retina, subconjunctival space, and orbit (most prominent, with resulting exophthalmos); keratitis, corneal ulcer; cataract.

Clinical

Increased capillary fragility with a tendency to hemorrhage in tissues throughout the body; poor wound healing; loose teeth; purpuric rash.

Laboratory

Laboratory tests are usually not helpful to ascertain a diagnosis of scurvy. Diagnosis is generally made by clinical findings and history.

Treatment

Dietary or pharmacologic doses of vitamin C is the standard treatment. Orange juice is a good choice to add to the diet.

BIBLIOGRAPHY

1. Goebel L, Buckler BS, Driscoll H, et al. (2013). Scurvy. [online] Available from www.emedicine.com/ped/TOPIC 2073.HTM. [Accessed August, 2013].

8.6. IRIS NEOVASCULARIZATION WITH PSEUDOEXFOLIATION SYNDROME

General

Anoxia secondary to iris vessel obstruction; electron microscopic studies reveal endothelial thickening with decreased lumen size and fenestration of vessel walls.

Ocular

Material found on posterior and anterior iris surface, anterior lens surface, ciliary processes, zonules, and anterior hyaloid membranes; neovascularization of iris stroma; increased permeability of iris vessels.

Clinical

None.

Laboratory

Diagnosis is made by clinical findings.

Treatment

Patients with pseudoexfoliation syndrome should have annual eye examinations for early detection of glaucoma.

BIBLIOGRAPHY

1. Pons ME, Eliassi-Rad B. (2011). Pseudoexfoliation glaucoma. [online] Available from www.emedicine.com/oph/topic140.htm. [Accessed August, 2013].

8.7C. JUVENILE XANTHOGRANULOMA (JXG; NEVOXANTHOENDOTHELIOMA)

General

Childhood disease; unknown etiology.

Ocular

Uveal tract tumor presenting as spontaneous hyphema; secondary glaucoma; uveitis; corneal, lid, and epibulbar tumors; proptosis; retinal and choroidal lesions (rare).

Clinical

Multiple benign tumors, primarily of the skin; usually appear in the first 3 years of life; lesions appear as yellow-to-brown papules or nodules.

Laboratory

Diagnostic techniques include biomicroscopy, high frequency ultrasound and cytologic examination of anterior chamber paracentesis material.

Treatment

Topical, subconjunctival, intralesional, and systemic corticosteroids are useful. Low-dose radiation may be the treatment of choice for diffuse uveal lesions. Glaucoma medications should be used in the setting of hyphema and increased IOP.

BIBLIOGRAPHY

1. Curtis T, Wheeler DT. (2012). Juvenile xanthogranuloma. [online] vailable from www.emedicine.com/oph/topic588.htm. [Accessed August, 2013].

8.7E. RETINOBLASTOMA

General

Malignant tumor arising in one or both retinas of young children, usually under the age of 2 years; usually unilateral; autosomal dominant; most common intraocular malignancy of childhood; incidence is one in 20,000 live births; origin is questionably neuroectodermal cells capable of multipotentiality; one third of patients have heritable (bilateral or have a positive family history) autosomal dominant and two thirds are sporadic; genetic transmission obeys two-mutation hypothesis of Knudson; trilateral retinoblastoma is bilateral retinoblastoma plus midline central nervous system tumor (most commonly pinealoma); most common second tumor is an osteogenic sarcoma (begins in 2nd decade).

Ocular

Hyphema; hypopyon; corneal tumor; lid edema; endophthalmitis; exophthalmos; intraocular calcification of globe; heterochromia; neovascularization of iris or retina; papilledema; panophthalmitis; retinoblastoma extension into orbit and choroid; cat's-eye reflex; leukocoria; mydriasis; vitreous hemorrhage tumor seeding; esotropia; exotropia; glaucoma; visual loss.

Clinical

Metastasis into the lymph system, bone marrow, and subarachnoid space; basal meningitis; death.

Laboratory

CT—calcification of lesion hallmark of disease; ultrasound—demonstrates calcification and MRI demonstrates presence and extent of extraocular disease.

Treatment

External beam radiation therapy is recommended on patients with significant vitreous seeding. Radioactive isotope plaques and chemotherapy are also an option. Removal of the tumor is the standard management for retinoblastoma.

BIBLIOGRAPHY

1. Isidro MA, Roque MR, Aaberg TM, et al. (2012). Retinoblastoma. [online] Available from www.emedicine.com/oph/TOPIC346.HTM. [Accessed August, 2013].

8.9. PUPILLARY MEMBRANE, PERSISTENT

General

Autosomal dominant.

Ocular

Remnants of pupillary membrane persist as strands and other irregular tissues in pupil; congenital cataract; corneal edema; Rieger syndrome; keratoconus.

Clinical

None.

Laboratory

Diagnosis is made by clinical findings.

Treatment

Cataract surgery may be necessary if vision is effected; steroids and Muro 128 may be used for corneal edema; keratoconus may be treated with spectacle correction, hard contacts, avoid eye rubbing. If hydrops occur, discontinue contact lens, use NaCl drops and ointment, patching, and short course of steroids. As disease advances, penetrating keratoplasty, deep anterior lamellar keratoplasty intacs with laser grooves or collagen stabilization of cornea.

BIBLIOGRAPHY

1. Duane TD. Clinical Ophthalmology. Philadelphia: JB Lippincott; 1987.
2. McKusick VA. Mendelian Inheritance in Man, 12th edition. Baltimore: The John Hopkins University Press; 1998.

⊟ 9. HYPHEMA (TRAUMATIC HYPHEMA)

General

Trauma although bleeding may occur spontaneously in conditions such as rubeosis iridis, leudemia, hemophilia, anticoagulation therapy, retinoblastoma or juvenile xanthogranuloma of iris.

Clinical

None.

Ocular

Tear and bleeding from the iris, ciliary body or elevated IOP may occur.

Laboratory

Diagnosis is made by clinical findings.

Treatment

Cycloplegics decreased the inflammation and discomfort associated with traumatic iritis. Topical beta-adrenergic antagonists are the therapy of choice for elevated IOP.

⊟ BIBLIOGRAPHY

1. Sheppard JD, Crouch ER, Williams PB, et al. (2011). Hyphema. [online] Available from www.emedicine.com/oph/TOP-IC765.HTM. [Accessed August, 2013].

⊟ 10. UGH SYNDROME (UVEITIS-GLAUCOMA-HYPHEMA SYNDROME) GLAUCOMA

General

It is caused by a defective anterior chamber lens; can be caused by toxic substance incorporated into the plastic of lens during manufacture or warped intraocular lens; syndrome may rarely occur after extracapsular cataract extraction (ECCE) with implantation of a posterior chamber intraocular lens.

Ocular

Uveitis-glaucoma-hyphema.

Clinical

None.

Laboratory

Diagnosis is made by clinical findings.

Treatment

Uveitis-glaucoma-hyphema medication should be the first plan of action. If medication is unsuccessful, a filtering surgical procedure with or without antimetabolites may be beneficial. Hyphema—cycloplegics decreased the inflammation and discomfort associated with traumatic iritis. Topical beta-adrenergic antagonists are the therapy of choice for elevated IOP; laser may be used to cauterize the bleeding vessel.

⊟ BIBLIOGRAPHY

1. Percival SP, Das SK. UGH syndrome after posterior chamber lens implantation. J Am Intraocul Implant Soc. 1983;9(2):200-1.
2. Masket S. Pseudophakic posterior iris chafing syndrome. J Cataract Refract Surg. 1986;12(3):252-6.
3. Van Liefferinge T, Van Oye R, Kestelyn P, et al. Uveitis-glaucoma-hyphema syndrome: a late complication of posterior chamber lenses. Bull Soc Belg Ophthalmol. 1994;252:61-5.

⊟ 11. HYPOPYON (PUS IN ANTERIOR CHAMBER)

1. Hypopyon ulcer: corneal ulcer with pus in the anterior chamber
   A. *Acanthamoeba*
   B. Acquired immunodeficiency syndrome (AIDS)
   C. *Aspergillus species*
   D. *Candida albicans*
   E. Chemical injury
   †F. *Diplococcus pneumoniae*
   G. *Escherichia coli*
   H. *Fusarium* species
   I. Herpes simplex
   J. Herpes zoster
   K. Measles
   L. Moraxella

M. *Neisseria gonorrhoeae*
N. *Proteus vulgaris*
O. *Pseudomonas aeruginosa*
†P. *Serratia* species
Q. Smallpox
†R. Spitting-cobra venom
S. *Staphylococcus*
T. *Streptococcus*
2. Severe acute iridocyclitis
 A. Behçet's disease
 †B. HLA-B27 positivity
 †C. Spondyloarthropathy
†3. Repeated corneal transplantation of human amniotic membrane
†4. Necrosis of intraocular tumors or metastasis
5. Retained intraocular foreign bodies, including toxic lens syndrome
†6. Endophthalmitis-at time of surgical treatment, accidental trauma, in drug users, or spontaneous occurrence
 A. *Acanthamoeba*
 B. Actinomycosis
 C. Amebiasis
 D. *Aspergillosis species*
 E. Bacterial including *Bacillus cereus*
 F. Behçet syndrome
 G. *Candida albicans*
 H. Coccidioidomycosis
 I. Coenurosis
 J. Cysticercosis
 K. *Fusarium* species
 L. Hydatid cyst
 M. Influenza
 N. *Listeria monocytogenes*
 O. Lockjaw (*Clostridium tetani*)
 P. Metastatic bacterial endophthalmitis
 Q. *Moraxella* species
 R. *Mucor* species
 †S. *Mycobacterium avium*
 *T. *Pseudomonas* species
 U. Relapsing fever
 †V. *Serratia marcescens*
 †W. Saprophytic fungi
 X. *Staphylococcus*
 *Y. *Streptoccus*
 Z. Sterile hypopyon
  1. Behçet syndrome (oculobuccogenital syndrome)
  †2. Endotoxin contamination of ultrasonic bath
  †3. Following cyanoacrylate sealing of a corneal perforation
  †4. Following refractive surgery

5. Histiocytosis X (Hand-Schüller-Christian syndrome)
†6. Intraocular lens or instrument polishing compounds or sterilization techniques
*7. Juvenile rheumatoid arthritis
†8. Laser iridotomy
9. Leukemia
*†10. Reaction to lens protein
†11. Rough intraocular lens edges
12. von Bechterev-Strumpel syndrome (rheumatoid spondylitis)
AA. Stevens-Johnson syndrome (dermatostomatitis)
BB. Tight contact lens or contact lens overwear syndrome
CC. Tuberculosis
DD. Weil disease (leptospirosis)
EE. Yersiniosis

Drugs, including the following:
- Benoxinate
- Butacaine
- Cocaine
- Colchicine
- Dibucaine
- Dyclonine
- Ferrocholinate
- Ferrous fumarate
- Ferrous gluconate
- Ferrous succinate
- Ferrous sulfate
- Iodide and iodine solutions and compounds
- Iron dextran
- Iron sorbitex
- Phenacaine
- Piperocaine
- Polysaccharide-iron complex
- Proparacaine
- Radioactive iodides
- Rifabutin
- Tetracaine urokinase
- Urokinase

†7. Vitreous "fluff-ball"
†8. Following refractive surgery
9. Pseudohypopyon
 A. Ghost cell glaucoma with khaki-colored cells
 †B. Accidental intraocular steroid injection
10. Acute angle-closure glaucoma
11. Non-Hodgkin lymphoma
†12. Pars plana vitrectomy and silicone oil injection

---

†Indicates a general entry and therefore has not been described in detail in the text

BIBLIOGRAPHY

1. Fraunfelder FT, Fraunfelder FW. Drug-induced ocular side effects. Woburn, MA: Butterworth-Heinemann; 2001.
2. Gabler B, Lohmann CP. Hypopyon after repeated transplantation of human amniotic membrane onto the corneal surface. Ophthalmology. 2000;107:1344-6.
3. Pau H. Differential diagnosis of eye diseases, 2nd edition. New York: Thieme Medical; 1988.
4. Recchia FM, Baumal CR, Sivalingam A, et al. Endophthalmitis after pediatric strabismus surgery. Arch Ophthalmol. 2000;118:939-44.
5. Roy FH. Ocular syndromes and systemic diseases, 5th edition. New Delhi, Jaypee Brothers Medical Publishers; 2013
6. Saran BR, Maguire AM, Nichols C, et al. Hypopyon uveitis in patients with acquired immunodeficiency syndrome treated for systemic Mycobacterium avium complex infection with rifabutin. Arch Ophthalmol. 1994;112;1159-61.
7. Zaidi AA, Ying GS, Daniel E, et.al. Hypopyon in patients with uveitis. Ophthalmology. 2010;117:366-72.

11.1A. ACANTHAMOEBA

General

It is caused by *Acanthamoeba polyphaga* and *Acanthamoeba cartel* (*see* Herpes Simplex Masquerade Syndrome); all types of contact lenses have been associated with Acanthamoeba keratitis, particularly daily-wear soft contact lenses.

Ocular

Hypopyon; uveitis; conjunctivitis and chemosis; keratitis; pannus; corneal ring abscess; papillitis; vitreitis; retinal perivasculitis; secondary glaucoma; post-keratoplasty *Acanthamoeba* keratitis may present as an infectious crystalline keratopathy in the periphery of the graft.

Clinical

Meningoencephalitis; meningitis; hemorrhagic encephalitis.

Laboratory

Polygonal double-walled cysts, under bright-field or phase-contrast microscopy or stained with hematoxylin and eosin, Gram, Giemsa or celluflor white.

Treatment

Medical therapy for *Acanthamoeba* infection is not well established. Topical antimicrobial agents that achieve high concentrations at the site of the infection can be considered. Treatment of keratitis consists of early diagnosis and aggressive surgical and medical therapies.

BIBLIOGRAPHY

1. Crum-Cianflone NF. (2013). Acanthamoeba. [online] Available from www.emedicine.com/med/TOPIC10.HTM. [Accessed August, 2013].
2. Wang JC, Ritterband DC. (2013). Herpes simplex keratitis. [online] Available from www.emedicine.com/oph/TOPIC100.HTM. [Accessed August, 2013].

11.1B. ACQUIRED IMMUNODEFICIENCY SYNDROME (AIDS; ACQUIRED CELLULAR IMMUNODEFICIENCY; ACQUIRED IMMUNODEFICIENCY)

General

Acquired breakdown of the immune system followed by disease that takes advantage of the body's collapsed defenses; acquired by shared drug needles or sexual intercourse; occurs most frequently in homosexually active men (75%), intravenous drug abusers (13%), and Haitian immigrants (6%).

Ocular

Retinal cotton-wool spots; cytomegalovirus (CMV) retinitis; retinal periphlebitis; conjunctival Kaposi sarcoma; necrotizing retinitis; retinal hemorrhages; conjunctivitis sicca; orbital Burkitt lymphoma; peripheral retinochoroiditis; vitreitis; fungal corneal ulcer; hypopyon; acute glaucoma; third nerve palsy; anterior uveitis; atypical retinitis; orbital pseudotumor; herpes zoster ophthalmicus; herpes simplex keratitis; bacterial keratitis; molluscum contagiosum; toxoplasma retinitis; acute retinal necrosis; human immunodeficiency virus (HIV) retinitis; syphilitic retinitis; *Pneumocystis carinii* choroiditis; fungal and bacterial endophthalmitis; fungal choroiditis; conjunctival microvasculopathy; keratitis sicca; subconjunctival hemorrhage.

Clinical

Because of lowered immunity, one-third develop Kaposi sarcoma; pneumonia caused by *P. carinii;* death.

Laboratory

ELISA test is used for screening, other tests are used to evaluate false-positive and false-negative test results.

Treatment

Medical consultations are required for systemic treatment. The treatment of CMV retinitis can include drugs such as ganciclovir, valganciclovir, fomivirsen, foscarnet and cidofovir. All of these drugs have specific adverse effects and complicate the decision to use for treatment.

⊟ BIBLIOGRAPHY

1. Dubin J. (2013). Rapid testing for HIV. [online] Available from www.emedicine.com/emerg/TOPIC253.HTM. [Accessed August, 2013].
2. Copeland RA, Phillpotts BA. (2011). Ocular manifestations of HIV infection. Available from www.emedicine.com/oph/TOPIC417.HTM. [Accessed August, 2013].

⊟ 11.1C. ASPERGILLOSIS

General

Systemic infection common in poultry farmers, feeders or breeders of pigeons, and persons who work with grains; should be considered in immunocompromised patients.

Ocular

Corneal ulcer; blepharitis; keratitis; scleritis; endophthalmitis; exophthalmos; retinal hemorrhages; retinal detachment; vitreitis; cataract; conjunctivitis; orbital cellulitis; paresis of extraocular muscles; secondary glaucoma; scleromalacia perforans; endogenous endophthalmitis; anterior chamber mass; invasion of choroid and anterior optic nerve.

Clinical

Pulmonary infections; invasive fungal disease.

Laboratory

Culture from superficial scrapings from bed of infection.

Treatment

Voriconazole is the drug of choice. Although disease outcomes substantially improve with antifungal treatment, patient survival and infection resolution depend on improved immunosuppression.

⊟ BIBLIOGRAPHY

1. Batra V. (2011). Pediatric Aspergillosis. [online] Available from www.emedicine.com/ped/TOPIC148.HTM. [Accessed August, 2013].

⊟ 11.1D. CANDIDIASIS

General

Yeast-like opportunistic fungal infection caused by *C. albicans.*

Ocular

Uveitis; hypopyon; conjunctivitis; keratitis; corneal ulcer; blepharitis; endophthalmitis; dacryocystitis; papillitis; retinal atrophy; Roth spot; vitreous abscess; retrobulbar abscess; retinal detachment; panophthalmitis; chorioretinitis; infectious crystalline keratopathy.

Clinical

C. albicans normally is present as an intestinal saprophyte in 35–75% of the human population; in situations of internal environmental change, however, *Candida* can become pathogenic (e.g. obesity, diabetes mellitus, malignancy, and other debilitating conditions).

Laboratory

Common yeast from up to 50% of healthy individuals isolate directly from the eye should be attempted to confirm the presence of organism. Blood agar and Sabouraud's dextrose agar may be used; polymerase chain reaction (PCR) for species identification.

Treatment

Mucocutaneous infection typically responds to topical therapy. Antifungal therapy should be started immediately after necessary cultures have been obtained from all suspected sites of infection. Infectious disease specialists are typically involved in cases of invasive candidiasis.

BIBLIOGRAPHY

1. Hedayati T. (2012). Candidiasis in emergency medicine. [online] Available from www.emedicine.com/emerg/TOPIC76.HTM. [Accessed July, 2013].

11.1E. ALKALINE INJURY OF THE EYE

General

A splash of alkaline solution causes the pH to rise and results in immediate damage to the external ocular tissues. These injuries are frequently seen from household chemicals or farming injuries from liquid ammonia used as fertilizer.

Ocular

Pain; lacrimation; blepharospasm; rise in IOP; rapid penetration of the cornea and sclera; chemical injury to iris, lens or ciliary body; symblepharon; phthisis bulbi; ankyloblepharon.

Laboratory

Diagnosis is made by clinical findings and history.

Treatment

Immediate copious irrigation, sticky paste of lime should be removed with a cotton-tipped applicator, mydriasis and topical antibiotics, pain medications, treatment of glaucoma with carbonic anhydrase inhibitors, patching and soft contact lenses may facilitate re-epithelialization, insertion of a methyl methacrylate ring may prevent fibrinous adhesions, lysis of adhesions with or without mucous membrane grafts, corneal stem cell transplantation, corneal transplantation, keratoprosthesis and conjunctival autographs.

BIBLIOGRAPHY

1. Roy FH, Fraunfelder FW, Fraunfelder FT. Roy and Fraunfelder's Current Ocular Therapy, 6th edition. London: Elsevier; 2008.

11.1G. ESCHERICHIA COLI

General

Gram-negative rod found in the gastrointestinal tract; urinary tract is the usual portal of entry.

Ocular

Uveitis; hyphema; hypopyon; gas bubbles in anterior chamber; purulent conjunctivitis; keratitis; corneal edema; panophthalmitis; endophthalmitis; glaucoma.

Clinical

Diarrhea; gastroenteritis; dehydration.

Laboratory

Anaerobic Gram-negative rod.

Treatment

Antibiotic therapy should start with ampicillin until sensitivity reports return.

BIBLIOGRAPHY

1. Suh DW. (2011). Ophthalmologic manifestations of Escherichia Coli. [online] Available from www.emedicine.com/oph/TOPIC496.HTM. [Accessed August, 2013].

⊟ 11.1H. FUSOBACTERIUM

General

Gram-negative; normal inhabitant of mouth and respiratory, intestinal, and urogenital tracts; usually secondary to an underlying disease, surgical procedure, or therapy that impairs the defense of the host; non-spore-forming, non-motile Gram-negative anaerobic bacilli.

Ocular

Conjunctivitis; dacryocystitis; orbital abscess; orbital cellulitis; corneal ulcer; tenonitis; lid edema; panophthalmitis; gangrene of conjunctiva; cavernous sinus thrombosis; cranial nerve palsy.

Clinical

Brain abscess; pneumonia; liver abscess; endocarditis; sepsis; tissue necrosis.

Laboratory

Gram stain of a smear of the specimen provides important preliminary information regarding types of organisms present.

Treatment

Patient's recovery from anaerobic infection depends on prompt and proper treatment according to the following principles: (1) neutralizing toxins produced by anaerobes, (2) preventing local bacterial proliferation by changing the environment, and (3) limiting the spread of bacteria.

⊟ BIBLIOGRAPHY

1. Brook I. (2012). Peptostreptococcus infection. [online] Available from www.emedicine.com/med/TOPIC1777.HTM. [Accessed August, 2013].

⊟ 11.1I. HERPES SIMPLEX

General

Large, complex deoxyribonucleic acid (DNA) virus.

Ocular

Conjunctivitis; keratitis; iridocyclitis; corneal ulcer; uveitis; hyphema; hypopyon; iris atrophy; cataract; scleritis; dacryoadenitis; blepharitis; acute retinal necrosis.

Clinical

Recurrent skin vesicles on lids, perioral area, nose and genitalia; meningitis, encephalitis.

Laboratory

Viral cultures.

Treatment

Antiviral therapy, topical or oral, is an effective treatment of epithelial herpes infection.

⊟ BIBLIOGRAPHY

1. Shaohui L, Pavan-Langston D, Colby KA. Pediatric herpes simplex of the anterior segment: characteristics, treatment, and outcomes. Ophthalmology. 2012;119:2003-8.
2. Wang JC. (2010). Ophthalmologic manifestations of herpes simplex keratitis. [online] Available from www.emedicine.com/oph/TOPIC100.HTM. [Accessed July, 2013].

⊟ 11.1J. HERPES ZOSTER

General

It is caused by varicella zoster virus; about 75% of cases occur in persons over age of 45 years; condition is more frequent with advancing age and in patients who are immunocompromised by drugs or disease; in particular, an increasing number of patients with herpes zoster ophthalmicus are immunosuppressed.

Ocular

Conjunctivitis; keratitis; recurrent corneal ulcer; neuralgia; zoster rash of eyelids; uveitis; iris atrophy; scleritis; cataract; optic neuritis; paralysis of third nerve; proptosis; paralysis of lids; orbital apex syndrome; retinitis; neurotrophic keratitis; acute retinal necrosis; progressive outer retinal necrosis; ocular motor nerve pareses; tonic pupil; encephalitis; vasculitis.

Clinical

Local lesions involving the posterior or root ganglia; nerve damage; tissue scarring.

Laboratory

Diagnosed mostly on the basis of the characteristic pain and appearance of the dermatomal rashes.

Treatment

Antiviral agents, systemic corticosteroids, antidepressants, and adequate pain control. Immunocompetent adults aged 60 years or older, benefit from receipt of the herpes zoster vaccine and have a lower incidence of herpes zoster.

BIBLIOGRAPHY

1. Diaz MM, Foster CS, Walton RC, et al. (2011). Herpes zoster ophthalmicus. [online] Available from www.emedicine.com/oph/TOPIC257.HTM. [Accessed August, 2013].
2. Ghaznawi N, Virdi A, Dayan A, et al. Herpes zoster ophthalmicus: comparison of disease in patients 60 years and older versus younger than 60 years. Ophthalmology. 2011;118(11):2242-50.
3. Ho J, Xirasagar S, Lin H. Increased risk of a cancer diagnosis after herpes zoster ophthalmicus: a nationwide population-based study. Ophthalmology. 2011;118(6):1076-81.
4. Tseng HF, Smith N, Harpaz R, et al. Herpes zoster vaccine in older adults and the risk of subsequent herpes zoster disease. JAMA. 2011;305(2):160-6.

11.1K. MEASLES (MORBILLI; RUBEOLA)

General

Acute, extremely communicable disease that affects young school-aged children; caused by paramyxovirus.

Ocular

Hypopyon; uveitis; conjunctivitis; Koplik (Hirschberg) spots of conjunctiva; keratitis; corneal ulcer; cellulitis of lid; dacryocystitis; congenital cataract; optic atrophy; opticneuritis; strabismus; pigmentary retinopathy; iris prolapse; hemianopsia; secondary glaucoma; central retinal artery occlusion; orbital cellulitis; accommodative spasm; paralysis of sixth nerve; keratoconus.

Clinical

Maculopapular rash; fever.

Laboratory

Diagnosis is made by clinical findings.

Treatment

Good hydration.

BIBLIOGRAPHY

1. Chen SS. (2011). Measles. [online] Available from www.emedicine.com/derm/TOPIC259.HTM. [Accessed July, 2013].

11.1L. MORAXELLA LACUNATA

General

Gram-negative rod; causes chronic angular blepharoconjunctivitis; without treatment, may persist for months or years; normally found in flora of respiratory tract; seen more frequently in alcoholics and those with poor sanitary habits; *Moraxella* organisms produce proteases, although those are not related directly to their pathogenetic mechanism.

Ocular

Catarrhal angular conjunctivitis; corneal ulcer; hypopyon; chronic blepharitis; eczema; lateral canthal skin erythema; iridocyclitis.

Clinical

Alcoholism; impaired nutrition; dermatitis.

Laboratory

Aerobic, oxidase positive, Gram-negative diplococcus or coccobacilli morphologically indistinguishable from *Neisseria*.

Treatment

Artificial tears, cold compresses, antibiotics.

⊟ BIBLIOGRAPHY

1. Baum J, Fedukowicz HB, Jordan A. A survey of Moraxella corneal ulcers in a derelict population. Am J Ophthalmol. 1980;90:476-80.
2. Burd EM. Bacterial keratitis and conjunctivitis. In: Smolin G, Thoft RA (Eds). The Cornea. Boston: Little, Brown and Company; 1994. pp. 20-1.
3. Roy FH, Fraunfelder FW, Fraunfelder's FT Roy and Fraunfelder's. Current Ocular Therapy, 6th edition. Philadelphia: WB Saunders; 2008.
4. van Bijsterveld OP. The incidence of Moraxella on mucous membranes and the skin. Am J Ophthalmol. 1972;74:72-6.

⊟ 11.1M. GONORRHEA

General

It is caused by *Neisseria gonorrhoeae*, which is transmitted sexually.

Ocular

Conjunctivitis; eyelid edema; keratitis; uveitis.

Clinical

Pelvic inflammatory disease; arthritis; dermatitis; carditis; meningitis.

Laboratory

Gram stain smear demonstrates Gram-negative diplococci with polymorphonuclear leukocytes in conjunctival exudates.

Treatment

Therapy consists of systemic antibiotics; topical antibiotics are relatively ineffective in the treatment of eye disease. It is important to treat all sexual partners simultaneously to prevent reinfection.

⊟ BIBLIOGRAPHY

1. Wong B. (2012). Gonorrhea. [online] Available from www.emedicine.com/oph/TOPIC497.HTM. [Accessed November, 2012].

⊟ 11.1N. PROTEUS INFECTIONS

General

Gram-negative bacilli found in water, soil and decaying organic substances.

Ocular

Conjunctivitis; keratitis; corneal ulcers; endophthalmitis; panophthalmitis; dacryocystitis; gangrene of eyelid; uveitis; hypopyon; paralysis of seventh nerve.

Clinical

Cutaneous infection after surgery; usually occurs as a secondary infection of the skin, ears, mastoid sinuses, eyes, peritoneal cavity, bone, urinary tract, meninges, lung, or bloodstream; meningitis; intracranial subdural and epidural empyema; brain abscess; intracranial septic thrombophlebitis affecting cavernous/lateral sinuses.

Laboratory

Proteus organisms are easily recovered through routine laboratory cultures. An ultrasound of the kidneys or a CT scan should be considered as part of a workup.

Treatment

Traditional treatment includes oral quinolone for 3 days or trimethoprim/sulfamethoxazole.

⊟ BIBLIOGRAPHY

1. Struble K. (2011). Proteus infections. [online] Available from www.emedicine.com/med/TOPIC1929.HTM. [Accessed August, 2013].

🗗 11.1O. PSEUDOMONAS AERUGINOSA

General

Gram-negative rod that is ubiquitous in water, soil and plants. Commonly found in hospital environment.

Clinical

None.

Ocular

Foreign body sensation, conjunctival injection and photophobia and corneal ulceration.

Laboratory

Gram-negative rod on Gram stain and Giemsa stain from corneal ulcer. Culturing contact lens and lens solutions may help to grow organisms.

Treatment

Fortified tobramycin and fortified cefazolin are drugs of choice.

🗗 BIBLIOGRAPHY

1. Roy FH, Fraunfelder FW, Fraunfelder FT. Roy & Fraunfelder's Current Ocular Therapy, 6th edition. London: Elsevier; 2008.

🗗 11.1Q. SMALLPOX (VARIOLA)

General

Highly contagious cutaneous disease caused by viral infection.

Ocular

Conjunctivitis; keratitis; corneal ulcer; hypopyon; endophthalmitis; congenital corneal clouding; albinotic spots on iris; choroiditis; vitreous opacities; papillitis; extraocular muscle palsies; entropion; dacryocystitis; chorioretinitis; optic neuritis; and vesicles of the eyelid; preauricular adenopathy; eyelid ulcerating pustules; several conditions predispose to the spread of vaccinia, including eczema, hypogammaglobulinemia, steroid therapy, and AIDS.

Clinical

Fever, headache and vomiting prior to appearance of the rash on the face, upper trunk, and down to the extremities.

Laboratory

Brick-shaped virions viewed with electron microscopy examination, virus culture from live cells, or DNA analysis using PCR and smallpox skin specimen should be collected.

Treatment

No known treatment is effective.

🗗 BIBLIOGRAPHY

1. Hussain AN, Hussain F, Alam M, et al. (2011). Smallpox. [online] Available from www.emedicine.com/med/TOPIC3545.HTM. [Accessed August, 2013].

🗗 11.1S. STAPHYLOCOCCUS

General

Gram-positive coccus *Staphylococcus aureus*; most common cause of suppurative infection in humans; more common in patients with a previous disorders, such as diabetes, thyroid disease, renal failure, or malnutrition; although most *S. aureus* isolates from other sources are encapsulated, capsules have not been noted in ocular isolates.

Ocular

Uveitis; hypopyon; conjunctivitis; keratitis; cellulitis of lid; meibomianitis; ptosis; blepharitis; endophthalmitis; dacryocystitis; increased IOP; orbital periosteitis.

Clinical

Tissues hypertonic, edematous, and painful; lesion liquefies, forming creamy yellow pus; fever; nausea; vomiting; cough; dyspnea; abdominal pain; diarrhea; bloody stools; dehydration; shock.

Laboratory

Aerobic Gram-positive cocci bacteria grow in grape-like clusters. Coagulase positive indicates pathogenicity.

Treatment

Specific antimicrobial therapy is chosen based on the site and severity of the infection and the antimicrobial sensitivities of the organism involved.

BIBLIOGRAPHY

1. Tolan RW. (2012). Staphylococcus Aureus infection. [online] Available from www.emedicine.com/ped/TOPIC2704.HTM. [Accessed August, 2013].

11.1T. STREPTOCOCCUS (SCARLET FEVER)

General

Gram-positive bacteria that can invade any tissue.

Ocular

Conjunctivitis; corneal ulcer; blepharitis; scarlatinal rash of lid; erysipelas dermatitis of lid; gangrene of lid; endophthalmitis; proptosis; dacryocystitis; optic neuritis; orbital cellulitis; uveitis; hypopyon; secondary glaucoma; paralysis of extraocular muscles; infectious crystalline keratopathy; scleritis.

Clinical

Pharyngitis; impetigo; scarlet fever; pneumonia; bacteremia; rheumatic fever; glomerulonephritis.

Laboratory

Gram-positive cocci growing in pairs or chains. Throat culture and sensitivity are useful.

Treatment

Penicillin is the drug of choice.

BIBLIOGRAPHY

1. Zabawski EJ. (2011). Scarlet fever. [online] Available from www.emedicine.com/emerg/TOPIC518.HTM. [Accessed August, 2013].

11.2A. BEHÇET SYNDROME (DERMATO-STOMATO-OPHTHALMIC SYNDROME; OCULOBUCCOGENITAL SYNDROME; GILBERT SYNDROME)

General

Virus infection; occurs in adults; chronic disease; complete remission is rare; etiology is unknown.

Ocular

Muscle palsies (occasional); nystagmus (occasional); conjunctivitis; hypopyon; iritis; recurrent uveitis; keratoconjunctivitis sicca; keratitis; vitreous hemorrhages; thrombophlebitis retinal veins (occasional); retinal hemorrhages; optic neuritis (occasional); macular edema; optic nerve atrophy; retinitis; secondary glaucoma; retinal vasculitis; disk edema; panophthalmitis; optic neuropathy; skin lesions, posterior uveitis and systemic complications have been associated with loss of vision with this disorder; corneal immune ring opacity.

Clinical

Aphthous lesions of mucous membranes of the mouth and genitalia; cerebellar signs; convulsions; paraplegia; skin erythema (multiforme bullosum); arthritis; urethritis; glossitis; recurrent fever.

Laboratory

Nonspecific human leukocyte antigen (HLA) B51 positive may help to support diagnosis.

Treatment

The goals of therapy are to suppress inflammation, to reduce the frequency and severity of recurrences, and to minimize involvement of the retina. To be effective, treatment must be started early. Extent of involvement and severity of disease determine the choice of medication. Treatment options include corticosteroids, cytotoxic agents, cyclosporine, and colchicine.

⊟ BIBLIOGRAPHY

1. Bashour M. (2012). Ophthalmologic manifestations of Behçet disease. [online] Available from www.emedicine.com/oph/TOPIC425.HTM. [Accessed August, 2013].

⊟ 11.5. TOXIC LENS SYNDROME (TOXIC ANTERIOR SEGMENT SYNDROME; TASS)

General

Syndrome occurs within a few days to several weeks of implantation of an IOL; with therapy, vision is restored in the majority of cases; increased incidence of disease caused by use of ethylene oxide sterilization (dry pack IOLs); toxic lens syndrome may be prevented by treating the lens with sodium hydroxide and by using modem lathe-cut or compression-molded lenses with polypropylene loops; risk factors include uveitis in history, pseudo-exfoliation syndrome, inadequate mydriasis at the start of surgery, problems with IOL implantation and pigment effusion during surgery.

Ocular

Pigment precipitation on the surface of IOL; hypopyon; vitreous opacification; chronic uveitis; secondary glaucoma.

Clinical

None.

Laboratory

Anterior chamber aspiration, vitreous tap and/or vitreous biopsy for Gram stain and microbiologic cultures.

Treatment

Topical steroids and nonsteroidal anti-inflammatory drugs (NSAIDs); patients should be evaluated the same or the next day to rule out infectious endophthalmitis, in which case, steroids would worsen the condition.

⊟ BIBLIOGRAPHY

1. Al-Ghoul AR, Charukamnoetkanok P, Dhaliwal DK. (2012). Toxic anterior segment syndrome. [online] Available from www.emedicine.com/oph/TOPIC779.HTM. [Accessed August, 2013].
2. Rishi E, Rishi P, Sengupta S, et al. Acute postoperative bacillus cereus endophthamitis mimicking Toxic Anterior Segment Syndrome. Ophthalmology. 2013:120:181-5.

⊟ 11.6A. ACANTHAMOEBA

General

It is caused by *Acanthamoeba polyphaga* and *Acanthamoeba cartel* (*see* Herpes Simplex Masquerade Syndrome); all types of contact lenses have been associated with Acanthamoeba keratitis, particularly daily-wear soft contact lenses.

Ocular

Hypopyon; uveitis; conjunctivitis and chemosis; keratitis; pannus; corneal ring abscess; papillitis; vitreitis; retinal perivasculitis; secondary glaucoma; post-keratoplasty

Acanthamoeba keratitis may present as an infectious crystalline keratopathy in the periphery of the graft.

Clinical

Meningoencephalitis; meningitis; hemorrhagic encephalitis.

Laboratory

Polygonal double-walled cysts, under bright-field or phase-contrast microscopy or stained with hematoxylin and eosin, Gram, Giemsa or celluflor white.

Treatment

Medical therapy for *Acanthamoeba* infection is not well established. Topical antimicrobial agents that achieve high concentrations at the site of the infection can be considered. Treatment of keratitis consists of early diagnosis and aggressive surgical and medical therapies.

⊟ BIBLIOGRAPHY

1. Crum-Cianflone NF. (2013). Acanthamoeba. [online] Available from www.emedicine.com/med/TOPIC10.HTM. [Accessed August, 2013].
2. Wang JC, Ritterband DC. (2013). Herpes simplex keratitis. [online] Available from www.emedicine.com/oph/TOPIC100.HTM. [Accessed August, 2013].

⊟ 11.6B. ACTINOMYCOSIS

General

Gram-positive *Actinomyces israelii*.

Ocular

Hypopyon; conjunctivitis; keratitis; corneal ulcer; proptosis; uveitis; dacryocystitis; yellow nodules on conjunctiva and eyelids; occlusion of nasolacrimal canaliculi; canaliculitis; orbital abscess; endophthalmitis (rare).

Clinical

Chronic inflammatory induration and sinus formation.

Laboratory

Canalicular discharge may be sent for Gram stain/Giemsa stain, cultures and sensitivities (i.e. blood agar, Sabouraud, anaerobic) and special stains (i.e. calcofluor white stain).

Treatment

Penicillins and cephalosporins are useful. Subconjunctival penicillin coadministered with systemic iodides and topical sulfacetamide or penicillin can be used.

⊟ BIBLIOGRAPHY

1. Roque MR, Roque BL, Foster CS. (2012). Actinomycosis in ophthalmology. [online] Available from www.emedicine.com/oph/TOPIC491.HTM. [Accessed August, 2013].

⊟ 11.6C. AMEBIASIS (AMEBIC DYSENTERY, ENTAMOEBA HISTOLYTICA)

General

It is caused by *Entamoeba histolytica*; *E. histolytica* cysts in stools are diagnostic.

Ocular

Conjunctivitis; iridocyclitis; hypopyon; central choroiditis; retinal hemorrhages; retinal perivasculitis; macular edema; corneal ulceration; granulomatous and non-granulomatous uveitis; vitreous hemorrhage.

Clinical

Chronic dysentery; abscesses of liver and brain; toxic megacolon.

Laboratory

Enzyme immunoassay (EIA): is the best test for making the specific diagnosis of *E. histolytica*.

Treatment

Metronidazole is considered the drug of choice for symptomatic, invasive disease. Asymptomatic intestinal infection may be treated with iodoquinol, paromomycin, or diloxanide furoate.

⊟ BIBLIOGRAPHY

1. Lacasse A, Cleveland KO, Cantey JR, et al. (2013). Amebiasis. [online] Available from www.emedicine.com/ped/TOPIC80.HTM. [Accessed August, 2013].

⮕ 11.6D. ASPERGILLOSIS

General

Systemic infection common in poultry farmers, feeders or breeders of pigeons, and persons who work with grains; should be considered in immunocompromised patients.

Ocular

Corneal ulcer; blepharitis; keratitis; scleritis; endophthalmitis; exophthalmos; retinal hemorrhages; retinal detachment; vitreitis; cataract; conjunctivitis; orbital cellulitis; paresis of extraocular muscles; secondary glaucoma; scleromalacia perforans; endogenous endophthalmitis; anterior chamber mass; invasion of choroid and anterior optic nerve.

Clinical

Pulmonary infections; invasive fungal disease.

Laboratory

Culture from superficial scrapings from bed of infection.

Treatment

Voriconazole is the drug of choice. Although disease outcomes substantially improve with antifungal treatment, patient survival and infection resolution depend on improved immunosuppression.

⮕ BIBLIOGRAPHY

1. Batra V. (2011). Pediatric Aspergillosis. [online] Available from www.emedicine.com/ped/TOPIC148.HTM. [Accessed August, 2013].

⮕ 11.6E. BACILLUS CEREUS

General

Highly virulent pathogen; most common contaminant of drug injection paraphernalia; usually enters the body as a result of penetrating trauma with a contaminated metallic foreign object; cause of food poisoning is toxin induced.

Ocular

Hypopyon; ring abscess of cornea; panophthalmitis; phthisis bulbi; orbital cellulitis; proptosis; vitreous abscess; necrosis of retina; endophthalmitis; keratitis.

Clinical

Fever; leukocytosis; septicemia; meningitis; endocarditis; osteomyelitis; wound infection.

Treatment

Most cases are self limited and treatment is not necessary. Oral rehydration is achieved by administering clear liquids and sodium-containing and glucose-containing solutions. Intravenous solutions are indicated in patients who are severely dehydrated or who have intractable vomiting. Ocular treatment includes antibiotics (intravitreal, topical and systemic) and vitrectomy surgery.

⮕ BIBLIOGRAPHY

1. Gamarra RM, Manuel D, Piper MH, et al. (2013). Food poisoning. [online] Available from www.emedicine.com/med/TOPIC807.HTM. [Accessed August, 2013].

⮕ 11.6F. BEHÇET SYNDROME (DERMATO-STOMATO-OPHTHALMIC SYNDROME; OCULOBUCCOGENITAL SYNDROME; GILBERT SYNDROME)

General

Virus infection; occurs in adults; chronic disease; complete remission is rare; etiology is unknown.

Ocular

Muscle palsies (occasional); nystagmus (occasional); conjunctivitis; hypopyon; iritis; recurrent uveitis; keratoconjunctivitis sicca; keratitis; vitreous hemorrhages; thrombophlebitis of retinal veins (occasional); retinal hemorrhages; optic neuritis (occasional); macular edema; optic nerve atrophy; retinitis; secondary glaucoma; retinal vasculitis; disk edema; panophthalmitis; optic neuropathy; skin lesions, posterior uveitis and systemic complications have been associated with loss of vision with this disorder; corneal immune ring opacity.

Clinical

Aphthous lesions of mucous membranes of the mouth and genitalia; cerebellar signs; convulsions; paraplegia; skin erythema (multiforme bullosum); arthritis; urethritis; glossitis; recurrent fever.

Laboratory

Nonspecific human leukocyte antigen (HLA) B51 positive may help to support diagnosis.

Treatment

The goals of therapy are to suppress inflammation, to reduce the frequency and severity of recurrences, and to minimize involvement of the retina. To be effective, treatment must be started early. Extent of involvement and severity of disease determine the choice of medication. Treatment options include corticosteroids, cytotoxic agents, cyclosporine, and colchicine.

BIBLIOGRAPHY

1. Bashour M. (2012). Ophthalmologic manifestations of Behçet disease. [online] Available from www.emedicine.com/oph/TOPIC425.HTM. [Accessed August, 2013].

11.6G. CANDIDIASIS

General

Yeast-like opportunistic fungal infection caused by *C. albicans.*

Ocular

Uveitis; hypopyon; conjunctivitis; keratitis; corneal ulcer; blepharitis; endophthalmitis; dacryocystitis; papillitis; retinal atrophy; Roth spot; vitreous abscess; retrobulbar abscess; retinal detachment; panophthalmitis; chorioretinitis; infectious crystalline keratopathy.

Clinical

C. albicans normally is present as an intestinal saprophyte in 35–75% of the human population; in situations of internal environmental change, however, Candida can become pathogenic (e.g. obesity, diabetes mellitus, malignancy, and other debilitating conditions).

Laboratory

Common yeast from up to 50% of healthy individuals isolate directly from the eye should be attempted to confirm the presence of organism. Blood agar and Sabouraud's dextrose agar may be used; PCR for species identification.

Treatment

Mucocutaneous infection typically responds to topical therapy. Antifungal therapy should be started immediately after necessary cultures have been obtained from all suspected sites of infection. Infectious disease specialists are typically involved in cases of invasive candidiasis.

BIBLIOGRAPHY

1. Hedayati T. (2012). Candidiasis in Emergency Medicine. [online] Available from www.emedicine.com/emerg/TOPIC76.HTM. [Accessed July, 2013].

11.6H. COCCIDIOIDOMYCOSIS (VALLEY FEVER, SAN JOAQUIN FEVER)

General

It is caused by fungus *Coccidioides immitis.*

Ocular

Conjunctivitis; choroiditis; uveitis; retinal hemorrhages; vitreal opacity; vitreal floaters; episcleritis; hypopyon; granulomatous lesion of optic nerve head; paralysis of sixth cranial nerve; secondary glaucoma; papilledema; mutton fat keratitic precipitates; necrotizing granulomatous conjunctivitis; iridocyclitis.

Clinical

Mild respiratory illness; cavity lung lesion.

Laboratory

Routine culture media, IgM antibody of acute, IgG antibody for present or past infection.

Treatment

Systemic fluconazole or amphotericin B is the treatment of choice. Ocular treatment includes topical amphotericin B and use of steroids sparingly.

BIBLIOGRAPHY

1. Hospenthal DR. (2011). Coccidioidomycosis. [online] Available from www.emedicine.com/ped/TOPIC423.HTM. [Accessed August, 2013].

11.6I. COENUROSIS (TAPEWORM)

General

Rare human infestation of the cystic larval stage of the dog tapeworm; usually infestation in the muscle, subcutaneous tissue, eye, nervous system, or brain; three species may be involved: (1) Multiceps taenia,(2) Multiceps serialis and (3) Multiceps glomeratus.

Ocular

Hypopyon; retinal detachment; retinal edema; anterior uveitis; conjunctivitis; proptosis; miosis; vitreal haze; increased IOP; coenurus cysts of the conjunctiva and iris.

Clinical

Ataxia; headache; loss of weight; somnolence; stiffness of neck and shoulders.

Laboratory

Perianal and stool examinations are useful.

Treatment

Anthelmintic drugs are used to rid the gastrointestinal (GI) tract of worms or systemically to rid the body of the helminth forms that invade organs and tissues

BIBLIOGRAPHY

1. Irizarry L. (2011). Tapeworm infestation. [online] Available from www.emedicine.com/emerg/TOPIC567.HTM. [Accessed August, 2013].

11.6J. CYSTICERCOSIS

General

It is caused by *Taenia solium.*

Ocular

Tenonitis; endophthalmitis; optic atrophy; papilledema; retinal detachment; retinal hemorrhages and exudates; vitreal hemorrhages; hypopyon; uveitis; paresis of extraocular muscles; periretinal proliferation; cysts may be present almost anywhere in or around the eye; orbital lesion; extraocular myositis; subretinal cysticercosis; acute preseptal cellulitis.

Clinical

Dead larvae may cause muscle pain; weakness; fever; eosinophilia; calcification of tissues.

Laboratory

The enzyme immunotransfer blot assay for the detection of serum and CSF antibodies to *T. solium* is the antibody test of choice. Diagnosis of neurocysticercosis is primarily based on CT scanning or MRI results.

Treatment

Medical treatment depends on the location of the cysts and the symptoms. Live parenchymal cysts can be treated with either albendazole or praziquantel, but corticosteroids and anti-seizure medications are often required in addition. Cases that do not respond to medical therapy, shunt placement, removal of large solitary cysts for decompression, and the removal of mobile cysts that cause ventricular obstruction should be considered.

BIBLIOGRAPHY

1. Ghadishah D, Burns MJ. (2012). Pediatric cysticercosis. [online] Available from www.emedicine.com/ped/TOPIC537.HTM. [Accessed August, 2013].

⊟ 11.6K. FUSOBACTERIUM

General

Gram-negative; normal inhabitant of mouth and respiratory, intestinal, and urogenital tracts; usually secondary to an underlying disease, surgical procedure, or therapy that impairs the defense of the host; non-spore-forming, non-motile Gram-negative anaerobic bacilli.

Ocular

Conjunctivitis; dacryocystitis; orbital abscess; orbital cellulitis; corneal ulcer; tenonitis; lid edema; panophthalmitis; gangrene of conjunctiva; cavernous sinus thrombosis; cranial nerve palsy.

Clinical

Brain abscess; pneumonia; liver abscess; endocarditis; sepsis; tissue necrosis.

Laboratory

Gram stain of a smear of the specimen provides important preliminary information regarding types of organisms present,

Treatment

Patient's recovery from anaerobic infection depends on prompt and proper treatment according to the following principles: (1) neutralizing toxins produced by anaerobes, (2) preventing local bacterial proliferation by changing the environment, and (3) limiting the spread of bacteria.

⊟ BIBLIOGRAPHY

1. Brook I. (2012). Peptostreptococcus infection. [online] Available from www.emedicine.com/med/TOPIC1777.HTM. [Accessed August, 2013].

⊟ 11.6L. HYDATID CYST (ECHINOCOCCOSIS)

General

It is caused by *Echinococcus granulosus* acquired by contact with a dog host.

Ocular

Conjunctivitis; keratitis; exophthalmos; phthisis bulbi; optic atrophy; optic neuritis; papilledema; abscesses of orbit and cornea; retinal detachment; retinal hemorrhages; cataract; hypopyon; secondary glaucoma; hydatid cysts of the conjunctiva, eyelid, orbit, and lacrimal system; acute visual loss; vitreous mass.

Clinical

Pruritus; urticaria; pulmonary cysts; brain cysts; anaphylactic shock; death.

Laboratory

Plain orbital radiographs may show enlarged orbital diameters and increased soft-tissue density. Ultrasonography demonstrates a cystic lesion without internal reflectivity; CT discloses a well-defined cystic mass.

Treatment

Echinococcosis is rare and can be severe. Refer patients to reference centers to confirm their diagnosis and to obtain advice on therapeutic strategy.

⊟ BIBLIOGRAPHY

1. Vuitton DA. (2011). Echinococcosis. [online] Available from www.emedicine.com/med/TOPIC326.HTM. [Accessed August, 2013].

🗗 11.6M. INFLUENZA

General

Acute respiratory infection of specific viral etiology which includes H1N1.

Ocular

Conjunctivitis; subconjunctival hemorrhages; keratitis; tenonitis; ptosis; cellulitis of orbit and lid; dacryocystitis; retinal hemorrhage; cataract; episcleritis; hypopyon; optic neuritis; uveitis; panophthalmitis; vitreal hemorrhage; paralysis of third or fourth nerve; uveitis following vaccination for influenza.

Clinical

Headache; fever; malaise; muscular aching; substernal soreness; nasal stuffiness; nausea.

Laboratory

The criterion standard for diagnosing influenza A and B is a viral culture of nasal-pharyngeal samples, throat samples, or both.

Treatment

Prevention is the most effective therapy. Two new drugs have been marketed recently for treatment of influenza A and B. These are the neuraminidase inhibitors, oseltamivir and zanamivir.

🗗 BIBLIOGRAPHY

1. Derlet RW. (2012). Influenza. [online] Available from www. emedicine.com/med/TOPIC1170.HTM. [Accessed August, 2013].

🗗 11.6N. LISTERELLOSIS (LISTERIOSIS)

General

It is caused by Gram-positive bacillus *Listeria monocytogenes*. High mortality among pregnant women, their fetuses, and immunocompromised persons with symptoms of abortion, neonatal death, septicemia, meningitis, brain abscesses, endocarditis.

Ocular

Conjunctivitis; keratitis; corneal abscess and ulcer; blepharitis; uveitis; endophthalmitis; cataract; secondary glaucoma.

Clinical

Vomiting; cardiorespiratory distress; diarrhea; hepatosplenomegaly; maculopapular skin lesions.

Laboratory

Histopathology and culture of rash, CT scanning or MRI may be useful in detecting abscesses in the brain or liver.

Treatment

Antibiotics as well as careful monitoring of the patient's temperature, respiratory system, fluid and electrolyte balance, nutrition, and cardiovascular support.

🗗 BIBLIOGRAPHY

1. Zach T, Anderson-Berry AL. (2013). Listeria infection. [online] Available from www.emedicine.com/ped/TOPIC1319.HTM. [Accessed August, 2013].

11.6O. LOCKJAW (TETANUS)

General

Acute infectious disease affecting nervous system; causative agent is *Clostridium tetani*; bacteria enters body through a puncture wound, abrasion, cut, or burn.

Ocular

Chemosis; keratitis; nystagmus; uveitis; corneal ulcer; cellulitis of orbit; hypopyon; panophthalmitis; pupil paralysis; pseudoptosis; blepharospasm; paralysis of third or seventh nerve; may occur following perforating ocular injuries.

Clinical

Severe muscle spasms; dysphagia; trismus; facial palsy; muscle stiffness; irritability.

Laboratory

Gram-positive spore-forming bacteria; laboratory studies are of little value.

Treatment

Passive immunization with human tetanus immune globulin shortens the course of tetanus and may lessen its severity. Benzodiazepines have emerged as the mainstay of symptomatic therapy for tetanus.

BIBLIOGRAPHY

1. Hinfey PB. (2012). Tetanus. [online] Available from www.emedicine.com/med/TOPIC2254.HTM. [Accessed November, 2012].

11.6P. METASTATIC BACTERIAL ENDOPHTHALMITIS

General

Causative agents usually of low pathogenicity (e.g. *Staphylococcus albus, Staphylococcus epidermidis*); occasionally organisms of greater pathogenicity (e.g. *P. aeruginosa, Diplococcus pneumoniae*); bilateral 45%; organisms originate in the body or are introduced by drug addicts using non-sterile needles.

Ocular

Conjunctival hemorrhages; conjunctivitis; Roth's spots; retinal arterial occlusion; uveitis; hypopyon; chorioretinitis; endophthalmitis; retinal hemorrhages.

Clinical

Manifestations are nonspecific.

Laboratory

Blood, sputum and urine cultures.

Treatment

Aggressive treatment is done with intravitreal and topical antibiotics, steroids and cycloplegics.

BIBLIOGRAPHY

1. Graham RH. (2012). Bacterial endophthalmitis. [online] Available from www.emedicine.com/oph/TOPIC393.HTM. [Accessed August, 2013].

11.6Q. MORAXELLA LACUNATA

General

Gram-negative rod; causes chronic angular blepharoconjunctivitis; without treatment, may persist for months or years; normally found in flora of respiratory tract; seen more frequently in alcoholics and those with poor sanitary habits; *Moraxella* organisms produce proteases, although those are not related directly to their pathogenetic mechanism.

Ocular

Catarrhal angular conjunctivitis; corneal ulcer; hypopyon; chronic blepharitis; eczema; lateral canthal skin erythema; iridocyclitis.

Clinical

Alcoholism; impaired nutrition; dermatitis.

Laboratory

Aerobic, oxidase positive, Gram-negative diplococcus or coccobacilli morphologically indistinguishable from *Neisseria*.

Treatment

Artificial tears, cold compresses, antibiotics.

BIBLIOGRAPHY

1. Baum J, Fedukowicz HB, Jordan A. A survey of Moraxella corneal ulcers in a derelict population. Am J Ophthalmol. 1980;90:476-80.
2. Burd EM. Bacterial keratitis and conjunctivitis. In: Smolin G, Thoft RA (Eds). The Cornea. Boston: Little, Brown and Company; 1994. pp. 20-1.
3. Roy FH, Fraunfelder FW, Fraunfelder's FT Roy and Fraunfelder's. Current Ocular Therapy, 6th edition.Philadelphia: WB Saunders; 2008.
4. van Bijsterveld OP. The incidence of Moraxella on mucous membranes and the skin. Am J Ophthalmol. 1972;74:72-6.

11.6R. MUCORMYCOSIS (PHYCOMYCOSIS)

General

Acute, often fatal infection caused by saprophytic fungi; associated with diabetes mellitus and ketoacidosis.

Ocular

Corneal ulcer; striate keratopathy; ptosis; panophthalmitis; proptosis; cellulitis of orbit; immobile pupil; retinitis; optic neuritis; paralysis of extraocular muscles; central retinal artery thrombosis.

Clinical

Epistaxis; nasal discharge; facial pain; facial palsies; anhidrosis; cranial nerve or peripheral motor and sensory nerve deficits may occur.

Laboratory

Tissue biopsy and culture of paranasal sinuses demonstrate the presence of the fungi, which appear as broad, irregular, nonseptate, branching hyphae on Hematoxylin and Eosin (H & E) stain.

Treatment

Amphotericin B.

BIBLIOGRAPHY

1. Crum-Cianflone NF. (2011). Mucormycosis. [online] Available from www.emedicine.com/oph/TOPIC225.HTM. [Accessed November, 2012].

11.6T. PSEUDOMONAS AERUGINOSA INFECTIONS

General

Gram-negative rod with secondary contaminant of superficial wounds; *Pseudomonas* organisms produce a variety of enzymes that cause pathologic changes, including hemolysins and exotoxins as well as a glycocalyx that increases adherence.

Ocular

Hypopyon; conjunctivitis; keratitis; ulcerative abscess of cornea; endophthalmitis; panophthalmitis.

Clinical

Local tissue damage and diminished host resistance, which may occur in ear, lung, skin, and urinary tract.

Laboratory

Complete blood count may reveal leukocytosis with a left shift and bandemia. Positive results on blood culture in the absence of extracardiac sites of infection may indicate pseudomonal endocarditis.

Treatment

Antimicrobials are the mainstay of therapy. Two-drug combination therapy such as an antipseudomonal beta-lactam antibiotic with an aminoglycoside.

BIBLIOGRAPHY

1. Klaus-Dieter L. (2012). Pseudomonas aeruginosa infections. [online] Available from www.emedicine.com/med/TOPIC1943.HTM. [Accessed November, 2012].

11.6U. RELAPSING FEVER (RECURRENT FEVER)

General

Acute infectious disease caused by *Borrelia* transmitted by lice; characterized by recurrent bouts of fever separated by relatively asymptomatic periods; there is an endemic form of rheumatic fever transmitted by tick vectors and spirochetes of the genus *Borrelia*.

Ocular

Extraocular muscle paralysis; uveitis; interstitial keratitis; hypopyon; conjunctivitis; optic nerve atrophy; subconjunctival and retinal hemorrhages; ptosis; mydriasis; retinal venous occlusion.

Clinical

Toxemia and febrile paroxysms are separated by afebrile periods.

Laboratory

Diagnosis is confirmed by bone marrow aspirates, cerebrospinal fluids or spirochetes in peripheral smears.

Treatment

The drugs of choice include doxycycline, penicillin G, chloramphenicol or erythromycin.

BIBLIOGRAPHY

1. Akhter K, Dorsainvil PA, Cunha BA. (2012). Relapsing fever. [online] Available from www.emedicine.com/med/TOPIC1999.HTM. [Accessed August, 2013].

11.6X. STAPHYLOCOCCUS

General

Gram-positive coccus *Staphylococcus aureus*; most common cause of suppurative infection in humans; more common in patients with a previous disorders, such as diabetes, thyroid disease, renal failure, or malnutrition; although most *S. aureus* isolates from other sources are encapsulated, capsules have not been noted in ocular isolates.

Ocular

Uveitis; hypopyon; conjunctivitis; keratitis; cellulitis of lid; Meibomianitis; ptosis; blepharitis; endophthalmitis; dacryocystitis; increased IOP; orbital periosteitis.

Clinical

Tissues hypertonic, edematous, and painful; lesion liquefies, forming creamy yellow pus; fever; nausea; vomiting; cough; dyspnea; abdominal pain; diarrhea; bloody stools; dehydration; shock.

Laboratory

Aerobic Gram-positive cocci bacteria grow in grape-like clusters. Coagulase positive indicates pathogenicity.

Treatment

Specific antimicrobial therapy is chosen based on the site and severity of the infection and the antimicrobial sensitivities of the organism involved.

BIBLIOGRAPHY

1. Tolan RW. (2012). Staphylococcus Aureus Infection. [online] Available from www.emedicine.com/ped/TOPIC2704.HTM. [Accessed August, 2013].

⊟ 11.6Y. STREPTOCOCCUS (SCARLET FEVER)

General

Gram-positive bacteria that can invade any tissue.

Ocular

Conjunctivitis; corneal ulcer; blepharitis; scarlatinal rash of lid; erysipelas dermatitis of lid; gangrene of lid; endophthalmitis; proptosis; dacryocystitis; optic neuritis; orbital cellulitis; uveitis; hypopyon; secondary glaucoma; paralysis of extraocular muscles; infectious crystalline keratopathy; scleritis.

Clinical

Pharyngitis; impetigo; scarlet fever; pneumonia; bacteremia; rheumatic fever; glomerulonephritis.

Laboratory

Gram-positive cocci growing in pairs or chains. Throat culture and sensitivity are useful.

Treatment

Penicillin is the drug of choice.

⊟ BIBLIOGRAPHY

1. Zabawski EJ. (2011). Scarlet Fever. [online] Available from www.emedicine.com/emerg/TOPIC518.HTM. [Accessed August, 2013].

⊟ 11.6Z(1). BEHÇET SYNDROME (DERMATO-STOMATO-OPHTHALMIC SYNDROME; OCULOBUCCOGENITAL SYNDROME; GILBERT SYNDROME)

General

Virus infection; occurs in adults; chronic disease; complete remission is rare; etiology is unknown.

Ocular

Muscle palsies (occasional); nystagmus (occasional); conjunctivitis; hypopyon; iritis; recurrent uveitis; keratoconjunctivitis sicca; keratitis; vitreous hemorrhages; thrombophlebitis retinal veins (occasional); retinal hemorrhages; optic neuritis (occasional); macular edema; optic nerve atrophy; retinitis; secondary glaucoma; retinal vasculitis; disk edema; panophthalmitis; optic neuropathy; skin lesions, posterior uveitis and systemic complications have been associated with loss of vision with this disorder; corneal immune ring opacity.

Clinical

Aphthous lesions of mucous membranes of the mouth and genitalia; cerebellar signs; convulsions; paraplegia; skin erythema (multiforme bullosum); arthritis; urethritis; glossitis; recurrent fever.

Laboratory

Nonspecific human leukocyte antigen (HLA) B51 positive may help to support diagnosis.

Treatment

The goals of therapy are to suppress inflammation, to reduce the frequency and severity of recurrences, and to minimize involvement of the retina. To be effective, treatment must be started early. Extent of involvement and severity of disease determine the choice of medication. Treatment options include corticosteroids, cytotoxic agents, cyclosporine, and colchicine.

⊟ BIBLIOGRAPHY

1. Bashour M. (2012). Ophthalmologic manifestations of Behçet disease. [online] Available from www.emedicine.com/oph/TOPIC425.HTM. [Accessed August, 2013].

11.6Z(5). HISTIOCYTOSIS X (HAND-SCHULLER-CHRISTIAN SYNDROME; LIPOID GRANULOMA; XANTHOMATOUS GRANULOMA SYNDROME; SCHULLER-CHRISTIAN-HAND SYNDROME; LETTERER-SIWE SYNDROME; ACUTE HISTIOCYTOSIS X; EOSINOPHILIC GRANULOMA; RETICULOENDOTHELIOSIS SYNDROME)

General

The term histiocytosis X has been proposed to include Letterer-Siwe disease, Hand-Schuller-Christian disease, and eosinophilic granuloma of bone; there are sufficient grounds to treat Hand-Schuller-Christian and Letterer-Siwe together as different phases of the same disease process; eosinophilic granuloma most likely represents a reaction pattern, sharing some histologic features with the first two but nonetheless carrying a more benign prognosis; Letterer-Siwe disease is referred to as acute differentiated histiocytosis; Hand-Schuller-Christian disease is referred to as subacute differentiated or chronic differentiated histiocytosis; Letterer-Siwe etiology is unknown, onset is in infancy and early childhood, and prognosis is generally poor; Hand-Schuller-Christian etiology is unknown, onset is in childhood, male preponderance is 2:1, and prognosis is chronic with remissions; eosinophil may play a contributory pathophysiologic role.

Ocular

Exophthalmos; ocular pulsations; orbital roof defects; xanthelasma; blepharitis; internal ophthalmoplegia; nystagmus; retinal hemorrhages; papilledema; optic atrophy; uveitis; hypopyon; pannus; bullous keratopathy; corneal ulcer; hypochromic heterochromia; retinal detachment; cataract; scleritis.

Clinical

Hepatosplenomegaly; lymphadenopathy; skin lesions with papular eruptions; ecchymosis; purpura; bone lesions; anemia; fatigue; anorexia; fever; xanthoma of the skin; diabetes insipidus; skull defects; lung fibrosis; cardiac insufficiency.

Laboratory

Diagnosis is made by clinical findings.

Treatment

Treatment is a combination of radiation and chemotherapy.

BIBLIOGRAPHY

1. Christian HA. Defects in Membranous Bones, Exophthalmos and Diabetes Insipidus, Volume I. New York: Paul B Hoeber; 1919. p. 390.
2. Duane TD. Clinical Ophthalmology. Philadelphia: JB Lippincott; 1987.
3. Roy FH, Fraunfelder FW, Fraunfelder FT. Roy and Fraunfelder's Current Ocular Therapy, 6th edition. Philadelphia: WB Saunders; 2008.
4. Hand A. Polyuria and tuberculosis. Arch Pediatr. 1893;10:673.
5. Mittelman D, Apple DJ, Goldberg MF. Ocular involvement in Letterer-Siwe disease. Am J Ophthalmol. 1973;75:261-5.
6. Pearlstone AD, Flom L. Letterer-Siwe's disease. J Pediatr Ophthalmol. 1970;77:103-5.
7. Petersen RA, Kuwabara T. Ocular manifestations of familial lymphohistiocytosis. Arch Ophthalmol. 1968;79:413-6.
8. Trocme SD, Aldave AJ. The eye and the eosinophil. Surv Ophthalmol. 1994;39:241-52.

11.6Z(7). JUVENILE RHEUMATOID ARTHRITIS (JRA; STILL DISEASE)

General

Onset before age 16 years; greater occurrence of systemic manifestations, monoarticular and oligoarticular joint involvement, and iridocyclitis.

Ocular

Hypopyon; band keratopathy; uveitis; cataract; papillitis; glaucoma; macular edema; ocular pain; vitreous cells; synechiae; scleritis; presumed to have an autoimmune etiology; antiocular antibodies, including iris protein antibodies, have been found in the sera of patients.

Clinical

Salmon pink macular rash; arthritis; hepatosplenomegaly; leukocytosis; chronic pain; joint swelling; low-grade fever; anemia; rheumatoid nodules.

Laboratory

Antinuclear antibody, rheumatoid factor, HLA B27, X-ray imaging of joints.

Treatment

Uveitis treated initially with topical corticosteroids. Systemic immunomodulatory agents may be useful for patients with limited or no response to topical or systemic corticosteroids.

BIBLIOGRAPHY

1. Roque MR, Roque BL, Miserocchi E, et al. (2012). Juvenile idiopathic arthritis uveitis. [online] Available from www.emedicine.com/oph/TOPIC675.HTM. [Accessed August, 2013].
2. Thorne JE, Woreta FA, Dunn JP, et al. Risk of cataract development among children with juvenile idiopathic arthritis-related uveitis treated with topical corticosteroids. Ophthalmology. 2010;117:1436-41.

11.6Z(9). LEUKEMIA

General

Acute or chronic blood disorder.

Ocular

Engorgement of conjunctival vessels; papillary hypertrophy; aggregations of tumor cells in conjunctiva, choroid, and orbit; secondary glaucoma; retinal venous engorgement and tortuosity with pronounced constrictions; retinal hemorrhages; retinal detachment; cotton-wool spots; macular edema; papilledema; optic atrophy; optic neuritis; paralysis of extraocular muscles; hypopyon; vitreous opacities; retinal sea fans; perilimbal subconjunctival infiltrates; corneal leukemic infiltration (rare); shallow serous retinal detachments; hyphema; iris neovascularization; central retinal vein occlusion; vitreous infiltrates.

Clinical

Frequent involvement of central nervous system; intracranial hemorrhage; thrombocytopenia; rising white cell count.

Laboratory

Complete blood count (CBC) and differential, bone marrow aspiration, immunophenotyping, chromosomal analysis.

Treatment

Chemotherapy with or without radiotherapy.

BIBLIOGRAPHY

1. Wu L, Evans T, Martinez J. (2012). Leukemias. [online]. Available from www.emedicine.com/oph/TOPIC489.HTM. [Accessed August, 2013].

11.6Z(12). VON BEKHTEREV-STRUMPELL SYNDROME (MARIE-STRUMPELL SPONDYLITIS; ANKYLOSING SPONDYLITIS; PIERRE-MARIE SYNDROME; BEKHTEREV DISEASE; RHEUMATOID SPONDYLITIS) OPTIC ATROPHY

General

Variant of rheumatoid arthritis; etiology unknown; autosomal dominant; male preponderance; onset at age 20–40 years; although genetic background determines susceptibility to uveitis, the disease pattern suggests the possibility of random environmental triggers unrelated to the course of the underlying rheumatologic disorder.

Ocular

Non-granulomatous anterior uveitis; optic nerve atrophy (occasionally); hypopyon; band keratopathy; spontaneous hyphema.

Clinical

Spondylitis of vertebra and sacroiliac joints; ankylosis; general arthralgia; kyphosis; scoliosis; displaced head and total rigidity of spine.

Laboratory

Histocompatibility antigen HLA-B27 and a negative rheumatoid factor and antinuclear antibody; X-ray evidence of narrowing of sacroiliac joint space and sclerosis.

Treatment

Oral NSAIDs, urethritis in Reiter's disease should be treated with tetracycline, topical steroids and cycloplegic agents.

🗗 BIBLIOGRAPHY

1. Vives MJ, Garfin SR. (2011). Rheumatoid arthritis of the cervical spine overview of rheumatoid spondylitis. [online] Available from www.emedicine.com/orthoped/TOPIC551. HTM. [Accessed August, 2013].

🗗 11.6AA. STEVENS-JOHNSON SYNDROME [DERMATOSTOMATITIS; ERYTHEMA MULTIFORME EXUDATIVUM; SYNDROMA MUCOCUTANEO-OCULARE; BAADER DERMATOSTOMATITIS SYNDROME; MUCOSAL-RESPIRATORY SYNDROME; FUCHS (2) SYNDROME; MUCOCUTANEOUS OCULAR SYNDROME]

General

Etiology unknown; affects all ages; most frequently seen in 1st and 3rd decades of life; prevalent in males; drugs are the most commonly identified etiologic factor in this condition.

Ocular

Hypopyon; iritis; keratitis; corneal ulcers; keratoconjunctivitis sicca; chemosis; conjunctivitis; widespread fibrinoid necrosis of conjunctival vessels; blepharitis; endophthalmitis; phthisis bulbi; uveitis; cataracts; pannus; optic neuritis; keratoconus; adenoviral conjunctivitis has been reported to have precipitated Stevens-Johnson syndrome; orbital cyst may be a complication.

Clinical

General malaise, headaches, chills, and fever; severe skin and mucous membrane eruptions (erythema multiforme); dorsa of hands and feet are most frequently affected; rhinitis; balanitis; vulvovaginitis; urethritis (nonspecific); cystitis; patients with AIDS are at higher risk of developing Stevens-Johnson syndrome.

Laboratory

No laboratory tests are specific to Stevens-Johnson syndrome. Diagnosis made from clinical findings.

Treatment

Systemic treatment with steroids is controversial. Antibiotics are used based on clinical course. Eyelid hygiene performed as needed.

🗗 BIBLIOGRAPHY

1. Plaza JA, Dronen SC, Foster J, et al. (2011). Erythema multiforme. [online] Available from www.emedicine.com/med/TOPIC727.HTM. [Accessed August, 2013].

🗗 11.6BB. NEOVASCULARIZATION, CORNEAL CONTACT LENS RELATED

General

Pathologic state in which new blood vessels extending in the corneal stroma from trauma, inflammation, infection, toxic insults secondary to contact lens usage.

Clinical

None.

Ocular

Vessel ingrowth into the cornea, ocular irritation.

Laboratory

Diagnosis is made by clinical findings.

Treatment

Observation, eliminate cause, topical steroid drops, reduced time for an individual using contact lens, corneal laser photocoagulation.

🗗 BIBLIOGRAPHY

1. Weissman BA, Yeung KK. (2011). Neovascularization, corneal, CL-related. [online] Available from emedicine.medscape.com/article/1195886-overview. [Accessed August, 2013].

⊟ 11.6CC. TUBERCULOSIS

General

Communicable disease caused by the acid-fast bacillus *Mycobacterium tuberculosis*.

Ocular

Conjunctivitis; subconjunctival nodules (tuberculomas); keratitis; pannus; corneal ulcer; blepharitis; cellulitis; meibomianitis; uveitis; dacryocystitis; chronic orbital cellulitis; retinitis; scleritis; scleral perforation; hypopyon; vitreous hemorrhages; optic neuritis; optic atrophy; tuberculous panophthalmitis; choroidal tubercles; intraorbital extraocular lesions.

Clinical

Pulmonary infection; pyuria; hematuria; epididymitis; dysuria; flank pain; distorted calyces; productive cough.

Laboratory

Acid-fast bacillus culture of body fluids including vitreous and aqueous. PCR is 89% positive for pulmonary infection.

Treatment

A course of chemotherapy (isoniazid, rifampin, pyrazinamide and ethambutol or streptomycin) for a period of 6 months is the recommended therapy.

⊟ BIBLIOGRAPHY

1. Collins JK. Handbook of Clinical Ophthalmology. New York: Masson; 1982.
2. D'Souza P, Garg R, Dhaliwal RS, et al. Orbital tuberculosis. Int Ophthalmol. 1994;18:149-52.
3. DeVoe AG, Locatcher-Khorazo D. The external manifestations of ocular tuberculosis. Trans Am Ophthalmol Soc. 1964;62:203-12.
4. Gupta V, Gupta A, Arora S, et al. Presumed tubercular serpiginous like choroiditis. Ophthalmology. 2003;110:1744-9.
5. Patkar S, Singhania BK, Agrawal A. Intraorbital extraocular tuberculosis: a report of three cases. Surg Neurol. 1994; 42:320-1.
6. Roy FH, Fraunfelder FW, Fraunfelder FT. Roy and Fraunfelder's. Current Ocular Therapy, 6th editon. Philadelphia: WB Saunders; 2008.
7. Tejada P, Mendez MJ, Negreira S. Choroidal tubercles with tuberculous meningitis. Int Ophthalmol. 1994;18:115-8.

⊟ 11.6DD. WEIL DISEASE (LEPTOSPIROSIS)

General

Acute severe infection caused by *Leptospira* transmitted by ingestion of food contaminated by the reservoir bacterium.

Ocular

Acute conjunctivitis; episcleritis; fibrinous iridocyclitis with vitreal haze; hypopyon; keratitis; pain on ocular movement; uveitis; optic neuritis; cataract; hemorrhagic retinitis; ptosis.

Clinical

Jaundice; fever; headaches; chills; vomiting; anemia; psychologic disturbances.

Laboratory

Complete blood count, urinalysis and isolation of organism in blood, urine or cerebrospinal fluid.

Treatment

Intravenous penicillin G for a week. Ceftriaxone can also be used.

⊟ BIBLIOGRAPHY

1. Hickey PW. (2012). Pediatric leptospirosis. [online] Available from www.emedicine.com/ped/TOPIC1298.HTM. [Accessed August, 2013].

🗗 11.6EE. YERSINIOSIS

General

Infection with one of the invasive rod-shaped *Yersinia* bacteria.

Clinical

Gastroenteritis, high fever, acute terminal ileitis.

Ocular

Corneal perforation, panophthalmitis, anterior uveitis, photophobia, lacrimation, pericorneal ciliary injection, aqueous flare and cell, keratic precipitates and macular edema.

Laboratory

Small, non-motile, Gram-negative coccobacilli found in stool samples and conjunctiva.

Treatment

Tetracycline or chloramphenicol is drug of choice.

🗗 BIBLIOGRAPHY

1. Roy FH, Fraunfelder FW, Fraunfelder FT. Roy and Fraunfelder's Current Ocular Therapy, 6th edition. London: Elsevier; 2008.

🗗 11.9A. GHOST CELL GLAUCOMA

General

Usually follows vitreous hemorrhage when the presence of blood debris in the anterior chamber clogs the trabecular meshwork resulting in elevated IOP.

Clinical

Vitreous hemorrhage sometimes is associated with diabetes.

Ocular

Elevated IOP, vitreous hemorrhage, corneal edema, decreased visual acuity, posterior vitreous detachment.

Laboratory

Cytologic examination of the aqueous humor, B-scan ultrasonography.

Treatment

Usually it involves surgical intervention with lavage of the anterior chamber or vitrectomy.

🗗 BIBLIOGRAPHY

1. Campbell DG, Essigmann EM. Hemolytic ghost cell glaucoma. Further studies. Arch Ophthalmol. 1979;97(11):2141-6.
2. Montenegro MH, Simmons RJ. Ghost cell glaucoma. Int Ophthalmol. 1994;34(1):111-5.
3. Rojas L, Ortiz G, Gutiérrez M, et al. Ghost cell glaucoma related to snake poisoning. Arch Ophthalmol. 2001;119(8):1212-3.

🗗 11.10. PRIMARY ANGLE-CLOSURE GLAUCOMA (PRIMARY CLOSED ANGLE GLAUCOMA)

General

Obstruction of aqueous humor outflow forms the anterior chamber which results from closure of the angle by the peripheral root of the iris.

Clinical

Pain, nausea.

Ocular

Flare in the anterior chamber, conjunctival chemosis, hyperemia, corneal epithelial edema, folds in Descemet's membrane, peripheral anterior synechiae, increased IOP, visual field defect.

Laboratory

Diagnosis is made by clinical findings.

Treatment

Systemic hyperosmotic agents, topical pilocarpine every 5 minutes, laser iridotomy and if IOP does not respond, filtering surgery may be necessary.

BIBLIOGRAPHY

1. Noecker RJ, Kahook MY. (2011). Glaucoma, angle closure, acute. [online] Available from www.emedicine.com/oph/TOPIC255.HTM. [Accessed August, 2013].
2. Tham CC, Ritch R. (2012). Glaucoma, angle closure, chronic. [online] Available from www.emedicine.com/oph/TOPIC122.HTM. [Accessed August, 2013].

11.11. RETICULUM CELL SARCOMA (NON-HODGKIN LYMPHOMA)

General

Autosomal recessive; large-cell lymphoma with chronic inflammation with a predominance of cells in vitreous cavity; average age at time of diagnosis is 60 years; female to male ratio is approximately 2:1; 80% bilateral (frequently asymmetrical).

Ocular

Chronic uveitis; chorioretinal lesions; mycosis fungoides; necrosis of orbital tissues; phthisis bulbi; endophthalmos; exophthalmos; exudative retinal detachment; iris neovascularization; glaucoma; branch retinal vein occlusion; macular edema; optic neuropathy; vitreous hemorrhage; partial cranial nerve III palsy; multiple retinal pigment epithelium masses.

Clinical

Lymphocytic hyperplasia; fever; anemia; thrombocytopenia; liver and spleen enlargement; associated with immune dysfunction states, such as AIDS, or following transplantation.

Laboratory

Computed tomography/MRI scan, HIV evaluation, CBC, lumbar puncture.

Treatment

Radiation, chemotherapy.

BIBLIOGRAPHY

1. Vinjamaram S, Estrada-Garcia DA, Hernandez-Ilizaliturri FJ, et al. (2012). Non-Hodgkin Lymphoma. [online] Available from emedicine.medscape.com/article/203399-overview. [Accessed August, 2013].

12. INTRAOCULAR EPITHELIAL CYSTS

General

Anterior chamber epithelial cyst develops when implanted epithelial cells proliferate centripetally.

Clinical

None.

Ocular

Perforated corneal ulcer, glaucoma and uveitis.

Laboratory

Diagnosis is made from clinical findings.

Treatment

Surgical intervention is required if complications obstruct the visual axis.

BIBLIOGRAPHY

1. Roy FH, Fraunfelder FW, Fraunfelder FT. Roy and Fraunfelder's Current Ocular Therapy, 6th edition. London: Elsevier; 2008.

13. MESODERMAL DYSGENESIS (ANTERIOR CHAMBER DYSGENESIS; DYSEMBRYOGENESIS; ANTERIOR SEGMENT OCULAR DYSGENESIS SYNDROME)

General

Mesodermal abnormalities, including oculocutaneous albinism; autosomal dominant.

Ocular

Capsular cataracts; external ophthalmoplegia; anterior chamber cleavage syndrome; atrophy of iris; ectropion; flat cornea; coloboma of iris and choroid; posterior embryotoxon; Axenfeld anomaly; Rieger anomaly; Peters anomaly; keratoconus; microphthalmos.

Clinical

None.

Laboratory/Ocular

Diagnosis is made by clinical findings.

Treatment/Ocular

Cataract surgery; filtration surgery to control IOP, genetic counseling, keratoplasty.

BIBLIOGRAPHY

1. Ferrell RE, Hittner HM, Kretzer FL, et al. Anterior segment mesenchymal dysgenesis: probable linkage to the MNS blood group on chromosome 4. Am J Hum Genet. 1982; 34:245-9.
2. Lubin JR. Oculocutaneous albinism associated with corneal mesodermal dysgenesis. Am J Ophthalmol. 1981; 91:347-50.
3. Lubin JR. Oculocutaneous albinism and corneal mesodermal dysgenesis. Am J Ophthalmol. 1981;92:587.
4. Ghose S, Singh NP, Kaur D, et al. Microphthalmos and anterior segment dysgenesis in a family. Ophthalmic Paediatr Genet. 1991;12:177-82.

14. NEOVASCULARIZATION OF ANTERIOR CHAMBER ANGLE (NEWLY FORMED VESSELS EXTEND INTO THE TRABECULAR MESHWORK)

†1. Anterior chamber angle
  A. Congenital pupillary iris lens membrane with goniodysgenesis
  B. Traumatic chamber angle
2. Iris tumors
  A. Hemangioma
  B. Melanoma
  †C. Metastatic carcinoma
3. Ocular vascular disease
  †*A. Central retinal artery thrombosis
  †*B. Central retinal vein thrombosis
  C. Hemiretinal branch vein occlusion (HBVO)
4. Postinflammatory
  †A. Anterior chamber implants
  B. Fungal endophthalmitis
  †C. Radiation
  D. Retinal detachment operation
  E. Uveitis, chronic

5. Proximal vascular disease
  A. Aortic arch syndrome (Takayasu syndrome)
  B. Carotid cavernous fistula
  †C. Carotid ligation
  †D. Carotid occlusive disease
  E. Cranial arteritis (temporal arteritis syndrome)
6. Retinal disease
  A. Coats disease (Leber miliary aneurysms)
  †*B. Diabetic retinopathy
  C. Eales disease (periphlebitis)
  †D. Glaucoma, chronic
  E. Melanoma of choroid
  F. Norrie disease (fetal iritis syndrome)
  †G. Persistent hyperplastic primary vitreous
  H. Retinal detachment
  I. Retinal hemangioma
  J. Retinal vessel occlusion
  K. Retinoblastoma
  L. Retrolental fibroplasia
  M. Sickle cell retinopathy (Herrick syndrome)

*Indicates most frequent
†Indicates a general entry and therefore has not been described in detail in the text

BIBLIOGRAPHY

1. Cibis GW, Waeltermann JM, Hurst E, et al. Congenital pupillary iris-lens membrane with goniodysgenesis. Ophthalmology. 1986;93:847-52.
2. Kimura R. Fluorescein gonioangiography of newly formed vessels in the anterior chamber angle. Tohoku J Exp Med. 1983;140:193-6.
3. Roy FH. Ocular syndromes and systemic diseases, 5th edition. New Delhi: Jaypee Brothers Medical Publishers; 2013.

14.2A. HEMANGIOMA

General

Hemangioma can occur throughout the body, but particularly in the head; primary intraosseous orbital hemangiomas are rare; capillary hemangioma of the orbit and eyelids generally is unilateral.

Ocular

Hemangiomas of lids or orbit; ptosis; strabismus; amblyopia; proptosis; optic atrophy; hypermetropia; cavernous hemangiomas are the most common benign orbital tumors of adults.

Clinical

Ipsilateral hemangiomas of the brain and meninges.

Laboratory

Neuroimaging can be of great assistance in making the diagnosis.

Treatment

Most of these lesions regress on their own; there is no need to intervention. If spontaneous regression does not occur, corticosteroids, in various formulations, may be considered. Topical application of timolol has been useful in some cases.

BIBLIOGRAPHY

1. Karmel M. Topical timolol for capillary hemangioma. Eyenet. 2010.
2. Seiff S, Zwick OM, DeAngelis DD, et al. (2011). Capillary hemangioma. [online] Available from www.emedicine.com/oph/TOPIC691.HTM. [Accessed August, 2013].

14.2B. IRIS MELANOMA

General

Malignant neoplasm.

Clinical

None.

Ocular

Iris melanoma, ectropion uvea, sector cataract, sentinel vessels, heterochromia, hyphema, chronic uveitis, glaucoma.

Laboratory

Diagnosis is made by clinical findings.

Treatment

Resection with iridectomy/iridocyclectomy or radiotherapy and enucleation.

BIBLIOGRAPHY

1. Waheed NK, Foster CS. (2012). Iris melanoma. [online] Available from www.emedicine.com/oph/TOPIC405.HTM. [Accessed August, 2013].

14.3C. RETINAL VENOUS OBSTRUCTION

General

Occlusion at the level of either the branch or central retinal venous system, causing a reduction in venous return.

Clinical

None.

Ocular

Painless visual loss, ischemic central retinal vein occlusion (CRVO), branch retinal vein occlusion.

Laboratory

Fluorescein angiography, optical coherence tomography (OCT) for assessment of macular edema.

Treatment

Anticoagulation, surgical adventitial shealthotomy, radial optic neurotomy, intravitreal injection of triamcinolone acetonide for macular edema. Vitrectomy may be necessary.

BIBLIOGRAPHY

1. Kooragayala LM. (2012). Central retinal vein occlusion. [online] Available from www.emedicine.com/oph/TOPIC388.HTM. [Accessed August, 2013].
2. Scott IU, van Velhuisen PC, Oden NL, et al. Baseline predictors of visual acuity and retinal thickness outcomes in patients with retinal vein occlusion: standard care versus corticosteroid for retinal vein occlusion study report 10. Ophthalmology. 2011;118:345-52.

14.4B. FUNGAL ENOPHTHALMITIS

General

Rare, intraocular fungal infection.

Clinical

None.

Ocular

Conjunctival injection; pain; mildly decreased vision; fibrinous membranes in anterior chamber; white fluffy retinal infiltrates.

Laboratory

Fungal tests are done on anterior chamber aspirates and vitreous cavity aspirates.

Treatment

Topical, subconjunctival, intravitreal antifungal agents; pars plana vitrectomy.

BIBLIOGRAPHY

1. Wu L, Evans T, García RA. (2012). Fungal endophthalmitis. [online] Available from www.emedicine.com/oph/TOPIC706.HTM. [Accessed August, 2013].

14.4D. RETINAL DETACHMENT, RHEGMATOGENOUS

General

Subretinal fluid accumulation in the space between the neurosensory retina and the underlying RPE. Most common type of retinal detachment and occurs with a retinal tear that allows liquefied vitreous to seep under the tear leading to the detachment.

Clinical

None.

Ocular

Vitreous traction, cut in visual field; vitreous floaters; decreased visual acuity; scleritis.

Laboratory

Diagnosis is generally made by clinical observation. Ultrasound may be necessary if the media is hazy.

Treatment

Scleral buckle, pneumatic retinopexy and vitrectomy are used for this type of detachment and the goal is to close all the breaks.

BIBLIOGRAPHY

1. Wu L, Evans T. (2011). Rhegmatogenous retinal detachment treatment and management. [online] Available from emedicine.medscape.com/article/1224737-treatment. [Accessed August, 2013].

14.4E. UVEITIS, ANTERIOR NONGRANULOMATOUS (IRITIS, CHRONIC)

General

Ocular inflammation. Etiology is idiopathic but certain systemic diseases may be the underlying cause.

Clinical

Human leukocyte antigen B27, Behçet disease, herpes zoster, sarcoidosis, syphilis, Lyme disease, JIA, Fuchs heterochromic iridocyclitis, tuberculosis.

Ocular

Photophobia, red eye, dull aching eye pain, perilimbal injection, keratic precipitates, flare and cell of anterior chamber, posterior synechiae, lenticular precipitates.

Laboratory

Diagnosis is made by clinical findings. If nongranulomatous iritis is recurrent, studies are necessary to determine the cause. HLA B27 typing, serologic testing for syphilis, sarcoidosis rheumatoid factor and Lyme disease may be indicated.

Treatment

Topical corticosteroids are the mainstay of therapy. Subconjunctival corticosteroids may be necessary in nonresponding cases. Cycloplegia is useful for controlling pain and photophobia.

BIBLIOGRAPHY

1. Levinson RD. (2012). Uveitis, anterior, nongranulomatous. [online] Available from www.emedicine.com/oph/TOPIC587.HTM. [Accessed August, 2013].

14.5A. TAKAYASU SYNDROME (MARTORELL SYNDROME; AORTIC ARCH SYNDROME; PULSELESS DISEASE; REVERSED COARCTATION SYNDROME)

General

Two types are: (1) occlusive inflammatory lesion (seen in young Japanese women) and (2) occlusive vascular disease without inflammation, associated with atherosclerosis and syphilis; onset between 5th decade and 6th decade; both sexes affected; can involve the aorta and its major branches as well as the coronary, hepatic, mesenteric, pulmonary, and renal arteries.

Ocular

Iris atrophy; cataracts; retinal microaneurysms; sausage-shaped venous dilations; reduced central retinal artery pressure; optic atrophy; cotton-wool spots; anterior segment ischemia; retinal arteriovenous shunts.

Clinical

Diminished or absent pulsation of arteries (head, neck, upper limbs); orthostatic syncope; facial atrophy; epileptiform seizures; intermittent claudication.

Laboratory

Arteriography, magnetic resonance angiography (MRA), MRI, CT scan, Gallium-67 radionuclide scan, or chest radiography.

Treatment

Corticosteroids, methotrexate or intravenous cyclophosphamide can be used in patients with glucocorticoid-resistant Takayasu arteritis (TA).

BIBLIOGRAPHY

1. Hom C. (2013). Pediatric Takayasu Arteritis. [online] Available from www.emedicine.com/ped/TOPIC1956.HTM. [Accessed August, 2013].

🗗 14.5B. CAROTID ARTERY SYNDROME (CAVERNOUS SINUS FISTULA SYNDROME; RED-EYED SHUNT SYNDROME)

General

Seventy-five percent of cases caused by trauma; others occur spontaneously or are congenital; fistula from carotid artery to cavernous sinus.

Ocular

Progressive, pulsating exophthalmos; distended pulsating superior orbital vein; venous congestion of lids; variable ophthalmoplegia, depending on involvement of cranial nerves III to VI; secondary glaucoma; congestion of conjunctiva with chemosis; corneal ulcerations; eversion of the lower lid; loss of corneal sensation; retinal edema; engorgement of retinal veins; papilledema; optic atrophy; ocular bruit that may be subjective and/or objective; diplopia; visual decrease; choroidal folds; dilated superior ophthalmic vein.

Clinical

Severe unilateral headache; buzzing noise.

Laboratory

Orbital ultrasonography, CT, six-vessel cranial digital subtraction angiography—characterization of the arterial supply and venous drainage of fistula.

Treatment

Use of intraocular lowering agent and topical lubrication is the ocular treatment of choice.

🗗 BIBLIOGRAPHY

1. Dailey EJ, Holloway JA, Murto RE, et al. Evaluation of ocular signs and symptoms in cerebral aneurysms. Arch Ophthalmol. 1964;71:463-74.
2. Duane TD. Clinical Ophthalmology. Philadelphia: JB Lippincott; 1987.
3. Flaharty PM, Lieb WE, Sergott RC, et al. Color Doppler imaging. A new noninvasive technique to diagnose and monitor carotid cavernous sinus fistulas. Arch Ophthalmol. 1991;109:522-6.
4. Gonshor LG, Kline LB. Choroidal folds and dural cavernous sinus fistula. Arch Ophthalmol. 1991;109:1065-6.
5. Phelps CD, Thompson HS, Ossoinig KC. The diagnosis and prognosis of atypical carotid cavernous fistula. Am J Ophthalmol. 1982;93:423-36.
6. Roy FH, Fraunfelder FW, Fraunfelder FT. Current Ocular Therapy, 6th edition. Philadelphia: WB Saunders; 2008.
7. Travers B. A case of aneurysm by anastomosis in the orbit, cured by ligation of common carotid artery. Med Chir Trans. 1917;2:1-420.

🗗 14.5E. TEMPORAL ARTERITIS SYNDROME (CRANIAL ARTERITIS SYNDROME; GIANT CELL ARTERITIS; HUTCHINSON-HORTON-MAGATH-BROWN SYNDROME)

General

Etiology unknown; mainly females; mainly Whites; ages 55–80 years; temporal artery shows inflammatory thickening; arteritis of the vessels supplying the optic nerve.

Ocular

Transient ptosis; partial or complete loss of vision on the affected side; retinal detachment; exudates and hemorrhages; narrowing of retinal vessels; obstruction of the central retinal artery; optic atrophy; ischemic optic neuropathy; acute decreased IOP; corneal hypesthesia; palsies of extraocular muscles; hemorrhagic glaucoma; diplopia; hemorrhages on or around the disk.

Clinical

Throbbing headache; hyperalgesia of the scalp; malaise; anorexia; weakness; weight loss; fever; nodular pulmonary nodules; cough; otitis with deafness.

Laboratory

Elevated ESR greater than 50 mm/hour, positive temporal artery biopsy.

Treatment

Systemic corticosteroids are the therapy of choice.

🗗 BIBLIOGRAPHY

1. Allen AW, Biega T, Varma MK. (2012). Temporal arteritis imaging. [online] Available from www.emedicine.com/radio/TOPIC675.HTM. [Accessed August, 2013].
2. Walvick MD, Walvick MP. Giant cell arteritis: laboratory predictors of a positive temporal artery biopsy. Ophthalmology. 2011;118(6):1201-4.

14.6A. COATS DISEASE (LEBER MILIARY ANEURYSM; RETINAL TELANGIECTASIA)

General

Exudative retinitis; rare; more common in males than females; 95% unilateral.

Ocular

Leukocoria; telangiectatic retinal vessels; solid gray-yellow retinal detachment; optic atrophy; vitreous hemorrhage; anterior uveitis; glaucoma; intraocular calcification (rare); fibro-osseous retinal nodules (atypical); hemorrhagic retinal macrocysts; cystoid macular edema.

Clinical

None.

Laboratory

Fluorescein angiography demonstrates large aneurysmal (light bulb) dilatation of the retinal vessels.

Treatment

Cryotherapy and vitrectomy can be used to obliterate the vascular abnormalities.

BIBLIOGRAPHY

1. Cameron JD, Yanoff M, Frayer WC. Coats' disease and Turner's syndrome. Am J Ophthalmol. 1974;78(5):852-4.
2. Senft SH, Hidayat AA, Cavender JC. Atypical presentation of Coats disease. Retina. 1994;14(1):36-8.

14.6C. EALES DISEASE (PERIPHLEBITIS)

General

Common; young adults.

Ocular

Sheathing of peripheral veins; hemorrhage in new vessels and later retinal detachment; retinal vascular tortuosity; microaneurysms of retina; post-neovascularization of vitreous; internuclear ophthalmoplegia.

Clinical

Epilepsy and hemiplegia have been reported; chronic encephalitis; ulcerative colitis; central nervous infarction.

Laboratory

Fluorescein angiography and tuberculosis screening test.

Treatment

Thyroid extract, osteogenic hormones, androgenic hormones and systemic steroids are recommended. The antioxidant vitamins A, C and E have been suggested as a possible therapy because antioxidizing enzymes are deficient in the vitreous samples.

BIBLIOGRAPHY

1. Roth DB, Fine HF. (2012). Eales disease. [online] Available from emedicine.medscape.com/article/1225636-overview. [Accessed August, 2013].

14.6E. MALIGNANT MELANOMA OF THE POSTERIOR UVEA (CHOROIDAL MELANOMA, CILIARY BODY MELANOMA, UVEAL MELANOMA, INTRAOCULAR MELANOMA)

General

Most common primary intraocular tumor in adults.

Clinical

Metastatic melanoma can appear in other parts of the body such as skin or liver.

Ocular

Intraocular tumors of the choroid, iris and ciliary body.

Laboratory

Ultrasonography, fluorescein angiography, indocyanine green angiography.

Treatment

Ocular therapy's goal is to eradicate the tumor before metastasis occurs. Diode laser, brachytherapy, stereotactic, local resection, enucleation and exenteration are all used to achieve this. Systemically intravenous therapy; intrahepatic chemoembolization has been used for isolated liver metastases. Proton beam is used to kill the tumor.

BIBLIOGRAPHY

1. Garcia-Valenzuela E, Pons ME, Puklin JE, et al. (2011). Choroidal Melanoma. [online] Available from www.emedicine.com/oph/TOPIC403.HTM [Accessed August, 2013].

14.6F. ANDERSEN-WARBURG SYNDROME (WHITNALL-NORMAN SYNDROME; OLIGOPHRENIA MICROPHTHALMOS SYNDROME; NORRIE DISEASE; ATROPHIA OCULI CONGENITAL FETAL IRITIS SYNDROME; CONGENITAL PROGRESSIVE OCULO-ACOUSTICO-CEREBRAL DYSPLASIA)

General

Sex-linked inheritance; gross deformation of both eyes; only males affected; onset at birth; putative gene for Norrie disease has been isolated and mapped to Xp11.3.

Ocular

Bilateral microphthalmos with extensive destruction of all ocular structures often resembling a pseudotumor; blindness at birth; iris atrophy; iritis; corneal opacification and lenticular destruction with a mass visible behind the lens as long as the lens is still clear; malformed retina and choroid with retinal pseudotumors; retinal detachment; retrolental vascular mass.

Clinical

Mental retardation ranging from imbecility to idiocy (may begin at any age) in about two-thirds of the cases; deafness of differing severity with onset between ages 9 and 45 years.

Laboratory

Diagnosis is made by clinical findings.

Treatment

Topical treatment for iritis; retinal detachment surgery and vitrectomy may be necessary. Immediate laser treatment is recommended following birth.

BIBLIOGRAPHY

1. Andersen SR, Warburg M. Norrie's disease: congenital bilateral pseudotumor of the retina with recessive X-chromosomal inheritance; Preliminary Report. Arch Ophthalmol. 1961;66(5):614-8.
2. Black G, Redmond RM. The molecular biology of Norrie's disease. Eye (Lond). 1994;8(5):491-6.
3. Chow CC, Kiernam DF, Chau FY, et al. Laser photocoagulation at birth prevents blindness in Norrie's disease diagnosed using amniocentesis. Ophthalmology. 2010;117(12):2402-6.

14.6H. RETINAL DETACHMENT, RHEGMATOGENOUS

General

Subretinal fluid accumulation in the space between the neurosensory retina and the underlying RPE. Most common type of retinal detachment and occurs with a retinal tear that allows liquefied vitreous to seep under the tear leading to the detachment.

Clinical

None.

Ocular

Vitreous traction, cut in visual field; vitreous floaters; decreased visual acuity; scleritis.

Laboratory

Diagnosis is generally made by clinical observation. Ultrasound may be necessary if the media is hazy.

Treatment

Scleral buckle, pneumatic retinopexy and vitrectomy are used for this type of detachment and the goal is to close all the breaks.

BIBLIOGRAPHY

1. Wu L, Evans T. (2011). Rhegmatogenous retinal detachment treatment and management. [online] Available from emedicine.medscape.com/article/1224737-treatment. [Accessed August, 2013].

14.6I. HEMANGIOMA

General

Hemangioma can occur throughout the body, but particularly in the head; primary intraosseous orbital hemangiomas are rare; capillary hemangioma of the orbit and eyelids generally is unilateral.

Ocular

Hemangiomas of lids or orbit; ptosis; strabismus; amblyopia; proptosis; optic atrophy; hypermetropia; cavernous hemangiomas are the most common benign orbital tumors of adults.

Clinical

Ipsilateral hemangiomas of the brain and meninges.

Laboratory

Neuroimaging can be of great assistance in making the diagnosis.

Treatment

Most of these lesions regress on their own; there is no need to intervention. If spontaneous regression does not occur, corticosteroids, in various formulations, may be considered. Topical application of timolol has been useful in some cases.

BIBLIOGRAPHY

1. Karmel M. Topical timolol for capillary hemangioma. Eyenet. 2010.
2. Seiff S, Zwick OM, DeAngelis DD, et al. (2011). Capillary hemangioma. [online] Available from www.emedicine.com/oph/TOPIC691.HTM. [Accessed August, 2013].

14.6J. RETINAL ARTERY OCCLUSION

General

This condition involves a sudden, painless visual loss.

Clinical

Temporal arteritis, jaw claudication, scalp tenderness.

Ocular

Ophthalmoscopic examination, a diffuse retinal pallor and a cherry-red spot in macula are noted.

Laboratory

To determine etiology; CBC to evaluate blood disorders, erythrocyte sedimentation rate (ESR), blood cultures, carotid ultrasound imaging, fluorescein angiogram.

Treatment

Intraocular pressure lowering medications, carbogen therapy, hyperbaric oxygen. Vitrectomy may be necessary.

BIBLIOGRAPHY

1. Graham RH, Ebrahim SA. (2012). Central retinal artery occlusion. [online] Available from www.emedicine.com/oph/TOPIC387.HTM. [Accessed August, 2013].

14.6K. RETINOBLASTOMA

General

Malignant tumor arising in one or both retinas of young children, usually under the age of 2 years; usually unilateral; autosomal dominant; most common intraocular malignancy of childhood; incidence is one in 20,000 live births; origin is questionably neuroectodermal cells capable of multipotentiality; one–third of patients have heritable (bilateral or have a positive family history) autosomal dominant and two thirds are sporadic; genetic transmission obeys two-mutation hypothesis of Knudson; trilateral retinoblastoma is bilateral retinoblastoma plus midline central nervous system tumor (most commonly pinealoma); most common second tumor is an osteogenic sarcoma (begins in 2nd decade).

Ocular

Hyphema; hypopyon; corneal tumor; lid edema; endophthalmitis; exophthalmos; intraocular calcification of globe; heterochromia; neovascularization of iris or retina; papilledema; panophthalmitis; retinoblastoma extension into orbit and choroid; cat's-eye reflex; leukocoria; mydriasis; vitreous hemorrhage tumor seeding; esotropia; exotropia; glaucoma; visual loss.

Clinical

Metastasis into the lymph system, bone marrow, and subarachnoid space; basal meningitis; death.

Laboratory

CT—calcification of lesion hallmark of disease; ultrasound—demonstrates calcification and MRI demonstrates presence and extent of extraocular disease.

Treatment

External beam radiation therapy is recommended on patients with significant vitreous seeding. Radioactive isotope plaques and chemotherapy are also an option. Removal of the tumor is the standard management for retinoblastoma.

BIBLIOGRAPHY

1. Isidro MA, Roque MR, Aaberg TM, et al. (2012). Retinoblastoma. [online] Available from www.emedicine.com/oph/TOPIC346.HTM. [Accessed August, 2013].

14.6L. RETROLENTAL FIBROPLASIA (RLF; RETINOPATHY OF PREMATURITY)

General

Bilateral disease seen primarily in premature infants with immature retinal vessels; excessive use of oxygen is responsible for the majority of cases, but disease is seen despite oxygen restrictions or even when no oxygen supplementation is used; known factors that correlate with degrees of retinopathy of prematurity are low birth weight, short gestational age, length of time with supplemental oxygen, length of time on a mechanical ventilator; role of excessive light in newborn nurseries also has been proposed.

Ocular

Anterior or posterior synechiae; neovascularization of iris; pallor of optic disk; dragged disk; attenuated vessels; retinal detachment; dilation of veins; retinal folds; retinal hemorrhage; retrolental mass; vascular tortuosity; vasoconstriction of retina; retinal pigmentary changes; vitreous haze; vitreous traction; vitreous hemorrhages; cataract; glaucoma; leukocoria; myopia; shallow anterior chamber; opaque retrolental membrane; ciliary body drawn anteriorly; ciliary process around dilated pupil; absent pupillary reflexes; keratoconus; associated strabismus; amblyopia.

Clinical

Low birth weight; prematurity.

Laboratory

Diagnosis is made by clinical findings.

Treatment

Cryotherapy and laser surgery can be effective. Vitrectomy may be necessary.

BIBLIOGRAPHY

1. Bashour M, Menassa J, Gerontis CC. (2013). Retinopathy of prematurity. [online] Available from www.emedicine.com/oph/TOPIC413.HTM. [Accessed August, 2013].

14.6M. HERRICK SYNDROME (DRESBACH SYNDROME; SICKLE CELL DISEASE; DREPANOCYTIC ANEMIA)

General

Usually occurs in members of the black race; poor prognosis.

Ocular

Secondary glaucoma; telangiectasia of conjunctival vessels; scleral icterus; vitreous hemorrhages; cataract; retinal hemorrhages; exudates, and neovascularization; retinitis proliferans; microaneurysms; thrombosis of retinal venules; retinal vascular sheathing; central vein occlusion; angioid streaks; retinopathy with "black sunburst sign" in patients with SS hemoglobin; "sea-fan sign" in patients with SC hemoglobin; comma signs of conjunctiva; fan-shaped neovascularization of iris; sector ischemic atrophy of iris; optic atrophy; white cotton mass of vitreous; retinal holes; color vision defects; central retinal artery obstruction; branch retinal artery obstruction; white without pressure; venous tortuosity; sickling maculopathy.

Clinical

Severe anemia with hemolytic crises; bone and joint aches; hemarthrosis; jaundice; hepatosplenomegaly.

Laboratory

Blood-sickling of red blood cells, newborn screening for hemoglobin disorders.

Treatment

Transfusion is required in an aplastic crisis; erythrocytapheresis is an automated red-cell exchange and bone marrow transplantation may be useful. Pain is the hallmark of sickle cell disease. While frequency and severity vary greatly, most patients have interval symptoms. Once pain has begun, no therapy reverses the process. Analgesics may provide a reasonable degree of comfort. While certain dosing guidelines are available, the amount of drug given should be titrated to the degree of pain experienced. Vitrectomy may be necessary.

BIBLIOGRAPHY

1. Maakaron JE, Taher A, Woermann UJ. (2012). Sickle cell anemia. [online] Available from www.emedicine.com/ped/TOPIC2096.HTM. [Accessed August, 2013].

15. SYNECHIAE, PERIPHERAL ANTERIOR

General

Consequence of altered anterior chamber anatomy and anterior chamber inflammation. Apposition of the iris against the trabecular meshwork as a result of pupil block without any inflammation can result in peripheral anterior synechiae. With inflammation or cellular proliferation, a membrane is formed between the iris and the trabecular meshwork, creating peripheral anterior synechiae.

Clinical

Inflammatory syndromes such as juvenile rheumatoid arthritis, intestinal keratitis, sarcoidosis, Posner-Schlossman syndrome, herpes simplex, herpes zoster, toxoplasmosis and syphilis.

Ocular

Primary angle-closure glaucoma, iris bombe, pupil block, posterior uveitis, central retinal vein occlusion (CRVO), nanophthalmos, suprachoroidal hemorrhage, ciliary block, posterior segment tumors, retinoblastoma, choroidal melanoma, retinopathy of prematurity.

Laboratory

Ultrasound biomicroscopy is helpful in evaluating the angle. Provocative testing is used to measure IOP while dilation and constriction of the pupil.

Treatment

No specific medical treatment exists. The following medications may be considered depending on the diagnosis: topical beta-blockers, alpha-agonists, carbonic anhydrase inhibitors, oral carbonic anhydrase inhibitors, topical prostaglandin analogs, miotics, cycloplegics, and topical corticosteroids.

Surgical

Yttrium aluminium garnet (YAG)/laser iridotomy, surgical iridotomy, argon laser peripheral iridoplasty, argon laser pupilloplasty, and glaucoma filtering procedures such as trabeculectomy, primary tube shunt.

BIBLIOGRAPHY

1. Khan BU, Hasanee K, Ahmed II. (2012). Peripheral anterior synechia. [online] Available from emedicine.medscape.com/article/1189962-diagnosis. [Accessed August, 2013].

16. PETERS ANOMALY

General

Autosomal recessive; may be morphologic entity with several eye syndromes, including Rieger syndrome, Mietens syndrome and fetal alcohol syndrome; may be due to a developmental field defect, a contiguous gene syndrome, or a defective homeotic gene controlling development of the eye and other body structures.

Ocular

Corneal opacification; lenticulocorneal adherence; iris adhesions; glaucoma; cataract; narrow lid fissures; colobomatous microphthalmia; persistent hyperplastic primary vitreous; retinal detachment; iris nodules.

Clinical

Short-limbed dwarfism; broad face; thin upper lip; hypoplastic columella; hypospadias; cleft lip and palate; craniofacial abnormalities; congenital heart disease; horseshoe kidney; polycystic kidneys; Wilms' tumor; mental retardation; external ear anomalies; camptodactyly.

Laboratory

Diagnosis is made by clinical findings.

Treatment

Glaucoma therapy, peripheral optical iridectomy, filtration surgery, cryoablation, or a tube shunt may be necessary if medications do not control the pressure. Corneal transplantation may be necessary if visual acuity is decreased.

BIBLIOGRAPHY

1. Giri G. (2012). Peters anomaly. [online] Available from www.emedicine.com/oph/TOPIC112.HTM. [Accessed August, 2013].

17. POSTOPERATIVE FLAT ANTERIOR CHAMBER

General

Flat anterior chamber following intraocular surgery.

Clinical

None.

Ocular

Corneal decompensation, cataract, intractable glaucoma.

Laboratory

Seidel test to demonstrate wound leak.

Treatment

Wound leaks usually require surgical repairs.

BIBLIOGRAPHY

1. Aquavella JV, Ford RM, McCormick GJ. (2012). Postoperative flat anterior chamber. [online] Available from www.emedicine.com/oph/TOPIC531.HTM. [Accessed August, 2013].

18. RECURRENT HYPHEMA

General

Trauma, although bleeding may occur spontaneously in conditions such as rubeosis iridis, leudemia, hemophilia, anticoagulation therapy, retinoblastoma or juvenile xanthogranuloma of iris. Recurrent hyphemas may be the result of iris nevus, rubbing of the iris on loops of older styles of intraocular lens or when the initial therapy for the traumatic hyphema is not adequate.

Clinical

None.

Ocular

Tear and bleeding from the iris, ciliary body or elevated IOP may occur.

Laboratory

Diagnosis is made by clinical findings.

Treatment

Cycloplegics decreased the inflammation and discomfort associated with traumatic iritis. Topical beta-adrenergic antagonists are the therapy of choice for elevated IOP. Recurrent hyphemas following an initial trauma may require bed rest and sometimes sedation (especially in active children). If the recurrent hyphema is due to an intraocular lens loop rubbing on an iris vessel, laser may be necessary to cauterize the vessel.

BIBLIOGRAPHY

1. Sheppard JD, Crouch ER, Williams PB, et al. (2011). Hyphema. [online] Available from www.emedicine.com/oph/TOPIC765.HTM. [Accessed August, 2013].

19. SHAKEN BABY SYNDROME (BATTERED-BABY SYNDROME; BATTERED-CHILD SYNDROME; CHILD ABUSE SYNDROME; SILVERMAN SYNDROME)

General

Associated with parental abuse or accidents.

Ocular

Exophthalmos with orbital hemorrhages; lid hematoma; lid edema; secondary glaucoma; hyphema; vitreous hemorrhages; retinal exudates and hemorrhages (Berlin edema); choroidal atrophy; retinal detachment; papilledema; optic nerve sheath hemorrhage; preretinal, intraretinal and subretinal hemorrhages; optic disk edema; choroidal hemorrhage.

Clinical

Soft tissue bruises; multiple fractures of long bones, ribs and skull; pharyngeal bruising, subdural hematoma; seizures; failure to thrive; vomiting associated with lethargy or drowsiness; respiratory irregularities; coma or death; intracranial hemorrhage.

Laboratory

CT of head to quantify degree of head trauma. MRI to define intraparenchymal brain lesions and subdural hematoma skeletal survey detects fractures of bones.

Treatment

- *Vitreous hemorrhage:* If possible the source of the bleeding needs to be isolated and treated with laser. Vitrectomy may be necessary.
- *Retinal detachment:* Scleral buckle, pneumatic retinopexy and vitrectomy may be used to close all the breaks.
- *Orbital hemorrhage:* Topical medication to lower IOP; lateral canthotomy and inferior cantholysis.

BIBLIOGRAPHY

1. Budenz DL, Farber MG, Mirchandani HG, et al. Ocular and optic nerve hemorrhages in abused infants with intracranial injuries. Ophthalmology. 1994;101(3):559-65.
2. Coody D, Brown M, Montgomery D, et al. Shaken baby syndrome: identification and prevention for nurse practitioners. J Pediatr Health Care. 1994;8(2):50-6.
3. Lambert SR, Johnson TE, Hoyt CS. Optic nerve sheath and retinal hemorrhages associated with the shaken baby syndrome. Arch Ophthalmol. 1986;104(10):1509-12.
4. Munger CE, Peiffer RL, Bouldin TW, et al. Ocular and associated neuropathologic observations in suspected whiplash shaken infant syndrome. A retrospective study of 12 cases. Am J Forensic Med Pathol. 1993;14(3):193-200.

🖿 20. SPONTANEOUS HYPHEMA

†1. Delayed following glaucoma surgery
2. Diseases of blood or blood vessels
   A. Hemophilia
   B. Leukemia
   C. Malignant lymphoma
   D. Purpura
   E. Scurvy
3. Fibrovascular membranes in retrolenticular or zonular area
   †A. Persistent primary vitreous
   B. Retinoschisis
   C. Retinopathy of prematurity
4. Systemic hypertension
†5. Hydrophthalmos
†6. Iatrogenic
†7. Intraocular neoplasms
*8. JXG-yellow nodules of skin and iris

9. Malignant exophthalmos
10. Microbial keratitis, especially Moraxella
†11. Occult trauma or trauma with late effect
12. Rubeosis iridis
13. Severe iritis with or without
    A. Behçet disease (dermatostomatoophthalmic syndrome)
    B. Diabetes mellitus (Willis disease)
    C. Gonococcal infection
    D. Herpes zoster or herpes simplex
†14. Use of warfarin, heparin, aspirin, or alcohol
†15. Vascular anomalies of iris
†16. Wound vascularization following cataract extraction

*Indicates most frequent
†Indicates a general entry and therefore has not been described in detail in the text

🖿 BIBLIOGRAPHY

1. Sheppard JD, Crouch ER, Williams PB, et al. (2011). Hyphema. [online] Available from emedicine.medscape.com/article/1190165-overview. [Accessed August, 2013].

🖿 20.2A. WERLHOF DISEASE (HEMOPHILIA AND THROMBOCYTOPENIC PURPURA)

General

Hemorrhagic disease of unknown etiology.

Ocular

Retinal hemorrhages; degeneration or severe intraocular hemorrhages with resultant retinitis proliferans.

Clinical

Petechiae and ecchymoses of skin and mucous membranes; tendency to bruise; decreased level of circulating platelets with a normal clotting time.

Laboratory

Diagnosis is made by clinical findings.

Treatment

See hematologist.

🖿 BIBLIOGRAPHY

1. Kobayashi H, Honda Y. Intraocular hemorrhage in a patient with hemophilia. Metab Ophthalmol. 1985;8:27-30.
2. Pau H. Differential diagnosis of eye diseases. New York: Thieme; 1987.
3. Werlhof PG. Disquisitio Medica et Philogica de Variolis et Anthracibus. Brunswick; 1735.

⏍ 20.2B. LEUKEMIA

General

Acute or chronic blood disorder.

Ocular

Engorgement of conjunctival vessels; papillary hypertrophy; aggregations of tumor cells in conjunctiva, choroid, and orbit; secondary glaucoma; retinal venous engorgement and tortuosity with pronounced constrictions; retinal hemorrhages; retinal detachment; cotton-wool spots; macular edema; papilledema; optic atrophy; optic neuritis; paralysis of extraocular muscles; hypopyon; vitreous opacities; retinal sea fans; perilimbal subconjunctival infiltrates; corneal leukemic infiltration (rare); shallow serous retinal detachments; hyphema; iris neovascularization; CRVO; vitreous infiltrates.

Clinical

Frequent involvement of central nervous system; intracranial hemorrhage; thrombocytopenia; rising white cell count.

Laboratory

CBC and differential, bone marrow aspiration, immunophenotyping, chromosomal analysis.

Treatment

Chemotherapy with or without radiotherapy.

⏍ BIBLIOGRAPHY

1. Wu L, Evans T, Martinez J. (2012). Leukemias. [online]. Available from www.emedicine.com/oph/TOPIC489.HTM. [Accessed August, 2013].

⏍ 20.2C. LYMPHOID HYPERPLASIA (REACTIVE LYMPHOID HYPERPLASIA; LYMPHOID TUMORS; MALIGNANT LYMPHOMA; PSEUDOLYMPHOMA; PSEUDO-TUMOR; BURKITT LYMPHOMA; NEOPLASTIC ANGIOENDOTHELIOMATOSIS)

General

Occurs in tropical Africa; young children; idiopathic orbital inflammation; systemic disease is rarely associated but occasionally occurs with either vasculitis or lymphomas; etiology of Burkitt lymphoma currently includes three factors: (1) Epstein-Barr virus, (2) malaria and (3) chromosomal translocations activating the c-Myc oncogene, which induces uncontrolled B-cell proliferation.

Ocular

Proptosis; extraocular motility disturbances; lesions of orbit, lacrimal gland, conjunctiva, and uvea; cortical blindness; retinal artery occlusion; retinal vascular and pigment epithelial alterations; vitreitis.

Clinical

Maxillary tumor; Epstein-Barr virus; cranial neuropathy.

Laboratory

Generally diagnosed with a lymph node biopsy.

Treatment

Chemotherapy, monoclonal antibody therapy and bone marrow or stem cell infusions may be chosen as therapy.

⏍ BIBLIOGRAPHY

1. Brooks HL, Downing J, McClure JA, et al. Orbital Buritt's lymphoma in a homosexual man with acquired immune deficiency. Arch Ophthalmol. 1984;102(10):1533-7.
2. Cheung MK, Martin DF, Chan CC, et al. Diagnosis of reactive lymphoid hyperplasia by chorioretinal biopsy. Am J Ophthalmol. 1994;118(4):457-62.

20.2D. HENOCH-SCHÖNLEIN PURPURA (PURPURA; ANAPHYLACTOID PURPURA)

General

Occurs chiefly in children, although it can affect persons of any age; frequently follows an upper respiratory tract infection within 3 weeks.

Ocular

Retinal hemorrhages; iritis; optic neuritis.

Clinical

Purpuric skin rash; concentrated on lower extremities; joint pain; abdominal pain; hematuria; central nervous system involvement.

Laboratory

Diagnosis is made by clinical findings.

Treatment

See hematologist.

BIBLIOGRAPHY

1. Harley RD (Ed). Pediatric Ophthalmology, 4th edition. Philadelphia: WB Saunders; 1998.
2. Lorentz WB, Weaver RG. Eye involvement in anaphylactoid purpura. Am J Dis Child. 1980;134:524-5.

20.2E. AVITAMINOSIS C (SCURVY; VITAMIN C DEFICIENCY)

General

Vitamin C deficiency.

Ocular

Hemorrhages of lids, anterior chamber, vitreous cavity, retina, subconjunctival space, and orbit (most prominent, with resulting exophthalmos); keratitis, corneal ulcer; cataract.

Clinical

Increased capillary fragility with a tendency to hemorrhage in tissues throughout the body; poor wound healing; loose teeth; purpuric rash.

Laboratory

Laboratory tests are usually not helpful to ascertain a diagnosis of scurvy. Diagnosis is generally made by clinical findings and history

Treatment

Dietary or pharmacologic doses of vitamin C is the standard treatment. Orange juice is a good choice to add to the diet.

BIBLIOGRAPHY

1. Goebel L, Buckler BS, Driscoll H, et al. (2013). Scurvy. [online] Available from www.emedicine.com/ped/TOPIC2073.HTM. [Accessed August, 2013].

20.3B. RETINOSCHISIS (RS)

General

Sex-linked; may not manifest until middle life.

Ocular

Intraretinal splitting due to degeneration or detachment of retina; retinal atrophy with sclerosis of the choroid; cystic maculopathy.

Clinical

None.

Laboratory

Optical coherence tomography provides high resolution of the macula region. Fluorescein angiography, ICGA and ERG are helpful tools in finding a diagnosis.

Treatment

No treatment is available.

BIBLIOGRAPHY

1. Small KW, McLellan CM, Song MK. (2012). Juvenile retinoschisis. [online] Available from www.emedicine.com/oph/TOPIC639.HTM. [Accessed August, 2013].

🗗 20.3C. RETROLENTAL FIBROPLASIA (RLF; RETINOPATHY OF PREMATURITY)

General

Bilateral disease seen primarily in premature infants with immature retinal vessels; excessive use of oxygen is responsible for the majority of cases, but disease is seen despite oxygen restrictions or even when no oxygen supplementation is used; known factors that correlate with degrees of retinopathy of prematurity are low birth weight, short gestational age, length of time with supplemental oxygen, length of time on a mechanical ventilator; role of excessive light in newborn nurseries also has been proposed.

Ocular

Anterior or posterior synechiae; neovascularization of iris; pallor of optic disk; dragged disk; attenuated vessels; retinal detachment; dilation of veins; retinal folds; retinal hemorrhage; retrolental mass; vascular tortuosity; vasoconstriction of retina; retinal pigmentary changes; vitreous haze; vitreous traction; vitreous hemorrhages; cataract; glaucoma; leukocoria; myopia; shallow anterior chamber; opaque retrolental membrane; ciliary body drawn anteriorly; ciliary process around dilated pupil; absent pupillary reflexes; keratoconus; associated strabismus; amblyopia.

Clinical

Low birth weight; prematurity.

Laboratory

Diagnosis is made by clinical findings.

Treatment

Cryotherapy and laser surgery can be effective. Vitrectomy may be necessary.

🗗 BIBLIOGRAPHY

1. Bashour M, Menassa J, Gerontis CC. (2013). Retinopathy of prematurity. [online] Available from www.emedicine.com/oph/TOPIC413.HTM. [Accessed August, 2013].

🗗 20.4. HYPERTENSION

General

Elevated blood pressure.

Ocular

Retinal arterial narrowing; arteriosclerosis; hemorrhages; retinal edema; cotton-wool spots; fatty exudates; optic disk edema; exudative retinal detachment; optic neuropathy; swollen optic nerve; CRVO; branch retinal vein occlusion; choroidal ischemia.

Clinical

Systemic hypertension; patchy loss of muscle tone in vessel walls; vascular decompensation.

Laboratory

Diagnosis is made from clinical findings; CBC, serum electrolytes, serum creatinine, serum glucose, uric acid and urinalysis, lipid profile (total cholesterol, low-density lipoprotein and high-density lipoprotein and triglycerides).

Treatment

Lifestyle modifications: Weight loss, stop smoking, exercise, reduce stress, limit alcohol intake, reduce sodium intake, maintain adequate calcium and potassium intake. Refer to internist for drug therapy.

🗗 BIBLIOGRAPHY

1. Madhur MS, Riaz K, Dreisbach AW, et al. (2012). Hypertension. [online] Available from www.emedicine.com/med/TOPIC1106.HTM. [Accessed August, 2013].

⊟ 20.8. JUVENILE XANTHOGRANULOMA (JXG; NEVOXANTHOENDOTHELIOMA)

General

Childhood disease; unknown etiology.

Ocular

Uveal tract tumor presenting as spontaneous hyphema; secondary glaucoma; uveitis; corneal, lid, and epibulbar tumors; proptosis; retinal and choroidal lesions (rare).

Clinical

Multiple benign tumors, primarily of the skin; usually appear in the first 3 years of life; lesions appear as yellow-to-brown papules or nodules.

Laboratory

Diagnostic techniques include biomicroscopy, high frequency ultrasound and cytologic examination of anterior chamber paracentesis material.

Treatment

Topical, subconjunctival, intralesional, and systemic corticosteroids are useful. Low-dose radiation may be the treatment of choice for diffuse uveal lesions. Glaucoma medications should be used in the setting of hyphema and increased IOP.

⊟ BIBLIOGRAPHY

1. Curtis T, Wheeler DT. (2012). Juvenile xanthogranuloma. [online] Available from www.emedicine.com/oph/topic 588.htm. [Accessed August, 2013].

⊟ 20.9. EXOPHTHALMOS (PROPTOSIS)

General

Abnormal protrusion of the eyeball. Etiology is varied and can include inflammatory, vascular or infections. Thyroid disease is the most frequent cause for both unilateral and bilateral exophthalmos.

Clinical

Thyroid disease, lymphoma, cavernous hemangiomas, leukemia, sinus disease.

Ocular

Proptosis, orbital cellulitis, orbital emphysema, lid retraction, punctate keratopathy, corneal ulcer, corneal perforation, diplopia.

Laboratory

Thyroid function studies, CT, MRI, ocular ultrasonography can all be used to determine the cause.

Treatment

Reversing the problem, which is causing the exophthalmos, is the treatment of choice and will minimize the ocular complications. Ocular lubricants are beneficial for controlling the corneal exposure.

⊟ BIBLIOGRAPHY

1. Mercandetti M, Cohen AJ. (2012). Exophthalmos. [online] Available from www.emedicine.com/oph/TOPIC616.HTM. [Accessed August, 2013].

⊟ 20.10. MORAXELLA LACUNATA

General

Gram-negative rod; causes chronic angular blepharoconjunctivitis; without treatment, may persist for months or years; normally found in flora of respiratory tract; seen more frequently in alcoholics and those with poor sanitary habits; *Moraxella* organisms produce proteases, although those are not related directly to their pathogenetic mechanism.

Ocular

Catarrhal angular conjunctivitis; corneal ulcer; hypopyon, chronic blepharitis; eczema; lateral canthal skin erythema; iridocyclitis.

Clinical

Alcoholism; impaired nutrition; dermatitis.

Laboratory

Aerobic, oxidase positive, Gram-negative diplococcus or coccobacilli morphologically indistinguishable from *Neisseria*.

Treatment

Artificial tears, cold compresses, antibiotics.

⎅ BIBLIOGRAPHY

1. Baum J, Fedukowicz HB, Jordan A. A survey of Moraxella corneal ulcers in a derelict population. Am J Ophthalmol. 1980;90:476-80.
2. Burd EM. Bacterial keratitis and conjunctivitis. In: Smolin G, Thoft RA (Eds). The Cornea. Boston: Little, Brown and Company; 1994. pp. 20-1.
3. Roy FH, Fraunfelder FW, Fraunfelder FT. Roy and Fraunfelder's Current Ocular Therapy, 6th edition. Philadelphia: WB Saunders; 2008.
4. van Bijsterveld OP. The incidence of Moraxella on mucous membranes and the skin. Am J Ophthalmol. 1972;74:72-6.

⎅ 20.12. RUBEOSIS IRIDIS

General

Neovascularization of the iris.

Clinical

None.

Ocular

Intractable type of secondary glaucoma, rubeosis iridis, diabetic retinopathy, retinal vein occlusion, carotid occlusive disease, iritis.

Laboratory

Diagnosis is made by clinical findings; check for diabetes.

Treatment

- Trabeculectomy with the antifibrotic agents, mitomycin-C and 5-fluorouracil (5-FU) is one modality. Trabeculectomy in neovascular glaucoma (NVG) has a significant failure rate. Using standard trabeculectomy (without antifibrosis), an IOP of less than 25 mm Hg on one medication or less has been reported to occur in 67–100% of patients in three studies. Using injections of 5-FU subconjunctivally in the postoperative period, the surgical success has been reported to be 68% over 3 years. Inject 0.1 mL of 5 mg/mL 5-FU subconjunctivally either superiorly above the bleb or inferiorly (just above the lower fornix). Mitomycin-C used intraoperatively has been shown to be more effective than 5-FU in routine trabeculectomies. No significant follow-up studies exist on the use of mitomycin-C with trabeculectomy in NVG.
- Valve implant surgery is another modality and is indicated when trabeculectomy fails or extensive conjunctival scarring exists, thereby preventing a standard filtering procedure. Molteno, Krupin and Ahmed valve implants commonly are used. One large series using the Krupin valve reported 79% of eyes with NVG had a 67% success rate in controlling IOP (< 24 mm Hg) with mean follow-up of 23 months. Long-term results are mixed. Using the Molteno implant, 60 eyes with NVG achieved a satisfactory IOP (< 21 mm Hg) and maintenance of visual acuity over 5 years of only 10.3%. If combined with the need for vitrectomy, consideration of pars plana tube—shunt insertion may reduce anterior segment complications.
- Avastin injections have shown some promise for the control of iris neovascularization.
- Complications include postoperative hypotony with associated complications, blockage of internal fistula, blockage of external filtration site (fibrosis of the filtering bleb) and corneal endothelial loss.

⎅ BIBLIOGRAPHY

1. Freudenthal J, Khan YA, Ahmed II, et al. (2011). Neovascular glaucoma. [online] Available from www.emedicine.com/oph/TOPIC135.HTM. [Accessed August, 2013].

20.13A. BEHÇET SYNDROME (DERMATO-STOMATO-OPHTHALMIC SYNDROME; OCULOBUCCOGENITAL SYNDROME; GILBERT SYNDROME)

General

Virus infection; occurs in adults; chronic disease; complete remission is rare; etiology is unknown.

Ocular

Muscle palsies (occasional); nystagmus (occasional); conjunctivitis; hypopyon; iritis; recurrent uveitis; keratoconjunctivitis sicca; keratitis; vitreous hemorrhages; thrombophlebitis retinal veins (occasional); retinal hemorrhages; optic neuritis (occasional); macular edema; optic nerve atrophy; retinitis; secondary glaucoma; retinal vasculitis; disk edema; panophthalmitis; optic neuropathy; skin lesions, posterior uveitis and systemic complications have been associated with loss of vision with this disorder; corneal immune ring opacity.

Clinical

Aphthous lesions of mucous membranes of the mouth and genitalia; cerebellar signs; convulsions; paraplegia; skin erythema (multiforme bullosum); arthritis; urethritis; glossitis; recurrent fever.

Laboratory

Nonspecific HLA B51 positive may help to support diagnosis.

Treatment

The goals of therapy are to suppress inflammation, to reduce the frequency and severity of recurrences, and to minimize involvement of the retina. To be effective, treatment must be started early. Extent of involvement and severity of disease determine the choice of medication. Treatment options include corticosteroids, cytotoxic agents, cyclosporine, and colchicine.

BIBLIOGRAPHY

1. Bashour M. (2012). Ophthalmologic manifestations of Behçet disease. [online] Available from www.emedicine.com/oph/TOPIC425.HTM. [Accessed August, 2013].

20.13B. DIABETES MELLITUS

General

Complex disorder of carbohydrate, lipid and protein metabolism characterized by hyperglycemia and a relative or total lack of insulin. Development is influenced by both genetic and environmental factors. Most commonly occurs in middle or late life (type II) and is seen most commonly in the obese. Diabetes can occur in the 1st or 2nd decade of life (type I) and usually involves the lack of insulin production by the pancreas and the need for insulin therapy.

Clinical

Atherosclerosis; nephropathy; neuropathy; polyuria; polydipsia; polyphagia; obesity; elevated plasma glucose and elevated glycated hemoglobin (A1C).

Ocular

Diabetic retinopathy; vitreous hemorrhage; macular edema; cataract; glaucoma; asteroid hyalosis; extraocular muscle paralysis; rubeosis iridis; corneal hypesthesia; optic nerve atrophy; papillopathy.

Laboratory

Diagnosis made by fasting plasma glucose of greater than 126 mg/dL and 2 hours post glucose load (75 g) plasma glucose of greater than 200 mg/dL and confirmed by repeat test.

Treatment

Goals include elimination of symptoms, by reduction of blood sugar and blood pressure. Smoking cessation, aspirin therapy, weight loss, exercise, diabetic diet as well as oral medication and/or insulin are all used in the treatment of diabetes. Diabetic retinopathy is most successfully treated with retinal photocoagulation. Pars plana vitrectomy is sometimes necessary to remove vitreous hemorrhage. Other ocular problems caused by diabetes such as cataracts and glaucoma are treated in traditional methods.

BIBLIOGRAPHY

1. Khardori R. (2012). Type 2 diabetes mellitus. [online] Available from emedicine.medscape.com/article/117853-overview. [Accessed August, 2013].
2. Ostri C, Lund-Andersen H, Sander B, et.al. Bilateral diabetic papillopathy and metabolic control. Ophthalmology. 2010; 117:2214-7.
3. Richter GM, Torres M, Choudhury F, et al. Risk factors for cortical, nuclear, posterior subcapsular, and mixed lens opacities: The Los Angeles Latino Eye Study. Ophthalmology. 2012;119:547-54.

20.13C. GONORRHEA

General

Caused by *Neisseria gonorrhoeae*, which is transmitted sexually.

Ocular

Conjunctivitis; eyelid edema; keratitis; uveitis.

Clinical

Pelvic inflammatory disease; arthritis; dermatitis; carditis; meningitis.

Laboratory

Gram stain smear demonstrates Gram-negative diplococci with polymorphonuclear leukocytes in conjunctival exudates.

Treatment

Therapy consists of systemic antibiotics; topical antibiotics are relatively ineffective in the treatment of eye disease. It is important to treat all sexual partners simultaneously to prevent reinfection.

BIBLIOGRAPHY

1. Wong B. (2013). Gonorrhea. [online] Available from www. emedicine.com/oph/TOPIC497.HTM. [Accessed August, 2013].

20.13D. HERPES ZOSTER

General

Caused by varicella zoster virus; about 75% of cases occur in persons over age of 45 years; condition is more frequent with advancing age and in patients who are immunocompromised by drugs or disease; in particular, an increasing number of patients with herpes zoster ophthalmicus are immunosuppressed.

Ocular

Conjunctivitis; keratitis; recurrent corneal ulcer; neuralgia; zoster rash of eyelids; uveitis; iris atrophy; scleritis; cataract; optic neuritis; paralysis of third nerve; proptosis; paralysis of lids; orbital apex syndrome; retinitis; neurotrophic keratitis; acute retinal necrosis; progressive outer retinal necrosis; ocular motor nerve pareses; tonic pupil; encephalitis; vasculitis.

Clinical

Local lesions involving the posterior or root ganglia; nerve damage; tissue scarring.

Laboratory

Diagnosed mostly on the basis of the characteristic pain and appearance of the dermatomal rashes.

Treatment

Antiviral agents, systemic corticosteroids, antidepressants, and adequate pain control. Immunocompetent adults aged 60 years or older, benefit from receipt of the herpes zoster vaccine and have a lower incidence of herpes zoster.

BIBLIOGRAPHY

1. Diaz MM, Foster CS, Walton RC, et al. (2011). Herpes zoster ophthalmicus. [online] Available from www.emedicine.com/oph/TOPIC257.HTM. [Accessed August, 2013].
2. Ghaznawi N, Virdi A, Dayan A, et al. Herpes zoster ophthalmicus: comparison of disease in patients 60 years and older versus younger than 60 years. Ophthalmology. 2011;118(11):2242-50.
3. Ho J, Xirasagar S, Lin H. Increased risk of a cancer diagnosis after herpes zoster ophthalmicus: a nationwide population-based study. Ophthalmology. 2011;118(6):1076-81.
4. Tseng HF, Smith N, Harpaz R, et al. Herpes zoster vaccine in older adults and the risk of subsequent herpes zoster disease. JAMA. 2011;305(2):160-6.

🗗 20.13D. HERPES SIMPLEX

General

Large, complex deoxyribonucleic acid (DNA) virus.

Ocular

Conjunctivitis; keratitis; iridocyclitis; corneal ulcer; uveitis; hyphema; hypopyon; iris atrophy; cataract; scleritis; dacryoadenitis; blepharitis; acute retinal necrosis.

Clinical

Recurrent skin vesicles on lids, perioral area, nose and genitalia; meningitis, encephalitis.

Laboratory

Viral cultures.

Treatment

Antiviral therapy, topical or oral, is an effective treatment of epithelial herpes infection.

🗗 BIBLIOGRAPHY

1. Liu S, Pavan-Langston D, Colby KA. Pediatric herpes simplex of the anterior segment: characteristics, treatment, and outcomes. Ophthalmology. 2012;119(10):2003-8.
2. Wang JC, Ritterband DC. (2012). Ophthalmologic manifestations of herpes simplex. [online] Available from www.emedicine.com/oph/TOPIC100.HTM. [Accessed August, 2013].

🗗 21. SPONTANEOUS HYPHEMA IN INFANTS

1. Acute rheumatoid iridocyclitis
2. Blood dyscrasias, such as anemia, leukemia, and disseminated intravascular coagulation
3. Iritis
*4. Juvenile xanthogranuloma
†5. Perinatal asphyxia
6. Persistent hyperplastic primary vitreous
7. Retinoblastoma
8. Retinoschisis
9. Retinopathy of prematurity
*†10. Trauma without history (consider child abuse)

*Indicates most frequent
†Indicates a general entry and therefore has not been described in detail in the text

🗗 BIBLIOGRAPHY

1. Appleboom T, Durso F. Retinoblastoma presenting as a total hyphema. Ann Ophthalmol. 1985;17:508-10.
2. Harley RD, Romayananda N, Chan GH. Juvenile xanthogranuloma. J Pediatr Ophthalmol Strabismus. 1982;19:33-9.

🗗 21.1. JUVENILE RHEUMATOID ARTHRITIS (JRA; STILL DISEASE)

General

Onset before age 16 years; greater occurrence of systemic manifestations, monarticular and oligoarticular joint involvement, and iridocyclitis.

Ocular

Hypopyon; band keratopathy; uveitis; cataract; papillitis; glaucoma; macular edema; ocular pain; vitreous cells; synechiae; scleritis; presumed to have an autoimmune etiology; antiocular antibodies, including iris protein antibodies, have been found in the sera of patients.

Clinical

Salmon pink macular rash; arthritis; hepatosplenomegaly; leukocytosis; chronic pain; joint swelling; low-grade fever; anemia; rheumatoid nodules.

Laboratory

Antinuclear antibody, rheumatoid factor, HLA B27, X-ray imaging of joints.

Treatment

Uveitis treated with initially with topical corticosteroids. Systemic immunomodulatory agents may be useful for patients with limited or no response to topical or systemic corticosteroids.

🗗 BIBLIOGRAPHY

1. Roque MR, Roque BL, Miserocchi E, et al. (2012). Juvenile idiopathic arthritis uveitis. [online] Available from www.emedicine.com/oph/TOPIC675.HTM. [Accessed August, 2013].
2. Thorne JE, Woreta FA, Dunn JP, et al. Risk of cataract development among children with juvenile idiopathic arthritis-related uveitis treated with topical corticosteroids. Ophthalmology. 2010;117:1436-41.

⊟ 21.2. ANEMIA

General

Ocular complications generally only seen in severe anemia.

Ocular

Palpebral conjunctival pallor; retinal hemorrhages; cotton-wool spots; retinal vein dilation; papilledema; ischemic optic neuropathy.

Clinical

Blood loss; excessive red blood cell destruction; inadequate red blood cell production; thrombocytopenia; leukemia.

Laboratory

CBC count, reticulocyte count, and review of the peripheral smear.

Treatment

Medical care consists of establishing the diagnosis and reason for the iron deficiency. In most patients, the iron deficiency should be treated with oral iron therapy, and the underlying etiology should be corrected so the deficiency does not recur.

⊟ BIBLIOGRAPHY

1. Inoue S, Lee MT. (2013). Pediatric acute anemia. [online] Available from www.emedicine.com/ped/TOPIC98.HTM. [Accessed August, 2013].

⊟ 21.2. LEUKEMIA

General

Acute or chronic blood disorder.

Ocular

Engorgement of conjunctival vessels; papillary hypertrophy; aggregations of tumor cells in conjunctiva, choroid, and orbit; secondary glaucoma; retinal venous engorgement and tortuosity with pronounced constrictions; retinal hemorrhages; retinal detachment; cotton-wool spots; macular edema; papilledema; optic atrophy; optic neuritis; paralysis of extraocular muscles; hypopyon; vitreous opacities; retinal sea fans; perilimbal subconjunctival infiltrates; corneal leukemic infiltration (rare); shallow serous retinal detachments; hyphema; iris neovascularization; CRVO; vitreous infiltrates.

Clinical

Frequent involvement of central nervous system; intracranial hemorrhage; thrombocytopenia; rising white cell count.

Laboratory

CBC and differential, bone marrow aspiration, immunophenotyping, chromosomal analysis.

Treatment

Chemotherapy with or without radiotherapy.

⊟ BIBLIOGRAPHY

1. Wu L, Evans T, Martinez J. (2012). Leukemias. [online]. Available from www.emedicine.com/oph/TOPIC489.HTM. [Accessed August, 2013].

⊟ 21.3. ANDERSEN-WARBURG SYNDROME (WHITNALL-NORMAN SYNDROME; OLIGOPHRENIA MICROPHTHALMOS SYNDROME; NORRIE DISEASE; ATROPHIA OCULI CONGENITAL FETAL IRITIS SYNDROME; CONGENITAL PROGRESSIVE OCULO-ACOUSTICO-CEREBRAL DYSPLASIA)

General

Sex-linked inheritance; gross deformation of both eyes; only males affected; onset at birth; putative gene for Norrie disease has been isolated and mapped to Xp11.3.

Ocular

Bilateral microphthalmos with extensive destruction of all ocular structures often resembling a pseudotumor; blindness at birth; iris atrophy; iritis; corneal opacification and lenticular destruction with a mass visible behind the lens as long as the lens is still clear; malformed retina and choroid with retinal pseudotumors; retinal detachment; retrolental vascular mass.

Clinical

Mental retardation ranging from imbecility to idiocy (may begin at any age) in about two-thirds of the cases; deafness of differing severity with onset between ages 9 and 45 years.

Laboratory

Diagnosis is made by clinical findings.

Treatment

Topical treatment for iritis; retinal detachment surgery and vitrectomy may be necessary. Immediate laser treatment is recommended following birth.

⊟ BIBLIOGRAPHY

1. Andersen SR, Warburg M. Norrie's disease: congenital bilateral pseudotumor of the retina with recessive X-chromosomal inheritance; Preliminary Report. Arch Ophthalmol. 1961;66(5):614-8.
2. Black G, Redmond RM. The molecular biology of Norrie's disease. Eye (Lond). 1994;8(5):491-6.
3. Chow CC, Kiernam DF, Chau FY, et al. Laser photocoagulation at birth prevents blindness in Norrie's disease diagnosed using amniocentesis. Ophthalmology. 2010;117(12):2402-6.
4. Enyedi LB, de Juan E, Gaitan A. Ultrastructural study of Norrie's disease. Am J Ophthalmol. l991;111(4):439-45.
5. Liberfarb RM, Eavey RD, De Long GR, et al. Norrie's disease: a study of two families. Ophthalmology. 1985;92(10):1445-51.
6. Norrie G. Causes of blindness in children; Twenty-five years' experience of Danish institutes for the blind. Acta Ophthalmologica. 1927;5(1-3):357-86.
7. Warburg M. Norrie's disease: differential diagnosis and treatment. Acta Ophthalmologica. 1975;53(2):217-36.
8. Wong F, Goldberg MF, Hao Y. Identification of a nonsense mutation at codon 128 of the Norrie's disease gene in a male infant. Arch Ophthalmol. 1993;111(11):1553-7.

⊟ 21.4. JUVENILE XANTHOGRANULOMA (JXG; NEVOXANTHOENDOTHELIOMA)

General

Childhood disease; unknown etiology.

Ocular

Uveal tract tumor presenting as spontaneous hyphema; secondary glaucoma; uveitis; corneal, lid, and epibulbar tumors; proptosis; retinal and choroidal lesions (rare).

Clinical

Multiple benign tumors, primarily of the skin; usually appear in the first 3 years of life; lesions appear as yellow-to-brown papules or nodules.

Laboratory

Diagnostic techniques include biomicroscopy, high frequency ultrasound and cytologic examination of anterior chamber paracentesis material.

Treatment

Topical, subconjunctival, intralesional, and systemic corticosteroids are useful. Low-dose radiation may be the treatment of choice for diffuse uveal lesions. Glaucoma medications should be used in the setting of hyphema and increased IOP.

BIBLIOGRAPHY

1. Curtis T, Wheeler DT. (2012). Juvenile xanthogranuloma. [online] Available from www.emedicine.com/oph/topic588.htm. [Accessed August, 2013].

21.6. PERSISTENT HYPERPLASTIC PRIMARY VITREOUS (PHPV, PERSISTENT FETAL VASCULATURE)

General

Congenital ocular disorder with the potential to affect the eye's anterior and posterior anatomy. Usually only affects one eye.

Clinical

Systemic abnormalities may include polydactyly, microcephaly, and cleft palate and lip as well as central nervous system abnormalities.

Ocular

Anterior PHPV includes engorged radial iris vessels, microcornea, Mittendorf dot, elongated ciliary processes, micro-ophthalmia, cataract.

Laboratory

Diagnosis is made by clinical findings.

Treatment

Monocular congenital cataract surgery and amblyopia therapy. Posterior transciliary for pars plana vitrectomy and removal of tissue.

BIBLIOGRAPHY

1. Roy FH, Fraunfelder FW, Fraunfelder FT. Roy and Fraunfelder's Current Ocular Therapy, 6th edition. London; Elsevier; 2008.

21.7. RETINOBLASTOMA

General

Malignant tumor arising in one or both retinas of young children, usually under the age of 2 years; usually unilateral; autosomal dominant; most common intraocular malignancy of childhood; incidence is one in 20,000 live births; origin is questionably neuroectodermal cells capable of multipotentiality; one third of patients have heritable (bilateral or have a positive family history) autosomal dominant and two thirds are sporadic; genetic transmission obeys two-mutation hypothesis of Knudson; trilateral retinoblastoma is bilateral retinoblastoma plus midline central nervous system tumor (most commonly pinealoma); most common second tumor is an osteogenic sarcoma (begins in 2nd decade).

Ocular

Hyphema; hypopyon; corneal tumor; lid edema; endophthalmitis; exophthalmos; intraocular calcification of globe; heterochromia; neovascularization of iris or retina; papilledema; panophthalmitis; retinoblastoma extension into orbit and choroid; cat's-eye reflex; leukocoria; mydriasis; vitreous hemorrhage tumor seeding; esotropia; exotropia; glaucoma; visual loss.

Clinical

Metastasis into the lymph system, bone marrow, and subarachnoid space; basal meningitis; death.

Laboratory

CT—calcification of lesion hallmark of disease; ultrasound—demonstrates calcification and MRI demonstrates presence and extent of extraocular disease.

Treatment

External beam radiation therapy is recommended on patients with significant vitreous seeding. Radioactive isotope plaques and chemotherapy are also an option. Removal of the tumor is the standard management for retinoblastoma.

BIBLIOGRAPHY

1. Isidro MA, Roque MR, Aaberg TM, et al. (2012). Retinoblastoma. [online] Available from www.emedicine.com/oph/TOPIC346.HTM. [Accessed August, 2013].

21.8. RETINOSCHISIS (RS)

General

Sex-linked; may not manifest until middle life.

Ocular

Intraretinal splitting due to degeneration or detachment of retina; retinal atrophy with sclerosis of the choroid; cystic maculopathy.

Clinical

None.

Laboratory

Optical coherence tomography provides high resolution of the macula region. Fluorescein angiography, ICGA and ERG are helpful tools in finding a diagnosis.

Treatment

No treatment is available.

BIBLIOGRAPHY

1. Small KW, McLellan CM, Song MK. (2012). Juvenile retinoschisis. [online] Available from www.emedicine.com/oph/TOPIC639.HTM. [Accessed August, 2013].

21.9. RETROLENTAL FIBROPLASIA (RLF; RETINOPATHY OF PREMATURITY)

General

Bilateral disease seen primarily in premature infants with immature retinal vessels; excessive use of oxygen is responsible for the majority of cases, but disease is seen despite oxygen restrictions or even when no oxygen supplementation is used; known factors that correlate with degrees of retinopathy of prematurity are low birth weight, short gestational age, length of time with supplemental oxygen, length of time on a mechanical ventilator; role of excessive light in newborn nurseries also has been proposed.

Ocular

Anterior or posterior synechiae; neovascularization of iris; pallor of optic disk; dragged disk; attenuated vessels; retinal detachment; dilation of veins; retinal folds; retinal hemorrhage; retrolental mass; vascular tortuosity; vasoconstriction of retina; retinal pigmentary changes; vitreous haze; vitreous traction; vitreous hemorrhages; cataract; glaucoma; leukocoria; myopia; shallow anterior chamber; opaque retrolental membrane; ciliary body drawn anteriorly; ciliary process around dilated pupil; absent pupillary reflexes; keratoconus; associated strabismus; amblyopia.

Clinical

Low birth weight; prematurity.

Laboratory

Diagnosis is made by clinical findings.

Treatment

Cryotherapy and laser surgery can be effective. Vitrectomy may be necessary.

BIBLIOGRAPHY

1. Bashour M, Menassa J, Gerontis CC. (2013). Retinopathy of prematurity. [online] Available from www.emedicine.com/oph/TOPIC413.HTM. [Accessed August, 2013].

⎙ 22. TOXIC LENS SYNDROME (TOXIC ANTERIOR SEGMENT SYNDROME; TASS)

General

Syndrome occurs within a few days to several weeks of implantation of an intraocular lens; with therapy, vision is restored in the majority of cases; increased incidence of disease caused by use of ethylene oxide sterilization (dry pack intraocular lenses); toxic lens syndrome may be prevented by treating the lens with sodium hydroxide and by using modem lathe-cut or compression-molded lenses with polypropylene loops; risk factors include uveitis in history, pseudoexfoliation syndrome, inadequate mydriasis at the start of surgery, problems with intraocular lens implantation, and pigment effusion during surgery.

Ocular

Pigment precipitation on the surface of an intraocular lens; hypopyon; vitreous opacification; chronic uveitis; secondary glaucoma.

Clinical

None.

Laboratory

Anterior chamber aspiration, vitreous tap, and/or vitreous biopsy for Gram stain and microbiologic cultures.

Treatment

Topical steroids and NSAIDs; patients should be evaluated the same or the next day to rule out infectious endophthalmitis, in which case, steroids would worsen the condition.

⎙ BIBLIOGRAPHY

1. Al-Ghoul AR, Charukamnoetkanok P, Dhaliwal DK. (2012). Toxic Anterior Segment Syndrome. [online] Available from www.emedicine.com/oph/TOPIC779.HTM. [Accessed August, 2013].

⎙ 23. WHITE MASS IN ANTERIOR CHAMBER

1. Endophthalmitis
2. Ocular aspergillosis
†3. Sterile inflammation following surgery or trauma
†4. Tumor

---

†Indicates a general entry and therefore has not been described in detail in the text

⎙ BIBLIOGRAPHY

1. Katz G, Winchester K, Lam S. Ocular aspergillosis isolated in the anterior chamber. Ophthalmology. 1993;100:1815-8.

⎙ 23.1. BACTERIAL ENDOPHTHALMITIS

General

Rare, intraocular bactria infection which can follow intraocular surgery or penetrating injury.

Clinical

None.

Ocular

Photophobia, pain, hypopyon, decreased vision.

Laboratory

Vitreous and anterior chamber specimens to determine organism.

Treatment

Systemic steroids, topical, intravitreal and subconjunctival antibiotics and vitrectomy.

⎙ BIBLIOGRAPHY

1. Graham RH. (2012). Bacterial endophthalmitis. [online] Available from www.emedicine.com/oph/TOPIC393.HTM. [Accessed August, 2013].

23.2. ASPERGILLOSIS

General

Systemic infection common in poultry farmers, feeders or breeders of pigeons, and persons who work with grains; should be considered in immunocompromised patients.

Ocular

Corneal ulcer; blepharitis; keratitis; scleritis; endophthalmitis; exophthalmos; retinal hemorrhages; retinal detachment; vitreitis; cataract; conjunctivitis; orbital cellulitis; paresis of extraocular muscles; secondary glaucoma; scleromalacia perforans; endogenous endophthalmitis; anterior chamber mass; invasion of choroid and anterior optic nerve.

Clinical

Pulmonary infections; invasive fungal disease.

Laboratory

Culture from superficial scrapings from bed of infection.

Treatment

Voriconazole is the drug of choice. Although disease outcomes substantially improve with antifungal treatment, patient survival and infection resolution depend on improved immunosuppression.

BIBLIOGRAPHY

1. Batra V. (2011). Pediatric Aspergillosis. [online] Available from www.emedicine.com/ped/TOPIC148.HTM. [Accessed August, 2013].

CHAPTER
17

Choroid

🗗 1. ANGIOID STREAKS

Angioid streaks are ruptures of Bruch membrane characterized ophthalmoscopically by brownish lines surrounding the disk and radiating toward the periphery.

†1. AC hemoglobinopathy

2. Acanthocytosis (abetalipoproteinemia, Bassen-Kornzweig syndrome)

†3. Acromegaly

†4. Acquired hemolytic anemia

5. Beta thalassemia minor

†6. Calcinosis

7. Chronic congenital idiopathic hyperphosphatemia

†8. Chronic familial hyperphosphatemia

†9. Cardiovascular disease with hypertension

†10. Cooley anemia

†11. Diffuse lipomatosis

†12. Dwarfism

†13. Epilepsy

†14. Facial angiomatosis

15. Fibrodysplasia hyperelastica (Ehlers-Danlos syndrome)

16. François dyscephalic syndrome (Hallermann-Streiff syndrome)

17. Hemochromatosis

18. Hereditary spherocytosis

†19. Hypercalcinosis

20. Idiopathic thrombocytic purpura

21. Lead poisoning

†22. Myopia

23. Neurofibromatosis

24. Ocular melanocytosis

25. Optic disk drusen

26. Osteitis deformans (Paget disease)

†27. Pituitary tumor

28. Previous choroidal detachment

*29. Pseudoxanthoma elasticum (Grönblad-Strandberg syndrome)

†30. Senile (actinic) elastosis of the skin

31. Sickle cell disease (Herrick syndrome)

32. Sturge-Weber syndrome

†33. Trauma

34. Tuberous sclerosis

†35. Thrombocytopenic purpura

🗗 BIBLIOGRAPHY

1. Aessopos A, Voskaridou E, Kavouklis E, et al. Angioid streaks in Sickle-thalassemia. Am J Ophthalmol. 1994;117:589-92.

2. Mansour AM. Is there an association between optic disc drusen and angioid streaks? Graefes Arch Clin Exp Ophthalmol. 1992;230:595-6.

3. Roy FH. Ocular Syndromes and Systemic Diseases, 5th edition. New Delhi: Jaypee Brothers Medical Publishers; 2013.

*Indicates most frequent
†Indicates a general entry and therefore has not been described in detail in the text

1.2. BASSEN-KORNZWEIG SYNDROME (ABETALIPOPROTEINEMIA; ACANTHOCYTOSIS; FAMILIAL HYPOLIPOPROTEINEMIA)

General

Inability to absorb and transport lipids; predominant in males; autosomal recessive inheritance; acanthocytosis, a peculiar burr cell malformation of the red blood cells; the basic defect is thought to be an inability to synthesize the apolipoprotein B peptide of low-density and very-low-density lipoproteins.

Ocular

Ptosis (may be present); nystagmus; progressive external ophthalmoplegia; retinitis pigmentosa (usually atypical); retinopathy develops with age after 10–14 years; optic atrophy occasionally; epicanthal folds; cataract; optic nerve pallor; hypopigmentation of retina; macular degeneration; dyschromatopsia.

Clinical

Steatorrhea; hypocholesterolemia; neurologic disorder with ataxia (similar to Friedreich ataxia); areflexia; Babinski sign; muscle weakness (facial, lingual; proximal and distal); slurred speech; lordosis; kyphosis.

Laboratory

Most patients will exhibit acanthocytosis on peripheral blood smear.

Treatment

Medical care is symptomatic and supportive.

BIBLIOGRAPHY

1. Van Gross K, Lorenzo N. (2012). Neuroacanthocytosis syndromes. [online] Available from www.emedicine.com/neuro/TOPIC502.HTM. [Accessed August, 2013].

1.5. COOLEY ANEMIA (THALASSEMIA; THALASSEMIA MAJOR; THALASSEMIA MINOR)

General

Autosomal dominant in synthesis of α or β chain of hemoglobin; most prevalent in Mediterranean and Oriental populations.

Ocular

Retinal hemorrhages; angioid streaks; macular vascular abnormalities; pigmented chorioretinal scars (black sunbursts); occlusion of peripheral retinal arteries; vitreous hemorrhages.

Clinical

Hemolytic anemia; hypochromic anemia.

Laboratory

Blood—hypochromic, microcystic anemia.

Treatment

Goals of medical therapy are correction of anemia, suppression of erythropoiesis, and inhibition of increased gastrointestinal (GI) iron.

BIBLIOGRAPHY

1. Takeshita K. (2012). Beta thalassemia. [online] Available from www.emedicine.com/med/TOPIC438.HTM. [Accessed August, 2013].

1.7. PAGET DISEASE (OSTEITIS DEFORMANS; CONGENITAL HYPERPHOS-PHATEMIA; HYPEROSTOSIS CORTICALIS DEFORMANS; POZZI SYNDROME; CHRONIC CONGENITAL IDIOPATHIC HYPERPHOSPHATEMIA; OSTEOCHALASIS DESMALIS FAMILIARIS; FAMILIAL OSTEOECTASIA)

General

Autosomal dominant; more frequent in men, but more severe in women; onset after age of 40 years; characterized by diffuse cortical thickening of involved bones with osteoporosis, bowing deformities and shortening of stature; osteogenic sarcoma not infrequent.

Ocular

Shallow orbits with progressive unilateral or bilateral proptosis palsy of extraocular muscles; corneal ring opacities; cataract; retinal hemorrhages; pigmentary retinopathy; macular changes resembling Kuhnt-Junius degeneration; angioid streaks; papilledema; optic nerve atrophy; blue sclera; exophthalmos.

Clinical

Skull deformities; kyphoscoliosis; hypertension and arteriosclerosis; muscle weakness; waddling gait; hearing impairment; osteoarthritis.

Laboratory

Bone-specific alkaline phosphatase (BSAP) levels, radiographs may demonstrate both osteolysis and excessive bone formation. Bone biopsies may be necessary for diagnostic purposes in rare cases.

Treatment

Medical therapy for Paget disease should include bisphosphonate treatment with serial monitoring of bone markers. Nonsteroidal anti-inflammatory drugs and acetaminophen may be effective for pain management. Chemotherapy, radiation, or both may be used to treat neoplasms arising from pagetic bone.

BIBLIOGRAPHY

1. Lohr KM, Driver K. (2011). Paget disease. [online] Available from emedicine.medscape.com/article/334607-overview. [Accessed August, 2013].

1.15. EHLERS-DANLOS SYNDROME (FIBRODYSPLASIA ELASTICA GENERALISATA; CUTIS HYPERELASTICA; MEEKEREN-EHLERS-DANLOS SYNDROME; INDIAN RUBBER MAN SYNDROME; CUTIS LAXA)

General

Present at birth; autosomal dominant; two groups: cutaneous and articular; syndrome is one of the three primary disorders of elastic tissue [other two disorders are pseudoxanthoma elasticum (Grönblad-Strandberg syndrome) and senile elastosis]; inherited disorder of collagen biosynthesis.

Ocular

Hyperelasticity of palpebral skin; easy eversion of upper lid; ptosis; epicanthal folds; hypotony of extraocular muscles; strabismus; microcornea; thinning of cornea with keratoconus; thinning of sclera (blue sclera); subluxation of lens; angioid streaks; chorioretinal hemorrhages; retinitis proliferans with secondary detachment; macular degeneration; myopia; ruptured globe after minor trauma; limbus-to-limbus corneal thinning; acute hydrops; cornea plana; keratoglobus.

Clinical

Cutaneous manifestations include thin, atrophic, fragile skin, cutaneous hyperelasticity and pseudomolluscoid tumors; articular manifestations include excessive articular laxity and luxations; hypermobile joints.

Laboratory

Biochemical studies can detect alterations in collagen molecules in cultured skin fibroblasts. Molecular [deoxyribonucleic acid (DNA)]-based testing is available. Diagnosis may by urinary analyte assay and clinical examination is the most common.

Treatment

Ascorbic acid therapy; in the event of skin lacerations seriously consider alternatives to sutures, including adhesive strips and wound glues; monitor for cardiac conditions and scoliosis.

⊞ BIBLIOGRAPHY

1. Steiner RD. (2011). Genetics of Ehlers-Danlos syndrome. [online] Available from www.emedicine.com/ped/TOPIC654.HTM. [Accessed January, 2013].

⊞ 1.16. HALLERMANN-STREIFF SYNDROME [DYSCEPHALIC-MANDIBULO-OCULO-FACIAL SYNDROME; OCULO-MANDIBULO-DYSCEPHALY; ULLRICH-FREMERY-DOHNA SYNDROME; FRANCOIS DYSCEPHALIC SYNDROME; MANDIBULO-OCULO-FACIAL DYSCEPHALY SYNDROME; FRANCOIS-HALLERMANN-STREIFF SYNDROME; HALLERMANN-STREIFF-FRANCOIS SYNDROME; AUDRY I SYNDROME; DOHNA SYNDROME; FRANCOIS SYNDROME (1); DYSCEPHALY- TEETH ABNORMALITY-DWARFISM; DYSCEPHALIA OCULOMANDIBULARIS-HYPOTRICHOSIS; MANDIBULO-OCULAR DYSCEPHALIA HYPOTRICHOSIS; FREMERY-DOHNA SYNDROME; OCULO-MANDIBULO-FACIAL DYSCEPHALY]

General

Rare; familial occurrence and consanguinity; males and females equally affected.

Ocular

Microphthalmos (bilateral); proptosis; nystagmus; strabismus; cataracts; bilateral optic atrophy; coloboma of optic disk, choroid, and iris; keratoglobus; microcornea; anti-Mongoloid slant; iris atrophy; uveitis; blue sclera; persistent pupillary membrane; secondary glaucoma.

Clinical

Malformations of skull (brachycephaly), facial skeleton, and jaws; erupted teeth at birth; diminished hair growth; hyperextensibility of joints; short stature; skin atrophy; mental deficiency; predisposition to upper airway compromise; obstructive sleep apnea.

Laboratory

Clinical.

Treatment

- *Cataract:* Change in glasses can sometimes improve a patient's visual function temporarily; however the most common treatment is cataract surgery.
- *Strabismus:* Equalized vision with correct refractive error; surgery may be helpful in patient with diplopia.
- *Uveitis:* Topical steroids and cycloplegic medication should be the initial treatment of choice. Oral steroids if not responsive to topical steroids, immunosuppressants if bilateral disease that does not respond to oral steroids, periocular steroids for unilateral or posterior uveitis. Vitrectomy can be used for severe vitreous opacification. Cryotherapy and laser photocoagulation may be used for localized pars plana exudates.
- *Glaucoma:* Glaucoma medication should be the first plan of action. If medication is unsuccessful, a filtering surgical procedure with or without antimetabotites may be beneficial.

⊞ BIBLIOGRAPHY

1. Francois J, Victoria-Troncoso V. Francois' dyscephalic syndrome and skin manifestations. Ophthalmologica. 1981;183:63-7.
2. Hallermann W. Vogelgesicht und Cataracta Congenita. Klin Monatsbl Augenheilkd. 1948;113:315.
3. Ronen S, Rozenmann Y, Isaacson M, et al. The early management of baby with Hallermann-Streiff-Francois syndrome. J Pediatr Ophthalmol Strabismus. 1979;16:119-21.
4. Roy FH, Fraunfelder FW, Fraunfelder FT. Roy and Fraunfelder's Current Ocular Therapy, 6th edition. Philadelphia: WB Saunders; 2008.
5. Spaepen A, Schrander-Stumpel C, Fryns JP, et al. Hallermann-Streiff syndrome: Clinical and psychological findings in children. Nosologic overlap with oculodentodigital dysplasia? Am J Med Genet. 1991;41:517-20.
6. Streiff EB. Dysmorphic Mandibulo-faciale (Tete d'Oiseau) et Alterations Oculaires. Ophthalmologica (Basel). 1950;120:79-83.

🗗 1.17. HEMOCHROMATOSIS

General

Iron metabolism disorder; genetically determined, but mode of inheritance is unknown; male preponderance 10:1; inheritance is autosomal recessive.

Ocular

Eyelid hyperpigmentation; diabetic retinopathy.

Clinical

Hemosiderin pigment deposition in many tissues; diabetes mellitus; cutaneous hyperpigmentation; cirrhosis of the liver; hypermelanotic pigmentation of skin; heart failure.

Laboratory

Detect iron metabolism defect.

Treatment

Diabetic retinopathy—glucose control with diet, exercise and medication, daily dose of aspirin (650 mg), laser photocoagulation, intravitreal injections of triamcinolone, Avastin and Lucentis can be used. The use of Avastin and Lucentis is off label. Vitrectomy and cryotherapy may also be necessary.

🗗 BIBLIOGRAPHY

1. Duchini A, Sfeir HE, Klachko DM. (2013). Hemochromatosis. [online] Available from www.emedicine.com/med/TOPIC975.HTM. [Accessed August, 2013].

🗗 1.18. CONGENITAL SPHEROCYTIC ANEMIA (CONGENITAL HEMOLYTIC JAUNDICE; HEREDITARY SPHEROCYTOSIS)

General

Hereditary deficiency of erythrocyte glucose-6-phosphate after exposure to certain drugs, chemicals, and foods such as fava beans.

Ocular

Congenital cataract; ring-shaped pigmentary deposits of cornea; tortuosity of retinal vessels; mongoloid palpebral aperture; microphthalmos.

Clinical

Leukemia; anemia.

Laboratory

The most sensitive test is the incubated osmotic fragility test performed after incubating RBCs for 18–24 hours under sterile conditions.

Treatment

The treatment involves presplenectomy care, splenectomy, and postsplenectomy complications.

🗗 BIBLIOGRAPHY

1. Gonzalez G, Eichner ER. (2012). Hereditary spherocytosis. [online] Available from www.emedicine.com/med/TOPIC2147.HTM. [Accessed August, 2013].

🗗 1.20. KASABACH-MERRITT SYNDROME (CAPILLARY ANGIOMA-THROMBOCYTOPENIA; HEMANGIOMA-THROMBOCYTOPENIA; THROMBOCYTOPENIA PURPURA-HEMANGIOMA)

General

Angioma causing sequestration of platelets and platelet deficiency.

Ocular

Capillary hemangiomas of the orbit; retinal detachments.

Clinical

Extraorbital hemangiomas found on trunk, extremities, and palate or in subglottic space; thrombocytopenia; found in infants; purpura and bleeding.

Laboratory

B-scan ultrasound, CT and MRI.

Treatment

Corticosteroids topical, injectable and systemic is the treatment of choice. Interferon α-2a has emerged as a new modality; laser surgery and incisional surgical techniques may be necessary.

BIBLIOGRAPHY

1. Seiff S. Zwick OM, DeAngelis DD, et al. (2011). Capillary Hemangioma. [online] Available from www.emedicine.com/oph/TOPIC691.HTM. [Accessed January, 2013].

1.21. LEAD POISONING

General

Now rare and mostly of industrial origin; cumulative poisoning; excreted slowly; absorption slow by any route; prolonged exposure required for development of symptoms; acute poisoning virtually nonexistent.

Ocular

Sclerosis and obliteration of choroidal vessels; retinal arterial spasms; retrobulbar neuritis; papilledema; optic atrophy; cortical blindness; divergence palsy; papillary paralysis; bilateral abducens paralysis; accommodative palsy; mechanism of ocular pathology with this condition is not well defined, although there is evidence pointing to the level of cyclic adenosine monophosphate.

Clinical

Loss of appetite; weight loss; colic; constipation; insomnia; headache; dizziness; irritability; moderate hypertension; albuminuria; anemia; blue line edge of gum; encephalopathy; peripheral neuropathy leading to paralysis; convulsions; mania; coma.

Laboratory

Whole blood lead level, radiograph of the abdomen.

Treatment

Eliminating the source of lead exposure is the treatment of choice. Chelation is used only when lead level does not drop fast enough or far enough or when the lead level is in the potentially encephalopathogenic level.

BIBLIOGRAPHY

1. Marcus S. (2013). Emergent management of lead toxicity. [online] Available from www.emedicine.com/emerg/TOPIC293.HTM. [Accessed August, 2013].

1.23. VON RECKLINGHAUSEN SYNDROME (NEUROFIBROMATOSIS TYPE I; NEURINOMATOSIS)

General

Dominant inheritance activated at puberty, during pregnancy and at menopause; strong evidence supports the existence of neurofibromatosis type I (NF-I) as a tumor suppressor gene.

Ocular

Proptosis; displacement of the globe; pulsation of the globe; ptosis; elephantiasis of the lids; pigment spots on lids; hydrophthalmos; nodular swelling of corneal nerves; cataracts; optic atrophy; choroidal melanoma; neurofibroma of the choroid, iris, eyelid and ciliary body; enlarged optic foramen; underdevelopment of orbital bones; café-au-lait spots on fundus; hamartoma of retina; congenital glaucoma; focal iris nodules; choroidal nevi; optic nerve gliomas; orbital neurofibroma; keratoconus.

Clinical

Café-au-lait skin pigmentations; fibroma molluscum; lipomas and sebaceous adenomas; schwannomas; growth abnormalities; spontaneous fractures; facial hemihypertrophy.

Laboratory

T2-weighted magnetic resonance imaging (MRI) images demonstrate multiple bright lesions in the basal ganglia, cerebellum, and brain in 80% optic nerve gliomas often develop perineural arachnoidal hyperplasia, which appears as an expanded cerebrospinal fluid (CSF) space around the nerve.

Treatment

Oral ketotifen may reduce the pain, tenderness and itchiness associated with neurofibromas.

⊟ BIBLIOGRAPHY

1. Dahl AA. (2011). Ophthalmologic manifestations of neurofibromatosis type. [online] Available from www.emedicine.com/oph/TOPIC338.HTM. [Accessed August, 2013].

⊟ 1.24. CONJUNCTIVAL MELANOTIC LESIONS (CONJUNCTIVAL NEVUS, CONJUNCTIVAL JUNCIONAL NEVUS, SUBEPITHELIAL NEVUS, COMPOUND NEVUS, BLUE NEVUS, MELANOSIS OCULI, CONJUNCTIVAL MELANOSIS, EPITHELIAL NELANOSIS, RACIAL MELANOSIS, SUB-EPITHELIAL MELANOCYTOSIS, CONGENITAL MELANOCYTOSIS, PRIMARY ACQUIRED MELANOSIS, MALIGNANT MELANOMA, CONJUNCTIVAL MELANOMA, CONJUNCTIVAL MALIGNANT MELANOMA)

General

Conjunctival lesions may be melanocytic or nonmelanocytic.

Clinical

None.

Ocular

Conjunctival lesion.

Laboratory

Photographic documentation and biopsy.

Treatment

Complete excision, with tumor-free margins of primary acquired melanosis with atypia. Cryotherapy, radiotherapy, topical mitomycin C or carbon dioxide CO_2 laser are useful adjunctive therapies.

⊟ BIBLIOGRAPHY

1. Roque MR, Roque BL, Foster CS. (2011). Conjunctival melanoma. [online] Available from www.emedicine.com/oph/TOPIC110.HTM. [Accessed January, 2013].

⊟ 1.25. PSEUDOPAPILLEDEMA (OPTIC NERVE HEAD DRUSEN)

General

Autosomal dominant; incidence in males and females is approximately the same; two thirds of the cases are bilateral; visual acuity is usually unaffected; it may cause slowly progressive visual field defect.

Ocular

Elevation of optic disk; drusen; injected conjunctiva; associated with retinitis pigmentosa, subretinal pigment epithelium hemorrhages (rare).

Clinical

None.

Laboratory

B-scan ultrasonography, fluorescein angiography.

Treatment

No treatment is needed for most causes of pseudopapilledema because they represent normal physiologic variants.

⊟ BIBLIOGRAPHY

1. Gossman MV, Giovannini J. (2011). Pseudopapilledema. [online] Available from www.emedicine.com/oph/TOPIC615.HTM. [Accessed January, 2013].

1.26. PAGET DISEASE (OSTEITIS DEFORMANS; CONGENITAL HYPERPHOS-PHATEMIA; HYPEROSTOSIS CORTICALIS DEFORMANS; POZZI SYNDROME; CHRONIC CONGENITAL IDIOPATHIC HYPERPHOSPHATEMIA; OSTEOCHALASIS DESMALIS FAMILIARIS; FAMILIAL OSTEOECTASIA)

General

Autosomal dominant; more frequent in men, but more severe in women; onset after age of 40 years; characterized by diffuse cortical thickening of involved bones with osteoporosis, bowing deformities and shortening of stature; osteogenic sarcoma not infrequent.

Ocular

Shallow orbits with progressive unilateral or bilateral proptosis palsy of extraocular muscles; corneal ring opacities; cataract; retinal hemorrhages; pigmentary retinopathy; macular changes resembling Kuhnt-Junius degeneration; angioid streaks; papilledema; optic nerve atrophy; blue sclera; exophthalmos.

Clinical

Skull deformities; kyphoscoliosis; hypertension and arteriosclerosis; muscle weakness; waddling gait; hearing impairment; osteoarthritis.

Laboratory

Bone-specific alkaline phosphatase (BSAP) levels, radiographs may demonstrate both osteolysis and excessive bone formation. Bone biopsies may be necessary for diagnostic purposes in rare cases.

Treatment

Medical therapy for Paget disease should include bisphosphonate treatment with serial monitoring of bone markers. Nonsteroidal anti-inflammatory drugs and acetaminophen may be effective for pain management. Chemotherapy, radiation, or both may be used to treat neoplasms arising from pagetic bone.

BIBLIOGRAPHY

1. Lohr KM, Driver K. (2011). Paget disease. [online] Available from emedicine.medscape.com/article/334607-overview. [Accessed February, 2013].

1.28. CHOROIDAL DETACHMENT (CILIOCHOROIDAL DETACHMENT)

General

Separation of the choroid and sclera created by a fluid accumulation between the two layers.

Clinical

Sturge-Weber syndrome, Vogt-Koyanagi-Harada syndrome.

Ocular

Scleritis, choriditis, orbital pseudotumor.

Laboratory

Diagnosis is made by clinical findings.

Treatment

Topical use of cycloplegic/mydriatic drops in addition to topical steroids when necessary.

BIBLIOGRAPHY

1. Traverso CE. (2012). Choroidal Detachment. [online] Available from www.emedicine.com/oph/TOPIC63.HTM. [Accessed August, 2013].

1.29. GRÖNBLAD-STRANDBERG SYNDROME (SYSTEMIC ELASTODYSTROPHY; PSEUDOXANTHOMA ELASTICUM; ELASTORRHEXIS; DARIER-GRÖNBLAD-STRANDBERG SYNDROME)

General

Autosomal recessive; female-to-male ratio of 2:1; inheritance is usually autosomal recessive, but it also has reported as autosomal dominant.

Ocular

"Angioid streaks" of the retina; macular hemorrhages and transudates not infrequent; choroidal sclerosis; retinal detachment; keratoconus; cataract; paralysis of extraocular muscles [secondary to vascular lesions of central nervous system (CNS)]; subluxation of lens; exophthalmos; optic atrophy; vitreous hemorrhages; Salmon spot multiple atrophic peripheral retinal pigment epithelium (RPE) lesions; reticular pigment dystrophy of the macula; optic disk drusen; multiple small crystalline bodies associated with atrophic RPE changes.

Clinical

Pseudoxanthoma elasticum with thickening, softening, and relaxation of the skin; skin changes are symmetrical in skin folds near large joints (axilla, elbow, inguinal region, lower abdomen, neck); flattening of the pulse curve and peripheral vascular disturbances; gastrointestinal hemorrhages.

Laboratory

Characteristic skin and retinal findings. Fluorescein angiography is done to detect angioid streaks and choroidal neovascular membranes.

Treatment

Dietary calcium and phosphorus restriction to minimum daily requirement levels has shown arrest in progression of the disease.

BIBLIOGRAPHY

1. Dahl AA, Calonje D, El-Harazi SM. (2012). Ophthalmologic manifestations of pseudoxanthoma elasticum. [online] Available from www.emedicine.com/oph/TOPIC475.HTM. [Accessed December, 2012].

1.31. HERRICK SYNDROME (DRESBACH SYNDROME; SICKLE CELL DISEASE; DREPANOCYTIC ANEMIA)

General

Usually occurs in members of the black race; poor prognosis.

Ocular

Secondary glaucoma; telangiectasis of conjunctival vessels; scleral icterus; vitreous hemorrhages; cataract; retinal hemorrhages, exudates, and neovascularization; retinitis proliferans; microaneurysms; thrombosis of retinal venules; retinal vascular sheathing; central vein occlusion; angioid streaks; retinopathy with "black sunburst sign" in patients with SS hemoglobin; "sea fan sign" in patients with SC hemoglobin; comma signs of conjunctiva; fan-shaped neovascularization of iris; sector ischemic atrophy of iris; optic atrophy; white cotton mass of vitreous; retinal holes; color vision defects; central retinal artery obstruction; branch retinal artery obstruction; white without pressure; venous tortuosity; sickling maculopathy.

Clinical

Severe anemia with hemolytic crises; bone and joint aches; hemarthrosis; jaundice; hepatosplenomegaly.

Laboratory

Blood-sickling of red blood cells, newborn screening for hemoglobin disorders.

Treatment

Transfusion is required in an aplastic crisis. Erythrocytapheresis is an automated red-cell exchange and bone marrow transplantation may be useful. Pain is the hallmark of sickle cell disease. While frequency and severity vary greatly, most patients have interval symptoms. Once pain has begun, no therapy reverses the process. Analgesics may provide a reasonable degree of comfort. While certain dosing guidelines are available, the amount of drug given should be titrated to the degree of pain experienced. Vitrectomy may be necessary.

BIBLIOGRAPHY

1. Maakaron JE, Taher AT. (2013). Sickle cell anemia. [online] Available from www.emedicine.com/ped/TOPIC2096.HTM. [Accessed August, 2013].

1.32. STURGE-WEBER SYNDROME (MENINGOCUTANEOUS SYNDROME; VASCULAR ENCEPHALOTRIGEMINAL SYNDROME; NEURO-OCULOCUTANEOUS ANGIOMATOSIS; ENCEPHALOFACIAL ANGIOMATOSIS; ENCEPHALOTRIGEMINAL SYNDROME)

General

Trisomy 22 or partial trisomy inheritance. Variations include Jahnke syndrome (neuro-oculocutaneous angiomatosis without glaucoma), Schirmer syndrome (oculocutaneous angiomatosis with early glaucoma), Lawford syndrome (oculocutaneous angiomatosis with late glaucoma and no increase in volume of globe) and Mille syndrome (oculocutaneous syndrome with choroidal angioma but no glaucoma).

Ocular

Unilateral hydrophthalmos; secondary glaucoma (late) conjunctival angiomata (telangiectases); iris decoloration; nevoid marks or vascular dilation of the episclera; glioma; serous retinal detachment; choroidal angiomata; deep anterior chamber angle; port-wine stain of eyelids; buphthalmos; optic nerve cupping; anisometropia; hemianopsia; increased corneal diameter; enophthalmos; exophthalmos; optic atrophy; choroidal hemangioma; anterior chamber angle vascularization.

Clinical

Vascular port-wine nevus (face, scalp, limbs, trunk, leptomeninges); acromegaly; facial hemihypertrophy; intracranial angiomas; convulsion; mental retardation; obesity; limb atrophy.

Laboratory

Neuroimaging studies and the clinical examination have been the procedures of choice to establish the diagnosis.

Treatment

Anticonvulsants for seizure control, symptomatic and prophylactic therapy for headache and glaucoma treatment to reduce the intraocular pressure (IOP).

BIBLIOGRAPHY

1. Del Monte MA, Taravella M. (2012). Sturge-Weber syndrome. [online] Available from www.emedicine.com/oph/TOPIC348.HTM. [Accessed August, 2013].
2. Takeoka M, Riviello JJ. (2010). Pediatric Sturge-Weber syndrome. [online] Available from www.emedicine.com/neuro/TOPIC356.HTM. [Accessed August, 2013].

1.34. BOURNEVILLE SYNDROME (BOURNEVILLE-PRINGLE SYNDROME; TUBEROUS SCLEROSIS; EPILOIA)

General

Irregular dominant inheritance; more frequent in females; most patients die before age 24 years.

Ocular

Vitreous often cloudy; lens opacities; retinal mushroom-like tumor of grayish-white color; yellowish-white plaques with small hemorrhages and cystic changes in retina; papilledema; disk drusen; cerebral astrocytoma; 40–50% of patients have normal intelligence.

Clinical

Grand mal, petit mal, or Jacksonian seizures (manifest first 2 years of life); mental changes from feeble mindedness to imbecility and idiocy; skin changes arranged usually about nose and cheeks (adenoma sebaceum); congenital tumors of kidney (hypernephroma or tubular adenoma) and heart (rhabdomyoma); cerebral astrocytoma.

Laboratory

Brain MRI is recommended for the detection and follow-up imaging of cortical tubers.

Treatment

A neurologist should be consulted to assist with seizure management and anticonvulsant medication.

🗗 BIBLIOGRAPHY

1. Schwartz RA, Jozwiak S, Pedersen R. (2012). Genetics of tuberous sclerosis. [online] Available from www.emedicine.com/ped/TOPIC2796.HTM. [Accessed August, 2013].

🗗 2. CENTRAL SEROUS CHORIORETINOPATHY

General

Disorder of the central macula.

Clinical

None.

Ocular

Decreased visual acuity, metamorphopsia, micropsia, central color vision deficiency, central scotoma.

Laboratory

Fluorescein angiopathy for "expansile dot" pattern, a "smokestack" pattern or diffuse hyperfluorescence.

Treatment

Observation in most cases. Thermal or photodynamic therapy is necessary in some cases.

🗗 BIBLIOGRAPHY

1. Oh KT. (2011). Central Serous Chorioretinopathy. [online] Available from www.emedicine.com/oph/TOPIC689.HTM. [Accessed August, 2013].

🗗 3. CHOROID COLOBOMA

1. Aicardi syndrome
2. Basal cell nevus syndrome (Gorlin syndrome)
3. Cat-eye syndrome (partial G-trisomy)
4. Charge association among coloboma, heart anomaly, choanal atresia, retardation, genital and ear anomalies
5. Doubtful association
   A. Crouzon syndrome (dysostosis craniofacialis)
   B. Ellis-van Creveld syndrome (chondroectodermal dysplasia)
   C. Hallerman-Streiff syndrome (dyscephalic mandibulo-oculofacial)
   D. Incontinentia pigmenti I (Bloch-Sulzberger syndrome)
   E. Kartagener syndrome (bronchiectasis-dextrocardia-sinusitis)
   F. Laurence-Moon-Bardet-Biedl syndrome (retinitis pigmentosa-poldactyly-adiposogenital syndrome)
   G. Pierre Robin syndrome (micrognathia-glossoptosis syndrome)
   H. Stickler syndrome (hereditary progressive arthro-ophthalmopathy)
   I. Tuberous sclerosis (Bourneville syndrome)
6. Goldenhar syndrome (oculoauriculovertebral dysplasia)
7. Goltz syndrome (focal dermal hypoplasia syndrome)
†8. Isolated, sporadic
9. Joubert syndrome with bilateral chorioretinal coloboma (coloboma, chorioretinal with cerebellar vermis aplasia)
10. Klinefelter syndrome (gynecomastia-aspermatogenesis syndrome)
11. Lenz microphthalmia syndrome
12. Linear sebaceous nevus syndrome
13. Median facial cleft syndrome

14. Meckel syndrome (dysencephalia splanchnocystic syndrome)
†15. Retinal astrocytoma
†16. Retinal dysplasia
17. Retinoblastoma
18. Rubinstein-Taybi syndrome (broad-thumbs syndrome)
19. Triploidy
20. Trisomy 18 (Edward syndrome)
21. Trisomy 13 (Patau syndrome)
22. Turner syndrome
23. Warburg syndrome

---

†Indicates a general entry and therefore has not been described in detail in the text

BIBLIOGRAPHY

1. Daufenbach DR, Ruttum MS, Pulido JS, et al. Chorioretinal colobomas in a pediatric population. Ophthalmology. 1998;105:1455-8.
2. Isenberg SJ. The eye in infancy. Chicago: Year Book Medical; 1989.
3. Ward JR, Saad de Owens C, Sierra IA. Upper-limb defect associated with developmental delay, unilateral poorly developed antihelix, hearing deficit, and bilateral choroid coloboma: a new syndrome. J Med Genet. 1992;29:589-91.

3.1. AICARDI SYNDROME

General

All symptoms present at birth; cause unknown; all findings progress with age; shows X-linked dominant inheritance.

Ocular

Microphthalmia; lid twitching; absent pupillary reflexes; round retinal lacunae up to disk size look like holes with retinal vessels crossing over them; funnel-shaped disk; chorioretinitis.

Clinical

Infantile spasms (tonic seizures in flexion); epileptic seizures; cyanosis; mental anomaly; vertebral anomalies; telangiectasia; hypotonia; head deformities with biparietal bossing, occipital flattening, and plagiocephaly; defects of corpus callosum; cortical heterotopia; characteristic electroencephalogram; dilated intracranial ventricle with leukomalacia.

Laboratory

Generally diagnosis is made by clinical findings. Neuroimaging can delineate the degree of CNS dysgenesis and help evaluate other potential etiologies of intractable epilepsy and developmental delay.

Treatment

Consultation with a child neurologist is recommended. Use of traditional epilepsy therapies for seizure manifestations is recommended.

BIBLIOGRAPHY

1. Davis RG, DiFazio MP. (2012). Aicardi syndrome. [online] Available from www.emedicine.com/ped/TOPIC58.HTM. [Accessed August, 2013].

3.2. BASAL CELL NEVUS SYNDROME (NEVOID BASAL CELL CARCINOMA SYNDROME; NEVOID BASALIOMA SYNDROME; GORLIN SYNDROME; GORLIN-GOLTZ SYNDROME; MULTIPLE BASAL CELL NEVI SYNDROME)

General

Autosomal dominant; onset of skin lesions in childhood, usually at puberty.

Ocular

Basal cell carcinomas of eyelids; strabismus; hypertelorism; congenital cataracts; choroidal colobomas; glaucoma; medullated nerve fibers; prominence of supraorbital ridges; corneal leukoma; basalioma of the skin; coloboma of the choroid and optic nerve.

Clinical

Basal cell tumors with facial involvement; shallow pits of the skin of the hands and feet; jaw cysts; rib anomalies;

kyphoscoliosis and fusion of vertebrae; medulloblastoma; frontal and temporoparietal bossing and broad nasal root.

Laboratory

Computed tomography (CT) scanning, ultrasonography, or magnetic resonance imaging (MRI) to evaluate neoplasms. Endoscopy to evaluate for the degree of polyposis and survey for malignant transformation is done.

Treatment

Patients may require medical attention for craniofacial, vertebral, dental and ophthalmologic abnormalities, in addition to diagnosis and treatment of potential neoplasia.

BIBLIOGRAPHY

1. Hsu EK, Mamula P, Ruchelli ED. (2011). Intestinal Polyposis Syndromes. [online] Available from www.emedicine.com/ped/TOPIC828.HTM. [Accessed January, 2013].

3.3. CAT'S-EYE SYNDROME (SCHACHENMANN SYNDROME; SCHMID-FRACCARO SYNDROME; PARTIAL TRISOMY G SYNDROME)

General

Causative factor is one extra chromosome, a G chromosome, which may be from a 13-15 or 21-22 chromosome; although the ocular findings of the syndrome are similar to the D 13-15 trisomy group, the systemic manifestations usually are less severe; this syndrome is associated with a supernumerary bisatellited marker chromosome derived from duplicated regions of 22pter'22q11.2; partial cat's-eye syndrome is characterized by the absence of coloboma.

Ocular

Hypertelorism; microphthalmos; anti-Mongoloid slant of palpebral fissures; strabismus; inferior vertical iris coloboma (cat eye); cataract; choroidal coloboma; epicanthal folds.

Clinical

Anal atresia; preauricular fistulae (bilateral); umbilical hernia; heart anomalies.

Laboratory

Chromosome analysis.

Treatment

- *Cataract:* Change in glasses can sometimes improve a patient's visual function temporarily; however, the most common treatment is cataract surgery.
- *Strabismus:* Equalized vision with correct refractive error; surgery may be helpful in patient with diplopia.

BIBLIOGRAPHY

1. Collins JF. Handbook of Clinical Ophthalmology. New York: Masson; 1982.
2. Cory CC, Jamison DL. The cat eye syndrome. Arch Ophthalmol. 1974;92:259-62.
3. Liehr T, Pfeiffer RA, Trautmann U. Typical and partial cat eye syndrome: identification of the marker chromosome by FISH. Clin Genet. 1992;42:91-6.
4. Mears AJ, Duncan AM, Budarf ML, et al. Molecular characterization of the marker chromosome associated with cat eye syndrome. Am J Hum Genet. 1994;55:134-43.
5. Peterson RA. Schmid-Fraccaro syndrome ("cat's eye" syndrome): partial trisomy of G chromosome. Arch Ophthalmol.1973;90:287.
6. Schachenmann G, Schmid W, Fraccaro M, et al. Chromosomes in coloboma and anal atresia. Lancet. 1965;2:290.
7. Walknowska J, Peakman D, Weleber RG. et al. Cytogenetic investigation of cat-eye syndrome. Am J Ophthalmol. 1977;84:477-86.

⊟ 3.4. CHARGE ASSOCIATION (MULTIPLE CONGENITAL ANOMALIES SYNDROME; COLOBOMA, HEART DISEASE, ATRESIA, RETARDED GROWTH, GENITAL HYPOPLASIA, EAR MALFORMATION ASSOCIATION)

General

Syndrome consists of four of six major manifestations of ocular coloboma, heart disease, atresia, retarded growth and development, genital hypoplasia, and ear malformations with or without hearing loss.

Ocular

Blepharoptosis; iris coloboma; optic nerve coloboma; macular hypoplasia; lacrimal canalicular atresia; nasolacrimal duct obstruction.

Clinical

Microcephaly; brachycephaly; malformed ear; bilateral finger contractures; heart disease; genital hypoplasia; heart disease; choanal atresia; retarded growth; hearing loss; facial nerve palsies; mental retardation.

Laboratory

CHD7 mutation analysis is diagnostic in 58–71% of individuals who meet the clinical criteria, head computed tomography (CT) and magnetic resonance imaging (MRI), cranial ultrasound.

Treatment

Secure airway, stabilize the patient, exclude major life-threatening congenital anomalies and transfer the individual with coloboma of the eye, heart defects, atresia of the nasal choanae, retardation of growth and/or development, genital and/or urinary abnormalities, and ear abnormalities and deafness (CHARGE) syndrome to a specialist center with pediatric otolaryngologist and other subspecialty services.

⊟ BIBLIOGRAPHY

1. Tegay DH, Yedowitz JC. (2012). CHARGE syndrome. [online] Available from www.emedicine.com/ped/TOPIC367.HTM. [Accessed January, 2013].

⊟ 3.5A. CROUZON SYNDROME (DYSOSTOSIS CRANIOFACIALIS; OXYCEPHALY; CRANIOFACIAL DYSOSTOSIS; PARROT-HEAD SYNDROME; MÖBIUS-CROUZON SYNDROME; HEREDITARY CRANIOFACIAL DYSOSTOSIS)

General

Autosomal dominant; manifestations present at birth.

Ocular

Bilateral exophthalmos; hypertelorism (wide interpupillary distance); obliquity of palpebral fissures with outer canthus slanting downward; nystagmus; exotropia; upper field defects due to pressure upon the optic nerve on its lower part; bluish sclera; exposure keratitis in extreme exophthalmos; cataract; papilledema; secondary optic atrophy; corneal dystrophy; ptosis; strabismus; keratoconus.

Clinical

Prognathism; maxillary hypoplasia with short upper lip; synostosis of coronal and lambda sutures; parrot-beaked nose (psittachosrhina); widening temporal fossae; headaches.

Laboratory

Skull, spine, and hand radiography is usually necessary to confirm the diagnosis.

Treatment

Neurosurgical procedure is recommended in cases of intracranial hypertension leading to further optic atrophy.

⊟ BIBLIOGRAPHY

1. Chen H. (2013). Genetics of Crouzon syndrome. [online] Available from www.emedicine.com/ped/TOPIC511.HTM. [Accessed August, 2013].

3.5B. ZOLLINGER-ELLISON SYNDROME (POLYGLANDULAR ADENOMATOSIS SYNDROME; MULTIPLE ENDOCRINE ADENOMATOSIS PARTIAL SYNDROME) OPTIC ATROPHY

General

Autosomal dominant; more frequent in males (2:1); etiology is islet cell adenoma of pancreas secreting a gastrin-like material; onset 3rd–5th decade (*see* Werner syndrome).

Ocular

Scotomata according to size and position of pituitary tumors; optic nerve atrophy; papilledema; bilateral extraocular muscle metastases.

Clinical

Enteritis and/or peptic ulcers; malignant or benign tumor of islet cell of pancreas; hypersecretion; vomiting; diarrhea; polyglandular adenomatosis; endocrine involvement.

Laboratory

Fasting serum gastrin levels, secretin stimulation test, levels of basal acid output, endoscopic ultrasonography.

Treatment

Proton pump inhibitors are the first line of treatment for Zollinger-Ellison syndrome (ZES).

BIBLIOGRAPHY

1. Guandalini S, Patton TJ. (2013). Pediatric Zollinger-Ellison syndrome. [online] Available from www.emedicine.com/ped/TOPIC2472.HTM. [Accessed August, 2013].

3.5C. HALLERMANN-STREIFF SYNDROME (DYSCEPHALIC-MANDIBULO-OCULO-FACIAL SYNDROME; OCULO-MANDIBULO-DYSCEPHALY; ULLRICH-FREMERY-DOHNA SYNDROME; FRANCOIS DYSCEPHALIC SYNDROME; MANDIBULO-OCULO-FACIAL DYSCEPHALY SYNDROME; FRANCOIS-HALLERMANN-STREIFF SYNDROME; HALLERMANN-STREIFF-FRANCOIS SYNDROME; AUDRY I SYNDROME; DOHNA SYNDROME; FRANCOIS SYNDROME (1); DYSCEPHALY- TEETH ABNORMALITY-DWARFISM; DYSCEPHALIA OCULOMANDIBULARIS-HYPOTRICHOSIS; MANDIBULO-OCULAR DYSCEPHALIA HYPOTRICHOSIS; FREMERY-DOHNA SYNDROME; OCULO-MANDIBULO-FACIAL DYSCEPHALY)

General

Rare; familial occurrence and consanguinity; males and females are equally affected.

Ocular

Microphthalmos (bilateral); proptosis; nystagmus; strabismus; cataracts; bilateral optic atrophy; coloboma of optic disk, choroid, and iris; keratoglobus; microcornea; antimongoloid slant; iris atrophy; uveitis; blue sclera; persistent pupillary membrane; secondary glaucoma.

Clinical

Malformations of skull (brachycephaly), facial skeleton and jaws; erupted teeth at birth; diminished hair growth; hyperextensibility of joints; short stature; skin atrophy; mental deficiency; predisposition to upper airway compromise; obstructive sleep apnea.

Laboratory

Diagnosis is made by clinical findings.

Treatment

- *Cataract:* Change in glasses can sometimes improve a patient's visual function temporarily; however the most common treatment is cataract surgery.
- *Strabismus:* Equalized vision with correct refractive error; surgery may be helpful in patients with diplopia.
- *Uveitis:* Topical steroids and cycloplegic medication should be the initial treatment of choice. Oral steroids should be given if not responsive to topical steroids, immunosuppressants if bilateral disease that does not respond to oral steroids, periocular steroids for unilateral or posterior uveitis. Vitrectomy can be used for severe vitreous opacification. Cryotherapy and laser photocoagulation may be used for localized pars plana exudates.
- *Glaucoma:* Glaucoma medication should be the first plan of action. If medication is unsuccessful, a filtering surgical procedure with or without antimetabolites may be beneficial.

BIBLIOGRAPHY

1. François J, Victoria-Troncoso V. François' dyscephalic syndrome and skin manifestations. Ophthalmologica. 1981;183(2):63-7.
2. Hallermann W. Vogelgesicht und Cataracta Congenita. Klin Monatsbl Augenheilkd. 1948;113:315-8.
3. Ronen S, Rozenmann Y, Isaacson M, et al. The early management of baby with Hallermann-Streiff-Francois syndrome. J Pediatr Ophthalmol Strabismus. 1979;16(2):119-21.
4. Roy FH, Fraunfelder FW, Fraunfelder FT. Roy and Fraunfelder's Current Ocular Therapy, 6th edition. Philadelphia, PA: WB Saunders; 2008.
5. Spaepen A, Schrander-Stumpel C, Fryns JP, et al. Hallermann-Streiff syndrome: clinical and psychological findings in children. Nosologic overlap with oculodentodigital dysplasia? Am J Med Genet. 1991;41(4):517-20.
6. Streiff EB. Dysmorphic Mandibulo-faciale (Tete d'Oiseau) et Alterations Oculaires. Ophthalmologica. 1950;120(1-2):79-83.

3.5D. BLOCH-SULZBERGER SYNDROME (INCONTINENTIA PIGMENTI; SIEMENS-BLOCH-SULZBERGER SYNDROME)

General

Familial disorder affecting ectoderm; manifestations at birth; female predominance; X-linked dominant phenotype; disturbance of skin pigmentation.

Ocular

Orbital mass; retrolental fibroplasia; pseudoglioma; strabismus; blue sclera; cataract; optic nerve atrophy; papillitis; nystagmus; chorioretinitis; anomalies of chamber angle; neovascularization of retina; retinal hemorrhages and edema; microphthalmia; tractional retinal detachment.

Clinical

Dental and skeletal anomalies common; neurologic abnormalities; recurrent inflammatory lesions; skin melanin pigmentation on the trunk (marble cake); occipital lobe infarct; neonatal infarction of the macula.

Laboratory

CT scan or MRI of the brain should be performed.

Treatment

No specific treatment. Lesions should be left intact and kept clean and meticulous dental care is very important.

BIBLIOGRAPHY

1. Chang CH. (2012). Neurologic manifestations of incontinentia pigmenti. [online] Available from www.emedicine.com/neuro/TOPIC169.HTM. [Accessed August, 2013].

3.5E. KARTAGENER SYNDROME (SINUSITIS-BRONCHIECTASIS-SITUS INVERSUS SYNDROME; BRONCHIECTASIS-DEXTROCARDIA-SINUSITIS; KARTAGENER TRIAD)

General

Autosomal recessive; onset in early infancy; occasionally dominant; finding of various structural defects in patients with this condition suggests that there are several genetic determinants.

Ocular

Myopia; glaucoma; conjunctival melanosis; iris coloboma; tortuous and dilated retinal vessels; retinal pigmentary degeneration; pseudopapillitis.

Clinical

Immotile cilia; situs inversus; bronchiectasis; sinusitis; various cardiovascular and renal abnormalities; dyspnea; productive cough; recurrent respiratory infections; palpitation; otitis media; nasal speech; conductive hearing loss; nasal polyps; situs inversus viscerum with hepatic dullness on left side.

Laboratory

High-resolution CT scan of the chest is the most sensitive modality for documenting early and subtle abnormalities within airways and pulmonary parenchyma when compared to routine chest radiographs.

Treatment

Antibiotics, intravenous or oral and continuous or intermittent, are used to treat upper and lower airway infections. Obstructive lung disease, if present, should be treated with inhaled bronchodilators and aggressive pulmonary toilet. Tympanostomy tubes are required to reduce conductive hearing loss and recurrent infections.

BIBLIOGRAPHY

1. Bent JP, Willis EB. (2013). Kartagener syndrome. [online] Available from www.emedicine.com/med/TOPIC1220.HTM. [Accessed August, 2013].

3.5F. LAURENCE-MOON-BARDET-BIEDL SYNDROME (BARDET-BIEDL SYNDROME; RETINITIS PIGMENTOSA-POLYDACTYLY-ADIPOSOGENITAL SYNDROME)

General

Recessive, autosomal dominant, and recessive sex-linked gene; male preponderance; onset in childhood; cases of Laurence-Moon-Bardet-Biedl belong to the group of heredoataxias.

Ocular

Ptosis; epicanthus; nystagmus; strabismus; night blindness; myopia; hypermetropia; iris coloboma; RP "bone corpuscles"; macular degeneration; attenuation of retinal vessels; choroidal atrophy; optic nerve atrophy; cataract; microphthalmia; keratoconus.

Clinical

Obesity (Fröhlich type); hypogenitalism; reduced intelligence and mental retardation; turricephaly; shortness of stature; atresia ani; genu valgum; congenital heart disease; polydactyly; body hair scant or absent; pseudogynecomastia.

Laboratory

Chromosomal analysis is recommended to confirm chromosomal sex and to evaluate for associated genetic syndromes.

Treatment

Consultation by pediatric endocrinologist and pediatric urologist is usually necessary.

BIBLIOGRAPHY

1. Telander DG, de Beus A, Small KW. (2012). Retinitis pigmentosa. [online] Available from www.emedicine.com/oph/TOPIC704.HTM. [Accessed August, 2013].

3.5G. PIERRE-ROBIN SYNDROME (ROBIN SYNDROME; MICROGNATHIA-GLOSSOPTOSIS SYNDROME)

General

Etiology unknown; manifestations at birth; pathogenesis based on arrested fetal development; history of intrauterine disturbance in early pregnancy (25% of cases); also increased incidence in offspring of mother's age 35 years or older; pathogenesis is thought to be incomplete development of the first brachial arch, which forms the maxilla and mandible.

Ocular

Microphthalmos; proptosis; ptosis; high myopia; glaucoma; cataract (rare); retinal disinsertion; megalocornea; iris atrophy; blue sclera; esotropia; conjunctivitis; distichiasis; vitreoretinal degeneration; retinal detachments.

Clinical

Micrognathia; cleft palate; glossoptosis; cyanosis; facial expression bird-like with flat base of nose and high-arched deformed palate with or without cleft; difficulty in breathing.

Laboratory

Diagnosis is made by clinical findings.

Treatment

Multidisciplinary approach is required to manage the complex features involved in the care of these children and their families.

🖥 BIBLIOGRAPHY

1. Tewfik TL, Trinh N, Teebi AS. (2012). Pierre Robin syndrome. [online] Available from www.emedicine.com/ent/TOPIC150.HTM. [Accessed August, 2013].

🖥 3.5H. STICKLER SYNDROME (HEREDITARY PROGRESSIVE ARTHROOPHTHALMOPATHY)

General

Autosomal dominant; onset in childhood; severe and debilitating connective tissue disorder inherited as an autosomal dominant syndrome with a variable phenotype; linkage analysis has provided statistical evidence for linkage of collagen type II (COL2A1) gene with this syndrome in some but not all families.

Ocular

Phthisis bulbi; glaucoma; chronic uveitis; keratopathy; complicated cataracts; chorioretinal degeneration; total retinal detachment during 1st decade of life; myopia; giant retinal tears.

Clinical

Bony enlargement of joints with abnormal development of the articular surfaces and premature degenerative changes; hypermobility of joints with abnormality in connective tissues supporting the joints; possible skeletal deformities.

Laboratory

Bone radiographs and a full genetic evaluation is appropriate.

Treatment

The primary concern is airway obstruction. Tracheotomy tube is effective in bypassing the obstruction. If feeding difficulties, special cleft nursing bottles are available. If this is not enough, gavage or feeding tubes can provide temporary nutrition.

🖥 BIBLIOGRAPHY

1. Tolarova MM. (2012). Pierre Robin malformation. [online] Available from www.emedicine.com/ped/TOPIC2680.HTM. [Accessed August, 2013].

🖥 3.5I. BOURNEVILLE SYNDROME (BOURNEVILLE-PRINGLE SYNDROME; TUBEROUS SCLEROSIS; EPILOIA)

General

Irregular dominant inheritance; more frequent in females; most patients die before age 24 years.

Ocular

Vitreous often cloudy; lens opacities; retinal mushroom-like tumor of grayish-white color; yellowish-white plaques with small hemorrhages and cystic changes in retina; papilledema; disk drusen; cerebral astrocytoma; 40–50% of patients have normal intelligence.

Clinical

Grand mal, petit mal, or Jacksonian seizures (manifest in first 2 years of life); mental changes from feeble minded-ness to imbecility and idiocy; skin changes arranged usually about nose and cheeks (adenoma sebaceum); congenital tumors of kidney (hypernephroma or tubular adenoma) and heart (rhabdomyoma); cerebral astrocytoma.

Laboratory

Brain MRI is recommended for the detection and follow-up imaging of cortical tubers.

Treatment

A neurologist should be consulted to assist with seizure management and anticonvulsant medication.

⊟ BIBLIOGRAPHY

1. Schwartz RA, Jozwiak S, Pedersen R. (2012). Genetics of tuberous sclerosis. [online] Available from www.emedicine.com/ped/TOPIC2796.HTM. [Accessed August, 2013].

⊟ 3.6. GOLDENHAR SYNDROME (OCULO-AURICULO-VERTEBRAL DYSPLASIA; GOLDENHAR-GORLIN SYNDROME)

General

Most cases have been sporadic, but cases of autosomal dominant and recessive inheritance have been reported; male preponderance (60%); present at birth.

Ocular

Anophthalmia; colobomata of choroid, iris, and eyelid; anti-Mongolian slant of lid fissure; epibulbar dermoid or lipodermoids of conjunctiva, cornea, and orbit; tilted optic disk; nerve hypoplasia; microphthalmia; macular heterotopia; tortuous retinal vessels.

Clinical

Frontal bulging of the skull; receding chin; malar hypoplasia; micrognathia and macrostomia; auricular appendices (single or multiple); multiple vertebral anomalies; preauricular fistulas; mental retardation.

Laboratory

Clinical.

Treatment

Dermoids—surgery for function or cosmesis.

⊟ BIBLIOGRAPHY

1. Tewfik TL, Al-Noury KI. (2013). Manifestations of craniofacial syndromes. [online] Available from www.emedicine.com/ent/TOPIC319.HTM. [Accessed August, 2013].

⊟ 3.7. GOLTZ SYNDROME (FOCAL DERMAL HYPOPLASIA SYNDROME)

General

X-linked dominant inheritance; lethal in males; skin manifestations present at birth.

Ocular

Microphthalmia; strabismus; coloboma of iris and/or choroid; epiphora; blue sclera; nystagmus; anophthalmos; keratoconus.

Clinical

Skin atrophy and linear pigmentation; telangiectasias of trunk and extremities; superficial, localized fatty skin deposits; multiple papillomas of mucous membranes and periorificial skin (oral, genital, anal); anomalies of extremities with syndactyly, oligodactyly, adactyly; hypohidrosis; paper-thin nails may be present; spina bifida; hypoplasia of right clavicle; umbilical or inguinal hernia.

Laboratory

Radiography may reveal osteopathia striata.

Treatment

Flashlamp-pumped pulse dye laser may ameliorate the pruritic symptoms that sometimes are noted in affected skin and improve the clinical appearance of the telangiectatic

and erythematous skin lesions. Papillomas frequently require repeated surgical intervention.

BIBLIOGRAPHY

1. Goltz RW, Castelo-Soccio L. (2012). Focal dermal hypoplasia syndrome. [online] Available from emedicine.medscape.com/article/1110936-overview. [Accessed February, 2013].

3.9. JOUBERT SYNDROME (FAMILIAL CEREBELLAR VERMIS AGENESIS)

General

Autosomal recessive; both sexes affected; onset in early infancy.

Ocular

Choroidal coloboma; nystagmus; ocular fibrosis, telecanthus.

Clinical

Episodic hyperpnea; apnea; ataxia; psychomotor retardation; rhythmic protrusion of tongue; mental retardation; micrognathia; complex cardiac malformation; cutaneous dimples over wrists and elbows.

Laboratory

Urine culture, renal ultrasonography, dimercaptosuccinic acid (DMSA) renal scanning.

Treatment

Lifetime follow-up is required whether or not involution has occurred or a nephrectomy.

BIBLIOGRAPHY

1. Swiatecka-Urban A. (2011). Multicystic renal dysplasia. [online] Available from www.emedicine.com/ped/TOPIC1493.HTM. [Accessed August, 2013].

3.10. KLINEFELTER SYNDROME (GYNECOMASTIA-ASPERMATOGENESIS SYNDROME; XXY SYNDROME; XXXY SYNDROME; XXYY SYNDROME; REIFENSTEIN-ALBRIGHT SYNDROME)

General

Occurrence in 1% of retarded males; phenotypically males with positive female sex chromatin; karyotype shows 47 chromosomes, 44 autosomes, and 3 sex chromosomes with the complement XXY.

Ocular

Anophthalmos; coloboma; corneal opacities.

Clinical

Testicular hypoplasia; sterility; gynecomastia; eunuchoid physique; mental retardation; association with progressive systemic sclerosis and systemic lupus erythematosus.

Laboratory

May be diagnosed prenatally based on cytogenetic analysis of a fetus. If not diagnosed prenatally, the 47, XXY karyotype may manifest as various subtle age-related clinical signs that may prompt chromosomal evaluation.

Treatment

Treatment should address three major facets of the disease: (1) hypogonadism, (2) gynecomastia, and (3) psychosocial problems.

BIBLIOGRAPHY

1. Chen H. (2013). Klinefelter syndrome. [online] Available from www.emedicine.com/ped/TOPIC1252.HTM. [Accessed August, 2013].

⊟ 3.11. LENZ MICROPHTHALMIA SYNDROME

General

X-linked recessive; female carriers.

Ocular

Microphthalmia; microcornea; ocular coloboma; colobomatous microphthalmia.

Clinical

Skeletal abnormalities of vertebral column, clavicles, and limbs; severe renal dysgenesis and hydroureters; dental anomalies; hypospadias and bilateral cryptorchidism; severe speech impairment; shortness of stature; long, cylindrical, and thin thorax; sloping shoulders; flat feet.

Laboratory

Diagnosis is made by clinical findings.

Treatment

None—ocular.

⊟ BIBLIOGRAPHY

1. Antoniades K, Tzouvelekis G, Doudou A, et al. A sporadic case of Lenz microphthalmia syndrome. Ann Ophthalmol. 1993;25:342-5.
2. Herrmann J, Optiz JM. The Lenz microphthalmia syndrome. Birth Defects. 1969;5:138-48.

⊟ 3.12. LINEAR NEVUS SEBACEUS OF JADASSOHN (NEVUS SEBACEUS OF JADASSOHN; JADASSOHN-TYPE ANETODERMA; ORGANOID NEVUS SYNDROME; SEBACEUS NEVUS SYNDROME)

General

Skin nevus caused by failure of separation of skin appendages from adjacent epithelium during the 3rd month of gestation.

Ocular

Proptosis; epibulbar lipodermoids; colobomata of eyelids, iris, and choroid; anti-Mongoloid fissures; ocular motor palsies; nystagmus; teratomas of orbit and aberrant lacrimal glands; corneal vascularization; vision defects; conjunctival dermolipomas; choristomas of conjunctiva, sclera; corneal vascularization/opacification; colobomas of uvea, retina, optic disk, and lids; optic nerve hypoplasia; microphthalmia; anophthalmia; hemangioma of the sclera/conjunctiva.

Clinical

Circumscribed lesions of the face and scalp with excessively large sebaceous glands; papillomatous epidermal hyperplasia; seizures; skeletal abnormalities, particularly in skull; failure to thrive; convulsion; mental retardation.

Laboratory

Epidermis shows papillomatous hyperplasia. In the dermis, the numbers of mature sebaceous glands are increased. Ectopic apocrine glands are often found in the deep dermis beneath sebaceous glands.

Treatment

Photodynamic therapy with topical aminolevulinic acid. Full-thickness skin excision is usually required, and topical destruction.

⊟ BIBLIOGRAPHY

1. Al Hammadi A, Lebwohl MG. (2012). Nevus sebaceous. [online] Available from www.emedicine.com/derm/TOPIC296.HTM. [Accessed August, 2013].

3.13. FRONTONASAL DYSPLASIA SYNDROME (MEDIAN CLEFT FACE SYNDROME)

General

Congenital disorder without genetic background; condition may present a variety of facial malformations, depending on the stage of embryonic development at which interference occurs.

Ocular

Hypertelorism; anophthalmia or microphthalmia; significant refractive errors; strabismus; nystagmus; eyelid ptosis; optic nerve hypoplasia; optic nerve colobomas; cataract; corneal dermoid; inflammatory retinopathy.

Clinical

Broad nasal root may be associated with median nasal groove and cleft of nose and/or upper lip; cleft of ala nasi (unilateral or bilateral); V-shaped hair prolongation into forehead.

Laboratory

CT, MRI and physical examination.

Treatment

Reconstruction surgery may be warranted.

BIBLIOGRAPHY

1. Kinsey JA, Streeten BW. Ocular abnormalities in the medial cleft face syndrome. Am J Ophthalmol. 1977;83:261-6.
2. Roarty JD, Pron GE, Siegel-Bartelt J, et al. Ocular manifestations of frontonasal dysplasia. Plast Reconstr Surg. 1994;93:25-30.
3. Sedano HO, Cohen MM, Jirasek J, et al. Frontonasal dysplasia. J Pediatr. 1970;76:906-13.
4. Weaver D, Bellinger D. Bifid nose associated with midline cleft of the upper lip: case report. Arch Otolaryngol. 1946;44:480-2.

3.14. MECKEL SYNDROME (DYSENCEPHALIA SPLANCHNOCYSTIC SYNDROME; GRUBER SYNDROME)

General

Autosomal recessive; ocular manifestations are similar to those of trisomy 13-15 syndrome.

Ocular

Cryptophthalmos; clinical anophthalmos; microphthalmos; Mongoloid slant of lid fissures; sclerocornea; microcornea; partial aniridia; cataract; retinal dysplasia; posterior staphyloma; optic nerve hypoplasia.

Clinical

Sloping forehead; posterior encephalocele; short neck; polydactyly and syndactyly (hands and feet); polycystic kidneys; cryptorchidism; cleft lip and palate; central nervous system abnormalities, including the Dandy-Walker malformation.

Laboratory

Chromosome analysis, MRI.

Treatment

Cardiac surgery may be warranted.

BIBLIOGRAPHY

1. Jayakar PB, Spiliopoulos M, Jayakar A. (2011). Meckel-Gruber syndrome. [online] Available from www.emedicine.com/ped/TOPIC1390.HTM. [Accessed August, 2013].

3.17. RETINOBLASTOMA

General

Malignant tumor arising in one or both retinas of young children, usually under the age of 2 years; usually unilateral; autosomal dominant; most common intraocular malignancy of childhood; incidence is 1 in 20,000 live births; origin is questionably neuroectodermal cells capable of multipotentiality; one-third of patients have heritable (bilateral or have a positive family history) autosomal dominant and two-thirds are sporadic; genetic transmission obeys two-mutation hypothesis of Knudson; trilateral retinoblastoma is bilateral retinoblastoma plus midline central nervous system tumor (most commonly pinealoma); most common second tumor is an osteogenic sarcoma (begins in 2nd decade).

Ocular

Hyphema; hypopyon; corneal tumor; lid edema; endophthalmitis; exophthalmos; intraocular calcification of globe; heterochromia; neovascularization of iris or retina; papilledema; panophthalmitis; retinoblastoma extension into orbit and choroid; cat's-eye reflex; leukocoria; mydriasis; vitreous hemorrhage; tumor seeding; esotropia; exotropia; glaucoma; visual loss.

Clinical

Metastasis into the lymph system, bone marrow and subarachnoid space; basal meningitis; death.

Laboratory

CT calcification of lesion: Hallmark of disease; ultrasound-demonstrates calcification and MRI demonstrates presence and extent of extraocular disease.

Treatment

External beam radiation therapy is recommended on patients with significant vitreous seeding. Radioactive isotope plaques and chemotherapy are also an option. Removal of the tumor is the standard management for retinoblastoma.

BIBLIOGRAPHY

1. Abramson DH, Dunkel IJ, Brodie SE, et al. Superselective ophthalmic artery chemotherapy as primary treatment for retinoblastoma (chemosurgery). Ophthalmology. 2010;117(8):1623-9.
2. Isidro MA, Roque MR. (2012). Retinoblastoma. [online] Available from www.emedicine.com/oph/TOPIC346.HTM. [Accessed January, 2013].

3.18. RUBINSTEIN-TAYBI SYNDROME (BROAD-THUMBS SYNDROME)

General

Inheritance polygenic or multifactorial; rare.

Ocular

Anti-Mongoloid slant of lid fissure; epicanthus; long eyelashes and highly arched brows; strabismus; myopia; hyperopia; iris coloboma; cataract; optic atrophy; ptosis; retinal detachment.

Clinical

Motor and mental retardation; broad thumbs and toes; highly arched palate; allergies; heart murmurs; anomalies of size, shape, and position of ears; dwarfism; cryptorchidism.

Laboratory

CT scan, MRI, chromosomal karyotype analysis, fluorescence in situ hybridization and CBP gene analysis.

Treatment

Physical therapy, speech and feeding therapy. Cardiothoracic intervention may be needed in patients with congenital heart defect.

BIBLIOGRAPHY

1. Mijuskovic ZP, Karadaglic D, Stojanov L. (2013). Dermatologic manifestations of Rubinstein-Taybi syndrome. Available from www.emedicine.com/derm/TOPIC711.HTM. [Accessed August, 2013].

3.19. TRIPLOIDY SYNDROME (IRIS COLOBOMA)

General

Extra set of chromosomes due to diandry or digyny; stillbirth or early neonatal death.

Ocular

Iris coloboma; microphthalmia; hypertelorism.

Clinical

Large placenta; prenatal growth deficits; large fontanels; syndactyly; heart defects; cleft lip; genital, brain, ear, and kidney malformations; meningomyelocele; micrognathia.

Laboratory/ocular

Diagnosis is made by clinical findings.

Treatment

None.

📖 BIBLIOGRAPHY

1. Arvidsson CG, Hamberg H, Johnsson H, et al. A boy with complete triploidy and unusually long survival. Acta Paediatr Scand. 1986;75:507-10.
2. Crane JP, Beaver HA, Cheung SW. Antenatal ultrasound findings in fetal triploidy syndrome. J Ultrasound Med. 1985;4:519-24.
3. Kaufman MH. New insights into triploidy and tetraploidy, from an analysis of model systems for these conditions. Hum Reprod. 1991;6:8-16.
4. Magalim SI, Scrascia E. Dictionary of Medical Syndromes, 2nd edition. Philadelphia: JB Lippincott; 1981.
5. O'Brien WF, Knuppel RA, Kousseff B, et al. Elevated maternal serum alpha-fetoprotein in triploidy. Obstet Gynecol. 1988;71:994-5.
6. Rubenstein JB, Swayne LC, Dise CA, et al. Placental changes in fetal triploidy syndrome. J Ultrasound Med. 1986;5:545-50.
7. Strobel SL, Brandt JT. Abnormal hematologic features in a live-born female with triploidy. Arch Pathol Lab Med. 1985;109:775-7.
8. Walker S, Andrews J, Gregson NM, et al. Three further cases of triploidy in man surviving to birth. J Med Genet. 1973;10:135-41.

📖 3.20. TRISOMY 18 SYNDROME (E SYNDROME; EDWARDS SYNDROME), CONGENITAL GLAUCOMA

General

Chromosome 18 present in triplicate; more common in females (3:1); age of mother over 40 years; onset from fetal life.

Ocular

Unilateral ptosis; epicanthal folds; congenital glaucoma; corneal opacities; lens opacities; optic atrophy.

Clinical

Low-set ears; micrognathia; high-arched palate; prominent occiput; cryptorchidism; failure to thrive; ventricular septal defect; hypertonicity with rigidity in flexion of limbs; mental retardation; umbilical and inguinal hernias.

Laboratory

Cytogenetic test, echocardiography, ultrasonography, and skeletal radiography are used to detect any abnormalities.

Treatment

Treat infections as appropriate. For feeding difficulties nasogastric and gastrostomy supplementation is recommended.

📖 BIBLIOGRAPHY

1. Chen H. (2013). Trisomy 18. [online] Availble from www.emedicine.com/ped/TOPIC652.HTM. [Accessed August, 2013].

📖 3.21. TRISOMY 13 SYNDROME (TRISOMY D1 SYNDROME, PATAU SYNDROME, REESE SYNDROME) IRIS COLOBOMA

General

Extra chromosome in the D group; fatal in the first few months of life; trisomy 13–15 resembles trisomy D1.

Ocular

Anophthalmia; microphthalmia; iris coloboma; cataracts; retinal dysplasia; optic nerve coloboma; optic atrophy; iris dyplasia; calcified lens; retinal detachment; optic nerve hypoplasia; orbital cysts.

Clinical

Apneic spells; developmental deficiency of the nervous system; seizures (minor motor); deafness; cleft lip and palate; hemangiomata; horizontal palmar creases; hyperconvex fingernails; interventricular septal defects; renal abnormalities; cardiovascular changes; respiratory involvement; gastrointestinal disease; urogenital involvement; cerebral hypoplasia with hydrocephalus; mental retardation.

Laboratory

Immediate conventional cytogenetic test. Ultrasonography for any anomalies. Trisomy 13 is best identified through cytogenetic study of amionic fluid.

Treatment

Surgical care is usually withheld for the first few months of life.

BIBLIOGRAPHY

1. Best RG, Gregg AR. (2012). Patau syndrome. [online] Available from www.emedicine.com/ped/TOPIC1745.HTM. [Accessed August, 2013].

3.22. TURNER SYNDROME (TURNER-ALBRIGHT SYNDROME; GONADAL DYSGENESIS; GENITAL DWARFISM SYNDROME; ULLRICH-TURNER SYNDROME; BONNEVIE-ULLRICH SYNDROME; PTERYGOLYMPHANGIECTASIA SYNDROME; ULLRICH-BONNEVIE SYNDROME) CATARACT, POSTERIOR

General

Ovarian or gonadal agenesis; 45 chromosomes with an XO sex-chromosome constitution; females; rare in males; onset in childhood.

Ocular

Exophthalmos; hypertelorism; ptosis; epicanthal folds; blue sclera; corneal nebulae; cataracts; conjunctival lymphedema; keratoconus.

Clinical

Webbed neck (pterygium colli); diminished growth; mandibulofacial disproportion; cubitus valgus; masculine chest and trunk; late appearance of pubic and axillary hair; congenital deafness; mental retardation; coarctation of aorta.

Laboratory

Karyotyping is needed for diagnosis. Y-chromosomal test; Luteinizing hormone (LH) and follicle-stimulating hormone (FSH) levels, thyroid function test, fasting glucose levels, echocardiography and MRI.

Treatment

Growth hormone therapy is used to prevent short stature. Estrogen replacement therapy is usually started by the age of 12–15 years.

BIBLIOGRAPHY

1. Postellon DC, Daniel MS. (2012). Turner syndrome. [online] Available from emedicine.medscape.com/article/949681-overview. [Accessed August, 2013].

3.23. WALKER-WARBURG SYNDROME (CEREBRO-OCULAR DYSPLASIA-MUSCULAR DYSTROPHY; WARBURG SYNDROME; COD-MD SYNDROME; FUKUYAMA CONGENITAL MUSCULAR DYSTROPHY; HARD + OR − E SYNDROME) CATARACT

General

Rare; encompassing a triad of brain, eye, and muscle abnormalities; probably autosomal recessive.

Ocular

Microphthalmia; cataract; immature anterior chamber angle; retinal dysplasia; retinal detachment; persistent hyperplastic primary vitreous; optic nerve hypoplasia; iris coloboma; opaque cornea; myopia; orbicularis weakness; irregular gray subretinal mottling; optic atrophy.

Clinical

Cerebral and cerebellar agyria-micropolygyria; cortical disorganization; glial mesodermal proliferation; neuronal heterotopias; hypoplasia of nerve tracts; hydrocephalus; encephalocele; muscular dystrophy; seizures; mental retardation; hypotonia; abnormal facies.

Laboratory

MRI, creatine kinases levels, electromyography and nerve conduction study.

Treatment

No specific treatment is available.

⊟ BIBLIOGRAPHY

1. Lopate G. (2013). Congenital Muscular Dystrophy. [online] Available from www.emedicine.com/neuro/TOPIC549. HTM. [Accessed August, 2013].

⊟ 4. CHOROIDAL DETACHMENT (CILIOCHOROIDAL DETACHMENT)

General

Separation of the choroid and sclera created by a fluid accumulation between the two layers.

Clinical

Sturge-Weber syndrome, Vogt-Koyanagi-Harada syndrome.

Ocular

Scleritis, choriditis, orbital pseudotumor.

Laboratory

Diagnosis is made by clinical findings.

Treatment

Topical use of cycloplegic/mydriatic drops in addition to topical steroids when necessary.

⊟ BIBLIOGRAPHY

1. Traverso CE. (2012). Choroidal Detachment. [online] Available from www.emedicine.com/oph/TOPIC63.HTM. [Accessed August, 2013].

⊟ 5. CHOROIDAL FOLDS

Choroidal folds are folds of the posterior pole, at the level of the choroid, with Hruby lens and pattern of alternating light lines on fluorescein angiography.

1. Choroidal tumor, such as a melanoma
2. Disciform degeneration
3. Exophthalmos
4. Graves disease (Basedow syndrome)
5. High hyperopia
†6. Idiopathic-no underlying pathologic state
†7. Infection of paranasal sinuses
†8. Long-standing orbital inflammation

†9. Massive cranioorbital hemangiopericytoma
10. Ocular hypotony
†11. Orbital mass
12. Papilledema
13. Posteriorly located choroidal detachment
†14. Postoperative condition, such as scleral buckle
15. Primary retinal detachment
†16. Subretinal neovascularization
17. Uveitis

---

†Indicates a general entry and therefore has not been described in detail in the text

⊟ BIBLIOGRAPHY

1. Traverso CE. (2012). Choroidal Detachment. [online] Available from www.emedicine.com/oph/TOPIC63.HTM. [Accessed August, 2013].

⏏ 5.1. MALIGNANT MELANOMA OF THE POSTERIOR UVEA (CHOROIDAL MELANOMA, CILIARY BODY MELANOMA, UVEAL MELANOMA, INTRAOCULAR MELANOMA)

General

Most common primary intraocular tumor in adults.

Clinical

Metastatic melanoma can appear in other parts of the body such as skin or liver.

Ocular

Intraocular tumors of the choroid, iris and ciliary body.

Laboratory

Ultrasonography, fluorescein angiography, indocyanine green angiography.

Treatment

Ocular therapy's goal is to eradicate the tumor before metastasis occurs. Diode laser, brachytherapy, stereotactic, local resection, enucleation and exenteration are all used to achieve this. Systemically intravenous therapy; intrahepatic chemoembolization has been used for isolated liver metastases. Proton beam is used to kill the tumor.

⏏ BIBLIOGRAPHY

1. Garcia-Valenzuela E, Pons ME, Puklin JE, et al. (2011). Choroidal Melanoma. [online] Available from www.emedicine.com/oph/TOPIC403.HTM. [Accessed August, 2013].

⏏ 5.2. JUNIUS-KUHNT SYNDROME [KUHNT-JUNIUS DISEASE; MACULAR SENILE DISCIFORM DEGENERATION (I); MACULA LUTEA JUVENILE DEGENERATION (2)]

General

Onset in advanced age or in juvenile period; etiology is unknown; possible autosomal dominant or recessive inheritance.

Ocular

Impairment of central vision; central scotoma; atrophic macular degeneration surrounded by retinal hemorrhages, resulting in mount-like lesion; exudative and atrophic reaction with deposit in and about macula.

Clinical

None.

Laboratory

Diagnosis is made by clinical findings.

Treatment

Macular degeneration: No treatment is available for non-neovascular age-related macular degeneration (AMD). Preventative therapy includes no smoking, control of hypertension, cholesterol and blood sugar, exercise and vitamins. Neovascular AMD treatment consists of laser, avastin and lucentis.

⏏ BIBLIOGRAPHY

1. Deutman AF. Hereditary dystrophies of the central retina and choroid. In: Winkelman JE, Crone RA (Eds). Perspectives in Ophthalmology. Amsterdam: Excerpta Medica; 1970.
2. Deutman AF. Macular dystrophies. In: Ryan SJ (Ed). Retina, 2nd edition. St. Louis: Mosby; 1994.
3. Kimura SJ, Caygill WM (Eds). Retinal Diseases. Philadelphia, PA: Lea & Febiger; 1966.

5.3. EXOPHTHALMOS (PROPTOSIS)

General

Abnormal protrusion of the eyeball. Etiology is varied and can include inflammatory, vascular or infections. Thyroid disease is the most frequent cause for both unilateral and bilateral exophthalmos.

Clinical

Thyroid disease, lymphoma, cavernous hemangiomas, leukemia, sinus disease.

Ocular

Proptosis, orbital cellulitis, orbital emphysema, lid retraction, punctate keratopathy, corneal ulcer, corneal perforation, diplopia.

Laboratory

Thyroid function studies, CT, MRI, ocular ultrasonography can all be used to determine the cause.

Treatment

Reversing the problem, which is causing the exophthalmos, is the treatment of choice and will minimize the ocular complications. Ocular lubricants are beneficial for controlling the corneal exposure.

BIBLIOGRAPHY

1. Mercandetti M, Cohen AJ. (2012). Exophthalmos. [online] Available from www.emedicine.com/oph/TOPIC616.HTM. [Accessed August, 2013].

5.4. BASEDOW SYNDROME (GRAVES DISEASE; HYPERTHYROIDISM; THYROTOXICOSIS; EXOPHTHALMIC GOITER; PARRY DISEASE)

General

Diffuse toxic goiter; inherited as a simple autosomal recessive; penetrance greater in females; however, dominant mode of inheritance and variable penetrance are possible; uncommon in either sex before the age of 15 years.

Ocular

Exophthalmos; swelling of eyelids and discoloration of upper eyelids; lid lag (von Graefe's sign); globe lag (Koeber's sign); lid trembling on gentle closure (Rosenbach's sign); reduced blinking (Stellwag's sign); retraction of upper lid; difficulty in everting upper lid (Gifford's sign); convergence weakness (Möbius's sign); impaired fixation on extreme lateral gaze (Suker's sign); possible external ophthalmoplegia (Ballet's sign); Dalrymple's sign (staring appearance); tearing; photophobia; epiphora; prolapse of lacrimal gland; neuroretinal edema; tortuous vessels; papilledema and papillitis; anisocoria; keratitis; increased IOP on upgaze; decreased visual acuity; enlargement of the extraocular muscles; increased volume of the extraorbital fat; superior rectus muscle enlargement; decreased venous outflow.

Clinical

Tachycardia; anxiety; insomnia; loss of weight; hyperhidrosis; restlessness; myocarditis (toxic); atrial fibrillation.

Laboratory

Visual field testing, forced duction testing for restrictive myopathy, CT, MRI, T4 and thyroid-stimulating hormone, thyroid-stimulating immunoglobulins.

Treatment

There is no immediate treatment; the disease is self-limited but prolonged course over 1 or more years. Five percent of patients may require surgical intervention which could be orbital decompression, strabismus surgery, lid-lengthening surgery or blepharoplasty.

BIBLIOGRAPHY

1. Ing E. (2012). Thyroid-associated orbitopathy. [online] Available from www.emedicine.com/oph/TOPIC237.HTM. [Accessed August, 2013].
2. Regensburg NI, Wiersinga WM, Berendschot TT, et al. Do subtypes of Graves' orbitopathy exist? Ophthalmology. 2011;118:191-6.

🗗 5.5. HYPEROPIA, HIGH

General

Defect in eyesight in which the focal point falls behind the retina, resulting in farsightedness; autosomal recessive; eye shorter than normal.

Ocular

Farsightedness.

Clinical

None.

Laboratory

Diagnosis is made by clinical findings.

Treatment

Glasses, contact lens, conductive keratoplasty, LASIK and phakic IOL.

🗗 BIBLIOGRAPHY

1. Roque MR, Roque BL, Limbonsiong R, et al. (2011). Conductive keratoplasty hyperopia and presbyopia. [online] Available from www.emedicine.com/oph/TOPIC736.HTM. [Accessed August, 2013].

🗗 5.10. OCULAR HYPOTONY

General

Low IOP resulting in anatomical or functional abnormalities to the eye.

Clinical

None.

Ocular

Thin corneas, corneal striae, aqueous flare, choroidal folds, effusion, macular folds, low IOP.

Laboratory

Diagnosis is made by clinical findings.

Treatment

Topical corticosteroids and cycloplegic agents are recommended.

🗗 BIBLIOGRAPHY

1. Roy FH, Fraunfelder FW, Fraunfelder FT. Roy and Fraunfelder's Current Ocular Therapy, 6th edition. London, UK: Elsevier; 2008.

🗗 5.12. PAPILLEDEMA

General

Papilledema is the swelling of the optic disk due to increased intracranial pressure.

Clinical

Holocranial headaches, neck and back pain, pulsatile tinnitus, nausea and vomiting.

Ocular

Visual loss, nerve fiber loss, intermittent or constant diplopia.

Laboratory

Lumbar puncture to determine if intracranial pressure is elevated.

Treatment

Underlying cause should be determined and treated. Systemic acetazolamide is the medical therapy of choice.

🗗 BIBLIOGRAPHY

1. Gossman MV, Giovannini J. (2012). Papilledema. [online] Available from www.emedicine.com/oph/TOPIC187.HTM. [Accessed August, 2013].

5.13. CHOROIDAL DETACHMENT (CILIOCHOROIDAL DETACHMENT)

General

Separation of the choroid and sclera created by a fluid accumulation between the two layers.

Clinical

Sturge-Weber syndrome, Vogt-Koyanagi-Harada syndrome.

Ocular

Scleritis, choriditis, orbital pseudotumor.

Laboratory

Diagnosis is made by clinical findings.

Treatment

Topical use of cycloplegic/mydriatic drops in addition to topical steroids when necessary.

BIBLIOGRAPHY

1. Traverso CE. (2012). Choroidal Detachment. [online] Available from www.emedicine.com/oph/TOPIC63.HTM. [Accessed January, 2013].

5.15. RETINAL DETACHMENT, RHEGMATOGENOUS

General

Subretinal fluid accumulation in the space between the neurosensory retina and the underlying RPE. Most common type of retinal detachment and occurs with a retinal tear that allows liquefied vitreous to seep under the tear leading to the detachment.

Clinical

None.

Ocular

Vitreous traction, cut in visual field; vitreous floaters; decreased visual acuity; scleritis.

Laboratory

Diagnosis is generally made by clinical observation. Ultrasound may be necessary if the media is hazy.

Treatment

Scleral buckle, pneumatic retinopexy and vitrectomy are used for this type of detachment and the goal is to close all the breaks.

BIBLIOGRAPHY

1. Wu L, Evans T. (2011). Rhegmatogenous retinal detachment treatment and management. [online] Available from emedicine.medscape.com/article/1224737-treatment. [Accessed August, 2013].

5.17. UVEITIS, ANTERIOR NONGRANULOMATOUS (IRITIS, CHRONIC)

General

Ocular inflammation. Etiology is idiopathic but certain systemic diseases may be the underlying cause.

Clinical

Human leukocyte antigen B27, Behçet disease, herpes zoster, sarcoidosis, syphilis, Lyme disease, JIA, Fuchs heterochromic iridocyclitis, tuberculosis.

Ocular

Photophobia, red eye, dull aching eye pain, perilimbal injection, keratic precipitates, flare and cell of anterior chamber, posterior synechiae, lenticular precipitates.

Laboratory

Diagnosis is made by clinical findings. If nongranulomatous iritis is recurrent, studies are necessary to determine the cause. HLA B27 typing, serologic testing for syphilis, sarcoidosis rheumatoid factor and Lyme disease may be indicated.

Treatment

Topical corticosteroids are the mainstay of therapy. Subconjunctival corticosteroids may be necessary in non-responding cases. Cycloplegia is useful for controlling pain and photophobia.

BIBLIOGRAPHY

1. Levinson RD. (2012). Uveitis, anterior, nongranulomatous. [online] Available from www.emedicine.com/oph/TOPIC587.HTM. [Accessed August, 2013].

6. CHOROIDAL HEMORRHAGE

1. Acutechoroiditis
*2. After glaucoma filtering procedure (especially with Sturge- Weber syndrome)
†3. Choroidal vascular aneurysm
†4. Choroidal vascular sclerosis, such as senile macular degeneration with hemorrhage (disciform degeneration of the macula)
5. General diseases
   A. Arteriosclerosis
   B. Blood dyscrasias
      1. Leukemia
      2. Pernicious anemia
      3. Purpura
      †4. Thrombocytopenia
   C. Diabetes mellitus (Willis disease)
   D. Ehlers-Danlos syndrome (fibrodysplasia elastica generalisata)
   E. Paget disease (osteitis deformans)
   F. Valsalva maneuver
†6. Myopia-accompanied by choroidal atrophy
†7. Papilledema-rare

*Indicates most frequent
†Indicates a general entry and therefore has not been described in detail in the text

BIBLIOGRAPHY

1. Traverso CE. (2012). Choroidal Detachment. [online] Available from www.emedicine.com/oph/TOPIC63.HTM. [Accessed August, 2013].

6.1. DOYNE HONEYCOMB CHOROIDITIS (DOMINANT ORBRUCH MEMBRANE DRUSEN; HUTCHINSON-TAYS CENTRAL GUTTATE CHOROIDITIS; HOLTHOUSE-BATTEN SUPERFICIAL CHOROIDITIS; MALATTIA-LEVENTINESE SYNDROME)

General

Autosomal dominant; represents early manifestation of senile macular degeneration; both sexes affected; onset in advanced age; patients present with drusen at an early age (2nd to 3rd year of life) with near-normal visual acuity in childhood.

Ocular

Drusen with multiple yellow lesions becoming calcified and presenting crystalline appearance.

Clinical

None.

Laboratory

Diagnosis is made by clinical findings.

Treatment

Vitamins, antioxidants, cessation of smoking and proper control of hypertension. There is evidence that patients with early or moderate dry macular degeneration should consume adequate quantities of antioxidants, including vitamin A, vitamin E, zinc and lutein. Prevention is the best treatment in this case because no satisfactory method exists.

BIBLIOGRAPHY

1. Maturi RK. (2012). Nonexudative ARMD. [online] Available from www.emedicine.com/oph/TOPIC383.HTM. [Accessed August, 2013].

🗗 6.2. STURGE-WEBER SYNDROME (MENINGOCUTANEOUS SYNDROME; VASCULAR ENCEPHALOTRIGEMINAL SYNDROME; NEURO-OCULOCUTANEOUS ANGIOMATOSIS; ENCEPHALOFACIAL ANGIOMATOSIS; ENCEPHALOTRIGEMINAL SYNDROME)

General

Trisomy 22 or partial trisomy inheritance. Variations include Jahnke syndrome (neuro-oculocutaneous angiomatosis without glaucoma), Schirmer syndrome (oculocutaneous angiomatosis with early glaucoma), Lawford syndrome (oculocutaneous angiomatosis with late glaucoma and no increase in volume of globe) and Mille syndrome (oculocutaneous syndrome with choroidal angioma but no glaucoma).

Ocular

Unilateral hydrophthalmos; secondary glaucoma (late) conjunctival angiomata (telangiectases); iris decoloration; nevoid marks or vascular dilation of the episclera; glioma; serous retinal detachment; choroidal angiomata; deep anterior chamber angle; port-wine stain of eyelids; buphthalmos; optic nerve cupping; anisometropia; hemianopsia; increased corneal diameter; enophthalmos; exophthalmos; optic atrophy; choroidal hemangioma; anterior chamber angle vascularization.

Clinical

Vascular port-wine nevus (face, scalp, limbs, trunk, leptomeninges); acromegaly; facial hemihypertrophy; intracranial angiomas; convulsion; mental retardation; obesity; limb atrophy.

Laboratory

Neuroimaging studies and the clinical examination have been the procedures of choice to establish the diagnosis.

Treatment

Anticonvulsants for seizure control, symptomatic and prophylactic therapy for headache and glaucoma treatment to reduce the IOP.

🗗 BIBLIOGRAPHY

1. Del Monte MA, Taravella M. (2012). Sturge-Weber syndrome. [online] Available from www.emedicine.com/oph/TOPIC348.HTM. [Accessed August, 2013].
2. Takeoka M, Riviello JJ. (2010). Pediatric Sturge-Weber syndrome. [online] Available from www.emedicine.com/neuro/TOPIC356.HTM. [Accessed August, 2013].

🗗 6.5A. ARTERIOSCLEROSIS

General

Thickening and induration of the arterial wall; prominent in the elderly.

Ocular

Increased arterial light reflex, copper/silver wire arteries; arteriovenous crossing changes; arterial caliber variation/irregularity; arterial straightening or tortuosity; intimal hyperplasia, medial atrophy, atherosclerotic fibrous plaques and calcifications of the internal elastic lamina observed in aged human orbital arteries.

Clinical

Increased collagen deposition in small- and medium-sized arteries with progressive replacement of the smooth muscle in the vessel walls; arterial wall changes at arteriovenous crossings.

Laboratory

Diagnosis is made by clinical findings.

Treatment

None.

🗗 BIBLIOGRAPHY

1. Büchi ER, Schiller P, Felice M, et al. Common histopathological changes in aged human orbital arteries. Int Ophthalmol. 1993;17:37-42.
2. Collins JF. Handbook of Clinical Ophthalmology. New York: Masson; 1982. p. 269.

⊟ 6.5B1. LEUKEMIA

General

Acute or chronic blood disorder.

Ocular

Engorgement of conjunctival vessels; papillary hypertrophy; aggregations of tumor cells in conjunctiva, choroid and orbit; secondary glaucoma; retinal venous engorgement and tortuosity with pronounced constrictions; retinal hemorrhages; retinal detachment; cotton-wool spots; macular edema; papilledema; optic atrophy; optic neuritis; paralysis of extraocular muscles; hypopyon; vitreous opacities; retinal sea fans; perilimbal subconjunctival infiltrates; corneal leukemic infiltration (rare); shallow serous retinal detachments; hyphema; iris neovascularization; central retinal vein occlusion; vitreous infiltrates.

Clinical

Frequent involvement of central nervous system; intracranial hemorrhage; thrombocytopenia; rising white cell count.

Laboratory

CBC and differential, bone marrow aspiration, immunophenotyping, chromosomal analysis.

Treatment

Chemotherapy with or without radiotherapy.

⊟ BIBLIOGRAPHY

1. Wu L, Evans T, Martinez J. (2012). Leukemias. [online] Available from www.emedicine.com/oph/TOPIC489.HTM. [Accessed August, 2013].

⊟ 6.5B2. ADDISON PERNICIOUS ANEMIA SYNDROME (PERNICIOUS ANEMIA SYNDROME; VITAMIN B12 DEFICIENCY ANEMIA; MACROCYTIC ANEMIA; BIERMER SYNDROME)

General

Autosomal dominant; female preponderance; onset between ages 30 years and 50 years; lack of intrinsic factor normally produced in the fundus of stomach and important for absorption of vitamin B12 in the intestinal tract; infrequent ocular involvement.

Ocular

Central scotoma, centrocecal scotomata, and field contractions in a few cases; retinal hemorrhages (round with white center) at the posterior pole; both retina and disk may have a whitish, hazy appearance; optic neuritis (ischemic); optic atrophy; palsies of extraocular muscles; ocular hypotony; cataract; bilateral, slowly progressive optic neuropathy, unclear etiology.

Clinical

Megaloblastic anemia (chronic and progressive); hypochlorhydria; glossitis; stomatitis; constipation or diarrhea; paresthesias and numbness; incoordination; ataxia; sphincter malfunction.

Laboratory

The peripheral blood usually shows a macrocytic anemia with a mild leukopenia and thrombocytopenia.

Treatment

The cause of the failure to absorb cobalamin should be determined. Vitamin B12 is available as either cyanocobalamin or hydroxocobalamin and each are useful in the treatment of vitamin B12 deficiency.

⊟ BIBLIOGRAPHY

1. Schick P, Conrad ME. (2013). Pernicious anemia. [online] Available from www.emedicine.com/med/TOPIC1799.HTM. [Accessed August, 2013].

6.5B3. KASABACH-MERRITT SYNDROME (CAPILLARY ANGIOMA-THROMBOCYTOPENIA; HEMANGIOMA-THROMBOCYTOPENIA; THROMBOCYTOPENIA PURPURA-HEMANGIOMA)

General

Angioma causing sequestration of platelets and platelet deficiency.

Ocular

Capillary hemangiomas of the orbit; retinal detachments.

Clinical

Extraorbital hemangiomas found on trunk, extremities and palate or in subglottic space; thrombocytopenia; found in infants; purpura and bleeding.

Laboratory

B-scan ultrasound, CT and MRI.

Treatment

Corticosteroids topical, injectable and systemic is the treatment of choice. Interferon alfa-2a has emerged as a new modality; laser surgery and incisional surgical techniques may be necessary.

BIBLIOGRAPHY

1. Seiff S, Zwick OM, DeAngelis DD, et al. (2011). Capillary Hemangioma. [online] Available from www.emedicine.com/oph/TOPIC691.HTM. [Accessed August, 2013].

6.5C. DIABETES MELLITUS

General

Complex disorder of carbohydrate, lipid and protein metabolism characterized by hyperglycemia and a relative or total lack of insulin. Development is influenced by both genetic and environmental factors. Most commonly occurs in middle or late life (type II) and is seen most commonly in the obese. Diabetes can occur in the 1st or 2nd decade of life (type I) and usually involves the lack of insulin production by the pancreas and the need for insulin therapy.

Clinical

Atherosclerosis; nephropathy; neuropathy; polyuria; polydipsia; polyphagia; obesity; elevated plasma glucose and elevated glycated hemoglobin (A1C).

Ocular

Diabetic retinopathy; vitreous hemorrhage; macular edema; cataract; glaucoma; asteroid hyalosis; extraocular muscle paralysis; rubeosis iridis; corneal hypesthesia; optic nerve atrophy; papillopathy.

Laboratory

Diagnosis made by fasting plasma glucose of greater than 126 mg/dL and 2 hours post glucose load (75 g) plasma glucose of greater than 200 mg/dL and confirmed by repeat test.

Treatment

Goals include elimination of symptoms, by reduction of blood sugar and blood pressure. Smoking cessation, aspirin therapy, weight loss, exercise, diabetic diet as well as oral medication and/or insulin are all used in the treatment of diabetes. Diabetic retinopathy is most successfully treated with retinal photocoagulation. Pars plana vitrectomy is sometimes necessary to remove vitreous hemorrhage. Other ocular problems caused by diabetes such as cataracts and glaucoma are treated in traditional methods.

BIBLIOGRAPHY

1. Khardori R. (2012). Type 2 diabetes mellitus. [online] Available from emedicine.medscape.com/article/117853-overview. [Accessed November, 2012].
2. Ostri C, Lund-Andersen H, Sander B, et al. Bilateral diabetic papillopathy and metabolic control. Ophthalmology. 2010;117:2214-7.
3. Richter GM, Torres M, Choudhury F, et al. Risk factors for cortical, nuclear, posterior subcapsular, and mixed lens opacities: The Los Angeles Latino Eye Study. Ophthalmology. 2012;119:547-54.

6.5D. EHLERS-DANLOS SYNDROME (FIBRODYSPLASIA ELASTICA GENERALISATA; CUTIS HYPERELASTICA; MEEKEREN-EHLERS-DANLOS SYNDROME; INDIAN RUBBER MAN SYNDROME; CUTIS LAXA)

General

Present at birth; autosomal dominant; two groups: cutaneous and articular; syndrome is one of the three primary disorders of elastic tissue [other two disorders are pseudoxanthoma elasticum (Grönblad-Strandberg syndrome) and senile elastosis]; inherited disorder of collagen biosynthesis.

Ocular

Hyperelasticity of palpebral skin; easy eversion of upper lid; ptosis; epicanthal folds; hypotony of extraocular muscles; strabismus; microcornea; thinning of cornea with keratoconus; thinning of sclera (blue sclera); subluxation of lens; angioid streaks; chorioretinal hemorrhages; retinitis proliferans with secondary detachment; macular degeneration; myopia; ruptured globe after minor trauma; limbus-to-limbus corneal thinning; acute hydrops; cornea plana; keratoglobus.

Clinical

Cutaneous manifestations include thin, atrophic, fragile skin, cutaneous hyperelasticity and pseudomolluscoid tumors; articular manifestations include excessive articular laxity and luxations; hypermobile joints.

Laboratory

Biochemical studies can detect alterations in collagen molecules in cultured skin fibroblasts. Molecular [deoxyribonucleic acid (DNA)]-based testing is available. Diagnosis may by urinary analyte assay and clinical examination is the most common.

Treatment

Ascorbic acid therapy, in the event of skin lacerations seriously consider alternatives to sutures, including adhesive strips and wound glues, monitor for cardiac conditions and scoliosis.

BIBLIOGRAPHY

1. Steiner RD. (2011). Genetics of Ehlers-Danlos syndrome. [online] Available from www.emedicine.com/ped/TOPIC654.HTM. [Accessed August, 2013].

6.5E. PAGET DISEASE (OSTEITIS DEFORMANS; CONGENITAL HYPERPHOSPHATEMIA; HYPEROSTOSIS CORTICALIS DEFORMANS; POZZI SYNDROME; CHRONIC CONGENITAL IDIOPATHIC HYPERPHOSPHATEMIA; OSTEOCHALASIS DESMALIS FAMILIARIS; FAMILIAL OSTEOECTASIA)

General

Autosomal dominant; more frequent in men, but more severe in women; onset after age of 40 years; characterized by diffuse cortical thickening of involved bones with osteoporosis, bowing deformities and shortening of stature; osteogenic sarcoma not infrequent.

Ocular

Shallow orbits with progressive unilateral or bilateral proptosis palsy of extraocular muscles; corneal ring opacities; cataract; retinal hemorrhages; pigmentary retinopathy; macular changes resembling Kuhnt-Junius degeneration; angioid streaks; papilledema; optic nerve atrophy; blue sclera; exophthalmos.

Clinical

Skull deformities; kyphoscoliosis; hypertension and arteriosclerosis; muscle weakness; waddling gait; hearing impairment; osteoarthritis.

Laboratory

Bone-specific alkaline phosphatase (BSAP) levels, radiographs may demonstrate both osteolysis and excessive bone formation. Bone biopsies may be necessary for diagnostic purposes in rare cases.

Treatment

Medical therapy for Paget disease should include bisphosphonate treatment with serial monitoring of bone markers. Nonsteroidal anti-inflammatory drugs and acetaminophen may be effective for pain management. Chemotherapy, radiation, or both may be used to treat neoplasms arising from pagetic bone.

BIBLIOGRAPHY

1. Lohr KM, Driver K. (2011). Paget disease. [online] Available from emedicine.medscape.com/article/334607-overview. [Accessed August, 2013].

6.5F. PURTSCHER SYNDROME (FAT EMBOLISM SYNDROME; TRAUMATIC RETINAL ANGIOPATHY; TRAUMATIC LIPORRHAGIA; VALSALVA RETINOPATHY OF DUANE; DUANE RETINOPATHY)

General

Most frequently seen in accidents associated with sudden rise in blood pressure and congestion in the head and chest; presence of fat embolism may be the causative factor; neurovascular changes in retina referred to as traumatic retinal angiopathy; several mechanisms have been proposed, including compressive trauma and post-traumatic fat embolism; most likely mechanism appears to be leukocyte aggregation by activated complement factor 5 (C5A), which can occur in diverse conditions such as trauma, acute pancreatitis, and connective tissue disease.

Ocular

Retinal and preretinal hemorrhages over entire fundus; cotton-wool exudates, mainly posterior aspect; retinal edema; posterior and macular serous detachment; venous congestion and engorgement; papilledema; usually bilateral, although unilateral causes have been reported.

Clinical

Multiple fractures (mainly extensive crushing); lung congestion; dyspnea; lymphorrhagia; pancreatitis; scleroderma; dermatomyositis; lupus erythematosus; childbirth.

Laboratory

Amylase level: Purtscher-like retinopathy is associated with acute pancreatitis; thus, an elevated amylase level may be diagnostic of this condition.

Treatment

In patients with retinopathy due to systemic vasculitis, steroid therapy is beneficial. Surgical care may be required for traumatic chest and head injuries.

BIBLIOGRAPHY

1. Chaum E. (2012). Purtscher retinopathy. [online] Available from www.emedicine.com/oph/topic419.HTM. [Accessed August, 2013].

7. PURTSCHER SYNDROME (FAT EMBOLISM SYNDROME; TRAUMATIC RETINAL ANGIOPATHY; TRAUMATIC LIPORRHAGIA; VALSALVA RETINOPATHY OF DUANE; DUANE RETINOPATHY)

General

Most frequently seen in accidents associated with sudden rise in blood pressure and congestion in the head and chest; presence of fat embolism may be the causative factor; neurovascular changes in retina referred to as traumatic retinal angiopathy; several mechanisms have been proposed, including compressive trauma and post-traumatic fat embolism; most likely mechanism appears to be leukocyte aggregation by activated complement factor 5 (C5A), which can occur in diverse conditions such as trauma, acute pancreatitis, and connective tissue disease.

Ocular

Retinal and preretinal hemorrhages over entire fundus; cotton-wool exudates, mainly posterior aspect; retinal edema; posterior and macular serous detachment; venous congestion and engorgement; papilledema; usually bilateral, although unilateral causes have been reported.

Clinical

Multiple fractures (mainly extensive crushing); lung congestion; dyspnea; lymphorrhagia; pancreatitis; scleroderma; dermatomyositis; lupus erythematosus; childbirth.

Laboratory

Amylase level: Purtscher-like retinopathy is associated with acute pancreatitis; thus, an elevated amylase level may be diagnostic of this condition.

Treatment

In patients with retinopathy due to systemic vasculitis, steroid therapy is beneficial. Surgical care may be required for traumatic chest and head injuries.

BIBLIOGRAPHY

1. Chaum E. (2012). Purtscher retinopathy. [online] Available from www.emedicine.com/oph/topic419.HTM. [Accessed August, 2013].

8. CHOROIDAL RUPTURES

General

Tearing of Bruch's membrane and the closely associated choriocapillaris and retinal pigment epithelium after contusive ocular injury.

Clinical

None.

Ocular

Subfoveal hemorrhage, pigmentary changes in the macula, angle recession.

Laboratory

Diagnosis is made by clinical findings.

Treatment

There is no treatment for choroidal rupture; however careful examinations are important to exclude other ocular complications.

BIBLIOGRAPHY

1. Wu L, Evans T. (2012). Choroidal Rupture. [online] Available from www.emedicine.com/oph/TOPIC533.HTM. [Accessed August, 2013].

9. CHOROIDEREMIA (TAPETOCHOROIDAL DYSTROPHY, PROGRESSIVE; CHOROIDAL SCLEROSIS)

General

Sex-linked; onset at early age; progressive; primary degeneration may be of the retina, retinal pigment epithelium, or choriocapillaris; pigment stippling or granularity also evident in female carriers who possess normal and abnormal cells, through Barr body inactivation of one X chromosome.

Ocular

Reduction of central vision; constriction of visual fields; night blindness; choroidal and retinal atrophy.

Clinical

None.

Laboratory

Diagnosis is made by clinical findings.

Treatment

Therapies are limited. Physicians should emphasize the therapies that are available to help patients. Perhaps, most importantly, it is essential to help patients maximize the vision they do have with refraction and low-vision evaluation. Vitamin A/beta-carotene may or may not be useful.

BIBLIOGRAPHY

1. Telander DG, Beus AD, Small KW. (2012). Retinitis Pigmentosa. [online] Available from www.emedicine.com/oph/TOPIC704.HTM. [Accessed August, 2013].

🖬 10. CHOROIDITIS (POSTERIOR UVEITIS)

1. Anterior and posterior uveitis
   A. Herpes simplex and zoster
   B. Peripheral uveitis (cyclitis)
   C. Sarcoidosis syndrome(Schaumann syndrome)
   D. Syphilis (acquired lues)
   E. Toxoplasmosis
   F. Tuberculosis
   †G. Unknown
   H. Vogt-Koyanagi-Harada syndrome (uveitis-vitiligo-alopecia-poliosis syndrome)
2. Acquired immunodeficiency syndrome (AIDS)
†3. Acute posterior multifocal placoid pigment epitheli-opathy
4. Behçet syndrome
5. Bird-shot choroidopathy
6. Candidiasis
7. Cat-scratch disease
8. Cryptococcosis
9. Cytomegalovirus (CMV) inclusion disease
10. Coccidioidomycosis
11. Epstein-Barr virus
12. Lyme disease
13. Histoplasmosis
†14. Multiple evanescent white dot syndrome
15. Multiple sclerosis
†16. *Pneumocystis carinii*
†17. Punctate inner choroidopathy
18. Sarcoidosis syndrome (Schaumann syndrome)
19. Serpiginous choroidopathy
20. Syphilis (acquired lues)
21. Systemic lupus erythematosus
22. Toxocariasis
*23. Toxoplasmosis
†24. Unknown
25. Varicella zoster

🖬 BIBLIOGRAPHY

1. Demiroğlu H, Barişta I, Dündar S. Risk factor assessment and prognosis of eye involvement in Behçet's disease in Turkey. Ophthalmology. 1997;104:701-5.
2. Kerrison JB, Flynn T, Green WR. Retinal pathologic changes in multiple sclerosis. Retina. 1994;14:445-51.
3. Ormerod LD, Skolnick KA, Menosky MM, et al. Retinal and choroidal manifestations of cat-scratch disease. Ophthalmology. 1998;105:1024-31.
4. Schubert HD, Greenebaum E, Neu HC. Cytologically proven seronegative Lyme choroiditis and vitreitis. Retina. 1994;14:39-41.

*Indicates most frequent
†Indicates a general entry and therefore has not been described in detail in the text

🖬 10.1A. HERPES SIMPLEX

General

Large, complex deoxyribonucleic acid (DNA) virus.

Ocular

Conjunctivitis; keratitis; iridocyclitis; corneal ulcer; uveitis; hyphema; hypopyon; iris atrophy; cataract; scleritis; dacryoadenitis; blepharitis; acute retinal necrosis.

Clinical

Recurrent skin vesicles on lids, perioral area, nose and genitalia; meningitis, encephalitis.

Laboratory

Viral cultures.

Treatment

Antiviral therapy, topical or oral, is an effective treatment of epithelial herpes infection.

🖬 BIBLIOGRAPHY

1. Wang JC. (2010). Ophthalmologic Manifestations of Herpes Simplex Keratitis. [online] Available from www.emedicine.com/oph/TOPIC100.HTM. [Accessed August, 2013].

⊟ 10.1A. HERPES ZOSTER

General

Caused by varicella zoster virus; about 75% of cases occur in persons over age of 45 years; condition is more frequent with advancing age and in patients who are immunocompromised by drugs or disease; in particular, an increasing number of patients with herpes zoster ophthalmicus are immunosuppressed.

Ocular

Conjunctivitis; keratitis; recurrent corneal ulcer; neuralgia; zoster rash of eyelids; uveitis; iris atrophy; scleritis; cataract; optic neuritis; paralysis of third nerve; proptosis; paralysis of lids; orbital apex syndrome; retinitis; neurotrophic keratitis; acute retinal necrosis; progressive outer retinal necrosis; ocular motor nerve pareses; tonic pupil; encephalitis; vasculitis.

Clinical

Local lesions involving the posterior or root ganglia; nerve damage; tissue scarring.

Laboratory

Diagnosed mostly on the basis of the characteristic pain and appearance of the dermatomal rashes.

Treatment

Antiviral agents, systemic corticosteroids, antidepressants, and adequate pain control. Immunocompetent adults aged 60 years or older, benefit from receipt of the herpes zoster vaccine and have a lower incidence of herpes zoster.

⊟ BIBLIOGRAPHY

1. Diaz MM, Foster CS, Walton RC, et al. (2011). Herpes zoster ophthalmicus. [online] Available from www.emedicine.com/oph/TOPIC257.HTM. [Accessed August, 2013].
2. Ghaznawi N, Virdi A, Dayan A, et al. Herpes zoster ophthalmicus: comparison of disease in patients 60 years and older versus younger than 60 years. Ophthalmology. 2011;118(11):2242-50.
3. Ho J, Xirasagar S, Lin H. Increased risk of a cancer diagnosis after herpes zoster ophthalmicus: a nationwide population-based study. Ophthalmology. 2011;118(6):1076-81.
4. Tseng HF, Smith N, Harpaz R, et al. Herpes zoster vaccine in older adults and the risk of subsequent herpes zoster disease. JAMA. 2011;305(2):160-6.

⊟ 10.1B. PARS PLANITIS (ANGIOHYALITIS, CHRONIC CYCLITIS, CYCLITIS PERPHERAL UVEITIS, PERIPHERAL UVEORETINITIS VITRITIS)

General

Idiopathic inflammatory condition.

Clinical

Sarcoidosis, multiple sclerosis, Lyme disease, toxocariasis, human T-lymphotropic virus (HTLV1).

Ocular

Cells and debris in the vitreous, vitritis, vascular sheathing, neovascularization, cystoid macular edema, vitreous hemorrhage, cataracts, glaucoma, retinal detachment, retinoschisis.

Laboratory

Diagnosis is made by clinical findings.

Treatment

Systemic corticosteroids, chlorambucil, azathioprine, cyclophosphamide, methotrexate, cyclosporine. Periocular corticosteroids are very effective. Cryotherapy is used on patients that are intolerant to corticosteroids.

⊟ BIBLIOGRAPHY

1. Roy FH, Fraunfelder FW, Fraunfelder FT. Roy and Fraunfelder's Current Ocular Therapy, 6th edition. London: Elsevier; 2008.

🔲 10.1C. SCHAUMANN SYNDROME (BESNIER-BOECK-SCHAUMANN SYNDROME; BOECK SARCOID; SARCOIDOSIS)

General

Etiology unknown; theories include tuberculosis, hypersensitivity to pine pollen, virus infection; affects blacks most often; chronic course with spontaneous remissions (*see* Heerfordt's syndrome); hilar or paratracheal nodes with erythema nodosum; onset most often in middle and old age; ocular involvement in 20–25% of all cases.

Ocular

Orbital granulomatous mass; bony defects; cutaneous and subcutaneous nodules; myogenic palsy; lacrimal gland adenopathy; decreased tear formation; secondary glaucoma; granulomatous uveitis with iris nodules, cells and flare; mutton fat keratic precipitates; keratitis sicca; vitreous floaters; band-shaped keratitis; complicated cataract; inflammatory retinal exudates; "candle wax drippings"; optic nerve atrophy; neuritis; eyelid nodules; ocular nerve enlargement (granuloma).

Clinical

Lymphadenopathy; hilar nodes; fatigue; cystic, punched-out or reticulated changes in small bones (mainly, hands and feet); muscle wasting; contractures; weakness in legs and arms.

Laboratory

Chest X-ray, CT scan, and MRI of the brain.

Treatment

Glucocorticoids are the treatment of choice.

🔲 BIBLIOGRAPHY

1. Sharma GD. (2011). Pediatric sarcoidosis. [online] Available from www.emedicine.com/ped/TOPIC2043.HTM. [Accessed August, 2013].

🔲 10.1D. ACQUIRED LUES (SYPHILIS; ACQUIRED SYPHILIS; LUES VENEREA; MALUM VENEREUM)

General

Causative agent, *Treponema pallidum*, usually transmitted sexually.

Ocular

Conjunctival chancroid; conjunctivitis; keratitis; blepharitis; ptosis; iris atrophy; hippus; dacryocystitis; optic nerve atrophy; optic neuritis; periostitis; episcleritis; scleritis; nystagmus; uveitis; vitreous hemorrhages; paralysis of sixth nerve; papilledema; retinal hemorrhages; retinitis proliferans; oculogyric crisis; neuroretinitis; papilledema (associated with aseptic meningitis); diffuse or multifocal chorioretinitis; vertical supranuclear gaze palsy; Benedikt syndrome.

Clinical

Primary lesion associated with regional lymphadenopathy; secondary bacteremic stage associated with generalized mucocutaneous lesions; tertiary stage characterized by destructive mucocutaneous, musculoskeletal, or parenchymal lesions, aortitis, or central nervous system disease; syphilis and human immunodeficiency virus (HIV) infection often coexist in the same patient who experiences a higher incidence and greater severity of neurologic and ocular manifestations; a significant percentage of patients infected with HIV-I and *T. pallidum* become seronegative to syphilis testing.

Laboratory

Serologic nontreponemal tests include Venereal Disease Research Laboratory (VDRL) and rapid plasma reagin (RPR).

Treatment

The goals are to reduce morbidity and to prevent complications. Penicillin is the antibiotic of choice for treating syphilis. Ocular syphilis should be treated the same as patients with neurosyphilis.

🔲 BIBLIOGRAPHY

1. Euerle B. (2012). Syphilis. [online] Available from www.emedicine.com/med/TOPIC2224.HTM. [Accessed August, 2013].
2. Majmudar PA. (2011). Interstitial Keratitis Overview of Interstitial Keratitis. [online] Available from www.emedicine.com/oph/TOPIC453.HTM. [Accessed August, 2013].

⊞ 10.1E. OCULAR TOXOPLASMOSIS (TOXOPLASMIC RETINOCHOROIDITIS; TOXOPLASMOSIS)

General

Parasite infestation caused by *Toxoplasma gondii*; cell-mediated immunity is believed to be the major defence mechanism against *Toxoplasma* infection; ocular toxoplasmosis occurs in approximately 1% of patients with AIDS; AIDS-related toxoplasma retinochoroiditis may have several atypical clinical manifestations.

Ocular

Keratitis; uveitis; optic atrophy; papillitis; anisocoria; persistent pupillary membrane; focal retinochoroiditis; scleritis; cataract; microphthalmos; myopia; nystagmus; esotropia.

Clinical

Cysts are seen in many organs, including brain and muscle; hydrocephalus; intracerebral calcification; various CNS complaints.

Laboratory

Serologic tests for anti-*T. gondii*. Antibodies are common.

Treatment

Triple drug therapy: pyrimethamine, sulfadiazine and prednisone. Pyrimethamine should be combined with folinic acid. Surgical care includes photocoagulation, cryotherapy or vitrectomy.

⊟ BIBLIOGRAPHY

1. Wuh L. (2011). Ophthalmologic Manifestations of Toxoplasmosis. [online] Available from www.emedicine.com/oph/TOPIC707.HTM. [Accessed August, 2013].
2. Lasave AF, Llopis MD, Muccioli C, et al. Intravitreal clindamycin and dexamethasone for zone 1 toxoplasmic retinochoroiditis at twenty-four months. Ophthalmology. 2010;1831-8.
3. Soheilian M, Ramezani A, Azimzadeh A, et al. Randomized trial of intravitreal clindamycin and dexamethasone versus pyrimethamine, sulfadiazine and prednisolone in treatment of ocular toxoplasmosis. Ophthalmology. 2011;118:134-41.

⊞ 10.1F. TUBERCULOSIS

General

Communicable disease caused by the acid-fast bacillus *Mycobacterium tuberculosis*.

Ocular

Conjunctivitis; subconjunctival nodules (tuberculomas); keratitis; pannus; corneal ulcer; blepharitis; cellulitis; meibomianitis; uveitis; dacryocystitis; chronic orbital cellulitis; retinitis; scleritis; scleral perforation; hypopyon; vitreous hemorrhages; optic neuritis; optic atrophy; tuberculous panophthalmitis; choroidal tubercles; intraorbital extraocular lesions.

Clinical

Pulmonary infection; pyuria; hematuria; epididymitis; dysuria; flank pain; distorted calyces; productive cough.

Laboratory

Acid-fast bacillus culture of body fluids including vitreous and aqueous. Polymerase chain reaction (PCR) is 89% positive for pulmonary infection.

Treatment

A course of chemotherapy (isoniazid, rifampin, pyrazinamide and ethambutol or streptomycin) for a period of 6 months is the recommended therapy.

⊟ BIBLIOGRAPHY

1. Collins JK. Handbook of Clinical Ophthalmology. New York: Masson; 1982.
2. D'Souza P, Garg R, Dhaliwal RS, et al. Orbital tuberculosis. Int Ophthalmol. 1994; 18:149-52.
3. DeVoe AG, Locatcher-Khorazo D. The external manifestations of ocular tuberculosis. Trans Am Ophthalmol Soc. 1964;62:203-12.
4. Roy FH, Fraunfelder FW, Fraunfelder FT. Roy and Fraunfelder's. Current Ocular Therapy, 6th editon. Philadelphia: WB Saunders; 2008.
5. Gupta V, Gupta A, Arora S, et al. Presumed tubercular serpiginous like choroiditis. Ophthalmology. 2003;110:1744-9.
6. Patkar S, Singhania BK, Agrawal A. Intraorbital extraocular tuberculosis: a report of three cases. Surg Neurol. 1994; 42:320-1.
7. Tejada P, Mendez MJ, Negreira S. Choroidal tubercles with tuberculous meningitis. Int Ophthalmol. 1994;18:115-8.

10.1H. VOGT-KOYANAGI-HARADA DISEASE (HARADA DISEASE; UVEITIS-VITILIGO-ALOPECIA-POLIOSIS SYNDROME)

General

Viral infection; occurs predominantly among Italian and Japanese individuals; young adults; chronic.

Ocular

White lashes; secondary glaucoma; bilateral uveitis; sympathetic ophthalmitis; exudative iridocyclitis; vitreous opacities; bilateral serous retinal detachment and edema with spontaneous reattachment after weeks; depigmentation and patches of scattered pigment later; bilateral acute diffuse exudative choroiditis; papilledema; macular hemorrhage; cataracts; phthisis bulbi; poliosis; scleromalacia; intraocular lymphoma.

Clinical

Poliosis; vitiligo; hearing defect; headache; vomiting; meningeal irritation; reported to occur rarely in children.

Laboratory

Immunohistochemistry specimens demonstrate infiltration of CD4+ T-cells, epithelioid cells and multinucleated giant cells.

Treatment

Systemic therapy involves the use of high-dose corticosteroids. Topical steroids may be needed in conjunction with the use of systemic steroids.

BIBLIOGRAPHY

1. Walton RC, Choczaj-Kukula A, Janniger CK. (2012). Vogt-Koyanagi-Harada Disease. [online] Available from www.emedicine.com/oph/TOPIC459.HTM. [Accessed August, 2013].

10.2. ACQUIRED IMMUNODEFICIENCY SYNDROME (AIDS; ACQUIRED CELLULAR IMMUNODEFICIENCY; ACQUIRED IMMUNODEFICIENCY)

General

Acquired breakdown of the immune system followed by disease that takes advantage of the body's collapsed defenses; acquired by shared drug needles or sexual intercourse; occurs most frequently in homosexually active men (75%), intravenous drug abusers (13%), and Haitian immigrants (6%).

Ocular

Retinal cotton-wool spots; cytomegalovirus retinitis; retinal periphlebitis; conjunctival Kaposi sarcoma; necrotizing retinitis; retinal hemorrhages; conjunctivitis sicca; orbital Burkitt lymphoma; peripheral retinochoroiditis; vitreitis; fungal corneal ulcer; hypopyon; acute glaucoma; third nerve palsy; anterior uveitis; atypical retinitis; orbital pseudotumor; herpes zoster ophthalmicus; herpes simplex keratitis; bacterial keratitis; molluscum contagiosum; cytomegalovirus retinitis; toxoplasma retinitis; acute retinal necrosis; HIV retinitis; syphilitic retinitis; *Pneumocystis carinii* choroiditis; fungal and bacterial endophthalmitis; fungal choroiditis; conjunctival microvasculopathy; keratitis sicca; subconjunctival hemorrhage.

Clinical

Because of lowered immunity, one third develops Kaposi sarcoma; pneumonia caused by *P. carinii*; death.

Laboratory

Enzyme-linked immunosorbent assay (ELISA) test is used for screening other tests are used to evaluate false-positive and false-negative test results.

Treatment

Medical consultations are required for systemic treatment. The treatment of CMV retinitis can include drugs such as ganciclovir, valganciclovir, fomivirsen, foscarnet and cidofovir. All of these drugs have specific adverse effects and complicate the decision to use for treatment.

BIBLIOGRAPHY

1. Dubin J. (2011). Rapid Testing for HIV. [online] Available from www.emedicine.com/emerg/TOPIC253.HTM. [Accessed August, 2013].
2. Copeland RA. (2011). Ocular Manifestations of HIV Infection. [online] Available from www.emedicine.com/oph/TOPIC417.HTM. [Accessed August, 2013].

10.4. BEHÇET SYNDROME (DERMATO-STOMATO-OPHTHALMIC SYNDROME; OCULOBUCCOGENITAL SYNDROME; GILBERT SYNDROME)

General

Virus infection; occurs in adults; chronic disease; complete remission is rare; etiology is unknown.

Ocular

Muscle palsies (occasional); nystagmus (occasional); conjunctivitis; hypopyon; iritis; recurrent uveitis; keratoconjunctivitis sicca; keratitis; vitreous hemorrhages; thrombophlebitis retinal veins (occasional); retinal hemorrhages; optic neuritis (occasional); macular edema; optic nerve atrophy; retinitis; secondary glaucoma; retinal vasculitis; disk edema; panophthalmitis; optic neuropathy; skin lesions, posterior uveitis and systemic complications have been associated with loss of vision with this disorder; corneal immune ring opacity.

Clinical

Aphthous lesions of mucous membranes of the mouth and genitalia; cerebellar signs; convulsions; paraplegia; skin erythema (multiforme, bullosum); arthritis; urethritis; glossitis; recurrent fever.

Laboratory

Nonspecific HLA B51 positive may help to support diagnosis.

Treatment

The goals of therapy are to suppress inflammation, to reduce the frequency and severity of recurrences, and to minimize involvement of the retina. To be effective, treatment must be started early. Extent of involvement and severity of disease determine the choice of medication. Treatment options include corticosteroids, cytotoxic agents, cyclosporine, and colchicine.

BIBLIOGRAPHY

1. Bashour M. (2012). Ophthalmologic manifestations of Behcet disease. [online] Available from www.emedicine.com/oph/TOPIC425.HTM. [Accessed August, 2013].

10.5. BIRDSHOT RETINOPATHY (VITILIGINOUS CHORIORETINITIS)

General

Uncommon; may relate to an inherited immune dysregulation but exact cause is unknown; average presenting age is 50 years; spots in the retina resemble the pattern seen with birdshot scatter from the shotgun.

Clinical

None.

Ocular

Gradual painless loss of vision; vitreous floaters; photopsia; vitritis; multiple ovoid spots that are orange to cream in color and hypopigmented in the posterior pole and in the mid periphery of the retina.

Laboratory

HLA-A29 blood testing; fluorescein angiography; indocyanine green angiography; optical coherence tomography; and electrophysiologic testing.

Treatment

Topical, systemic and regional steroids may be useful. Cyclosporine, ketoconazole and other immunomodulatory therapies may also be necessary.

BIBLIOGRAPHY

1. Samson CM, Ali AM, Foster CS. (2011). Birdshot Retinopathy. [online] Available from emedicine.medscape.com/article/1223257-overview. [Accessed August, 2013].

🖻 10.6. CANDIDIASIS

General

Yeast-like opportunistic fungal infection caused by *Candida albicans*.

Ocular

Uveitis; hypopyon; conjunctivitis; keratitis; corneal ulcer; blepharitis; endophthalmitis; dacryocystitis; papillitis; retinal atrophy; Roth spot; vitreous abscess; retrobulbar abscess; retinal detachment; panophthalmitis; chorioretinitis; infectious crystalline keratopathy.

Clinical

C. albicans normally is present as an intestinal saprophyte in 35–75% of the human population; in situations of internal environmental change, however, *Candida* can become pathogenic (e.g. obesity, diabetes mellitus, malignancy, and other debilitating conditions).

Laboratory

Common yeast from up to 50% of healthy individuals isolate directly from the eye should be attempted to confirm the presence of organism. Blood agar and Sabouraud's dextrose agar may be used; PCR for species identification.

Treatment

Mucocutaneous infection typically responds to topical therapy. Antifungal therapy should be started immediately after necessary cultures have been obtained from all suspected sites of infection. Infectious disease specialists are typically involved in cases of invasive candidiasis.

🖻 BIBLIOGRAPHY

1. Hedayati T. (2012). Candidiasis in Emergency Medicine. [online] Available from www.emedicine.com/emerg/TOPIC76.HTM. [Accessed August, 2012].

🖻 10.7. PARINAUD OCULOGLANDULAR SYNDROME (PARINAUD CONJUNCTIVA-ADENITIS SYNDROME; CATSCRATCH OCULOGLANDULAR SYNDROME; CATSCRATCH DISEASE; BARTONELLA HENSELAE)

General

Most frequently seen in children; incubation period 7–10 days; caused by small pleomorphic Gram-negative bacillus; good prognosis; affects both sexes; about 90% of patients with this condition have serologic evidence of infection by *Rochalimaea henselae*.

Ocular

Conjunctivitis; retrotarsal conjunctival granulations; formation of granulomata in anterior segment about 3 mm high and 2–6 mm in diameter; inferior fornix usually affected; ulceration common; neuroretinitis; optic neuritis.

Clinical

Tender, red papule at the site of a catscratch; regional preauricular and cervical lymphadenitis (often only one gland involved); irregular fever for 4–5 days and malaise; fever; parotid gland swelling.

Laboratory

Histopathology of biopsied lymph node of Warthin-Starry silver stain.

Treatment

Symptomatic treatment includes warm compresses, analgesics and antipyretics. Aspiration of lymph node if distension causes pain. Antibiotics may be necessary in severe cases.

🖻 BIBLIOGRAPHY

1. Chi SL, Stinnett S, Eggenberger E, et al. Clinical characteristics in 53 patients with cat scratch optic neuropathy. Ophthalmology. 2012;119(1):183-7.
2. Nervi SJ, Ressner RA, Drayton JR, et al. (2011). Catscratch disease. [online] Available from www.emedicine.com/med/TOPIC304.HTM. [Accessed August, 2013].

🔲 10.8. CRYPTOCOCCOSIS (TORULOSIS)

General

A pulmonary infection caused by *Cryptococcus neoformans*, a saprophyte found in weathered pigeon droppings, soil, and unpasteurized cow's milk; infection acquired through respiratory system and usually manifests as meningoencephalitis; higher incidence in patients with AIDS.

Ocular

Blurred or poor vision; diplopia; uveitis; papilledema; retinal detachment; retinal hemorrhage and exudates; secondary glaucoma; vitreous reaction; retinitis; proptosis; a mass over the optic nerve head; disease process can be bilateral or unilateral; cranial nerve VI palsy; visual loss; conjunctivitis.

Clinical

Severe headache; dizziness; ataxia; vomiting; tinnitus; memory disturbances; Jacksonian convulsions; fever usually is absent; occurs frequently in patients with leukemia or lymphoma.

Laboratory

The diagnosis is based on skin biopsy findings evaluated after fungal staining and culture.

Treatment

The goal of pharmacotherapy is either to terminate the infection when possible or to control the infection and to reduce morbidity when cure is not possible.

🔲 BIBLIOGRAPHY

1. King JW, DeWitt ML. (2013). Cryptococcosis. [online] Available from www.emedicine.com/med/TOPIC482.HTM. [Accessed August, 2013].

🔲 10.9. CYTOMEGALIC INCLUSION DISEASE (CYTOMEGALOVIRUS; CONGENITAL CYTOMEGALIC INCLUSION DISEASE)

General

Cytomegalovirus passes transplacentally from an asymptomatic mother to fetus.

Ocular

Uveitis; cataract; optic atrophy; inclusion bodies in the aqueous humor; severe conjunctivitis; corneal opacities; microphthalmos; strabismus; dacryoadenitis; chorioretinitis; CMV retinitis (most common cause of acquired viral retinitis, primarily because of the AIDS virus); glaucoma.

Clinical

Cerebral calcifications; microcephaly; mental retardation; inclusion bodies in the urine; spastic diplegia; seizures; cerebellar hypoplasia; intraventricular hemorrhage; hydrocephalus.

Laboratory

Antigen testing, qualitative and quantitative polymerase chain reaction, shell vial assay.

Treatment

Ganciclovir, foscarnet, acyclovir and cidofovir.

🔲 BIBLIOGRAPHY

1. Akhter K, Wills TS. (2013). Cytomegalovirus. [online] Available from www.emedicine.com/med/TOPIC504.HTM. [Accessed August, 2013].

10.10. COCCIDIOIDOMYCOSIS (VALLEY FEVER, SAN JOAQUIN FEVER)

General

Caused by fungus *Coccidioides immitis*.

Ocular

Conjunctivitis; choroiditis; uveitis; retinal hemorrhages; vitreal opacity; vitreal floaters; episcleritis; hypopyon; granulomatous lesion of optic nerve head; paralysis of sixth cranial nerve; secondary glaucoma; papilledema; mutton fat keratitic precipitates; necrotizing granulomatous conjunctivitis; iridocyclitis.

Clinical

Mild respiratory illness; cavity lung lesion.

Laboratory

Routine culture media, IgM antibody of acute, IgG antibody for present or past infection.

Treatment

Systemic fluconazole or amphotericin B is the treatment of choice. Ocular treatment includes topical amphotericin B and use of steroids sparingly.

BIBLIOGRAPHY

1. Hospenthal DR. (2011) Coccidioidomycosis. [online] Available from www.emedicine.com/ped/TOPIC423.HTM. [Accessed November, 2012].

10.11. INFECTIOUS MONONUCLEOSIS (MONONUCLEOSIS; EPSTEIN-BARR VIRUS, ACUTE; ACUTE EPSTEIN-BARR VIRUS, GLANDULAR FEVER)

General

Asymptomatic in childhood; manifested in late adolescence of early adulthood; associated with Burkitt lymphoma and nasopharyngeal carcinoma.

Ocular

Conjunctivitis; ptosis; hippus; dacryocystitis; episcleritis; hemianopsia; nystagmus; retinal and subconjunctival hemorrhages; optic neuritis; orbital edema; scotoma; paralysis of extraocular muscles; uveitis; peripheral choroiditis; keratitis; papilledema; scleritis; retrobulbar neuritis, Sjögren syndrome; retinitis, choroiditis.

Clinical

Fever; widespread lymphadenopathy; pharyngitis; hepatic involvement; presence of atypical lymphocytes and heterophile antibodies in the blood; fatigue.

Treatment

A self-limited illness that does not usually require specific therapy. Splenic rupture is an acute abdominal emergency that usually requires surgical intervention.

BIBLIOGRAPHY

1. Cunha BA. (2011). Infectious Mononucleosis. [online] Available from www.emedicine.com/med/TOPIC1499.HTM. [Accessed August, 2013].

10.12. LYME DISEASE

General

Caused by tick bite; symptoms resolve after treatment.

Ocular

Keratitis may occur up to 5 years after the first episode; diplopia; photophobia; ischemic optic neuropathy; iritis; panophthalmitis; conjunctivitis; exudative retinal detachment; choroiditis; vitreitis; multiple cranial nerve palsies; association with acute, posterior, multifocal, placoid, pigment epitheliopathy; branch retinal artery occlusion.

Clinical

Arthritis; increased intracranial pressure; effusion of knees; swelling of wrists.

Laboratory

Immunofluorescent assay (IFA) and ELISA.

Treatment

Oral antibiotics for 2–3 weeks: tetracycline 500 mg four times a day, doxycycline 100 mg two times a day, phenoxy-methyl penicillin 500 mg four times a day, or amoxicillin 500 mg three to four times a day.

BIBLIOGRAPHY

1. Zaidman GW. (2011). Ophthalmic Aspects of Lyme Disease Overview of Lyme Disease. [online] Available from www.emedicine.com/oph/TOPIC262.HTM. [Accessed August, 2013].

10.13. HISTOPLASMOSIS (HISTOPLASMOSIS CHOROIDITIS; HISTOPLASMOSIS MACULOPATHY; PRESUMED OCULAR HISTOPLASMOSIS SYNDROME)

General

Fungal infection caused by *Histoplasma capsulatum*.

Ocular

Circumpapillary atrophy; maculopathy; scattered yellow "histo" spots; optic disk edema; disseminated choroiditis (immunocompromised patients); vitreous hemorrhage; punched-out chorioretinal lesions; choroidal neovascular membrane; exogenous endophthalmitis (isolated report).

Clinical

Pulmonary infection; fever; malaise.

Laboratory

Sixty percent of the adult population from the Ohio and Mississippi river valleys have a positive histoplasmin skin test; therefore clinic course is most helpful.

Treatment

Although the diagnosis is clinical, certain ancillary tests help in confirming it. Fluorescein angiography, human leukocyte antigen (HLA) typing B7 and DRw2 may be indicated.

BIBLIOGRAPHY

1. Wu L. (2012). Presumed Ocular Histoplasmosis Syndrome. [online] Available from www.emedicine.com/oph/TOPIC406.HTM. [Accessed August, 2013].

10.15. DISSEMINATED SCLEROSIS (MULTIPLE SCLEROSIS)

General

Disseminated demyelination affecting white matter of the brain, spinal cord, and optic nerves; etiology is unknown.

Ocular

Nystagmus; ptosis; myokymia; optic atrophy; papillitis; optic neuritis; anisocoria; Argyll Robertson pupil; Marcus Gunn pupil; hippus, decreased or absent papillary reaction to light; periphlebitis; visual field defects; gaze palsy; paralysis of third or sixth nerve; uveitis; oscillopsia; Uhthoff symptom (reduction of visual acuity with exercise or ocular hyperthermia); pars planitis; retinal venous sheathing; retinitis; granulomatous uveitis.

Clinical

Incoordination; paresthesia; spasticity; tic douloureux; urinary frequency and infections; progressive disability; paralysis; death.

Laboratory

MRI, CSF positive for oligoclonal band, albumin and immunoglobulin G (IgG) index; brainstem auditory-evoked response (BAER) and somatosensory-evoked potentials (SEP).

Treatment

Patients with MS may require multiple consultations to rule out other causes for their symptoms. Drugs such as immunomodulators, immunosuppressors, antiparkinson agents, CNS stimulants are all used in the management of the disease.

BIBLIOGRAPHY

1. Luzzio C, Dangond F. (2012). Multiple sclerosis. [online] Available from www.emedicine.com/neuro/topic228.HTM. [Accessed January, 2013].

10.18. SCHAUMANN SYNDROME (BESNIER-BOECK-SCHAUMANN SYNDROME; BOECK SARCOID; SARCOIDOSIS)

General

Etiology unknown; theories include tuberculosis, hypersensitivity to pine pollen, virus infection; affects blacks most often; chronic course with spontaneous remissions (*see* Heerfordt's syndrome); hilar or paratracheal nodes with erythema nodosum; onset most often in middle and old age; ocular involvement in 20–25% of all cases.

Ocular

Orbital granulomatous mass; bony defects; cutaneous and subcutaneous nodules; myogenic palsy; lacrimal gland adenopathy; decreased tear formation; secondary glaucoma; granulomatous uveitis with iris nodules, cells and flare; mutton fat keratic precipitates; keratitis sicca; vitreous floaters; band-shaped keratitis; complicated cataract; inflammatory retinal exudates; "candle wax drippings"; optic nerve atrophy; neuritis; eyelid nodules; ocular nerve enlargement (granuloma).

Clinical

Lymphadenopathy; hilar nodes; fatigue; cystic, punched-out or reticulated changes in small bones (mainly, hands and feet); muscle wasting; contractures; weakness in legs and arms.

Laboratory

Chest X-ray, CT scan, and MRI of the brain.

Treatment

Glucocorticoids are the treatment of choice.

BIBLIOGRAPHY

1. Sharma GD. (2011). Pediatric sarcoidosis. [online] Available from www.emedicine.com/ped/TOPIC2043.HTM. [Accessed December, 2012].

10.19. SERPIGINOUS CHOROIDOPATHY

General

Etiology unknown; more frequently in men; onset between 4th decade and 5th decade of life; usually bilateral; rare in Crohn's disease, sarcoidosis and periarteritis nodosa; indistinguishable from tuberculosis (TB).

Ocular

Over half have scars in other eye which presents with decreased vision, metamorphopsia. Three types of ocular: (1) peripapillary geographic choroiditis, 80%; (2) macular serpiginous choroiditis, 10% and (3) relentless placoid chorioretinitis, 10%.

Laboratory

Diagnosis is made by clinical findings.

Treatment

Responds well to corticosteroid and immunomodulatory therapy. Periocular steroids may be useful; intravitreal triamcinolone if macula is threatened.

BIBLIOGRAPHY

1. Mansour SE, Cook GR. (2012). Multifocal Choroidopathy Syndromes. [online] Available from www.emedicine.medscape.com/article/1190935-overview. [Accessed August, 2013].

10.20. ACQUIRED LUES (SYPHILIS; ACQUIRED SYPHILIS; LUES VENEREA; MALUM VENEREUM)

General

Causative agent, *T. pallidum*, usually transmitted sexually.

Ocular

Conjunctival chancroid; conjunctivitis; keratitis; blepharitis; ptosis; iris atrophy; hippus; dacryocystitis; optic nerve atrophy; optic neuritis; periostitis; episcleritis; scleritis; nystagmus; uveitis; vitreous hemorrhages; paralysis of sixth nerve; papilledema; retinal hemorrhages; retinitis proliferans; oculogyric crisis; neuroretinitis; papilledema (associated with aseptic meningitis); diffuse or multifocal chorioretinitis; vertical supranuclear gaze palsy; Benedikt syndrome.

Clinical

Primary lesion associated with regional lymphadenopathy; secondary bacteremic stage associated with generalized mucocutaneous lesions; tertiary stage characterized by destructive mucocutaneous, musculoskeletal, or parenchymal lesions, aortitis, or central nervous system disease; syphilis and HIV infection often coexist in the same patient who experiences a higher incidence and greater severity of neurologic and ocular manifestations; a significant percentage of patients infected with HIV-I and *T. pallidum* become seronegative to syphilis testing.

Laboratory

Serologic nontreponemal tests include VDRL and RPR.

Treatment

The goals are to reduce morbidity and to prevent complications. Penicillin is the antibiotic of choice for treating syphilis. Ocular syphilis should be treated the same as patients with neurosyphilis.

BIBLIOGRAPHY

1. Euerle B. (2012). Syphilis. [online] Available from www.emedicine.com/med/TOPIC2224.HTM. [Accessed August, 2013].
2. Majmudar PA. (2011). Interstitial Keratitis Overview of Interstitial Keratitis. [online] Available from www.emedicine.com/oph/TOPIC453.HTM. [Accessed August, 2013].

10.21. DISSEMINATED LUPUS ERYTHEMATOSUS (SYSTEMIC LUPUS ERYTHEMATOSUS; LUPUS ERYTHEMATOSUS; KAPOSI-LIBMAN-SACK SYNDROME, SLE)

General

Possible etiology includes viral infections and genetic predisposition; immunologic abnormalities.

Ocular

Keratitis; keratoconjunctivitis sicca; corneal ulcer; optic nerve atrophy; optic neuritis; papilledema; arteritis; central retinal vein occlusion; retinal detachment; microaneurysm; scleritis; uveitis; ptosis; conjunctivitis; paralysis of third nerve; homonymous hemianopsia; multifocal microinfarcts; mydriasis; nystagmus; proptosis; orbital myositis; pseudoretinitis pigmentosa; photophobia.

Clinical

Polyarthritis; morning stiffness; fever; malaise; fatigue; polyserositis; renal disease; central nervous system disease; anemia; leukopenia; maculopapular rash in a "butterfly" distribution over malar region; alopecia.

Laboratory

Antibodies to double-stranded DNA or the Smith (Sm) antigen or a false-positive serology test for syphilis; positive antinuclear antibody test that is caused by a medication.

Treatment

Fever, rash, musculoskeletal, and serositis manifestations respond to hydroxychloroquine and NSAIDs. Low-to-moderate dose steroids are necessary for acute flares. CNS involvement and renal disease constitute more serious disease and often require high-dose steroids and other immunosuppression agents. Diffuse proliferative lupus nephritis has been treated with cyclophosphamide induction therapy.

BIBLIOGRAPHY

1. Bartles CM, Muller D. (2012). Systemic erythematosus lupus. [online] Available from www.emedicine.com/med/TOPIC2228.HTM. [Accessed November, 2012].

🖻 10.22. NEMATODE OPHTHALMIA SYNDROME (VISCERAL LARVA MIGRANS SYNDROME; TOXOCARIASIS)

General

Usually found in children; invasion by larvae of *Toxocara canis* and *Toxocara cati* of viscera and eyes; pronounced eosinophilia; as many as 30% of asymptomatic children demonstrate serologic evidence of prior *Toxocara infestations.*

Ocular

Leukocoria; uveitis; cataract; marked vitreous reaction with large floaters; choroiditis; large, cyst-like white masses extending into vitreous; optic neuritis; papillitis; strabismus; hemorrhagic, exudative, or granulomatous retinitis; retinal detachment; endophthalmitis; larvae present in the cornea.

Clinical

Hepatosplenomegaly; pulmonary infiltration; fever; cough; lack of appetite.

Laboratory

Eosinophilia in patients with visceral disease. ELISA test is best to document systemic or ocular infection with *T. canis.*

Treatment

Treatment is by case-by-case basis; in most cases no treatment is needed; systemic anthelmintic agents; vitrectomy may be necessary.

🖻 BIBLIOGRAPHY

1. Biglan AW, Glickman LT, Lobes LA. Serum and vitreous Toxocara antibody in nematode endophthalmitis. Am J Ophthalmol. 1979;88:898-901.
2. Fraunfelder FT, Roy FH. Current Ocular Therapy, 5th edition. Philadelphia: WB Saunders; 2000.
3. Maguire AM, Green WR, Michels RG, et al. Recovery of intraocular Toxocara Canis by pars plana vitrectomy. Ophthalmology. 1990;97:675-80.
4. Raistrick ER, Hart JC. Ocular toxocariasis in adults. Br J Ophthalmol. 1976;60:365-70.
5. Wilder HC. Nematode endophthalmitis. Trans Am Acad Ophthalmol Otolaryngol. 1950;55:99.
6. Wilkinson C. Ocular toxocariasis. In: Ryan SJ (Ed). Retina, 2nd edition. St. Louis: Mosby; 1994. pp. 1545-52

🖻 10.23. OCULAR TOXOPLASMOSIS (TOXOPLASMIC RETINOCHOROIDITIS; TOXOPLASMOSIS)

General

Parasite infestation caused by *T. gondii*; cell-mediated immunity is believed to be the major defence mechanism against *Toxoplasma* infection; ocular toxoplasmosis occurs in approximately 1% of patients with AIDS; AIDS-related toxoplasma retinochoroiditis may have several atypical clinical manifestations.

Ocular

Keratitis; uveitis; optic atrophy; papillitis; anisocoria; persistent pupillary membrane; focal retinochoroiditis; scleritis; cataract; microphthalmos; myopia; nystagmus; esotropia.

Clinical

Cysts are seen in many organs, including brain and muscle; hydrocephalus; intracerebral calcification; various CNS complaints.

Laboratory

Serologic tests for anti-*T. gondii*. Antibodies are common.

Treatment

Triple drug therapy: pyrimethamine, sulfadiazine and prednisone. Pyrimethamine should be combined with folinic acid. Surgical care includes photocoagulation, cryotherapy or vitrectomy.

🖻 BIBLIOGRAPHY

1. Wuh L. (2011). Ophthalmologic Manifestations of Toxoplasmosis. [online] Available from www.emedicine.com/oph/TOPIC707.HTM. [Accessed August, 2013].
2. Lasave AF, Llopis MD, Muccioli C, et al. Intravitreal clindamycin and dexamethasone for zone 1 toxoplasmic retinochoroiditis at twenty-four months. Ophthalmology. 2010;1831-8.
3. Soheilian M, Ramezani A, Azimzadeh A, et al. Randomized trial of intravitreal clindamycin and dexamethasone versus pyrimethamine, sulfadiazine and prednisolone in treatment of ocular toxoplasmosis. Ophthalmology. 2011;118:134-41.

🗗 10.25. CHICKENPOX (VARICELLA)

General

Acute exanthematous disease; highly contagious; children ages between 2 years and 8 years.

Ocular

Conjunctival ulcer; corneal ulcer; descemetocele; corneal opacity; keratitis; paresis of third, fourth, and sixth nerves; optic neuritis; papilledema; retinitis; hemorrhagic retinopathy; uveitis; cataract; paralytic mydriasis; phthisis bulbi; unifocal choroiditis; dendritic keratitis; acute retinal necrosis (in a patient with AIDS); disciform keratitis.

Clinical

Fever; malaise; rash; pruritus.

Laboratory

Diagnosis is made by clinical findings.

Treatment

Isolation oral antihistamines, such as diphenhydramine and hydroxyzine, are used for severe pruritus and acetaminophen is recommended for use for the reduction of fever.

🗗 BIBLIOGRAPHY

1. Bechtel KA. (2011). Pediatric Chickenpox. [online] Available from www.emedicine.com/emerg/TOPIC367.HTM. [Accessed August, 2013].

🗗 11. CHOROIDITIS (POSTERIOR UVEITIS) IN CHILDREN

1. Ankylosing spondylitis
2. Anterior and posterior uveitis
   A. Sarcoidosis syndrome (Schaumann syndrome)
   B. Sympathetic ophthalmia
   C. Vogt-Koyanagi-Harada syndrome
†3. Arteritis
4. Behçet disease (dermatostomatoophthalmic syndrome)
†5. Chorioretinitis of unknown cause
   †A. Disseminated chorioretinitis
   B. Juxtapapillary chorioretinitis
6. Cytomegalovirus inclusion disease (cytomegalovirus)
7. Diffuse unilateral subacute neuroretinitis
8. Herpes simplex chorioretinitis
9. Human immunodeficiency virus retinopathy
†10. Inability of leukocytes to kill microorganisms
11. Intermediate uveitis
12. Juvenile psoriatic arthritis
13. Juvenile rheumatoid arthritis
14. Nematode (Toxocara) retinochoroiditis
15. Reiter disease* (idiopathic blennorrheal arthritis syndrome)
16. Reticulum cell sarcoma of brain
17. Rubella
18. Subacute sclerosing panencephalitis
19. Syphilitic retinochoroiditis
*20. Toxoplasmic retinochoroiditis
21. Tuberculosis

🗗 BIBLIOGRAPHY

1. Kanski JJ, Shun-Shin A. Systemic uveitis syndrome in childhood: an analysis of cases. Ophthalmology. 1984;91: 1247-51.
2. Kraus-Mackiw E. O'Connor GR (Ed). Uveitis: Pathophysiology and Therapy, 2nd edition. New York: Thieme; 1986.
3. Okada AA, Foster CS. Posterior uveitis in the pediatric population. Int Ophthalmol Clin. 1992;32:121-52.

*Indicates most frequent
†Indicates a general entry and therefore has not been described in detail in the text

11.1. VON BEKHTEREV-STRUMPELL SYNDROME (MARIE-STRUMPELL SPONDYLITIS; ANKYLOSING SPONDYLITIS; PIERRE-MARIE SYNDROME; BEKHTEREV DISEASE; RHEUMATOID SPONDYLITIS) OPTIC ATROPHY

General

Variant of RA; etiology unknown; autosomal dominant; male preponderance; onset at age 20–40 years; although genetic background determines susceptibility to uveitis, the disease pattern suggests the possibility of random environmental triggers unrelated to the course of the underlying rheumatologic disorder.

Ocular

Nongranulomatous anterior uveitis; optic nerve atrophy (occasionally); hypopyon; band keratopathy; spontaneous hyphema.

Clinical

Spondylitis of vertebra and sacroiliac joints; ankylosis; general arthralgia; kyphosis; scoliosis; displaced head and total rigidity of spine.

Laboratory

Histocompatibility antigen HLA-B27 and a negative rheumatoid factor and ANA; X-ray evidence of narrowing of sacroiliac joint space and sclerosis.

Treatment

Oral NSAIDs, urethritis in Reiter's disease should be treated with tetracycline, topical steroids and cycloplegic agents.

BIBLIOGRAPHY

1. Vives MJ, Garfin SR. (2011). Rheumatoid arthritis of the cervical spine overview of rheumatoid spondylitis. [online] Available from www.emedicine.com/orthoped/TOPIC551. HTM. [Accessed August, 2013].

11.2A. SCHAUMANN SYNDROME (BESNIER-BOECK-SCHAUMANN SYNDROME; BOECK SARCOID; SARCOIDOSIS)

General

Etiology unknown; theories include tuberculosis, hypersensitivity to pine pollen, virus infection; affects blacks most often; chronic course with spontaneous remissions (*see* Heerfordt's syndrome); hilar or paratracheal nodes with erythema nodosum; onset most often in middle and old age; ocular involvement in 20–25% of all cases.

Ocular

Orbital granulomatous mass; bony defects; cutaneous and subcutaneous nodules; myogenic palsy; lacrimal gland adenopathy; decreased tear formation; secondary glaucoma; granulomatous uveitis with iris nodules, cells and flare; mutton fat keratic precipitates; keratitis sicca; vitreous floaters; band-shaped keratitis; complicated cataract; inflammatory retinal exudates; "candle wax drippings"; optic nerve atrophy; neuritis; eyelid nodules; ocular nerve enlargement (granuloma).

Clinical

Lymphadenopathy; hilar nodes; fatigue; cystic, punched-out or reticulated changes in small bones (mainly, hands and feet); muscle wasting; contractures; weakness in legs and arms.

Laboratory

Chest X-ray, CT scan, and MRI of the brain.

Treatment

Glucocorticoids are the treatment of choice.

BIBLIOGRAPHY

1. Sharma GD. (2011). Pediatric sarcoidosis. [online] Available from www.emedicine.com/ped/TOPIC2043.HTM. [Accessed August, 2013].

11.2B. SYMPATHETIC OPHTHALMIA

General

Trauma or injury to one eye and later onset of inflammation in the other eye.

Ocular

Iridocyclitis (acute inflammation of iris, ciliary body and anterior chamber); choroiditis; chronic persistent keratitic precipitates; posterior synechiae; phthisis bulbi; it has been reported following laser cyclocoagulation.

Clinical

None.

Laboratory

Diagnosis is made by clinical findings.

Treatment

Aggressive treatment is done with steroids and nonsteroids.

BIBLIOGRAPHY

1. Bechrakis NE, Müller-Stolzenburg NW, Helbig H, et al. Sympathetic ophthalmia following laser cyclocoagulation. Arch Ophthalmol. 1994;112(1):80-4.
2. Boniuk V, Boniuk M. The incidence of phthisis bulbas a complication of cataract surgery in the congenital rubella syndrome. Trans Am Acad Ophthalmol Otolaryngol. 1970;74(2):360-8.
3. Duane TD. Clinical Ophthalmology. Philadelphia, PA: JB Lippincott; 1987.

11.2C. VOGT-KOYANAGI-HARADA DISEASE (HARADA DISEASE; UVEITIS-VITILIGO-ALOPECIA-POLIOSIS SYNDROME)

General

Viral infection; occurs predominantly among Italian and Japanese individuals; young adults; chronic.

Ocular

White lashes; secondary glaucoma; bilateral uveitis; sympathetic ophthalmitis; exudative iridocyclitis; vitreous opacities; bilateral serous retinal detachment and edema with spontaneous reattachment after weeks; depigmentation and patches of scattered pigment later; bilateral acute diffuse exudative choroiditis; papilledema; macular hemorrhage; cataracts; phthisis bulbi; poliosis; scleromalacia; intraocular lymphoma.

Clinical

Poliosis; vitiligo; hearing defect; headache; vomiting; meningeal irritation; reported to occur rarely in children.

Laboratory

Immunohistochemistry specimens demonstrate infiltration of CD4+ T-cells, epithelioid cells and multinucleated giant cells.

Treatment

Systemic therapy involves the use of high-dose corticosteroids. Topical steroids may be needed in conjunction with the use of systemic steroids.

BIBLIOGRAPHY

1. Walton RC, Choczaj-Kukula A, Janniger CK. (2012). Vogt-Koyanagi-Harada Disease. [online] Available from www.emedicine.com/oph/TOPIC459.HTM. [Accessed August, 2013].

11.4. BEHÇET SYNDROME (DERMATO-STOMATO-OPHTHALMIC SYNDROME; OCULOBUCCOGENITAL SYNDROME; GILBERT SYNDROME)

General

Virus infection; occurs in adults; chronic disease; complete remission is rare; etiology is unknown.

Ocular

Muscle palsies (occasional); nystagmus (occasional); conjunctivitis; hypopyon; iritis; recurrent uveitis; keratoconjunctivitis sicca; keratitis; vitreous hemorrhages; thrombophlebitis retinal veins (occasional); retinal hemorrhages; optic neuritis (occasional); macular edema; optic nerve atrophy; retinitis; secondary glaucoma; retinal vasculitis; disk edema; panophthalmitis; optic neuropathy; skin lesions, posterior uveitis and systemic complications have been associated with loss of vision with this disorder; corneal immune ring opacity.

Clinical

Aphthous lesions of mucous membranes of the mouth and genitalia; cerebellar signs; convulsions; paraplegia; skin erythema (multiforme bullosum); arthritis; urethritis; glossitis; recurrent fever.

Laboratory

Nonspecific HLA B51 positive may help to support diagnosis.

Treatment

The goals of therapy are to suppress inflammation, to reduce the frequency and severity of recurrences, and to minimize involvement of the retina. To be effective, treatment must be started early. Extent of involvement and severity of disease determine the choice of medication. Treatment options include corticosteroids, cytotoxic agents, cyclosporine, and colchicine.

BIBLIOGRAPHY

1. Bashour M. (2012). Ophthalmologic manifestations of Behcet disease. [online] Available from www.emedicine.com/oph/TOPIC425.HTM. [Accessed August, 2013].

11.5B. JENSEN DISEASE (JUXTAPAPILLARY RETINOPATHY)

General

Etiology is unknown.

Ocular

Circumscribed inflammatory changes of the choroid; field defect.

Clinical

None.

Laboratory

Diagnosis is made by clinical findings.

Treatment

None—ocular.

BIBLIOGRAPHY

1. Harley RD, Nelson LB, Olitsky SE (Eds). Harley's Pediatric Ophthalmology, 5th illustrated edition. Philadelphia, PA: Lippincott Williams & Wilkins; 2005.
2. Magalini SI, Scrascia E. Dictionary of Medical Syndromes, 2nd edition. Philadelphia, PA: JB Lippincott; 1981.

11.6. CYTOMEGALIC INCLUSION DISEASE (CYTOMEGALOVIRUS; CONGENITAL CYTOMEGALIC INCLUSION DISEASE)

General

Cytomegalovirus passes transplacentally from an asymptomatic mother to fetus.

Ocular

Uveitis; cataract; optic atrophy; inclusion bodies in the aqueous humor; severe conjunctivitis; corneal opacities; microphthalmos; strabismus; dacryoadenitis; chorioretinitis; CMV retinitis (most common cause of acquired viral retinitis, primarily because of the AIDS virus); glaucoma.

Clinical

Cerebral calcifications; microcephaly; mental retardation; inclusion bodies in the urine; spastic diplegia; seizures; cerebellar hypoplasia; intraventricular hemorrhage; hydrocephalus.

Laboratory

Antigen testing, qualitative and quantitative polymerase chain reaction, shell vial assay.

Treatment

Ganciclovir, foscarnet, acyclovir and cidofovir.

BIBLIOGRAPHY

1. Akhter K, Wills TS. (2013). Cytomegalovirus. [online] Available from www.emedicine.com/med/TOPIC504.HTM. [Accessed August, 2013].

11.7. DIFFUSE UNILATERAL SUBACUTE NEURORETINITIS SYNDROME (DUSN; UNILATERAL WIPEOUT SYNDROME; WIPEOUT SYNDROME)

General

It is caused by a nematode that is not *T. canis*, i.e. at least two nematodes of different sizes; usually occurs in children or young adults; nematode may remain viable in the eye for 3 years or longer.

Ocular

Vitreitis; papillitis; gray-white lesions of retina; optic atrophy; retinal vessel narrowing; diffuse pigment epithelial degeneration; endophthalmitis; nematode in fundus; the pathognomonic finding in DUSN is the presence of a motile intraocular nematode.

Clinical

Weight loss; lack of appetite; cough; fever; pulmonary infiltration; hepatomegaly; leukocytosis; persistent eosinophilia.

Laboratory

Electroretinopathy, enzyme-linked immunosorbent assays for individual nematode species.

Treatment

Direct laser photocoagulation of the nematode is the treatment of choice for DUSN; surgical transvitreal removal of the nematode may be indicated in selected cases.

BIBLIOGRAPHY

1. Kooragayala LM. (2011). Diffuse unilateral subacute neuroretinitis. [online] Available from emedicine.medscape.com/article/1226931-overview. [Accessed February, 2013].

🔲 11.8. HERPES SIMPLEX

General

Large, complex DNA virus.

Ocular

Conjunctivitis; keratitis; iridocyclitis; corneal ulcer; uveitis; hyphema; hypopyon; iris atrophy; cataract; scleritis; dacryoadenitis; blepharitis; acute retinal necrosis.

Clinical

Recurrent skin vesicles on lids, perioral area, nose and genitalia; meningitis, encephalitis.

Laboratory

Viral cultures.

Treatment

Antiviral therapy, topical or oral, is an effective treatment of epithelial herpes infection.

🔲 BIBLIOGRAPHY

1. Wang JC. (2010). Ophthalmologic Manifestations of Herpes Simplex Keratitis. [online] Available from www.emedicine.com/oph/TOPIC100.HTM. [Accessed August, 2013].
2. Shaohui L, Pavan-Langston D, Colby KA. Pediatric herpes simplex of the anterior segment: characteristics, treatment, and outcomes. Ophthalmology. 2012;119:2003-8.

🔲 11.9. ACQUIRED IMMUNODEFICIENCY SYNDROME (AIDS; ACQUIRED CELLULAR IMMUNODEFICIENCY; ACQUIRED IMMUNODEFICIENCY)

General

Acquired breakdown of the immune system followed by disease that takes advantage of the body's collapsed defenses; acquired by shared drug needles or sexual intercourse; occurs most frequently in homosexually active men (75%), intravenous drug abusers (13%), and Haitian immigrants (6%).

Ocular

Retinal cotton-wool spots; CMV retinitis; retinal periphlebitis; conjunctival Kaposi sarcoma; necrotizing retinitis; retinal hemorrhages; conjunctivitis sicca; orbital Burkitt lymphoma; peripheral retinochoroiditis; vitreitis; fungal corneal ulcer; hypopyon; acute glaucoma; third nerve palsy; anterior uveitis; atypical retinitis; orbital pseudotumor; herpes zoster ophthalmicus; herpes simplex keratitis; bacterial keratitis; molluscum contagiosum; toxoplasma retinitis; acute retinal necrosis; HIV retinitis; syphilitic retinitis; *P. carinii* choroiditis; fungal and bacterial endophthalmitis; fungal choroiditis; conjunctival microvasculopathy; keratitis sicca; subconjunctival hemorrhage.

Clinical

Because of lowered immunity, one third develops Kaposi sarcoma; pneumonia caused by *P. carinii*; death.

Laboratory

Enzyme-linked immunosorbent assay test is used for screening other tests are used to evaluate false-positive and false-negative test results.

Treatment

Medical consultations are required for systemic treatment. The treatment of CMV retinitis can include drugs such as ganciclovir, valganciclovir, fomivirsen, foscarnet and cidofovir. All of these drugs have specific adverse effects and complicate the decision to use for treatment.

🔲 BIBLIOGRAPHY

1. Dubin J. (2011). Rapid Testing for HIV. [online] Available from www.emedicine.com/emerg/TOPIC253.HTM. [Accessed August, 2013].
2. Copeland RA. (2011). Ocular Manifestations of HIV Infection. [online] Available from www.emedicine.com/oph/TOPIC417.HTM. [Accessed August, 2013].

11.11. UVEITIS (IRITIS, IRIDOCYSTITIS, INTERMEDIATE AND POSTERIOR UVEITIS, NONINFECTIOUS CHORIORETINITIS)

General

Mostly idiopathic or post-traumatic but other causes include infections, malignancies, autoimmune diseases and pharmaceutical.

Ocular

Photophobia, ciliary flush, decreased vision.

Clinical

None.

Laboratory

Chest X-ray—sarcoid; purified protein derivative (PPD), fluorescent treponemal antibody-absorption (FTA-ABS)—syphilis; Lyme C6 peptide—Lyme disease.

Treatment

Oral steroids should be given if not responsive to topical steroids; immunosuppressants if bilateral disease that does not respond to oral steroids; periocular steroids for unilateral or posterior uveitis. Vitrectomy can be used for severe vitreous opacification. Cryotherapy and laser photocoagulation may be used for localized pars plana exudates. Fluocinolone acetonide intravitreal implants may also be useful.

BIBLIOGRAPHY

1. Levinson RD. (2012). Uveitis, anterior, granulomatous. [online] Available from www.emedicine.com/oph/TOPIC586.HTM. [Accessed August, 2013].
2. Levinson RD. (2012). Uveitis, anterior, nongranulomatous. [online] Available from www.emedicine.com/oph/TOPIC587.HTM. [Accessed August, 2013].
3. Walton RC. (2012). Uveitis, anterior, childhood. [online] Available from www.emedicine.com/oph/TOPIC585.HTM. [Accessed August, 2013].

11.12. PSORIATIC ARTHRITIS

General

Chronic skin disease of unknown etiology; both sexes affected; onset at any age; disease peaks at puberty.

Ocular

Conjunctivitis; iritis; keratitis; uveitis.

Clinical

Rash; spondylitis; inflammatory bowel disease; diarrhea; degenerative disease of spine.

Laboratory

The differentiation of psoriatic arthritis from rheumatoid arthritis and gout can be facilitated by the absence of the typical laboratory findings of those conditions. Joint X-rays can facilitate the diagnosis of psoriatic arthritis.

Treatment

The simplest treatment of psoriasis is daily sun exposure, sea bathing, topical moisturizers, and relaxation. Moisturizers, such as petrolatum jelly, are helpful. Anthralin, coal or wood tar, corticosteroids, salicylic acid, phenolic compounds, and calcipotriene (a vitamin D analog) also may be effective. Ocular lubricants and punctal occlusion, oral and topical corticosteroids are sometimes beneficial.

BIBLIOGRAPHY

1. Lambert JR, Wright V. Eye inflammation in psoriatic arthritis. Ann Rheum Dis. 1976;35:354-6.

⊟ 11.13. JUVENILE RHEUMATOID ARTHRITIS (JRA; STILL DISEASE)

General

Onset before age of 16 years; greater occurrence of systemic manifestations, monoarticular and oligoarticular joint involvement, and iridocyclitis.

Ocular

Hypopyon; band keratopathy; uveitis; cataract; papillitis; glaucoma; macular edema; ocular pain; vitreous cells; synechiae; scleritis; presumed to have an autoimmune etiology; antiocular antibodies, including iris protein antibodies, have been found in the sera of patients.

Clinical

Salmon pink macular rash; arthritis; hepatosplenomegaly; leukocytosis; chronic pain; joint swelling; low-grade fever; anemia; rheumatoid nodules.

Laboratory

Antinuclear antibody, rheumatoid factor, HLA-B27, X-ray imaging of joints.

Treatment

Uveitis is treated initially with topical corticosteroids. Systemic immunomodulatory agents may be useful for patients with limited or no response to topical or systemic corticosteroids.

⊟ BIBLIOGRAPHY

1. Roque MR, Roque BL, Miserocchi E, et al. (2012). Juvenile idiopathic arthritis uveitis. [online] Available from www.emedicine.com/oph/TOPIC675.HTM. [Accessed August, 2013].
2. Thorne JE, Woreta FA, Dunn JP, et al. Risk of cataract development among children with juvenile idiopathic arthritis-related uveitis treated with topical corticosteroids. Ophthalmology. 2010;117:1436-41.

⊟ 11.14. NEMATODE OPHTHALMIA SYNDROME (VISCERAL LARVA MIGRANS SYNDROME; TOXOCARIASIS)

General

Usually found in children; invasion by larvae of *T. canis* and *T. cati* of viscera and eyes; pronounced eosinophilia; as many as 30% of asymptomatic children demonstrate serologic evidence of prior *Toxocara* infestations.

Ocular

Leukocoria; uveitis; cataract; marked vitreous reaction with large floaters; choroiditis; large, cyst-like white masses extending into vitreous; optic neuritis; papillitis; strabismus; hemorrhagic, exudative, or granulomatous retinitis; retinal detachment; endophthalmitis; larvae present in the cornea.

Clinical

Hepatosplenomegaly; pulmonary infiltration; fever; cough; lack of appetite.

Laboratory

Eosinophilia in patients with visceral disease. ELISA test is best to document systemic or ocular infection with *T. canis*.

Treatment

Treatment is by case-by-case basis; in most cases no treatment is needed; systemic anthelmintic agents; vitrectomy may be necessary.

⊟ BIBLIOGRAPHY

1. Biglan AW, Glickman LT, Lobes LA. Serum and vitreous Toxocara antibody in nematode endophthalmitis. Am J Ophthalmol. 1979;88:898-901.
2. Roy FH, Fraunfelder FW, Fraunfelder FT ROY and Fraunfelder's. Current Ocular Therapy, 6th edition. Philadelphia: WB Saunders; 2008.
3. Maguire AM, Green WR, Michels RG, et al. Recovery of intraocular Toxocara Canis by pars plana vitrectomy. Ophthalmology. 1990;97:675-80.
4. Raistrick ER, Hart JC. Ocular toxocariasis in adults. Br J Ophthalmol. 1976;60:365-70.
5. Wilder HC. Nematode endophthalmitis. Trans Am Acad Ophthalmol Otolaryngol. 1950;55:99.
6. Wilkinson C. Ocular toxocariasis. In: Ryan SJ (Ed). Retina, 2nd edition. St. Louis: Mosby; 1994. pp. 1545-52.

11.15. REITER SYNDROME (FIESSINGER-LEROY SYNDROME; CONJUNCTIVO-URETHRO-SYNOVIAL SYNDROME; IDIOPATHIC BLENNORRHEAL ARTHRITIS SYNDROME; POLYARTHRITIS ENTERICA)

General

Etiology unknown; males; onset ages 16–42 years; probably a combined infectious/autoimmune pathogenetic mechanism; reactive arthritis probably associated with infection with many different species of microorganisms; HLA-B27 confers disease susceptibility to infection.

Ocular

Sterile mucopurulent conjunctivitis, usually bilateral; photophobia; epiphora; iritis; keratitis; uveitis; paralysis of extraocular muscles; optic neuritis; secondary glaucoma; hypopyon; hyphema.

Clinical

Skin erythema; genital ulcerations; urethritis with discharge; cystitis with dysuria, abacterial pyuria, and hematuria; arthritis with pain, swelling, heat, and effusion; fever; weight loss; fatigue; malaise; fever; diarrhea; oral mucosal lesions; arthralgia.

Laboratory

Giemsa stain may reveal Gram-negative intracellular diplococci associated with gonorrhea. Stool cultures may also be helpful for enteric pathogens. HLA-B27 antigen testing will not provide a diagnosis but may be useful.

Treatment

Systemic antibiotics are useful. Topical corticosteroids and mydriatics should be administered early to minimize tissue damage. NSAIDs may help reduce ocular inflammation.

BIBLIOGRAPHY

1 Bashour M. (2012). Ophthalmologic manifestations of reactive arthritis. [online] Available from www.emedicine.com/oph/TOPIC524.HTM. [Accessed August, 2013].

11.16. RETICULUM CELL SARCOMA (NON-HODGKIN LYMPHOMA)

General

Autosomal recessive; large-cell lymphoma with chronic inflammation with a predominance of cells in vitreous cavity; average age at time of diagnosis is 60 years; female to male ratio is approximately 2:1; 80% bilateral (frequently asymmetrical).

Ocular

Chronic uveitis; chorioretinal lesions; mycosis fungoides; necrosis of orbital tissues; phthisis bulbi; endophthalmos; exophthalmos; exudative retinal detachment; iris neovascularization; glaucoma; branch retinal vein occlusion; macular edema; optic neuropathy; vitreous hemorrhage; partial cranial nerve III palsy; multiple retinal pigment epithelium masses.

Clinical

Lymphocytic hyperplasia; fever; anemia; thrombocytopenia; liver and spleen enlargement; associated with immune dysfunction states, such as AIDS, or following transplantation.

Laboratory

CT/MRI scan, HIV evaluation, complete blood count (CBC), lumbar puncture.

Treatment

Radiation, chemotherapy.

BIBLIOGRAPHY

1. Vinjamaram S, Estrada-Garcia DA, Hernandez-Ilizaliturri FJ, et al. (2012). Non-Hodgkin Lymphoma. [online] Available from emedicine.medscape.com/article/203399-overview. [Accessed August, 2013].

⊟ 11.17. RUBELLA SYNDROME (CONGENITAL RUBELLA SYNDROME; GERMAN MEASLES; GREGG SYNDROME)

General

Rubella infection of the mother during first trimester of pregnancy; ocular disease is the most commonly found abnormality in patients with congenital rubella syndrome (75%), multiorgan disease is common (greater than 75%); no significant association has been found between gestational age and time of maternal infection and incidence of individual ocular conditions.

Ocular

Nystagmus; glaucoma; corneal haziness; cataracts; retinal pigmentary changes; appearance and central distribution of lesions are quite distinguishable from retinitis pigmentosa; retinopathy is not progressive and has little, if any, effect on vision; waxy atrophy of optic disk; conjunctivitis; megalocornea or microcornea; buphthalmos; microphthalmos; uveitis; iris atrophy; spherophakia; strabismus.

Clinical

Low-birth weight; diarrhea; pneumonia; urinary infection; hearing loss; heart disease; hepatosplenomegaly; mental retardation; inguinal hernias; ataxia; cardiac abnormalities.

Laboratory

Diagnosis is made by clinical findings. If in doubt, a rising titer of IgM will indicate a recent infection.

Treatment

Treatment for rubella of the eye centers on glaucoma and cataract.

⊟ BIBLIOGRAPHY

1. Lombardo PC. (2011). Dermatologic Manifestations of Rubella. [online] Available from www.emedicine.com/derm/TOPIC380.HTM. [Accessed August, 2013].

⊟ 11.18. DAWSON DISEASE (DAWSON ENCEPHALITIS; SUBACUTE SCLEROSING PANENCEPHALITIS; INCLUSION-BODY ENCEPHALITIS)

General

Sclerosing panencephalitis classified as a degenerative, progressive neurologic disorder caused by a measles virus infection of the CNS.

Ocular

Nystagmus; ptosis; papilledema; optic neuritis; macular pigmentation and degeneration; focal retinitis; ocular motor palsies; optic atrophy; preretinal vitreous membrane; exophthalmos; visual agnosia; chorioretinitis; retinal vasculitis; macular chorioretinitis.

Clinical

Chronic inflammation of brain with neuronal degeneration; gliosis; eosinophilic inclusion bodies in brain tissue; decline in intellect; behavioral changes; slurred speech; drooling; motor abnormalities; disorientation; seizures; death.

Laboratory

Refer to neurologist.

Treatment

- *Ptosis:* If visual acuity is affected most cases require surgical correction and there are several procedures that may be used including levator resection, repair or advancement and Fasanella-Servat.
- *Optic neuritis:* Intravenous steroids may be used with optic neuritis or ischemic neuropathy. Stem cell treatment may be the future treatment of choice.

⊟ BIBLIOGRAPHY

1. Fenichel GM (Ed). Subacute sclerosing panencephalitis. Clinical Pediatric Neurology, 2nd edition. Philadelphia: WB Saunders; 1993. p. 137.

2. Gravina RF, Nakanishi AS, Faden A. Subacute sclerosing panencephalitis. Am J Ophthalmol. 1978;86:106-9.

3. Johnston HM, Wise GA, Henry JG. Visual deterioration as presentation of subacute sclerosing panencephalitis. Arch Dis Child. 1980;55:899-90l.

4. Kovacs B, Vastag O. Fluoroangiographic picture of the acute stage of the retinal lesion in subacute sclerosing panencephalitis. Ophthalmologica. 1978;177:264-9.

5. Meyer E, Majlin M, Zonis S. Subacute sclerosing panencephalitis: clinicopathological study of the eyes. J Pediatr Ophthalmol Strabismus. 1978;15:19-23.

6. Miller JR, Jubelt B. Viral infections. In: Rowland LP (Ed). Merritt's Textbook of Neurology, 9th edition. Baltimore: Williams & Wilkins; 1995. pp. 164-5.

7. Miller NR (Ed). SSPE. Walsh and Hoyt's Clinical Neuro-Ophthalmology (Vol. 5), 4th edition. Baltimore: Williams & Wilkins; 1995. pp. 4048-58.

8. Salmon JF, Pan EL, Murray AD. Visual loss with dancing extremities and mental disturbances. Surv Ophthalmol. 1991;35:299-306.

9. Takayama S, Iwasaki Y, Yamanouchi H, et al. Characteristic Clinical features in a case of fulminant subacute sclerosing panencephalitis. Brain Dev. 1994;16:132-5.

10. Vignaendra V, Lim CL, Chen ST. Subacute sclerosing panencephalitis with unusual ocular movements: polygraphic studies. Neurology. 1978;28:1052-6.

11. Zagami AS, Lethlean AK. Chorioretinitis as a possible very early manifestation of subacute sclerosing panencephalitis. Aust N Z J Med. 1991;21:350-2.

⊟ 11.19. ACQUIRED LUES (SYPHILIS; ACQUIRED SYPHILIS; LUES VENEREA; MALUM VENEREUM)

General

Causative agent, *T. pallidum*, usually transmitted sexually.

Ocular

Conjunctival chancroid; conjunctivitis; keratitis; blepharitis; ptosis; iris atrophy; hippus; dacryocystitis; optic nerve atrophy; optic neuritis; periostitis; episcleritis; scleritis; nystagmus; uveitis; vitreous hemorrhages; paralysis of sixth nerve; papilledema; retinal hemorrhages; retinitis proliferans; oculogyric crisis; neuroretinitis; papilledema (associated with aseptic meningitis); diffuse or multifocal chorioretinitis; vertical supranuclear gaze palsy; Benedikt syndrome.

Clinical

Primary lesion associated with regional lymphadenopathy; secondary bacteremic stage associated with generalized mucocutaneous lesions; tertiary stage characterized by destructive mucocutaneous, musculoskeletal, or parenchymal lesions, aortitis, or central nervous system disease; syphilis and HIV infection often coexist in the same patient who experiences a higher incidence and greater severity of neurologic and ocular manifestations; a significant percentage of patients infected with HIV-I and *T. pallidum* become seronegative to syphilis testing.

Laboratory

Serologic nontreponemal tests include VDRL and RPR.

Treatment

The goals are to reduce morbidity and to prevent complications. Penicillin is the antibiotic of choice for treating syphilis. Ocular syphilis should be treated the same as patients with neurosyphilis.

⊟ BIBLIOGRAPHY

1. Euerle B. (2012). Syphilis. [online] Available from www.emedicine.com/med/TOPIC2224.HTM. [Accessed August, 2013].

2. Majmudar PA. (2011). Interstitial keratitis: overview of interstitial keratitis. [online] Available from www.emedicine.com/oph/TOPIC453.HTM. [Accessed August, 2013].

11.20. OCULAR TOXOPLASMOSIS (TOXOPLASMIC RETINOCHOROIDITIS; TOXOPLASMOSIS)

General

Parasite infestation caused by *T. gondii*; cell-mediated immunity is believed to be the major defence mechanism against *Toxoplasma* infection; ocular toxoplasmosis occurs in approximately 1% of patients with AIDS; AIDS-related toxoplasma retinochoroiditis may have several atypical clinical manifestations.

Ocular

Keratitis; uveitis; optic atrophy; papillitis; anisocoria; persistent pupillary membrane; focal retinochoroiditis; scleritis; cataract; microphthalmos; myopia; nystagmus; esotropia.

Clinical

Cysts are seen in many organs, including brain and muscle; hydrocephalus; intracerebral calcification; various CNS complaints.

Laboratory

Serologic tests for anti-*T. gondii*. Antibodies are common.

Treatment

Triple drug therapy pyrimethamine, sulfadiazine and prednisone. Pyrimethamine should be combined with folinic acid. Surgical care includes photocoagulation, cryotherapy or vitrectomy.

BIBLIOGRAPHY

1. Lasave AF, Llopis MD, Muccioli C, et al. Intravitreal clindamycin and dexamethasone for zone 1 toxoplasmic retinochoroiditis at twenty-four months. Ophthalmology. 2010;1831-8.
2. Wuh L. (2011). Ophthalmologic Manifestations of Toxoplasmosis. [online] Available from www.emedicine.com/oph/TOPIC707.HTM. [Accessed August, 2013].

11.21. TUBERCULOSIS

General

Communicable disease caused by the acid-fast bacillus *Mycobacterium tuberculosis*.

Ocular

Conjunctivitis; subconjunctival nodules (tuberculomas); keratitis; pannus; corneal ulcer; blepharitis; cellulitis; meibomianitis; uveitis; dacryocystitis; chronic orbital cellulitis; retinitis; scleritis; scleral perforation; hypopyon; vitreous hemorrhages; optic neuritis; optic atrophy; tuberculous panophthalmitis; choroidal tubercles; intraorbital extraocular lesions.

Clinical

Pulmonary infection; pyuria; hematuria; epididymitis; dysuria; flank pain; distorted calyces; productive cough.

Laboratory

Acid-fast bacillus culture of body fluids including vitreous and aqueous. PCR is 89% positive for pulmonary infection.

Treatment

A course of chemotherapy (isoniazid, rifampin, pyrazinamide and ethambutol or streptomycin) for a period of 6 months is the recommended therapy.

BIBLIOGRAPHY

1. Collins JK. Handbook of Clinical Ophthalmology. New York: Masson; 1982.
2. DeVoe AG, Locatcher-Khorazo D. The external manifestations of ocular tuberculosis. Trans Am Ophthalmol Soc. 1964;62:203-12.
3. D'Souza P, Garg R, Dhaliwal RS, et al. Orbital tuberculosis. Int Ophthalmol. 1994;18:149-52.
4. Gupta V, Gupta A, Arora S, et al. Presumed tubercular serpiginous like choroiditis. Ophthalmology. 2003;110:1744-9.
5. Patkar S, Singhania BK, Agrawal A. Intraorbital extraocular tuberculosis: a report of three cases. Surg Neurol 1994; 42:320-1.
6. Roy FH, Fraunfelder FW, Fraunfelder FT. Roy and Fraunfelder's. Current Ocular Therapy, 6th editon. Philadelphia: WB Saunders; 2008.
7. Tejada P, Mendez MJ, Negreira S. Choroidal tubercles with tuberculous meningitis. Int Ophthalmol. 1994;18:115-8.

⊟ 12. CHOROIDORETINAL DEGENERATION WITH RETINAL REFLEX IN HETEROZYGOUS WOMEN

General

Sex-linked; chorioretinal degeneration differentiated by presence in heterozygous women of a tapetal-like retinal reflex; there is probably more than one X-linked locus leading to a retinitis pigmentosa type of picture.

Ocular

Retinitis pigmentosa; golden-hued, patchy appearance around macula.

Clinical

None.

Laboratory

Diagnosis is made by clinical findings.

Treatment

Retinitis pigmentosa: Vitamin A 15,000 IU/day is thought to slow the decline of retinal function, dark sunglasses for outdoor use, surgery for cataract, genetic counseling.

⊟ BIBLIOGRAPHY

1. McKusick VA. Mendelian Inheritance in Man, A Catalog of Human Genes and Genetic Disorders, 12th edition. Baltimore, MD: The Johns Hopkins University Press; 1998.
2. Musarella MA, Anson-Cartwright L, Leal SM, et al. Multipoint linkage analysis and heterogeneity testing in 20 X-linked retinitis pigmentosa families. Genomics. 1990;8(2):286-96.
3. Nussbaum RL, Lewis RA, Lesko JG, et al. Mapping X-linked ophthalmic diseases: linkage relationship of X-linked retinitis pigmentosa to X chromosomal short arm markers. Hum Genet. 1985;70(1):45-50.
4. Online Mendelian Inheritance in Man, OMIM. McKusick-Nathans Institute for Genetic Medicine, Johns Hopkins University and National Center for Biotechnology Information, National Library of Medicine, February 12, 2007. [online] Available from www.ncbi.nlm.nih.gov/omim. [Accessed August, 2013].

⊟ 13. CHOROIDORETINAL DYSTROPHY

General

Sex-linked; similar to retinitis pigmentosa with absence of annular scotoma and little vascular change.

Ocular

Early poor central vision; retinitis pigmentosa; night blindness.

Clinical

None.

Laboratory

Diagnosis is made by clinical findings.

Treatment

Retinitis pigmentosa: Vitamin A 15,000 IU/day is thought to slow the decline of retinal function, dark sunglasses for outdoor use, surgery for cataract, genetic counseling.

⊟ BIBLIOGRAPHY

1. Hoare GW. Choroido-retinal dystrophy. Br J Ophthalmol. 1965;49(9):449-59.
2. McKusick VA. Mendelian Inheritance in Man, A Catalog of Human Genes and Genetic Disorders, 12th edition. Baltimore, MD: The Johns Hopkins University Press; 1998.

14. CROWDED DISK SYNDROME (BILATERAL CHOROIDAL FOLDS AND OPTIC NEUROPATHY)

Ocular

Bilateral choroidal folds; optic disk congestion; optic atrophy; hyperopia; shortened axial length.

Clinical

Elevated intracranial pressure is ruled out.

Laboratory

Fluorescein angiogram, CT or MRI when orbital tumor or inflammation suspected; ultrasonography when posterior scleritis is suspected.

Treatment

Reversal of underlying cause is the therapy of choice.

BIBLIOGRAPHY

1. Kim JW, Lee DK, Cooper T. (2011). Compressive Optic Neuropathy. [online] Available from www.emedicine.com/oph/TOPIC167.HTM. [Accessed August, 2013].
2. Younge BR. (2012). Anterior Ischemic Optic Neuropathy. [online] Available from www.emedicine.com/oph/TOPIC161.HTM. [Accessed August, 2013].

15. CYTOMEGALIC INCLUSION DISEASE (CYTOMEGALOVIRUS; CONGENITAL CYTOMEGALIC INCLUSION DISEASE)

General

Cytomegalovirus passes transplacentally from an asymptomatic mother to fetus.

Ocular

Uveitis; cataract; optic atrophy; inclusion bodies in the aqueous humor; severe conjunctivitis; corneal opacities; microphthalmos; strabismus; dacryoadenitis; chorioretinitis; CMV retinitis (most common cause of acquired viral retinitis, primarily because of the AIDS virus); glaucoma.

Clinical

Cerebral calcifications; microcephaly; mental retardation; inclusion bodies in the urine; spastic diplegia; seizures; cerebellar hypoplasia; intraventricular hemorrhage; hydrocephalus.

Laboratory

Antigen testing, qualitative and quantitative polymerase chain reaction, shell vial assay.

Treatment

Ganciclovir, foscarnet, acyclovir and cidofovir.

BIBLIOGRAPHY

1. Akhter K, Wills TS. (2013). Cytomegalovirus. [online] Available from www.emedicine.com/med/TOPIC504.HTM. [Accessed August, 2013].

16. DOYNE HONEYCOMB CHOROIDITIS (DOMINANT ORBRUCH MEMBRANE DRUSEN; HUTCHINSON-TAYS CENTRAL GUTTATE CHOROIDITIS; HOLTHOUSE-BATTEN SUPERFICIAL CHOROIDITIS; MALATTIA-LEVENTINESE SYNDROME)

General

Autosomal dominant; represents early manifestation of senile macular degeneration; both sexes affected; onset in advanced age; patients present with drusen at an early age (2nd to 3rd year of life) with near-normal visual acuity in childhood.

Ocular

Drusen with multiple yellow lesions becoming calcified and presenting crystalline appearance.

Clinical

None.

Laboratory

Diagnosis is made by clinical findings.

Treatment

Vitamins, antioxidants, cessation of smoking and proper control of hypertension. There is evidence that patients with early or moderate dry macular degeneration should consume adequate quantities of antioxidants, including vitamin A, vitamin E, zinc and lutein. Prevention is the best treatment in this case because no satisfactory method exists.

⊟ BIBLIOGRAPHY

1. Maturi RK. (2012). Nonexudative ARMD. [online] Available from www.emedicine.com/oph/TOPIC383.HTM. [Accessed August, 2013].

⊟ 17. EXPULSIVE CHOROIDAL HEMORRHAGE

General

Separation of the choroid and sclera created by a fluid accumulation between the two layers caused by a rupture of the choroidal vessels. Generally, it is associated with ocular trauma and during or following ocular surgery. Postoperative hypotony is the most common causative factor. It is seen more frequently in individuals with short axial length.

Clinical

Hypertension; diffuse arteriosclerosis; sickle cell anemia; tachycardia.

Ocular

Pain, visual loss, ciliochoroidal edema/detachment; increased IOP; extrusion of eye contents; shallow anterior chamber; vitreous hemorrhage; retinal detachment.

Laboratory

B-scan ultrasonography.

Treatment

Topical use of cycloplegic/mydriatic drops in addition to topical steroids when necessary. If IOP is elevated, glaucoma medications may be useful. If the hemorrhage causes a detachment which persist longer than 1 week, drainage of the suprachoroidal fluid should be considered.

⊟ BIBLIOGRAPHY

1. Traverso CE. (2012). Choroidal Detachment. [online] Available from www.emedicine.medscape.com/article/1190349-overview. [Accessed August, 2013].

⊟ 18. HISTOPLASMOSIS (HISTOPLASMOSIS CHOROIDITIS; HISTOPLASMOSIS MACULOPATHY; PRESUMED OCULAR HISTOPLASMOSIS SYNDROME)

General

Fungal infection caused by *Histoplasma capsulatum*.

Ocular

Circumpapillary atrophy; maculopathy; scattered yellow "histo" spots; optic disk edema; disseminated choroiditis (immunocompromised patients); vitreous hemorrhage; punched-out chorioretinal lesions; choroidal neovascular membrane; exogenous endophthalmitis (isolated report).

Clinical

Pulmonary infection; fever; malaise.

Laboratory

Sixty percent of the adult population from the Ohio and Mississippi river valleys have a positive histoplasmin skin test; therefore clinic course is most helpful.

Treatment

Although the diagnosis is clinical, certain ancillary tests help in confirming it. Fluorescein angiography, HLA typing B7 and DRw2 may be indicated.

⊟ BIBLIOGRAPHY

1. Wu L. (2012). Presumed Ocular Histoplasmosis Syndrome. [online] Available from www.emedicine.com/oph/TOPIC406.HTM. [Accessed August, 2013].

⊟ 19. MALIGNANT MELANOMA OF THE POSTERIOR UVEA (CHOROIDAL MELANOMA, CILIARY BODY MELANOMA, UVEAL MELANOMA, INTRAOCULAR MELANOMA)

General

Most common primary intraocular tumor in adults.

Clinical

Metastatic melanoma can appear in other parts of the body such as skin or liver.

Ocular

Intraocular tumors of the choroid, iris and ciliary body.

Laboratory

Ultrasonography, fluorescein angiography, indocyanine green angiography.

Treatment

Ocular therapy's goal is to eradicate the tumor before metastasis occurs. Diode laser, brachytherapy, stereotactic, local resection, enucleation and exenteration are all used to achieve this. Systemically intravenous therapy; intrahepatic chemoembolization has been used for isolated liver metastases. Proton beam is used to kill the tumor.

⊟ BIBLIOGRAPHY

1. Garcia-Valenzuela E, Pons ME, Puklin JE, et al. (2011). Choroidal Melanoma. [online] Available from www.emedicine.com/oph/TOPIC403.HTM. [Accessed August, 2013].

⊟ 20. OCULAR TOXOPLASMOSIS (TOXOPLASMIC RETINOCHOROIDITIS; TOXOPLASMOSIS)

General

Parasite infestation caused by *T. gondii*; cell-mediated immunity is believed to be the major defence mechanism against *Toxoplasma* infection; ocular toxoplasmosis occurs in approximately 1% of patients with AIDS; AIDS-related toxoplasma retinochoroiditis may have several atypical clinical manifestations.

Ocular

Keratitis; uveitis; optic atrophy; papillitis; anisocoria; persistent pupillary membrane; focal retinochoroiditis; scleritis; cataract; microphthalmos; myopia; nystagmus; esotropia.

Clinical

Cysts are seen in many organs, including brain and muscle; hydrocephalus; intracerebral calcification; various CNS complaints.

Laboratory

Serologic tests for anti-*T. gondii*. Antibodies are common.

Treatment

Triple drug therapy pyrimethamine, sulfadiazine and prednisone. Pyrimethamine should be combined with folinic acid. Surgical care includes photocoagulation, cryotherapy or vitrectomy.

⊟ BIBLIOGRAPHY

1. Wuh L. (2011). Ophthalmologic Manifestations of Toxoplasmosis. [online] Available from www.emedicine.com/oph/TOPIC707.HTM. [Accessed August, 2013].
2. Lasave AF, Llopis MD, Muccioli C, et al. Intravitreal clindamycin and dexamethasone for zone 1 toxoplasmic retinochoroiditis at twenty-four months. Ophthalmology. 2010;1831-8.
3. Soheilian M, Ramezani A, Azimzadeh A, et al. Randomized trial of intravitreal clindamycin and dexamethasone versus pyrimethamine, sulfadiazine and prednisolone in treatment of ocular toxoplasmosis. Ophthalmology. 2011;118:134-41.

21. PARS PLANITIS (ANGIOHYALITIS, CHRONIC CYCLITIS, CYCLITIS PERIPHERAL UVEITIS, PERIPHERAL UVEORETINITIS VITRITIS)

General

Idiopathic inflammatory condition.

Clinical

Sarcoidosis, multiple sclerosis, Lyme disease, toxocariasis, human T-lymphotropic virus (HTLV1).

Ocular

Cells and debris in the vitreous, vitritis, vascular sheathing, neovascularization, cystoid macular edema, vitreous hemorrhage, cataracts, glaucoma, retinal detachment, retinoschisis.

Laboratory

Diagnosis is made by clinical findings.

Treatment

Systemic corticosteroids, chlorambucil, azathioprine, cyclophosphamide, methotrexate, cyclosporine. Periocular corticosteroids are very effective. Cryotherapy is used on patients that are intolerant to corticosteroids.

BIBLIOGRAPHY

1. Roy FH, Fraunfelder FW, Fraunfelder FT. Roy and Fraunfelder's Current Ocular Therapy, 6th edition. London: Elsevier; 2008.
2. Soheilian M, Ramezani A, Azimzadeh A, et al. Randomized trial of intravitreal clindamycin and dexamethasone versus pyrimethamine, sulfadiazine and prednisolone in treatment of ocular toxoplasmosis. Ophthalmology. 2011;118:134-41.

22. SERPIGINOUS CHOROIDOPATHY

General

Etiology unknown; more frequently in men; onset between 4th decade and 5th decade of life; usually bilateral; rare in Crohn's disease, sarcoidosis and periarteritis nodosa; indistinguishable from TB.

Ocular

Over half have scars in other eye which presents with decreased vision, metamorphopsia. Three types of ocular: (1) peripapillary geographic choroiditis, 80%; (2) macular serpiginous choroiditis, 10% and (3) relentless placoid chorioretinitis, 10%.

Laboratory

Diagnosis is made by clinical findings.

Treatment

Responds well to corticosteroid and immunomodulatory therapy. Periocular steroids may be useful; intravitreal triamcinolone if macula is threatened.

BIBLIOGRAPHY

1. Mansour SE, Cook GR. (2012). Multifocal Choroidopathy Syndromes. [online] Available from www.emedicine.medscape.com/article/1190935-overview. [Accessed August, 2013].

23. SYMPATHETIC OPHTHALMIA

General

Trauma or injury to one eye and later onset of inflammation in the other eye.

Ocular

Iridocyclitis (acute inflammation of iris, ciliary body and anterior chamber); choroiditis; chronic persistent keratic precipitates; posterior synechiae; phthisis bulbi; it has been reported following laser cyclocoagulation.

Clinical

None.

Laboratory

Diagnosis is made by clinical findings.

Treatment

Aggressive treatment with steroids and nonsteroids.

BIBLIOGRAPHY

1. Bechrakis NE, Müller-Stolzenburg NW, Helbig H, et al. Sympathetic ophthalmia following laser cyclocoagulation. Arch Ophthalmol. 1994;112(1):80-4.

2. Boniuk V, Boniuk M. The incidence of phthisis bulbi as a complication of cataract surgery in congenital rubella syndrome. Trans Am Acad Ophthalmol Otolaryngol. 1970;74(2):360-8.

3. Duane TD. Clinical Ophthalmology. Philadelphia: JB Lippincott; 1987.

24A. GIANT CELL ARTERITIS (TEMPORAL ARTERITIS SYNDROME; CRANIAL ARTERITIS SYNDROME; HUTCHINSON-HORTON-MAGATH-BROWN SYNDROME)

General

Etiology unknown; mainly females; mainly whites; ages 55–80 years; temporal artery shows inflammatory thickening; arteritis of the vessels supplying the optic nerve.

Ocular

Transient ptosis; partial or complete loss of vision on the affected side; retinal detachment; exudates and hemorrhages; narrowing of retinal vessels; obstruction of the central retinal artery; optic atrophy; ischemic optic neuropathy; acute decreased IOP; corneal hypesthesia; palsies of extraocular muscles; hemorrhagic glaucoma; diplopia; hemorrhages on or around the disk.

Clinical

Throbbing headache; hyperalgesia of the scalp; malaise; anorexia; weakness; weight loss; fever; nodular pulmonary nodules; cough; otitis with deafness.

Laboratory

Elevated erythrocyte sedimentation rate (ESR) greater than 50 mm/hour, positive temporal artery biopsy.

Treatment

Systemic corticosteroids are the therapy of choice.

BIBLIOGRAPHY

1. Allen AW, Biega T, Varma MK. (2012). Temporal Arteritis Imaging. [online] Available from www.emedicine.com/radio/TOPIC675.HTM [Accessed January, 2013].

2. Walvick MD, Walvick MP. Giant cell arteritis: laboratory predictors of a positive temporal artery biopsy. Ophthalmology. 2011;118(6):1201-4.

24B. DISSEMINATED LUPUS ERYTHEMATOSUS (SYSTEMIC LUPUS ERYTHEMATOSUS; LUPUS ERYTHEMATOSUS; KAPOSI-LIBMAN-SACK SYNDROME, SLE)

General

Possible etiology includes viral infections and genetic predisposition; immunologic abnormalities.

Ocular

Keratitis; keratoconjunctivitis sicca; corneal ulcer; optic nerve atrophy; optic neuritis; papilledema; arteritis; central retinal vein occlusion; retinal detachment; microaneurysm; scleritis; uveitis; ptosis; conjunctivitis; paralysis of third nerve; homonymous hemianopsia; multifocal microinfarcts; mydriasis; nystagmus; proptosis; orbital myositis; pseudoretinitis pigmentosa; photophobia.

Clinical

Polyarthritis; morning stiffness; fever; malaise; fatigue; polyserositis; renal disease; central nervous system disease; anemia; leukopenia; maculopapular rash in a "butterfly" distribution over malar region; alopecia.

Laboratory

Antibodies to double-stranded DNA or the Smith (Sm) antigen or a false-positive serology test for syphilis; positive antinuclear antibody test that is caused by a medication.

Treatment

Fever, rash, musculoskeletal, and serositis manifestations respond to hydroxychloroquine and NSAIDs. Low-to-moderate dose steroids are necessary for acute flares. CNS involvement and renal disease constitute more serious disease and often require high-dose steroids and other immunosuppression agents. Diffuse proliferative lupus nephritis has been treated with cyclophosphamide induction therapy.

BIBLIOGRAPHY

1. Bartles CM, Muller D. (2012). Systemic erythematosus lupus. [online] Available from www.emedicine.com/med/TOPIC2228.HTM. [Accessed August, 2013].

24C. KUSSMAUL DISEASE (KUSSMAUL-MAIER DISEASE; NECROTIZING ANGIITIS; PAN; POLYARTERITIS NODOSA)

General

Progressive process of vascular inflammation and necrosis, manifested by numerous nodules along the course of small and medium-sized arteries; lesions are segmental in distribution, have a predilection for bifurcation and involve all but the pulmonary arteries; arteries in gastrointestinal tract, kidneys, and muscles are particularly affected; affects primarily males between ages 20 and 50 years.

Ocular

Retinal detachment; cotton-wool patches; polyarteritis nodosa lesion of arteries; pseudoretinitis pigmentosa; conjunctivitis; corneal ulcer; tenonitis; ptosis; exophthalmos; uveitis; optic atrophy; cataract; scleritis; paralysis of extraocular muscles; neuroretinitis; macular star; peripheral ulcerative keratitis; retinal vasculitis; pseudotumor of the orbit; central retinal artery occlusion.

Clinical

Fever; myalgia; hypertension; gastrointestinal disorders; neuropathy; respiratory infection; weight loss; anginal pain; hemiplegia; convulsion; acute brain syndrome; skin lesions; diffuse erythema; purpura; urticaria; gangrene; tachycardia; pericarditis; aortitis; painful facial swelling; diplopia.

Laboratory

Diagnosis is made by clinical findings.

Treatment

- *Retinal detachment:* Scleral buckle, pneumatic retinopexy and vitrectomy may be used to close all the breaks.
- *Corneal ulcer:* Corneal cultures may be taken and treatment is initiated. Treatment includes a broad spectrum of antibiotics and cycloplegic drops.
- *Uveitis:* Topical steroids and cycloplegic medication should be the initial treatment of choice. Oral steroids if not responsive to topical steroids, immunosuppressants if bilateral disease that does not respond to oral steroids, periocular steroids for unilateral or posterior uveitis. Vitrectomy can be used for severe vitreous opacification. Cryotherapy and laser photocoagulation may be used for localized pars plana exudates.

BIBLIOGRAPHY

1. Akova YA, Jabbur NS, Foster CS. Ocular presentation of polyarteritis nodosa. Clinical course and management with steroid and cytotoxic therapy. Ophthalmology. 1993;100(12):1775-81.
2. Kussmaul A, Maier R. Ueber Eine Bisher Nicht Beschriebene Eigenthumliche Artenener Krankung (Periarteritis Nodosa), die Mit Morbus Brightii und Rapid Fortschreitender Allgemeiner Muskellahumung Einhergeht. Dtsch Arch Klin Med. 1866;1:484-518.
3. Matsuda A, Chin S, Ohashi T. A case of neuroretinitis associated with long-standing polyarteritis nodosa. Ophthalmologica. 1994;208(3):168-71.
4. Roy FH, Fraunfelder FW. Roy and Fraunfelder's Current Ocular Therapy, 5th edition. Philadelphia: WB, Saunders; 2008.
5. Solomon SM, Solomon JH. Bilateral central retinal artery occlusions in polyarteritis nodosa. Ann Ophthalmol. 1978;10(5):567-9.

24D. RHEUMATOID ARTHRITIS (ADULT)

General

Systemic disease of unknown cause; more common in women (3:1); thought to have a strong autoimmune pathogenesis with positive immunoglobulins M, G, and A directed against the Fc portion of immunoglobulin G.

Ocular

Sjögren syndrome; episcleritis; scleritis; keratitis; corneal ulcers; corneal perforation; uveitis; motility disorders; dry eyes; posterior scleritis (rare).

Clinical

Synovitis; stiffness; swelling; cartilaginous hypertrophy; joint pain; fibrous ankylosis; malaise; weight loss; vasomotor disturbance.

Laboratory

About 80% are positive for rheumatoid factor but is also found in systemic lupus erythematosus, Sjögren syndrome, sarcoidosis, hepatitis B and tuberculosis.

Treatment

Nonsteroidal anti-inflammatory drugs, disease-modifying anti-rheumatologic drugs (DMARDs), corticosteroids and immunosuppressants can be used.

BIBLIOGRAPHY

1. Temprano KK, Smith HR. (2013). Rheumatoid arthritis. [online] Available from www.emedicine.com/emerg/TOP-IC48.HTM. [Accessed August, 2013].

24E. WEGENER SYNDROME (WEGENER GRANULOMATOSIS)

General

Etiology unknown; occurs between 4th decade and 5th decade of life; persistent rhinitis or sinusitis; three characteristic features are: (1) necrotizing granulomatous lesions in the respiratory tract, (2) generalized focal arthritis and (3) necrotizing thrombotic glomerulitis.

Ocular

Exophthalmos; lid and conjunctival chemosis; papillitis; conjunctivitis; corneal ulcer; corneal abscess; optic atrophy; optic neuritis; orbital cellulitis; episcleritis; sclerokeratitis; cataract; peripheral ring corneal ulcers; ptosis; dacryocystitis; retinal periphlebitis; cotton-wool spots; retinal and vitreous hemorrhages; rubeosis iridis; neovascular glaucoma.

Clinical

Severe sinusitis; pulmonary inflammation; arteritis; weakness; fever; weight loss; bony destruction; granulomatous vasculitis of the upper and lower respiratory tracts; glomerulonephritis; diffuse pulmonary infiltrates; lymphadenopathy; diffuse pulmonary hemorrhage; overlap with giant cell arteritis.

Laboratory

Histopathology: necrotizing, granulomatous vasculitis with infiltrating neutrophils, lymphocytes and giant cells; urine—proteinuria, hematuria and urinary casts.

Treatment

Topical eye lubricants, ophthalmic antibiotic solution or ointment and corticosteroid drops may prove to be beneficial. Orbital decompression needed when medical treatment is unresponsive to treat optic nerve compression.

BIBLIOGRAPHY

1. Collins JF. Handbook of Clinical Ophthalmology. New York: Masson; 1982.
2. Flach AJ. Ocular manifestations of Wegener's granulomatosis. JAMA. 1995;274(15):1199-200.
3. Haynes BF, Fishman ML, Fauci AS, et al. The ocular manifestations of Wegener's granulomatosis. Fifteen years' experience and review of the literature. Am J Med. 1977;63(1):131-41.
4. Leavitt RY, Fauci AS. Less common manifestations and presentations of Wegener's granulomatosis. Curr Opin Rheumatol. 1992;4(1):16-22.
5. Robinson MR, Lee SS, Sneller MC, et al. Tarsal-conjunctival disease associated with Wegener's granulomatosis. Ophthalmology. 2003;110(9):1770-80.
6. Roy FH, Fraunfelder, FW, Fraunfelder FT. Roy and Fraunfelder's Current Ocular Therapy, 6th edition. Philadelphia: WB Saunders; 2008.
7. Straatsma BR. Ocular manifestations of Wegener's granulomatosis. Am J Ophthalmol. 1957;44(6):789-99.

25. UVEAL EFFUSION

Uveal effusion involves leaking of fluid from the choriocapillaris into the choroid or subretinal space or both.

1. Hydrostatic
   A. Dural arteriovenous fistula
   †B. Hypotony, wound leak
   †C. Nanophthalmos
†2. Idiopathic
†3. Inflammatory
   †A. After panretinal photocoagulation

---

†Indicates a general entry and therefore has not been described in detail in the text

†B. HIV
†C. Scleritis, infected scleral buckle
D. Systemic lupus erythematosus
†E. Trauma, intraocular surgery
F. Uveitis, sympathetic ophthalmia, Harada disease

BIBLIOGRAPHY

1. Uyama M, Takahashi K, Kozaki J, et al. Uveal effusion syndrome. Ophthalmology. 2000;107:441-9.
2. Wisotsky BJ, Magat-Gordon CB, Puklin JE. Angle closure glaucoma as an initial presentation of systemic lupus erythematosus. Ophthalmology. 1998;105:1170-2.

25.1A. ARTERIOVENOUS FISTULA (ARTERIOVENOUS ANEURYSM; ARTERIOVENOUS ANGIOMA; ARTERIOVENOUS MALFORMATION; CIRSOID ANEURYSM; RACEMOSE HEMANGIOMA; VARICOSE ANEURYSM)

General

Abnormal communications between arteries and veins that allow arterial blood to enter the vein directly without traversing a capillary network; may be congenital or secondary to penetrating trauma or blunt trauma.

Ocular

Uveitis; chemosis and neovascularization of conjunctiva; bullous keratopathy; eyelid edema; ptosis; exophthalmos; iris atrophy; papilledema; retinal hemorrhages; cataract; paresis of third or sixth nerves; glaucoma; upper lid tumor; total choroidal detachment; leaking retinal macroaneurysms; central retinal vein occlusion; iris neovascularization.

Clinical

Cerebral hemorrhage; death; substernal pain; dyspnea; varicose veins.

Laboratory

Orbital ultrasonography, CT and six-vessel cranial digital subtraction angiography.

Treatment

Obtain emergent neurosurgical consultation for definitive treatment.

BIBLIOGRAPHY

1. Zebian RC, Kazzi AA. (2013). Emergent management of subarachnoid hemorrhage. [online] Available from www.emedicine.com/emerg/TOPIC559.HTM. [Accessed August, 2013].

25.3D. DISSEMINATED LUPUS ERYTHEMATOSUS (SYSTEMIC LUPUS ERYTHEMATOSUS; LUPUS ERYTHEMATOSUS; KAPOSI-LIBMAN-SACK SYNDROME, SLE)

General

Possible etiology includes viral infections and genetic predisposition; immunologic abnormalities.

Ocular

Keratitis; keratoconjunctivitis sicca; corneal ulcer; optic nerve atrophy; optic neuritis; papilledema; arteritis;

central retinal vein occlusion; retinal detachment; microaneurysm; scleritis; uveitis; ptosis; conjunctivitis; paralysis of third nerve; homonymous hemianopsia; multifocal microinfarcts; mydriasis; nystagmus; proptosis; orbital myositis; pseudoretinitis pigmentosa; photophobia.

Clinical

Polyarthritis; morning stiffness; fever; malaise; fatigue; polyserositis; renal disease; central nervous system disease; anemia; leukopenia; maculopapular rash in a "butterfly" distribution over malar region; alopecia.

Laboratory

Antibodies to double-stranded DNA or the Smith (Sm) antigen or a false-positive serology test for syphilis; positive antinuclear antibody test that is caused by a medication.

Treatment

Fever, rash, musculoskeletal, and serositis manifestations respond to hydroxychloroquine and NSAIDs. Low-to-moderate dose steroids are necessary for acute flares. CNS involvement and renal disease constitute more serious disease and often require high-dose steroids and other immunosuppression agents. Diffuse proliferative lupus nephritis has been treated with cyclophosphamide induction therapy.

BIBLIOGRAPHY

1. Bartles CM, Muller D. (2012). Systemic erythematosus lupus. [online] Available from www.emedicine.com/med/TOPIC2228.HTM. [Accessed November, 2012].

25.3F. UVEITIS, ANTERIOR NONGRANULOMATOUS (IRITIS, CHRONIC)

General

Ocular inflammation. Etiology is idiopathic but certain systemic diseases may be the underlying cause.

Clinical

Human leukocyte antigen B27, Behçet disease, herpes zoster, sarcoidosis, syphilis, Lyme disease, JIA, Fuchs heterochromic iridocyclitis, tuberculosis.

Ocular

Photophobia, red eye, dull aching eye pain, perilimbal injection, keratic precipitates, flare and cell of anterior chamber, posterior synechiae, lenticular precipitates.

Laboratory

Diagnosis is made by clinical findings. If nongranulomatous iritis is recurrent, studies are necessary to determine the cause. HLA B27 typing, serologic testing for syphilis, sarcoidosis rheumatoid factor and Lyme disease may be indicated.

Treatment

Topical corticosteroids are the mainstay of therapy. Subconjunctival corticosteroids may be necessary in non-responding cases. Cycloplegia is useful for controlling pain and photophobia.

BIBLIOGRAPHY

1. Levinson RD. (2012). Uveitis, anterior, nongranulomatous. [online] Available from www.emedicine.com/oph/TOPIC587.HTM. [Accessed August, 2013].

25.3F. SYMPATHETIC OPHTHALMIA

General

Trauma or injury to one eye and later onset of inflammation in the other eye.

Ocular

Iridocyclitis (acute inflammation of iris, ciliary body and anterior chamber); choroiditis; chronic persistent keratitic precipitates; posterior synechiae; phthisis bulbi; it has been reported following laser cyclocoagulation.

Clinical

None.

Laboratory

Diagnosis is made by clinical findings.

Treatment

Aggressive treatment is done with steroids and nonsteroids.

BIBLIOGRAPHY

1. Bechrakis NE, Müller-Stolzenburg NW, Helbig H, et al. Sympathetic ophthalmia following laser cyclocoagulation. Arch Ophthalmol. 1994;112(1):80-4.
2. Boniuk V, Boniuk M. The incidence of phthisis bulb as a complication of cataract surgery in the congenital rubella syndrome. Trans Am Acad Ophthalmol Otolaryngol. 1970;74(2):360-8.
3. Duane TD. Clinical Ophthalmology. Philadelphia, PA: JB Lippincott; 1987.

25.3F. VOGT-KOYANAGI-HARADA DISEASE (HARADA DISEASE; UVEITIS-VITILIGO-ALOPECIA-POLIOSIS SYNDROME)

General

Viral infection; occurs predominantly among Italian and Japanese individuals; young adults; chronic.

Ocular

White lashes; secondary glaucoma; bilateral uveitis; sympathetic ophthalmitis; exudative iridocyclitis; vitreous opacities; bilateral serous retinal detachment and edema with spontaneous reattachment after weeks; depigmentation and patches of scattered pigment later; bilateral acute diffuse exudative choroiditis; papilledema; macular hemorrhage; cataracts; phthisis bulbi; poliosis; scleromalacia; intraocular lymphoma.

Clinical

Poliosis; vitiligo; hearing defect; headache; vomiting; meningeal irritation; reported to occur rarely in children.

Laboratory

Immunohistochemistry specimens demonstrate infiltration of CD4+ T-cells, epithelioid cells and multinucleated giant cells.

Treatment

Systemic therapy involves the use of high-dose corticosteroids. Topical steroids may be needed in conjunction with the use of systemic steroids.

BIBLIOGRAPHY

1. Walton RC, Choczaj-Kukula A, Janniger CK. (2012). Vogt-Koyanagi-Harada Disease. [online] Available from www.emedicine.com/oph/TOPIC459.HTM. [Accessed August, 2013].

26. COCCIDIOIDOMYCOSIS (VALLEY FEVER, SAN JOAQUIN FEVER)

General

Caused by fungus *Coccidioides immitis*.

Ocular

Conjunctivitis; choroiditis; uveitis; retinal hemorrhages; vitreal opacity; vitreal floaters; episcleritis; hypopyon; granulomatous lesion of optic nerve head; paralysis of sixth cranial nerve; secondary glaucoma; papilledema; mutton fat keratitic precipitates; necrotizing granulomatous conjunctivitis; iridocyclitis.

Clinical

Mild respiratory illness; cavity lung lesion.

Laboratory

Routine culture media, IgM antibody of acute, IgG antibody for present or past infection.

Treatment

Systemic fluconazole or amphotericin B is the treatment of choice. Ocular treatment includes topical amphotericin B and use of steroids sparingly.

BIBLIOGRAPHY

1. Hospenthal DR. (2011) Coccidioidomycosis. [online] Available from www.emedicine.com/ped/TOPIC423.HTM. [Accessed August, 2013].

27. VITREORETINOCHOROIDOPATHY (VRCP; AUTOSOMAL DOMINANT VITREORETINOCHOROIDOPATHY; ADVIRC) CHOROIDAL ATROPHY

General

Autosomal dominant.

Ocular

Chorioretinal hypopigmentation or hyperpigmentation; preretinal punctate opacities; retinal arteriolar narrowing and occlusion; choroidal atrophy; diffuse retinal vascular incompetence; cystoid macular edema; presenile cataracts; fibrillar condensation and moderate pleocytosis of vitreous; myopia; optically empty vitreous; lattice degeneration; retinal breaks; retinal detachment; glaucoma; spontaneous vitreous hemorrhage.

Clinical

None.

Laboratory

Diagnosis is made by clinical findings.

Treatment

Cataract: Change in glasses can sometimes improve a patient's visual function temporarily; however the most common treatment is cataract surgery.

BIBLIOGRAPHY

1. Blair NP, Goldberg MF, Fishman GA, et al. Autosomal dominant vitreoretinochoroidopathy. Br J Ophthalmol. 1984;68(1):2-9.
2. McKusick VA. Mendelian Inheritance in Man, A Catalog of Human Genes and Genetic Disorders, 12th edition. Baltimore: The Johns Hopkins University Press; 1998.
3. Online Mendelian Inheritance in Man, OMIM. McKusick-Nathans Institute for Genetic Medicine, Johns Hopkins University and National Center for Biotechnology Information, National Library of Medicine, February 12, 2007. [online] Available from www.ncbi.nlm.nih.gov/omim [Accessed January, 2013].
4. Traboulsi EL, Payne JW. Autosomal dominant vitreoretinopathy. Report of the third family. Arch Ophthalmol. 1993;111(2):194-6.

CHAPTER
18

Ciliary Body

⊟ 1. ACCOMMODATIVE SPASM

General

Episodic excessive contraction of the ciliary muscle.

Clinical

Posterior fossa tumor, central nervous system (CNS) infection, head trauma, cerebrovascular injuries.

Ocular

Diplopia, esotropia, accommodation, convergence, miosis.

Laboratory

Computed tomography (CT) and magnetic resonance imaging (MRI).

Treatment

Cycloplegics to break the accommodative component; refractive correction for distance with reading addition.

⊟ BIBLIOGRAPHY

1. Roy FH, Fraunfelder FW, Fraunfelder FT. Roy and Fraunfelder's Current Ocular Therapy, 6th edition. London: Elsevier; 2008.

⊟ 2. CILIARY BODY CONCUSSIONS AND LACERATIONS

General

Trauma which can frequently result in damage to other structures of the eye as well as the ciliary body. Choroid can be separated from the sclera and allow aqueous to drain into the suprachoroidal space.

Ocular

Hypotony, iris atrophy, angle-closure glaucoma, cataract, loss of retinal pigment epithelium, choroidal folds, cystoid macular edema, optic atrophy, phthisis bulbi.

Laboratory

Diagnosis is made by clinical findings.

Treatment

Topical steroids and cyclopentolate; surgery—sodium hyaluronate into the anterior chamber to close the cyclodialysis cleft, argon laser photocoagulation.

⊟ BIBLIOGRAPHY

1. Roy FH, Fraunfelder FW, Fraunfelder FT. Roy and Fraunfelder's Current Ocular Therapy, 6th edition. London: Elsevier; 2008.

3. CILIARY BODY DETACHMENT (*SEE* HYPOTONY)

- Eye surgery
- Myotonic dystrophy
- Trauma

BIBLIOGRAPHY

1. Rosa N, Lanza M, Borrelli M, et al. Low intraocular pressure resulting from ciliary body detachment in patients with myotonic dystrophy. Ophthalmology. 2011;118:260-4.

4. LONG CILIARY PROCESSES EXTENDING TO DILATED PUPILLARY SPACE

1. Aniridia
2. Anterior rotation of ciliary processes
   - †A. After scleral buckling operation
   - B. Angle closure
   - †C. Anterior choroidal separation
   - D. Cyst or tumor behind iris
   - E. Dislocated lens
   - †F. From adherence to limbal scar
   - G. Plateau iris
3. †Extreme mydriasis
4. Falciform detachment of the retina
5. Incontinentia pigmenti (Bloch-Sulzberger syndrome)
6. Norrie disease (atrophia oculi congenita)
7. Persistent hyperplastic primary vitreous (PHPV)
8. †Retinal dysplasia
9. Retrolental fibroplasia (RLF)
10. †Surgical coloboma
11. Trisomy 13 (trisomy D)

BIBLIOGRAPHY

1. Epstein DL. Chandler and Grant's Glaucoma, 3rd edition. Philadelphia: Lea & Febiger; 1986.
2. Hansen AC. Norrie's disease. Am J Ophthalmol. 1963;66: 320-32.

†Indicates a general entry and therefore has not been described in detail in the text

4.1. ANIRIDIA (CONGENITAL ANIRIDIA, HEREDITARY ANIRIDIA)

General

Hereditary, recessive (two-thirds of cases), can be dominant, sporadic or traumatic; absence of the iris; rare; usually bilateral unless due to trauma.

Ocular

Absence of iris; subluxed lens; iridodialysis; cataract; glaucoma; corneal scarring, vascularization, and edema; iris colobomata; round eccentric pupils; keratoconus.

Clinical

Cerebellar ataxia; mental retardation; Wilms' tumor (WT).

Laboratory

Chromosomal deletion, cytogenic analysis, submicroscopic deletions of WT gene with fluorescence in situ hybridization (FISH) technique, polymerase chain reaction (PCR) genotyping haplotypes across paired box gene 6 (PAX6)-WT1 region provides evidence of a chromosomal deletion.

Treatment

Systemic or topical glaucoma therapy.

BIBLIOGRAPHY

1. François J, Coucke D, Coppieters R. Aniridia-Wilms' tumor syndrome. Ophthalmologica. 1977;174(1):35-9.
2. Johns KJ, O'Day DM. Posterior chamber intraocular lenses after extracapsular cataract extraction in patients with aniridia. Ophthalmology. 1991;98(11):1698-702.
3. Kremer I, Rajpal RK, Rapuano CJ, et al. Results of penetrating keratoplasty in aniridia. Am J Ophthalmol. 1993;115(3): 317-20.
4. Magalini SI, Scrascia E. Dictionary of Medical Syndromes, 2nd edition. Philadelphia, PA: JB Lippincott; 1981.
5. Mintz-Hittner HA, Ferrell RE, Lyons LA, et al. Criteria to detect minimal expressivity within families with autosomal dominant aniridia. Am J Ophthalmol. 1992;114(6):700-7.
6. Nelson LB, Spaeth GL, Nowinski TS, et al. Aniridia. A review. Surv Ophthalmol. 1984;28(6):621-42.
7. Skeens HM, Brooks BP, Holland EJ. Congenital aniridia variant: minimally abnormal irides with severe limbal stem cell deficiency. Ophthalmology. 2011;118(7):1260-4.

⊟ 4.2B. CHRONIC ANGLE CLOSURE GLAUCOMA

General

Portion of the anterior chamber angle is closed with peripheral anterior synechiae; five types: (1) chronic angle-closure glaucoma, (2) combined mechanism, (3) mixed mechanism, (4) plateau iris and (5) miotic-induced angle-closure glaucoma.

Clinical

Asymptomatic due to the slow onset of the disease.

Ocular

Elevated intraocular pressure (IOP); peripheral anterior synechiae; deposits of pigment in the angle; plateau iris.

Laboratory

Measurement of IOP; gonioscopy; optic nerve head and retinal nerve fiber layer assessments; visual field testing and slit-lamp examination.

Treatment

Iridotomy is the treatment of choice. Argon laser peripheral iridoplasty and goniosynechialysis may be necessary.

⊟ BIBLIOGRAPHY

1. Tham CC, Ritch R. (2012). Glaucoma, angle closure, chronic. [online] Available from emedicine.medscape.com/article/1205154-overview. [Accessed January, 2013].

⊟ 4.2D. IRIS CYSTS

General

Intraepithelial cyst originating between the epithelial layers and stromal cysts that are congenital or caused by surgery or trauma.

Clinical

None.

Ocular

Keratopathy, iridocyclitis, glaucoma, iris cysts.

Laboratory

Diagnosis is made by clinical findings.

Treatment

Chemical cauterization, laser photocoagulation, diathermy, cryocoagulation and block excision with cornea sclera transplant.

⊟ BIBLIOGRAPHY

1. Roy FH, Fraunfelder FW, Fraunfelder FT. Roy and Fraunfelder's Current Ocular Therapy, 6th edition. London: Elsevier; 2008.

⊟ 4.2E. DISLOCATION OF THE LENS

General

Ectopia lentis, occurs when the lens is not in its normal position.

Clinical

Marfan syndrome, Weill-Marchesani syndrome, sulfite-oxidase deficiency.

Laboratory

Diagnosis is made by clinical findings.

Treatment

Careful phacoemulsification; topical steroids should be given to control ocular inflammation.

⊟ BIBLIOGRAPHY

1. Eifrig CW. (2011). Ectopia lentis. [online] Available from www.emedicine.com/oph/TOPIC55.HTM. [Accessed August, 2013].

🗗 4.2G. PLATEAU IRIS SYNDROME

General

Rare; occurs in younger age group; presumably due in part to an anterior insertion of the iris; pupillary block is not a significant part of the mechanism leading to angle closure.

Ocular

Spontaneous or mydriasis-induced angle closure despite a patent iridectomy; anterior chamber is of normal depth axially and the iris plane is flat, but a peripheral roll of iris can close the angle either when the pupil dilates spontaneously or after mydriatic drugs are administered.

Clinical

Nausea; vomiting.

Laboratory

Indentation gonioscopy.

Treatment

Iridotomy.

🗗 BIBLIOGRAPHY

1. Wang JC, Lee PS, Ritch R, et al. (2012). Plateau iris glaucoma. [online] Available from www.emedicine.com/oph/TOPIC574.HTM. [Accessed August, 2013].

🗗 4.4. FALCIFORM DETACHMENT

General

Autosomal dominant or recessive; preperinatally acquired; characterized by ocular signs only; falciform detachment and congenital total detachment may alternate in affected siblings; falciform detachment and folds; retina projects as a wedge-shaped fold from the posterior pole of eye into the vitreous, occasionally as far anterior as the lens; less typical fold flattens and tapers out in the mid-periphery of the retina.

Ocular

Falciform folds; retinal detachment; RLF.

Clinical

None.

Laboratory

Diagnosis is made by clinical findings

Treatment

Encircling buckle, gas injection, vitrectomy and peeling the tractional (falciform) fold.

🗗 BIBLIOGRAPHY

1. McKusick VA. Mendelian Inheritance in Man, A Catalog of Human Genes and Genetic Disorders, 12th edition. Baltimore, MD: The Johns Hopkins University Press; 1998.

🗗 4.5. BLOCH-SULZBERGER SYNDROME (INCONTINENTIA PIGMENTI; SIEMENS-BLOCH-SULZBERGER SYNDROME)

General

Familial disorder affecting ectoderm; manifestations at birth; female predominance; X-linked dominant phenotype; disturbance of skin pigmentation.

Ocular

Orbital mass; RLF; pseudoglioma; strabismus; blue sclera; cataract; optic nerve atrophy; papillitis; nystagmus; chorioretinitis; anomalies of chamber angle; neovascularization of retina; retinal hemorrhages and edema; microphthalmia; tractional retinal detachment.

Clinical

Dental and skeletal anomalies common; neurologic abnormalities; recurrent inflammatory lesions; skin melanin pigmentation on the trunk: (marble cake); occipital lobe infarct; neonatal infarction of the macula.

Laboratory

CT scan or MRI of the brain should be performed.

Treatment

No specific treatment. Lesions should be left intact and kept clean and meticulous dental care is very important.

BIBLIOGRAPHY

1. Chang CH. (2012). Neurologic manifestations of incontinentia pigmenti. [online] Available from www.emedicine.com/neuro/TOPIC169.HTM. [Accessed August, 2013].

4.6. ANDERSEN-WARBURG SYNDROME (WHITNALL-NORMAN SYNDROME; OLIGOPHRENIA MICROPHTHALMOS SYNDROME; NORRIE DISEASE; ATROPHIA OCULI CONGENITAL FETAL IRITIS SYNDROME; CONGENITAL PROGRESSIVE OCULO-ACOUSTICO-CEREBRAL DYSPLASIA)

General

Sex-linked inheritance; gross deformation of both eyes; only males affected; onset at birth; putative gene for Norrie disease has been isolated and mapped to Xp11.3.

Ocular

Bilateral microphthalmos with extensive destruction of all ocular structures often resembling a pseudotumor; blindness at birth; iris atrophy; iritis; corneal opacification and lenticular destruction with a mass visible behind the lens as long as the lens is still clear; malformed retina and choroid with retinal pseudotumors; retinal detachment; retrolental vascular mass.

Clinical

Mental retardation ranging from imbecility to idiocy (may begin at any age) in about two-thirds of the cases; deafness of differing severity with onset between ages 9 and 45 years.

Laboratory

Diagnosis is made by clinical findings.

Treatment

Topical treatment for iritis; retinal detachment surgery and vitrectomy may be necessary. Immediate laser treatment is recommended following birth.

BIBLIOGRAPHY

1. Andersen SR, Warburg M. Norrie's disease: congenital bilateral pseudotumor of the retina with recessive X-chromosomal inheritance; Preliminary Report. Arch Ophthalmol. 1961;66(5):614-8.
2. Black G, Redmond RM. The molecular biology of Norrie's disease. Eye (Lond). 1994;8(5):491-6.
3. Chow CC, Kiernam DF, Chau FY, et al. Laser photocoagulation at birth prevents blindness in Norrie's disease diagnosed using amniocentesis. Ophthalmology. 2010;117(12):2402-6.
4. Enyedi LB, de Juan E, Gaitan A. Ultrastructural study of Norrie's disease. Am J Ophthalmol. l991;111(4):439-45.
5. Liberfarb RM, Eavey RD, De Long GR, et al. Norrie's disease: a study of two families. Ophthalmology. 1985;92(10): 1445-51.
6. Norrie G. Causes of blindness in children; Twenty-five years' experience of Danish institutes for the blind. Acta Ophthalmologica. 1927;5(1-3):357-86.
7. Warburg M. Norrie's disease: differential diagnosis and treatment. Acta Ophthalmologica. 1975;53(2):217-36.
8. Wong F, Goldberg MF, Hao Y. Identification of a nonsense mutation at codon 128 of the Norrie's disease gene in a male infant. Arch Ophthalmol. 1993;111(11):1553-7.

4.7. PERSISTENT HYPERPLASTIC PRIMARY VITREOUS (PHPV, PERSISTENT FETAL VASCULATURE)

General

Spectrum of conditions caused by failure of apoptosis of the primary hyaloidal vasculature system, incomplete ocular neurovascular development.

Ocular

Amblyopia, persistent hyaloid stalk; PHPV; cataract; progressive retinal detachment; vitreous hemorrhage; ciliary body detachment; decreased visual acuity.

Laboratory

Diagnosis is based on clinical findings.

Treatment

Surgical procedure may be necessary to eliminate media opacities and relieve tractional forces.

REFERENCES

1. Roy FH, Fraunfelder FW, Fraunfelder FT. Roy and Fraunfelder's Current Ocular Therapy, 6th edition. London: Elsevier; 2008.

4.9. RETROLENTAL FIBROPLASIA (RLF; RETINOPATHY OF PREMATURITY)

General

Bilateral disease seen primarily in premature infants with immature retinal vessels; excessive use of oxygen is responsible for the majority of cases, but disease is seen despite oxygen restrictions or even when no oxygen supplementation is used; known factors that correlate with degrees of retinopathy of prematurity are low birth weight, short gestational age, length of time with supplemental oxygen, length of time on a mechanical ventilator; role of excessive light in newborn nurseries also has been proposed.

Ocular

Anterior or posterior synechiae; neovascularization of iris; pallor of optic disk; dragged disk; attenuated vessels; retinal detachment; dilation of veins; retinal folds; retinal hemorrhage; retrolental mass; vascular tortuosity; vasoconstriction of retina; retinal pigmentary changes; vitreous haze; vitreous traction; vitreous hemorrhages; cataract; glaucoma; leukocoria; myopia; shallow anterior chamber; opaque retrolental membrane; ciliary body drawn anteriorly; ciliary process around dilated pupil; absent pupillary reflexes; keratoconus; associated strabismus; amblyopia.

Clinical

Low birth weight; prematurity.

Laboratory

Diagnosis is made by clinical findings.

Treatment

Cryotherapy and laser surgery can be effective. Vitrectomy may be necessary.

BIBLIOGRAPHY

1. Bashour M, Menassa J, Gerontis CC. (2013). Retinopathy of prematurity. [online] Available from www.emedicine.com/oph/TOPIC413.HTM. [Accessed August, 2013].

4.11. TRISOMY 13 SYNDROME (TRISOMY DL SYNDROME, PATAU SYNDROME, REESE SYNDROME) IRIS COLOBOMA

General

Extra chromosome in the D group; fatal in the first few months of life; trisomy 13–15 resembles trisomy D1.

Ocular

Anophthalmia; microphthalmia; iris coloboma; cataracts; retinal dysplasia; optic nerve coloboma; optic atrophy; iris dysplasia; calcified lens; retinal detachment; optic nerve hypoplasia; orbital cysts.

Clinical

Apneic spells; developmental deficiency of the nervous system; seizures (minor motor); deafness; cleft lip and palate; hemangiomata; horizontal palmar creases; hyperconvex fingernails; interventricular septal defects; renal abnormalities; cardiovascular changes; respiratory involvement; gastrointestinal disease; urogenital involvement; cerebral hypoplasia with hydrocephalus; mental retardation.

Laboratory

Immediate conventional cytogenetic test. Ultrasonography for any anomalies. Trisomy 13 is best identified through cytogenetic study of amniotic fluid.

Treatment

Surgical care is usually withheld for the first few months of life.

BIBLIOGRAPHY

1 Best RG, Gregg AR. (2012). Patau syndrome. [online] Available from www.emedicine.com/ped/TOPIC1745.HTM. [Accessed August, 2013].

5. MALIGNANT MELANOMA OF THE POSTERIOR UVEA (CHOROIDAL MELANOMA, CILIARY BODY MELANOMA, UVEAL MELANOMA, INTRAOCULAR MELANOMA)

General

Most common primary intraocular tumor in adults.

Clinical

Metastatic melanoma can appear in other parts of the body such as skin or liver.

Ocular

Intraocular tumors of the choroid, iris and ciliary body.

Laboratory

Ultrasonography, fluorescein angiography, indocyanine green angiography.

Treatment

Ocular therapy's goal is to eradicate the tumor before metastasis occurs. Diode laser, brachytherapy, stereotactic, local resection, enucleation and exenteration are all used to achieve this. Systemically intravenous therapy; intrahepatic chemoembolization has been used for isolated liver metastases. Proton beam is used to kill the tumor.

BIBLIOGRAPHY

1. Garcia-Valenzuela E, Pons ME, Puklin JE, et al. (2011). Choroidal Melanoma. [online] Available from www.emedicine.com/oph/TOPIC403.HTM [Accessed August, 2013].

6. PARS PLANITIS (PERIPHERAL UVEITIS)

In pars planitis, inferior exudates in the peripheral retina, ora, pars plana, and peripheral vitreous, vitreous ray and cells, posterior cortical cataract, perivasculitis, partial thrombosis of central retinal vein, glaucoma, peripheral retinal hemorrhages, and retinal detachment may be present.

†1. Dental infection
†2. Hereditary
*†3. Idiopathic
4. Multiple sclerosis (disseminated sclerosis)
†5. Nematodiases
6. Rheumatic disease
7. Sarcoidosis syndrome (Schaumann syndrome)

_____
*Indicates most frequent

†8. Sinus infection
†9. Streptococcal hypersensitivity
10. Syphilis (acquired lues)
11. Toxoplasmosis
12. Ulcerative colitis (inflammatory bowel disease)

---

†Indicates a general entry and therefore has not been described in detail in the text

REFERENCES

1. Josephberg RG, Kanter ED, Jaffee RM. A fluorescein angiographic study of patients with pars planitis and peripheral exudation (snowbanking) before and after cryopexy. Ophthalmology. 1994;101:262-6.
2. Phillips WB, Bergren RL, McNamara JA. Pars planitis presenting with vitreous hemorrhage. Ophthalmic Surg Lasers. 1993;24:630-1.

6.4. DISSEMINATED SCLEROSIS (MULTIPLE SCLEROSIS)

General

Disseminated demyelination affecting white matter of the brain, spinal cord, and optic nerves; etiology is unknown.

Ocular

Nystagmus; ptosis; myokymia; optic atrophy; papillitis; optic neuritis; anisocoria; Argyll Robertson pupil; Marcus Gunn pupil; hippus, decreased or absent papillary reaction to light; periphlebitis; visual field defects; gaze palsy; paralysis of third or sixth nerve; uveitis; oscillopsia; Uhthoff symptom (reduction of visual acuity with exercise or ocular hyperthermia); pars planitis; retinal venous sheathing; retinitis; granulomatous uveitis.

Clinical

Incoordination; paresthesia; spasticity; tic douloureux; urinary frequency and infections; progressive disability; paralysis; death.

Laboratory

MRI, cerebrospinal fluid positive for oligoclonal band, albumin and immunoglobulin G (IgG) index; brainstem auditory-evoked response (BAER) and somatosensory-evoked potentials (SEP).

Treatment

Patients with multiple sclerosis may require multiple consultations to rule out other causes for their symptoms. Drugs such as immunomodulators, immunosuppressors, antiparkinson agents, CNS stimulants are all used in the management of the disease.

BIBLIOGRAPHY

1. Luzzio C, Dangond F. (2012). Multiple sclerosis. [online] Available from www.emedicine.com/neuro/topic228.htm. [Accessed August, 2013].

6.6. RHEUMATOID ARTHRITIS (ADULT)

General

Systemic disease of unknown cause; more common in women (3:1); thought to have a strong autoimmune pathogenesis with positive immunoglobulins M, G, and A directed against the Fc portion of immunoglobulin G.

Ocular

Sjögren syndrome; episcleritis; scleritis; keratitis; corneal ulcers; corneal perforation; uveitis; motility disorders; dry eyes; posterior scleritis (rare).

Clinical

Synovitis; stiffness; swelling; cartilaginous hypertrophy; joint pain; fibrous ankylosis; malaise; weight loss; vasomotor disturbance.

Laboratory

About 80% are positive for rheumatoid factor but is also found in systemic lupus erythematosus, Sjögren syndrome, sarcoidosis, hepatitis B and tuberculosis.

Treatment

Nonsteroidal anti-inflammatory drugs (NSAIDs), disease-modifying anti-rheumatologic drugs (DMARDs), corticosteroids and immunosuppressants can be used.

BIBLIOGRAPHY

1. Temprano KK, Smith HR. (2013). Rheumatoid arthritis. [online] Available from www.emedicine.com/emerg/TOPIC48.HTM. [Accessed August, 2013].

⊟ 6.7. SCHAUMANN SYNDROME (BESNIER-BOECK-SCHAUMANN SYNDROME; BOECK SARCOID; SARCOIDOSIS)

General

Etiology unknown; theories include tuberculosis, hypersensitivity to pine pollen, virus infection; affects blacks most often; chronic course with spontaneous remissions (*see* Heerfordt's syndrome); hilar or paratracheal nodes with erythema nodosum; onset most often in middle and old age; ocular involvement in 20–25% of all cases.

Ocular

Orbital granulomatous mass; bony defects; cutaneous and subcutaneous nodules; myogenic palsy; lacrimal gland adenopathy; decreased tear formation; secondary glaucoma; granulomatous uveitis with iris nodules, cells and flare; mutton fat keratic precipitates; keratitis sicca; vitreous floaters; band-shaped keratitis; complicated cataract; inflammatory retinal exudates; "candle wax drippings"; optic nerve atrophy; neuritis; eyelid nodules; ocular nerve enlargement (granuloma).

Clinical

Lymphadenopathy; hilar nodes; fatigue; cystic, punched-out or reticulated changes in small bones (mainly, hands and feet); muscle wasting; contractures; weakness in legs and arms.

Laboratory

Chest X-ray, CT scan, and MRI of the brain.

Treatment

Glucocorticoids are the treatment of choice.

⊟ BIBLIOGRAPHY

1. Sharma GD. (2011). Pediatric sarcoidosis. [online] Available from www.emedicine.com/ped/TOPIC2043.HTM. [Accessed August, 2013].

⊟ 6.10. ACQUIRED LUES (SYPHILIS; ACQUIRED SYPHILIS; LUES VENEREA; MALUM VENEREUM)

General

Causative agent, *Treponema pallidum*, usually transmitted sexually.

Ocular

Conjunctival chancroid; conjunctivitis; keratitis; blepharitis; ptosis; iris atrophy; hippus; dacryocystitis; optic nerve atrophy; optic neuritis; periostitis; episcleritis; scleritis; nystagmus; uveitis; vitreous hemorrhages; paralysis of sixth nerve; papilledema; retinal hemorrhages; retinitis proliferans; oculogyric crisis; neuroretinitis; papilledema (associated with aseptic meningitis); diffuse or multifocal chorioretinitis; vertical supranuclear gaze palsy; Benedikt syndrome.

Clinical

Primary lesion associated with regional lymphadenopathy; secondary bacteremic stage associated with generalized mucocutaneous lesions; tertiary stage characterized by destructive mucocutaneous, musculoskeletal, or parenchymal lesions, aortitis, or CNS disease; syphilis and human immunodeficiency virus (HIV) infection often coexist in the same patient who experiences a higher incidence and greater severity of neurologic and ocular manifestations; a significant percentage of patients infected with HIV-I and *T. pallidum* become seronegative to syphilis testing.

Laboratory

Serologic non-treponemal tests include Venereal Disease Research Laboratory (VDRL) and rapid plasma reagin (RPR).

Treatment

The goals are to reduce morbidity and to prevent complications. Penicillin is the antibiotic of choice for treating syphilis. Ocular syphilis should be treated the same as patients with neurosyphilis.

BIBLIOGRAPHY

1. Euerle B. (2012). Syphilis. [online] Available from www.emedi-cine.com/med/TOPIC2224.HTM. [Accessed August, 2013].

2. Majmudar PA. (2011). Interstitial keratitis overview of interstitial keratitis. [online] Available from www.emedi-cine.com/oph/TOPIC453.HTM. [Accessed August, 2013].

6.11. OCULAR TOXOPLASMOSIS (TOXOPLASMIC RETINOCHOROIDITIS; TOXOPLASMOSIS)

General

Parasite infestation caused by *Toxoplasma gondii*; cell-mediated immunity is believed to be the major defence mechanism against *Toxoplasma* infection; ocular toxoplasmosis occurs in approximately 1% of patients with acquired immunodeficiency syndrome (AIDS); AIDS-related toxoplasma retinochoroiditis may have several atypical clinical manifestations.

Ocular

Keratitis; uveitis; optic atrophy; papillitis; anisocoria; persistent pupillary membrane; focal retinochoroiditis; scleritis; cataract; microphthalmos; myopia; nystagmus; esotropia.

Clinical

Cysts are seen in many organs, including brain and muscle; hydrocephalus; intracerebral calcification; various CNS complaints.

Laboratory

Serologic tests for anti-*T. gondii*. Antibodies are common.

Treatment

Triple drug therapy: pyrimethamine, sulfadiazine and prednisone. Pyrimethamine should be combined with folinic acid. Surgical care includes photocoagulation, cryotherapy or vitrectomy.

BIBLIOGRAPHY

1. Wuh L. (2011). Ophthalmologic manifestations of toxoplasmosis. [online] Available from www.emedicine.com/oph/TOPIC707.HTM. [Accessed August, 2013].

2. Lasave AF, Llopis MD, Muccioli C, et al. Intravitreal clindamycin and dexamethasone for zone 1 toxoplasmic retinochoroiditis at twenty-four months. Ophthalmology. 2010;1831-8.

3. Soheilian M, Ramezani A, Azimzadeh A, et al. Randomized trial of intravitreal clindamycin and dexamethasone versus pyrimethamine, sulfadiazine and prednisolone in treatment of ocular toxoplasmosis. Ophthalmology. 2011;118:134-41.

6.12. ULCERATIVE COLITIS (REGIONAL ENTERITIS; INFLAMMATORY BOWEL DISEASE)

General

Chronic inflammatory disease of unknown etiology; both sexes affected; onset at all ages, most frequently between ages of 20 years and 40 years; usually abrupt onset; psychosomatic pathogenesis possible.

Ocular

Iritis; uveitis; episcleritis; papillomatous changes of palpebral conjunctiva; scleritis; serous retinal detachment; choroidal infiltrates; retrobulbar neuritis; papillitis; retinal pigment epithelium disturbance; choroidal folds.

Clinical

Abdominal pain; cramps; diarrhea; arthritis; weight loss; erythema nodosum; aphthous stomatitis; pallor; tenderness over colon; nutritional deficiency; carcinoma; associations with Sjögren syndrome and Takayasu disease have been reported.

Laboratory

Elevated white blood count and erythrocyte sedimentation rate. Radiography demonstrates the "sting sign" of narrowed lumen in the terminal ileum.

Treatment

Systemic corticosteroids, metronidazole, pain medication and antispasmodic drugs give relief.

BIBLIOGRAPHY

1. Khan AN, Sheen AJ, Varia H. (2011). Ulcerative colitis imaging. [online] Available from www.emedicine.com/radio/TOPIC785.HTM. [Accessed August, 2013].

7. PIGMENTED CILIARY BODY LESIONS

†1. Ciliary body cyst
†2. Diffuse iris melanotic lesion
†3. Drugs including the following:
  • Adrenal cortex injection
  • Aldosterone
  • Betamethasone
  • Cortisone
  • Demecarium
  • Desoxycorticosterone
  • Dexamethasone
  • Echothiophate
  • Edrophonium
  • Epinephrine
  • Fludrocortisone
  • Fluprednisolone
  • Hydrocortisone
  • Isoflurophate
  • Meprednisone
  • Methylprednisolone
  • Neostigmine
  • Paramethasone
  • Physostigmine
  • Pilocarpine
  • Prednisolone
  • Prednisone
  • Triamcinolone
4. Malignant melanoma
†5. Melanocytoma of ciliary body
†6. Peripheral uveal detachment
†7. Posttraumatic pigmentary migration

BIBLIOGRAPHY

1. Biswas J, D'Souza C, Shanmugam MP. Diffuse melanotic lesion of the iris as a presenting feature of ciliary body melanocytoma: report of a case and review of the literature. Surv Ophthalmol. 1998;42:378-83.
2. Fraunfelder FT, Fraunfelder FW. Drug-induced Ocular Side Effects. Woburn, MA: Butterworth-Heinemann; 2001.
3. Lois N, Shields CL, Shields JA, et al. Cavitary melanoma of the ciliary body. Ophthalmology. 1998;105:1091-8.

†Indicates a general entry and therefore has not been described in detail in the text

7.4. MALIGNANT MELANOMA OF THE POSTERIOR UVEA (CHOROIDAL MELANOMA, CILIARY BODY MELANOMA, UVEAL MELANOMA, INTRAOCULAR MELANOMA)

General

Most common primary intraocular tumor in adults.

Clinical

Metastatic melanoma can appear in other parts of the body such as skin or liver.

Ocular

Intraocular tumors of the choroid, iris and ciliary body.

Laboratory

Ultrasonography, fluorescein angiography, indocyanine green angiography.

Treatment

Ocular therapy's goal is to eradicate the tumor before metastasis occurs. Diode laser, brachytherapy, stereotactic, local resection, enucleation and exenteration are all used to achieve this. Systemically intravenous therapy; intrahepatic chemoembolization has been used for isolated liver metastases. Proton beam is used to kill the tumor.

BIBLIOGRAPHY

1. Garcia-Valenzuela E, Pons ME, Puklin JE, et al. (2011). Choroidal Melanoma. [online] Available from www.emedicine.com/oph/TOPIC403.HTM [Accessed August, 2013].

CHAPTER
19

Conjunctiva

1. ACUTE FOLLICULAR CONJUNCTIVITIS (ADENOVIRAL CONJUNCTIVITIS; PHARYNGOCONJUNCTIVAL FEVER; SYNDROME OF BEAL)

General

It is an infectious disease produced by adenovirus; serotypes 3, 4, 7, 8, 19, 37 and several others may cause acute conjunctivitis with or without upper respiratory tract involvement; epidemic keratoconjunctivitis has been reported worldwide associated with 11 virus serotypes, with serotypes 8, 11 and 19 being the most commonly responsible.

Ocular

Conjunctivitis; chemosis; keratitis; blepharitis; blepharospasm.

Clinical

Fever; pharyngitis; lymph node enlargement; malaise; myalgia; headache; diarrhea.

Laboratory

Laboratory test is generally not useful. Cell cultures from infected areas and adenoviral antibody titer allow for precise identification of serotype.

Treatment

Symptomatic control may include cold compresses, artificial tears; nonsteroidal and occasionally steroidal drops to relieve itching.

BIBLIOGRAPHY

1. Scott IU. (2012). Pharyngoconjunctival fever. [online] Available from www.emedicine.com/oph/TOPIC501.HTM. [Accessed September, 2013].

2. ACUTE HEMORRHAGIC CONJUNCTIVITIS (AHC; EPIDEMIC HEMORRHAGIC KERATOCONJUNCTIVITIS, APOLLO 11 DISEASE)

General

First reported in 1969, first epidemic in United States in 1981; enterovirus; explosive onset; usually bilateral; coxsackievirus A24 and enterovirus 70 have been implicated in the most recent outbreaks.

Ocular

Chemosis; follicular conjunctivitis; petechial bulbar hemorrhages; seromucous discharge; keratitis; lacrimation; lid edema; photophobia; preauricular lymphadenopathy.

Clinical

Systemic symptoms are rare, although several cases of lumbosacral radiculomyelitis have occurred late in the course of the disease; polio-like paralysis (associated with enterovirus 70).

Laboratory

Antisera have been used with good results. These are being supplanted by polymerase chain reaction (PCR) methods, which reduce the time needed for viral typing.

Treatment

Very contagious with transmitted eye to hand to eye contact. Self-limited course; generally no treatment is necessary.

BIBLIOGRAPHY

1. Plechaty G. (2011). Acute hemorrhagic conjunctivitis. [online] Available from www.emedicine.com/oph/TOPIC492.HTM. [Accessed September, 2013].

3. ACUTE MUCOPURULENT CONJUNCTIVITIS

This type of conjunctivitis is epidemic pink eye, marked hyperemia and a mucopurulent discharge, which tends toward spontaneous recovery.

1. Gram-positive group
   A. Pneumococcus
   B. Staphylococcus-eyelid lesions and punctate staining of the lower cornea may occur
2. Gram-negative group
   A. *Haemophilus aegyptius* (Koch-Weeks bacillus)
   †B. *Haemophilus influenzae*
3. Associated with exanthems and viral infections
   A. German measles (Greig syndrome)
   B. Measles (rubeola)
   C. Mumps
   *D. Reiter syndrome (conjunctivourethrosynovial syndrome)
   E. Scarlet fever
4. Fungus
   A. *Candida albicans*
   †B. Leptothrix
5. Lyell disease-toxic epidermal necrolysis or scalded-skin syndrome
6. Relapsing polychondritis
7. Sjögren syndrome (secretoinhibitor syndrome)
8. Etiology obscure in many cases

BIBLIOGRAPHY

1. Fedukowicz HB. External Infections of the Eye: Bacterial, Viral, and Mycotic, 3rd edition. New York: Appleton-Century-Crofts; 1984.
2. Okumoto M, Smolin G. Pneumococcal infections of the eye. Am J Ophthalmol. 1974;77:346-52.
3. Roy FH. Ocular Syndromes and Systemic Diseases, 5th edition. New Delhi, India: Jaypee Brothers Medical Publishers; 2012.

†Indicates a general entry and therefore has not been described in detail in the text

3.1A. PNEUMOCOCCAL INFECTIONS (STREPTOCOCCUS PNEUMONIAE INFECTIONS)

General

Gram-positive diplococcus *Streptococcus pneumoniae;* some strains are encapsulated while others are not; ocular infections usually are caused by the encapsulated strains; conjunctivitis and corneal scarring produced in an animal model have been attributed to a hemolytic cytolytic exopeptidase.

Ocular

Hypopyon; conjunctivitis; keratitis; corneal ulcer; endophthalmitis; dacryocystitis; uveitis; orbital cellulitis; secondary glaucoma; ophthalmia neonatorum.

Clinical

Upper respiratory infection; chills; sharp pain in hemithorax; cough with sputum production; fever; headache; gastrointestinal symptoms.

Laboratory

Gram stain demonstrates Gram-positive cocci in pairs. The unattached end of each cocci is slightly pointed outward.

Treatment

Impetigo, oral antibiotics and topical antibiotic ointment; preseptal cellulitis, oral antibiotics; orbital celluliti, need team of infectious diseases, otolaryngology and ophthalmology to develop plan of therapy; dacryocystitis, oral and topical antibiotics, dacryocystorhinostomy may be necessary; conjunctivitis, topical antibiotic; keratitis, topical antibiotics; poststreptococcal reactive arthritis can occur with uveitis, topical steroids and cycloplegics; endophthalmitis, prompt and aggressive therapy with topical, intravitreal and sometimes systemic antibiotics and pars plana vitrectomy; post-refractive surgery keratitis, flap raised, cultured and treated. Occasionally the flap should be amputated.

BIBLIOGRAPHY

1. Muench DF. (2012). Pneumococcal infections. [online] Available from www.emedicine.com/med/TOPIC1848. HTM. [Accessed September, 2013].

3.1B. STAPHYLOCOCCUS

General

Gram-positive coccus *Staphylococcus aureus;* most common cause of suppurative infection in humans; more common in patients with a previous disorders, such as diabetes, thyroid disease, renal failure, or malnutrition; although most *S. aureus* isolates from other sources are encapsulated, capsules have not been noted in ocular isolates.

Ocular

Uveitis; hypopyon; conjunctivitis; keratitis; cellulitis of lid; meibomianitis; ptosis; blepharitis; endophthalmitis; dacryocystitis; increased intraocular pressure (IOP) orbital periosteitis.

Clinical

Tissues hypertonic, edematous, and painful; lesion liquefies, forming creamy yellow pus; fever; nausea; vomiting; cough; dyspnea; abdominal pain; diarrhea; bloody stools; dehydration; shock.

Laboratory

Aerobic Gram-positive cocci bacteria grow in grape-like clusters. Coagulase positive indicates pathogenicity.

Treatment

Specific antimicrobial therapy is chosen based on the site and severity of the infection and the antimicrobial sensitivities of the organism involved.

BIBLIOGRAPHY

1. Tolan RW. (2012). Staphylococcus Aureus Infection. [online] Available from www.emedicine.com/ped/TOPIC2704.HTM. [Accessed September, 2013].

3.2A. HAEMOPHILUS AEGYPTIUS (KOCH-WEEKS BACILLUS)

General

Caused by Gram-negative Koch-Weeks bacillus in warm climate regions; characterized by a 24- to 48-hour incubation period; now classified as *H. influenzae* biotype III; *H. influenzae* is divided into biotypes based on biochemical reactions (indole production, urease activity, ornithine decarboxylase activity) and into serotypes based on their capsular polysaccharides; common cause of purulent conjunctivitis and preseptal cellulitis in children.

Ocular

Conjunctivitis; corneal opacity; corneal ulcer; phlyctenular keratoconjunctivitis; keratitis; cellulitis of lid; pseudoptosis; uveitis; petechial subconjunctival hemorrhages.

Clinical

Coryza; systemic symptoms are rare.

Laboratory

Poorly staining Gram-negative bacilli or coccobacilli. Culture on chocolate agar.

Treatment

Antibiotics are the mainstay of treatment. Invasive and serious infections are best treated with an intravenous third-generation cephalosporin until antibiotic sensitivities are available.

🗗 BIBLIOGRAPHY

1. Devarajan VR. (2012) Haemophilus Influenzae Infections. [online] Available from. www.emedicine.com/med/TOPIC936.HTM. [Accessed September, 2013].

🗗 3.3A. RUBELLA SYNDROME (CONGENITAL RUBELLA SYNDROME; GERMAN MEASLES; GREGG SYNDROME)

General

Rubella infection of the mother during first trimester of pregnancy; ocular disease is the most commonly found abnormality in patients with congenital rubella syndrome (75%), multiorgan disease is common (greater than 75%); no significant association has been found between gestational age and time of maternal infection and incidence of individual ocular conditions.

Ocular

Nystagmus; glaucoma; corneal haziness; cataracts; retinal pigmentary changes; appearance and central distribution of lesions are quite distinguishable from retinitis pigmentosa; retinopathy is not progressive and has little, if any, effect on vision; waxy atrophy of optic disk; conjunctivitis; megalocornea or microcornea; buphthalmos; microphthalmos; uveitis; iris atrophy; spherophakia; strabismus.

Clinical

Low-birth weight; diarrhea; pneumonia; urinary infection; hearing loss; heart disease; hepatosplenomegaly; mental retardation; inguinal hernias; ataxia; cardiac abnormalities.

Laboratory

Diagnosis is made by clinical findings. If in doubt, a rising titer of immunoglobulin M will indicate a recent infection.

Treatment

Treatment for rubella of the eye centers on glaucoma and cataract.

🗗 BIBLIOGRAPHY

1. Lombardo PC. (2011). Dermatologic manifestations of rubella. [online] Available from www.emedicine.com/derm/TOPIC380.HTM. [Accessed September, 2013].

🗗 3.3B. MEASLES (MORBILLI; RUBEOLA)

General

Acute, extremely communicable disease that affects young school-aged children; caused by paramyxovirus.

Ocular

Hypopyon; uveitis; conjunctivitis; Koplik (Hirschberg) spots of conjunctiva; keratitis; corneal ulcer; cellulitis of lid; dacryocystitis; congenital cataract; optic atrophy; optic neuritis; strabismus; pigmentary retinopathy; iris prolapse; hemianopsia; secondary glaucoma; central retinal artery occlusion; orbital cellulitis; accommodative spasm; paralysis of sixth nerve; keratoconus.

Clinical

Maculopapular rash; fever.

Laboratory

Diagnosis is made by clinical findings.

Treatment

Good hydration.

BIBLIOGRAPHY

1. Chen SSP. (2011). Measles. [online] Available from www.zemedicine.com/derm/TOPIC259.HTM. [Accessed September, 2013].

3.3C. MUMPS

General

Viral infection.

Ocular

Conjunctivitis; keratitis; corneal ulcer; tenonitis; exophthalmos; microphthalmos; optic atrophy; optic neuritis; papillitis; scleritis; uveitis; cortical blindness; congenital punctal occlusion; paralysis of extraocular muscles; dacryoadenitis; iritis; paralysis of accommodation; internal and external ophthalmoparesis.

Clinical

Affects the parotid glands, but infection of other glandular tissue occurs, including the lacrimal gland and testicles; encephalitis; meningitis.

Laboratory

Mumps virus by acute serologic studies.

Treatment

Generous hydration and alimentation, analgesics for headaches. No antiviral agent is available.

BIBLIOGRAPHY

1. Defendi GL. (2012). Mumps. [online] Available from www.emedicine.com/ped/TOPIC1503.HTM. [Accessed September, 2013].

3.3D. REITER SYNDROME (FIESSINGER-LEROY SYNDROME; CONJUNCTIVO-URETHRO-SYNOVIAL SYNDROME; IDIOPATHIC BLENNORRHEAL ARTHRITIS SYNDROME; POLYARTHRITIS ENTERICA)

General

Etiology unknown; males; onset ages 16–42 years; probably a combined infectious/autoimmune pathogenetic mechanism; reactive arthritis probably associated with infection with many different species of microorganisms; HLA-B27 confers disease susceptibility to infection.

Ocular

Sterile mucopurulent conjunctivitis, usually bilateral; photophobia; epiphora; iritis; keratitis; uveitis; paralysis of extraocular muscles; optic neuritis; secondary glaucoma; hypopyon; hyphema.

Clinical

Skin erythema; genital ulcerations; urethritis with discharge; cystitis with dysuria, abacterial pyuria, and hematuria; arthritis with pain, swelling, heat, and effusion; fever; weight loss; fatigue; malaise; fever; diarrhea; oral mucosal lesions; arthralgia.

Laboratory

Giemsa stain may reveal Gram-negative intracellular diplococci associated with gonorrhea. Stool cultures may also be helpful for enteric pathogens. HLA-B27 antigen testing will not provide a diagnosis but may be useful.

Treatment

Systemic antibiotics are useful. Topical corticosteroids and mydriatics should be administered early to minimize tissue damage. Nonsteroidal anti-inflammatory drugs (NSAIDs) may help reduce ocular inflammation.

BIBLIOGRAPHY

1. Bashour M. (2012). Ophthalmologic manifestations of reactive arthritis. [online] Available from www.emedicine.com/oph/TOPIC524.HTM. [Accessed September, 2013]

3.3E. STREPTOCOCCUS (SCARLET FEVER)

General

Gram-positive bacteria that can invade any tissue.

Ocular

Conjunctivitis; corneal ulcer; blepharitis; scarlatinal rash of lid; erysipelas dermatitis of lid; gangrene of lid; endophthalmitis; proptosis; dacryocystitis; optic neuritis; orbital cellulitis; uveitis; hypopyon; secondary glaucoma; paralysis of extraocular muscles; infectious crystalline keratopathy; scleritis.

Clinical

Pharyngitis; impetigo; scarlet fever; pneumonia; bacteremia; rheumatic fever; glomerulonephritis.

Laboratory

Gram-positive cocci growing in pairs or chains. Throat culture and sensitivity are useful.

Treatment

Penicillin is the drug of choice.

BIBLIOGRAPHY

1. Zabawski EJ, Grace GW, Young M. (2011). Scarlet fever. [online] Available from www.emedicine.com/emerg/TOPIC518.HTM. [Accessed September, 2013].

3.4A. CANDIDIASIS

General

Yeast-like opportunistic fungal infection caused by *C. albicans*.

Ocular

Uveitis; hypopyon; conjunctivitis; keratitis; corneal ulcer; blepharitis; endophthalmitis; dacryocystitis; papillitis; retinal atrophy; Roth spot; vitreous abscess; retrobulbar abscess; retinal detachment; panophthalmitis; chorioretinitis; infectious crystalline keratopathy.

Clinical

C. albicans normally is present as an intestinal saprophyte in 35–75% of the human population; in situations of internal environmental change, however, *Candida* can become pathogenic (e.g. obesity, diabetes mellitus, malignancy, and other debilitating conditions).

Laboratory

Common yeast from up to 50% of healthy individuals isolate directly from the eye should be attempted to confirm the presence of organism. Blood agar and Sabouraud's dextrose agar may be used; PCR for species identification.

Treatment

Mucocutaneous infection typically responds to topical therapy. Antifungal therapy should be started immediately after necessary cultures have been obtained from all suspected sites of infection. Infectious disease specialists are typically involved in cases of invasive candidiasis.

BIBLIOGRAPHY

1. Hedayati T. (2012). Candidiasis in emergency medicine. [online] Available from www.emedicine.com/emerg/TOPIC76.HTM. [Accessed September, 2013].

3.5. FUCHS-LYELL SYNDROME (DEBRÉ-LAMY-LYELL SYNDROME; TOXIC EPIDERMAL NECROLYSIS)

General

Allergic reaction with severe manifestations; similar to Fuchs-Salzmann-Terrien syndrome (*see* Fuchs-Salzmann-Terrien Syndrome); may result as a reaction to *S. aureus* toxin in children or associated with certain medications, including penicillin, sulfa drugs, nonsteroidal anti-inflammatory agents, and allopurinol.

Ocular

Obstruction of nasolacrimal duct; cicatricial changes in conjunctiva and cornea; conjunctivitis; symblepharon; corneal ulceration and possible perforation.

Clinical

Inflammation of mucous membrane with ulcerations; general epidermolysis; cicatricial changes, especially of orifices.

Laboratory

Hematology studies, chemistry to assess fluid and electrolyte losses, liver enzyme tests, coagulation studies.

Treatment

Management requires prompt detection and withdrawal of all potential causative agents, evaluation, and largely supportive care.

BIBLIOGRAPHY

1. Cohen V, Jellinek SP, Schwartz RA. (2013). Toxic epidermal necrolysis. [online] Available from www.emedicine.com/med/TOPIC2291.HTM. [Accessed September, 2013].

3.6. RELAPSING POLYCHONDRITIS (JAKSCH WARTENHOST SYNDROME; MEYENBURG-ALTHERZ-VEHLINGER SYNDROME; VON MEYENBERG II SYNDROME)

General

Episodic, yet generally progressive; onset usually in middle life; possibly caused by lysosomal labilizing factor of endogenous or exogenous toxic nature or immunologic reactions; possible association with Reiter's syndrome.

Ocular

Conjunctivitis; corneal ulcer; exophthalmos; panophthalmitis; phthisis bulbi; proptosis; optic neuritis; papilledema; retinal detachment; blue sclera; episcleritis; scleromalacia; vitreous opacity; cataracts; nystagmus; retinal artery thrombosis; keratoconjunctivitis sicca; secondary glaucoma; scotoma; uveitis; paresis of third or sixth nerve; conjunctival mass (salmon patch); chorioretinitis.

Clinical

Destruction of cartilage and eventual replacement with connective tissue; polyarthritis; chondritis; tracheal collapse; bronchial collapse; anemia; liver dysfunction; death; malaise; fever; dyspnea; changes in pitch of voice; hearing impairment; vertigo; deformed ears; aortic valve insufficiency.

Laboratory

No specific serologic markers.

Treatment

No therapy.

BIBLIOGRAPHY

1. Compton N, Buckner JH, Harp KI, et al. (2012). Polychondritis. [online] Available from emedicine.medscape.com/article/331475-overview. [Accessed September, 2013].

3.7. SJÖGREN SYNDROME (GOUGEROT-SJÖGREN SYNDROME; SECRETOINHIBITOR SYNDROME; SICCA SYNDROME)

General

Etiology unknown; autosomal recessive; occurs in women over age 40 years; failure of the lacrimal and conjunctival glands to maintain adequate secretion; similarities exist with Mikulicz syndrome; insidious onset; associated with collagen disorders; Epstein-Barr virus infection.

Ocular

Blepharoconjunctivitis; tears show no lysozyme; kerato-conjunctivitis sicca; superficial corneal ulcers; thready, tenacious, yellow-white discharge of the conjunctiva; hypertrophy of lacrimal gland; decreased tear secretion with cellular and mucous debris in tear film; cicatrization of cornea and conjunctiva.

Clinical

Dryness of mouth and other mucous membranes; enlarged salivary glands; dysphagia; painless swelling of joints; polyarthritis; dental cavities; vaginitis; laryngitis; rhinitis sicca; hepatomegaly; focal myositis; alopecia; splenomegaly.

Laboratory

Tear osmolarity, fluorecein clearance test and tear function index. Parotid flow rate may determine xerostomia.

Treatment

Artificial tears and lubricating ointments are the treatment of choice. Topical autologous serum eye drops also provide therapeutic benefit.

BIBLIOGRAPHY

1. Aquavella JV, Williams ZR, Boghani S, et al. (2011). Ophthalmologic manifestations of Sjögren syndrome. [online] Available from www.emedicine.com/oph/TOPIC477.HTM. [Accessed September, 2013].

4. ALLERGIC CONJUNCTIVITIS (ALLERGIC RHINOCONJUNCTIVITIS, HAY FEVER CONJUNCTIVITIS, ATOPIC KERATOCONJUNCTIVITIS, ALLERGIC CONJUNCTIVITIS, GIANT PAPILLARY CONJUNCTIVITIS)

General

Exposure of sensitive individuals to specific allergens, recurrent, seasonal (spring and summer due to pollens) or house dust and animal dander.

Clinical

None.

Ocular

Itching, conjunctival erythema and chemosis, papillary hypertrophy.

Laboratory

Diagnosis is made by clinical findings.

Treatment

Artificial tears, cool compresses, vasoconstrictors, antihistamines, mast cell stabilizers, nonsteroidal anti-inflammatories, steroids and systemic antihistamines.

BIBLIOGRAPHY

1. Ventocilla M, Bloomenstein MR, Majmudar PA. (2012). Allergic conjunctivitis. [online] Available from www.emedicine.com/oph/TOPIC85.HTM. [Accessed September, 2013].

5. AMYLOIDOSIS OF GINGIVA AND CONJUNCTIVA, WITH MENTAL RETARDATION (PRIMARY SYSTEMIC AMYLOIDOSIS)

General

Autosomal recessive; primary amyloidosis differs from secondary by the mesodermal tissues being affected and nodular form of deposits; no pre-existing medical condition; preferential involvement of mesenchymal tissues; variable staining of deposits.

Ocular

Conjunctivitis with deposits; corneal leukoma; waxy eyelid papules with purpura; proptosis; diplopia; decreased vision; ptosis; keratitis sicca; upper lid mass; tonic pupil; accommodative paresis; diffuse yellow conjunctival mass.

Clinical

Hyperplastic gingivitis, tongue, skin and muscles; lungs with icing-like coating; mental retardation; peripheral neuropathy; congestive heart failure; polyarthropathy; spontaneous, incidental purpura; macroglossia; bleeding diathesis; idiopathic carpal tunnel syndrome.

Laboratory

Echocardiography is valuable in the evaluation of amyloid heart disease. Doppler studies are useful and may show abnormal relaxation early in the course of the disease. Advanced involvement is characterized by restrictive hemodynamics.

Treatment

The treatment is often unsatisfactory. No reliable method for the accurate assessment of the total amount of amyloid in the body exists. The similarity with multiple myeloma suggests that chemotherapy may be useful. Using different regimens of intermittent oral melphalan and prednisone may also be useful.

BIBLIOGRAPHY

1. Nyirady J, Schwartz RA. (2012). Primary systemic amyloidosis. [online] Available from www.emedicine.com/derm/TOPIC19.HTM. [Accessed September, 2013].

6. ANGELUCCI SYNDROME (CRITICAL ALLERGIC CONJUNCTIVITIS SYNDROME)

General

Etiology unknown; pruriginous cutaneous and mucous reactions that appear and cease rather suddenly.

Ocular

Chemosis; conjunctivitis (papillary type); severe itching and burning; photophobia.

Clinical

Tachycardia; vasomotor lability; excitability; allergies asthma, urticaria, edema); dystrophic conditions and endocrine disorders are frequently associated findings.

Laboratory

Diagnosis is made by clinical findings.

Treatment

Symptomatic control may include cold compresses, artificial tears; nonsteroidal and occasionally steroidal drops to relieve itching.

BIBLIOGRAPHY

1. Angelucci A. Di una Sindrome Sconoscita Negli Infermi di Cattarro Primaverile. Arch Ottal Palermo. 1898;4:270-6.
2. Geeraets WJ. Ocular Syndromes, 3rd edition. Philadelphia, PA: Lea & Febiger; 1976.
3. Magalini SI, Scrascia E. Dictionary of Medical Syndromes, 2nd edition. Philadelphia, PA: Lippincott Williams and Wilkins; 1981.

⊟ 7. ANGULAR CONJUNCTIVITIS (MORAX-AXENFELD BACILLUS)

General

It is caused by *Moraxella lacunata*, which frequently inhabits the nose.

Ocular

Conjunctivitis; hypopyon; keratitis; uveitis; corneal marginal ulcer.

Laboratory

Diagnosis is made by clinical findings.

Treatment

- *Conjunctivitis:* Antibiotic medication should be used to treat the infection.
- *Corneal ulcer:* Corneal cultures may be taken and treatment is initiated. Treatment includes a broad spectrum of antibiotics and cycloplegic drops.

- *Uveitis:* Topical steroids and cycloplegic medication should be the choice of initial treatment. Oral steroids should be given if not responsive to topical steroids, immunosuppressants if bilateral disease that does not respond to oral steroids, and periocular steroids for unilateral or posterior uveitis. Vitrectomy can be used for severe vitreous opacification. Cryotherapy and laser photocoagulation may be used for localized pars plana exudates.

⊟ BIBLIOGRAPHY

1. Jones DB. Early diagnosis and therapy of bacterial corneal ulcers. Int Ophthalmol Clin. 1973;13(4):1-29.
2. Marioneaux SJ, Cohen EJ, Arentsen JJ, et al. Moraxella keratitis. Cornea. 1991;10(1):21-4.
3. van Bijsterveld OP. Bacterial proteases in Moraxella angular conjunctivitis. Am J Ophthalmol. 1971;72(1):181-4.

⊟ 8. BACTERIAL CONJUNCTIVITIS (INFECTIVE CONJUNCTIVITIS, MUCOPURULENT CONJUNCTIVITIS)

General

Most common in children and occasionally seen in elderly, usually acute and hand to eye. The most important microorganisms are *S. pneumoniae, S. aureus* and *H. influenzae.*

Clinical

None.

Ocular

Conjunctival erythema, mattering of the conjunctiva and chemosis.

Laboratory

Swab for blood agar plate, chocolate agar plate and Gram's stain; antimicrobial susceptibility testing.

Treatment

Systemic gonococcus, single intramuscular (IM) dose of ceftriaxone; hemophilus, oral amoxicillin for children and adults. Typical Gram positive, use bacitracin ointment and Gram negative—gentamicin or tobramycin drops.

⊟ BIBLIOGRAPHY

1. Yeung KK, Marlin DS. (2011). Bacterial conjunctivitis. [online] Available from www.emedicine.com/oph/TOP-IC88.HTM. [Accessed September, 2013].

9. BENIGN MUCOSAL PEMPHIGOID (CHRONIC CICATRICIAL CONJUNCTIVITIS; CICATRICIAL PEMPHIGOID; ESSENTIAL SHRINKAGE OF THE CONJUNCTIVA; MEMBRANE PEMPHIGUS; OCULAR PEMPHIGOID)

General

Etiology unknown; involving older age group, especially over 70 years; chronic autoimmune disorder characterized by fibrosis beneath the conjunctival epithelium; associated with the major histocompatibility complex class I alleles, which confer susceptibility to the disease; likely due to a multigene effect and associated with environmental factors; incidence in women is twice as frequent as men, no geographic or racial predilection.

Ocular

Conjunctivitis; absence of goblet cells of conjunctiva; conjunctival ulcer; pannus and keratitis; corneal opacity; entropion; trichiasis; cicatrization of lacrimal ducts; corneal perforation; symblepharon; dry eyes; bilateral involvement (may be asymmetrical); ocular shrinkage; xerosis; conjunctival and corneal bullae.

Clinical

Subepidermal and subepithelial blistering of mucous membranes; blisters may occur in pharyngeal, laryngeal, nasal, anal and genital mucosa.

Laboratory

Diagnosis is made by clinical findings.

Treatment

Subconjunctival injections of steroid or mitomycin may be helpful. Systemic immunomodulators are the major therapeutic plan.

BIBLIOGRAPHY

1. Foster CS, Hamam R, Letko E. (2011). Ophthalmologic manifestations of cicatricial pemphigoid. [online] Available from www.emedicine.com/oph/TOPIC83.HTM. [Accessed September, 2013].

10. BITOT SPOTS

Bitot spots are small gray or white, sharply outlined areas, cheese-like or foamy, occurring on either side of the limbus but especially in the temporal area.

1. Associated with coloboma of lid
2. Associated with corectopia, nystagmus, and absent foveal reflexes
3. Associated with Rieger anomaly
†4. Congenital anomaly
5. Corneal snowflake dystrophy
†6. Exposure
†7. Idiopathic
8. Keratosis follicularis (Darier-White disease) associated with retinitis pigmentosa
†9. Pellagra or other poor nutritional states
10. Vitamin A deficiency

BIBLIOGRAPHY

1. Daicker B. Ocular involvement in keratosis follicularis associated with retinitis pigmentosa. Ophthalmologica. 1995;209:47-51.

†Indicates a general entry and therefore has not been described in detail in the text

10.1. EYELID COLOBOMA

General

Full thickness lid defect generally in the junction of the medial and middle third of the upper lid; causes include trauma, surgical accident or a congenital defect. Most constant feature of Treacher Collins syndrome.

Clinical

Treacher Collins syndrome.

Ocular

Full thickness lid defect; dry eye syndrome; corneal defects.

Laboratory

Diagnosis is made by clinical observation.

Treatment

Temporary treatment involves articial tears, ointment, bandage contact lens and bedtime patching until surgery can be performed. Surgical treatment usually involves direct closure.

BIBLIOGRAPHY

1. Bashour M. (2012). Eyelid coloboma. [online] Available from emedicine.medscape.com/article/1213581-overview. [Accessed September, 2013].

10.2. NYSTAGMUS

General

A repetitive involuntary eye movement that often indicates an underlying ocular or neurologic disorder.

Ocular

Oscillopsia, vertical and/or torsional diplopia, superior oblique myokymia.

Clinical

Vertigo.

Laboratory

Diagnosis is made by clinical findings.

Treatment

- *Nystagmus*
  - *Seesaw nystagmus:* Visual field to consider neoplastic or vascular etiologies.
  - *Upbeat nystagmus:* It may indicate multiple sclerosis, cerebellar degeneration, tumors or infarcts. Treatment is directed toward the identification and resolution of underlying cause.
  - *Downbeat nystagmus:* It affects the cerebellum or craniocervical junction including Arnold-Chiari malformation, multiple sclerosis, trauma, tumor, infarction and many toxic metabolic entities. MRI may indicate a surgically correctable lesion. Periodic alternating nystagmus is continuous horizontal nystagmus from stroke, tumor, multiple sclerosis, trauma, infection and drug intoxication. It can occur from cataract, vitreous hemorrhage or optic atrophy.

BIBLIOGRAPHY

1. Bardorf CM, Stavern GV, Garcia-Valenzuela E. (2012). Acquired nystagmus. [online] Available from www.emedicine.com/oph/TOPIC339.HTM. [Accessed September, 2013].

10.3. RIEGER SYNDROME (AXENFELD-RIEGER SYNDROME; DYSGENESIS MESODERMALIS CORNEAE ET IRIDES; DYSGENESIS MESOSTROMALIS; AXENFELD POSTERIOR EMBRYOTOXON-JUVENILE GLAUCOMA)

General

Autosomal dominant; neural crest abnormality; 50% of patients develop glaucoma.

Ocular

Microphthalmia; congenital glaucoma; iris hypoplasia; deformed and acentric pupil; anterior synechiae; aniridia; microcornea; corneal opacities in Descemet's membrane parallel to the limbus; dislocated lens; optic atrophy; cataract; strabismus; ptosis; hypertelorism; keratoconus; posterior embryotoxon; broad iris processes to embryotoxon; iris stromal hypoplasia; corectopia; polycoria; secondary glaucoma.

Clinical

Face wide; hypodontia; underdeveloped maxilla; teeth deformities; myotonic dystrophy; facial anomalies: maxillary hypoplasia, protrusion of the lower lip, broad, flat nose; dental anomalies include absent teeth, pig-like incisors and decreased crown size; hypospadias.

Laboratory

Diagnosis is made by clinical findings.

Treatment/ocular

Congenital glaucoma can be treated with beta-blockers, prostaglandin analogs and carbonic anhydrase inhibitors. Surgery such as goniotomy or trabeculectomy can be used if IOP is not controlled.

BIBLIOGRAPHY

1. Eagle RC. Congenital, developmental and degenerative disorders of the iris and ciliary body. In: Albert DM, Jakobiec FA (Eds). Albert & Jakobiec's Principles and Practice of Ophthalmology: Clinical Practice, 3rd edition. Philadelphia, PA: WB Saunders; 1994. pp. 367-87.
2. Montes JG, Montes JC. Syndrome de Rieger, anomalie de axenfeld con glaucoma Juvenil familiar. Arch Soc Ophth Hisp Am. 1967;27:93.
3. Rieger H. Beitrage zur Kenntnis seltener Missbildungen der Iris. Graefes Arch Clin Esp Ophthalmol. 1935;133:602.
4. Wesley RK, Baker JD, Golnick AL. Rieger's syndrome: (oligodontia and primary mesodermal dysgenesis of the iris) clinical features and report of an isolated case. J Pediatr Ophthalmol Strabismus. 1978;15(2):67-70.

10.5. CORNEAL SNOWFLAKE DYSTROPHY

General

Autosomal dominant; prevalence of green irides.

Ocular

Star-shaped chromatophore-like cells attached to anterior lens capsule; Bitot's spots; white flecks on endothelium and Descemet's membrane.

Clinical

Lactose intolerance; malabsorption of fat; vitamin A deficiency; dry skin; nevi; freckles.

Laboratory

Diagnosis is made by clinical findings.

Treatment

Sodium chloride drops or ointment.

BIBLIOGRAPHY

1. Meretoja J. Inherited corneal snowflake dystrophy with oculocutaneous pigmentation disturbances and other symptoms. Ophthalmologica. 1985;191(4):197-205.
2. Meretoja J. Inherited syndrome with corneal snowflake dystrophy, oculocutaneous pigmentary disturbances, pseudoexfoliation and malabsorption. Statistical data of some symptoms. Ophthalmic Res. 1987;19(5):245-54.

10.8. DARIER-WHITE SYNDROME (KERATOSIS FOLLICULARIS; DYSKERATOSIS FOLLICULARIS SYNDROME; PSOROSPERMOSIS)

General

Unknown etiology; defect in the synthesis, organization, and maturation of tonofilament-desmosome complex; irregular dominant inheritance; both sexes equally affected, with onset in childhood; chronic but relatively benign and more aggravated in the summer.

Ocular

Conjunctival keratosis; bilateral corneal subepithelial infiltrations and sometimes corneal ulceration; cataract formation (rare).

Clinical

Confluent flesh-colored keratotic papules on head, neck, back, abdomen, and groin; small stature; mild mental retardation; hair loss; genital hypoplasia; oral-mucosal lesions; hypertrophic flexural involvement; acral signs.

Laboratory

The *ATP2A2* gene sequencing and skin biopsy can be used to confirm the diagnosis.

Treatment

Systemic antibiotics, acyclovir, contraceptives, retinoids. Topical emollients, retinoids and 5-fluorouracil. Dermabrasion.

BIBLIOGRAPHY

1. Pui-Yan K, Wong JW, Bhutani T, et al. (2012). Keratosis follicularis (Darier disease). [online] Available from www.emedicine.com/derm/TOPIC209.HTM. [Accessed September, 2013].

10.10 VITAMIN A DEFICIENCY

General

Worldwide cause of blindness; onset in childhood; dietary vitamin A insufficiency; interference of absorption from the intestinal tract and transport or storage in the liver, as with diarrhea or vomiting; most frequent in young children.

Ocular

Bitot spots; conjunctival xerosis; corneal xerosis; keratomalacia with perforation; photophobia; enlarged tarsal glands; corneal ulcer; nyctalopia; hemeralopia; obstruction of the tear ducts.

Clinical

Diarrhea; malabsorption syndrome; follicular hyperkeratosis; lesions on buttocks, legs, and arms; xerosis of skin; tracheitis; bronchitis; pneumonia; chronic obstruction of pancreatic or biliary ducts; increased infant mortality.

Laboratory

Serum retinol study, serum RBP study, zinc levels, CBC, electrolyte evaluation and liver function studies.

Treatment

Vitamin A rich foods such as beef, chicken, sweet potatoes, mangoes, carrots, eggs, fortified milk, and leafy green vegetables.

BIBLIOGRAPHY

1. Ansstas G, Thakore J, Gopalswamy N. (2012). Vitamin A deficiency. [online] Available from www.emedicine.com/med/TOPIC2381.HTM. [Accessed September, 2013].

11. BLEPHAROCONJUNCTIVITIS

General

Chronic blepharitis caused by *Staphylococcus*, seborrheic, meibomian seborrhea or seborrheic with secondary meibomianitis.

Clinical

Seborrheic dermatitis.

Ocular

Blepharitis, keratoconjunctivitis.

Laboratory

Eyelid and conjunctival cultures.

Treatment

Ocular: Warm compresses to lids, eyelid scrubs, bacitracin ointment, ocular lubricants and rarely topical steroids. Systemic antibiotics are sometimes necessary in severe cases.

BIBLIOGRAPHY

1. Roy FH, Fraunfelder FW, Fraunfelder FT. Roy and Fraunfelder's Current Ocular Therapy, 6th edition. London, UK: Elsevier; 2008.

🗗 12. LESIONS OF CARUNCLE

†1. Apocrine hydrocystoma
*2. Basal cell carcinoma
 3. Capillary hemangioma
†4. Chronic inflammation
 5. Dermoid
†6. Ectopic lacrimal gland
†7. Epithelial inclusion cyst
†8. Foreign-body granuloma
†9. Granular cell myeloblastoma
†10. Histiocytic lymphoma
†11. Lipogranuloma
†12. Lymphangiectasis
 13. Malignant melanoma
†14. Nevus
†15. Normal caruncle

†*16. Oncocytoma
 17. Papilloma
†18. Pilar cyst
†19. Plasmacytoma
†20. Pyogenic granuloma
 21. Reactive lymphoid hyperplasia
†22. Sebaceous gland hyperplasia
†*23. Sebaceous gland adenoma
 24. Seborrheic keratosis
 25. Squamous cell carcinoma

*Indicates most frequent
†Indicates a general entry and therefore has not been described in detail in the text

🗗 BIBLIOGRAPHY

1. Rennie IG. Oncocytomas of the lacrimal caruncle. Br J Ophthalmol. 1980;64:935.
2. Shields CL, Shields JA, White D, et al. Types and frequency of lesions of the caruncle. Am J Ophthalmol 1986;102:771-8.
3. Shields CL, Shields JA. Tumors of the caruncle. Int Ophthalmol Clin. 1993;33:31-6.

🗗 12.2. BASAL CELL CARCINOMA

General

Most common malignant neoplasm of lids; it can occasionally occur as a primary basal cell cancer of the conjunctiva and in the lacrimal canaliculus.

Ocular

Neoplasm most common on lower lid and medial canthus; lacrimation.

Clinical

Tumors of skin and other regions, including sinuses.

Laboratory

Typical histology findings. Imaging studies only for invading or deep tumor in the medial canthus.

Treatment

Surgery involves local excision; advanced and recurrent tumors are best managed by a multidisciplinary approach involving head and neck surgical oncologists. Photodynamic therapy and cryosurgery are also effective.

🗗 BIBLIOGRAPHY

1. Bader RS, Santacroce L, Diomede L, et al. (2012). Basal Cell Carcinoma. [online] Available from www.emedicine.com/ent/TOPIC722.HTM. [Accessed September, 2013].

🗗 12.3. HEMANGIOMA, CAPILLARY

General

Benign orbital tumors of infancy, rapid growth; thought to be of placental origin due to a unique microvascular phenotype shared by juvenile hemangiomas and human placenta.

Clinical

Kasabach-Merritt syndrome; congestive heart failure; nasopharyngeal obstruction; thrombocytopenia; hemolytic anemia.

Ocular

Red, thickened spot in the periorbital area, lid or brow; amblyopia; anisometropia.

Laboratory

Neuroimaging studies are useful to establish the diagnosis; CT, MRI and ultrasound may be beneficial.

Treatment

Corticosteroids topically, systemically and injected are the first line of treatment. Interferon may also be used in resistant cases. Laser and incisional surgical techniques have had variable success.

⊟ BIBLIOGRAPHY

1. Al Dhaybi R, Superstein R, Milet A, et. al. Treatment of periocular infantile hemangiomas with propranolol: case series of 18 children. Ophthalmology. 2011;118(6):1184-8.
2. Seiff S, Zwick OM, DeAngelis DD, et al. (2011). Capillary Hemangioma. [online] Available from emedicine.medscape.com/article/1218805-overview. [Accessed September, 2013].

⊟ 12.5. DERMOID (DERMOID CHORISTOMA; DERMOID CYST; DERMOLIPOMA; LIPODERMOID)

General

Benign tumors composed of epidermal tissue, dermal adnexal structures, skin appendages, hair follicles, sebaceous gland and sweat glands; slowly growing.

Ocular

Dermoid of conjunctiva, cornea and lids; keratitis; extraocular muscle paralysis; exophthalmos; astigmatism; visual loss; orbital lesions causing diplopia and proptosis; may be connected with the lacrimal canaliculum.

Clinical

Subcutaneous dermoids of the skin; aplasia cutis congenita possibly associated with strabismus has been reported.

Laboratory

Radiographs of the orbit reveal the deeper orbital cysts; CT is commonly used to image orbital cysts; MRI of dermoid cyst is especially valuable in deeper orbital lesions.

Treatment

Surgery for function or cosmesis.

⊟ BIBLIOGRAPHY

1. Schwartz RA, Ruszczak Z. (2012). Dermoid cyst. [online] Available from www.emedicine.com/derm/TOPIC686.HTM. [Accessed September, 2013].

⊟ 12.13. MALIGNANT MELANOMA OF THE POSTERIOR UVEA (CHOROIDAL MELANOMA, CILIARY BODY MELANOMA, UVEAL MELANOMA, INTRAOCULAR MELANOMA)

General

Most common primary intraocular tumor in adults.

Clinical

Metastatic melanoma can appear in other parts of the body such as skin or liver.

Ocular

Intraocular tumors of the choroid, iris and ciliary body.

Laboratory

Ultrasonography, fluorescein angiography, indocyanine green angiography.

Treatment

Ocular therapy's goal is to eradicate the tumor before metastasis occurs. Diode laser, brachytherapy, stereotactic, local resection, enucleation and exenteration are all used to achieve this. Systemically intravenous therapy; intra hepatic chemoembolization has been used for isolated liver metastases. Proton beam is used to kill the tumor.

BIBLIOGRAPHY

1. Garcia-Valenzuela E, Pons ME, Puklin JE, et al. (2011). Choroidal Melanoma. [online] Available from www.emedicine.com/oph/TOPIC403.HTM [Accessed September, 2013].

12.17. PAPILLOMA (WART; VERRUCA)

General

Cutaneous or mucosal tumor of proliferating epithelial and fibrovascular tissues; viral etiology or noninfectious.

Ocular

Papillary conjunctivitis; pseudopterygium; corneal opacity; epithelial keratitis; corneal vascularization; lid ulcers; lacrimal system obstruction; hemorrhages of conjunctiva, lids and lacrimal system.

Clinical

Mulberry or cauliflower-like tumors that may occur on any cutaneous or mucosal surface.

Laboratory

Histologic evaluation is diagnostic.

Treatment

Salicylic acid is a first-line therapy used to treat warts, intralesional immunotherapy using injections, cryosurgery, carbon dioxide lasers, electrodesiccation and curettage or surgical excision.

BIBLIOGRAPHY

1. Shenefelt PD. (2012). Nongenital warts. [online] Available from www.emedicine.com/derm/TOPIC457.HTM. [Accessed September, 2013].

12.21. LYMPHOID HYPERPLASIA (REACTIVE LYMPHOID HYPERPLASIA; LYMPHOID TUMORS; MALIGNANT LYMPHOMA; PSEUDOLYMPHOMA; PSEUDO-TUMOR; BURKITT LYMPHOMA; NEOPLASTIC ANGIOENDOTHELIOMATOSIS)

General

Occurs in tropical Africa; young children; idiopathic orbital inflammation; systemic disease is rarely associated but occasionally occurs with either vasculitis or lymphomas; etiology of Burkitt lymphoma currently includes three factors: (1) Epstein-Barr virus, (2) malaria, and (3) chromosomal translocations activating the *c-myc* oncogene, which induces uncontrolled B-cell proliferation.

Ocular

Proptosis; extraocular motility disturbances; lesions of orbit, lacrimal gland, conjunctiva, and uvea; cortical blindness; retinal artery occlusion; retinal vascular and pigment epithelial alterations; vitreitis.

Clinical

Maxillary tumor; Epstein-Barr virus; cranial neuropathy.

Laboratory

Generally diagnosed with a lymph node biopsy.

Treatment

Chemotherapy, monoclonal antibody therapy and bone marrow or stem cell infusions may be chosen as therapy.

BIBLIOGRAPHY

1. Brooks HL, Downing J, McClure JA, et al. Orbital Buritt's lymphoma in a homesexual man with cquired immune deficiency. Arch Ophthalmol. 1984;102:1533-7.
2. Cheung MK, Martin DF, Chan CC, et al. Diagnosis of reactive lymphoid hyperplasia by chorioretinal biopsy. Am J Ophthalmol. 1994;118:457-62.

⊟ 12.24. ACTINIC AND SEBORRHEIC KERATOSIS

General

Actinic keratosis is a precancerous lesion that occurs most commonly on sunlight-exposed areas of the skin. Seborrheic keratosis is a benign epithelial tumor that appears predominantly on the trunk and head.

Clinical

Lupus.

Ocular

Eyebrow and eyelids lesions.

Laboratory

Diagnosis is made by clinical findings.

Treatment

Cryosurgery is the treatment of choice.

⊟ BIBLIOGRAPHY

1. Roy FH, Fraunfelder FW, Fraunfelder FT. Roy and Fraunfelder's Current Ocular Therapy, 6th edition. London: Elsevier; 2008.

⊟ 12.25. SQUAMOUS CELL CARCINOMA, CONJUNCTIVAL

General

Malignant epithelial neoplasm characterized by basement membrane invasion or distant metastasis. Believed to arise from limbal stem cells and present as a mass in the interpalpebral fissure. Seen more frequently in Caucasians and individuals with exposure to sunlight but multiple infectious agents may play a role in the development. Human papillomavirus, human immunodeficiency virus (HIV), actinic exposure, the use of petroleum products and cigarette smoking may also be factors.

Clinical

Human papillomavirus, HIV, actinic exposure, the use of petroleum products, cigarette smokers.

Ocular

Gelatinous and velvety papilliform or leukoplakic mass on the nasal or temporal limbal area; irritation, chronic conjunctivitis.

Laboratory

Excisional biopsy is used to make positive diagnosis.

Treatment

Excisional biopsy is the treatment of choice. Careful monitoring is necessary to look for orbital invasion. Oncologist should be consulted if metastatic disease is suspected.

⊟ BIBLIOGRAPHY

1. Monroe M. (2012). Head and neck cutaneous squamous Cell carcinoma. [online] Available from emedicine.medscape.com/article/1192041-overview. [Accessed September, 2013].

⊟ 13. CHRONIC FOLLICULAR CONJUNCTIVITS (CONJUNCTIVITIS GIANT PAPILLARY) LYMPHOID FOLLICLES COBBLESTONING OF CONJUNCTIVA WITH LONG-TERM COURSE

†1. Chronic follicular conjunctivitis—Axenfeld's type (orphan's) frequently found in institutionalized children; almost asymptomatic; long duration (to months or longer); no keratitis; cause unknown.

†*2. Chronic follicular conjunctivitis, toxic type
   A. Bacterial origin, such as that due to a diplobacillus or other microorganism

* Indicates most frequent

B. Drugs, including the following:
- Acyclovir
- Adenine arabinoside
- Amphotericin B
- Apraclonidine
- Atropine
- Carbachol
- Clonidine
- Demecarium
- Diatrizoate meglumine and sodium
- Di-isopropyl fluorophosphate
- Dipivefrin
- DPE
- Echothiophate
- Eserine
- F3t
- Framycetinz
- Gentamicin
- Homatropine
- Hyaluronidase
- Idoxuridine
- Isoflurophate
- Ketorolac tromethamine
- Methscopolamine
- Neomycin
- Neostigmine
- Physostigmine
- Pilocarpine
- Scopolamine
- Sulfacetamide
- Sulfamethizole
- Sulfisoxazole
- Trifluorothymidine
- Trifluridine
- Vidarabine

†3. Chronic follicular conjunctivitis with epithelial keratitis; differentiated from Axenfeld type by shorter duration (to months) and by epithelial keratitis involving upper third of cornea; epidemic in schools; can be transmitted by mascara pencil; cause unknown.

4. Ectodermal syndrome (Rothmund syndrome)

5. Folliculosis-associated general lymphoid hypertrophy

†*6. Molluscum contagiosum conjunctivitis

†7. Neurocutaneous syndrome (ectodermal dysgenesis)

†8. Parinaud syndrome-chronic fever and regional lymphadenopathy, frequently cat-scratch fever

†*9. Postoperative penetrating keratoplasty or cataract surgery sutures

†10. Sebaceous carcinoma with papillary conjunctivitis

†11. Trachoma: Stages to 3

†12. Use of hard and soft contact lens

†*14. Use of ocular prostheses

†15. With generalized lymphadenopathy.

Treatment

Identify cause.
- May have complication with contact lenses (CLs).
- Topical mast cell stabilizers and antihistamine combination solutions (e.g. olopatadine, Elestat).
- Cool compresses.
- Refractive surgery to avoid CLs.

⊡ BIBLIOGRAPHY

1. Weissman BA, Yeung KK. (2013). Giant papillary conjunctivitis. [online] Available from www.emedicine.com/oph/TOPIC87.HTM. [Accessed September, 2013].

---

†Indicates a general entry and therefore has not been described in detail in the text

⊡ 13.4. ROTHMUND SYNDROME (ROTHMUND-THOMSON SYNDROME; TELANGIECTASIA-PIGMENTATION-CATARACT SYNDROME; ECTODERMAL SYNDROME; CONGENITAL POIKILODERMA WITH JUVENILE CATARACT) KERATOCONUS

General

Autosomal recessive; more common in females (2:1); Werner syndrome in adults has certain similarities to this syndrome; inflammatory phase progresses to atrophy and telangiectasia; onset at age from 3 months to 6 months.

Ocular

Eyebrows may be sparse or absent; hypertelorism; cilia sometimes are diminished or absent; trichiasis; epiphora; cataracts (anterior subcapsular, posterior stellate, or perinuclear type); corneal lesions; retinal hyperpigmentation; keratoconus; strabismus; epibulbar dermoids.

Clinical

Poikiloderma; hypogonadism; hypomenorrhea; head deformity (enlarged with depressed nasal bridge as well as microcephaly); small stature, with short or malformed distal phalanges; aplasia cutis congenita (congenital absence of skin in one or more areas); alopecia.

Laboratory

Skeletal radiograph by age 5 years.

Treatment

Sun blocker with UVA and UVB should be use often. Keratolytics and retinoids are use to treat hyperkeratotic lesions.

BIBLIOGRAPHY

1. Hsu S, George SJ. (2012). Rothmund-Thomson syndrome. [online] Available from www.emedicine.com/derm/TOPIC379.HTM. [Accessed September, 2013].

13.5. LYMPHOID HYPERPLASIA (REACTIVE LYMPHOID HYPERPLASIA; LYMPHOID TUMORS; MALIGNANT LYMPHOMA; PSEUDOLYMPHOMA; PSEUDOTUMOR; BURKITT LYMPHOMA; NEOPLASTIC ANGIOENDOTHELIOMATOSIS)

General

Occurs in tropical Africa; young children; idiopathic orbital inflammation; systemic disease is rarely associated but occasionally occurs with either vasculitis or lymphomas; etiology of Burkitt lymphoma currently includes three factors: (1) Epstein-Barr virus, (2) malaria and (3) chromosomal translocations activating the c-Myc oncogene, which induces uncontrolled B-cell proliferation.

Ocular

Proptosis; extraocular motility disturbances; lesions of orbit, lacrimal gland, conjunctiva, and uvea; cortical blindness; retinal artery occlusion; retinal vascular and pigment epithelial alterations; vitreitis.

Clinical

Maxillary tumor; Epstein-Barr virus; cranial neuropathy.

Laboratory

Generally diagnosed with a lymph node biopsy.

Treatment

Chemotherapy, monoclonal antibody therapy and bone marrow or stem cell infusions may be chosen as therapy.

BIBLIOGRAPHY

1. Brooks HL, Downing J, McClure JA, et al. Orbital Buritt's lymphoma in a homosexual man with acquired immune deficiency. Arch Ophthalmol. 1984;102(10):1533-7.
2. Cheung MK, Martin DF, Chan CC, et al. Diagnosis of reactive lymphoid hyperplasia by chorioretinal biopsy. Am J Ophthalmol. 1994;118(4):457-62.

14. CHRONIC MUCOPURULENT CONJUNCTIVITIS (MUCOPURULENT DISCHARGE, MODERATE HYPEREMIA WITH A CHRONIC COURSE)

1. Infective element-lids or lacrimal apparatus
   †A. *Monilia* species
   B. Morax-Axenfeld diplobacillus (angular conjunctivitis)
   †*C. Pneumococcus
   D. Pubic lice
   E. Staphylococcus
   †F. *Streptothrix foersteri*

†2. *Allergic*: Cosmetics
3. Irritative
   †A. Associated infections or irritation of lids, lacrimal apparatus, nose, or skin
   †B. Deficiency of lacrimal secretions
   †C. Direct irritants: Foreign body, mascara, dust, wind, smog, insecticides, chlorinated water, and many others

D. Exposure: Ectropion, facial paralysis, exophthalmos, and others.

†E. Eyestrain

†F. Metabolic conditions: Gout, alcoholism, or prolonged digestive disturbances

†G. Overtreatment by drugs: Antibiotics, miotics, mydriatics.

---

†Indicates a general entry and therefore has not been described in detail in the text

⊟ BIBLIOGRAPHY

1. Fedukowicz HB. External infections of the eye: Bacterial, Viral, and Mycotic, 3rd edition. New York: Appleton-Century-Crofts; 1984.
2. Geyer O, Neudorfer M, Lazar M. Phenylephrine prodrug. Ophthalmology. 1991;98:1483.
3. Okumoto M, Smolin G. Pneumococcal infections of the eye. Am J Ophthalmol. 1974;77:346-52.
4. Roy FH. Ocular Syndromes and systemic diseases, 5th edition. New Delhi: Jaypee Brothers; 2013.

⊟ 14.1B. ANGULAR CONJUNCTIVITIS (MORAX-AXENFELD BACILLUS)

General

It is caused by *M. lacunata*, which frequently inhabits the nose.

Ocular

Conjunctivitis; hypopyon; keratitis; uveitis; corneal marginal ulcer.

Laboratory

Diagnosis is made by clinical findings.

Treatment

- *Conjunctivitis:* Antibiotic medication should be used to treat the infection.
- *Corneal ulcer:* Corneal cultures may be taken and treatment is initiated. Treatment includes a broad spectrum of antibiotics and cycloplegic drops.
- *Uveitis:* Topical steroids and cycloplegic medication should be the choice of initial treatment. Oral steroids should be given if not responsive to topical steroids, immunosuppressants if bilateral disease that does not respond to oral steroids, and periocular steroids for unilateral or posterior uveitis. Vitrectomy can be used for severe vitreous opacification. Cryotherapy and laser photocoagulation may be used for localized pars plana exudates.

⊟ BIBLIOGRAPHY

1. Jones DB. Early diagnosis and therapy of bacterial corneal ulcers. Int Ophthalmol Clin. 1973;13(4):1-29.
2. Marioneaux SJ, Cohen EJ, Arentsen JJ, et al. Moraxella keratitis. Cornea. 1991;10(1):21-4.
3. van Bijsterveld OP. Bacterial proteases in Moraxella angular conjunctivitis. Am J Ophthalmol. 1971;72(1):181-4.

⊟ 14.1D. PEDICULOSIS AND PHTHIRIASIS

General

Infestation of lice on head, body, or pubic area.

Ocular

Conjunctivitis; keratitis; infestation of lice or nits glued to shafts of eyelashes and eyebrow.

Clinical

Pruritus; skin excoriation; impetigo; pyoderma with lymphadenitis and febrile episodes.

Laboratory

Removal from hair shaft and examination under microscope.

Treatment

Treatments involve spreading an ointment at the base of the eyelashes at night to trap mites as they emerge from their burrow and/or move from one follicle to another.

⊟ BIBLIOGRAPHY

1. Guenther L. (2012). Pediculosis (Lice). [online] Available from www.emedicine.com/med/TOPIC1769.HTM. [Accessed September, 2013].

🗗 14.1E. STAPHYLOCOCCUS

General

Gram-positive coccus *S. aureus;* most common cause of suppurative infection in humans; more common in patients with a previous disorders, such as diabetes, thyroid disease, renal failure, or malnutrition; although most *S. aureus* isolates from other sources are encapsulated, capsules have not been noted in ocular isolates.

Ocular

Uveitis; hypopyon; conjunctivitis; keratitis; cellulitis of lid; meibomianitis; ptosis; blepharitis; endophthalmitis; dacryocystitis; increased IOP; orbital periosteitis.

Clinical

Tissues hypertonic, edematous, and painful; lesion liquefies, forming creamy yellow pus; fever; nausea; vomiting; cough; dyspnea; abdominal pain; diarrhea; bloody stools; dehydration; shock.

Laboratory

Aerobic Gram-positive cocci bacteria grow in grape-like clusters. Coagulase positive indicates pathogenicity.

Treatment

Specific antimicrobial therapy is chosen based on the site and severity of the infection and the antimicrobial sensitivities of the organism involved.

🗗 BIBLIOGRAPHY

1. Tolan RW. (2012). Staphylococcus Aureus Infection. [online] Available from www.emedicine.com/ped/TOPIC2704.HTM. [Accessed September, 2013].

🗗 14.3D. ECTROPION

General

Outward turning of eyelid which can be congenital or acquired.

Clinical

Facial abnormalities.

Ocular

Eyelid turning outward, exposure keratopathy, ocular irritation or infection.

Laboratory

Diagnosis is made by clinical findings.

Treatment

- Topical ocular lubricants.
- *Congenital*: Full thickness skin graft with canthal tendon tightening.
- *Involutional*: Tighten the lid by resecting full-thickness wedge-medial spindle procedure for punctal eversion. Paralytic may require a fascia lata sling procedure if it does not resolve in 3–6 months.

🗗 BIBLIOGRAPHY

1. Ing E. (2012). Ectropion. [online] Available from www.emedicine.com/oph/TOPIC211.HTM. [Accessed September, 2013].

🗗 15. CICATRICIAL CONJUNCTIVITIS (CICATRICIAL PEMPHIGOID) SCARRING OF CONJUNCTIVA

*1. *General*: A postinfectious type of membranous conjunctivitis such as *C. diphtheriae, Streptococcal* conjunctivitis, autoimmune or presumably autoimmune sarcoidosis, scleroderma, pemphigoid, lichen planus, atopic blepharoconjunctivitis, miscellaneous causes and linear IgA dermatosis.

2. Upper lid
   A. Trachoma

3. Lower lid
 *A. Acne rosacea (ocular rosacea)
 B. Chemical (especially alkali)
 C. *Chlamydia* organisms (psittacosis-lymphogranu-loma group)
 †D. Chronic cicatricial conjunctivitis-occurs in the elderly; has a chronic course; may have concurrent skin and mucous membrane lesions
 *E. Congenital syphilis
 F. Dermatitis herpetiformis
 G. Epidemic keratoconjunctivitis
 H. Epidermolysis acuta toxica (Lyell syndrome)
 I. Epidermolysis bullosa
 *J. Erythema multiforme (Stevens-Johnson disease)
 K. Erythroderma ichthyosiforme
 L. Exfoliative dermatitis
 M. Fuchs-Lyell syndrome
 N. Hydroa vacciniforme
 O. Impetigo
 P. Lamellar ichthyoses
 Q. Ocular pemphigoid
 R. Paraneoplastic lichen planus
 †S. Radium burns
 T. Reiter syndrome (conjunctivourethrosynovial syndrome)
 U. Sjögren syndrome (secretoinhibitor syndrome)
 V. Staphylococcal granuloma
 W. Syphilis (acquired lues)
 X. Systemic scleroderma (progressive systemic sclerosis)
 Y. Vaccinia
†*4. Drugs
 A. Demecarium bromide
 *B. Echothiophate iodide
 C. Idoxuridine
 D. Penicillamine
 E. Pilocarpine
 F. Practolol
 G. Thiabendazole
 H. Timolol
 I. Topical ocular epinephrine

Treatment

- No topical agent is effective in stopping ocular pemphigoid (OCP) activity.

---

*Indicates most frequent
†Indicates a general entry and therefore has not been described in detail in the text

- Systemic corticosteroids can control the activity of the disease.
- Long-term use (> 1 year) of systemic immunomodulators is the major therapeutic strategy in treating OCP.
  - For mild-to-moderate inflammation, diaminodiphenylsulfone (Dapsone) is the first-line agent, provided the patient is not glucose-6-phosphate dehydrogenase deficient.
  - For severe inflammation, initially use cyclophosphamide, and add systemic prednisone with rapid taper for a limited period of time.
  - Perform ocular surgical procedures when the inflammation is completely under control, and use systemic corticosteroids perioperatively, when the procedure involves the conjunctiva or the cornea.
  - Epilation.
  - Punctal occlusion.
  - Lid surgery.
  - Fornix reconstruction.
  - Corneal surgery.
  - Cataract surgery
- Consult an appropriate specialist in case of skin involvement or involvement of other mucous membranes. Patients who have difficulty swallowing or breathing require an immediate endoscopic examination.
- Patients receiving chemotherapy may require regular consultations with a chemotherapeutist.
- Refer patients to an ear, nose, and throat specialist for laryngoscopy in case of recent onset of hoarseness, which may be caused by laryngeal stenosis and tracheal scarring. These patients are in a medical emergency because of the risk of mucous accumulation and subsequent fatal asphyxiation. A statim laryngoscopy is essential, and it may be a life-saving procedure.

BIBLIOGRAPHY

1. Foster CS, Hamam R, Letko E. (2011). Ophthalmologic manifestations of cicatricial pemphigoid. [online] Available from www.emedicine.com/oph/TOPIC83.HTM. [Accessed September, 2013].
2. Klein PA, Callen JP. (2012). Linear IgA dermatosis. [online] Available from www.emedicine.com/derm/TOPIC240.HTM. [Accessed September, 2013].
3. Graham RH. (2012). Trichiasis. [online] Available from www.emedicine.com/oph/TOPIC609.HTM. [Accessed September, 2013].
4. Camara JG, Worak SR, Bengzon AU. (2012). Obstruction nasolacrimal duct. [online] http://www.emedicine.com/oph/TOPIC465.HTM. [Accessed September, 2013].

5. Foster CS, Yuksel E, Anzaar F, et al. (2012). Dry eye syndrome. [online] Available from emedicine.medscape.com/article/1210417-overview. [Accessed September, 2013].
6. Rostami S. (2011). Distichiasis. [online] Available from www.emedicine.com/oph/TOPIC603.HTM. [Accessed September, 2013].
7. Ventocilla M, Bloomenstein MR, Majmudar PA. (2012). Allergic conjunctivitis. [online] Available from www.emedicine.com/oph/TOPIC85.HTM. [Accessed September, 2013].

🗗 15.1. DIPHTHERIA

General

Acute infectious disease caused by *Corynebacterium diphtheriae;* severity is dependent upon the amount of exotoxin absorbed prior to initiation of specific therapy.

Ocular

Conjunctivitis; xerophthalmia; keratitis; corneal ulcer; blepharitis; cellulitis of lid; meibomianitis; ptosis; dacryocystitis; cataract; central retinal artery occlusion; optic neuritis; accommodative spasm or paralysis; convergence paralysis; divergence paralysis; paralysis of third, fourth, or sixth nerve; paralysis of accommodation (in children); ocular motor nerve paresis; choroiditis; cranial neuropathies involving the trigeminal, vagus, and hypoglossal cranial nerves; myocarditis.

Clinical

Local inflammatory lesion, with effect on heart, kidneys, and nervous system.

Laboratory

Gram-positive rods commonly affect children younger than 10 years.

Treatment

Systemic treatment involves use of diphtheria antitoxin and antibiotics. Ocular treatment includes diphtheria antitoxin and high titer y-globulin preparation. Topical penicillin-G ointment helps to eradicate the bacilli.

🗗 BIBLIOGRAPHY

1. Demirci CS. (2011). Pediatric diphtheria. [online] Available from www.emedicine.com/ped/TOPIC596.HTM. [Accessed September, 2013].

🗗 15.1. STREPTOCOCCUS (SCARLET FEVER)

General

Gram-positive bacteria that can invade any tissue.

Ocular

Conjunctivitis; corneal ulcer; blepharitis; scarlatinal rash of lid; erysipelas dermatitis of lid; gangrene of lid; endophthalmitis; proptosis; dacryocystitis; optic neuritis; orbital cellulitis; uveitis; hypopyon; secondary glaucoma; paralysis of extraocular muscles; infectious crystalline keratopathy; scleritis.

Clinical

Pharyngitis; impetigo; scarlet fever; pneumonia; bacteremia; rheumatic fever; glomerulonephritis.

Laboratory

Gram-positive cocci growing in pairs or chains. Throat culture and sensitivity are useful.

Treatment

Penicillin is the drug of choice.

🗗 BIBLIOGRAPHY

1. Zabawski EJ. (2011). Scarlet fever. [online] Available from www.emedicine.com/emerg/TOPIC518.HTM. [Accessed September, 2013].

15.1. SCHAUMANN SYNDROME (BESNIER-BOECK-SCHAUMANN SYNDROME; BOECK SARCOID; SARCOIDOSIS)

General

Etiology unknown; theories include tuberculosis, hypersensitivity to pine pollen, virus infection; affects blacks most often; chronic course with spontaneous remissions (*see* Heerfordt's syndrome); hilar or paratracheal nodes with erythema nodosum; onset most often in middle and old age; ocular involvement in 20–25% of all cases.

Ocular

Orbital granulomatous mass; bony defects; cutaneous and subcutaneous nodules; myogenic palsy; lacrimal gland adenopathy; decreased tear formation; secondary glaucoma; granulomatous uveitis with iris nodules, cells and flare; mutton fat keratic precipitates; keratitis sicca; vitreous floaters; band-shaped keratitis; complicated cataract; inflammatory retinal exudates; "candle wax drippings"; optic nerve atrophy; neuritis; eyelid nodules; ocular nerve enlargement (granuloma).

Clinical

Lymphadenopathy; hilar nodes; fatigue; cystic, punched-out or reticulated changes in small bones (mainly, hands and feet); muscle wasting; contractures; weakness in legs and arms.

Laboratory

Chest X-ray, CT scan, and magnetic resonance imaging (MRI) of the brain.

Treatment

Glucocorticoids are the treatment of choice.

BIBLIOGRAPHY

1. Sharma GD. (2011). Pediatric sarcoidosis. [online] Available from www.emedicine.com/ped/TOPIC2043.HTM. [Accessed December, 2012].

15.1. PROGRESSIVE SYSTEMIC SCLEROSIS (SCLERODERMA; SYSTEMIC SCLERODERMA)

General

Chronic connective tissue disease of unknown etiology; chronic and usually progressive disorder; typical onset is in 3rd to 5th decade; ratio of women to men is 4:1; primary sites of pathology are the arterioles and capillaries of affected organs.

Ocular

Marginal corneal ulcers; shortened fornices of the conjunctiva; ptosis; cotton-wool patches of retina; papilledema; retinal hemorrhages; cicatrization of conjunctiva and cornea; blepharitis; blepharospasm; thready, tenacious yellow-white conjunctival discharge; hypertrophy of lacrimal gland; episcleritis; ocular myositis; Sjögren syndrome; uveitis; vitreous haze; keratitis sicca; decreased corneal sensation; iritis; ischemic choroidopathy; iris sectorial atrophy; blepharophimosis; heterochromia; keratoconus; central retinal vein occlusion; branch retinal vein occlusion.

Clinical

Vascular insufficiency; Raynaud's phenomenon; malaise; weight loss; stiffness; fever; polyarticular arthritis; diffuse edema of the hands; calcinosis; esophageal involvement; sclerodactyly; telangiectasis; esophageal stricture; renal failure; diffuse interstitial fibrosis.

Laboratory

No specific test establishes diagnosis. Hypergammaglobulinemia—50% of cases ANA increased in 40–70% cases.

Treatment

Skin thickening can be treated with D-penicillamine and other experimental drugs. Pruritus can be treated with moisturizers and histamine. Raynaud's phenomenon can be treated with calcium channel blockers. Renal crisis episodes are best prevented and treated with the aggressive use of angiotensin-converting enzyme (ACE) inhibitors. Myositis may be treated cautiously with steroids.

BIBLIOGRAPHY

1. Jimenez SA, Cronin PM, Koenig AS, et al. (2012). Scleroderma. [online] Available from www.emedicine.com/med/TOPIC2076.HTM. [Accessed December, 2012].

15.1. BENIGN MUCOSAL PEMPHIGOID (CHRONIC CICATRICIAL CONJUNCTIVITIS; CICATRICIAL PEMPHIGOID; ESSENTIAL SHRINKAGE OF THE CONJUNCTIVA; MEMBRANE PEMPHIGUS; OCULAR PEMPHIGOID)

General

Etiology unknown; involving older age group, especially over 70 years; chronic autoimmune disorder characterized by fibrosis beneath the conjunctival epithelium; associated with the major histocompatibility complex class I alleles, which confer susceptibility to the disease; likely due to a multigene effect and associated with environmental factors; incidence in women is twice as frequent as men, no geographic or racial predilection.

Ocular

Conjunctivitis; absence of goblet cells of conjunctiva; conjunctival ulcer; pannus and keratitis; corneal opacity; entropion; trichiasis; cicatrization of lacrimal ducts; corneal perforation; symblepharon; dry eyes; bilateral involvement (may be asymmetrical); ocular shrinkage; xerosis; conjunctival and corneal bullae.

Clinical

Subepidermal and subepithelial blistering of mucous membranes; blisters may occur in pharyngeal, laryngeal, nasal, anal and genital mucosa.

Laboratory

Diagnosis is made by clinical findings.

Treatment

Subconjunctival injections of steroid or mitomycin may be helpful. Systemic immunomodulators are the major therapeutic plan.

BIBLIOGRAPHY

1. Foster CS, Hamam R, Letko E. (2011). Ophthalmologic manifestations of cicatricial pemphigoid. [online] Available from www.emedicine.com/oph/TOPIC83.HTM. [Accessed September, 2013].

15.1. LICHEN PLANUS

General

Conjunctival disorder associated with dermatologic disorder; disappears spontaneously.

Ocular

Conjunctivitis; cicatrizing conjunctivitis; keratin plaque on bulbar conjunctiva.

Clinical

Grayish-white papules; oral lesions may precede skin lesions.

Laboratory

Diagnosis is made by clinical findings.

Treatment

Topical and systemic corticosteroids, systemic immunomodulators.

BIBLIOGRAPHY

1. Foster CS, Hamam R, Letko E. (2011). Ophthalmologic manifestations of cicatricial pemphigoid. [online] Available from www.emedicine.com/oph/TOPIC83.HTM. [Accessed September, 2013].

15.1. BLEPHAROCONJUNCTIVITIS

General

Chronic blepharitis caused by *Staphylococcus,* seborrheic, meibomian seborrhea or seborrheic with secondary meibomianitis.

Clinical

Seborrheic dermatitis.

Ocular

Blepharitis, keratoconjunctivitis.

Laboratory

Eyelid and conjunctival cultures.

Treatment

Ocular: Warm compresses to lids, eyelid scrubs, bacitracin ointment, ocular lubricants and rarely topical steroids. Systemic antibiotics are sometimes necessary in severe cases.

BIBLIOGRAPHY

1. Roy FH, Fraunfelder FW, Fraunfelder FT. Roy and Fraunfelder's Current Ocular Therapy, 6th edition. London, UK: Elsevier; 2008.

15.1. LINEAR IgA DISEASE

General

Bullous dermatosis with pruritic urticarial lesions with overlying vesicles or bullae; skin lesions heal without scarring; homogeneous deposition of immunoglobulin A (IgA) at the dermal-epidermal junction and rarely, deposition of other immunoglobulin present; heterogeneous disease with regard to its clinical features, target antigens, and immunogenetics; association with HLA-B8, DR3, Cw7, and the linked rare tumor necrosis factor-a allele; may be induced by amiodarone.

Ocular

Chronic conjunctivitis; subconjunctival fibrosis; symblepharon; chronic progressive conjunctival cicatrization.

Clinical

Recurrent blistering skin disorder consisting of urticarial macules and plaques with vesicular eruptions on trunk and extremities; subepidermal vesiculation.

Laboratory

Diagnosis is made by clinical findings.

Treatment

Conjunctivitis: Symptomatic control may include cold compresses, artificial tears; NSAIDs and occasionally steroidal drops to relieve itching.

BIBLIOGRAPHY

1. Foster CS, Hamam R, Letko E. (2011). Ophthalmologic manifestations of cicatricial pemphigoid. [online] Available from www.emedicine.com/oph/TOPIC83.HTM. [Accessed September, 2013].

15.2A. TRACHOMA

General

Most common in rural communities of the Middle East, Africa, Asia, and South and Central America; caused by *C. trachomatis*; associated with poor sanitation and medical care.

Ocular

Chronic keratoconjunctivitis; papillae follicles; keratitis; opacities of cornea; scars of palpebral conjunctiva; ptosis; tearing; entropion.

Clinical

Rhinitis; otitis media; upper respiratory tract infection.

Laboratory

Most endemic areas, lab tests are unavailable. Commercial PCR based assay has high sensitivity and specificity.

Treatment

Tetracycline eye ointment for 6 weeks or a single dose azithromycin systemically.

🗗 BIBLIOGRAPHY

1. Solomon AW. (2011). Trachoma. [online] Available from www.emedicine.com/oph/TOPIC118.HTM. [Accessed September, 2013].
2. Biebesheimer JB, House J, Hong KC, et al. Complete local elimination of infectious trachoma from severely affected communitieis after six biannual mass azithromycin distributions. Ophthalmology. 209;116:2047-50.

🗗 15.3A. ACNE ROSACEA (ACNE ERYTHEMATOSA; OCULAR ROSACEA)

General

Etiology unknown; usually occurs in women 30–50 years of age; pathogenetic mechanism remains unclear.

Ocular

Conjunctivitis; corneal neovascularization (wedge-shaped); keratitis; meibomianitis; blepharitis; recurrent chalazion; conjunctival hyperemia; superficial punctate keratopathy; corneal vascularization, thinning, perforation, and scarring; episcleritis; scleritis; iritis; nodular conjunctivitis.

Clinical

Symmetrical erythema; papules; pustules; telangiectasia; sebaceous gland hypertrophy of the forehead, malar eminences, and nose.

Laboratory

Diagnosis is made from clinical findings.

Treatment

Systemic antibiotics are useful in most cases.

🗗 BIBLIOGRAPHY

1. Banasikowaska AK, Singh S. (2012). Rosacea. [online] Available from www.emedicine.com/derm/TOPIC377.HTM. [Accessed September, 2013].

🗗 15.3B. ALKALINE INJURY OF THE EYE

General

A splash of alkaline solution causes the pH to rise and results in immediate damage to the external ocular tissues. These injuries are frequently seen from household chemicals or farming injuries from liquid ammonia used as fertilizer.

Ocular

Pain; lacrimation; blepharospasm; rise in IOP; rapid penetration of the cornea and sclera; chemical injury to iris, lens or ciliary body; symblepharon; phthisis bulbi; ankyloblepharon.

Laboratory

Diagnosis is made by clinical findings and history.

Treatment

Immediate copious irrigation, sticky paste of lime should be removed with a cotton-tipped applicator, mydriasis and topical antibiotics, pain medications, treatment of glaucoma with carbonic anhydrase inhibitors, patching and soft contact lenses may facilitate re-epithelialization, insertion of a methyl methacrylate ring may prevent fibrinous adhesions, lysis of adhesions with or without mucous membrane grafts, corneal stem cell transplantation, corneal transplantation, keratoprosthesis and conjunctival autographs.

BIBLIOGRAPHY

1. Roy FH, Fraunfelder FW, Fraunfelder FT. Roy and Fraunfelder's Current Ocular Therapy, 6th edition. London: Elsevier; 2008.

15.3C. CHLAMYDIA (INCLUSION CONJUNCTIVITIS; PARATRACHOMA)

General

Organism that infects the epithelium of mucoid surfaces; sexually transmitted; major cause of non-gonococcal urethritis in men and cervicitis in women; major cause of neonatal ophthalmia; *Chlamydia trachomatis* is an intracellular bacterium lacking respiratory enzymes that has an affinity for mucosal epithelium; serotypes A through C have been epidemiologically associated with trachoma; serotypes E through K have been associated with genital infection and keratoconjunctivitis in sexually active adults and neonates; other serotypes have been associated with lymphogranuloma venereum and Reiter syndrome.

Ocular

Follicular conjunctivitis; corneal opacities; keratitis; corneal ulcer; lid edema; uveitis.

Clinical

Pneumonia; gastrointestinal disturbances; genital discharge.

Laboratory

Giemsa stain, cell culture—time intensive, direct fluorescent monoclonal antibiotics to stain smears.

Treatment

Three to six weeks of oral tetracycline (500 mg qid), oral doxycycline (100 mg bid), or oral erythromycin stearate (500 mg qid). Simultaneous treatment of all sexual partners is important to prevent reinfection.

BIBLIOGRAPHY

1. Bashour M. (2012) Ophthalmologic manifestations of Chlamydia. [online] Available from www.emedicine.com/oph/TOPIC494.HTM. [Accessed September, 2013].

15.3E. CONGENITAL LUES (CONGENITAL SYPHILIS)

General

Caused by intrauterine transplacental infection of fetus by *T. pallidum* (*see* Syphilis).

Ocular

Conjunctivitis; keratitis; dacryocystitis; optic nerve atrophy; periostitis; anisocoria; Argyll Robertson pupil; retinal degeneration; nystagmus; gumma of conjunctiva, eyelids, and orbit; paresis of extraocular muscles; secondary glaucoma; uveitis; iridoschisis.

Clinical

Cutaneous and mucous membrane lesions; periostitis; anemia; hepatosplenomegaly; ectodermal defects; central nervous system involvement; gummatous lesions.

Laboratory

Fluorescent treponemal antibody-absorption (FTA-ABS) and microhemagglutination assay (MHA-TP) are the standard test. All patients with syphilis should also be tested for HIV.

Treatment

Parenteral penicillin is the preferred treatment for all stages of syphilis. The treatment varies from primary and secondary syphilis, late latent syphilis, tertiary syphilis and neurosyphilis. Ocular treatment includes topical steroids and cycloplegics and it can relieve the symptoms of anterior uveitis and interstitial keratitis. Subconjunctival steroids have been used to relieve recurrent anterior segment inflammation. Severe corneal opacification may require keratoplasty, however, with recurrent inflammation and graft rejection.

BIBLIOGRAPHY

1. Waseem M. (2011). Pediatric syphilis. [online] Available from www.emedicine.com/ped/TOPIC2193.HTM. [Accessed September, 2013].

15.3F. DERMATITIS HERPETIFORMIS (DUHRING-BROCQ DISEASE)

General

Malignant; atypical; does not respond well to sulfone or sulfapyridine therapy; uncommon; autoimmune blistering dermatosis; pruritic eruption involving the scalp, buttocks, lower back, and extensor surface of arms; autoantibody is generally of immunoglobulin A class causing deposition at the dermal-epidermal junction.

Ocular

Bullae of conjunctiva, skin, and mucous membranes; blisters are intraepithelial (acantholysis) and usually do not leave scars; epithelium desquamates in patches; corneal and conjunctival vascularization; symblepharon; cataract.

Clinical

Vesicles; erythema; pruritus; burning; eruption classically involves extensor surface of the knees, elbows, buttocks, sacrum, scapula, and scalp.

Laboratory

Diagnosis is made by clinical findings and skin biopsy.

Treatment

Dapsone and sulfapyridine are the primary medications used for therapy. Avoidance of gluten is also helpful.

BIBLIOGRAPHY

1. Miller JL, Zaman SA. (2013). Dermatitis herpetiformis. [online] Available from www.emedicine.com/derm/TOPIC95.HTM. [Accessed September, 2013].

15.3G. EPIDEMIC KERATOCONJUNCTIVITIS

General

Highly communicable; adenovirus types 8 and 19; usually bilateral; epidemic keratoconjunctivitis has been reported worldwide associated with 11 virus serotypes, with serotypes 8, 11, and 19 being the most common responsible ones.

Ocular

Follicular or membranous conjunctivitis; chemosis; subconjunctival hemorrhages; corneal opacity; punctate epithelial keratitis; corneal ulcer; blepharospasm; lid edema; serous discharge; uveitis; epiphora.

Clinical

Submaxillary and cervical lymphadenopathy.

Laboratory

Viral isolation on cell culture from conjunctival scrapings.

Treatment

No effective topical or systemic treatment available. Topical steroids may be used if epithelial keratitis occurs.

BIBLIOGRAPHY

1. Bawazeer A. (2011). Epidemic keratoconjunctivitis. [online] Available from www.emedicine.com/oph/TOPIC677.HTM. [Accessed September, 2013].

15.3H. SCALDED SKIN SYNDROME (TOXIC EPIDERMAL NECROLYSIS; RITTER DISEASE; TOXIC EPIDERMAL NECROLYSIS OF LYELL; STAPHYLOCOCCAL SCALDED SKIN SYNDROME; LYELL SYNDROME; EPIDERMOLYSIS ACUTA TOXICA; TOXIC EPIDERMAL NECROLYSIS) SYMBLEPHARON

General

Generalized exfoliative dermatitis frequently affecting neonates and resulting from an initial focal staphylococcal infection (i.e. Staphylococcal ophthalmia neonatorum); toxic epidermal necrolysis usually refers to manifestation in the adult secondary to a drug reaction but affects all ages; immunopathogenetic mechanisms probably initiated with drug-skin binding with aberrant immune responses, including complement and immunoglobulin G deposition with the epidermis and mucosa; recent reports suggest that patients with the acquired immunodeficiency syndrome (AIDS) are at higher risk for developing mucocutaneous reactions, such as toxic epidermal necrolysis; mortality rate approximately 30%.

Ocular

Necrotic areas of lids, conjunctiva, and cornea; symblepharon; loss of corneal epithelium; corneal ulcer; leukoma; perforation of globe; abolition of lacrimal secretion; conjunctival chemosis; blepharitis; entropion; periorbital swelling; trichiasis; distichiasis; fornix shortening.

Clinical

Widespread reddening and tenderness of the skin followed by the exfoliation of large areas of skin; in children, erythema starts usually around the mouth and spreads over the entire body within hours, followed by blisters and large exudative lesions; fever; shock.

Laboratory

Culture and biopsy of the lesion.

Treatment

Intravenous penicillinase-resistant and antistaphylococcal antibiotics. Cloxacillin is the treatment of choice.

BIBLIOGRAPHY

1. Lopez-Garcia JS, Jara LR, Garcia-Lozano CI, et al. Ocular features and histopathologic changes during follow-up of toxic epidermal necrolysis. Ophthalmology. 2011;118:265-71.
2. Kim JH, Benson P. (2012). Dermatologic manifestations of staphylococcal scalded skin syndrome. [online] Available from www.emedicine.com/derm/TOPIC402.HTM. [Accessed September, 2013].

15.3I. GOLDSCHEIDER SYNDROME (WEBER-COCKAYNE SYNDROME; EPIDERMOLYSIS BULLOSA; DOMINANT EPIDERMOLYSIS BULLOSA DYSTROPHIEA ALBOPAPULOIDEA)

General

Rare; Weber-Cockayne syndrome, inherited as an autosomal dominant trait, is actually a milder form without scar formation, whereas Goldscheider syndrome, inherited either autosomal dominant or recessive, shows dystrophic changes with scarring; consanguinity frequent.

Ocular

Blepharitis; shrinkage of conjunctiva; pseudomembrane formation with symblepharon; conjunctivitis; bullous keratitis and subepithelial blisters lead to erosions with subsequent ulcerations and corneal opacities or even perforation; sclera may be similarly involved; lagophthalmos, cicatricial lacrimal stenosis; retinal detachment; cataract; pannus.

Clinical

Vesicular and bullous skin lesions and similar lesions of mucous membranes occur spontaneously or after mild trauma; keloid scars and contraction after healing are common in the dystrophic forms, whereas in the mild form the lesions heal without scarring but may leave some skin pigmentation; growth and mental retardation may be present in the group with recessive inheritance; stenosis of the larynx due to scarring may occur.

Laboratory

Obtain a skin biopsy following a thorough history and physical examination.

Treatment

Wound healing and prevention of infection is the preferred strategy. Esophageal lesions can be managed with phenytoin and oral steroid elixirs to reduce the symptoms of dysphagia. In addition, if oral candidiasis is present, an anticandidal medication is helpful. Patients can experience recurrent blepharitis in one or both eyes along with bullous lesions of the conjunctiva, corneal ulcerations, corneal scarring, obliteration of tear ducts, eyelid lesions and cicatricial conjunctivitis. Corneal erosions are treated with antibiotic ointment and use of cycloplegic agents to reduce ciliary spasm and provide comfort. Avoid using tape to patch the eye because of frequent blistering of the skin under the adhesive. Chronic blepharitis can result in cicatricial ectropion and exposure keratitis. Moisture chambers and ocular lubricants are used commonly for management. This disorder also has been treated with full-thickness skin grafting to the upper eyelid.

BIBLIOGRAPHY

1. Marinkovich MP. (2012). Epidermolysis bullosa. [online] Available from www.emedicine.com/derm/TOPIC124. HTM. [Accessed September, 2013].

15.3J. STEVENS-JOHNSON SYNDROME [DERMATOSTOMATITIS; ERYTHEMA MULTIFORME EXUDATIVUM; SYNDROMA MUCOCUTANEO-OCULARE; BAADER DERMATOSTOMATITIS SYNDROME; MUCOSAL-RESPIRATORY SYNDROME; FUCHS (2) SYNDROME; MUCOCUTANEOUS OCULAR SYNDROME]

General

Etiology unknown; affects all ages; most frequently seen in 1st and 3rd decades of life; prevalent in males; drugs are the most commonly identified etiologic factor in this condition.

Ocular

Hypopyon; iritis; keratitis; corneal ulcers; keratoconjunctivitis sicca; chemosis; conjunctivitis; widespread fibrinoid necrosis of conjunctival vessels; blepharitis; endophthalmitis; phthisis bulbi; uveitis; cataracts; pannus; optic neuritis; keratoconus; adenoviral conjunctivitis has been reported to have precipitated Stevens-Johnson syndrome; orbital cyst may be a complication.

Clinical

General malaise, headaches, chills, and fever; severe skin and mucous membrane eruptions (erythema multiforme); dorsa of hands and feet are most frequently affected; rhinitis; balanitis; vulvovaginitis; urethritis (nonspecific); cystitis; patients with AIDS are at higher risk of developing Stevens-Johnson syndrome.

Laboratory

No laboratory tests are specific to Stevens-Johnson syndrome. Diagnosis is made from clinical findings.

Treatment

Systemic treatment with steroids is controversial. Antibiotics are used based on clinical course. Eyelid hygiene performed as needed.

BIBLIOGRAPHY

1. Plaza JA, Dronen SC, Foster J, et al. (2011). Erythema multiforme. [online] Available from www.emedicine.com/med/TOPIC727.HTM. [Accessed September, 2013].

15.3K. BULLOUS ICHTHYOSIFORM ERYTHRODERMA (COLLODION BABY; CONGENITAL ICHTHYOSIS; EPIDERMOLYTIC HYPERKERATOSIS; ICHTHYOSIS; ICHTHYOSIS VULGARIS; LAMELLAR ICHTHYOSIS; NONBULLOUS ICHTHYOSIFORM ERYTHRODERMA; XERODERMA; X-LINKED ICHTHYOSIS)

General

Autosomal inherited disorder; affects both sexes; normal at birth; onset within first 7 days; X-linked; pathogenesis may be secondary to physicochemical changes of corneal tissues including accumulation of cholesterol sulfate.

Ocular

Keratopathy; corneal scarring; keratitis; conjunctivitis; lagophthalmos; photophobia; ectropion; lid erythema; lacrimation; keratoconus; deep corneal punctate/filiform lesions.

Clinical

At birth, the skin surface is moist, red, and tender; within several days, thick scales form.

Laboratory

Diagnosis is made by clinical findings.

Treatment

Genetic counseling and prenatal diagnosis also can be offered. Newborns with denuded skin are at increased risk for infection, secondary sepsis, and electrolyte imbalance and should be transferred to the neonatal intensive care unit (NICU) to be monitored and treated as needed.

BIBLIOGRAPHY

1. Chen TS, Metz BJ. (2012). Epidermolytic Hyperkeratosis (Bullous Congenital Ichthyosiform Erythroderma). [online] www.emedicine.com/derm/TOPIC590.HTM. [Accessed September, 2013].

15.3L. CONTACT DERMATITIS (DERMATITIS VENENATA)

General

Reaction of skin due to contact with foreign material; inflammatory disorder of the skin that may result from immunologic hypersensitivity (allergic contact dermatitis) or cutaneous injury not involving immunologic mechanisms (irritant contact dermatitis) from offending topical agents.

Ocular

Keratoconjunctivitis; chemosis; leukoma; corneal ulcer; pruritus of lids.

Clinical

Dermatitis; itching, erythema; vesiculation; edema with weeping and crusting.

Laboratory

Diagnosis is made by clinical findings.

Treatment

Adequate hygiene and avoidance of the contactant may be helpful. Many cases of localized mild contact dermatitis respond well to cool compresses and adequate wound care. Antibiotic therapy may be necessary for secondary infection. Low-strength topical steroids, such as hydrocortisone may be effective in decreasing inflammation and symptoms associated with very mild contact dermatitis. Systemic steroids are the mainstay of therapy in acute episodes of severe extensive allergic contact dermatitis.

BIBLIOGRAPHY

1. Crowe MA. (2011). Pediatric contact dermatitis. [online] Available from www.emedicine.com/ped/TOPIC2569.HTM. [Accessed September, 2013].

⊟ 15.3M. FUCHS-LYELL SYNDROME (DEBRÉ-LAMY-LYELL SYNDROME; TOXIC EPIDERMAL NECROLYSIS)

General

Allergic reaction with severe manifestations; similar to Fuchs-Salzmann-Terrien syndrome (*see* Fuchs-Salzmann-Terrien Syndrome); may result as a reaction to *S. aureus* toxin in children or associated with certain medications, including penicillin, sulfa drugs, nonsteroidal anti-inflammatory agents, and allopurinol.

Ocular

Obstruction of nasolacrimal duct; cicatricial changes in conjunctiva and cornea; conjunctivitis; symblepharon; corneal ulceration and possible perforation.

Clinical

Inflammation of mucous membrane with ulcerations; general epidermolysis; cicatricial changes, especially of orifices.

Laboratory

Hematology studies, chemistry to assess fluid and electrolyte losses, liver enzyme tests, coagulation studies.

Treatment

Management requires prompt detection and withdrawal of all potential causative agents, evaluation, and largely supportive care.

⊟ BIBLIOGRAPHY

1. Cohen V, Jellinek SP, Schwartz RA. (2013). Toxic epidermal necrolysis. [online] Available from www.emedicine.com/med/TOPIC2291.HTM. [Accessed September, 2013].

⊟ 15.3N. HYDROA VACCINIFORME

General

Sensitivity to sunlight.

Ocular

Conjunctivitis; corneal vesiculae; keratitis; cicatricial ectropion.

Clinical

Vesicular skin eruptions in areas exposed to sunlight.

Laboratory

Repetitive, broad-spectrum, UV-A phototesting.

Treatment

Consult a dermatologist for evaluation and management of Hydroa vacciniforme (HV).

⊟ BIBLIOGRAPHY

1. Sebastian QL, Del Rosario R. (2011). Hydroa vacciniforme. [online] Available from www.emedicine.com/derm/TOPIC181.HTM. [Accessed September, 2013].

⊟ 15.3O. IMPETIGO

General

Superficial primary pyoderma caused by streptococci and *S. aureus*.

Ocular

Pustular, crusting lesions of lids and brows; conjunctivitis; corneal ulcer; cicatricial ankyloblepharon.

Clinical

Thin-roofed vesicles that develop a thin amber crust occur on face and exposed areas of the extremities; extremely common skin infections caused by *S. aureus* in patients infected with HIV.

Laboratory

Diagnosis is made by clinical findings.

Treatment

Antibiotics are the mainstay of therapy and the chosen agent must provide coverage against both *S. aureus* and *S. pyogenes*. Topical antibiotics are used in patients with small or few lesions.

🗗 BIBLIOGRAPHY

1. Lewis LS, Friedman AD. (2013). Impetigo. [online] Available from www.emedicine.com/derm/TOPIC195.HTM. [Accessed September, 2013].

🗗 15.3P. BULLOUS ICHTHYOSIFORM ERYTHRODERMA (COLLODION BABY; CONGENITAL ICHTHYOSIS; EPIDERMOLYTIC HYPERKERATOSIS; ICHTHYOSIS; ICHTHYOSIS VULGARIS; LAMELLAR ICHTHYOSIS; NONBULLOUS ICHTHYOSIFORM ERYTHRODERMA; XERODERMA; X-LINKED ICHTHYOSIS)

General

Autosomal inherited disorder; affects both sexes; normal at birth; onset within first 7 days; X-linked; pathogenesis may be secondary to physicochemical changes of corneal tissues including accumulation of cholesterol sulfate.

Ocular

Keratopathy; corneal scarring; keratitis; conjunctivitis; lagophthalmos; photophobia; ectropion; lid erythema; lacrimation; keratoconus; deep corneal punctate/filiform lesions.

Clinical

At birth, the skin surface is moist, red, and tender; within several days, thick scales form.

Laboratory

Diagnosis is made by clinical findings.

Treatment

Genetic counseling and prenatal diagnosis also can be offered. Newborns with denuded skin are at increased risk for infection, secondary sepsis, and electrolyte imbalance and should be transferred to the NICU to be monitored and treated as needed.

🗗 BIBLIOGRAPHY

1. Chen TS, Metz BJ. (2012). Epidermolytic hyperkeratosis (Bullous Congenital Ichthyosiform Erythroderma). [online] www.emedicine.com/derm/TOPIC590.HTM. [Accessed September, 2013].

🗗 15.3Q. BENIGN MUCOSAL PEMPHIGOID (CHRONIC CICATRICIAL CONJUNCTIVITIS; CICATRICIAL PEMPHIGOID; ESSENTIAL SHRINKAGE OF THE CONJUNCTIVA; MEMBRANE PEMPHIGUS; OCULAR PEMPHIGOID)

General

Etiology unknown; involving older age group, especially over 70 years; chronic autoimmune disorder characterized by fibrosis beneath the conjunctival epithelium; associated with the major histocompatibility complex class I alleles, which confer susceptibility to the disease; likely due to a multigene effect and associated with environmental factors; incidence in women is twice as frequent as men, no geographic or racial predilection.

Ocular

Conjunctivitis; absence of goblet cells of conjunctiva; conjunctival ulcer; pannus and keratitis; corneal opacity; entropion; trichiasis; cicatrization of lacrimal ducts; corneal perforation; symblepharon; dry eyes; bilateral involvement (may be asymmetrical); ocular shrinkage; xerosis; conjunctival and corneal bullae.

Clinical

Subepidermal and subepithelial blistering of mucous membranes; blisters may occur in pharyngeal, laryngeal, nasal, anal and genital mucosa.

Laboratory

Diagnosis is made by clinical findings.

Treatment

Subconjunctival injections of steroid or mitomycin may be helpful. Systemic immunomodulators are the major therapeutic plan.

BIBLIOGRAPHY

1. Foster CS, Hamam R, Letko E. (2011). Ophthalmologic manifestations of cicatricial pemphigoid. [online] Available from www.emedicine.com/oph/TOPIC83.HTM. [Accessed September, 2013].

15.3R. LICHEN PLANUS

General

Conjunctival disorder associated with dermatologic disorder; disappears spontaneously.

Ocular

Conjunctivitis; cicatrizing conjunctivitis; keratin plaque on bulbar conjunctiva.

Clinical

Grayish-white papules; oral lesions may precede skin lesions.

Laboratory

Diagnosis is made by clinical findings.

Treatment

Topical and systemic corticosteroids, systemic immunomodulators.

BIBLIOGRAPHY

1. Foster CS, Hamam R, Letko E. (2011). Ophthalmologic manifestations of cicatricial pemphigoid. [online] Available from www.emedicine.com/oph/TOPIC83.HTM. [Accessed September, 2013].

15.3T. REITER SYNDROME (FIESSINGER-LEROY SYNDROME; CONJUNCTIVO-URETHRO-SYNOVIAL SYNDROME; IDIOPATHIC BLENNORRHEAL ARTHRITIS SYNDROME; POLYARTHRITIS ENTERICA)

General

Etiology unknown; males; onset ages 16–42 years; probably a combined infectious/autoimmune pathogenetic mechanism; reactive arthritis probably associated with infection with many different species of microorganisms; HLA-B27 confers disease susceptibility to infection.

Ocular

Sterile mucopurulent conjunctivitis, usually bilateral; photophobia; epiphora; iritis; keratitis; uveitis; paralysis of extraocular muscles; optic neuritis; secondary glaucoma; hypopyon; hyphema.

Clinical

Skin erythema; genital ulcerations; urethritis with discharge; cystitis with dysuria, abacterial pyuria, and hematuria; arthritis with pain, swelling, heat, and effusion; fever; weight loss; fatigue; malaise; fever; diarrhea; oral mucosal lesions; arthralgia.

Laboratory

Giemsa stain may reveal Gram-negative intracellular diplococci associated with gonorrhea. Stool cultures may also be helpful for enteric pathogens. HLA-B27 antigen testing will not provide a diagnosis but may be useful.

Treatment

Systemic antibiotics are useful. Topical corticosteroids and mydriatics should be administered early to minimize tissue damage. NSAIDs may help to reduce ocular inflammation.

BIBLIOGRAPHY

1. Bashour M. (2012). Ophthalmologic manifestations of reactive arthritis. [online] Available from www.emedicine.com/oph/TOPIC524.HTM. [Accessed September, 2013].

15.3U. SJÖGREN SYNDROME (GOUGEROT-SJÖGREN SYNDROME; SECRETOINHIBITOR SYNDROME; SICCA SYNDROME)

General

Etiology unknown; autosomal recessive; occurs in women over age 40 years; failure of the lacrimal and conjunctival glands to maintain adequate secretion; similarities exist with Mikulicz syndrome; insidious onset; associated with collagen disorders; Epstein-Barr virus infection.

Ocular

Blepharoconjunctivitis; tears show no lysozyme; keratoconjunctivitis sicca; superficial corneal ulcers; thready, tenacious, yellow-white discharge of the conjunctiva; hypertrophy of lacrimal gland; decreased tear secretion with cellular and mucous debris in tear film; cicatrization of cornea and conjunctiva.

Clinical

Dryness of mouth and other mucous membranes; enlarged salivary glands; dysphagia; painless swelling of joints; polyarthritis; dental cavities; vaginitis; laryngitis; rhinitis sicca; hepatomegaly; focal myositis; alopecia; splenomegaly.

Laboratory

Tear osmolarity, fluorecein clearance test and tear function index. Parotid flow rate may determine xerostomia.

Treatment

Artificial tears and lubricating ointments are the treatment of choice. Topical autologous serum eye drops also provide therapeutic benefit.

BIBLIOGRAPHY

1. Aquavella JV, Williams ZR, Boghani S, et al. (2011). Ophthalmologic manifestations of Sjogren syndrome. [online] Available from www.emedicine.com/oph/TOPIC477.HTM. [Accessed September, 2013].

15.3V. STAPHYLOCOCCUS

General

Gram-positive coccus *S. aureus*; most common cause of suppurative infection in humans; more common in patients with a previous disorders, such as diabetes, thyroid disease, renal failure, or malnutrition; although most *S. aureus* isolates from other sources are encapsulated, capsules have not been noted in ocular isolates.

Ocular

Uveitis; hypopyon; conjunctivitis; keratitis; cellulitis of lid; meibomianitis; ptosis; blepharitis; endophthalmitis; dacryocystitis; increased IOP; orbital periosteitis.

Clinical

Tissues hypertonic, edematous, and painful; lesion liquefies, forming creamy yellow pus; fever; nausea; vomiting; cough; dyspnea; abdominal pain; diarrhea; bloody stools; dehydration; shock.

Laboratory

Aerobic Gram-positive cocci bacteria grow in grape-like clusters. Coagulase positive indicates pathogenicity.

Treatment

Specific antimicrobial therapy is chosen based on the site and severity of the infection and the antimicrobial sensitivities of the organism involved.

BIBLIOGRAPHY

1. Tolan RW. (2012). Staphylococcus Aureus infection. [online] Available from www.emedicine.com/ped/TOPIC2704.HTM. [Accessed September, 2013].

15.3W. ACQUIRED LUES (SYPHILIS; ACQUIRED SYPHILIS; LUES VENEREA; MALUM VENEREUM)

General

Causative agent, *Treponema pallidum*, usually transmitted sexually.

Ocular

Conjunctival chancroid; conjunctivitis; keratitis; blepharitis; ptosis; iris atrophy; hippus; dacryocystitis; optic nerve atrophy; optic neuritis; periostitis; episcleritis; scleritis; nystagmus; uveitis; vitreous hemorrhages; paralysis of sixth nerve; papilledema; retinal hemorrhages; retinitis proliferans; oculogyric crisis; neuroretinitis; papilledema (associated with aseptic meningitis); diffuse or multifocal chorioretinitis; vertical supranuclear gaze palsy; Benedikt syndrome.

Clinical

Primary lesion associated with regional lymphadenopathy; secondary bacteremic stage associated with generalized mucocutaneous lesions; tertiary stage characterized by destructive mucocutaneous, musculoskeletal, or parenchymal lesions, aortitis, or central nervous system disease; syphilis and HIV infection often coexist in the same patient who experiences a higher incidence and greater severity of neurologic and ocular manifestations; a significant percentage of patients infected with HIV-I and *T. pallidum* become seronegative to syphilis testing.

Laboratory

Serologic nontreponemal tests include Venereal Disease Research Laboratory (VDRL) and rapid plasma reagin (RPR).

Treatment

The goals are to reduce morbidity and to prevent complications. Penicillin is the antibiotic of choice for treating syphilis. Ocular syphilis should be treated the same as patients with neurosyphilis.

BIBLIOGRAPHY

1. Majmudar PA. (2011). Interstitial keratitis overview of interstitial Keratitis. [online] Available from www.emedicine.com/oph/TOPIC453.HTM. [Accessed September, 2013].

15.3X. PROGRESSIVE SYSTEMIC SCLEROSIS (SCLERODERMA; SYSTEMIC SCLERODERMA)

General

Chronic connective tissue disease of unknown etiology; chronic and usually progressive disorder; typical onset is in 3rd-5th decade; ratio of women to men is 4:l; primary sites of pathology are the arterioles and capillaries of affected organs.

Ocular

Marginal corneal ulcers; shortened fornices of the conjunctiva; ptosis; cotton-wool patches of retina; papilledema; retinal hemorrhages; cicatrization of conjunctiva and cornea; blepharitis; blepharospasm; thready, tenacious yellow-white conjunctival discharge; hypertrophy of lacrimal gland; episcleritis; ocular myositis; Sjögren syndrome; uveitis; vitreous haze; keratitis sicca; decreased corneal sensation; iritis; ischemic choroidopathy; iris sectorial atrophy; blepharophimosis; heterochromia; keratoconus; central retinal vein occlusion; branch retinal vein occlusion.

Clinical

Vascular insufficiency; Raynaud's phenomenon; malaise; weight loss; stiffness; fever; polyarticular arthritis; diffuse edema of the hands; calcinosis; esophageal involvement; sclerodactyly; telangiectasis; esophageal stricture; renal failure; diffuse interstitial fibrosis.

Laboratory

No specific test establishes diagnosis. Hypergammaglobulinemia—50% of cases, ANA increased in 40–70% cases.

Treatment

Skin thickening can be treated with D-penicillamine and other experimental drugs. Pruritus can be treated with moisturizers and histamine. Raynaud's phenomenon can be treated with calcium channel blockers. Renal crisis episodes are best prevented and treated with the aggressive use of ACE inhibitors. Myositis may be treated cautiously with steroids.

⊟ BIBLIOGRAPHY

1. Jimenez SA, Cronin PM, Koenig AS, et al. (2012). Scleroderma. [online] Available from www.emedicine.com/med/TOPIC2076.HTM. [Accessed September, 2013].

⊟ 15.3Y. VACCINIA (KERATITIS)

General

Laboratory virus used for vaccination against smallpox.

Ocular

Pustules of lids; edema of lids; conjunctivitis; orbital cellulitis; keratitis; pannus; corneal perforation; iridocyclitis; central serous retinopathy; perivasculitis; pseudoretinitis pigmentosa; ocular palsies papillitis; optic atrophy.

Clinical

Vesicles; pustules; erythema; fever; malaise; axillary lymphadenopathy; necrosis of skin; vaccinia gangrenosa; encephalomyelitis; drowsiness; vomiting; coma; death.

Laboratory

Immune deficiency workup should be considered as well as imaging studies.

Treatment

VIG can be helpful in selected patients.

⊟ BIBLIOGRAPHY

1. Lee JJ, Diven D, Poonawalla TA, et al. (2012). Vaccinia. [online] Available from www.emedicine.com/med/TOPIC2356.HTM. [Accessed Sepetember, 2013].

⊟ 16. CONJUNCTIVAL MELANOTIC LESIONS (CONJUNCTIVAL NEVUS, CONJUNCTIVAL JUNCIONAL NEVUS, SUBEPITHELIAL NEVUS, COMPOUND NEVUS, BLUE NEVUS, MELANOSIS OCULI, CONJUNCTIVAL MELANOSIS, EPITHELIAL NELANOSIS, RACIAL MELANOSIS, SUB-EPITHELIAL MELANOCYTOSIS, CONGENITAL MELANOCYTOSIS, PRIMARY ACQUIRED MELANOSIS, MALIGNANT MELANOMA, CONJUNCTIVAL MELANOMA, CONJUNCTIVAL MALIGNANT MELANOMA)

General

Conjunctival lesions may be melanocytic or nonmelanocytic.

Clinical

None.

Ocular

Conjunctival lesion.

Laboratory

Photographic documentation and biopsy.

Treatment

Complete excision, with tumor-free margins of primary acquired melanosis with atypia. Cryotherapy, radiotherapy, topical mitomycin C or carbon dioxide (CO_2) laser are useful adjunctive therapies.

⊟ BIBLIOGRAPHY

1. Roque MR, Roque BL, Foster CS. (2011). Conjunctival melanoma. [online] Available from www.emedicine.com/oph/TOPIC110.HTM. [Accessed September, 2013].

⊟ 17. CONJUNCTIVAL XEROSIS (DRYNESS OF CONJUNCTIVA)

†1. Absence of blinking
†2. Drugs, including the following:
   - Acebutolol
   - Amiodarone
   - Atenolol
   - Betaxolol
   - Busulfan
   - Chlorambucil
   - Clonidine
   - Cyclophosphamide
   - Doxepin
   - Ibuprofen
   - Ketoprofen
   - Labetalol
   - Levobunolol
   - Methyldopa
   - Metoprolol
   - Nadolol
   - Naproxen
   - Oxprenolol
   - Perhexiline
   - Pindolol
   - Practolol
   - Primidone
   - Propanolol
   - Propoxyphene
   - Quinidine
   - Sulindac
   - Thiabendazole
   - Timolol
   - Vinblastine
3. Following cicatricial conjunctivitis
†4. Illness or coma
*†5. Lack of closure of lids in sleep
6. Result of exposure of conjunctiva to air
   †A. Deficient closure of lids, such as with paralysis of orbicularis, as part of facial palsy, spasms of the levator, or ectropion
   B. Excessive proptosis, such as in exophthalmic goiter or orbital tumor

*Indicates most frequent
†Indicates a general entry and therefore has not been described in detail in the text

*7. Vitamin A deficiency
   A. Dietary deficiencies, including malnutrition, cystic fibrosis, anorexia nervosa, and bulimia
   B. Digestive tract disorders
      1. Colitis and enteritis
      2. In pancreas-chronic pancreatitis
      †3. In stomach-achlorhydria, chronic gastritis or diarrhea, peptic ulcer
   C. Hookworm disease
   D. *Liver disease, such as chronic cirrhosis
   E. Malaria
   F. Pregnancy
   G. Pulmonary tuberculosis
   H. Skin disorders, such as pityriasis rubra pilaris
   I. *Thyroid gland disorder, such as hyperthyroidism
   J. Uyemura syndrome (fundus albipunctatus with hemeralopia and xerosis)
8. Decreased tear production
   A. Congenital alacrima
   B. Keratoconjunctivitis sicca
   C. Riley-Day syndrome (familial dysautonomia)
   D. Sjögren syndrome
   †E. Surgical excision of the lacrimal and accessory lacrimal glands
   †F. X-irradiation of the lacrimal gland
†9. Following x-irradiation of the conjunctiva

Treatment

- Identify cause
- Treat cause
- *Dry eyes*: Avoid ceiling fans, heat, medications for sinus and allergy. The use of over-the-counter eye drops and ointments is helpful.

⊟ BIBLIOGRAPHY

1. Fraunfelder FT, Fraunfelder FW. Drug-induced ocular side effects. Woburn, MA: Butterworth-Heinemann; 2001.
2. Gilbert JM, Weiss JS, Sattler AL, et al. Ocular manifestations and impression cytology of anorexia nervosa. Ophthalmology. 1990;97:1001.
3. Newell FW. Ophthalmology: Principles and Concepts, 7th edition. St. Louis: CV Mosby; 1991.
4. Roy FH. Ocular Syndromes and Systemic Diseases, 5th edition. Jaypee Brother's: New Delhi; 2014.

🗗 17.3. BENIGN MUCOSAL PEMPHIGOID (CHRONIC CICATRICIAL CONJUNCTIVITIS; CICATRICIAL PEMPHIGOID; ESSENTIAL SHRINKAGE OF THE CONJUNCTIVA; MEMBRANE PEMPHIGUS; OCULAR PEMPHIGOID)

General

Etiology unknown; involving older age group, especially over 70 years; chronic autoimmune disorder characterized by fibrosis beneath the conjunctival epithelium; associated with the major histocompatibility complex class I alleles, which confer susceptibility to the disease; likely due to a multigene effect and associated with environmental factors; incidence in women is twice as frequent as men, no geographic or racial predilection.

Ocular

Conjunctivitis; absence of goblet cells of conjunctiva; conjunctival ulcer; pannus and keratitis; corneal opacity; entropion; trichiasis; cicatrization of lacrimal ducts; corneal perforation; symblepharon; dry eyes; bilateral involvement (may be asymmetrical); ocular shrinkage; xerosis; conjunctival and corneal bullae.

Clinical

Subepidermal and subepithelial blistering of mucous membranes; blisters may occur in pharyngeal, laryngeal, nasal, anal and genital mucosa.

Laboratory

Diagnosis is made by clinical findings.

Treatment

Subconjunctival injections of steroid or mitomycin may be helpful. Systemic immunomodulators are the major therapeutic plan.

🗗 BIBLIOGRAPHY

1. Foster CS, Hamam R, Letko E. (2011). Ophthalmologic manifestations of cicatricial pemphigoid. [online] Available from www.emedicine.com/oph/TOPIC83.HTM. [Accessed September, 2013].

🗗 17.6B. EXOPHTHALMOS (PROPTOSIS)

General

Abnormal protrusion of the eyeball. Etiology is varied and can include inflammatory, vascular or infections. Thyroid disease is the most frequent cause for both unilateral and bilateral exophthalmos.

Clinical

Thyroid disease, lymphoma, cavernous hemangiomas, leukemia, sinus disease.

Ocular

Proptosis, orbital cellulitis, orbital emphysema, lid retraction, punctate keratopathy, corneal ulcer, corneal perforation, diplopia.

Laboratory

Thyroid function studies, CT, MRI, ocular ultrasonography can all be used to determine the cause.

Treatment

Reversing the problem, which is causing the exophthalmos, is the treatment of choice and will minimize the ocular complications. Ocular lubricants are beneficial for controlling the corneal exposure.

🗗 BIBLIOGRAPHY

1. Mercandetti M, Cohen AJ. (2012). Exophthalmos. [online] Available from www.emedicine.com/oph/TOPIC616.HTM. [Accessed September, 2013].

⊟ 17.7. VITAMIN A DEFICIENCY

General

Worldwide cause of blindness; onset in childhood; dietary vitamin A insufficiency; interference of absorption from the intestinal tract and transport or storage in the liver, as with diarrhea or vomiting; most frequent in young children.

Ocular

Bitot spots; conjunctival xerosis; corneal xerosis; keratomalacia with perforation; photophobia; enlarged tarsal glands; corneal ulcer; nyctalopia; hemeralopia; obstruction of the tear ducts.

Clinical

Diarrhea; malabsorption syndrome; follicular hyperkeratosis; lesions on buttocks, legs, and arms; xerosis of skin; tracheitis; bronchitis; pneumonia; chronic obstruction of pancreatic or biliary ducts; increased infant mortality.

Laboratory

Serum retinol study, serum retinol binding protein (RBP) study, zinc levels, CBC, electrolyte evaluation and liver function studies.

Treatment

Vitamin A rich foods such as beef, chicken, sweet potatoes, mangoes, carrots, eggs, fortified milk, and leafy green vegetables.

⊟ BIBLIOGRAPHY

1. Ansstas G, Thakore J, Gopalswamy N. (2012). Vitamin A deficiency. [online] Available from www.emedicine.com/med/TOPIC2381.HTM. [Accessed September, 2013].

⊟ 17.7A. CYSTIC FIBROSIS SYNDROME (FIBROCYSTIC DISEASE OF PANCREAS)

General

Autosomal recessive; Caucasians; lungs, pancreas, and salivary glands are mainly involved.

Ocular

Ischemic retinopathy caused by carbon dioxide retention and chronic respiratory insufficiency; vein congestion and capillary dilation around the optic nerve; retinal hemorrhages; macular degeneration; papilledema; optic atrophy; xerosis of conjunctiva; optic neuritis; abnormal pupillary responses; decreased contrast sensitivity.

Clinical

Failure to gain weight properly; recurrent pulmonary infections; salty skin; pancreatic insufficiency with malabsorption; abdominal cramps; diarrhea; increased appetite; dyspnea; chronic cough; production of viscous tenacious sputum; fever; retarded growth; delayed puberty; distended abdomen; hyper-resonant chest; depressed diaphragm; clubbing of fingers.

Laboratory

The diagnosis is based on pulmonary and/or gastrointestinal tract manifestations, a family history, and positive results on sweat test.

Treatment

Because of the complex and multisystemic involvement the need for care by specialists, treatment and follow-up care at specialty centers with multidisciplinary care teams is recommended.

⊟ BIBLIOGRAPHY

1. Sharma GD. (2013). Cystic fibrosis. [online] Available from www.emedicine.com/ped/TOPIC535.HTM. [Accessed September, 2013].

⊟ 17.7A. ANOREXIA NERVOSA (APEPSIA HYSTERICCI)

General

Compulsive neurosis; refusal to eat; occurs in adolescent to young adult females; symptomatic recovery or chronic course.

Ocular

Cataract; central retinal vein occlusion; myopathy of orbicularis oculi (weakness of eye closure).

Clinical

Severe cachexia; loss of hair; nausea; constipation; diarrhea; depression; vigorous activity; weight loss; menstrual disturbance.

Laboratory

No definitive diagnostic tests are available; however, given the multiorgan system effects of starvation, a thorough medical evaluation is warranted.

Treatment

Initial therapy should be stabilization for any life-threatening conditions. Metabolic abnormalities should be corrected as needed, with oral or parenteral treatment depending on the patient's mental status and decision to cooperate.

⊟ BIBLIOGRAPHY

1. Cushing TA, Jacoby LE. (2013). Emergent management of anorexia nervosa. [online] Available from www.emedicine.com/emerg/TOPIC34.HTM. [Accessed September, 2013].

⊟ 17.7B1. CROHN DISEASE (GRANULOMATOUS ILEOCOLITIS)

General

Autoimmune or hypersensitivity inflammatory change; slight prevalence in males; Jewish people most frequently affected; onset at any age; more severe in young people; remission; relapses.

Ocular

Recurrent conjunctivitis; marginal corneal ulcers; keratitis; blepharitis; dry eye; scleritis; episcleritis; iris atrophy; uveitis; pupil immobility and dilatation; macular edema; macular hemorrhages; extraocular muscles palsy; vitreal haze; retinal vasculitis; subconjunctival nodules; conjunctival ulcer; pannus; acute dacryoadenitis; orbital pseudotumor.

Clinical

Inflammatory bowel disease; abdominal distention; tenderness of abdomen; mass in right lower quadrant of abdomen; diarrhea; abdominal cramps; bloating; flatulence; weight loss; nervousness; tension; depression; pyoderma gangrenosum.

Laboratory

Test result positive for anti-*Saccharomyces cerevisiae* antibodies (ASCA) and negative for perinuclear anti-neutrophil cytoplasmic antibody (p-ANCA) antigen suggests the presence of Crohn's disease. CT, MRI, barium contrast studies, colonoscopy and upper endoscopy may also be useful.

Treatment

Treat diarrhea; antibiotic and anti-inflammatory drugs, antimetabolites, anti-tumor necrosis factor antibody, immunosuppressive agents; surgical correction for fibrostenotic obstruction may be necessary.

⊟ BIBLIOGRAPHY

1. Rangasamy P, Yung-Hsin C, Coash ML, et al. (2011). Crohn Disease. [online] Available from www.emedicine.com/med/TOPIC477.HTM. [Accessed September, 2013].

🗗 17.7B1. ULCERATIVE COLITIS (REGIONAL ENTERITIS; INFLAMMATORY BOWEL DISEASE)

General

Chronic inflammatory disease of unknown etiology; both sexes affected; onset at all ages, most frequently between ages of 20 and 40 years; usually abrupt onset; psychosomatic pathogenesis possible.

Ocular

Iritis; uveitis; episcleritis; papillomatous changes of palpebral conjunctiva; scleritis; serous retinal detachment; choroidal infiltrates; retrobulbar neuritis; papillitis; retinal pigment epithelium disturbance; choroidal folds.

Clinical

Abdominal pain; cramps; diarrhea; arthritis; weight loss; erythema nodosum; aphthous stomatitis; pallor; tenderness over colon; nutritional deficiency; carcinoma; associations with Sjögren syndrome and Takayasu disease have been reported.

Laboratory

Elevated white blood count and erythrocyte sedimentation rate. Radiography demonstrates the "sting sign" of narrowed lumen in the terminal ileum.

Treatment

Systemic corticosteroids, metronidazole, pain medication and antispasmodic drugs give relief.

🗗 BIBLIOGRAPHY

1. Khan AN, Sheen AJ, Varia H. (2011). Ulcerative colitis imaging. [online] Available from www.emedicine.com/radio/TOPIC785.HTM. [Accessed September, 2013].

🗗 17.7B2. PANCREATITIS

General

Inflammation of pancreas.

Ocular

Xerosis; night blindness; multiple branch retinal artery occlusions; cotton-wool patches; retinal edema; striate and blot hemorrhages; retinopathy of pancreatitis has been considered to indicate multiple-organ failure and poor prognosis in severe acute pancreatitis; mechanism may be secondary to granulocyte aggregation and leukoembolization due to activated complement.

Clinical

Chronic pancreatitis; lipid emboli; malabsorption; vitamin A deficiency.

Laboratory

Pancreatic function tests, diagnosis of chronic pancreatitis requires morphologic abnormalities to appear on imaging procedures.

Treatment

The goals of medical treatment are to modify behaviors that may exacerbate the disease, to enable the pancreas to heal itself, to determine the cause of abdominal pain and alleviate it, to detect pancreatic exocrine insufficiency and restore digestion and absorption to normal, and to diagnose and treat endocrine insufficiency. Cessation of alcohol consumption and tobacco smoking are important. Endoscopic treatment is sometimes necessary.

🗗 BIBLIOGRAPHY

1. Huffman JL, Obideen K, Wehbi M. (2012). Chronic pancreatitis. [online] Available from www.emedicine.com/med/TOPIC1721.HTM. [Accessed September, 2013].

17.7C. ANKYLOSTOMIASIS (HOOKWORM DISEASE)

General

Causative agents include *Necator americanus, Ancylostoma duodenale, Ancylostoma braziliense,* and *Ancylostoma caninum*; final diagnosis depends upon finding eggs in feces.

Ocular

Retinal hemorrhages around optic disk; diplopia; conjunctival xerosis; visual field defects; cataract.

Clinical

Maculopapules; localized erythema; microcytic hypochromic anemia.

Laboratory

Stool examination for ova and parasites usually reveals oval eggs with thin, colorless shells that can be seen 2 months after exposure.

Treatment

Imidazoles are the most effective drugs to treat hookworm. Albendazole or mebendazole is the drug of choice.

BIBLIOGRAPHY

1. Haburchak DR. (2011). Hookworms. [online] Available from www.emedicine.com/med/TOPIC1028.HTM. [Accessed September, 2013].

17.7D. MOSSE SYNDROME (POLYCYTHEMIA-HEPATIC CIRRHOSIS SYNDROME)

General

Unknown etiology.

Ocular

Scleral icterus; marked retinal venous tortuosity and dilation; retinal artery occlusion (occasionally); papilledema.

Clinical

Thrombosis of portal vein secondary to polycythemia; hepatosplenomegaly; ascites; clinical features of liver cirrhosis.

Laboratory

Clinical.

Treatment

- *Retinal artery occlusion:* Intraocular pressure lowering medications, carbogen therapy, hyperbaric oxygen. Vitrectomy may be necessary.
- *Papilledema:* Underlying cause should be determined and treated. Systemic acetazolamide is the medical therapy of choice.

BIBLIOGRAPHY

1. Barbas AP. Surgical problems associated with polycythemia. Br J Hosp Med. 1980;23:289-90, 92, 94.
2. Geeraets WJ. Ocular Syndromes, 3rd edition. Philadelphia: Lea & Febiger; 1976.
3. Mosse M. Uber Policythamie mit Urobilinikterus und Milztumor. Dtsch Med Wochenschr. 1907;33:2175.

17.7E. MALARIA

General

Caused by *Plasmodium*, which is transmitted by mosquito bite, blood transfusion, or contaminated needles and syringes.

Ocular

Proliferative retinitis; vascular embolism; keratitis; ocular herpes simplex; blepharitis; optic atrophy; papilledema; papillitis; optic neuritis; anisocoria; Argyll Robertson pupil;

vitreal hemorrhages and opacity; cataract; myopia; strabismus; uveitis; scleral icterus; scotoma; lagophthalmos; ptosis; subconjunctival hemorrhages; paralysis of third, fourth, or sixth nerve; epibulbar hemorrhage involving the conjunctiva, episclera, tendinous insertion of the medial rectus.

Clinical

Fever; anemia; splenomegaly; death.

Laboratory

Blood smear.

Treatment

Consult infectious disease specialist.

⊟ BIBLIOGRAPHY

1. Perez-Jorge EV, Herchline TE. (2013). Malaria. [online] Available from www.emedicine.com/med/TOPIC1385.HTM. [Accessed September, 2013].

⊟ 17.7F. PREGNANCY

General

Pregnancy results in hormonal changes that produce ocular effects; symptoms resolve at end of pregnancy term.

Ocular

Myopia; visual field defects; corneal edema; acute ischemic optic neuropathy; central serous retinopathy; glaucoma; ptosis; diabetic retinopathy; Krukenberg spindles; transient blindness; serous retinal detachment; retinal artery occlusion; retinal vein occlusion; disseminated intravascular coagulopathy; uveal melanoma.

Clinical

Nausea; headaches; hypertension; benign intracranial hypertension; pre-eclampsia; toxemia; fluid retention.

Laboratory

Home pregnancy test that utilize the modern immuno-metric assay. Transvaginal ultrasound and transabdominal ultrasound are also useful.

Treatment

Most ocular symptoms resolve at the end of pregnancy. Obstetrician should be consulted before topical medications are prescribed.

⊟ BIBLIOGRAPHY

1. Somani S, Bhatti A, Ahmed II. (2011). Pregnancy special considerations. [online] Available from www.emedicine.com/oph/TOPIC747.HTM. [Accessed September, 2013].

⊟ 17.7G. TUBERCULOSIS

General

Communicable disease caused by the acid-fast bacillus *Mycobacterium tuberculosis*.

Ocular

Conjunctivitis; subconjunctival nodules (tuberculomas); keratitis; pannus; corneal ulcer; blepharitis; cellulitis; meibomianitis; uveitis; dacryocystitis; chronic orbital cellulitis; retinitis; scleritis; scleral perforation; hypopyon; vitreous hemorrhages; optic neuritis; optic atrophy; tuberculous panophthalmitis; choroidal tubercles; intraorbital extraocular lesions.

Clinical

Pulmonary infection; pyuria; hematuria; epididymitis; dysuria; flank pain; distorted calyces; productive cough.

Laboratory

Acid-fast bacillus culture of body fluids including vitreous and aqueous. PCR is 89% positive for pulmonary infection.

Treatment

A course of chemotherapy (isoniazid, rifampin, pyrazinamide and ethambutol or streptomycin) for a period of 6 months is the recommended therapy.

🖭 BIBLIOGRAPHY

1. Collins JK. Handbook of clinical ophthalmology. New York: Masson; 1982.
2. D'Souza P, Garg R, Dhaliwal RS, et al. Orbital tuberculosis. Int Ophthalmol. 1994; 18:149-52.
3. DeVoe AG, Locatcher-Khorazo D. The external manifestations of ocular tuberculosis. Trans Am Ophthalmol Soc. 1964;62:203-12.
4. Roy, FH, Fraunfelder FT, Fraunfelder FH. Roy and Fraunfelders's Current Ocular Therapy, 6th editon. Philadelphia: WB Saunders; 2008.
5. Gupta V, Gupta A, Arora S, et al. Presumed tubercular serpiginous like choroiditis. Ophthalmology. 2003;110:1744-9.
6. Patkar S, Singhania BK, Agrawal A. Intraorbital extraocular tuberculosis: a report of three cases. Surg Neurol 1994; 42:320-1.
7. Tejada P, Mendez MJ, Negreira S. Choroidal tubercles with tuberculous meningitis. Int Ophthalmol. 1994;18:115-8.

🖭 17.7H. PITYRIASIS RUBRA PILARIS [KAPOSI DISEASE (2); DEVERGIE DISEASE; HEBRA DISEASE; TARRAL-BESNIER DISEASE; LICHEN RUBER; LICHEN RUBER ACUMINATUS; PITYRIASIS PILARIS]

General

Abnormal keratinization of unknown etiology; hereditary and acquired forms have been described in the literature; hereditary form tends to be less severe and more limited in extent.

Ocular

Papules on bulbar conjunctiva; keratitis; ectropion; pannus; corneal ulceration.

Clinical

Cutaneous manifestations; erythema; follicular papules.

Laboratory

The diagnosis is usually made on the basis of a correlation between clinical and histologic findings.

Treatment

Topical medications; calcipotriol is a vitamin D analog; emollients; extracorporeal photochemotherapy.

🖭 BIBLIOGRAPHY

1. Shenefelt PD. (2012). Pityriasis Rubra Pilaris. [online] Available from www.emedicine.com/derm/TOPIC337.HTM. [Accessed September, 2013].

🖭 17.7I. BASEDOW SYNDROME (GRAVES DISEASE; HYPERTHYROIDISM; THYROTOXICOSIS; EXOPHTHALMIC GOITER; PARRY DISEASE)

General

Diffuse toxic goiter; inherited as a simple autosomal recessive; penetrance greater in females; however, dominant mode of inheritance and variable penetrance are possible; uncommon in either sex before the age of 15 years.

Ocular

Exophthalmos; swelling of eyelids and discoloration of upper eyelids; lid lag (von Graefe's sign); globe lag (Koeber's sign); lid trembling on gentle closure (Rosenbach's sign); reduced blinking (Stellwag's sign); retraction of upper lid; difficulty in everting upper lid (Gifford's sign); convergence weakness (Möbius's sign); impaired fixation on extreme lateral gaze (Suker's sign); possible external ophthalmoplegia (Ballet's sign); Dalrymple's sign (staring appearance); tearing; photophobia; epiphora; prolapse of lacrimal gland; neuroretinal edema; tortuous vessels; papilledema and papillitis; anisocoria; keratitis; increased IOP on upgaze; decreased visual acuity; enlargement of the extraocular muscles; increased volume of the extraorbital fat; superior rectus muscle enlargement; decreased venous outflow.

Clinical

Tachycardia; anxiety; insomnia; loss of weight; hyperhidrosis; restlessness; myocarditis (toxic); atrial fibrillation.

Laboratory

Visual field testing, forced duction testing for restrictive myopathy, CT, MRI, T4 and thyroid-stimulating hormone, thyroid-stimulating immunoglobulins.

Treatment

There is no immediate treatment; the disease is self-limited but prolonged course over 1 or more years. Five percent of patients may require surgical intervention which could be orbital decompression, strabismus surgery, lid-lengthening surgery or blepharoplasty.

BIBLIOGRAPHY

1. Regensburg NI, Wiersinga WM, Berendschot TT, et al. Do subtypes of Graves' orbitopathy exist? Ophthalmology. 2011;118:191-6.
2. Ing E. (2012). Thyroid-associated orbitopathy. [online] Available from www.emedicine.com/oph/TOPIC237.HTM. [Accessed September, 2013].

17.7J. UYEMURA SYNDROME (FUNDUS ALBIPUNCTATUS WITH HEMERALOPIA AND XEROSIS) NIGHT BLINDNESS

General

Rare; resembles retinitis punctata albescens, fundus albipunctatus, and congenital idiopathic night blindness or Oguchi disease; avitaminosis A; affects both sexes.

Ocular

Night blindness; conjunctival xerosis; Bitot spots; white spots on the fundus.

Clinical

None.

Laboratory

Clinical.

Treatment

None.

BIBLIOGRAPHY

1. Krill AE, Martin D. Photopic abnormalities in congenital stationary nightblindness. Invest Ophthalmol. 1971;10:625-36.
2. Uyemura M. Uber eine Merkwurdige Augenhintergrundsveranderung bei zwei Fallen von Idiopathischer Hemeralopie. Klin Monatsbl Augenheilkd. 1928;81:471.
3. Venkataswamy G. Ocular manifestations of vitamin A deficiency. Br J Ophthalmol. 1967;51:854-9.

17.8A. ALACRIMA

General

Autosomal recessive; wide spectrum of lacrimal secretory disorders that are mostly congenital in origin. Symptoms of these disorders can range from a complete absence of tears to hyposecretion of tears; symptoms of rarer disorders include a selective absence of tearing in response to emotional stimulation but a normal secretory response to mechanical stimulation. It may be associated with syndromes such as Riley-Day, anhidrotic ectodermal dysplasia, Sjögren and Allgrove.

Clinical

Decreased salivation and sweating; osteoporosis; short stature; adrenocortical insufficiency.

Ocular

Foreign body sensation; photophobia, decreased visual acuity; absence of tears; chronic blepharoconjunctivitis; hyperemia; thick mucoid discharge; keratinization; pannus; corneal ulcers or perforation; tonic pupils; optic atrophy.

Laboratory

CT scan of orbits to determine aplastic lacrimal glands; Schirmer testing; conjunctival and lacrimal gland biopsy.

Treatment

Artificial tears, gels and ointments are used as the primary treatment. Permanent or temporary punctal occlusion can be effective. Tarsorrhaphy may be necessary if the corneal health has been compromised.

BIBLIOGRAPHY

1. DeAngelis DD, Hurwitz J. (2012). Alacrima. [online] Available from emedicine.medscape.com/article/1210539-overview. [Accessed September, 2013].

17.8B. KERATOCONJUNCTIVITIS SICCA AND SJÖGREN'S SYNDROME

General

Autoimmune disease, seen more frequently in females.

Clinical

Xerostomia (dry mouth), dry nasal and genital mucosa.

Ocular

Severe dry eyes, corneal ulceration, corneal perforation, corneal scarring and vascularization.

Laboratory

Biopsy of lip and lachrymal gland positive, anti-nuclear antibody rheumatoid factor (RF) and anti-ro (Sjögren's specific A) and anti-La (Sjögren specific B). Elevated IgG level positive—predication for positive biopsy.

Treatment

Severe cases—immunosuppressive agents as cyclosporin A and corticosteroids. Frequent application of tear substitutes, steroids, punctal plugs, bandage contacts and partial tarsorrhaphy.

BIBLIOGRAPHY

1. Foster CS, Yuksel E, Anzaar F, et al. (2013). Dry eye syndrome. [online] Available from www.emedicine.com/oph/TOPIC597.HTM. [Accessed September, 2013].

17.8C. RILEY-DAY SYNDROME (CONGENITAL FAMILIAL DYSAUTONOMIA)

General

It is autosomal recessive; it occurs in Ashkenazi Jewish population; impaired catechol metabolism; manifested in first few days of life; it is characterized by developmental loss of neurons from the sensory and autonomic nervous systems.

Ocular

Congenital failure of tear production; corneal anesthesia; neuroparalytic keratitis; keratitis sicca; corneal ulcers; optic atrophy.

Clinical

Excessive salivation; failure to thrive; recurrent respiratory infections; diarrhea; insensitivity to pain; spontaneous fractures; pandysautonomia; orthostatic hypotension; gastrointestinal paresis; decreased fungiform papillae on the tongue.

Laboratory

Deoxyribonucleic acid (DNA) test is used to confirm the diagnosis.

Treatment

Artificial drops and/or gels are useful in any dry eye condition. Tarsorrhaphy is an effective treatment of the decompensated neurotrophic cornea.

BIBLIOGRAPHY

1. D'Amico RA, Axelrod FB. (2011). Familial dysautonomia. [online] Available from www.emedicine.com/oph/TOPIC678.HTM. [Accessed September, 2013].

🖶 17.8D SJÖGREN SYNDROME (GOUGEROT-SJÖGREN SYNDROME; SECRETOINHIBITOR SYNDROME; SICCA SYNDROME)

General

Etiology is unknown; autosomal recessive; it occurs in women over age of 40 years; failure of the lacrimal and conjunctival glands to maintain adequate secretion; similarities exist with Mikulicz syndrome (*see* Mikulicz-Radecki syndrome); insidious onset; it is associated with collagen disorders; Epstein-Barr virus infection.

Ocular

Blepharoconjunctivitis; tears show no lysozyme; keratoconjunctivitis sicca; superficial corneal ulcers; thready, tenacious, yellow-white discharge of the conjunctiva; hypertrophy of lacrimal gland; decreased tear secretion with cellular and mucous debris in tear film; cicatrization of cornea and conjunctiva.

Clinical

Dryness of mouth and other mucous membranes; enlarged salivary glands; dysphagia; painless swelling of joints; polyarthritis; dental cavities; vaginitis; laryngitis; rhinitis sicca; hepatomegaly; focal myositis; alopecia; splenomegaly.

Laboratory

Tear osmolarity, fluorescein clearance test and tear function index. Parotid flow rate may determine xerostomia.

Treatment

Artificial tears and lubricating ointments are the treatment of choice. Topical autologous serum eye drops also provide therapeutic benefit.

🖶 BIBLIOGRAPHY

1. Aquavella JV, Williams ZR, Boghani S, et al. (2011). Ophthalmologic manifestations of Sjögren syndrome. [online] Available from www.emedicine.com/oph/TOPIC477.HTM. [Accessed September, 2013].

🖶 18. CONJUNCTIVITIS, LIGNEOUS

General

Autosomal recessive; palpebral conjunctiva becomes the site of dense woody membrane that has global shape; associated with systemic use of tranexamic acid.

Ocular

Corneal scarring; dense membrane of the conjunctiva; may occur as a complication following strabismus surgery.

Clinical

None.

Laboratory

Clinical.

Treatment

Surgical excision of conjunctiva membrane followed by cautery, cryoplexy and grafting of conjunctiva or sclera.

🖶 BIBLIOGRAPHY

1. Bierly JR, Blandford DL, Weeks JA, et al. Ligneous conjunctivitis as a complication following strabismus surgery. J Pediatr Ophthalmol Strabismus. 1994;31:99-103.
2. Diamond JP, Chandna A, Williams C, et al. Tranexamic acid-associated ligneous conjunctivitis with gingival and peritoneal lesions. Br J Ophthalmol. 1991;75:753-4.
3. McKusick VA. Mendelian Inheritance in Man; A Catalog of Human Genes and Genetic Disorders, 12th edition. Baltimore: The Johns Hopkins University Press; 1998.
4. Online Mendelian Inheritance in Man, OMIM. McKusick-Nathans Institute for Genetic Medicine, Johns Hopkins University and National Center for Biotechnology Information, National Library of Medicine, February 12, 2007. Available from www.ncbi.nlm.nih.gov/omim. [Accessed September, 2013].
5. Pavan-Langston D. Cornea and external disease. Ligneous conjunctivitis. In: Pavan-Langston D (Ed). Manual of Ocular Diagnosis and Therapy, 4th edition. Boston: Little, Brown and Company; 1995. p. 103.

19. CORNEAL AND CONJUNCTIVAL CALCIFICATIONS

General

Eye calcium may occur as isolated conditions or in association with a variety of disease entities.

Clinical

None.

Ocular

Calcific band keratopathy, calcium deposits of conjunctiva, chronic uveitis causes deposits, ocular trauma.

Laboratory

Diagnosis is made by clinical findings.

Treatment

Symptomatic treatment includes chelation of calcium salt deposit with ethylenediaminetetraacetic acid (EDTA).

BIBLIOGRAPHY

1. Taravella M. (2012). Band keratopathy. [online] Available from www.emedicine.com/oph/TOPIC105.HTM. [Accessed September, 2013].

20. CHLAMYDIA (INCLUSION CONJUNCTIVITIS; PARATRACHOMA)

General

Organism that infects the epithelium of mucoid surfaces; sexually transmitted; major cause of non-gonococcal urethritis in men and cervicitis in women; major cause of neonatal ophthalmia; *C. trachomatis* is an intracellular bacterium lacking respiratory enzymes that has an affinity for mucosal epithelium; serotypes A through C have been epidemiologically associated with trachoma; serotypes E through K have been associated with genital infection and keratoconjunctivitis in sexually active adults and neonates; other serotypes have been associated with lymphogranuloma venereum and Reiter syndrome.

Ocular

Follicular conjunctivitis; corneal opacities; keratitis; corneal ulcer; lid edema; uveitis.

Clinical

Pneumonia; gastrointestinal disturbances; genital discharge.

Laboratory

Giemsa stain, cell culture—time intensive, direct fluorescent monoclonal antibiotics to stain smears.

Treatment

Three to six weeks of oral tetracycline (500 mg qid), oral doxycycline (100 mg bid), or oral erythromycin stearate (500 mg qid). Simultaneous treatment of all sexual partners is important to prevent reinfection.

BIBLIOGRAPHY

1. Bashour M. (2012) Ophthalmologic manifestations of Chlamydia. [online] Available from www.emedicine.com/oph/TOPIC494.HTM. [Accessed September, 2013].

21. CONJUNCTIVITIS, VIRAL

General

Characterized commonly by an acute follicular conjunctival reaction and preauricular adenopathy. Adenovirus is the most common cause but can be result of herpes simplex, molluscum, vaccina, HIV and others. Generally self-limited and benign but tends to follow a longer course than bacterial. It may last for 2–4 weeks.

Clinical

Herpes simplex virus (HSV), varicella-zoster virus, picornavirus, poxvirus, and HIV. Rarely Epstein-Barr virus, paramyxovirus, rubella and HIV.

Ocular

Foreign body sensation, tearing, itching, photophobia, redness, HSV keratoconjunctivitis, vesicular stomatitis virus (VSV) keratoconjunctivitis, ocular chlamydia, vernal keratoconjunctivitis, blepharoconjunctivitis, epithelial keratitis.

Laboratory

Diagnosis is made by clinical findings. If inflammation is severe or chronic, culture and smear for viral identity should be considered.

Treatment

No evidence exists that demonstrates efficacy of antiviral agents. It is recommended for patients to use cold compresses and artificial tears for comfort. Topical steroids may be used when subepithelial infiltrates impair vision.

BIBLIOGRAPHY

1. Scott IU, Luu K. (2011). Viral conjunctivitis. [online] Available from emedicine.medscape.com/article/1191370-diagnosis. [Accessed September, 2013].

22. CONJUNCTIVOCHALASIS (CCH)

General

Relaxation of conjunctiva; redundant loose nonedematous inferior bulbar conjunctiva; associated with disruption of the tear meniscus; causative agent not yet determined but may be associated with age-related elastotic degeneration and chronic inflammation.

Ocular

Dry eye; punctal occlusion; delayed tear clearance; age-related elastotic degeneration; chronic inflammation; epiphora.

Laboratory

Diagnosis is determined by clinical observation.

Treatment

High-frequency radio wave electrosurgery has proven to be beneficial.

BIBLIOGRAPHY

1. Youm DJ, Kim JM, Choi CY. Simple surgical approach with high-frequency radio-wave electrosurgery for conjunctivochalasis. Ophthalmology. 2010;117(11):2129-33.

23. DRY EYE SYNDROME

General

Multifactorial disease of the tears and the ocular surface that result in symptoms of discomfort, visual disturbance and tear film instability with potential damage to the ocular surface by increased osmolarity of the tear film and inflammation of the ocular surface. The most common cause is aqueous tear deficiency. Keratoconjunctivitis sicca, which is an ocular surface disorder, may also be a cause. It is associated with connective tissue diseases such as rheumatoid arthritis and systemic sclerosis; postmenopausal women; pregnant women; and individuals taking oral contraceptives and hormone replacement therapy.

Clinical

Rheumatoid arthritis; systemic sclerosis; menopause; pregnancy, prostate disease.

Ocular

Foreign body sensation; burning; itching; photophobic; blurred vision; excessive tearing; irregular corneal surface; decreased tear break-up time; punctate epithelial keratopathy; debris in the tear film; corneal ulcer.

Laboratory

Diagnosis is generally made by clinical observation; careful history; tear break-up test; Schirmer test and the use of Rose Bengal and fluorescein to check for staining is useful. Additional testing can be used to determine the tear components. These include conjunctival biopsy, tear function index, tear ferning test, impression cytology and meibometry.

Treatment

Environmental and dietary modifications; elimination of systemic medications if possible; artificial tears, gels and ointments; anti-inflammatory agents such as topical corticosteroids, cyclosporine A and omega-3 fatty acids; and tetracyclines for meibomianitis. Punctal plugs; moisture chamber spectacles and autologous serum tears may be necessary if the symptoms persist. Sometimes systemic anti-inflammatory agents, tarsorrhaphy, mucous membrane grafting; amniotic membrane transplantation and salivary gland duct transposition may be necessary in the worst cases.

🔖 BIBLIOGRAPHY

1. Foster CS, Yuksel E, Anzaar F, et al. (2012). Dry eye syndrome. [online] Available from emedicine.medscape.com/article/1210417-overview. [Accessed January, 2013].

2. Liang L, Sheha H, Fu Y, et al. Ocular surface morbidity in eyes with senile sunken upper eyelids. Ophthalmology. 2011;118(12):2487-92.

🔖 24. ELSCHNIG SYNDROME I (MEIBOMIAN CONJUNCTIVITIS)

General

Chronic inflammations; characteristic foamy secretion; benign.

Ocular

Conjunctivitis; foamy secretion; ocular irritation; photophobia; minimal visual impairment.

Clinical

Hyperplasia of tarsal glands.

Laboratory

Diagnosis is made by clinical findings.

Treatment

Symptomatic control may include cold compresses, artificial tears; nonsteroidal and occasionally steroidal drops to relieve itching.

🔖 BIBLIOGRAPHY

1. Elschnig A. Belt ray Artiologie und Therapie der chronischen Conjunctivitis. Dtsch Med Wochenschr. 1908;34: 1133-5.
2. Magalini SI, Scrascia E. Dictionary of Medical Syndromes, 2nd edition. Philadelphia, PA: Lippincott Williams & Wilkins; 1981.

🔖 25. EPIDEMIC KERATOCONJUNCTIVITIS

General

Highly communicable; adenovirus types 8 and 19; usually bilateral; epidemic keratoconjunctivitis has been reported worldwide associated with 11 virus serotypes, with serotypes 8, 11 and 19 being the most common responsible ones.

Ocular

Follicular or membranous conjunctivitis; chemosis; subconjunctival hemorrhages; corneal opacity; punctate epithelial keratitis; corneal ulcer; blepharospasm; lid edema; serous discharge; uveitis; epiphora.

Clinical

Submaxillary and cervical lymphadenopathy.

Laboratory

Viral isolation on cell culture from conjunctival scrapings.

Treatment

No effective topical or systemic treatment is available. Topical steroids may be used if epithelial keratitis occurs.

🔖 BIBLIOGRAPHY

1. Bawazeer A, Hodge WG. (2011). Epidemic keratoconjunctivitis. [online] Available from www.emedicine.com/oph/TOPIC677.HTM. [Accessed September, 2013].

☐ 26. FILTERING BLEBS AND ASSOCIATED PROBLEMS

General

Elevation of conjunctiva and Tenon's capsule from anterior chamber fistula caused by antimetabolite/antifibrotic usage, trabeculectomy, bleb leaks or overfiltering blebs.

Clinical

None.

Ocular

Overfiltering blebs, overhanging blebs, bleb dysesthesia. Complications include: hypotony, flat anterior chamber, corneal edema, choroidal effusion, endophthalmitis, dellen, uncontrolled glaucoma, astigmatism, cataract and suprachoroidal hemorrhage.

Laboratory

Diagnosis is made by clinical findings and Seidel test.

Treatment

Conservative treatment includes pressure patching, large diameter bandage contact lens. Cryotherapy, laser thermotherapy and autologous blood injection, cyanoacrylate to dry conjunctiva to close leaking bleb and compression sutures may be used if conservative therapy does not resolve the problem.

☐ BIBLIOGRAPHY

1. Traverso CE. (2012). Filtering bleb complications. [online] Available from www.emedicine.com/oph/TOPIC541.HTM. [Accessed September, 2013].

☐ 27. HERPES SIMPLEX

General

Large, complex DNA virus.

Ocular

Conjunctivitis; keratitis; iridocyclitis; corneal ulcer; uveitis; hyphema; hypopyon; iris atrophy; cataract; scleritis; dacryoadenitis; blepharitis; acute retinal necrosis.

Clinical

Recurrent skin vesicles on lids, perioral area, nose and genitalia; meningitis, encephalitis.

Laboratory

Viral cultures.

Treatment

Antiviral therapy, topical or oral, is an effective treatment of epithelial herpes infection.

☐ BIBLIOGRAPHY

1. Wang JC, Ritterband DC. (2012). Ophthalmologic manifestations of herpes simplex. [online] Available from www.emedicine.com/oph/TOPIC100.HTM. [Accessed September, 2013].

☐ 28. HERPES ZOSTER

General

Caused by varicella zoster virus; about 75% of cases occur in persons over age of 45 years; condition is more frequent with advancing age and in patients who are immunocompromised by drugs or disease; in particular, an increasing number of patients with herpes zoster ophthalmicus are immunosuppressed.

Ocular

Conjunctivitis; keratitis; recurrent corneal ulcer; neuralgia; zoster rash of eyelids; uveitis; iris atrophy; scleritis; cataract; optic neuritis; paralysis of third nerve; proptosis; paralysis of lids; orbital apex syndrome; retinitis; neurotrophic keratitis; acute retinal necrosis; progressive outer retinal necrosis; ocular motor nerve pareses; tonic pupil; encephalitis; vasculitis.

Clinical

Local lesions involving the posterior or root ganglia; nerve damage; tissue scarring.

Laboratory

Diagnosed mostly on the basis of the characteristic pain and appearance of the dermatomal rashes.

Treatment

Antiviral agents, systemic corticosteroids, antidepressants, and adequate pain control. Immunocompetent adults aged 60 years or older, benefit from receipt of the herpes zoster vaccine and have a lower incidence of herpes zoster.

BIBLIOGRAPHY

1. Diaz MM, Foster CS, Walton RC, et al. (2011). Herpes zoster ophthalmicus. [online] Available from www.emedicine.com/oph/TOPIC257.HTM. [Accessed January, 2013].
2. Ghaznawi N, Virdi A, Dayan A, et al. Herpes zoster ophthalmicus: comparison of disease in patients 60 years and older versus younger than 60 years. Ophthalmology. 2011;118(11):2242-50.
3. Ho J, Xirasagar S, Lin H. Increased risk of a cancer diagnosis after herpes zoster ophthalmicus: a nationwide population-based study. Ophthalmology. 2011;118(6):1076-81.
4. Tseng HF, Smith N, Harpaz R, et al. Herpes zoster vaccine in older adults and the risk of subsequent herpes zoster disease. JAMA. 2011;305(2):160-6.

29. GIANT PAPILLARY CONJUNCTIVITIS SYNDROME

General

Commonly associated with contact lenses (hard and soft), foreign bodies, and ocular prosthesis; immunologic in origin.

Ocular

Ocular irritation; itching of the eye; decreased visual acuity; increased mucous production; papillary changes of the upper tarsal conjunctiva; contact lens coatings; may appear after a lens change from one style to another or by replacement of the previous design; aging of a lens, particularly of a soft contact lens, may be associated; usually bilateral, although it can be markedly asymmetrical.

Clinical

None.

Laboratory

Diagnosis is made by clinical findings.

Treatment

Stop wearing contact lens for 4 weeks, replace contact lens every 6–12 months, topical lubricants and nonsteroidal anti-inflammatory drops.

BIBLIOGRAPHY

1. Weissman BA, Yeung KK. (2011). Giant papillary conjunctivitis. [online] Available from www.emedicine.com/oph/TOPIC87.HTM. [Accessed September, 2013].

30. CONJUNCTIVAL LACERATIONS

General

Usually not serious; however, they may mask an underlying ocular injury or retain foreign body.

Clinical

None.

Ocular

Subconjunctival hemorrhage, symblepharon.

Laboratory

Diagnosis is made by clinical findings.

Treatment

Surgical repair is rarely necessary. Ice packs may be used to minimize swelling.

BIBLIOGRAPHY

1. Roy FH, Fraunfelder FW, Fraunfelder FT. Roy and Fraunfelder's Current Ocular Therapy, 6th edition. London, UK: Elsevier; 2008.

🔁 31. LIGNEOUS CONJUNCTIVITIS

General

Rare form of recurrent conjunctivitis, usually bilateral in infants or children.

Clinical

None.

Ocular

Inflammation characterized by formation of thick membranes and pseudomembranes to the lid.

Laboratory

Histology, plasminogen activity and plasminogen antigen levels.

Treatment

Surgical excision of conjunctival membrane followed by cautery, cryopexy and grafting with conjunctiva or sclera.

🔁 BIBLIOGRAPHY

1. Roy FH, Fraunfelder FW, Fraunfelder FT. Roy and Fraunfelder's Current Ocular Therapy, 6th edition. London, UK: Elsevier; 2008.

🔁 32. MEMBRANOUS CONJUNCTIVITIS

Exudate permeates epithelium to such an extent that removal of membrane is difficult and a raw bleeding surface results. Membranous conjunctivitis can lead to symblepharon, ankyloblepharon, and entropion with trichiasis.

1. Chemical irritants
   A. Acids, such as acetic or lactic
   *B. Alkali, such as ammonia or lime
   †C. Metallic salts, such as silver nitrate or copper sulfate
2. *C. diphtheriae*
3. Ligneous conjunctivitis-chronic, cause unknown

---

*Indicates most frequent
†Indicates a general entry and therefore has not been described in detail in the text

4. Pneumococcus
5. Streptococcus
6. Uncommon-actinomyces, glandular fever, measles, *variola, Pseudomonas aeruginosa, herpes simplex,* and epidemic keratoconjunctivitis (type adenovirus)

🔁 BIBLIOGRAPHY

1. Fedukowicz HB. External Infections of the Eye: Bacterial, Viral, and Mycotic, 3rd edition. New York: Appleton-Century-Crofts; 1984.
2. Roy FH. Ocular Syndromes and Systemic Diseases, 5th edition. New Delhi: Jaypee Brothers Medical Publishers; 2013.

🔁 32.1A. ACID BURNS OF THE EYE

General

Acid injuries of the eyes are characterized by protein coagulation and precipitation with the anion. Direct tissue damage produced by the hydrogen ion.

Clinical

None.

Ocular

Chemosis, corneal epithelial defects, limbal blanching, corneal clouding, photophobia, corneal neovascularization, symblepharon formation.

Laboratory

Diagnosis is made from clinical history and findings.

Treatment

Immediate irrigation, topical antibiotics for bacterial infection if needed, contact lenses aid in re-epithelialization of the cornea.

🔁 BIBLIOGRAPHY

1. Roy FH, Fraunfelder FW, Fraunfelder FT. Roy and Fraunfelder's Current Ocular Therapy, 6th edition. London: Elsevier; 2008.

32.1B. ALKALINE INJURY OF THE EYE

General

A splash of alkaline solution causes the pH to rise and results in immediate damage to the external ocular tissues. These injuries are frequently seen from household chemicals or farming injuries from liquid ammonia used as fertilizer.

Ocular

Pain; lacrimation; blepharospasm; rise in IOP; rapid penetration of the cornea and sclera; chemical injury to iris, lens or ciliary body; symblepharon; phthisis bulbi; ankyloblepharon.

Laboratory

Diagnosis is made by clinical findings and history.

Treatment

Immediate copious irrigation, sticky paste of lime should be removed with a cotton-tipped applicator, mydriasis and topical antibiotics, pain medications, treatment of glaucoma with carbonic anhydrase inhibitors, patching and soft contact lenses may facilitate re-epithelialization, insertion of a methyl methacrylate ring may prevent fibrinous adhesions, lysis of adhesions with or without mucous membrane grafts, corneal stem cell transplantation, corneal transplantation, keratoprosthesis and conjunctival autographs.

BIBLIOGRAPHY

1. Roy FH, Fraunfelder FW, Fraunfelder FT. Roy and Fraunfelder's Current Ocular Therapy, 6th edition. London: Elsevier; 2008.

32.2. DIPHTHERIA

General

Acute infectious disease caused by *C. diphtheriae;* severity is dependent upon the amount of exotoxin absorbed prior to initiation of specific therapy.

Ocular

Conjunctivitis; xerophthalmia; keratitis; corneal ulcer; blepharitis; cellulitis of lid; meibomianitis; ptosis; dacryocystitis; cataract; central retinal artery occlusion; optic neuritis; accommodative spasm or paralysis; convergence paralysis; divergence paralysis; paralysis of third, fourth, or sixth nerve; paralysis of accommodation (in children); ocular motor nerve paresis; choroiditis; cranial neuropathies involving the trigeminal, vagus, and hypoglossal cranial nerves; myocarditis.

Clinical

Local inflammatory lesion, with effect on heart, kidneys, and nervous system.

Laboratory

Gram-positive rods commonly affect children younger than 10 years.

Treatment

Systemic treatment involves use of diphtheria antitoxin and antibiotics. Ocular treatment includes diphtheria antitoxin and high titer y-globulin preparation. Topical penicillin-G ointment helps to eradicate the bacilli.

BIBLIOGRAPHY

1. Demirci CS. (2011). Pediatric diphtheria. [online] Available from www.emedicine.com/ped/TOPIC596.HTM. [Accessed September, 2013].

🗗 32.3. LIGNEOUS CONJUNCTIVITIS

General

Rare form of recurrent conjunctivitis, usually bilateral in infants or children.

Clinical

None.

Ocular

Inflammation characterized by formation of thick membranes and pseudomembranes to the lid.

Laboratory

Histology, plasminogen activity and plasminogen antigen levels.

Treatment

Surgical excision of conjunctival membrane followed by cautery, cryopexy and grafting with conjunctiva or sclera.

🗗 BIBLIOGRAPHY

1. Roy FH, Fraunfelder FW, Fraunfelder FT. Roy and Fraunfelder's Current Ocular Therapy, 6th edition. London, UK: Elsevier; 2008.

🗗 32.4. PNEUMOCOCCAL INFECTIONS (STREPTOCOCCUS PNEUMONIAE INFECTIONS)

General

Gram-positive diplococcus *S. pneumoniae*; some strains are encapsulated while others are not; ocular infections usually are caused by the encapsulated strains; conjunctivitis and corneal scarring produced in an animal model have been attributed to a hemolytic cytolytic exopeptidase.

Ocular

Hypopyon; conjunctivitis; keratitis; corneal ulcer; endophthalmitis; dacryocystitis; uveitis; orbital cellulitis; secondary glaucoma; ophthalmia neonatorum.

Clinical

Upper respiratory infection; chills; sharp pain in hemithorax; cough with sputum production; fever; headache; gastrointestinal symptoms.

Laboratory

Gram stain demonstrates Gram-positive cocci in pairs. The unattached end of each cocci is slightly pointed outward.

Treatment

Impetigo, oral antibiotics and topical antibiotic ointment; preseptal cellulitis, oral antibiotics; orbital celluliti, need team of infectious disease specialist, otolaryngologist and ophthalmologist to develop plan of therapy; dacryocystitis, oral and topical antibiotics, dacryocystorhinostomy may be necessary; conjunctivitis, topical antibiotic; keratitis, topical antibiotics; poststreptococcal reactive arthritis can occur with uveitis, topical steroids and cycloplegics; endophthalmitis, prompt and aggressive therapy with topical, intravitreal and sometimes systemic antibiotics and pars plana vitrectomy; post-refractive surgery keratitis, flap raised, cultured and treated. Occasionally the flap should be amputated.

🗗 BIBLIOGRAPHY

1. Muench DF. (2012). Pneumococcal infections. [online] Available from www.emedicine.com/med/TOPIC1848. HTM. [Accessed September, 2013].

🗗 32.5. STREPTOCOCCUS (SCARLET FEVER)

General

Gram-positive bacteria that can invade any tissue.

Ocular

Conjunctivitis; corneal ulcer; blepharitis; scarlatinal rash of lid; erysipelas dermatitis of lid; gangrene of lid; endophthalmitis; proptosis; dacryocystitis; optic neuritis; orbital cellulitis; uveitis; hypopyon; secondary glaucoma; paralysis of extraocular muscles; infectious crystalline keratopathy; scleritis.

Clinical

Pharyngitis; impetigo; scarlet fever; pneumonia; bacteremia; rheumatic fever; glomerulonephritis.

Laboratory

Gram-positive cocci growing in pairs or chains. Throat culture and sensitivity are useful.

Treatment

Penicillin is the drug of choice.

🗗 BIBLIOGRAPHY

1. Zabawski EJ. (2011). Scarlet Fever. [online] Available from www.emedicine.com/emerg/TOPIC518.HTM. [Accessed September, 2013].

🗗 32.6. ACTINOMYCOSIS

General

Gram-positive *Actinomyces israelii.*

Ocular

Hypopyon; conjunctivitis; keratitis; corneal ulcer; proptosis; uveitis; dacryocystitis; yellow nodules on conjunctiva and eyelids; occlusion of nasolacrimal canaliculi; canaliculitis; orbital abscess; endophthalmitis (rare).

Clinical

Chronic inflammatory induration and sinus formation.

Laboratory

Canalicular discharge may be sent for Gram stain/Giemsa stain, cultures and sensitivities (i.e. blood agar, Sabouraud, anaerobic) and special stains (i.e. calcofluor white stain).

Treatment

Penicillins and cephalosporins are useful. Subconjunctival penicillin coadministered with systemic iodides and topical sulfacetamide or penicillin can be used.

🗗 BIBLIOGRAPHY

1. Roque MR, Roque BL, Foster CS. (2012). Actinomycosis in ophthalmology. [online] Available from www.emedicine.com/oph/TOPIC491.HTM. [Accessed September, 2013].

🗗 32.6. MEASLES (MORBILLI; RUBEOLA)

General

Acute, extremely communicable disease that affects young school-aged children; caused by paramyxovirus.

Ocular

Hypopyon; uveitis; conjunctivitis; Koplik (Hirschberg) spots of conjunctiva; keratitis; corneal ulcer; cellulitis of lid; dacryocystitis; congenital cataract; optic atrophy; optic neuritis; strabismus; pigmentary retinopathy; iris prolapse; hemianopsia; secondary glaucoma; central retinal artery occlusion; orbital cellulitis; accommodative spasm; paralysis of sixth nerve; keratoconus.

Clinical

Maculopapular rash; fever.

Laboratory

Diagnosis is made by clinical findings.

Treatment

Good hydration.

BIBLIOGRAPHY

1. Chen SS. (2011). Measles. [online] Available from www.emedicine.com/derm/TOPIC259.HTM. [Accessed September, 2013].

32.6. SMALLPOX (VARIOLA)

General

Highly contagious cutaneous disease caused by viral infection.

Ocular

Conjunctivitis; keratitis; corneal ulcer; hypopyon; endophthalmitis; congenital corneal clouding; albinotic spots on iris; choroiditis; vitreous opacities; papillitis; extraocular muscle palsies; entropion; dacryocystitis; chorioretinitis; optic neuritis; and vesicles of the eyelid; preauricular adenopathy; eyelid ulcerating pustules; several conditions predispose to the spread of vaccinia, including eczema, hypogammaglobulinemia, steroid therapy, and AIDS.

Clinical

Fever, headache, and vomiting prior to appearance of the rash on the face, upper trunk, and down to the extremities.

Laboratory

Brick-shaped virions viewed with electron microscopy examination, virus culture from live cells, or DNA analysis using PCR and smallpox skin specimen should be collected.

Treatment

No known treatment is effective.

BIBLIOGRAPHY

1. Hussain AN, Hussain F, Alam M, et al. (2011). Smallpox. [online] Available from www.emedicine.com/med/TOPIC3545.HTM. [Accessed September, 2013].

32.6. PSEUDOMONAS AERUGINOSA

General

Gram-negative rod that is ubiquitous in water, soil and plants. Commonly found in hospital environment.

Clinical

None.

Ocular

Foreign body sensation, conjunctival infection, and photophobia, and corneal ulceration.

Laboratory

Gram-negative rod on Gram stain and Giemsa stain from corneal ulcer. Culturing contact lens and lens solutions may help to grow organisms.

Treatment

Fortified tobramycin and fortified cefazolin are drugs of choice.

BIBLIOGRAPHY

1. Roy FH, Fraunfelder FW, Fraunfelder FT. Current Ocular Therapy, 6th edition. London: Elsevier; 2008.

⊟ 32.6. HERPES SIMPLEX

General

Large, complex DNA virus.

Ocular

Conjunctivitis; keratitis; iridocyclitis; corneal ulcer; uveitis; hyphema; hypopyon; iris atrophy; cataract; scleritis; dacryoadenitis; blepharitis; acute retinal necrosis.

Clinical

Recurrent skin vesicles on lids, perioral area, nose and genitalia; meningitis, encephalitis.

Laboratory

Viral cultures.

Treatment

Antiviral therapy, topical or oral, is an effective treatment of epithelial herpes infection.

⊟ BIBLIOGRAPHY

1. Shaohui L, Pavan-Langston D, Colby KA. Pediatric herpes simplex of the anterior segment. Ophthalmology. 2012;119:2003-8.
2. Wang JC, Ritterband DC. (2012). Ophthalmologic manifestations of herpes simplex. [online] Available from www.emedicine.com/oph/TOPIC100.HTM. [Accessed September, 2013].

⊟ 32.6. EPIDEMIC KERATOCONJUNCTIVITIS

General

Highly communicable; adenovirus types 8 and 19; usually bilateral; epidemic keratoconjunctivitis has been reported worldwide associated with 11 virus serotypes, with serotypes 8, 11, and 19 being the most common responsible ones.

Ocular

Follicular or membranous conjunctivitis; chemosis; subconjunctival hemorrhages; corneal opacity; punctate epithelial keratitis; corneal ulcer; blepharospasm; lid edema; serous discharge; uveitis; epiphora.

Clinical

Submaxillary and cervical lymphadenopathy.

Laboratory

Viral isolation on cell culture from conjunctival scrapings.

Treatment

No effective topical or systemic treatment available. Topical steroids may be used if epithelial keratitis occurs.

⊟ BIBLIOGRAPHY

1. Bawazeer A. (2011). Epidemic keratoconjunctivitis. [online] Available from www.emedicine.com/oph/TOPIC677.HTM. [Accessed September, 2013].

⊟ 33. MENINGOCOCCEMIA (NEISSERIA MENINGITIDES; MENINGITIS)

General

Systemic bacterial infection caused by *Neisseria meningitides;* can be present chronically in patients with immune deficiencies including deficient complement levels.

Ocular

Photophobia; conjunctivitis; chemosis; keratitis; uveitis; panophthalmitis; retinal endophlebitis; macular edema; papillitis; optic neuritis; paresis of sixth or seventh nerve; nystagmus; miosis; hippus; cortical blindness; papilledema (rare); conjunctival petechiae; strabismus.

Clinical

Meningitis; fever; malaise; joint pain; splenic enlargement.

Laboratory

Cultures from blood, spinal fluid, or joint fluid.

Treatment

Treat with antibiotics promptly.

⊟ BIBLIOGRAPHY

1. Javid MH, Ahmed SH. (2012). Meningococcemia. [online] Available from www.emedicine.com/med/TOPIC1445. HTM. [Accessed September, 2013].

⊟ 34. MUCOUS MEMBRANE PEMPHIGOID

General

Immune-mediated disease characterized by autoantibodies to the basement membrane zone at the subepithelial junction of mucous membranes.

Ocular

Progressive cicatrizing conjunctivitis; symblepharon; corneal clouding.

Clinical

Nasal and oral mucosa cicatrization; trachea and esophagus cicatrization.

Laboratory

Diagnosis is made by clinical findings.

Treatment

No topical agent is effective. Systemic corticosteroids can control the progression of the disease. Surgeries such as marginal rotation of the eyelid, mucous membrane grafting, retractor placation, fornix reconstruction.

⊟ BIBLIOGRAPHY

1. Foster CS, Hamam R, Letko E. (2011). Ophthalmologic manifestations of cicatricial pemphigoid. [online] Available from www.emedicine.com/oph/TOPIC83.HTM. [Accessed September, 2013].

⊟ 35. OPHTHALMIA NEONATORUM (CONJUNCTIVITIS OCCURRING IN NEWBORNS)

*†1. Chemical conjunctivitis, such as from silver nitrate instillation

*†2. *C. trachomatis*

3. Bacteria

   A. Gram positive
   1. *C. diphtheriae*
   2. *S. aureus*
   †3. *Staphylococcus epidermidis*
   4. Streptococcus group D
   5. *S. pneumoniae*
   †6. *Streptococcus viridans*

   B. Gram negative
   1. Coliform bacillus, such as *Escherichia coli*
   †2. *Enterobacter cloacae*
   3. *H. influenzae*
   †4. *Haemophilus parainfluenzae*
   †5. *K. pneumoniae*
   †6. Meningococcus
   7. *Mima polymorpha*—Gram negative
   8. *N. gonorrhoeae and N. catarrhalis*
   9. *Neisseria* organisms
   †10. Pneumonococcus
   11. *Proteus mirabilis*
   12. *P. aeruginosa*
   †13. *Pseudomonas pyocyanea*
   †14. S. *marcescens*

4. Virus
   A. Herpes simplex
   †B. *Streptococcus viridans*
   †C. Coxsackie A
   †D. TRIC virus

5. Other
   A. *Acinetobacter* species
   †B. *Branhamella catarrhalis*
   †C. C. *albicans*
   †D. *Citrobacter feundi*
   E. *Clostridium perfringens*
   †F. Inclusion blennorrhea
   G. Listeriosis (*L. monocytogenes*)
   H. *Moraxella species*

---

*Indicates most frequent
†Indicates a general entry and therefore has not been described in detail in the text

†I.   *Mycoplasma* organisms
†J.   *Peptococcus prevotii*
K.   *Propionibacterium* species
†L.   *Trichomonas vaginalis*

⊟ BIBLIOGRAPHY

1. McCourt EA, Enzenauer RW, Jatla KK, et al. (2013). Neonatal conjunctivitis. [online] Available from www.emedicine.com/oph/TOPIC325.HTM. [Accessed September, 2013].

⊟ 35.3A1. DIPHTHERIA

General

Acute infectious disease caused by *C. diphtheriae;* severity is dependent upon the amount of exotoxin absorbed prior to initiation of specific therapy.

Ocular

Conjunctivitis; xerophthalmia; keratitis; corneal ulcer; blepharitis; cellulitis of lid; meibomianitis; ptosis; dacryocystitis; cataract; central retinal artery occlusion; optic neuritis; accommodative spasm or paralysis; convergence paralysis; divergence paralysis; paralysis of third, fourth, or sixth nerve; paralysis of accommodation (in children); ocular motor nerve paresis; choroiditis; cranial neuropathies involving the trigeminal, vagus, and hypoglossal cranial nerves; myocarditis.

Clinical

Local inflammatory lesion, with effect on heart, kidneys, and nervous system.

Laboratory

Gram-positive rods commonly affect children younger than 10 years.

Treatment

Systemic treatment involves use of diphtheria antitoxin and antibiotics. Ocular treatment includes diphtheria antitoxin and high titer y-globulin preparation. Topical penicillin-G ointment helps to eradicate the bacilli.

⊟ BIBLIOGRAPHY

1. Demirci CS. (2011). Pediatric diphtheria. [online] Available from www.emedicine.com/ped/TOPIC596.HTM. [Accessed September, 2013].

⊟ 35.3A2. STAPHYLOCOCCUS

General

Gram-positive coccus *S. aureus;* most common cause of suppurative infection in humans; more common in patients with a previous disorders, such as diabetes, thyroid disease, renal failure, or malnutrition; although most *S. aureus* isolates from other sources are encapsulated, capsules have not been noted in ocular isolates.

Ocular

Uveitis; hypopyon; conjunctivitis; keratitis; cellulitis of lid; meibomianitis; ptosis; blepharitis; endophthalmitis; dacryocystitis; increased IOP; orbital periosteitis.

Clinical

Tissues hypertonic, edematous, and painful; lesion liquefies, forming creamy yellow pus; fever; nausea; vomiting; cough; dyspnea; abdominal pain; diarrhea; bloody stools; dehydration; shock.

Laboratory

Aerobic Gram-positive cocci bacteria grow in grape-like clusters. Coagulase positive indicates pathogenicity.

Treatment

Specific antimicrobial therapy is chosen based on the site and severity of the infection and the antimicrobial sensitivities of the organism involved.

⊟ BIBLIOGRAPHY

1. Tolan RW. (2012). Staphylococcus Aureus infection. [online] Available from www.emedicine.com/ped/TOPIC2704.HTM. [Accessed September, 2013].

⊟ 35.3A4. STREPTOCOCCUS (SCARLET FEVER)

General

Gram-positive bacteria that can invade any tissue.

Ocular

Conjunctivitis; corneal ulcer; blepharitis; scarlatinal rash of lid; erysipelas dermatitis of lid; gangrene of lid; endophthalmitis; proptosis; dacryocystitis; optic neuritis; orbital cellulitis; uveitis; hypopyon; secondary glaucoma; paralysis of extraocular muscles; infectious crystalline keratopathy; scleritis.

Clinical

Pharyngitis; impetigo; scarlet fever; pneumonia; bacteremia; rheumatic fever; glomerulonephritis.

Laboratory

Gram-positive cocci growing in pairs or chains. Throat culture and sensitivity are useful.

Treatment

Penicillin is the drug of choice.

⊟ BIBLIOGRAPHY

1. Zabawski EJ. (2011). Scarlet fever. [online] Available from www.emedicine.com/emerg/TOPIC518.HTM. [Accessed September, 2013].

⊟ 35.3A5. PNEUMOCOCCAL INFECTIONS (STREPTOCOCCUS PNEUMONIAE INFECTIONS)

General

Gram-positive diplococcus *S. pneumoniae;* some strains are encapsulated while others are not; ocular infections usually are caused by the encapsulated strains; conjunctivitis and corneal scarring produced in an animal model have been attributed to a hemolytic cytolytic exopeptidase.

Ocular

Hypopyon; conjunctivitis; keratitis; corneal ulcer; endophthalmitis; dacryocystitis; uveitis; orbital cellulitis; secondary glaucoma; ophthalmia neonatorum.

Clinical

Upper respiratory infection; chills; sharp pain in hemithorax; cough with sputum production; fever; headache; gastrointestinal symptoms.

Laboratory

Gram stain demonstrates Gram-positive cocci in pairs. The unattached end of each cocci is slightly pointed outward.

Treatment

Impetigo, oral antibiotics and topical antibiotic ointment; preseptal cellulitis, oral antibiotics; orbital cellulitis, need team of infectious disease specialist, otolaryngologist and ophthalmologist to develop plan of therapy; dacryocystitis, oral and topical antibiotics, dacryocystorhinostomy may be necessary; conjunctivitis, topical antibiotic; keratitis, topical antibiotics; poststreptococcal reactive arthritis can occur with uveitis, topical steroids and cycloplegics; endophthalmitis, prompt and aggressive therapy with topical, intravitreal and sometimes systemic antibiotics and pars plana vitrectomy; post-refractive surgery keratitis, flap raised, cultured and treated. Occasionally the flap should be amputated.

⊟ BIBLIOGRAPHY

1. Muench DF. (2012). Pneumococcal infections. [online] Available from www.emedicine.com/med/TOPIC1848.HTM. [Accessed September, 2013].

⊟ 35.3B1. ESCHERICHIA COLI

General

Gram-negative rod found in the gastrointestinal tract; urinary tract is the usual portal of entry.

Ocular

Uveitis; hyphema; hypopyon; gas bubbles in anterior chamber; purulent conjunctivitis; keratitis; corneal edema; panophthalmitis; endophthalmitis; glaucoma.

Clinical

Diarrhea; gastroenteritis; dehydration.

Laboratory

Anaerobic Gram-negative rod.

Treatment

Antibiotic therapy should start with ampicillin until sensitivity reports return.

⊟ BIBLIOGRAPHY

1. Suh DW. (2011). Ophthalmologic manifestations of Escherichia Coli. [online] Available from www.emedicine.com/oph/TOPIC496.HTM. [Accessed September, 2013].

⊟ 35.3B3. HAEMOPHILUS INFLUENZAE

General

Gram-negative rod.

Ocular

Conjunctivitis; cellulitis; tenonitis; uveitis; vitreous opacity; pannus; corneal opacity.

Clinical

Pharyngitis; epiglottitis; laryngotracheitis; pneumonia; bronchitis; otitis media; meningitis; cellulitis; septic arthritis; sinusitis.

Laboratory

Gram-negative coccobacillus with eight biotypes and six serotypes. Gram stain and culture.

Treatment

Antibiotics are the mainstay of treatment. Invasive and serious infections are best treated with an intravenous third-generation cephalosporin until antibiotic sensitivities are available.

⊟ BIBLIOGRAPHY

1. Devarajan VR. (2012). Haemophilus influenzae infections. [online] Available from www.emedicine.com/med/TOPIC936.HTM. [Accessed September, 2013].

⊟ 35.3B7. ACINETOBACTER (MIMA POLYMORPHA; ACINETOBACTER IWOFFI)

General

Gram-negative pleomorphic bacillus *Mima;* generally occurs in patient with lowered resistance.

Ocular

Conjunctivitis and chemosis; corneal ulcer; blepharitis; iris prolapse; endophthalmitis.

Clinical

Meningitis; pneumonitis; endocarditis; urethritis; vaginitis; arthritis; dermatitis; intracranial abscess; subdural empyema.

Laboratory

Culture of the appropriate body fluid that is properly transported, plated, and incubated grows *Acinetobacter baumannii.*

Treatment

An infectious disease specialist should be consulted to differentiate colonization from infection and for antibiotic recommendations.

⊟ BIBLIOGRAPHY

1. Cunha BA. (2011). Acinetobacter. [online] Available from www.emedicine.com/med/TOPIC3456.HTM. [Accessed September, 2013].

⊟ 35.3B8. GONORRHEA

General

Caused by *Neisseria gonorrhoeae*, which is transmitted sexually.

Ocular

Conjunctivitis; eyelid edema; keratitis; uveitis.

Clinical

Pelvic inflammatory disease; arthritis; dermatitis; carditis; meningitis.

Laboratory

Gram stain smear demonstrates Gram-negative diplococci with polymorphonuclear leukocytes in conjunctival exudates.

Treatment

Therapy consists of systemic antibiotics; topical antibiotics are relatively ineffective in the treatment of eye disease. It is important to treat all sexual partners simultaneously to prevent reinfection.

⊟ BIBLIOGRAPHY

1. Wong B. (2012). Gonorrhea. [online] Available from www.emedicine.com/oph/TOPIC497.HTM. [Accessed September, 2013].

⊟ 35.3B9. MENINGOCOCCEMIA (NEISSERIA MENINGITIDES; MENINGITIS)

General

Systemic bacterial infection caused by *N. meningitides;* can be present chronically in patients with immune deficiencies including deficient complement levels.

Ocular

Photophobia; conjunctivitis; chemosis; keratitis; uveitis; panophthalmitis; retinal endophlebitis; macular edema; papillitis; optic neuritis; paresis of sixth or seventh nerve; nystagmus; miosis; hippus; cortical blindness; papilledema (rare); conjunctival petechiae; strabismus.

Clinical

Meningitis; fever; malaise; joint pain; splenic enlargement.

Laboratory

Cultures from blood, spinal fluid, or joint fluid.

Treatment

Treat with antibiotics promptly.

⊟ BIBLIOGRAPHY

1. Javid MH, Ahmed SH. (2012). Meningococcemia. [online] Available from www.emedicine.com/med/TOPIC1445.HTM. [Accessed September, 2013].

35.3B11. PROTEUS INFECTIONS

General

Gram-negative bacilli found in water, soil and decaying organic substances.

Ocular

Conjunctivitis; keratitis; corneal ulcers; endophthalmitis; panophthalmitis; dacryocystitis; gangrene of eyelid; uveitis; hypopyon; paralysis of seventh nerve.

Clinical

Cutaneous infection after surgery; usually occurs as a secondary infection of the skin, ears, mastoid sinuses, eyes, peritoneal cavity, bone, urinary tract, meninges, lung, or bloodstream; meningitis; intracranial, subdural and epidural empyema; brain abscess; intracranial septic thrombophlebitis affecting cavernous/lateral sinuses.

Laboratory

Proteus organisms are easily recovered through routine laboratory cultures. An ultrasound of the kidneys or a CT scan should be considered as part of a workup.

Treatment

Traditional treatment includes oral quinolone for 3 days or trimethoprim/sulfamethoxazole.

BIBLIOGRAPHY

1. Struble K. (2011). Proteus infections. [online] Available from www.emedicine.com/med/TOPIC1929.HTM. [Accessed September, 2013].

35.3B12. PSEUDOMONAS AERUGINOSA

General

Gram-negative rod that is ubiquitous in water, soil and plants. Commonly found in hospital environment.

Clinical

None.

Ocular

Foreign body sensation, conjunctival injection, and photophobia, and corneal ulceration.

Laboratory

Gram-negative rod on Gram stain and Giemsa stain from corneal ulcer. Culturing contact lens and lens solutions may help to grow organisms.

Treatment

Fortified tobramycin and fortified cefazolin are drugs of choice.

BIBLIOGRAPHY

1. Roy FH, Fraunfelder FW, Fraunfelder FT. Roy and Fraunfelder's Current Ocular Therapy, 6th edition. London: Elsevier; 2008.

35.4A. HERPES SIMPLEX

General

Large, complex DNA virus.

Ocular

Conjunctivitis; keratitis; iridocyclitis; corneal ulcer; uveitis; hyphema; hypopyon; iris atrophy; cataract; scleritis; dacryoadenitis; blepharitis; acute retinal necrosis.

Clinical

Recurrent skin vesicles on lids, perioral area, nose and genitalia; meningitis, encephalitis.

Laboratory

Viral cultures.

Treatment

Antiviral therapy, topical or oral, is an effective treatment of epithelial herpes infection.

⊟ BIBLIOGRAPHY

1. Shaohui L, Pavan-Langston D, Colby KA. Pediatric herpes simplex of the anterior segment. Ophthalmology. 2012;119: 2003-8.

2. Wang JC, Ritterband DC. (2012). Ophthalmologic manifestations of herpes simplex. [online] Available from www.emedicine.com/oph/TOPIC100.HTM. [Accessed September, 2013].

⊟ 35.5A. ACINETOBACTER

General

Cutaneous flora found in wet zones such as groin, axilla, mouth, throat, nose, conjunctiva, bladder and rectum.

Clinical

Pneumonia, septicemia, urinary tract infection, meningitis, skin and wound infections.

Ocular

Endophthalmitis, keratitis; corneal ulcers and corneal abscesses.

Laboratory

Culture usually on broth media.

Treatment

Fluoroquinolones (third or fourth generation) is the treatment of choice.

⊟ BIBLIOGRAPHY

1. Roy FH, Fraunfelder FW, Fraunfelder FT. Roy and Fraunfelder's Current Ocular Therapy, 6th edition. London; Elsevier; 2008.

⊟ 35.5E. CLOSTRIDIUM PERFRINGENS

General

Gram-positive rod; most important cause of gas gangrene infection.

Ocular

Hypopyon; gas bubbles in anterior chamber; endophthalmitis; proptosis; glaucoma; coffee-colored discharge; eyelid edema; severe ocular pain; endophthalmitis after penetrating trauma or metastatic.

Clinical

Traumatized ischemic skeletal muscle, abdominal wall, or uterus; hemolytic anemia; shock; death.

Laboratory

ELISA of the wound exudate, tissue samples, or serum can confirm diagnosis.

Treatment

Antibiotic therapy and hyperbaric oxygen may be useful. In more severe cases fasciotomy, debridement, and amputation may be necessary.

⊟ BIBLIOGRAPHY

1. Ho H, Figueroa-Casas JB, Maxfield DG, et al. [online] Available from www.emedicine.com/med/TOPIC843.HTM. [Accessed September, 2013].

⊟ 35.5G. LISTERELLOSIS (LISTERIOSIS)

General

Caused by Gram-positive bacillus *Listeria monocytogenes*. High mortality among pregnant women, their fetuses, and immunocompromised persons with symptoms of abortion, neonatal death, septicemia, meningitis, brain abscesses, endocarditis.

Ocular

Conjunctivitis; keratitis; corneal abscess and ulcer; blepharitis; uveitis; endophthalmitis; cataract; secondary glaucoma.

Clinical

Vomiting; cardiorespiratory distress; diarrhea; hepatosplenomegaly; maculopapular skin lesions.

Laboratory

Histopathology and culture of rash, CT scanning or MRI may be useful in detecting abscesses in the brain or liver.

Treatment

Antibiotics as well as careful monitoring of the patient's temperature, respiratory system, fluid and electrolyte balance, nutrition, and cardiovascular support.

⊟ BIBLIOGRAPHY

1. Zach T, Anderson-Berry AL. (2013). Listeria infection. [online] Available from www.emedicine.com/ped/TOPIC1319.HTM. [Accessed September, 2013].

⊟ 35.5H. MORAXELLA LACUNATA

General

Gram-negative rod; causes chronic angular blepharoconjunctivitis; without treatment, may persist for months or years; normally found in flora of respiratory tract; seen more frequently in alcoholics and those with poor sanitary habits; *Moraxella* organisms produce proteases, although those are not related directly to their pathogenetic mechanism.

Ocular

Catarrhal angular conjunctivitis; corneal ulcer; hypopyon; chronic blepharitis; eczema; lateral canthal skin erythema; iridocyclitis.

Clinical

Alcoholism; impaired nutrition; dermatitis.

Laboratory

Aerobic, oxidase positive, Gram-negative diplococcus or coccobacilli morphologically indistinguishable from *Neisseria*.

Treatment

Artificial tears, cold compresses, antibiotics.

⊟ BIBLIOGRAPHY

1. Baum J, Fedukowicz HB, Jordan A. A survey of Moraxella corneal ulcers in a derelict population. Am J Ophthalmol. 1980;90:476-80.
2. Burd EM. Bacterial keratitis and conjunctivitis. In: Smolin G, Thoft RA (Eds). The Cornea. Boston: Little, Brown and Company; 1994. pp. 20-1.
3. Roy FH, Fraunfelder FW. Roy and Fraunfelder's Current Ocular Therapy, 6th edition. Philadelphia: WB Saunders; 2008.
4. van Bijsterveld OP. The incidence of Moraxella on mucous membranes and the skin. Am J Ophthalmol. 1972;74:72-6.

⊟ 35.5K. PROPIONIBACTERIUM ACNES

General

Gram-positive, pleomorphic, non-spore forming bacillus that is considered part of the normal eyelid and conjunctival anaerobic flora. Pathogenic if introduced intraocular.

Clinical

None.

Ocular

Chronic keratitis, endophthalmitis, vitritis.

Laboratory

Aerobic and anaerobic cultures must be incubated for 14 days. Capsular biopsy may demonstrate Gram-positive, plemorphic, non-spore forming bacillus or Gram stain.

Treatment

Vancomycin, intravitreal or systemic

BIBLIOGRAPHY

1. Roy FH, Fraunfelder FW, Fraunfelder FT. Roy and Fraunfelder's Current Ocular Therapy, 6th edition. London: Elsevier; 2008.

36. PARINAUD OCULOGLANDULAR SYNDROME (PARINAUD CONJUNCTIVA-ADENITIS SYNDROME; CATSCRATCH OCULOGLANDULAR SYNDROME; CATSCRATCH DISEASE; BARTONELLA HENSELAE)

General

Most frequently seen in children; incubation time 7–10 days; caused by small pleomorphic Gram-negative bacillus; good prognosis; affects both sexes; about 90% of patients with this condition have serologic evidence of infection by *Rochalimaea henselae*.

Ocular

Conjunctivitis; retrotarsal conjunctival granulations; formation of granulomata in anterior segment about 3 mm high and 2–6 mm in diameter; inferior fornix usually affected; ulceration common; neuroretinitis; optic neuritis.

Clinical

Tender, red papule at the site of a cat scratch; regional preauricular and cervical lymphadenitis (often only one gland involved); irregular fever for 4–5 days and malaise; fever; parotid gland swelling.

Laboratory

Histopathology of biopsied lymph node of Warthin-Starry silver stain.

Treatment

Symptomatic treatment includes warm compresses, analgesics and antipyretics. Aspiration of lymph node if distention causes pain. Antibiotics may be necessary in severe cases.

BIBLIOGRAPHY

1. Chi SL, Stinnett S, Eggenberger E, et al. Clinical characteristics in 53 patients with cat scratch optic neuropathy. Ophthalmology. 2012;119:183-7.
2. Nervi SJ. (2011). Catscratch disease. [online] Available from www.emedicine.com/med/TOPIC304.HTM. [Accessed September, 2013].

37. PETZETAKIS-TAKOS SYNDROME (PHLYCTENULAR KERATOCONJUNCTIVITIS)

General

Malnutrition; lack of hygiene.

Ocular

Superficial keratitis; palpebral edema; cornea hyperesthesia; photophobia; blepharospasm; decreased pupillary response; xerophthalmia.

Clinical

Lymph node hypertrophy.

Laboratory

Diagnosis is made by clinical findings.

Treatment

Topical antihistamines, NSAIDs and corticosteroids may be useful.

⊟ BIBLIOGRAPHY

1. Magalini SI, Scrascia E. Dictionary of Medical Syndromes, 2nd edition. Philadelphia, PA: Lippincott Williams & Wilkins; 1981.

2. Petzetakis M. Les Troubles Oculaires Pendant la Trophopenie et l'Epidemic de la Pellagre. La Keratopathie Superficielle Trophopenique. Presse Med. 1950;58:1082-4.

⊟ 38. PSEUDOMEMBRANOUS CONJUNCTIVITIS

In pseudomembranous conjunctivitis, the fibrin network is easily peeled off, leaving the conjunctiva intact; it forms on the conjunctiva.

1. Bacteria
   A. *C. diphtheriae*
   *B. Gonococcus
   *C. Meningococcus
   D. Pneumococcus
   E. Staphylococcus
   *F. Streptococcus
   G. Uncommon: *H. aegyptius, H. influenzae, Moraxella catarrhalis, Pseudomonas aeruginosa, E. coli, Bacillus subtilis, Shigella, Salmonella paratyphi* B, *M. tuberculosis,* and *T. pallidum.*

2. Viral
   *A. Epidemic keratoconjunctivitis (type adenovirus)
   *B. Herpes simplex
   C. Herpes zoster
   D. Reiter syndrome (conjunctivourethrosynovial syndrome)
   E. Vaccina

3. Fungal: *C. albicans.* Allergic-vernal conjunctivitis.

*4. Toxic
   *A. Stevens-Johnson syndrome can be caused by drugs, including the following:
   - Acetazolamide
   - Acetohexamide
   - Acetophenazine
   - Allobarbital
   - Allopurinol
   - Amidone
   - Aminosalicylate
   - Aminosalicylic acid
   - Amithiozone
   - Amobarbital
   - Amodiaquine
   - Amoxicillin
   - Ampicillin

- Antipyrine
- Aprobarbital
- Aspirin
- Auranofin
- Aurothioglucose
- Aurothioglycanide
- Barbital
- Belladonna
- Bendroflumethiazide
- Benzathine penicillin G
- Benzthiazide
- Bromide
- Bromisovalum
- Butabarbital
- Butalbital
- Butallylonal
- Butaperazine
- Butethal
- Captopril
- Carbamazepine
- Carbenicillin
- Carbromal
- Carisoprodol
- Carphenazine
- Cefaclor
- Cefadroxil
- Cefamandole
- Cefazolin
- Cefonicid
- Cefoperazone
- Ceforanide
- Cefotaxime
- Cefotetan
- Cefoxitin
- Cefsulodin
- Ceftazidime
- Ceftizoxime
- Ceftriaxone
- Cefuroxime
- Cephalexin

---

* Indicates most frequent

- Cephaloglycin
- Cephaloridine
- Cephalothin
- Cephapirin
- Cephradine
- Chloroquine
- Chlorothiazide
- Chlorpromazine
- Chlorpropamide
- Chlortetracycline
- Chlorthalidone
- Cimetidine
- Clindamycin
- Cloxacillin
- Cyclobarbital
- Cyclopentobarbital
- Cyclothiazide
- Danazol
- Demeclocycline
- Dichlorphenamide
- Dicloxacillin
- Diethazine
- Diphenylhydantoin
- Doxycycline
- Enalapril
- Erythromycin
- Ethopropazine
- Ethosuximide
- Ethotoin
- Ethoxzolamide
- Fenoprofen
- Fluphenazine
- Furosemidc
- Gentamicin
- Glyburide
- Gold Au 198
- Gold sodium thiomalate
- Gold sodium thiosulfate
- Heptabarbital
- Hetacillin
- Hexethal
- Hexobarbital
- Hydrabamine penicillin V
- Hydrochlorothiazide
- Hydroflumethiazide
- Hydroxychloroquine
- Ibuprofen
- Indapamide
- Indomethacin

- Isoniazid
- Lincomycin
- Mephenytoin
- Mephobarbital
- Meprobamate
- Mesoridazine
- Methacycline
- Metharbital
- Methazolamide
- Methdilazine
- Methicillin
- Methitural
- Methohexital
- Methotrimeprazine
- Methsuximide
- Methyclothiazide
- Methylphenidate
- Metolazone
- Minocycline
- Minoxidil
- Moxalactam
- Nafcillin
- Naproxen
- Oxacillin
- Oxyphenbutazone
- Oxytetracycline
- Paramethadione
- Penicillin
- Pentobarbital
- Perazine
- Pericyazine
- Perphenazine
- Phenacetin
- Phenobarbital
- Phenoxymethyl penicillin
- Phensuximide
- Phenylbutazone
- Phenytoin
- Piperacetazine
- Piproxen
- Polythiazide
- Potassium penicillin g
- Potassium penicillin v
- Potassium phenethicillin
- Potassium phenoxymethyl
- Primidone
- Probarbital
- Procaine penicillin g
- Prochlorperazine

- Promazine
- Promethazine
- Proparacaine
- Propiomazine
- Propranolol
- Quinethazone
- Quinine
- Rifampin
- Secobarbital
- Smallpox vaccine
- Sodium salicylate
- Sulfacetamide
- Sulfachlorpyridazine
- Sulfacytine
- Sulfadiazine
- Sulfadimethoxine
- Sulfamerazine
- Sulfameter
- Sulfamethazine
- Sulfamethizole
- Sulfamethoxazole
- Sulfamethoxypyridazine
- Sulfanilamide
- Sulfaphenazole
- Sulfapyridine
- Sulfasalazine
- Sulfathiazole
- Sulfisoxazole
- Sulindac
- Sulthiame
- Talbutal
- Tetracycline
- Thiabendazole
- Thiamylal
- Thiethylperazine
- Thiopental
- Thiopropazate
- Thioproperazine
- Thioridazine
- Tolazamide
- Tolbutamide
- Trichlormethiazide
- Trifluoperazine
- Triflupromazine
- Trimeprazine
- Trimethadione
- Vancomycin
- Vinbarbital

†*B. Benign mucous membrane pemphigoid can be caused by drugs, including the following:
- Carbamazepine
- Carbimazole
- Diphenylhydantoin
- Ethosuximide
- Griseofulvin
- Hydralazine
- Isoniazid
- Methimazole
- Methsuximide
- Methylthiouracil
- Paramethadione
- Phensuximide
- Practolol
- Propylthiouracil
- Streptomycin
- Trimethadione

C. Lyell disease (toxic epidermal necrolysis or scalded-skin syndrome) can be caused by drugs, including the following:
- Acetaminophen
- Acetanilide
- Acetazolamide
- Acid bismuth sodium tartrate
- Adrenal cortex injection
- Aldosterone
- Allobarbital
- Amobarbital
- Amoxapine
- Amoxicillin
- Ampicillin
- Antipyrine
- Aprobarbital
- Aurothioglucose
- Aurothioglycanide
- Barbital
- Bendroflumethiazide
- Benzathine penicillin G
- Benzthiazide
- Betamethasone
- Bismuth oxychloride
- Bismuth sodium
- Bismuth sodium
- Bismuth sodium tartrate
- Busulfan
- Butabarbital
- Butalbital

- Butallylonal
- Butethal
- Carbamazepine
- Carbenicillin
- Carbimazole
- Chlorambucil
- Chlorthiazide
- Chlortetracycline
- Chlorthalidone
- Clomipramine
- Cloxacillin
- Cortisone
- Cyclobarbital
- Cyclopentobarbital
- Cyclophosphamide
- Cyclothiazide
- Dapsone
- Demeclocycline
- Desoxycorticosterone
- Dexamethasone
- Dichlorphenamide
- Dicloxacillin
- Diltiazem
- Diphenylhydantoin
- Doxepin
- Doxycycline
- Erythromycin
- Ethambutol
- Ethotoin
- Ethoxzolamide
- Fludrocortisone
- Fluprednisolone
- Gold Au 198
- Gold sodium thiomalate
- Heptabarbital
- Hetacillin
- Hexethal
- Hexobarbital
- Hydrabamine penicillin V
- Hydrochlorothiazide
- Hydrocortisone
- Ibuprofen
- Indapamide
- Indomethacin
- Isoniazid
- Kanamycin
- Mechlorethamine
- Melphalan
- Mephenytoin
- Mephobarbital
- Meprednisone
- Methacycline
- Metharbital
- Methazolamide
- Methicillin
- Methitural
- Methohexital
- Methotrexate
- Methyclothiazide
- Methylprednisolone
- Metolazone
- Minocycline
- Nafcillin
- Nitrofurantoin
- Oxacillin
- Oxyphenbutazone
- Oxytetracycline
- Paramethadione
- Paramethasone
- Penicillamine
- Pentobarbital
- Phenobarbital
- Phenoxymethyl penicillin
- Phenylbutazone
- Phenytoin
- Piroxicam
- Poliovirus vaccine
- Polythiazide
- Potassium penicillin G
- Potassium penicillin V
- Potassium phenethicillin
- Prednisolone
- Prednisone
- Primidone
- Probarbital
- Procaine penicillin G
- Procarbazine
- Quinethazone
- Secobarbital
- Smallpox vaccine
- Sodium salicylate
- Streptomycin
- Sulfacetamide
- Sulfachlorpyridazine
- Sulfadiazine
- Sulfadimethoxine
- Sulfamerazine
- Sulfameter

- Sulfamethazine
- Sulfamethizole
- Sulfamethoxazole
- Sulfamethoxypyridazine
- Sulfanilamide
- Sulfaphenazole
- Sulfapyridine
- Sulfasalazine
- Sulfathiazole
- Sulfisoxazole
- Sulindac
- Talbutal
- Tetracycline
- Thiabendazole
- Thiamylal
- Thioglycollate
- Thiopental
- Triamcinolone
- Trichlormethiazide
- Triethylene-melamine
- Triglycollamate
- Trimethadione
- Trimipramine
- Uracil mustard
- Vinbarbital

  D. Pemphigus vulgaris

†E. Hereditary epidermolysis bullosa
5. Chemical irritants
   A. Acids, such as acetic or lactic
  *B. Alkalis, such as ammonia or lime
  †C. Metallic salts, such as silver nitrate or copper sulfate
  †D. Vegetable and animal irritants
6. Acute graft-versus-host disease
7. Hoof-and-mouth disease
8. Koch-Weeks bacillus
9. Ligneous conjunctivitis: Chronic, cause unknown
10. Lipoid proteinosis (Urbach-Wiethe disease)
*11. Superior limbic keratoconjunctivitis
†12. Traumatic or operative healing of wounds
13. Wegener granulomatosis

BIBLIOGRAPHY

1. Barthelemy H, Mauduit G, Kanitakis J, et al. Lipoid proteinosis with pseudomembranous conjunctivitis. J Am Acad Dermatol. 1986;14:367-71.
2. Fraunfelder FT, Fraunfelder FW. Drug-induced ocular side effects. Woburn, MA: Butterworth-Heinemann; 2001.
3. Pau H. Differential diagnosis of eye diseases, 2nd edition. New York: Thieme Medical; 1988.

---

†Indicates a general entry and therefore has not been described in detail in the text

38.1A. DIPHTHERIA

General

Acute infectious disease caused by *C. diphtheriae;* severity is dependent upon the amount of exotoxin absorbed prior to initiation of specific therapy.

Ocular

Conjunctivitis; xerophthalmia; keratitis; corneal ulcer; blepharitis; cellulitis of lid; meibomianitis; ptosis; dacryocystitis; cataract; central retinal artery occlusion; optic neuritis; accommodative spasm or paralysis; convergence paralysis; divergence paralysis; paralysis of third, fourth, or sixth nerve; paralysis of accommodation (in children); ocular motor nerve paresis; choroiditis; cranial neuropathies involving the trigeminal, vagus, and hypoglossal cranial nerves; myocarditis.

Clinical

Local inflammatory lesion, with effect on heart, kidneys, and nervous system.

Laboratory

Gram-positive rods commonly affect children younger than 10 years.

Treatment

Systemic treatment involves use of diphtheria antitoxin and antibiotics. Ocular treatment includes diphtheria antitoxin and high titer y-globulin preparation. Topical penicillin-G ointment helps to eradicate the bacilli.

BIBLIOGRAPHY

1. Demirci CS. (2011). Pediatric Diphtheria. [online] Available from www.emedicine.com/ped/TOPIC596.HTM. [Accessed September, 2013].

⊞ 38.1B. GONORRHEA

General

Caused by *N. gonorrhoeae*, which is transmitted sexually.

Ocular

Conjunctivitis; eyelid edema; keratitis; uveitis.

Clinical

Pelvic inflammatory disease; arthritis; dermatitis; carditis; meningitis.

Laboratory

Gram stain smear demonstrates Gram-negative diplococci with polymorphonuclear leukocytes in conjunctival exudates.

Treatment

Therapy consists of systemic antibiotics; topical antibiotics are relatively ineffective in the treatment of eye disease. It is important to treat all sexual partners simultaneously to prevent reinfection.

⊞ BIBLIOGRAPHY

1. Wong B. (2012). Gonorrhea. [online] Available from www.emedicine.com/oph/TOPIC497.HTM. [Accessed September, 2013].

⊞ 38.1C. MENINGOCOCCEMIA (NEISSERIA MENINGITIDES; MENINGITIS)

General

Systemic bacterial infection caused by *N. meningitides*; can be present chronically in patients with immune deficiencies including deficient complement levels.

Ocular

Photophobia; conjunctivitis; chemosis; keratitis; uveitis; panophthalmitis; retinal endophlebitis; macular edema; papillitis; optic neuritis; paresis of sixth or seventh nerve; nystagmus; miosis; hippus; cortical blindness; papilledema (rare); conjunctival petechiae; strabismus.

Clinical

Meningitis; fever; malaise; joint pain; splenic enlargement.

Laboratory

Cultures from blood, spinal fluid, or joint fluid.

Treatment

Treat with antibiotics promptly.

⊞ BIBLIOGRAPHY

1. Javid MH, Ahmed SH. (2012). Meningococcemia. [online] Available from www.emedicine.com/med/TOPIC1445.HTM. [Accessed September, 2013].

⊞ 38.1D. PNEUMOCOCCAL INFECTIONS (STREPTOCOCCUS PNEUMONIAE INFECTIONS)

General

Gram-positive diplococcus *S. pneumoniae;* some strains are encapsulated while others are not; ocular infections usually are caused by the encapsulated strains; conjunctivitis and corneal scarring produced in an animal model have been attributed to a hemolytic cytolytic exopeptidase.

Ocular

Hypopyon; conjunctivitis; keratitis; corneal ulcer; endophthalmitis; dacryocystitis; uveitis; orbital cellulitis; secondary glaucoma; ophthalmia neonatorum.

Clinical

Upper respiratory infection; chills; sharp pain in hemithorax; cough with sputum production; fever; headache; gastrointestinal symptoms.

Laboratory

Gram stain demonstrates Gram-positive cocci in pairs. The unattached end of each cocci is slightly pointed outward.

Treatment

Impetigo, oral antibiotics and topical antibiotic ointment; preseptal cellulitis, oral antibiotics; orbital celluliti, need team of infectious disease specialist, otolaryngologist and ophthalmologist to develop plan of therapy; dacryocystitis, oral and topical antibiotics, dacryocystorhinostomy may be necessary; conjunctivitis, topical antibiotic; keratitis, topical antibiotics; poststreptococcal reactive arthritis can occur with uveitis, topical steroids and cycloplegics; endophthalmitis, prompt and aggressive therapy with topical, intravitreal and sometimes systemic antibiotics and pars plana vitrectomy; post-refractive surgery keratitis, flap raised, cultured and treated. Occasionally the flap should be amputated.

BIBLIOGRAPHY

1. Muench DF. (2012). Pneumococcal infections. [online] Available from www.emedicine.com/med/TOPIC1848.HTM. [Accessed September, 2013].

38.1E. STAPHYLOCOCCUS

General

Gram-positive coccus *S. aureus;* most common cause of suppurative infection in humans; more common in patients with a previous disorders, such as diabetes, thyroid disease, renal failure, or malnutrition; although most *S. aureus* isolates from other sources are encapsulated, capsules have not been noted in ocular isolates.

Ocular

Uveitis; hypopyon; conjunctivitis; keratitis; cellulitis of lid; meibomianitis; ptosis; blepharitis; endophthalmitis; dacryocystitis; increased IOP; orbital periosteitis.

Clinical

Tissues hypertonic, edematous, and painful; lesion liquefies, forming creamy yellow pus; fever; nausea; vomiting; cough; dyspnea; abdominal pain; diarrhea; bloody stools; dehydration; shock.

Laboratory

Aerobic Gram-positive cocci bacteria grow in grape-like clusters. Coagulase positive indicates pathogenicity.

Treatment

Specific antimicrobial therapy is chosen based on the site and severity of the infection and the antimicrobial sensitivities of the organism involved.

BIBLIOGRAPHY

1. Tolan RW. (2012). Staphylococcus aureus infection. [online] Available from www.emedicine.com/ped/TOPIC2704.HTM. [Accessed September, 2013].

38.1F. STREPTOCOCCUS (SCARLET FEVER)

General

Gram-positive bacteria that can invade any tissue.

Ocular

Conjunctivitis; corneal ulcer; blepharitis; scarlatinal rash of lid; erysipelas dermatitis of lid; gangrene of lid; endophthalmitis; proptosis; dacryocystitis; optic neuritis; orbital cellulitis; uveitis; hypopyon; secondary glaucoma; paralysis of extraocular muscles; infectious crystalline keratopathy; scleritis.

Clinical

Pharyngitis; impetigo; scarlet fever; pneumonia; bacteremia; rheumatic fever; glomerulonephritis.

Laboratory

Gram-positive cocci growing in pairs or chains. Throat culture and sensitivity are useful.

Treatment

Penicillin is the drug of choice.

BIBLIOGRAPHY

1. Zabawski EJ. (2011). Scarlet fever. [online] Available from www.emedicine.com/emerg/TOPIC518.HTM. [Accessed September, 2013].

38.1G. HAEMOPHILUS AEGYPTIUS (KOCH-WEEKS BACILLUS)

General

Caused by Gram-negative Koch-Weeks bacillus in warm climate regions; characterized by a 24- to 48-hour incubation period; now classified as *H. influenzae* biotype III; *H. influenzae* is divided into biotypes based on biochemical reactions (indole production, urease activity, ornithine decarboxylase activity) and into serotypes based on their capsular polysaccharides; common cause of purulent conjunctivitis and preseptal cellulitis in children.

Ocular

Conjunctivitis; corneal opacity; corneal ulcer; phlyctenular keratoconjunctivitis; keratitis; cellulitis of lid; pseudoptosis; uveitis; petechial subconjunctival hemorrhages.

Clinical

Coryza; systemic symptoms are rare.

Laboratory

Poorly staining Gram-negative bacilli or coccobacilli. Culture on chocolate agar.

Treatment

Antibiotics are the mainstay of treatment. Invasive and serious infections are best treated with an intravenous third-generation cephalosporin until antibiotic sensitivities are available.

BIBLIOGRAPHY

1. Devarajan VR. (2012) Haemophilus influenzae infections. [online] Available from. www.emedicine.com/med/TOPIC936.HTM. [Accessed September, 2013].

38.1G. HAEMOPHILUS INFLUENZAE

General

Gram-negative rod.

Ocular

Conjunctivitis; cellulitis; tenonitis; uveitis; vitreous opacity; pannus; corneal opacity.

Clinical

Pharyngitis; epiglottitis; laryngotracheitis; pneumonia; bronchitis; otitis media; meningitis; cellulitis; septic arthritis; sinusitis.

Laboratory

Gram-negative coccobacillus with eight biotypes and six serotypes. Gram stain and culture.

Treatment

Antibiotics are the mainstay of treatment. Invasive and serious infections are best treated with an intravenous third-generation cephalosporin until antibiotic sensitivities are available.

BIBLIOGRAPHY

1. Devarajan VR. (2012). Haemophilus influenzae infections. [online] Available from www.emedicine.com/med/TOPIC936.HTM. [Accessed September, 2013].

⊟ 38.1G. PSEUDOMONAS AERUGINOSA

General

Gram-negative rod that is ubiquitous in water, soil and plants. Commonly found in hospital environment.

Clinical

None.

Ocular

Foreign body sensation, conjunctival injection, and photophobia, and corneal ulceration.

Laboratory

Gram-negative rod on Gram stain and Giemsa stain from corneal ulcer. Culturing contact lens and lens solutions may help to grow organisms.

Treatment

Fortified tobramycin and fortified cefazolin are drugs of choice.

⊟ BIBLIOGRAPHY

1. Roy FH, Fraunfelder FW, Fraunfelder FT. Roy and Fraunfelder's Current Ocular Therapy, 6th edition. London: Elsevier; 2008.

⊟ 38.1G. ESCHERICHIA COLI

General

Gram-negative rod found in the gastrointestinal tract; urinary tract is the usual portal of entry.

Ocular

Uveitis; hyphema; hypopyon; gas bubbles in anterior chamber; purulent conjunctivitis; keratitis; corneal edema; panophthalmitis; endophthalmitis; glaucoma.

Clinical

Diarrhea; gastroenteritis; dehydration.

Laboratory

Anaerobic Gram-negative rod.

Treatment

Antibiotic therapy should start with ampicillin until sensitivity reports return.

⊟ BIBLIOGRAPHY

1. Suh DW. (2011). Ophthalmologic manifestations of Escherichia coli. [online] Available from www.emedicine.com/oph/TOPIC496.HTM. [Accessed September, 2013].

⊟ 38.1G. BACILLUS SUBTILIS (HAY BACILLUS)

General

Gram-positive rod found in air, soil, dust, water, milk, and hay; frequently seen in people who work near hay.

Ocular

Conjunctivitis; ring abscess of cornea; corneal ulcer; endophthalmitis; panophthalmitis; dacryocystitis; orbit abscess.

Clinical

Fever; leukocytosis.

Laboratory

Diagnosis is made by clinical findings.

Treatment

- *Conjunctivitis:* Antibiotic medication should be used to treat the infection.
- *Corneal ulcer:* Corneal cultures may be taken and treatment initiated. Treatment includes a broad spectrum of antibiotics and cycloplegic drops.

38.1G. SHIGELLOSIS (BACILLARY DYSENTERY)

General

Caused by *Shigella*; frequently passed through food and via food handlers; more commonly seen in countries with poor sanitation; evidence suggests that the ability of *Shigella* to invade and multiply within the corneal epithelium is similar to the invasion in the intestinal epithelium.

Ocular

Scleroconjunctivitis; severe uveitis; conjunctival xerosis.

Clinical

Fever; abdominal pain; diarrhea; intestinal perforation; toxic megacolon; dehydration; there has been one case reported of an association with the Klüver-Bucy syndrome.

Laboratory

Stool culture and blood cultures.

Treatment

Oral rehydration and antibiotic treatment.

BIBLIOGRAPHY

1. Kroser JA. (2013). Shigellosis. [online] Available from www.emedicine.com/med/TOPIC2112.HTM. [Accessed September, 2013].
2. Farber HJ, Guillerman RP. (2012). Pediatric hypersensitivity pneumonitis. [online] Available from www.emedicine.com/ped/TOPIC2577.HTM. [Accessed September, 2013].

38.1G. TUBERCULOSIS

General

Communicable disease caused by the acid-fast bacillus *Mycobacterium tuberculosis*.

Ocular

Conjunctivitis; subconjunctival nodules (tuberculomas); keratitis; pannus; corneal ulcer; blepharitis; cellulitis; meibomianitis; uveitis; dacryocystitis; chronic orbital cellulitis; retinitis; scleritis; scleral perforation; hypopyon; vitreous hemorrhages; optic neuritis; optic atrophy; tuberculous panophthalmitis; choroidal tubercles; intraorbital extraocular lesions.

Clinical

Pulmonary infection; pyuria; hematuria; epididymitis; dysuria; flank pain; distorted calyces; productive cough.

Laboratory

Acid-fast bacillus culture of body fluids including vitreous and aqueous. PCR is 89% positive for pulmonary infection.

Treatment

A course of chemotherapy (isoniazid, rifampin, pyrazinamide and ethambutol or streptomycin) for a period of 6 months is the recommended therapy.

BIBLIOGRAPHY

1. Collins JK. Handbook of Clinical Ophthalmology. New York: Masson; 1982.
2. D'Souza P, Garg R, Dhaliwal RS, et al. Orbital tuberculosis. Int Ophthalmol. 1994;18:149-52.
3. DeVoe AG, Locatcher-Khorazo D. The external manifestations of ocular tuberculosis. Trans Am Ophthalmol Soc. 1964;62:203-12.
4. Roy, FH, Fraunfelder FT, Fraunfelder FH. Roy and Fraunfeldr's Current Ocular Therapy, 6th editon. London: Elseuier 2008.
5. Gupta V, Gupta A, Arora S, et al. Presumed tubercular serpiginous like choroiditis. Ophthalmology. 2003;110:1744-9.
6. Patkar S, Singhania BK, Agrawal A. Intraorbital extraocular tuberculosis: a report of three cases. Surg Neurol. 1994;42:320-1.
7. Tejada P, Mendez MJ, Negreira S. Choroidal tubercles with tuberculous meningitis. Int Ophthalmol. 1994;18:115-8.

38.2A. EPIDEMIC KERATOCONJUNCTIVITIS

General

Highly communicable; adenovirus types 8 and 19; usually bilateral; epidemic keratoconjunctivitis has been reported worldwide associated with 11 virus serotypes, with serotypes 8, 11 and 19 being the most common responsible ones.

Ocular

Follicular or membranous conjunctivitis; chemosis; subconjunctival hemorrhages; corneal opacity; punctate epithelial keratitis; corneal ulcer; blepharospasm; lid edema; serous discharge; uveitis; epiphora.

Clinical

Submaxillary and cervical lymphadenopathy.

Laboratory

Viral isolation on cell culture from conjunctival scrapings.

Treatment

No effective topical or systemic treatment is available. Topical steroids may be used if epithelial keratitis occurs.

BIBLIOGRAPHY

1. Bawazeer A, Hodge WG. (2011). Epidemic keratoconjunctivitis. [online] Available from www.emedicine.com/oph/TOPIC677.HTM. [Accessed September, 2013].

38.2B. HERPES SIMPLEX

General

Large, complex DNA virus.

Ocular

Conjunctivitis; keratitis; iridocyclitis; corneal ulcer; uveitis; hyphema; hypopyon; iris atrophy; cataract; scleritis; dacryoadenitis; blepharitis; acute retinal necrosis.

Clinical

Recurrent skin vesicles on lids, perioral area, nose and genitalia; meningitis, encephalitis.

Laboratory

Viral cultures.

Treatment

Antiviral therapy, topical or oral, is an effective treatment of epithelial herpes infection.

BIBLIOGRAPHY

1. Shaohui L, Pavan-Langston D, Colby KA. Pediatric herpes simplex of the anterior segment. Ophthalmology. 2012;119: 2003-8.
2. Wang JC, Ritterband DC. (2012). Ophthalmologic manifestations of herpes simplex. [online] Available from www.emedicine.com/oph/TOPIC100.HTM. [Accessed September, 2013].

38.2C HERPES ZOSTER

General

Caused by varicella zoster virus; about 75% of cases occur in persons over age of 45 years; condition is more frequent with advancing age and in patients who are immunocompromised by drugs or disease; in particular, an increasing number of patients with herpes zoster ophthalmicus are immunosuppressed.

Ocular

Conjunctivitis; keratitis; recurrent corneal ulcer; neuralgia; zoster rash of eyelids; uveitis; iris atrophy; scleritis; cataract; optic neuritis; paralysis of third nerve; proptosis; paralysis of lids; orbital apex syndrome; retinitis; neurotrophic keratitis; acute retinal necrosis; progressive outer retinal necrosis; ocular motor nerve pareses; tonic pupil; encephalitis; vasculitis.

Clinical

Local lesions involving the posterior or root ganglia; nerve damage; tissue scarring.

Laboratory

Diagnosed mostly on the basis of the characteristic pain and appearance of the dermatomal rashes.

Treatment

Antiviral agents, systemic corticosteroids, antidepressants, and adequate pain control. Immunocompetent adults aged 60 years or older, benefit from receipt of the herpes zoster vaccine and have a lower incidence of herpes zoster.

🗗 BIBLIOGRAPHY

1. Ghaznawi N, Virdi A, Dayan A, et al. Herpes zoster ophthalmicus: comparison of disease in patients 60 years and older versus younger than 60 years. Ophthalmology. 2011;118:2242-50.
2. Ho J, Xirasagar S, Lin H. Increased risk of a cancer diagnosis after herpes zoster ophthalmicus: a nationwide population-based study. Ophthalmology. 2011;118:1076-81.
3. Tseng HF, Smith N, Harpaz R, et al. Herpes zoster vaccine in older adults and the risk of subsequent herpes zoster disease. JAMA. 2011;305:160-6.

🗗 38.2D. REITER SYNDROME (FIESSINGER-LEROY SYNDROME; CONJUNCTIVO-URETHRO-SYNOVIAL SYNDROME; IDIOPATHIC BLENNORRHEAL ARTHRITIS SYNDROME; POLYARTHRITIS ENTERICA)

General

Etiology unknown; males; onset ages 16–42 years; probably a combined infectious/autoimmune pathogenetic mechanism; reactive arthritis probably associated with infection with many different species of microorganisms; HLA-B27 confers disease susceptibility to infection.

Ocular

Sterile mucopurulent conjunctivitis, usually bilateral; photophobia; epiphora; iritis; keratitis; uveitis; paralysis of extraocular muscles; optic neuritis; secondary glaucoma; hypopyon; hyphema.

Clinical

Skin erythema; genital ulcerations; urethritis with discharge; cystitis with dysuria, abacterial pyuria, and hematuria; arthritis with pain, swelling, heat, and effusion; fever; weight loss; fatigue; malaise; fever; diarrhea; oral mucosal lesions; arthralgia.

Laboratory

Giemsa stain may reveal Gram-negative intracellular diplococci associated with gonorrhea. Stool cultures may also be helpful for enteric pathogens. HLA-B27 antigen testing will not provide a diagnosis but may be useful.

Treatment

Systemic antibiotics are useful. Topical corticosteroids and mydriatics should be administered early to minimize tissue damage. NSAIDs may help to reduce ocular inflammation.

🗗 BIBLIOGRAPHY

1. Bashour M. (2012). Ophthalmologic manifestations of reactive arthritis. [online] Available from www.emedicine.com/oph/TOPIC524.HTM. [Accessed September, 2013].

🗗 38.2E. VACCINIA (KERATITIS)

General

Laboratory virus used for vaccination against smallpox.

Ocular

Pustules of lids; edema of lids; conjunctivitis; orbital cellulitis; keratitis; pannus; corneal perforation; iridocyclitis; central serous retinopathy; perivasculitis; pseudoretinitis pigmentosa; ocular palsies papillitis; optic atrophy.

Clinical

Vesicles; pustules; erythema; fever; malaise; axillary lymphadenopathy; necrosis of skin; vaccinia gangrenosa; encephalomyelitis; drowsiness; vomiting; coma; death.

Laboratory

Immune deficiency workup should be considered as well as imaging studies.

Treatment

VIG can be helpful in selected patients.

⊟ BIBLIOGRAPHY

1. Lee JJ, Diven D, Poonawalla TA, et al. (2012). Vaccinia. [online] Available from www.emedicine.com/med/TOP-IC2356.HTM. [Accessed Sepetember, 2013].

⊟ 38.3. CANDIDIASIS

General

Yeast-like opportunistic fungal infection caused by *C. albicans.*

Ocular

Uveitis; hypopyon; conjunctivitis; keratitis; corneal ulcer; blepharitis; endophthalmitis; dacryocystitis; papillitis; retinal atrophy; Roth spot; vitreous abscess; retrobulbar abscess; retinal detachment; panophthalmitis; chorioretinitis; infectious crystalline keratopathy.

Clinical

C. albicans normally is present as an intestinal saprophyte in 35–75% of the human population; in situations of internal environmental change, however, *Candida* can become pathogenic (e.g. obesity, diabetes mellitus, malignancy, and other debilitating conditions).

Laboratory

Common yeast from up to 50% of healthy individuals isolated directly from the eye should be attempted to confirm the presence of organism. Blood agar and Sabouraud's dextrose agar may be used; PCR for species identification.

Treatment

Mucocutaneous infection typically responds to topical therapy. Antifungal therapy should be started immediately after necessary cultures have been obtained from all suspected sites of infection. Infectious disease specialists are typically involved in cases of invasive candidiasis.

⊟ BIBLIOGRAPHY

1. Hedayati T. (2012). Candidiasis in emergency medicine. [online] Available from www.emedicine.com/emerg/TOP-IC76.HTM. [Accessed September, 2013].

⊟ 38.4A. STEVENS-JOHNSON SYNDROME [DERMATOSTOMATITIS; ERYTHEMA MULTIFORME EXUDATIVUM; SYNDROMA MUCOCUTANEO-OCULARE; BAADER DERMATOSTOMATITIS SYNDROME; MUCOSAL-RESPIRATORY SYNDROME; FUCHS (2) SYNDROME; MUCOCUTANEOUS OCULAR SYNDROME]

General

Etiology unknown; affects all ages; most frequently seen in 1st and 3rd decades of life; prevalent in males; drugs are the most commonly identified etiologic factor in this condition.

Ocular

Hypopyon; iritis; keratitis; corneal ulcers; keratoconjunctivitis sicca; chemosis; conjunctivitis; widespread fibrinoid necrosis of conjunctival vessels; blepharitis; endophthalmitis; phthisis bulbi; uveitis; cataracts; pannus; optic neuritis; keratoconus; adenoviral conjunctivitis has been reported to have precipitated Stevens-Johnson syndrome; orbital cyst may be a complication.

Clinical

General malaise, headaches, chills, and fever; severe skin and mucous membrane eruptions (erythema multiforme); dorsa of hands and feet are most frequently affected; rhinitis; balanitis; vulvovaginitis; urethritis (nonspecific); cystitis; patients with AIDS are at higher risk of developing Stevens-Johnson syndrome.

Laboratory

No laboratory tests are specific to Stevens-Johnson syndrome. Diagnosis is made from clinical findings.

Treatment

Systemic treatment with steroids is controversial. Antibiotics are used based on clinical course. Eyelid hygiene performed as needed.

⊟ BIBLIOGRAPHY

1. Plaza JA, Dronen SC, Foster J, et al. (2011). Erythema multiforme. [online] Available from www.emedicine.com/med/TOPIC727.HTM. [Accessed September, 2013].

⊟ 38.4C SCALDED SKIN SYNDROME (TOXIC EPIDERMAL NECROLYSIS; RITTER DISEASE; TOXIC EPIDERMAL NECROLYSIS OF LYELL; STAPHYLOCOCCAL SCALDED SKIN SYNDROME; LYELL SYNDROME; EPIDERMOLYSIS ACUTA TOXICA; TOXIC EPIDERMAL NECROLYSIS) SYMBLEPHARON

General

Generalized exfoliative dermatitis frequently affecting neonates and resulting from an initial focal staphylococcal infection (i.e. staphylococcal ophthalmia neonatorum); toxic epidermal necrolysis usually refers to manifestation in the adult secondary to a drug reaction but affects all ages; immunopathogenetic mechanisms probably initiated with drug-skin binding with aberrant immune responses, including complement and immunoglobulin G deposition with the epidermis and mucosa; recent reports suggest that patients with the AIDS are at higher risk for developing mucocutaneous reactions, such as toxic epidermal necrolysis; mortality rate approximately 30%.

Ocular

Necrotic areas of lids, conjunctiva, and cornea; symblepharon; loss of corneal epithelium; corneal ulcer; leukoma; perforation of globe; abolition of lacrimal secretion; conjunctival chemosis; blepharitis; entropion; periorbital swelling; trichiasis; distichiasis; fornix shortening.

Clinical

Widespread reddening and tenderness of the skin followed by the exfoliation of large areas of skin; in children, erythema starts usually around the mouth and spreads over the entire body within hours, followed by blisters and large exudative lesions; fever; shock.

Laboratory

Culture and biopsy of the lesion.

Treatment

Intravenous penicillinase-resistant and antistaphylococcal antibiotics. Cloxacillin is the treatment of choice.

⊟ BIBLIOGRAPHY

1. Lopez-Garcia JS, Jara LR, Garcia-Lozano CI, et al. Ocular features and histopathologic changes during follow-up of toxic epidermal necrolysis. Ophthalmology. 2011;118:265-71.
2. Kim JH, Benson P. (2012). Dermatologic manifestations of staphylococcal scalded skin syndrome. [online] Available from www.emedicine.com/derm/TOPIC402.HTM. [Accessed September, 2013].

⊟ 38.4D. PEMPHIGUS VULGARIS

General

Primarily in middle-aged people; prognosis varies, from poor to chronic; generalized bullous eruption; blistering autoimmune disease that affects the skin and mucous membranes; association between particular HLA-DR4 and pemphigus vulgaris has been reported.

Ocular

Conjunctival bullae; catarrhal conjunctivitis; scarring and adhesions of conjunctiva.

Clinical

Cutaneous blisters, which may be clear, pustular, or hemorrhagic.

Laboratory

Histopathology from the edge of a blister, indirect immunofluorescence (IDIF) using the patient's serum if direct immunofluorescence (DIF) is positive.

Treatment

Corticosteroids, and immunosuppressive drugs are useful.

BIBLIOGRAPHY

1. Zeina B, Sakka N, Mansoor S. (2013). Pemphigus vulgaris. [online] Available from www.emedicine.com/derm/TOPIC319.HTM. [Accessed September, 2013].

38.5A. ACID BURNS OF THE EYE

General

Acid injuries of the eyes are characterized by protein coagulation and precipitation with the anion. Direct tissue damage produced by the hydrogen ion.

Clinical

None.

Ocular

Chemosis, corneal epithelial defects, limbal blanching, corneal clouding, photophobia, corneal neovascularization, symblepharon formation.

Laboratory

Diagnosis is made from clinical history and findings.

Treatment

Immediate irrigation, topical antibiotics for bacterial infection if needed, contact lenses aid in re-epithelialization of the cornea.

BIBLIOGRAPHY

1. Roy FH, Fraunfelder FW, Fraunfelder FT. Roy and Fraunfelder's Current Ocular Therapy, 6th edition. London: Elsevier; 2008.

38.5B. ALKALINE INJURY OF THE EYE

General

A splash of alkaline solution causes the pH to rise and results in immediate damage to the external ocular tissues. These injuries are frequently seen from household chemicals or farming injuries from liquid ammonia used as fertilizer.

Ocular

Pain; lacrimation; blepharospasm; rise in IOP; rapid penetration of the cornea and sclera; chemical injury to iris, lens or ciliary body; symblepharon; phthisis bulbi; ankyloblepharon.

Laboratory

Diagnosis is made by clinical findings and history.

Treatment

Immediate copious irrigation, sticky paste of lime should be removed with a cotton-tipped applicator, mydriasis and topical antibiotics, pain medications, treatment of glaucoma with carbonic anhydrase inhibitors, patching and soft contact lenses may facilitate re-epithelialization, insertion of a methyl methacrylate ring may prevent fibrinous adhesions, lysis of adhesions with or without mucous membrane grafts, corneal stem cell transplantation, corneal transplantation, keratoprosthesis and conjunctival autographs.

BIBLIOGRAPHY

1. Roy FH, Fraunfelder FW, Fraunfelder FT. Roy and Fraunfelder's Current Ocular Therapy, 6th edition. London: Elsevier; 2008.

38.6. GRAFT VERSUS HOST DISEASE

General

Major complication of bone marrow transplantation; donor T lymphocytes attack recipient's cells; targets are skin, liver, intestine, oral mucosa, conjunctiva, lacrimal gland, vaginal mucosa, and esophageal mucosa.

Ocular

Keratoconjunctivitis; photophobia; hemorrhagic conjunctivitis; proptosis; intraretinal hemorrhages; nerve palsy; herpes simplex/herpes zoster manifestations; uveitis; corneal epithelial denudement; conjunctival scarring; dry eye syndrome; corneal melt; dacryoadenitis; keratoconjunctivitis sicca; cataract; retinitis.

Clinical

Leukemia; aplastic anemia; exanthematous dermatitis; hepatitis; enteritis; scleroderma-like involvement of skin; chronic liver dysfunction; recurrent bacterial infections.

Laboratory

Diagnosis is made by clinical findings.

Treatment

- *Keratoconjunctivitis:* Ocular lubricants, nonsteroidal anti-inflammatory and steroid drops, oral nonsteroidal anti-inflammatory or steroids. Supratarsol steroids. Surgical excision, cryotherapy and beta irradiation of papillae.
- *Proptosis:* Reversing the problem which is causing the exophthalmos is the treatment of choice and will minimize the ocular complications. Ocular lubricants are beneficial for control of the corneal exposure.

BIBLIOGRAPHY

1. Chang-Godinich A, Raizman MB. (2013). Atopic keratoconjunctivitis. [online] Available from www.emedicine.com/oph/TOPIC102.HTM. [Accessed September, 2013].

38.7. HOOF AND MOUTH DISEASE

General

Viral etiology.

Ocular

Conjunctival painful red blisters.

Clinical

Mucous membranes develop painful red blisters; lymph glands swollen; preauricular lymphadenopathy.

Laboratory

Clinical features include the classic corneal dendrites of HSV infection and follicular conjunctivitis, and preauricular adenopathy associated with adenoviral infection.

Treatment

Cold compresses and lubricants, such as artificial tears, for comfort; antibiotic may be used to prevent bacterial superinfection. Topical steroids may be used for pseudomembranes.

BIBLIOGRAPHY

1. Pau H. Differential Diagnosis of Eye Disease. New York: Thieme; 1987.

38.8. HAEMOPHILUS AEGYPTIUS (KOCH-WEEKS BACILLUS)

General

It is caused by Gram-negative Koch-Weeks bacillus in warm climate regions; characterized by a 24- to 48-hour incubation period; now classified as *H. influenzae* biotype III; *H. influenzae* is divided into biotypes based on biochemical reactions (indole production, urease activity, ornithine decarboxylase activity) and into serotypes based on their capsular polysaccharides; common cause of purulent conjunctivitis and preseptal cellulitis in children.

Ocular

Conjunctivitis; corneal opacity; corneal ulcer; phlyctenular keratoconjunctivitis; keratitis; cellulitis of lid; pseudoptosis; uveitis; petechial subconjunctival hemorrhages.

Clinical

Coryza; systemic symptoms are rare.

Laboratory

Poorly staining Gram-negative bacilli or coccobacilli. Culture on chocolate agar.

Treatment

Antibiotics are the mainstay of treatment. Invasive and serious infections are best treated with an intravenous third-generation cephalosporin until antibiotic sensitivities are available.

BIBLIOGRAPHY

1. Devarajan VR. (2012) Haemophilus influenzae infections. [online] Available from. www.emedicine.com/med/TOPIC936.HTM. [Accessed September, 2013].

38.9. LIGNEOUS CONJUNCTIVITIS

General

Rare form of recurrent conjunctivitis, usually bilateral in infants or children.

Clinical

None.

Ocular

Inflammation characterized by formation of thick membranes and pseudomembranes to the lid.

Laboratory

Histology, plasminogen activity and plasminogen antigen levels.

Treatment

Surgical excision of conjunctival membrane followed by cautery, cryopexy and grafting with conjunctiva or sclera.

BIBLIOGRAPHY

1. Roy FH, Fraunfelder FW, Fraunfelder FT. Roy and Fraunfelder's Current Ocular Therapy, 6th edition. London, UK: Elsevier; 2008.

38.10. URBACH-WIETHE SYNDROME (ROSSLE-URBACH-WIETHE SYNDROME; LIPOPROTEINOSIS; HYALINOSIS CUTIS ET MUCOSAE; LIPOID PROTEINOSIS; PROTEINOSIS-LIPOIDOSIS) DRY EYES

General

Rare autosomal recessive disorder in which hyaline material is deposited in the skin, mucous membranes, and brain; both sexes affected; onset in infancy; relatively benign progressive course; association with diabetes mellitus.

Ocular

Margin of eyelids may show bead-like excrescences with loss of cilia; itching of eyes; dry eyes.

Clinical

Skin about face covered with small, yellowish-white, waxy nodules; alopecia; hoarseness of voice at birth or within first few years of life; tongue large, thick; hyperkeratotic lesions on knees, elbows, and fingers; inability to cry; dry mouth.

Laboratory

Erythrocyte sedimentation rate, polymerase chain amplification and direct nucleotide sequence of the ECM1 gene.

Treatment

No cure is known.

BIBLIOGRAPHY

1. Cordoro KM, Osleber MF, De Leo VA. (2013). Lipoid proteinosis. [online] Available from www.emedicine.com/derm/TOPIC241.HTM. [Accessed September, 2013].

🖭 38.11. SUPERIOR LIMBIC KERATOCONJUNCTIVITIS (THEODORES SUPERIOR LIMBIC KERATOCONJUNCTIVITIS, SLK)

General

Corneal disease affecting the superior limbus.

Clinical

None.

Ocular

Hyperemia, thickened upper bulbar conjunctiva in a "corridor-like" distribution, fine papillary inflammation of superior palpebral conjunctival, punctuate erosion over the superior and perilimbal cornea and superior filamentary keratopathy.

Laboratory

Giemsa-stained scraping of upper conjunctiva demonstrates keratinized cells.

Treatment

Topical lubricants and mast cells stabilizers, punctal plugs, silver nitrate treatment on upper tarsal and bulbar conjunctiva, bandage contact lens, brief focal applications of thermal cautery and recession of involved superior bulbar conjunctiva.

🖭 BIBLIOGRAPHY

1. Oakman JH. (2011). Superior limbic keratoconjunctivitis. [online] Available from www.emedicine.com/oph/TOPIC103.HTM. [Accessed September, 2013].

🖭 38.13. WEGENER SYNDROME (WEGENER GRANULOMATOSIS)

General

Etiology unknown; occurs in 4th and 5th decades of life; persistent rhinitis or sinusitis; three characteristic features are: (1) necrotizing granulomatous lesions in the respiratory tract, (2) generalized focal arthritis, and (3) necrotizing thrombotic glomerulitis.

Ocular

Exophthalmos; lid and conjunctival chemosis; papillitis; conjunctivitis; corneal ulcer; corneal abscess; optic atrophy; optic neuritis; orbital cellulitis; episcleritis; sclerokeratitis; cataract; peripheral ring corneal ulcers; ptosis; dacryocystitis; retinal periphlebitis; cotton-wool spots; retinal and vitreous hemorrhages; rubeosis iridis; neovascular glaucoma.

Clinical

Severe sinusitis; pulmonary inflammation; arteritis; weakness; fever; weight loss; bony destruction; granulomatous vasculitis of the upper and lower respiratory tracts; glomerulonephritis; diffuse pulmonary infiltrates; lymphadenopathy; diffuse pulmonary hemorrhage; overlap with giant cell arteritis.

Laboratory

Histopathology: necrotizing, granulomatous vasculitis with infiltrating neutrophils, lymphocytes and giant cells; urine—proteinuria, hematuria and urinary casts.

Treatment

Topical eye lubricants, ophthalmic antibiotic solution or ointments and corticosteroid drops may prove to be beneficial. Orbital decompression is needed when medical treatment is unresponsive to treat optic nerve compression.

🖭 BIBLIOGRAPHY

1. Collins JF. Handbook of Clinical Ophthalmology. New York, Chicago: Year Book Medical Publication Masson; 1982.
2. Flach AJ. Ocular manifestations of Wegener's granulomatosis [Letter]. JAMA. 1995;274(15):1199-200.

3. Haynes BF, Fishman ML, Fauci AS, et al. The ocular manifestations of Wegener's Wegener's granulomatosis. Fifteen years' experience and review of the literature. Am J Med. 1977;63(1):131-141.

4. Leavitt RY, Fauci AS. Less common manifestations and presentations of Wegener's Wegener's granulomatosis. Curr Opin Rheumatol. 1992;4(1):16-22.

5. Robinson MR, Lee SS, Sneller MC, et al. Tarsal-conjunctival disease associated with Wegener's granulomatosis. Ophthalmology. 2003;110(9): 1770-1780.

6. Roy FH, Fraunfelder FW, Fraunfelder FT. Roy and Fraunfelder's Current Ocular Therapy, 6th edition. Philadelphia: WB Saunders; 2008.

7. Straatsma BR. Ocular manifestations of Wegener granulomatosis. Am J Ophthalmol. 1957;44(6):789-99.

🖽 39. PTERYGIUM OF CONJUNCTIVA AND CORNEA

General

Autosomal dominant; more frequent in people who work outdoors; occurs late in life.

Ocular

Wing-shaped thickening in the conjunctiva, usually nasal, in the interpalpebral fissure area; alterations in corneal topography can cause a reduction in visual acuity.

Clinical

None.

Laboratory

Diagnosis is made by clinical findings.

Treatment

Patients with pterygia can be observed unless the lesions exhibit growth toward the center of the cornea or the patient exhibits symptoms of significant redness, discomfort, or alterations in visual function. Surgery for excision of pterygia is beneficial if visual function is disturbed.

🖽 BIBLIOGRAPHY

1. Fisher JP, Trattler WB. (2011). Pterygium. [online] Available from www.emedicine.com/oph/TOPIC542.HTM. [Accessed September, 2013].

🖽 40. PURULENT CONJUNCTIVITIS

Purulent conjunctivitis is characterized as violent acute conjunctival inflamation, great swelling of lids, copious secretion of pus, and a marked tendency to corneal involvement and even possible loss of the eye.

1. Gram-positive group
   - †A. Bacillus of Doderlein (*Lactobacillus* sp.)
   - †B. *Listeria monocytogenes*
   - *C. Pneumococcus
   - D. Staphylococcus
   - *E. Streptococcus
2. Gram-negative group
   - †A. *Aerobacter aerogenes*
   - B. Enterobacteriaceae
   - C. *E. coli*
   - *D. *H. influenzae* biotype III
   - E. *Klebsiella*
   - F. *M. lacunata*
   - *G. *N. gonorrhoeae*
   - H. *N. meningitidis*
   - I. *Proteus* species
   - J. *Pseudomonas* species
   - †K. *Serratia marcescens*
3. Vaccinia virus
4. Fungus
   - A. *Actinomyces* species
   - B. *Candida* species
   - *C. *Nocardia* species
5. Wiskott-Aldrich syndrome: X-linked

---

*Indicates most frequent
†Indicates a general entry and therefore has not been described in detail in the text

BIBLIOGRAPHY

1. Fedukowicz HB. External infections of the eye: Bacterial, Viral, Mycotic, 3rd edition. New York: Appleton-Century-Crofts; 1984.

2. Roy FH. Ocular Syndromes and Systemic Diseases, 5th edition. New Delhi: Jaypee Brothers Medical Publishers; 2013.
3. Snead JW, Stern WH, Whitcher JP, et al. Listeria monocytogenes endophthalmitis. Am J Ophthalmol. 1977; 84:337-44.

40.1C. PNEUMOCOCCAL INFECTIONS (STREPTOCOCCUS PNEUMONIAE INFECTIONS)

General

Gram-positive diplococcus *S. pneumoniae;* some strains are encapsulated while others are not; ocular infections usually are caused by the encapsulated strains; conjunctivitis and corneal scarring produced in an animal model have been attributed to a hemolytic cytolytic exopeptidase.

Ocular

Hypopyon; conjunctivitis; keratitis; corneal ulcer; endophthalmitis; dacryocystitis; uveitis; orbital cellulitis; secondary glaucoma; ophthalmia neonatorum.

Clinical

Upper respiratory infection; chills; sharp pain in hemithorax; cough with sputum production; fever; headache; gastrointestinal symptoms.

Laboratory

Gram stain demonstrates Gram-positive cocci in pairs. The unattached end of each cocci is slightly pointed outward.

Treatment

Impetigo, oral antibiotics and topical antibiotic ointment; preseptal cellulitis, oral antibiotics; orbital cellulitis, need team of infectious diseases, otolaryngology and ophthalmology to develop plan of therapy; dacryocystitis, oral and topical antibiotics, dacryocystorhinostomy may be necessary; conjunctivitis, topical antibiotic; keratitis, topical antibiotics; poststreptococcal reactive arthritis can occur with uveitis, topical steroids and cycloplegics; endophthalmitis, prompt and aggressive therapy with topical, intravitreal and sometimes systemic antibiotics and pars plana vitrectomy; post-refractive surgery keratitis, flap raised, cultured and treated. Occasionally the flap should be amputated.

BIBLIOGRAPHY

1. Muench DF. (2012). Pneumococcal infections. [online] Available from www.emedicine.com/med/TOPIC1848.HTM. [Accessed September, 2013].

40.1D. STAPHYLOCOCCUS

General

Gram-positive coccus *S. aureus;* most common cause of suppurative infection in humans; more common in patients with a previous disorders, such as diabetes, thyroid disease, renal failure, or malnutrition; although most *S. aureus* isolates from other sources are encapsulated, capsules have not been noted in ocular isolates.

Ocular

Uveitis; hypopyon; conjunctivitis; keratitis; cellulitis of lid; meibomianitis; ptosis; blepharitis; endophthalmitis; dacryocystitis; increased IOP; orbital periosteitis.

Clinical

Tissues hypertonic, edematous, and painful; lesion liquefies, forming creamy yellow pus; fever; nausea; vomiting; cough; dyspnea; abdominal pain; diarrhea; bloody stools; dehydration; shock.

Laboratory

Aerobic Gram-positive cocci bacteria grow in grape-like clusters. Coagulase positive indicates pathogenicity.

Treatment

Specific antimicrobial therapy is chosen based on the site and severity of the infection and the antimicrobial sensitivities of the organism involved.

BIBLIOGRAPHY

1. Tolan RW. (2012). Staphylococcus aureus infection. [online] Available from www.emedicine.com/ped/TOPIC2704.HTM. [Accessed September, 2013].

40.1E. STREPTOCOCCUS (SCARLET FEVER)

General

Gram-positive bacteria that can invade any tissue.

Ocular

Conjunctivitis; corneal ulcer; blepharitis; scarlatinal rash of lid; erysipelas dermatitis of lid; gangrene of lid; endophthalmitis; proptosis; dacryocystitis; optic neuritis; orbital cellulitis; uveitis; hypopyon; secondary glaucoma; paralysis of extraocular muscles; infectious crystalline keratopathy; scleritis.

Clinical

Pharyngitis; impetigo; scarlet fever; pneumonia; bacteremia; rheumatic fever; glomerulonephritis.

Laboratory

Gram-positive cocci growing in pairs or chains. Throat culture and sensitivity are useful.

Treatment

Penicillin is the drug of choice.

BIBLIOGRAPHY

1. Zabawski EJ. (2011). Scarlet fever. [online] Available from www.emedicine.com/emerg/TOPIC518.HTM. [Accessed September, 2013].

40.2B. ENTEROBIASIS (OXYURIASIS; PINWORM; SEATWORM)

General

Intestinal infection caused by *Enterobius vermicularis*; worm's head attached to cecal mucosa, appendix, or parts of bowel; worms travel anal canal and deposit eggs on perianal skin; eggs infective for 10–20 days; airborne transmission; common in children; extraintestinal pinworm infection has been reported.

Ocular

Palpebral edema; blepharitis; keratoconjunctivitis; macular edema.

Clinical

Pruritus; eczema; pyogenic infection; vaginal discharge; chronic granulomatous salpingitis; endometritis.

Laboratory

Wide (2 inch) transparent tape is pressed against the perineum at night or in the morning before the patient bathes to capture eggs. Three such specimens are usually consecutively collected. Diagnosis is made by identifying eggs under the low-power lens of microscope. Dilute sodium hydroxide or toluene should be added to the slide.

Treatment

Mebendazole or albendazole are recommended as first-line treatment of pinworms. Simultaneously treating all household members may be reasonable.

BIBLIOGRAPHY

1. Wolfram W, Curry JL, Indra S. (2013). Enterobiasis. [online] Available from www.emedicine.com/ped/TOPIC684.HTM. [Accessed September, 2013].

40.2C. ESCHERICHIA COLI

General

Gram-negative rod found in the gastrointestinal tract; urinary tract is the usual portal of entry.

Ocular

Uveitis; hyphema; hypopyon; gas bubbles in anterior chamber; purulent conjunctivitis; keratitis; corneal edema; panophthalmitis; endophthalmitis; glaucoma.

Clinical

Diarrhea; gastroenteritis; dehydration.

Laboratory

Anaerobic Gram-negative rod.

Treatment

Antibiotic therapy should start with ampicillin until sensitivity reports return.

⊟ BIBLIOGRAPHY

1. Suh DW. (2011). Ophthalmologic manifestations of Escherichia coli. [online] Available from www.emedicine.com/oph/TOPIC496.HTM. [Accessed September, 2013].

⊟ 40.2D. HAEMOPHILUS INFLUENZAE

General

Gram-negative rod.

Ocular

Conjunctivitis; cellulitis; tenonitis; uveitis; vitreous opacity; pannus; corneal opacity.

Clinical

Pharyngitis; epiglottitis; laryngotracheitis; pneumonia; bronchitis; otitis media; meningitis; cellulitis; septic arthritis; sinusitis.

Laboratory

Gram-negative coccobacillus with eight biotypes and six serotypes. Gram stain and culture.

Treatment

Antibiotics are the mainstay of treatment. Invasive and serious infections are best treated with an intravenous third-generation cephalosporin until antibiotic sensitivities are available.

⊟ BIBLIOGRAPHY

1. Devarajan VR. (2012). Haemophilus influenzae infections. [online] Available from www.emedicine.com/med/TOPIC936.HTM. [Accessed September, 2013].

⊟ 40.2E. RHINOSCLEROMA (KLEBSIELLA RHINOSCLEROMATIS)

General

Chronic granulomatous disease; Gram-negative bacillus; cicatricial deformities; chronic progressive granulomatous infection of the upper airways caused by the bacterium *Klebsiella rhinoscleromatis*.

Ocular

Conjunctivitis; chronic dacryocystitis; lid inflammation.

Clinical

Granulomas affecting nose and upper respiratory tract causing sclerosis and deformities; airway obstruction; leprosy; paracoccidioidomycosis; sarcoidosis; basal cell carcinoma; Wegener granulomatosis; also may occur in immunocompromised HIV patients.

Laboratory

Culturing in MacConkey agar is positive in only 50–60% of patients. CT scan and MRI are useful.

Treatment

Bronchoscopy can be used as the initial treatment. Long-term antimicrobial and in cases there were obstruction in suspected cases; surgical intervention may be necessary.

⊟ ADDITIONAL RESOURCES

1. Schwartz RA, Goriniene E. (2012). Rhinoscleroma. [online] Available from www.emedicine.com/derm/TOPIC831.HTM. [Accessed September, 2013].

⊟ 40.2F. MORAXELLA LACUNATA

General

Gram-negative rod; causes chronic angular blepharoconjunctivitis; without treatment, may persist for months or years; normally found in flora of respiratory tract; seen more frequently in alcoholics and those with poor sanitary habits; *Moraxella* organisms produce proteases, although those are not related directly to their pathogenetic mechanism.

Ocular

Catarrhal angular conjunctivitis; corneal ulcer; hypopyon; chronic blepharitis; eczema; lateral canthal skin erythema; iridocyclitis.

Clinical

Alcoholism; impaired nutrition; dermatitis.

Laboratory

Aerobic, oxidase positive, Gram-negative diplococcus or coccobacilli morphologically indistinguishable from *Neisseria.*

Treatment

Artificial tears, cold compresses, antibiotics.

⊟ BIBLIOGRAPHY

1. Baum J, Fedukowicz HB, Jordan A. A survey of Moraxella corneal ulcers in a derelict population. Am J Ophthalmol. 1980;90:476-80.
2. Burd EM. Bacterial keratitis and conjunctivitis. In: Smolin G, Thoft RA (Eds). The Cornea. Boston: Little, Brown and Company; 1994. pp. 20-1.
3. Roy FH, Fraunfelder FW. Current Ocular Therapy, 6th edition. Philadelphia: WB Saunders; 2008.
4. van Bijsterveld OP. The incidence of Moraxella on mucous membranes and the skin. Am J Ophthalmol. 1972;74:72-6.

⊟ 40.2G. GONORRHEA

General

Caused by *N. gonorrhoeae*, which is transmitted sexually.

Ocular

Conjunctivitis; eyelid edema; keratitis; uveitis.

Clinical

Pelvic inflammatory disease; arthritis; dermatitis; carditis; meningitis.

Laboratory

Gram stain smear demonstrates Gram-negative diplococci with polymorphonuclear leukocytes in conjunctival exudates.

Treatment

Therapy consists of systemic antibiotics; topical antibiotics are relatively ineffective in the treatment of eye disease. It is important to treat all sexual partners simultaneously to prevent reinfection.

⊟ BIBLIOGRAPHY

1. Wong B. (2012). Gonorrhea. [online] Available from www.emedicine.com/oph/TOPIC497.HTM. [Accessed September, 2013].

⊟ 40.2H. MENINGOCOCCEMIA (NEISSERIA MENINGITIDES; MENINGITIS)

General

Systemic bacterial infection caused by *N. meningitides*; can be present chronically in patients with immune deficiencies including deficient complement levels.

Ocular

Photophobia; conjunctivitis; chemosis; keratitis; uveitis; panophthalmitis; retinal endophlebitis; macular edema; papillitis; optic neuritis; paresis of sixth or seventh nerve;

nystagmus; miosis; hippus; cortical blindness; papilledema (rare); conjunctival petechiae; strabismus.

Clinical

Meningitis; fever; malaise; joint pain; splenic enlargement.

Laboratory

Cultures from blood, spinal fluid, or joint fluid.

Treatment

Treat with antibiotics promptly.

BIBLIOGRAPHY

1. Javid MH, Ahmed SH. (2012). Meningococcemia. [online] Available from www.emedicine.com/med/TOPIC1445.HTM. [Accessed September, 2013].

40.2I. PROTEUS INFECTIONS

General

Gram-negative bacilli found in water, soil and decaying organic substances.

Ocular

Conjunctivitis; keratitis; corneal ulcers; endophthalmitis; panophthalmitis; dacryocystitis; gangrene of eyelid; uveitis; hypopyon; paralysis of seventh nerve.

Clinical

Cutaneous infection after surgery; usually occurs as a secondary infection of the skin, ears, mastoid sinuses, eyes, peritoneal cavity, bone, urinary tract, meninges, lung, or bloodstream; meningitis; intracranial subdural and epidural empyema; brain abscess; intracranial septic thrombophlebitis affecting cavernous/lateral sinuses.

Laboratory

Proteus organisms are easily recovered through routine laboratory cultures. An ultrasound of the kidneys or a CT scan should be considered as part of a workup.

Treatment

Traditional treatment includes oral quinolone for 3 days or trimethoprim/sulfamethoxazole.

BIBLIOGRAPHY

1. Struble K. (2011). Proteus infections. [online] Available from www.emedicine.com/med/TOPIC1929.HTM. [Accessed September, 2013

40.2J. PSEUDOMONAS AERUGINOSA

General

Gram-negative rod that is ubiquitous in water, soil and plants. Commonly found in hospital environment.

Clinical

None.

Ocular

Foreign body sensation, conjunctival injection, and photophobia, and corneal ulceration.

Laboratory

Gram-negative rod on Gram stain and Giemsa stain from corneal ulcer. Culturing contact lens and lens solutions may help to grow organisms.

Treatment

Fortified tobramycin and fortified cefazolin are drugs of choice.

BIBLIOGRAPHY

1. Roy FH, Fraunfelder FW, Fraunfelder FT. Roy and Fraunfelder's Current Ocular Therapy, 6th edition. London: Elsevier; 2008.

🗗 40.3. VACCINIA (KERATITIS)

General

Laboratory virus used for vaccination against smallpox.

Ocular

Pustules of lids; edema of lids; conjunctivitis; orbital cellulitis; keratitis; pannus; corneal perforation; iridocyclitis; central serous retinopathy; perivasculitis; pseudoretinitis pigmentosa; ocular palsies papillitis; optic atrophy.

Clinical

Vesicles; pustules; erythema; fever; malaise; axillary lymphadenopathy; necrosis of skin; vaccinia gangrenosa; encephalomyelitis; drowsiness; vomiting; coma; death.

Laboratory

Immune deficiency workup should be considered as well as imaging studies.

Treatment

VIG can be helpful in selected patients.

🗗 BIBLIOGRAPHY

1. Lee JJ, Diven D, Poonawalla TA, et al. (2012). Vaccinia. [online] Available from www.emedicine.com/med/TOPIC2356.HTM. [Accessed Sepetember, 2013].

🗗 40.4A. ACTINOMYCOSIS

General

Gram-positive *Actinomyces israelii.*

Ocular

Hypopyon; conjunctivitis; keratitis; corneal ulcer; proptosis; uveitis; dacryocystitis; yellow nodules on conjunctiva and eyelids; occlusion of nasolacrimal canaliculi; canaliculitis; orbital abscess; endophthalmitis (rare).

Clinical

Chronic inflammatory induration and sinus formation.

Laboratory

Canalicular discharge may be sent for Gram stain/Giemsa stain, cultures and sensitivities (i.e. blood agar, Sabouraud, anaerobic) and special stains (i.e. calcofluor white stain).

Treatment

Penicillins and cephalosporins are useful. Subconjunctival penicillin coadministered with systemic iodides and topical sulfacetamide or penicillin can be used.

🗗 BIBLIOGRAPHY

1. Roque MR, Roque BL, Foster CS. (2012). Actinomycosis in ophthalmology. [online] Available from www.emedicine.com/oph/TOPIC491.HTM. [Accessed September, 2013].

🗗 40.4B. CANDIDIASIS

General

Yeast-like opportunistic fungal infection caused by *C. albicans.*

Ocular

Uveitis; hypopyon; conjunctivitis; keratitis; corneal ulcer; blepharitis; endophthalmitis; dacryocystitis; papillitis; retinal atrophy; Roth spot; vitreous abscess; retrobulbar abscess; retinal detachment; panophthalmitis; chorioretinitis; infectious crystalline keratopathy.

Clinical

C. albicans normally is present as an intestinal saprophyte in 35–75% of the human population; in situations of internal environmental change, however, *Candida* can become pathogenic (e.g. obesity, diabetes mellitus, malignancy, and other debilitating conditions).

Laboratory

Common yeast from up to 50% of healthy individuals isolate directly from the eye should be attempted to confirm the presence of organism. Blood agar and Sabouraud's dextrose agar may be used; PCR for species identification.

Treatment

Mucocutaneous infection typically responds to topical therapy. Antifungal therapy should be started immediately after necessary cultures have been obtained from all suspected sites of infection. Infectious disease specialists are typically involved in cases of invasive candidiasis.

🗗 BIBLIOGRAPHY

1. Hedayati T. (2012). Candidiasis in emergency medicine. [online] Available from www.emedicine.com/emerg/TOPIC76.HTM. [Accessed September, 2013].

🗗 40.4C. NOCARDIOSIS

General

Aerobic Actinomycetaceae that may cause a chronic suppurative process; aerobic Gram-positive filamentous bacteria with branching pattern which resemble fungi.

Ocular

Conjunctivitis; keratitis; corneal ulcer; uveitis; lid involvement; orbital cellulitis; endophthalmitis; glaucoma; external ophthalmoplegia; scleritis; canaliculitis; preseptal cellulitis.

Clinical

Granuloma; draining sinuses; brain abscess; meningitis.

Laboratory

Gram-positive filamentous structures with an intermittent or a beaded staining pattern, weakly acid-fast. Organism culture from the infection (i.e. respiratory secretion, skin biopsies, or aspirates from abscesses).

Treatment

Antimicrobial therapy is the treatment of choice.

🗗 BIBLIOGRAPHY

1. DeCroos FC, Garg P, Reddy AK, et al. Optimizing diagnosis and management of nocardia keratitis, scleritis, and endophthalmitis: 11 year microbial and clinical overview. Ophthalmology. 2011;118:1193-200.
2. Greenfield RA. (2011). Nocardiosis. [online] Available from www.emedicine.com/med/TOPIC1644.HTM. [Accessed November, 2012].

🗗 40.5. WISKOTT-ALDRICH SYNDROME (CORNEAL ULCER)

General

Sex-linked recessive; early infancy with death in the 1st decade of life; abnormal immune responses; expression of CD43 is defective in this X-chromosome-linked immunodeficiency disorder, suggesting that CD43 might have a role in T-cell activation.

Ocular

Periorbital hemorrhages; vesicular skin eruptions; blepharitis; lid nodules; episcleritis; scleral icterus; conjunctival hemorrhages and purulent discharge; corneal ulcers; retinal hemorrhages; papilledema; peripapillary hemorrhages.

Clinical

Eczema; epistaxis; purpura; hematemesis; bloody diarrhea; otitis media.

Laboratory

CBC, delayed-type hypersensitivity (DTH) skin test and chest radiographs.

Treatment

Stem cell reconstitution is the main stream of therapy.

🖶 BIBLIOGRAPHY

1. Schwartz RA, Siperstein R. (2013). Pediatric Wiskott-Aldrich syndrome. [online] Available from www.emedicine.com/ped/TOPIC2443.HTM. [Accessed September, 2013].

🖶 41. STEVENS-JOHNSON SYNDROME [DERMATOSTOMATITIS; ERYTHEMA MULTIFORME EXUDATIVUM; SYNDROMA MUCOCUTANEO-OCULARE; BAADER DERMATOSTOMATITIS SYNDROME; MUCOSAL-RESPIRATORY SYNDROME; FUCHS (2) SYNDROME; MUCOCUTANEOUS OCULAR SYNDROME]

General

Etiology unknown; affects all ages; most frequently seen in 1st and 3rd decades of life; prevalent in males; drugs are the most commonly identified etiologic factor in this condition.

Ocular

Hypopyon; iritis; keratitis; corneal ulcers; keratoconjunctivitis sicca; chemosis; conjunctivitis; widespread fibrinoid necrosis of conjunctival vessels; blepharitis; endophthalmitis; phthisis bulbi; uveitis; cataracts; pannus; optic neuritis; keratoconus; adenoviral conjunctivitis has been reported to have precipitated Stevens-Johnson syndrome; orbital cyst may be a complication.

Clinical

General malaise, headaches, chills and fever; severe skin and mucous membrane eruptions (erythema multiforme); dorsa of hands and feet are most frequently affected; rhinitis; balanitis; vulvovaginitis; urethritis (nonspecific); cystitis; patients with AIDS are at higher risk of developing Stevens-Johnson syndrome.

Laboratory

No laboratory tests are specific to Stevens-Johnson syndrome. Diagnosis made from clinical findings.

Treatment

Systemic treatment with steroids is controversial. Antibiotics are used based on clinical course. Eyelid hygiene performed as needed.

🖶 BIBLIOGRAPHY

1. Plaza JA, Dronen SC, Foster J, et al. (2011). Erythema multiforme. [online] Available from www.emedicine.com/med/TOPIC727.HTM. [Accessed September, 2013].

🖶 42. SUPERIOR LIMBIC KERATOCONJUNCTIVITIS (THEODORES SUPERIOR LIMBIC KERATOCONJUNCTIVITIS, SLK)

General

Corneal disease affecting the superior limbus.

Clinical

None.

Ocular

Hyperemia, thickened upper bulbar conjunctiva in a "corridor-like" distribution, fine papillary inflammation of superior palpebral conjunctival, punctate erosion over the superior and perilimbal cornea and superior filamentary keratopathy.

Laboratory

Giemsa-stained scraping of upper conjunctiva demonstrates keratinized cells.

Treatment

Topical lubricants and mast cells stabilizers, punctual plugs, silver nitrate treatment on upper tarsal and bulbar conjunctiva, bandage contact lens, brief focal applications of thermal cautery and recession of involved superior bulbar conjunctiva.

⊟ BIBLIOGRAPHY

1. Oakman JH. (2011). Superior limbic keratoconjunctivitis. [online] Available from www.emedicine.com/oph/TOPIC103.HTM. [Accessed September, 2013].

⊟ 43. TUMORS OF THE CONJUNCTIVA

1. Epithelial tumors
   A. Keratoacanthoma
   B. Dyskeratosis
      1. Epithelial plaques-leukoplakia, hereditary benign intraepithelial dyskeratosis
      2. Intraepithelial epithelioma (Bowen disease) (61N)
   †C. Metastatic uveal melanoma
   †D. Papilloma-including virus types 11, 16, and 18
   †E. Epithelioma
   †F. Adenoma
      1. Papillary cystadenoma lymphomatosum (Warthin tumor)
      2. Oncocytoma (oxyphil-cell adenoma)
      3. Pleomorphic adenoma of Krause glands
†2. Mesoblastic tumors
   A. Inflammatory hyperplasias
      1. Granuloma
      2. Plasmoma
   B. Connective tissue tumors
      1. Fibroma
      2. Lipoma
      3. Myxoma
†3. The reticuloses
   A. Lymphoma
   B. Lymphosarcoma
   C. Mycosis fungoides
†4. Vascular tumors-angiomas
   A. Polymorphous hemangioma, telangiectatic granuloma, granuloma pyogenicum
   B. Lymphangioma
   C. Angiosarcoma monomorphous angioma, Kaposi (hemorrhagic) sarcoma
†5. Pigmented tumors
   A. Nevus
   B. Malignant melanoma
   C. Intraepithelial melanoma-precancerous melanosis
6. Peripheral nerve tumors
   †A. Neurofibroma
      1. Neurilemmoma (neurinoma, schwannoma)
      2. Malignant schwannoma (neurogenic sarcoma; neurofibrosarcoma)
      3. Plexiform neurofibromatosis
   B. Tuberous sclerosis (Bourneville disease)
   †C. Intrascleral nerve loops
†7. Amyloidosis
†8. Metastatic renal cell carcinoma
†9. Trematode-induced granulomas
10. Hypertrophic discoid lupus erythematosus

⊟ BIBLIOGRAPHY

1. Crawford JB, Howes EL Jr, Char DH. Combined nevi of the conjunctiva. Arch Ophthalmol. 1999;117:1121-7.
2. Duong HQ, Copeland RA. (2013). Conjunctival papilloma. [online] Available from www.emedicine.com/oph/TOPIC611.HTM. [Accessed September, 2013].
3. Grossniklaus HE, Green WR, Wolff SM, et al. Hemangiopericytoma of the conjunctiva. Ophthalmology. 1986;93:265-7.
4. Jay V, Font RL. Conjunctival amelanotic malignant melanoma arising in primary acquired melanosis sine pigmento. Ophthalmology. 1998;105:191-4.
5. Marsh WM, Streeten BW, Hoepner JA, et al. Localized conjunctival with amyloidosis associated with extranodal lymphoma. Ophthalmology. 1987;94:61-4.
6. Monroe M. (2013). Head and neck cutaneous squamous cell carcinoma. [online] Available from www.emedicine.com/oph/TOPIC116.HTM. [Accessed September, 2013].
7. Odrich MG, Jakobiec FA, Lancaster WD, et al. A spectrum of bilateral squamous conjunctival tumors associated with the human papillomavirus type 16. Ophthalmology. 1991;98:628-35.
8. Peter J, Hidayat AA. Myxomas of the conjunctiva. Am J Ophthalmol. 1986;102:80-6.
9. Rathinam S, Fritsche TR, Srinivasan M, et al. An outbreak of trematode-induced granulomas of the conjunctiva. Ophthalmology. 2001;108:1223-9.
10. Roque MR, Roque BL, Foster CS. (2011). Conjunctival melanoma. [online] Available from www.emedicine.com/oph/TOPIC110.HTM. [Accessed September, 2013].
11. Sagerman RH, Abramson DH. Tumors of the eye and ocular adnexae. New York: Pergamon Press; 1982.
12. Uy HS, Pineda R, Shore JW, et al. Hypertrophic discoid lupus erythematosus of the conjunctiva. Am J Ophthalmol. 1999;127:604-5.
13. Ware GT, Haik BG, Morris WR. Renal cell carcinoma with involvement of iris and conjunctiva. Am J Ophthalmol. 1999;127.4:458-9.
14. Winward KE, Curtin VT. Conjunctival squamous cell carcinoma in a patient with human immunodeficiency virus infection. Am J Ophthalmol. 1989;107:554-5.

†Indicates a general entry and therefore has not been described in detail in the text

🗗 43.1A. KERATOACANTHOMA

General

Benign epithelial tumor that arises on hair follicles in exposed skin of Caucasians.

Clinical

Keratoacanthoma can occur in other parts of the body.

Ocular

Conjunctival nodules may result in foreign body sensation and tearing.

Laboratory

Biopsy of lesion can be diagnostic.

Treatment

Excisional biopsy, curettage, cryotherapy, radiation.

🗗 BIBLIOGRAPHY

1. Roy FH, Fraunfelder FW, Fraunfelder FT. Roy and Fraunfelder's Current Ocular Therapy. 6th edition. London: Elsevier; 2008.

🗗 43.1B. BOWEN DISEASE (INTRAEPITHELIAL EPITHELIOMA; CARCINOMA IN SITU; DYSKERATOSIS)

General

Squamous cell carcinomas *in situ* of the skin or conjunctiva.

Ocular

Dysplastic epithelium, intraepithelial epithelioma, or invasive squamous cell carcinoma of conjunctiva or cornea; infiltration of lacrimal system and sclera.

Laboratory

Ocular—Full thickness conjunctival biopsy which should include basement membrane.

Treatment

The goals of therapy are to reduce morbidity and to prevent complications. Simple excision with conventional margins surgery is the most common and preferred treatment for smaller lesions and those not in problematic areas.

🗗 BIBLIOGRAPHY

1. Eid MP, Anderson BE. (2012). Bowen disease. [online] Available from www.emedicine.com/derm/TOPIC59.HTM. [Accessed September, 2013].

🗗 43.6B. BOURNEVILLE SYNDROME (BOURNEVILLE-PRINGLE SYNDROME; TUBEROUS SCLEROSIS; EPILOIA)

General

Irregular dominant inheritance; more frequent in females; most patients die before age of 24 years.

Ocular

Vitreous often cloudy; lens opacities; retinal mushroom-like tumor of grayish-white color; yellowish-white plaques with small hemorrhages and cystic changes in retina; papilledema; disk drusen; cerebral astrocytoma; 40–50% of patients have normal intelligence.

Clinical

Grand mal, petit mal, or Jacksonian seizures (manifest in first 2 years of life); mental changes from feeble mindedness to imbecility and idiocy; skin changes arranged usually about nose and cheeks (adenoma sebaceum); congenital tumors of kidney (hypernephroma or tubular adenoma) and heart (rhabdomyoma); cerebral astrocytoma.

Laboratory

Brain MRI is recommended for the detection and follow-up imaging of cortical tubers.

Treatment

A neurologist should be consulted to assist with seizure management and anticonvulsant medication.

⌗ BIBLIOGRAPHY

1. Schwartz RA, Jozwiak S, Pedersen R. (2012). Genetics of tuberous sclerosis. [online] Available from www.emedicine.com/ped/TOPIC2796.HTM. [Accessed September, 2013].

⌗ 44. VERNAL KERATOCONJUNCTIVITIS (ATOPIC KERATOCONJUNCTIVITIS, ALLERGIC CONJUNCTIVITIS, GIANT PAPILLARY CONJUNCTIVITIS)

General

Bilateral, chronic, severe allergy, more frequent in young males and during the spring time.

Clinical

Atopy present in half of the cases.

Ocular

Giant papillae conjunctivitis.

Laboratory

Diagnosis is made by clinical findings.

Treatment

Ocular lubricants, nonsteroidal anti-inflammatory and steroid drops, oral nonsteroidal anti-inflammatory or steroids. Supratarsal steroids. Surgical excision, cryotherapy and beta-irradiation of papillae.

⌗ BIBLIOGRAPHY

1. Ventocilla M, Bloomenstein MR, Majmudar PA. (2012). Allergic conjunctivitis. [online] Available from www.emedicine.com/oph/TOPIC85.HTM. [Accessed September, 2013].

CHAPTER

20

Cornea

⊟ 1. DEGENERATION

⊟ 1A. ANTERIOR EMBRYOTOXON (ARCUS)

In this condition, white or gray substance is deposited at level of the Descemet membrane and Bowman membrane initially and then in the stroma with a clear limbal interval.

1. *Age:* May be present normally in a white patient older than 40 years of age or in a black patient older than 35 years of age
2. Alagille syndrome
3. Alport syndrome (hereditary nephritis)
4. Associated with corneal disease, such as interstitial keratitis
5. Contralateral carotid occlusive disease—when unilateral
6. Familial hypercholesterolemia [type II, familial beta-lipoproteins and type III, familial hyper-beta and pre-beta lipoproteins (carbohydrate-induced hyperlipemia)]
7. *Hereditary*: Autosomal dominant or autosomal recessive inheritance
8. Isolated phenomenon
9. Long exposure to irritating dust or chemicals
10. Ocular anomaly association, such as blue sclera, megalocornea, or aniridia
11. Secondary to ocular disease, such as large corneal scars, sclerokeratitis, limbal dermoid, nevus, or epithelial cyst
12. Schnyder crystalline dystrophy.

⊟ BIBLIOGRAPHY

1. Bagla SK, Golden RL. Unilateral arcus corneae senilis and carotid occlusive disease. JAMA. 1975;233:450.
2. Chavis RM, Groshong T. Corneal arcus in Alport's syndrome. Am J Ophthalmol. 1973;75:793-4.
3. Hingorani M, Nischal KK, Davies A, et al. Ocular abnormalities in Alagille syndrome. Ophthalmology. 1999;106:330-7.
4. Wu R, Wong TY, Saw SM, et al. Effect of corneal arcus on central corneal thickness, intraocular pressure, and primary open-angle glaucoma: the Singapore Malay Eye Study. Arch Ophthalmol. 2010;128:1455-61.
* "Corneal arcus was associated with higher intraocular pressure (IOP) and lower central corneal thickness (CCT) independent of age, sex, and ocular factors".

1A2. ALAGILLE SYNDROME (AGS; ALAGILLE-WATSON SYNDROME, AWS; CHOLESTASIS WITH PERIPHERAL PULMONARY STENOSIS; ARTERIOHEPATIC DYSPLASIA, AHD; HEPATIC DUCTULAR HYPOPLASIA, SYNDROMATIC)

General

May be associated with 20p 11.2 deletion and four distinct coding mutations in *Jag 1* gene.

Ocular

Posterior embryotoxon and retinal pigmentary changes; anterior chamber anomalies, associated with eccentric or ectopic pupils.

Clinical

Neonatal jaundice; prominent forehead and chin; pulmonic valvular stenosis as well as peripheral arterial stenosis; abnormal vertebrae (butterfly vertebrae) and decrease in interpediculate distance in the lumbar spine; absent deep tendon reflexes and poor school performance; in the facies, broad forehead, pointed mandible, and bulbous tip of the nose; and in the fingers, varying degrees of foreshortening.

Laboratory

Liver biopsy specimens typically exhibit features suggestive of chronic cholestasis and paucity of interlobular bile ducts. The majority of biopsies (wedge or needle) reveal features of bile duct paucity.

Treatment

Subspecialty consultation may facilitate diagnosis and provide long-term care. Consultation with an ophthalmologist may provide the diagnosis. A pediatric hepatologist can assist with management of chronic cholestatic liver disease. Cardiology consultation can assist with the diagnosis and therapy for intracardiac disease, as well as other vascular abnormalities. Nephrology consultations are useless when structural renal disease is present or if suspicions of evolving renal insufficiency arise.

BIBLIOGRAPHY

1. Scheimann A. (2012). Alagille syndrome. [online] Available from www.emedicine.com/ped/TOPIC60.HTM. [Accessed September, 2013].

1A3. ALPORT SYNDROME (HEREDITARY FAMILIAL CONGENITAL HEMORRHAGIC NEPHRITIS; HEREDITARY NEPHRITIS; FAMILIAL NEPHRITIS)

General

Autosomal dominant inheritance; early death in males; normal life span in females.

Ocular

Anterior lenticonus (bilateral progressive); subcapsular cataracts; thinning of lens capsule; fundus albipunctatus; retinopathy similar to juvenile macular degeneration; hyaline bodies of optic nerve head; vesicles in Descemet membrane affecting basement membrane collagen; anterior and polar cataracts.

Clinical

Hemorrhagic nephritis; progressive nerve deafness; deafness (high tone, sensorineural); most often transmitted as an X-linked dominant trait, although dominant and recessive transmission has been reported.

Laboratory

Urinalysis reveals microscopic or gross hematuria. Renal ultrasonography is indicated for children with persistent microscopic hematuria.

Treatment

There is no treatment to prevent progression. Renal transplantation is the treatment of choice.

BIBLIOGRAPHY

1. Devarajan P. (2011). Pediatric Alport syndrome. [online] Available from www.emedicine.com/ped/TOPIC74.HTM. [Accessed September, 2013].

⊟ 1A12. SCHNYDER'S CRYSTALLINE CORNEAL DYSTROPHY

General

Rare, autosomal dominant disorder with abnormal bilateral deposition of cholesterol and lipid in the cornea.

Clinical

Hypercholesterolemia and genu valgam.

Ocular

Central corneal haze, subepithelial cholesterol crystal deposition, midperipheral, panstromal haze and arcus lipoides.

Laboratory

Serum lipid analysis because hyperlipidemia.

Treatment

Phototherapeutic keratectomy (PTK) can be used to treat subepithelial crystals and penetrating keratoplasty (PK) may be necessary.

⊟ BIBLIOGRAPHY

1. Weiss JS, Spagnolo B. (2011). Crystalline dystrophy. [online] Available from www.emedicine.com/oph/topic548.HTM. [Accessed September, 2013].

⊟ 1B. BAND-SHAPED KERATOPATHY

This type of corneal opacification extends horizontally over the cornea, at the level of the Bowman membrane, in the exposed part of the palpebral aperture.

1. Anterior mosaic dystrophy, primary type
   A. Episkopi (sex-linked recessive)
   †B. Labrador keratopathy
2. Chemical fume related as mercury vapor or calcium bichromate vapor
†3. Cyclosporine as eyedrops
4. De Barsy syndrome
5. Discoid lupus erythematosus
†6. Dysproteinemia
7. Gout (hyperuricemia)
†8. High levels of visible electromagnetic radiation, such as xenon arc photocoagulation and laser causing acute severe anterior uveitis
9. Hypercalcemia
   A. Excessive vitamin D as with oral intake, Boeck sarcoid with liver involvement, acute osteoporosis, Heerfordt syndrome.
   B. Hyperparathyroidism
   C. Hypophosphatasia (phosphoethanolaminuria)
   D. Idiopathic hypercalcemia
   E. Milk-alkali syndrome
   F. Paget syndrome (osteitis deformans)
   G. Renal failure, such as that associated with Fanconi syndrome (cystinosis)
10. Ichthyosis vulgaris
11. Local degenerative diseases, including chronicuveitis, phthisis bulbi, absolute glaucoma, infantile polyarthritis (Still disease), rheumatoid arthritis (RA), interstitial keratitis, Felty syndrome.
†12. Long-term miotic therapy
†13. Long-term steroid phosphate preparations
14. Progressive facial hemiatrophy (Parry-Romberg syndrome)
†15. Rothmund syndrome (ectodermal syndrome)
†16. Silicone oil in anterior chamber
17. Tuberous sclerosis (Bourneville syndrome)
†18. Tumoral calcinosis
†19. Viscoat usage
20. Wagner syndrome (hyaloideoretinal degeneration)

Treatment

- Low serum calcium levels along with high phosphate levels are observed with renal failure, hypoparathyroidism, and pseudohypoparathyroidism.
- High serum calcium and high phosphate levels are observed with vitamin D intoxication and milk-alkali syndrome.
- Band keratopathy is the result of precipitation of calcium salts on the corneal surface (directly under the epithelium). Serum and normal body fluids (e.g. tears, aqueous humor) contain calcium and phosphate in concentrations that approach their solubility product.

---

†Indicates a general entry and therefore has not been described in detail in the text

Evaporation of tears tends to concentrate solutes and increase the tonicity of tears; it is especially true in the intrapalpebral area where the greatest exposure of the corneal surface to ambient air occurs. Elevated serum calcium or serum phosphate can tip the balance in favor of precipitation. Topical medications that contain phosphates also may contribute to this problem. Finally, elevation of the surface pH out of the physiologic range changes the solubility product and favors precipitation. This type of tissue pH change can be seen in chronically inflamed eyes and may explain, in part, why patients with uveitis are at risk for the development of this problem.

- Endothelial function may play a role in the formation of calcium deposition. Compromise of endothelial function and corneal edema are sometimes seen in patients who have silicone oil inside the eye when it comes into contact with the posterior cornea. Although this association has been noted, the exact reasons remain uncertain.

BIBLIOGRAPHY

1. Agraharkar M, Dellinger OD, Gangakhedkar AK. (2012). Hypercalcemia. [online] Available from www.emedicine.com/med/TOPIC1068.HTM. [Accessed September, 2013].
2. Dahl AA, DeBarge LR. (2013). Ophthalmologic manifestations of sarcoidosis. [online] Available from www.emedicine.com/oph/TOPIC451.HTM. [Accessed September, 2013].
3. Herndon L, Choplin NT, Law SK, et al. (2012). Uveitic glaucoma. [online] Available from www.emedicine.com/oph/TOPIC145.HTM. [Accessed September, 2013].
4. Janigian RH, Filippopoulos T, Welcome BA. (2013). Intermediate uveitis. [online] Available from www.emedicine.com/oph/TOPIC445.HTM. [Accessed September, 2013].
5. Lederer E, Ouseph R, Nayak V. (2012). Hyperphosphatemia. [online] Available from www.emedicine.com/med/TOPIC1097.HTM. [Accessed September, 2013].
6. Rothschild BM, Miller AV, Francis ML. (2013). Gout and pseudogout. www.emedicine.com/oph/TOPIC506.HTM. [Accessed September, 2013].
7. Taravella M. (2012). Band keratopathy treatment and management. [online] Available from emedicine.medscape.com/article/1194813-treatment. [Accessed September, 2013].
8. Walton RC. (2012). Uveitis, anterior, childhood. [online] Available from www.emedicine.com/oph/TOPIC585.HTM. [Accessed September, 2013].

1B1A. EPISKOPI BLINDNESS

General

Sex-linked; confined to male members of Greek Cypriot family group, most of whom live in Episkopi.

Ocular

Microphthalmia; corneal opacities; transverse corneal band; iritis; cataract; retrolental opacities; retinitis pigmentosa; Leber optic atrophy; amaurosis.

Clinical

None.

Laboratory

Clinical.

Treatment

- *Cataract*: Change in glasses can sometimes improve a patient's visual function temporarily; however the most common treatment is cataract surgery.

- *Retinitis pigmentosa*: Vitamin A 15,000 IU/day is thought to slow the decline of retinal function, dark sunglasses for outdoor use, surgery for cataract, genetic counseling.

- *Iritis*: Oral steroids if not responsive to topical steroids, immunosuppressants if bilateral disease that does not respond to oral steroids, periocular steroids for unilateral or posterior uveitis. Vitrectomy can be used for severe vitreous opacification. Cryotherapy and laser photocoagulation may be used for localized pars plana exudates.

BIBLIOGRAPHY

1. Roy FH. Ocular Differential Diagnosis, 9th edition. New Delhi: Jaypee Brothers Medical Publishers; 2012.
2. Taylor PJ, Coates T, Newhouse ML. Episkopi blindness: hereditary blindness in a Greek Cypriot family. Br J Ophthalmol. 1959;43:340-4.

1B2. MERCURY POISONING (MINAMATA SYNDROME)

General

Both sexes affected; onset several weeks or months after ingestion of fish from contaminated water or animals fed with contaminated grain; symptoms may be mild to severe.

Ocular

Constriction of visual fields; blindness.

Clinical

Paresthesia of mouth, tongue, and extremity; hearing loss; asthenia; fatigue; inability to concentrate; dysarthria; tremors; persistent vegetative state; peripheral neuropathy; cerebella ataxia; gait disturbance; sensory impairment; anosmia; loss of taste; bladder disturbance; mental deterioration.

Laboratory

Mercury levels, complete blood count (CBC) and serum chemistries, urine mercury levels.

Treatment

Oxygen, hemodialysis only in severe cases, chelating agents.

BIBLIOGRAPHY

1. Olson DA. (2013). Mercury toxicity. [online] Available from www.emedicine.com/emerg/TOPIC813.HTM. [Accessed September, 2013].

1B4. DE BARSY SYNDROME

General

Rare progeroid syndrome associated with characteristic ocular, facial, skeletal, dermatologic, and neurologic abnormalities.

Ocular

Congenital corneal opacification (loss of Bowman layer); cataracts.

Clinical

Short stature, pectus excavatum, skeletal dysplasia with short legs, multiple joint dislocations, especially involving the hands; skin redundancy (as seen in cutis laxa); midface hypoplasia; thin transparent skin with prominent superficial veins; frontal bossing and aged, progeroid facies; early death; hypotonia; mental retardation; brisk deep tendon reflexes.

Laboratory

None.

Treatment

- *Corneal opacification:* Check for elevated intraocular pressure (IOP). Medical treatment includes the use of hyperosmotic drops, non-steroidal and steroid eye drops. Corneal transplant may be necessary.
- *Cataracts*: Change in glasses can sometimes improve a patient's visual function temporarily; however the most common treatment is cataract surgery.

BIBLIOGRAPHY

1. Aldave AJ, Eagle RC, Streeten BW, et al. Congenital corneal opacification in DeBarsy syndrome. Arch Ophthalmol. 2001;119:285-8.
2. Bartsocas CS, Dimitriou J, Kavadias A, et al. De Barsy syndrome. Prog Clin Biol Res. 1982;104:157-60.
3. de Barsy AM, Moens E, Dierckx L. Dwarfism, oligophrenia and degeneration of the elastic tissue in skin and corne1B5a: a new syndrome. Helv Paediatr Acta. 1968;3:305-13.

⊟ 1B5. DISSEMINATED LUPUS ERYTHEMATOSUS (SYSTEMIC LUPUS ERYTHEMATOSUS; LUPUS ERYTHEMATOSUS; KAPOSI-LIBMAN-SACK SYNDROME, SLE)

General

Possible etiology includes viral infections and genetic predisposition; immunologic abnormalities.

Ocular

Keratitis; keratoconjunctivitis sicca; corneal ulcer; optic nerve atrophy; optic neuritis; papilledema; arteritis; central retinal vein occlusion; retinal detachment; microaneurysm; scleritis; uveitis; ptosis; conjunctivitis; paralysis of third nerve; homonymous hemianopsia; multifocal microinfarcts; mydriasis; nystagmus; proptosis; orbital myositis; pseudoretinitis pigmentosa; photophobia.

Clinical

Polyarthritis; morning stiffness; fever; malaise; fatigue; polyserositis; renal disease; central nervous system (CNS) disease; anemia; leukopenia; maculopapular rash in a "butterfly" distribution over malar region; alopecia.

Laboratory

Antibodies to double-stranded DNA or the Smith (Sm) antigen or a false-positive serology test for syphilis; positive antinuclear antibody (ANA) test that is caused by a medication.

Treatment

Fever, rash, musculoskeletal, and serositis manifestations respond to hydroxychloroquine and nonsteroidal anti-inflammatory drugs (NSAIDs). Low-to-moderate dose steroids are necessary for acute flares. CNS involvement and renal disease constitute more serious disease and often require high-dose steroids and other immunosuppression agents. Diffuse proliferative lupus nephritis has been treated with cyclophosphamide induction therapy.

⊟ BIBLIOGRAPHY

1. Bartles CM, Muller D. (2012). Systemic erythematosus lupus. [online] Available from www.emedicine.com/med/TOPIC2228.HTM. [Accessed September, 2013].

⊟ 1B7. GOUT (HYPERURICEMIA)

General

Genetic disease of purine metabolism and renal excretion of uric acid.

Ocular

Conjunctivitis; episcleritis; posterior scleritis; ocular motor disturbances; iritis; band keratopathy; interpalpebral paralimbal nodules.

Clinical

Acute inflammatory arthritis; accumulation of sodium urate deposits; uric acid nephrolithiasis; renal failure; tophi in any body tissue; marked swelling of feet and ankles.

Laboratory

Serum uric acid is used in diagnosing this condition and in monitoring the treatment process.

Treatment

Treatment is directed at reducing both hyperuricemia and ocular inflammation. Treatment involves hydration, colchicine for prevention and acute treatment, nonsteroidal and steroidal anti-inflammatory drugs, uricosuric agents (e.g. probenecid), and antihyperuricemic drugs.

⊟ BIBLIOGRAPHY

1. Rothschild BM, Miller AV, Francis ML. (2013). Gout and pseudogout. www.emedicine.com/oph/TOPIC506.HTM. [Accessed September, 2013].

1B9. WILLIAMS-BEUREN SYNDROME (SUPRAVALVULAR AORTIC STENOSIS; BEUREN ELFIN FACE; HYPERCALCEMIA SUPRAVALVULAR AORTIC STENOSIS; HYPERCALCEMIC FACE) HYPERTELORISM

General

Onset at birth or early infancy; occurs in both sexes; etiology unknown; possible abnormality of vitamin D metabolism.

Ocular

Bilateral corneal opacities; hypertelorism; prominent epicanthal folds; strabismus.

Clinical

Anorexia; slow weight gain; retarded physical and mental development; Elfin face; absent aortic systolic click; harsh ejection systolic murmur; tooth enamel hypoplasia; malocclusion; cavities.

Laboratory

Fluorescence in situ hybridization (FISH) for the 7q11.23 elastin gene deletion, serum calcium, blood urea nitrogen (BUN), and creatine levels. Thyroid stimulating hormone levels, baseline echocardiogram, and renal ultrasound.

Treatment

Treatment is done on a patient-to-patient basis with multiple health care prefessionals are involved.

BIBLIOGRAPHY

1. Khan A, Caluseriu O, Huang LH, et al. (2012). Williams syndrome. [online] Available from www.emedicine.com/ped/TOPIC2439.HTM. [Accessed September, 2013].

1B9A. SCHAUMANN SYNDROME (BESNIER-BOECK-SCHAUMANN SYNDROME; BOECK SARCOID; SARCOIDOSIS)

General

Etiology unknown; theories include tuberculosis, hypersensitivity to pine pollen, virus infection; affects blacks most often; chronic course with spontaneous remissions (*see* Heerfordt's syndrome); hilar or paratracheal nodes with erythema nodosum; onset most often in middle and old age; ocular involvement in 20–25% of all cases.

Ocular

Orbital granulomatous mass; bony defects; cutaneous and subcutaneous nodules; myogenic palsy; lacrimal gland adenopathy; decreased tear formation; secondary glaucoma; granulomatous uveitis with iris nodules, cells and flare; mutton fat keratic precipitates; keratitis sicca; vitreous floaters; band-shaped keratitis; complicated cataract; inflammatory retinal exudates; "candle wax drippings"; optic nerve atrophy; neuritis; eyelid nodules; ocular nerve enlargement (granuloma).

Clinical

Lymphadenopathy; hilar nodes; fatigue; cystic, punched-out or reticulated changes in small bones (mainly, hands and feet); muscle wasting; contractures; weakness in legs and arms.

Laboratory

Chest X-ray, CT scan, and MRI of the brain.

Treatment

Glucocorticoids are the treatment of choice.

BIBLIOGRAPHY

1 Sharma GD. (2011). Pediatric sarcoidosis. [online] Available from www.emedicine.com/ped/TOPIC2043.HTM. [Accessed September, 2013].

🗗 1B9A. HEERFORDT SYNDROME (UVEOPAROTID FEVER; UVEOPAROTITIS; UVEOPAROTITIC PARALYSIS)

General

It occurs in young adults, more frequently in females than in males; usual cause is sarcoidosis.

Ocular

Band keratopathy; keratoconjunctivitis sicca; uveitis; optic atrophy; papilledema; episcleritis; snowball opacity of vitreous; retinal vasculitis; proptosis; cataract; paralysis of seventh nerve; sarcoid nodules of eyelid, iris, ciliary body, choroid, and sclera; dacryoadenitis.

Clinical

Parotid gland swelling; facial paralysis; lymphadenopathy; splenomegaly; cutaneous nodules; facial nerve palsy.

Laboratory

Biopsy of liver, skin, lymph nodes or conjunctiva show non-caseating epithelioid cell follicles; X-ray shows lung changes; low tuberculin sensitivity; elevated angiotensin-converting enzyme level.

Treatment

Systemic corticosteroids are the treatment of choice.

🗗 BIBLIOGRAPHY

1. Dahl AA. (2011). Ophthalmologic manifestations of sarcoidosis. [online] Available from www.emedicine.com/oph/TOPIC451.HTM. [Accessed September, 2013].

🗗 1B9B. HYPERPARATHYROIDISM

General

Increased secretion of parathyroid hormone (PTH).

Ocular

Glass-like crystals of conjunctiva; band keratopathy; optic atrophy; papilledema; vascular engorgement of retina; ptosis; scleral thinning; ectopic calcifications in the choroid and sclera; unilateral visual loss; ischemic optic neuropathy.

Clinical

Hypercalcemia; hypophosphatemia; brown tumor.

Laboratory

Diagnosis is made based on hypercalcemia and elevated PTH levels. Other abnormal laboratory findings may include elevated BUN and creatinine levels, hyperchloremic acidosis, reduced serum bicarbonate levels due to renal bicarbonate casting, hypophosphatemia, elevated alkaline phosphatase levels and hypercalciuria.

Treatment

Surgical removal of the pathologic gland or glands. Medical management of hyperparathyroidism is generally reserved for patients with poor medical conditions.

🗗 BIBLIOGRAPHY

1. LaBagnara J. (2011). Hyperparathyroidism in otolaryngology and facial plastic surgery. [online] Available from www.emedicine.com/ent/TOPIC299.HTM. [Accessed September, 2013].

1B9C. HYPOPHOSPHATASIA (PHOSPHOETHANOLAMINURIA)

General

Hypophosphatasia (phosphoethanolaminuria) is an inborn error of metabolism that entails increased urinary excretion of phosphoethanolamine (PEA) and associated low alkaline phosphatase and hypercalcemia; it is prevalent in females; may result from absence or abnormal circulating factor regulating expression of alkaline phosphatase.

Ocular

Papilledema; optic atrophy; exophthalmos; blue sclera; conjunctival calcification; lid retraction; cataract; corneal subepithelial calcifications.

Clinical

Defect in true bone formation associated with widespread skeletal abnormalities; low serum alkaline phosphatase activity; hypercalcemia; nausea; vomiting; bowing of legs; convulsions; premature loss of teeth.

Laboratory

Assess the alkaline phosphatase levels. The levels are low in all types of hypophosphatasia. Fasting laboratory evaluations should include levels of calcium, phosphorus, magnesium, alkaline phosphatase, creatinine, PTH, serum 25-hydroxyvitamin D [25(OH)D] and 1, 25-dihydroxyvitamin D [1,25(OH)(2)D]. Levels of pyridoxal-5′-phosphate (PLP), inorganic pyrophosphate (PPi) and PEA in serum and urine determine the diagnosis.

Treatment

No medical therapy is available. Supportive care is necessary to decrease the morbidity associated with hypophosphatasia. Regularly examine infants and children to check for evidence of increased intracranial pressure. Observe fractures closely. Adult pseudofractures may require orthopedic care to heal properly. A dentist should closely monitor all individuals with hypophosphatasia.

BIBLIOGRAPHY

1. Plotkin H, Anadiotis GA. (2012). Hypophosphatasia. [online] Available from www.emedicine.com/ped/TOPIC1126.HTM. [Accessed September, 2013].

1B9D. DRUMMOND SYNDROME (IDIOPATHIC HYPERCALCEMIA; BLUE DIAPER SYNDROME)

General

Autosomal recessive; manifests itself in infancy; defective intestinal transport of tryptophan, which oxidizes to indigo blue and stains the diaper blue.

Ocular

Sclerosis of optic foramina (occasionally); prominent epicanthal folds; nystagmus; strabismus; peripheral retinal atrophy; papilledema; optic atrophy; microcornea; hypoplasia of the optic nerve; abnormal eye movements.

Clinical

Dwarfism; osteosclerosis; craniostenosis; depressed bridge of nose; "elfin-like" face; mental retardation; anorexia; vomiting; constipation.

Laboratory

Measurement of serum phosphate, alkaline phosphatase, serum chloride, serum bicarbonate, and urinary calcium.

Treatment

Treatment depends on the severity of symptoms and the underlying cause.

BIBLIOGRAPHY

1. Agraharkar M, Dellinger OD, Gangakhedkar AK. (2012). Hypercalcemia. [online] Available from www.emedicine.com/med/TOPIC1068.HTM. [Accessed September, 2013].

🗗 1B9E. BURNETT SYNDROME (MILK DRINKER SYNDROME; MILK-ALKALI SYNDROME)

General

Characterized by alkalosis, hypercalcemia, and transient renal insufficiency with azotemia; develops during milk-alkali therapy for peptic ulcer; seen in excessive intake of milk or soluble alkali, as in therapy for peptic ulcer.

Ocular

Band-shaped keratopathy; conjunctivitis with calcification.

Clinical

Nausea, vomiting; headache; irritability; dizziness; depression; confusion.

Laboratory

Diagnosing the etiology of hypercalcemia is difficult. Much of the laboratory workup should be guided by the history and physical examination and may include renal imaging, X-ray and serology.

Treatment

Initial treatment involves hydration to improve urinary calcium output. The addition of diuretics inhibits tubular reabsorption of calcium.

🗗 BIBLIOGRAPHY

1. Claudius IA, Fattal O, Nakamoto J, et al. (2013). Pediatric Hypercalcemia. [online] Available from www.emedicine.com/ped/TOPIC1062.HTM. [Accessed September, 2013].

🗗 1B9F. PAGET DISEASE (OSTEITIS DEFORMANS; CONGENITAL HYPERPHOS-PHATEMIA; HYPEROSTOSIS CORTICALIS DEFORMANS; POZZI SYNDROME; CHRONIC CONGENITAL IDIOPATHIC HYPERPHOSPHATEMIA; OSTEOCHALASIS DESMALIS FAMILIARIS; FAMILIAL OSTEOECTASIA)

General

Autosomal dominant; more frequent in men, but more severe in women; onset after age of 40 years; characterized by diffuse cortical thickening of involved bones with osteoporosis, bowing deformities and shortening of stature; osteogenic sarcoma not infrequent.

Ocular

Shallow orbits with progressive unilateral or bilateral proptosis palsy of extraocular muscles; corneal ring opacities; cataract; retinal hemorrhages; pigmentary retinopathy; macular changes resembling Kuhnt-Junius degeneration; angioid streaks; papilledema; optic nerve atrophy; blue sclera; exophthalmos.

Clinical

Skull deformities; kyphoscoliosis; hypertension and arteriosclerosis; muscle weakness; waddling gait; hearing impairment; osteoarthritis.

Laboratory

Bone-specific alkaline phosphatase (BSAP) levels, radiographs may demonstrate both osteolysis and excessive bone formation. Bone biopsies may be necessary for diagnostic purposes in rare cases.

Treatment

Medical therapy for Paget disease should include bisphosphonate treatment with serial monitoring of bone markers. NSAIDs and acetaminophen may be effective for pain management. Chemotherapy, radiation, or both may be used to treat neoplasms arising from pagetic bone.

🗗 BIBLIOGRAPHY

1. Lohr KM, Driver K. (2011). Paget disease. [online] Available from emedicine.medscape.com/article/334607-overview. [Accessed September, 2013].

⌗ 1B9G. LIGNAC-FANCONI SYNDROME (FANCONI-LIGNAC SYNDROME; CYSTINOSIS SYNDROME; CYSTINE STORAGE-AMINOACIDURIA-DWARFISM SYNDROME; RENAL RICKETS; NEPHROPATHIC CYSTINOSIS)

General

Autosomal recessively inherited storage disorder in which non-protein cystine accumulates within cellular lysosomes; occurs primarily in children; prognosis in children with renal tubular insufficiency and dwarfism poor, with survival past age 10 years rare without renal transplant.

Ocular

Cystine crystals located in conjunctiva, cornea, sclera, iris, ciliary body, lens, and perhaps choroid; general clouding of cornea caused by dense deposition of cystine crystals; pupillary block glaucoma; photophobia; band keratopathy; posterior synechiae with thickened stroma of iris; decreased visual function; patchy retinopathy; visual field constriction.

Clinical

Fanconi syndrome with rickets; dwarfism; glomerular dystrophy; renal failure; oral motor dysfunction.

Laboratory

The diagnosis is made based on tests that document the excessive loss of substances in the urine (e.g. amino acids, glucose, phosphate, bicarbonate) in the absence of high plasma concentrations.

Treatment

Replacement of substances lost in the urine. Liver transplantation is sometimes necessary.

⌗ BIBLIOGRAPHY

1. Fathallah-Shaykh S, Spitzer A. (2013). Fanconi syndrome. [online] Available from www.emedicine.com/ped/TOPIC756.HTM. [Accessed September, 2013].

⌗ 1B10. BULLOUS ICHTHYOSIFORM ERYTHRODERMA (COLLODION BABY; CONGENITAL ICHTHYOSIS; EPIDERMOLYTIC HYPERKERATOSIS; ICHTHYOSIS; ICHTHYOSIS VULGARIS; LAMELLAR ICHTHYOSIS; NONBULLOUS ICHTHYOSIFORM ERYTHRODERMA; XERODERMA; X-LINKED ICHTHYOSIS)

General

Autosomal inherited disorder; affects both sexes; normal at birth; onset within first 7 days; X-linked; pathogenesis may be secondary to physicochemical changes of corneal tissues including accumulation of cholesterol sulfate.

Ocular

Keratopathy; corneal scarring; keratitis; conjunctivitis; lagophthalmos; photophobia; ectropion; lid erythema; lacrimation; keratoconus; deep corneal punctate/filiform lesions.

Clinical

At birth, the skin surface is moist, red, and tender; within several days, thick scales form.

Laboratory

Diagnosis is made by clinical findings.

Treatment

Genetic counseling and prenatal diagnosis also can be offered. Newborns with denuded skin are at increased risk for infection, secondary sepsis, and electrolyte imbalance and should be transferred to the neonatal intensive care unit (NICU) to be monitored and treated as needed.

⌗ BIBLIOGRAPHY

1. Chen TS, Metz BJ. (2012). Epidermolytic hyperkeratosis (Bullous Congenital Ichthyosiform Erythroderma).[online] www.emedicine.com/derm/TOPIC590.HTM. [Accessed September, 2013].

🗗 1B11. PHTHISIS BULBI

General

Shrunken, not functional eye secondary to trauma, infection, radiation or other ocular abnormalities.

Clinical

None.

Ocular

Scared swollen cornea; low IOP; distorted globe; cataract; ocular pain; blind.

Laboratory

Diagnosis is made by clinical observation.

Treatment

No treatment is available to improve. Alcohol injection can sometimes be used to reduce pain. Enucleation may also be necessary to eliminate the pain.

🗗 BIBLIOGRAPHY

1. University of Utah Health Care—Moran Eye Center. Phthisis bulbi. [online] Available from uuhsc.utah.edu/Moran EyeCenter/opatharch/uvea/phthisis_bubli.htm. [Accessed September, 2013].

🗗 JUVENILE RHEUMATOID ARTHRITIS (JRA; STILL DISEASE)

General

Onset before age of 16 years; greater occurrence of systemic manifestations, monoarticular and oligoarticular joint involvement, and iridocyclitis.

Ocular

Hypopyon; band keratopathy; uveitis; cataract; papillitis; glaucoma; macular edema; ocular pain; vitreous cells; synechiae; scleritis; presumed to have an autoimmune etiology; antiocular antibodies, including iris protein antibodies, have been found in the sera of patients.

Clinical

Salmon pink macular rash; arthritis; hepatosplenomegaly; leukocytosis; chronic pain; joint swelling; low-grade fever; anemia; rheumatoid nodules.

Laboratory

Antinuclear antibody, rheumatoid factor, HLA-B27, X-ray imaging of joints.

Treatment

Uveitis is treated initially with topical corticosteroids. Systemic immunomodulatory agents may be useful for patients with limited or no response to topical or systemic corticosteroids.

🗗 BIBLIOGRAPHY

1. Roque MR, Roque BL, Miserocchi E, et al. (2012). Juvenile idiopathic arthritis uveitis. [online] Available from www.emedicine.com/oph/TOPIC675.HTM. [Accessed September, 2013].

🗗 RHEUMATOID ARTHRITIS (ADULT)

General

Systemic disease of unknown cause; more common in women (3:1); thought to have a strong autoimmune pathogenesis with positive IgM, IgG and IgA directed against the fragment crystallizable (Fc) portion of IgG.

Ocular

Sjögren syndrome; episcleritis; scleritis; keratitis; corneal ulcers; corneal perforation; uveitis; motility disorders; dry eyes; posterior scleritis (rare).

Clinical

Synovitis; stiffness; swelling; cartilaginous hypertrophy; joint pain; fibrous ankylosis; malaise; weight loss; vasomotor disturbance.

Laboratory

About 80% are positive for rheumatoid factor but it is also found in systemic lupus erythematosus (SLE), Sjögren syndrome, sarcoidosis, hepatitis B and tuberculosis.

Treatment

Nonsteroidal anti-inflammatory drugs, disease-modifying antirheumatic drugs (DMARDs), corticosteroids and immunosuppressant can be used.

BIBLIOGRAPHY

1. Temprano KK, Smith HR. (2012). Rheumatoid arthritis. [online] Available from www.emedicine.com/emerg/TOPIC48.HTM. [Accessed September, 2013].

INTERSTITIAL KERATITIS

General

Nonsuppurative inflammation characterized by cellular infiltrates, usually caused by syphilis but can be secondary to bacterial, viral, parasitic and autoimmune causes.

Clinical

Syphilis; tuberculosis; leprosy; lyme disease; acathamoeba; leishmania; Epstein-Barr; mumps; Cogan syndrome.

Ocular

Decreased vision; photophobia; tearing; blepharospasm; dense, white stromal necrosis of the cornea.

Laboratory

Clinical findings; serologic testing to determine the cause.

Treatment

Treat the underlying disorder. Ocular—topical corticosteroids; if permanent corneal opacity occurs, corneal transplant may be necessary.

BIBLIOGRAPHY

1. Majmudar PA. (2013). Interstitial keratitis. [online] Available from emedicine.medscape.com/article/1194376-overview. [Accessed September, 2013].

FELTY SYNDROME (CHAUFFARD-STILL SYNDROME; PRIMARY SPLENIC NEUTROPENIA WITH ARTHRITIS; RHEUMATOID ARTHRITIS WITH HYPERSPLENISM; STILL-CHAUFFARD SYNDROME; UVEITIS-RHEUMATOID ARTHRITIS SYNDROME)

General

Etiology not fully understood, possibly infection or allergy; onset in middle-aged patients or children; prognosis poor; collagen disorder; occasionally can occur without articular disease.

Ocular

Decreased tear formation; scleromalacia perforans; keratoconjunctivitis; chronic anterior uveitis; scleritis; vitreous opacities; macular edema; choroidal inflammation; papillitis; keratic precipitates; band-shaped keratopathy.

Clinical

Rheumatoid arthritis; splenomegaly; leukopenia; anemia (mild); oral lesion with ulcers and atrophy.

Laboratory

CBC with differential, CT, erythrocyte sedimentation rate (ESR) and serum immunoglobulin (Ig) levels invariably are elevated.

Treatment

Control the underlying RA with immunosuppressive therapy for RA often improves granulocytopenia and splenomegaly.

⊟ BIBLIOGRAPHY

1. Keating RM. (2012). Felty syndrome. [online] Available from www.emedicine.com/med/TOPIC782.HTM. [Accessed September, 2012].

⊟ 1B14. ROMBERG SYNDROME (PARRY-ROMBERG SYNDROME; PROGRESSIVE HEMIFACIAL ATROPHY; PROGRESSIVE FACIAL HEMIATROPHY; FACIAL HEMIATROPHY) ENOPHTHALMUS

General

Autosomal dominant; irritation in the peripheral trophic sympathetic system; onset in 2nd decade; both sexes affected.

Ocular

Enophthalmos; outer canthus lowered; absence of nasal portion of eyebrow; ptosis; paresis of ocular muscles; miosis; iritis; iridocyclitis; heterochromia iridis; keratitis; neuroparalytic keratitis; cataracts; choroiditis; Fuchs heterochromic cyclitis; retinal vascular abnormalities; association with Coats syndrome and exudative stellate neuroretinopathy; scleral melting.

Clinical

Atrophy of soft tissue on one side of the face, including tongue; trigeminal neuralgia and/or paresthesia; alopecia and poliosis not uncommon.

Laboratory/Ocular

Neuroimaging, CT scan of the orbits, MRI and bone scans.

Treatment/Ocular

Chemotherapy, ionizing radiation or immunosuppressive treatments.

⊟ BIBLIOGRAPHY

1. Aracena T, Roca FP, Barragan M. Progressive hemifacial atrophy (Parry-Romberg syndrome): report of two cases. Ann Ophthalmol. 1979;11:953-8.
2. Gass JD, Harbin TS, Del Piero EJ. Exudative stellate neuroretinopathy and Coats' syndrome in patients with progressive hemifacial atrophy. Eur J Ophthalmol. 1991; 1:2-10.
3. Hoang-Xuan T, Foster CS, Jakobiec FA, et al. Romberg's progressive hemifacial atrophy: an association with scleral melting. Cornea. 1991;10:361-6.
4. La Hey E, Baarsma GS. Fuchs' heterochromic cyclitis and retinal vascular abnormalities in progressive hemifacial atrophy. Eye. 1993;7:426-8.
5. Parry CH. Collections from unpublished papers, Volume 1. London: Underwood; 1825.
6. Romberg MH. Trophoneurosen, Klin Ergebn. Berlin: A. Forster; 1846.

⊟ 1B17. BOURNEVILLE SYNDROME (BOURNEVILLE-PRINGLE SYNDROME; TUBEROUS SCLEROSIS; EPILOIA)

General

Irregular dominant inheritance; more frequent in females; most patients die before age 24 years.

Ocular

Vitreous often cloudy; lens opacities; retinal mushroom-like tumor of grayish-white color; yellowish-white plaques with small hemorrhages and cystic changes in retina; papilledema; disk drusen; cerebral astrocytoma; 40–50% of patients have normal intelligence.

Clinical

Grand mal, petit mal, or Jacksonian seizures (manifest in first 2 years of life); mental changes from feeble mindedness to imbecility and idiocy; skin changes arranged usually about nose and cheeks (adenoma sebaceum); congenital tumors of kidney (hypernephroma or tubular adenoma) and heart (rhabdomyoma); cerebral astrocytoma.

Laboratory

Brain MRI is recommended for the detection and follow-up imaging of cortical tubers.

Treatment

A neurologist should be consulted to assist with seizure management and anticonvulsant medication.

BIBLIOGRAPHY

1. Schwartz RA, Jozwiak S, Pedersen R. (2013). Genetics of tuberous sclerosis. [online] Available from www.emedicine. com/ped/TOPIC2796.HTM. [Accessed September, 2013].

1B20. WAGNER SYNDROME (HYALOIDEORETINAL DEGENERATION; HEREDITARY HYALOIDEORETINAL DEGENERATION AND PALATOSCHISIS; CLEFTING SYNDROME; GOLDMANN-FAVRE SYNDROME; FAVRE HYALOIDEORETINAL DEGENERATION; RETINOSCHISIS WITH EARLY HEMERALOPIA) NYSTAGMUS

General

Irregular dominant inheritance; both sexes are affected.

Ocular

Epicanthus; nystagmus; myopia; iris atrophy; vitreous opacities with dense streaks and folds in posterior hyaloid membrane; corneal degeneration, including band-shaped keratopathy; cataracts; hyaloideoretinal degeneration (usually apparent after 15 years of age); narrowing of retinal vessels; pigmentary changes; type of retinal degeneration varies from case to case; retinal detachment and avascular preretinal membranes; marked choroidal sclerosis; pale optic disk; Bergmeister's papilla.

Clinical

Palatoschisis; genua valga; facial anomalies; hypoplastic maxilla; saddle nose; hyperextensible fingers, elbows and knees; tapering fingers.

Laboratory

Diagnosis is made by clinical findings.

Treatment

- *Seesaw nystagmus:* Visual field to consider neoplastic or vascular etiologies.
- *Upbeat nystagmus:* It may indicate multiple sclerosis, cerebellar degeneration, tumors or infarcts. Treatment is directed toward identification and resolution of underlying cause.
- *Downbeat nystagmus:* It affects the cerebellum or craniocervical junction including Arnold-Chiari malformation, multiple sclerosis, trauma, tumor, infection and many toxic metabolic entities. MRI may indicate a surgically correctable lesion. Periodic alternating nystagmus is continuous horizontal nystagmus from stroke, tumor, multiple sclerosis, trauma, infection, drug intoxication. It can occur from cataract, vitreous hemorrhage or optic atrophy.
- *Corneal opacity:* Medical treatment includes the use of hyperosmotic drops, nonsteroidal and steroid eye drops. Corneal transplant may be necessary.
- *Cataract:* Change in glasses can sometimes improve a patient's visual function temporarily; however, the most common treatment is cataract surgery.

BIBLIOGRAPHY

1. Black GC, Perveen R, Wiszniewski W, et al. A novel hereditary developmental vitreoretinopathy with multiple ocular abnormalities localizing to a 5-cM region of chromosome 5q13-q14. Ophthalmology. 1999;106(11):2074-81.
2. Frandsen E. Hereditary hyaloideoretinal degeneration (Wagner) in a Danish family. Arch Ophthalmol (Kbh). 1966;74:223.
3. Hirose T, Lee KY, Schepens CL. Wagner's hereditary vitreoretinal degeneration and retinal detachment. Arch Ophthalmol. 1973;89(3):176-85.
4. Kaiser-Kupfer M. Ectrodactyly, ectodermal dysplasia, and clefting syndrome. Am J Ophthalmol. 1973;76(6):992-8.
5. Wagner H. Ein Bisher Unbekanntes Erbleiden des Auges (Degeneratio Hyaloideo Hereditaria), Beobachtet im Kanton Zurich. Klin Monatsbl Augenheilkd. 1938;100:840.

1C. BIETTI DISEASE (BIETTI MARGINAL CRYSTALLINE DYSTROPHY)

General

Autosomal recessive; metabolic disturbance; histopathologic studies demonstrated advanced panchorioretinal atrophy with crystals and complex lipid inclusions seen in choroidal fibroblasts.

Ocular

Marginal corneal crystalline dystrophy with retinitis punctata albescens; panchorioretinal atrophy.

Clinical

Asymptomatic.

Laboratory

Diagnosis is made by clinical findings.

Treatment

Mild cases can be observed and soft contact lenses are helpful; PK may be necessary; graft recurrences are treated by superficial keratectomy, PTK or repeat PK.

BIBLIOGRAPHY

1. Bernauer W, Daicker B. Bietti's corneal-retinal dystrophy. A 16-year progression. Retina. 1992;12(1):18-20.
2. Kaiser-Kupfer MI, Chan CC, Markello TC, et al. Clinical biochemical and pathologic correlations in Bietti's crystalline dystrophy. Am J Ophthalmol. 1994;118(5):569-82.
3. Mauldin WM, O'Connor PS. Crystalline retinopathy (Bietti's tapetoretinal degeneration without marginal corneal dystrophy). Am J Ophthalmol. 1981;92(5):640-6.
4. Welch RB. Bietti's tapetoretinal degeneration with marginal corneal dystrophy crystalline retinopathy. Trans Am Ophthalmol Soc. 1977;75:164-79.

1D. EROSION SYNDROME

General

It is caused by imperfect adherence of corneal epithelium due to abnormalities in the basement membrane; abnormalities may be inherent, induced by trauma or both; disease is not vision threatening.

Ocular

Disabling episodes of pain; stabbing pain in the eye like that from a foreign body, most frequent on awakening; lesser forms of irritation; blurring of vision; drying associated with a stinging in the eyes; irregular astigmatism; corneal findings include anterior membrane dystrophies (epithelial and subepithelial dot, map or fingerprint-type changes).

Clinical

None.

Laboratory

Diagnosis is made by clinical findings.

Treatment

Goal of therapy is regenerating or repairing the epithelial basement membrane to restore thc adhesion between the epithelium and the anterior stroma, topical lubrication therapy, bandage soft contact lenses, debridement of the epithelium and basement membrane, or anterior stromal micropuncture may be useful.

BIBLIOGRAPHY

1. Verma A, Ehrenhaus MP. (2012). Recurrent corneal erosion. [online] Available from www.emedicine.com/oph/TOPIC113.HTM. [Accessed September, 2013].

🗗 1E. PTERYGIUM OF CONJUNCTIVA AND CORNEA

General

Autosomal dominant; more frequent in people who work outdoors; occurs late in life.

Ocular

Wing-shaped thickening in the conjunctiva, usually nasal, in the interpalpebral fissure area; alterations in corneal topography can cause a reduction in visual acuity.

Clinical

None.

Laboratory

Diagnosis is made by clinical findings.

Treatment

Patients with pterygia can be observed unless the lesions exhibit growth toward the center of the cornea or the patient exhibits symptoms of significant redness, discomfort, or alterations in visual function. Surgery for excision of pterygia is beneficial if visual function is disturbed.

🗗 BIBLIOGRAPHY

1. Fisher JP, Trattler WB. (2011). Pterygium. [online] Available from www.emedicine.com/oph/TOPIC542.HTM. [Accessed September, 2013].

🗗 1F. FUCHS-SALZMANN-TERRIEN SYNDROME

General

Features similar to those of Fuchs-Lyell syndrome; both are based on drug allergies (antibiotics, sulfonamides, arsenic preparations) (*see* Fuchs-Lyell syndrome).

Ocular

Features of Salzmann nodular dystrophy; superficial punctate keratitis; marginal degeneration of the cornea; intraocular hemorrhages; choroidal hemorrhages.

Clinical

Allergic cutaneous lesions with erythema and degrees of exfoliative dermatitis.

Laboratory

Hematology studies, chemistry to assess fluid and electrolyte losses, liver enzyme tests, coagulation studies.

Treatment

Management requires prompt detection and withdrawal of all potential causative agents, evaluation, and largely supportive care.

🗗 BIBLIOGRAPHY

1. Duke-Elder S (Ed). System of ophthalmology, Volume VIII. St. Louis: CV Mosby; 1965.
2. Fuchs E. Uber knotchenformige Hornhauttrubung. Graefes Arch Clin Exp Ophthalmol. 1902;53:423.

🗗 1H. TERRIEN DISEASE (TERRIEN MARGINAL DEGENERATION; GUTTER DYSTROPHY; PERIPHERAL FURROW KERATITIS; SENILE MARGINAL ATROPHY)

General

Rare; no known cause; 75% of patients are males from the age 10–70 years.

Ocular

Usually bilateral; may be asymmetrical; peripheral, fine, yellow-white, punctate stromal opacities associated with mild, superficial corneal vascularization; progressive thinning leads to peripheral gutter formation; decrease in visual acuity; loss of Bowman membrane and anterior stromal lamella with partial replacement of these tissues by a vascularized connective tissue; fatty deposits; thin stroma; thickness changes in Descemet's membrane; regular recurring attacks of pain and inflammation; keratoconus; reported association with Terrien's marginal degeneration.

Clinical

None.

Laboratory

Diagnosis is made by clinical findings.

Treatment/Ocular

Mild cases can be observed and soft contact lenses are helpful; PK may be necessary; graft recurrences are treated by superficial keratectomy, PTK or repeat PK.

BIBLIOGRAPHY

1. Ashenhurst M, Slomovic A. Corneal hydrops in Terrien's marginal degeneration: an unusual complication. Can J Ophthalmol. 1987;22(6):328-30.
2. Austin P, Brown SI. Inflammatory Terrien's marginal corneal disease. Am J Ophthalmol. 1981;92(2):189-92.
3. Friedlaender MH. Allergy and Immunology of the Eye, Illustrated edition. Hagerstown, MD: Harper & Row; 1979. p. 190.
4. Kremer I. Terrien's marginal degeneration associated with vernal conjunctivitis. Am J Ophthalmol. 1991;111(4):517-8.
5. Lopez JS, Price FW, Whitcup SM, et al. Immunohistochemistry of Terrien's and Mooren's corneal degeneration. Arch Ophthalmol. 1991;109(7):988-92.

2. DYSTROPHY

2A1. COGAN-GUERRY SYNDROME (MICROCYSTIC CORNEAL DYSTROPHY; MAP-DOT FINGERPRINT DYSTROPHY)

General

Etiology obscure; condition benign and asymptomatic; females predominantly affected; ultrastructural studies show discontinuous multilaminar thickened basement membrane under abnormal epithelium; the primary defect appears to be synthesis of abnormal basement membrane and adhesion complexes by the dystrophic epithelium.

Ocular

Reduced vision mainly with the involvement of center of cornea; very fine wavy lines resembling fingerprints within or very close to corneal epithelium and best seen on biomicroscopy with retroillumination; fine grayish spheres (0.1–0.5 mm in diameter) in superficial corneal epithelium; map-like irregular borderlined slightly grayish area.

Clinical

None.

Laboratory

Diagnosis is made by clinical findings.

Treatment

Pain suppression with pressure patch and antibiotic ointment; recurrence suppression with Muro drops or ointment; persistent erosion may be helped by mechanical debridement, local cycloplegics and a diamond burr to polish Bowman's membrane; anterior stromal puncture in resistant erosion and PTK may be useful.

BIBLIOGRAPHY

1. Verdier D. (2012). Map-dot-fingerprint dystrophy. [online] Available from emedicine.medscape.com/article/1193945-overview. [Accessed September, 2013].

2A2. CORNEAL DYSTROPHY, MEESMANN EPITHELIAL (MEESMANN EPITHELIAL DYSTROPHY OF CORNEA)

General

Autosomal dominant; rare; onset 1st year of life; possible that a disturbance of the cytoplasmic ground substance results in cellular homogenization with cyst formation.

Ocular

Myriads of fine punctate opacities in epithelium and Bowman membrane of cornea; thickening of the epithelial basement membrane of cornea; keratoconus.

Clinical

None.

Laboratory

Diagnosis is made by clinical findings.

Treatment

Usually not treatment. Bandage contact lens can be used to reduce discomfort and reduce visual loss.

◫ BIBLIOGRAPHY

1. Tremblay M, Dubé I. Meesmann's corneal dystrophy: ultrastructural features. Can J Ophthalmol. 1982;17:24-8.
2. Fine BS, Yanoff M, Pitts E, et al. Meesmann's epithelial dystrophy of cornea. Am J Ophthalmol. 1977;83:633-42.
3. McKusick VA. Mendelian Inheritance in Man; A Catalog of Human Genes and Genetic Disorders, 12th edition. Baltimore: The Johns Hopkins University Press; 1998.
4. Online Mendelian Inheritance in Man, OMIM. McKusick-Nathans Institute for Genetic Medicine, Johns Hopkins University and National Center for Biotechnology Information, National Library of Medicine, February 12, 2007. Available from www.ncbi.nlm.nih.gov/omim. [Accessed September, 2013].
5. Cogan DG, Donaldson DD, Kuwabara T, et al. Microcystic dystrophy of the corneal epithelium. Trans Am Ophthalmol Soc. 1964;62:213-25.

◫ 2A3. THYGESON SYNDROME (KERATITIS SUPERFICIALIS PUNCTATA)

General

Etiology is probably of viral origin; recurrence every 3–4 years.

Ocular

Punctate lesions of cornea; keratitis.

Clinical

None.

Laboratory/ocular

Diagnosis is made by clinical findings.

Treatment/ocular

Keratitis: Local treatment is used for prevention and reduction of corneal damage. Systemic therapy is used for controlling the underlying disease. Tissue adhesives may be necessary for impending perforation. Keratectomy, conjunctival resection, amniotic membrane transplantation and keratoplasty may be necessary.

◫ BIBLIOGRAPHY

1. Magalini SI, Scrascia E. Dictionary of Medical Syndromes, 2nd edition. Philadelphia, PA: Lippincott Williams and Wilkins; 1981.
2. Thygeson P. Superficial punctate keratitis. J Am Med Assoc. 1950;144(18):1544-9.

◫ 2B1. REIS-BUCKLERS CORNEAL DYSTROPHY (CORNEAL DYSTROPHY OF BOWMAN'S LAYER, SUPERFICIAL VARIANT OF GRANULAR DYSTROPHY, GRANULAR CORNEAL DYSTROPHY TYPE III)

General

Bilateral, progressive, autosomal dominant corneal dystrophy, manifests in early childhood.

Clinical

None.

Ocular

Recurrent corneal epithelial erosions, corneal scarring, opacification at level of Bowman's layer and superficial stroma.

Laboratory

Mutation in TGFBI gene on chromosome 5q31 in many cases.

Treatment

Ocular lubricants, topical antibiotics, cycloplegic agents and hyperosmotic agents are useful. Debridement of loose epithelium, therapeutic contact lens, anterior stromal micropuncture, PTK, lamellar keratoplasty or PK may be necessary.

BIBLIOGRAPHY

1. Afshari N, Trattler WB, Clark WL. (2012). Granular dystrophy. [online] Available from www.emedicine.com/oph/TOPIC92.HTM. [Accessed September, 2013].

2B2. FRANCOIS (1) DYSTROPHY (FRANCOIS-NEETENS SYNDROME; CENTRAL CLOUDY DYSTROPHY; CLOUDY CENTRAL CORNEAL DYSTROPHY)

General

Autosomal dominant; etiology unknown; not progressive; isolated keratocytes contain elevated amounts of glycosaminoglycans and lipids.

Ocular

Bilateral dystrophy of central third of cornea; snowflake patches covering the pupil; lesions show no definite structure or limits; more dense near Descemet membrane and becoming less toward the anterior surface toward the periphery; associated with central cloudy dystrophy; keratoconus; limbal dermoid; pseudoxanthoma elasticum; lenticular opacities; reduced corneal sensation.

Laboratory

Diagnosis is made by clinical findings.

Treatment

Treatment is primarily surgical. Treatment of amblyopia and optical therapy can be helpful.

BIBLIOGRAPHY

1. Scheinfeld NS, Freilich BD, Freilich J. (2013). Congenital clouding of the cornea. [online] Available from www.emedicine.com/oph/TOPIC771.HTM. [Accessed September, 2013].

2B3. GRANULAR CORNEAL DYSTROPHY

General

Autosomal dominant inheritance affecting the corneal stroma.

Clinical

None.

Ocular

Corneal dystrophy can be divided into four types: (1) Granular corneal dystrophy (GCD) -I, classic, Groenouw; GCD-II, Avellino dystrophy, combined lattice/granular; GCD-III, superficial, Reis Bucklers' corneal dystrophy, affecting the Bowman's layer; GCD-IV, French variant similar to GCD-III.

Laboratory

Diagnosis is made by clinical findings.

Treatment

Mild cases—observation and recurrent erosion therapy; soft contact lenses are helpful; PK may be necessary; graft recurrences treated by superficial keratectomy; PTK or repeat PK.

BIBLIOGRAPHY

1. Afshari N, Trattler WB, Clark WL. (2012). Granular dystrophy. [online] Available from www.emedicine.com/oph/TOPIC92.HTM. [Accessed September, 2013].

🖥 2B4. LATTICE CORNEAL DYSTROPHY (LATTICE DYSTROPHY TYPE I, LATTICE DYSTROPHY TYPE II, LATTICE DYSTROPHY TYPE III, LCD-I, LCD-II, LCD-III, MERETOJA'S SYNDROME, BIBER-HAAB-DIMMER DYSTROPHY, FAMILIAL MYLOID POLYNEUROPATHY TYPE IV, AVELLINO DYSTROPHY)

General

Lattice corneal dystrophy (LCD)-I, autosomal dominant; LCD-II, autosomal dominant onset 3rd decade (Scandinavia); LCD-III, autosomal dominant, onset 3rd decade (Japan).

Clinical

None.

Ocular

Corneal dystrophy, thin lines in corneal stroma.

Laboratory

Diagnosis is made by clinical diagnosis.

Treatment

- *Topical*: Lubricants, soft contacts, pressure patching.
- *Surgical*: PTK may be useful in superficial lesions. PK may be necessary.

🖥 BIBLIOGRAPHY

1. Roy FH. Ocular Differential Diagnosis, 9th edition. New Delhi: Jaypee Brothers Medical Publishers; 2012.

🖥 2B5. CORNEAL DYSTROPHY, MACULAR TYPE (GROENOUW TYPE II CORNEAL DYSTROPHY)

General

Autosomal recessive; onset in 1st decade, between 5 and 9 years; progressive; acid mucopolysaccharides found in corneal fibroblasts; it has been suggested that the defect may not be limited to the cornea.

Ocular

Minute gray, punctate opacities; reduced corneal sensitivity; photophobia; foreign body sensations; recurrent corneal erosions; keratoconus.

Clinical

Defect in metabolism of glycoprotein processing.

Laboratory

Diagnosis is made by clinical findings.

Treatment

Once the acute episode of recurrent corneal erosion resolves, preventive treatment may include sodium chloride (NaCl) 5% drops or artificial tear lubricating drops during the day and NaCl 5% ointment or lubricating ointment at bedtime. Excessive corneal erosions or a mild visual decrease can be treated with excimer laser PTK. If visual acuity drops and the opacities are deep, lamellar or full-thickness corneal transplantation can be performed.

🖥 BIBLIOGRAPHY

1. Afshari N, Trattler WB, Clark WL. (2012). Macular dystrophy. [online] Available from www.emedicine.com/oph/TOPIC94. HTM. [Accessed September, 2013].

2C1. FUCHS' CORNEAL DYSTROPHY (FUCHS' ENDOTHELIAL DYSTROPHY OF THE CORNEA, COMBINED DYSTROPHY OF FUCHS', ENDOTHELIAL DYSTROPHY OF THE CORNEA, EPITHELIAL DYSTROPHY OF FUCHS', FUCHS' EPITHELIAL-ENDOTHELIAL DYSTROPHY)

General

Bilateral, slowly progressive, primary corneal disease, which results in vision loss due to corneal edema. Autosomal dominant and usually not clinically evident until the 4th or 5th decade of life.

Clinical

None.

Ocular

Central corneal guttae; gray, thickened appearance of Descemet's membrane; stromal edema; subepithelial edema; decreased visual acuity.

Laboratory

Diagnosis is made by clinical findings. The characteristics include endothelium producing an abnormal, banded, posterior layer of Descemet's membrane with characteristics of central guttae excrescences which are a hallmark of this disease.

Treatment

Early intervention includes NaCl 5% solution or ointment and the use of a hair dryer on low heat setting for tear film evaporation and corneal deturgescence. Surgical intervention includes corneal transplantation, endothelial keratoplasty (EK), deep lamellar endothelial keratoplasty (DLEK) and Descemet's stripping endothelial keratoplasty (DSEK).

BIBLIOGRAPHY

1. Singh D, Mittal V. (2012). Fuchs endothelial dystrophy. [online] Available from www.emedicine.com/oph/TOPIC91.HTM. [Accessed September, 2013].

2C2. POSTERIOR POLYMORPHOUS DYSTROPHY

General

Rare, bilateral corneal disorder of Descemet's membrane. Autosomal dominant associated with Alport's syndrome and keratoconus.

Clinical

None.

Ocular

Corneal edema which usually develops in midlife, open or closed angle glaucoma.

Laboratory

Specular microscopy shows dark rings with scalloped-edges around a light center.

Treatment

Sodium chloride drops or ointment, glaucoma therapy (medical or surgical) and PK may be necessary.

BIBLIOGRAPHY

1. Roy FH, Fraunfelder FW, Fraunfelder FT. Roy and Fraunfelder's Current Ocular Therapy, 6th edition. London, UK: Elsevier; 2008.

2C3. CORNEAL SNOWFLAKE DYSTROPHY

General

Autosomal dominant; prevalence of green irides.

Ocular

Star-shaped chromatophore-like cells attached to anterior lens capsule; Bitot's spots; white flecks on endothelium and Descemet's membrane.

Clinical

Lactose intolerance; malabsorption of fat; vitamin A deficiency; dry skin; nevi; freckles.

Laboratory

Diagnosis is made by clinical findings.

Treatment

Sodium chloride drops or ointment.

BIBLIOGRAPHY

1. Meretoja J. Inherited corneal snowflake dystrophy with oculocutaneous pigmentation disturbances and other symptoms. Ophthalmologica. 1985;191(4):197-205.
2. Meretoja J. Inherited syndrome with corneal snowflake dystrophy, oculocutaneous pigmentary disturbances, pseudoexfoliation and malabsorption. Statistical data of some symptoms. Ophthalmic Res. 1987;19(5):245-54.

2D1. SCHNYDER'S CRYSTALLINE CORNEAL DYSTROPHY

General

Rare, autosomal dominant disorder with abnormal bilateral deposition of cholesterol and lipid in the cornea.

Clinical

Hypercholester: olemia and genu valgum.

Ocular

Central corneal haze, subepithelial cholesterol crystal deposition, midperipheral, panstromal haze and arcus lipoides.

Laboratory

Serum lipid analysis due to hyperlipidemia.

Treatment

Phototherapeutic keratectomy can be used to treat subepithelial crystals and PK may be necessary.

BIBLIOGRAPHY

1. Weiss JS, Spagnolo B. (2011). Crystalline dystrophy. [online] Available from www.emedicine.com/oph/TOPIC548.HTM. [Accessed September, 2013].

3A. KERATOCONUS (CONICAL CORNEA)

Keratoconus is characterized by noninflammatory ectasia of the cornea in its axial part, with considerable visual impairment because of development of a high degree of irregular myopic astigmatism. Keratoconus may be associated with:

[†]1. Acute hydrops of the cornea
2. Alagille syndrome
[†]3. Anteoderma and bilateral subcapsular cataracts
4. Aniridia
5. Apert syndrome (acrodysplasia)
6. Asthma, hay fever
[*]7. Atopic dermatitis, keratosis plantaris, and palmaris
[†]8. Autographism
9. Avellino dystrophy
10. Blue sclerotics, including van der Hoeve syndrome (osteogenesis imperfecta)
11. Chandler syndrome (iridocorneal endothelial syndrome)
[†]12. Congenital hip dysplasia
13. Wearing of contact lens
14. Crouzon syndrome

* Indicates most frequent

†15. Deep filiform corneal dystrophy
16. Ehlers-Danlos syndrome (fibrodysplasia elastica gen-eralisata, cutis hyperelastica)
†17. Essential iris atrophy
†18. Facial hemiatrophy
†*19. Familial
†20. False chordae tendineae of left ventricle
†21. Fleck corneal dystrophy
22. Floppy eyelid syndrome
23. Focal dermal hypoplasia (Goltz syndrome)
24. Fuchs corneal endothelial dystrophy
25. Grönblad-Strandberg syndrome (pseudoxanthoma elasticum)
†26. Hereditary history
†27. Hyperextensible joints and mitral valve prolapse
†28. Hyperornithemia
29. Infantile tapetoretinal degeneration of Leber
†30. Iridocorneal dysgenesis
†31. Iridoschisis
†32. Joint hypermobility
33. Kuru syndrome
34. Laurence-Moon-Bardet-Biedl syndrome (retinitis-polydactyly-adiposogenital syndrome)
35. Little syndrome (nail-patella syndrome)
36. Lymphogranuloma venereum
37. Marfan syndrome (arachnodactyly dystrophia meso-dermalis congenita)
38. Measles retinopathy
†39. Microcornea
40. Mongolism (Down syndrome)
41. Mulvihill-Smith syndrome
†42. Neurocutaneous angiomatosis
43. Neurodermatitis
44. Neurofibromatosis (von Recklinghausen syndrome)
45. Noonan syndrome (male Turner syndrome)
46. Ocular hypertension
47. Pellucid marginal corneal degeneration
†48. Posterior ectasia following laser in situ keratomileusis (generally if stromal bed less than 250 ì)
49. Posterior lenticonus
50. Posterior polymorphous dystrophy
51. Retinal disinsertion syndrome
52. Retinitis pigmentosa
53. Retinopathy of prematurity
54. Rieger syndrome
55. Tourette disease
†*56. Trauma, such as rubbing of eyes, birth injury, or con-tusion
†57. Vernal catarrh
†58. Vernal conjunctivitis

Treatment

The use of gas permeable contact lenses (CLs) is usually the first choice, but there still other options that may be beneficial to treat the condition.

🗗 BIBLIOGRAPHY

1. Weissman BA, Yeung KK. (2013). Keratoconus. [online] Available from www.emedicine.com/oph/TOPIC104.HTM. [Accessed September, 2013].

†Indicates a general entry and therefore has not been described in detail in the text

🗗 3A2. ALAGILLE SYNDROME (AGS; ALAGILLE-WATSON SYNDROME, AWS; CHOLESTASIS WITH PERIPHERAL PULMONARY STENOSIS; ARTERIOHEPATIC DYSPLASIA, AHD; HEPATIC DUCTULAR HYPOPLASIA, SYNDROMATIC)

General

May be associated with 20p 11.2 deletion and four distinct coding mutations in Jag 1 gene.

Ocular

Posterior embryotoxon and retinal pigmentary changes; anterior chamber anomalies, associated with eccentric or ectopic pupils.

Clinical

Neonatal jaundice; prominent forehead and chin; pulmonic valvular stenosis as well as peripheral arterial stenosis; abnormal vertebrae (butterfly vertebrae) and decrease in interpediculate distance in the lumbar spine; absent deep tendon reflexes and poor school performance; in the facies, broad forehead, pointed mandible, and bulbous tip of the nose; and in the fingers, varying degrees of fore-shortening.

Laboratory

Liver biopsy specimens typically exhibit features suggestive of chronic cholestasis and paucity of interlobular bile ducts. The majority of biopsies (wedge or needle) reveal features of bile duct paucity.

Treatment

Subspecialty consultation may facilitate diagnosis and provide long-term care. Consultation with an ophthalmologist may provide the diagnosis. A pediatric hepatologist can assist with management of chronic cholestatic liver disease. Cardiology consultation can assist with the diagnosis and therapy for intracardiac disease, as well as other vascular abnormalities. Nephrology consultations are useless when structural renal disease is present or if suspicions of evolving renal insufficiency arise.

🗗 BIBLIOGRAPHY

1. Scheimann A. (2012). Alagille syndrome. [online] Available from www.emedicine.com/ped/TOPIC60.HTM. [Accessed September, 2013].

🗗 3A4. ANIRIDIA (CONGENITAL ANIRIDIA, HEREDITARY ANIRIDIA)

General

Hereditary, recessive (two-thirds of cases), can be dominant, sporadic or traumatic; absence of the iris; rare; usually bilateral unless due to trauma.

Ocular

Absence of iris; subluxed lens; iridodialysis; cataract; glaucoma; corneal scarring, vascularization, and edema; iris colobomata; round eccentric pupils; keratoconus.

Clinical

Cerebellar ataxia; mental retardation; Wilms' tumor (WT).

Laboratory

Chromosomal deletion, cytogenic analysis, submicroscopic deletions of WT gene with FISH technique, polymerase chain reaction (PCR) genotyping halotypes across paired box gene 6 (PAX6)-WT1 region provides evidence of a chromosomal deletion.

Treatment

Systemic or topical glaucoma therapy.

🗗 BIBLIOGRAPHY

1. François J, Coucke D, Coppieters R. Aniridia-Wilms' tumor syndrome. Ophthalmologica. 1977;174(1):35-9.
2. Johns KJ, O'Day DM. Posterior chamber intraocular lenses after extracapsular cataract extraction in patients with aniridia. Ophthalmology. 1991;98(11):1698-702.
3. Kremer I, Rajpal RK, Rapuano CJ, et al. Results of penetrating keratoplasty in aniridia. Am J Ophthalmol. 1993;115(3):317-20.
4. Magalini SI, Scrascia E. Dictionary of Medical Syndromes, 2nd edition. Philadelphia, PA: JB Lippincott; 1981.
5. Mintz-Hittner HA, Ferrell RE, Lyons LA, et al. Criteria to detect minimal expressivity within families with autosomal dominant aniridia. Am J Ophthalmol. 1992;114(6):700-7.
6. Nelson LB, Spaeth GL, Nowinski TS, et al. Aniridia. A review. Surv Ophthalmol. 1984;28(6):621-42.
7. Skeens HM, Brooks BP, Holland EJ. Congenital aniridia variant: minimally abnormal irides with severe limbal stem cell deficiency. Ophthalmology. 2011;118(7):1260-4.

🗗 3A5. APERT SYNDROME (ACROCEPHALOSYNDACTYLISM SYNDROME; ACROCRANIO-DYSPHALANGIA; ACRODYSPLASIA; SPHENOACROCRANIO-SYNDACTYLY; ABSENT-DIGITS-CRANIAL-DEFECTS SYNDROME)

General

Inherited; most often recessive, sometimes dominant; an extreme form of Apert syndrome has been described as Carpenter syndrome, with the latter being familial and transmitted as an autosomal recessive.

Ocular

Shallow orbit; exophthalmos; hypertelorism; ptosis; strabismus; nystagmus; ophthalmoplegia; hyperopia; exposure keratitis; cataracts; ectopia lentis; medullated nerve fibers; retinal detachment; papilledema with subsequent optic atrophy; keratoconus.

Clinical

Oxycephaly (tower skull); syndactyly (symmetrically); synostoses and synarthroses of shoulder and elbows frequent; agenesis of spinal bones and limbs; headaches; hypertelorism; hypoplastic maxilla; acrocephaly; abnormality of sutures.

Laboratory

CT is the most useful radiological examination in identifying skull shape and presence or absence of involved sutures. MRI reveals the anatomy of the soft-tissue structures and associated brain abnormalities.

Treatment

Medical treatment involves fitting patient with hearing aids, providing airway management and psychological counseling. Surgical care involves early release of the coronal suture and fronto-orbital advancement and reshaping to reduce dysmorphic and unwanted skull growth changes.

BIBLIOGRAPHY

1. Chen H. (2013). Apert syndrome. [online] Available from www.emedicine.com/ped/TOPIC122.HTM. [Accessed September, 2013].

3A6. ASTHMA (HAYFEVER)

General

Asthma characterized by paroxysms of expiratory dyspnea and wheezing, overinflation of the lungs, cough, and rhonchi; causes include allergy to external inhaled allergens, respiratory infections, and psychophysiologic reaction to stress. Hayfever (allergic asthma) characterized by sneezing, rhinorrhea, swelling of nasal mucosa, and itchy eyes; caused by spread of pollens in air or exposure to antigens; seasonal; occurs most frequently in young persons.

Ocular

Lacrimation; allergic conjunctivitis; periocular xanthogranulomas.

Clinical

Rhinorrhea; sneezing; mucosal swelling with occlusion of airway; insomnia; nasal polyps; wheezing; cough; headache; rhinitis.

Laboratory

Testing for reaction to specific allergens can be helpful to confirm the diagnosis of allergic rhinitis and to determine specific allergic triggers.

Treatment

The management involves allergen avoidance, pharmacological management, and immunotherapy. Symptoms can be treated with oral antihistamines, decongestants, or both.

BIBLIOGRAPHY

1. Morris MJ. (2013). Asthma. [online] Available from www.emedicine.com/emerg/TOPIC43.HTM. [Accessed September, 2013].

3A7. ATOPIC DERMATITIS (ATOPIC ECZEMA; BESNIER PRURIGO)

General

Highly specific disease resulting from heredity determined lowered cutaneous threshold to pruritus and characterized by intense itching; elevated total and specific immunoglobulin E.

Ocular

Keratoconjunctivitis; keratoconus; cataract; atopic dermatitis of lid; secondary glaucoma; uveitis; possible association with retinal detachment; pannus; blepharoconjunctivitis; corneal scarring; suppurative keratitis.

Clinical

In infants, it involves the face with dry or oozing erythematous patches; in children and adolescents, itching localized in the neck, antecubital spaces, popliteal folds, and ears; seborrheic changes.

Laboratory

Diagnosis is made by clinical findings.

Treatment

Topical corticosteroids are the mainstay of treatment. Adequate rehydration will minimize the direct effects of irritants and allergens on the skin and maximize the effect of topically applied therapies, thus decreasing the need for topical steroids.

BIBLIOGRAPHY

1. Schwartz RA. (2013). Pediatric atopic dermatitis. [online] Available from www.emedicine.com/ped/TOPIC2567.HTM. [Accessed September, 2013].

3A9. LATTICE CORNEAL DYSTROPHY (LATTICE DYSTROPHY TYPE I, LATTICE DYSTROPHY TYPE II, LATTICE DYSTROPHY TYPE III, LCD-I, LCD-II, LCD-III, MERETOJA'S SYNDROME, BIBER-HAAB-DIMMER DYSTROPHY, FAMILIAL MYLOID POLYNEUROPATHY TYPE IV, AVELLINO DYSTROPHY)

General

LCD-I, autosomal dominant; LCD-II, autosomal dominant onset 3rd decade (Scandinavia); LCD-III, autosomal dominant, onset 3rd decade (Japan).

Clinical

None.

Ocular

Corneal dystrophy, thin lines in corneal stroma.

Laboratory

Diagnosis is made by clinical diagnosis.

Treatment

- *Topical*: Lubricants, soft contacts, pressure patching.
- *Surgical*: PTK may be useful in superficial lesions. PK may be necessary.

BIBLIOGRAPHY

1. Roy FH. Ocular Differential Diagnosis, 9th edition. New Delhi: Jaypee Brothers Medical Publishers; 2012.

3A10. VAN DER HOEVE SYNDROME (OSTEOGENESIS IMPERFECTA; OSTEOPSATHYROSIS; EKMAN SYNDROME; LOBSTEIN SYNDROME; SPURWAY SYNDROME; VROLIK SYNDROME; EDDOWES SYNDROME; BRITTLE BONE DISEASE) GLAUCOMA

General

Autosomal dominant.

Ocular

Glaucoma; blue sclera; keratoconus; cataract; optic nerve atrophy; retinopathy; retinal detachment.

Clinical

Brittle bones; deafness; hyperflexibility of ligaments; dental defects; developmental delay.

Laboratory

DNA blood test, analysis of type I, III and V collagens synthesized by fibroblast, prenatal sonography.

Treatment

Synthetic analogs of pyrophosphate, cyclic intravenous pamidronate, growth hormone.

BIBLIOGRAPHY

1. Ramachandran M, Achan P, Jones DH, et al. (2012). Osteogenesis imperfecta. [online] Available from www.emedicine.com/orthoped/TOPIC530.HTM. [Accessed September, 2013].

3A11. IRIS NEVUS SYNDROME (COGAN-REESE SYNDROME; CHANDLER SYNDROME; IRIDOCORNEAL ENDOTHELIAL SYNDROME; ICE SYNDROME)

General

Usually unilateral but may be bilateral; usually in young adult women; nonfamilial; cause unknown; Chandler, Cogan-Reese, and iridocorneal endothelial (ICE) syndromes have been considered as three separate syndromes but they are now recognized as a single spectrum of diseases.

Ocular

Unilateral glaucoma in eyes with peripheral anterior synechiae; multiple iris nodules; ectopic Descemet's membrane; corneal edema; stromal iris atrophy; iris pigment epithelial atrophy; ectropion uveae; ectopic pupil; keratoconus; herpes simplex virus deoxyribonucleic acid (DNA) has been detected in patients with ICE syndrome from corneal specimens.

Clinical

Glass-like membrane covering the anterior iris surface; corneal endothelial degeneration and accompanying ectopic endothelial membranes are responsible for occlusion of the filtration meshwork and subsequent pressure increase.

Laboratory

Diagnosis is made by clinical findings.

Treatment

This disease does not usually respond to medications and trabeculectomy operations. Glaucoma drainage devices create an alternate aqueous pathway by channeling aqueous from the anterior chamber through a tube to an equatorial plate inserted under the conjunctiva that promotes bleb formation.

BIBLIOGRAPHY

1. Alvarado JA, Underwood JL, Green WR, et al. Detection of herpes simplex viral DNA in the iridocorneal endothelial syndrome. Arch Ophthalmol. 1994;112(12):1601-9.
2. Buckley RJ. Pathogenesis of the ICE syndrome. Br J Ophthalmol. 1994;78(8):595-6.
3. Chandler PA. Atrophy of the stroma of the iris; endothelial dystrophy, corneal edema, and glaucoma. Am J Ophthalmol. 1956;41(4):607-15.
4. Cogan DG, Reese AB. A syndrome of iris nodules, ectopic Descemet's membrane, and unilateral glaucoma. Doc Ophthalmol. 1969;26:424-33.
5. Radius RL, Herschler J. Histopathology in the iris-nevus (Cogan-Reese) syndrome. Am J Ophthalmol. 1980;89(6):780-6.
6. Rodrigues MM, Stulting RD, Waring GO. Clinical, electron microscopic, and immunohistochemical study of the corneal endothelium and Descemet's membrane in the iridocorneal endothelial syndrome. Am J Ophthalmol. 1986;101(1):16-27.

3A13. NEOVASCULARIZATION, CORNEAL CONTACT LENS RELATED

General

Pathologic state in which new blood vessels extending in the corneal stroma from trauma, inflammation, infection, toxic insults secondary to contact lens usage.

Clinical

None.

Ocular

Vessel ingrowth into the cornea, ocular irritation.

Laboratory

Diagnosis is made by clinical findings.

Treatment

Observation, eliminate cause, topical steroid drops, reduced time for an individual using contact lens, corneal laser photocoagulation.

BIBLIOGRAPHY

1. Weissman BA, Yeung KK. (2011). Neovascularization, corneal, CL-related. [online] Available from emedicine.medscape.com/article/1195886-overview. [Accessed September, 2013].

3A14. CROUZON SYNDROME (DYSOSTOSIS CRANIOFACIALIS; OXYCEPHALY; CRANIOFACIAL DYSOSTOSIS; PARROT-HEAD SYNDROME; MÖBIUS-CROUZON SYNDROME; HEREDITARY CRANIOFACIAL DYSOSTOSIS)

General

Autosomal dominant; manifestations present at birth.

Ocular

Bilateral exophthalmos; hypertelorism (wide interpupillary distance); obliquity of palpebral fissures with outer canthus slanting downward; nystagmus; exotropia; upper field defects due to pressure upon the optic nerve on its lower part; bluish sclera; exposure keratitis in extreme exophthalmos; cataract; papilledema; secondary optic atrophy; corneal dystrophy; ptosis; strabismus; keratoconus.

Clinical

Prognathism; maxillary hypoplasia with short upper lip; synostosis of coronal and lambda sutures; parrot-beaked nose (psittachosrhina); widening temporal fossae; headaches.

Laboratory

Skull, spine, and hand radiography is usually necessary to confirm the diagnosis.

Treatment

Neurosurgical procedure is recommended in cases of intracranial hypertension leading to further optic atrophy.

BIBLIOGRAPHY

1. Chen H. (2013). Genetics of Crouzon syndrome. [online] Available from www.emedicine.com/ped/TOPIC511.HTM. [Accessed September, 2013].

3A16. EHLERS-DANLOS SYNDROME (FIBRODYSPLASIA ELASTICA GENERALISATA; CUTIS HYPERELASTICA; MEEKEREN-EHLERS-DANLOS SYNDROME; INDIAN RUBBER MAN SYNDROME; CUTIS LAXA)

General

Present at birth; autosomal dominant; two groups: cutaneous and articular; syndrome is one of the three primary disorders of elastic tissue [other two disorders are pseudoxanthoma elasticum (Grönblad-Strandberg syndrome) and senile elastosis]; inherited disorder of collagen biosynthesis.

Ocular

Hyperelasticity of palpebral skin; easy eversion of upper lid; ptosis; epicanthal folds; hypotony of extraocular muscles; strabismus; microcornea; thinning of cornea with keratoconus; thinning of sclera (blue sclera); subluxation of lens; angioid streaks; chorioretinal hemorrhages; retinitis proliferans with secondary detachment; macular degeneration; myopia; ruptured globe after minor trauma; limbus-to-limbus corneal thinning; acute hydrops; cornea plana; keratoglobus.

Clinical

Cutaneous manifestations include thin, atrophic, fragile skin, cutaneous hyperelasticity and pseudomolluscoid tumors; articular manifestations include excessive articular laxity and luxations; hypermobile joints.

Laboratory

Biochemical studies can detect alterations in collagen molecules in cultured skin fibroblasts. Molecular (DNA) based testing is available. Diagnosis may by urinary analyte assay and clinical examination is the most common.

Treatment

Ascorbic acid therapy, in the event of skin lacerations seriously consider alternatives to sutures, including adhesive strips and wound glues, monitor for cardiac conditions and scoliosis.

BIBLIOGRAPHY

1. Steiner RD. (2011). Genetics of Ehlers-Danlos syndrome. [online] Available from www.emedicine.com/ped/TOPIC654.HTM. [Accessed September, 2013].

3A22. FLOPPY EYELID SYNDROME

General

Origin unknown; more common in males; overweight; X-chromosome-linked inheritance pattern or possible hormonal influence; it has been postulated that the degenerative changes in the tarsus may result from the combination of local pressure-induced lid ischemia and systemic hypoventilation.

Ocular

Easily everted, floppy upper eyelid and papillary conjunctivitis of the upper palpebral conjunctiva; upper eyelid everts during sleep, resulting in irritation, papillary conjunctivitis and conjunctival keratinization; most distinct feature is rubbery, malleable upper tarsus; keratoconus; punctate keratopathy; blepharoptosis; lash ptosis.

Clinical

Obesity; sleep apnea.

Laboratory

Conjunctival scrapings reveal keratinized epithelial cells. Bacterial cultures are important.

Treatment

Full-thickness upper and lower eyelid resection.

BIBLIOGRAPHY

1. Ezra DG, Beaconsfield M, Sira M, et al. Long-term outcomes of surgical approaches to the treatment of floppy eyelid syndrome. Ophthalmology. 2010;117(4):839-46.
2. Ezra DG, Beaconsfield M, Sira M, et al. The associations of floppy eyelid syndrome: a case control study. Ophthalmology. 2010;117(4):831-8.

3A23. GOLTZ SYNDROME (FOCAL DERMAL HYPOPLASIA SYNDROME)

General

X-linked dominant inheritance; lethal in males; skin manifestations present at birth.

Ocular

Microphthalmia; strabismus; coloboma of iris and/or choroid; epiphora; blue sclera; nystagmus; anophthalmos; keratoconus.

Clinical

Skin atrophy and linear pigmentation; telangiectasias of trunk and extremities; superficial, localized fatty skin deposits; multiple papillomas of mucous membranes and periorificial skin (oral, genital, anal); anomalies of extremities with syndactyly, oligodactyly, adactyly; hypohidrosis; paper-thin nails may be present; spina bifida; hypoplasia of right clavicle; umbilical or inguinal hernia.

Laboratory

Radiography may reveal osteopathia striata.

Treatment

Flashlamp-pumped pulse dye laser may ameliorate the pruritic symptoms that sometimes are noted in affected skin and improve the clinical appearance of the telangiectatic and erythematous skin lesions. Papillomas frequently require repeated surgical intervention.

BIBLIOGRAPHY

1. Goltz RW, Castelo-Soccio L. (2012). Focal dermal hypoplasia syndrome. [online] Available from emedicine.medscape.com/article/1110936-overview. [Accessed September, 2013].

3A24. FUCHS' CORNEAL DYSTROPHY (FUCHS' ENDOTHELIAL DYSTROPHY OF THE CORNEA, COMBINED DYSTROPHY OF FUCHS, ENDOTHELIAL DYSTROPHY OF THE CORNEA, EPITHELIAL DYSTROPHY OF FUCHS, FUCHS' EPITHELIAL-ENDOTHELIAL DYSTROPHY)

General

Bilateral, slowly progressive, primary corneal disease, which results in vision loss due to corneal edema. Autosomal dominant and usually not clinically evident until the 4th or 5th decade of life.

Clinical

None.

Ocular

Central corneal guttae; gray, thickened appearance of Descemet's membrane; stromal edema; subepithelial edema; decreased visual acuity.

Laboratory

Diagnosis is made by clinical findings. The characteristics include endothelium producing an abnormal, banded, posterior layer of Descemet's membrane with characteristics of central guttae excrescences which are a hallmark of this disease.

Treatment

Early intervention includes NaCl 5% solution or ointment and the use of a hair dryer on low heat setting for tear film evaporation and corneal deturgescence. Surgical intervention includes corneal transplantation, EK, DLEK and DSEK.

BIBLIOGRAPHY

1. Singh D, Mittal V. (2012). Fuchs endothelial dystrophy. [online] Available from www.emedicine.com/oph/TOPIC91.HTM. [Accessed September, 2013].

3A25. GRÖNBLAD-STRANDBERG SYNDROME (SYSTEMIC ELASTODYSTROPHY; PSEUDOXANTHOMA ELASTICUM; ELASTORRHEXIS; DARIER-GRÖNBLAD-STRANDBERG SYNDROME)

General

Autosomal recessive; female-to-male ratio of 2:1; inheritance is usually autosomal recessive, but it also has reported as autosomal dominant.

Ocular

"Angioid streaks" of the retina; macular hemorrhages and transudates not infrequent; choroidal sclerosis; retinal detachment; keratoconus; cataract; paralysis of extraocular muscles (secondary to vascular lesions of CNS); subluxation of lens; exophthalmos; optic atrophy; vitreous hemorrhages; Salmon spot multiple atrophic peripheral retinal pigment epithelium (RPE) lesions; reticular pigment dystrophy of the macula; optic disk drusen; multiple small crystalline bodies associated with atrophic RPE changes.

Clinical

Pseudoxanthoma elasticum with thickening, softening, and relaxation of the skin; skin changes are symmetrical in skin folds near large joints (axilla, elbow, inguinal region, lower abdomen, neck); flattening of the pulse curve and peripheral vascular disturbances; gastrointestinal hemorrhages.

Laboratory

Characteristic skin and retinal findings. Fluorescein angiography is done to detect angioid streaks and choroidal neovascular membranes.

Treatment

Dietary calcium and phosphorus restriction to minimum daily requirement levels has shown arrest in progression of the disease.

BIBLIOGRAPHY

1. Dahl AA, Calonje D, El-Harazi SM. (2012). Ophthalmologic manifestations of pseudoxanthoma elasticum. [online] Available from www.emedicine.com/oph/TOPIC475.HTM. [Accessed September, 2013].

3A29. LEBER TAPETORETINAL DYSTROPHY SYNDROME (AMAUROSIS CONGENITA; RETINAL APLASIA; RETINAL ABIOTROPHY; PIGMENTARY RETINITIS WITH CONGENITAL AMAUROSIS; DYSGENESIS NEUROEPITHELIALIS RETINAE; ALSTROM-OLSEN SYNDROME)

General

Autosomal recessive inheritance; consanguinity; occurs from teens to 30 years of age.

Ocular

Nystagmus; keratoconus; narrow retinal arteries; yellowish-brown or gray macular lesions; grayish atrophic retinal lesions; salt-and-pepper-like retinal pigmentation or typical "bone corpuscle" pigmentary changes; keratoglobus.

Clinical

Mental retardation; microcephaly; mongoloid appearance; oculodigital sign; association with Down syndrome has been reported; hypoplasia of the cerebellar vermis; mild-to-moderate ventriculomegaly.

Laboratory

Diagnosis is made by clinical findings.

Treatment

Keratoconus: Spectacle correction, hard contacts, avoid eye rubbing. If hydrops occur, discontinue contact lens, use NaCl drops and ointment, patching, and short course of steroids. As disease advances PK, deep anterior lamellar keratoplasty intacs with laser grooves or collagen stabilization of cornea.

BIBLIOGRAPHY

1. Elder MJ. Leber congenital amaurosis and its association with keratoconus and keratoglobus. J Pediatr Ophthalmol Strabismus. 1994;31:38-40.
2. Firat T. Clinical and genetic investigations in Leber' tapetoretinal dystrophy. Ann Ophthalmol. 1970;2:664.
3. Hayasaka S, Noda S, Setogawa T, et al. Leber congenital amaurosis in an infant with Down syndrome. Ann Ophthalmol. 1992;24:250-2.
4. Lambert SR, Sherman S, Taylor D, et al. Concordance and recessive inheritance of Leber congenital amaurosis. Am J Med Genet. 1993;4:275-7.
5. Leber T. Uber Retinitis Pigmentosa und Angeborene Amaurose. Arch F Ophthalmol (Berlin). 1869;15:1.
6. Magalini SI, Scrascia E. Dictionary of Medical Syndromes, 2nd edition. Philadelphia: JB Lippincott; 1981.
7. Pau H. Differential Diagnosis of Eye Diseases. New York: Thieme; 1987.
8. Steinberg A, Ronen S, Zlotogorski Z, et al. Central nervous involvement in Leber congenital amaurosis. J Pediatr Ophthalmol Strabismus. 1992;29:224-7.

⊟ 3A33. KURU SYNDROME (LAUGHING DEATH)

General

Restricted to Fore tribe of eastern New Guinea; prevalent in children and adult women; etiology unknown, possibly related to the tribe's practice of cannibalism; uncertain whether significant genetic factors also are involved.

Ocular

Strabismus; nystagmus.

Clinical

Ataxia; trembling leg muscles; incoordination; exaggeration of voluntary movements; jerks; slurred speech; fecal incontinence; aphonia; dysphagia.

Laboratory

Diagnosis is made by clinical findings.

Treatment

- *Seesaw nystagmus*: Visual field to consider neoplastic or vascular etiologies.
- *Upbeat nystagmus*: May indicate multiple sclerosis, cerbellar degeneration, tumors or infarcts. Treatment is directed towards identification and resolution of underlying cause.
- *Downbeat*: Affects the cerebellum or craniocervical junction including Arnold-Chiari malformation, multiple sclerosis, trauma, tumor, infarction and many toxic metabolic entities. MRI may indicate a surgically correctable lesion. Periodic alternating nystagmus is continous horizontal nystagmus from stroke, tumor, multiple sclerosis, trauma, infection, drug intoxication. It can occur from cataract, vitreous hemorrhage or optic atrophy.

⊟ BIBLIOGRAPHY

1. Khan ZZ, Huycke MM, Janson PA, et al. (2012). Kuru. [online] Available from www.emedicine.com/med/TOPIC1248.HTM. [Accessed September, 2013].

⊟ 3A34. LAURENCE-MOON-BARDET-BIEDL SYNDROME (BARDET-BIEDL SYNDROME; RETINITIS PIGMENTOSA-POLYDACTYLY-ADIPOSOGENITAL SYNDROME)

General

Recessive, autosomal dominant, and recessive sex-linked gene; male preponderance; onset in childhood; cases of Laurence-Moon belong to the group of heredoataxias.

Ocular

Ptosis; epicanthus; nystagmus; strabismus; night blindness; myopia; hypermetropia; iris coloboma; RP "bone corpuscles"; macular degeneration; attenuation of retinal vessels; choroidal atrophy; optic nerve atrophy; cataract; microphthalmia; keratoconus.

Clinical

Obesity (Fröhlich type); hypogenitalism; reduced intelligence and mental retardation; turricephaly; shortness of stature; atresia ani; genu valgum; congenital heart disease; polydactyly; body hair scant or absent; pseudogynecomastia.

Laboratory

Chromosomal analysis is recommended to confirm chromosomal sex and to evaluate for associated genetic syndromes.

Treatment

Consultation by pediatric endocrinologist and pediatric urologist is usually necessary.

⊟ BIBLIOGRAPHY

1. Telander DG, de Beus A, Small KW. (2012). Retinitis pigmentosa. [online] Available from www.emedicine.com/oph/TOPIC704.HTM. [Accessed September, 2013].

🖵 3A35. LITTLE SYNDROME (NAIL-PATELLA SYNDROME; HEREDITARY OSTEO-ONYCHO-DYSPLASIA; HOOD SYNDROME)

General

Inherited as autosomal dominant; affects males and females equally.

Ocular

Hypertelorism; ptosis; epicanthus; microcornea; keratoconus; sclerocornea; cataract; microphakia; light pigmentation of iris root with dark pigmented "clover-leaf" spots, referred to as the Lester line, not seen in all cases.

Clinical

Absent or hypoplastic patella; hypoplastic or dislocated head of radius; exostosis of skull bones; bilateral horns of iliac crests; longitudinal ridging of fingernails; glomerulonephritis; renal involvement; bilateral antecubital pterygia; arthrogryposis; disorder has been mapped to the long arm of chromosome 9; sensorineural hearing loss.

Laboratory

Conduct urinalysis, along with a microscopic analysis, to check for proteinuria and hematuria. Radiography findings reveal iliac horns. MRI to identify abnormal muscle insertions; renal biopsy.

Treatment

Renal dialysis and transplantation are necessary.

🖵 BIBLIOGRAPHY

1. Hoover-Fong J, McIntosh I, Sweeney E. (2012). Genetics of nail-patella syndrome. [online] Available from www.emedicine.com/ped/TOPIC1546.HTM. [Accessed September, 2013].

🖵 3A36. LYMPHOGRANULOMA VENEREUM (NICOLAS-FAVRE DISEASE; TROPICAL BUBO LGV; LYMPHOGRANULOMA INGUINALE)

General

Venereally transmitted infection caused by chlamydia.

Ocular

Conjunctivitis; chronic lid edema; keratitis; pannus; corneal ulcer; keratoconus; episcleritis; uveitis; tortuosity of retinal vessels; retinal hemorrhages.

Clinical

Enlargement of inguinal lymph nodes; lymphadenitis; lymphogranuloma.

Laboratory

CSF evaluation including cell count and differential and glucose and protein levels, CT MRI.

Treatment

Management is supportive. Administer adequate analgesia.

🖵 BIBLIOGRAPHY

1. Arsove P, Edwards B. (2012). Lymphogranuloma venereum. [online] Available from emedicine.medscape.com/article/220869-overview. [Accessed September, 2013].

🖵 3A37. MARFAN SYNDROME (DOLICHOSTENOMELIA; ARACHNODACTYLY; HYPERCHONDROPLASIA; DYSTROPHIA MESODERMALIS CONGENITA)

General

Hypoplastic form of dystrophia mesodermalis congenita; autosomal dominant; affects both sexes. It has been demonstrated that an abnormality of the gene coding for the connective tissue protein fibrillin is responsible for chronic Marfan syndrome.

Ocular

Exotropia; nystagmus; paralysis of accommodation; myopia (axial or lenticular); iridodonesis; miosis; persistent pupillary membrane; blue sclera; spherophakia; lens dislocation; cataract; megalocornea; retinal detachment (less frequently); pigmentary retinopathy; colobomata of macula, iris, optic nerve, and uveal tract (less frequently); keratoconus; central retinal artery occlusion; rhegmatogenous retinal detachment; syringoma.

Clinical

Arachnodactyly; skeletal anomalies; asymmetric thorax; dolichocephaly and high-arched palate; dissecting aneurysm; mitral valve prolapse; prominent ears; kyphoscoliosis; pectus excavatum; flat feet; hammer toes; pulmonary and kidney defects.

Laboratory

Genetic testing, molecular studies.

Treatment

- *Keratoconus*: Spectacle correction, hard contacts, avoid eye rubbing. If hydrops occur, discontinue contact lens, use sodium chloride (NaCl) drops and ointment, patching, and short course of steroids. As disease advances, PK, deep anterior lamellar keratoplasty intacs with laser grooves or collagen stabilization of cornea.
- *Cataract*: Change in glasses can sometimes improve a patient's visual function temporarily; however the most common treatment is cataract surgery.
- *Glaucoma*: Glaucoma medication should be the first plan of action. If medication is unsuccessful, a filtering surgical procedure with or without antimetabolites may be beneficial.
- *Strabismus*: Equalized vision with correct refractive error; surgery may be helpful in patient with diplopia.

BIBLIOGRAPHY

1. Chen H. (2011). Genetics of Marfan syndrome. [online] Available from www.emedicine.com/ped/TOPIC1372.HTM. [Accessed September, 2013].

3A38. MEASLES (MORBILLI; RUBEOLA)

General

Acute, extremely communicable disease that affects young school-aged children; caused by paramyxovirus.

Ocular

Hypopyon; uveitis; conjunctivitis; Koplik (Hirschberg) spots of conjunctiva; keratitis; corneal ulcer; cellulitis of lid; dacryocystitis; congenital cataract; optic atrophy; optic neuritis; strabismus; pigmentary retinopathy; iris prolapse; hemianopsia; secondary glaucoma; central retinal artery occlusion; orbital cellulitis; accommodative spasm; paralysis of sixth nerve; keratoconus.

Clinical

Maculopapular rash; fever.

Laboratory

Diagnosis is made by clinical findings.

Treatment

Good hydration.

BIBLIOGRAPHY

1. Chen SS. (2011). Measles. [online] Available from www.emedicine.com/derm/TOPIC259.HTM. [Accessed September, 2013].

3A40. DOWN SYNDROME (MONGOLISM)

General

Trisomy of chromosome 21.

Ocular

Hypertelorism; epicanthus; blepharitis; ectropion; nystagmus; esotropia; high myopia (30%); hyperopia; color blindness; yellow spots on the iris; hypoplasia of the iris; blepharoconjunctivitis; lens opacities (50%); keratoconus (may be acute); corneal hydrops; corneal ectasia; corneal edema; leukoma; lateral displacement of canaliculi and puncta; megaloblepharon; euryblepharon; decreased accommodation; Leber congenital amaurosis.

Clinical

Mental retardation; skeletal abnormalities; overextension of joints; deformed and low-set ears; short fifth finger; transverse palmar crease; fissured tongue; heart anomalies.

Laboratory

Amniocentesis during second trimester to check mothers who have low α-fetoprotein serum values, prenatal echography, craniofacial X-ray to check features and echocardiography.

Treatment

Primary care provider should coordinate the multisystemic evaluation. Awareness of systemic and ocular findings is essential for managing patients.

⊟ BIBLIOGRAPHY

1. Izquierdo NJ, Townsend W. (2011). Ophthalmologic manifestations of down syndrome. [online] Available from www.emedicine.com/oph/TOPIC522.HTM. [Accessed August, 2013].

⊟ 3A41. MULVIHILL-SMITH SYNDROME

General

Progeroid disorder.

Ocular

Keratoconus; conjunctivitis.

Clinical

Patients have short stature, microcephaly, unusual facies, numerous pigmented nevi, hypodontia, sensorineural hearing loss, immunodeficiency (low IgG), and a high-pitched voice.

Laboratory

Diagnosis is made by clinical findings.

Treatment

Keratoconus: Spectacle correction, hard contacts, avoid eye rubbing. If hydrops occur, discontinue contact lens, use NaCl drops and ointment, patching, and short course of steroids. As disease advances, PK, deep anterior lamellar keratoplasty, intacs with laser grooves or collagen stabilization of cornea.

⊟ BIBLIOGRAPHY

1. Bartsch O, Tympner KD, Schwinger E, et al. Mulvihill-Smith syndrome: case report and review. J Med Genet. 1994;31:707-11.
2. Ohashi H, Tsukahara M, Murano I, et al. Premature aging and immunodeficiency: Mulvihill-Smith syndrome? Am J Med Genet. 1997;45:597-600.
3. Rau S, Duncker GI. Keratoconus in Mulvihill-Smith syndrome. Klin Monatsbl Augenheilkd. 1994;205:44-6.

⊟ 3A43. NEURODERMATITIS (LICHEN SIMPLEX CHRONICUS)

General

Skin altered due to chronic rubbing or scratching.

Ocular

Keratoconjunctivitis; lid edema; lid pigmentation; lid lichenification; atopic cataracts; keratoconus.

Clinical

Pruritus; dermatitis; seborrheic dermatitis; contact dermatitis; lichenification of skin; skin hyperpigmentation.

Laboratory

Serum immunoglobulin E level, potassium hydroxide examination, skin biopsy.

Treatment

Topical steroids are the treatment of choice.

⊟ BIBLIOGRAPHY

1. Hogan DJ, Mason SH, Bower SM. (2012). Lichen simplex chronicus. [online] Available from www.emedicine.com/derm/TOPIC236.HTM. [Accessed September, 2013].

3A44. VON RECKLINGHAUSEN SYNDROME (NEUROFIBROMATOSIS TYPE I; NEURINOMATOSIS)

General

Dominant inheritance activated at puberty, during pregnancy and at menopause; strong evidence supports the existence of neurofibromatosis type I (NF-I) as a tumor suppressor gene.

Ocular

Proptosis; displacement of the globe; pulsation of the globe; ptosis; elephantiasis of the lids; pigment spots on lids; hydrophthalmos; nodular swelling of corneal nerves; cataracts; optic atrophy; choroidal melanoma; neurofibroma of the choroid, iris, eyelid and ciliary body; enlarged optic foramen; underdevelopment of orbital bones; café-au-lait spots on fundus; hamartoma of retina; congenital glaucoma; focal iris nodules; choroidal nevi; optic nerve gliomas; orbital neurofibroma; keratoconus.

Clinical

Café-au-lait skin pigmentations; fibroma molluscum; lipomas and sebaceous adenomas; schwannomas; growth abnormalities; spontaneous fractures; facial hemihypertrophy.

Laboratory

T2-weighted MRI images demonstrate multiple bright lesions in the basal ganglia, cerebellum, and brain in 80% optic nerve gliomas often develop perineural arachnoidal hyperplasia, which appears as an expanded cerebrospinal fluid (CSF) space around the nerve.

Treatment

Oral ketotifen may reduce the pain, tenderness and itchiness associated with neurofibromas.

BIBLIOGRAPHY

1. Dahl AA. (2011). Ophthalmologic manifestations of neurofibromatosis type. [online] Available from www.emedicine.com/oph/TOPIC338.HTM. [Accessed August, 2013].

3A45. NOONAN SYNDROME (MALE TURNER SYNDROME)

General

Similar to Turner syndrome, but with normal chromosomal analysis; X-linked dominant inheritance; X-linked dominant phenotype.

Ocular

Hypertelorism; exophthalmos; ptosis (unilateral or bilateral); antimongoloid-slanting palpebral fissure; myopia; keratoconus; optic disk coloboma.

Clinical

Valvular pulmonary stenosis; short stature; webbed neck; low hairline in the back; cubitus valgus; deformed chest wall; micrognathia; low-set ears; mild mental retardation.

Laboratory

Xl deficiency, bleeding diatheses, karyotyping test, cardiac examination.

Treatment

Growth hormone therapy.

BIBLIOGRAPHY

1. Ibrahim J, McGovern MM. (2013). Noonan syndrome. [online] Available from www.emedicine.com/ped/TOPIC1616.HTM. [Accessed September, 2013].

🖵 3A46. OCULAR HYPERTENSION

General

Elevated IOP without any evidence of glaucomatous optic neuropathy.

Clinical

None.

Ocular

Normal eye examination with elevated IOP.

Laboratory

Diagnosis is made by clinical findings.

Treatment

If abnormalities occur in cup/disk ratio or visual field with serial examinations, start on monotherapy as topical beta-blocker.

🖵 BIBLIOGRAPHY

1. Chang-Godinich A. (2013). Ocular hypertension. [online] Available from www.emedicine.com/oph/TOPIC578.HTM. [Accessed September, 2013].

🖵 3A47. PELLUCID MARGINAL DEGENERATION

General

Progressive, rare, non-inflammatory peripheral corneal thinning disorder.

Clinical

None.

Ocular

Inferior corneal thinning.

Laboratory

Videokeratography detects small amount of change.

Treatment

Contact lens, peripheral lamellar crescentic keratoplasty followed in a few months by a central PK.

🖵 BIBLIOGRAPHY

1. Rasheed K, Rabinowitz Y. (2012). Pellucid marginal degeneration. [online] Available from www.emedicine.com/oph/TOPIC551.HTM. [Accessed September, 2013].

🖵 3A49. LENTICONUS AND LENTIGLOBUS

General

Lenticonus is a circumscribed conical bulge of the anterior or more commonly, posterior lens capsule and cortex. In lentiglobus, the entire posterior capsule has a globular shape.

Clinical

Alport's syndrome, Waardenburg's syndrome.

Ocular

Oil droplet appearance, amblyopia, strabismus.

Laboratory

Diagnosis is made by clinical findings.

Treatment

Lens extraction with irrigation-aspiration.

🖵 BIBLIOGRAPHY

1. Roy FH, Fraunfelder FW, Fraunfelder FT. Roy and Fraunfelder's Current Ocular Therapy, 6th edition. London, UK: Elsevier; 2008.

⊟ 3A50. POSTERIOR POLYMORPHOUS DYSTROPHY

General

Rare, bilateral corneal disorder of Descemet's membrane. Autosomal dominant associated with Alport's syndrome and keratoconus.

Clinical

None.

Ocular

Corneal edema which usually develops in midlife, open or closed angle glaucoma.

Laboratory

Specular microscopy shows dark rings with scalloped-edges around a light center.

Treatment

Sodium chloride drops or ointment, glaucoma therapy (medical or surgical) and PK may be necessary.

⊟ BIBLIOGRAPHY

1. Roy FH, Fraunfelder FW, Fraunfelder FT. Roy and Fraunfelder's Current Ocular Therapy, 6th edition. London, UK: Elsevier; 2008.

⊟ 3A51. RETINAL DISINSERTION SYNDROME (KERATOCONUS)

General

None.

Ocular

Subluxation of the lens; microphthalmos; bilateral keratoconus; retinal detachment.

Clinical

None.

Laboratory

Diagnosis is made by clinical findings.

Treatment

Spectacle correction, hard contacts, avoid eye rubbing. If hydrops occur, discontinue contact lens, use NaCl drops and ointment, patching, and short course of steroids. As disease advances, PK, deep anterior lamellar keratoplasty intacs with laser grooves or collagen stabilization of cornea. Subluxation of the lens—careful phacoemulsification, topical steroids to control ocular inflammation.

⊟ BIBLIOGRAPHY

1. Ryan SJ (Ed). Retina (Volume III), 2nd edition. St. Louis: Mosby; 1994.
2. Hovland KR, Schepens CL, Freeman HM. Developmental giant retinal tears associated with lens coloboma. Arch Ophthalmol. 1968;80:325-31.
3. Shammas HJ, McGaughey AS. Retinal disinsertion syndrome: report of a case. J Pediatr Ophthalmol Strabismus. 1979;16:284-6.

⊟ 3A52. RETINITIS PIGMENTOSA

General

Inherited progressive retinal disorder may have changes in ear or kidney.

Clinical

Hearing defect and kidney defect can be associated with the disease.

Ocular

Waxy-pole optic nerve, bonespickle pigmentation, posterior subcapsular cataract, visual field defect.

Laboratory

Diagnosis is made by clinical findings. A diagnostic genetic test is available and differentiates between simplex retinitis pigmentosa (RP) and autosomal recessive RP.

Treatment

Vitamin A 15,000 IU/day is thought to slow the decline of retinal function, dark sunglasses for outdoor use, surgery for cataract, genetic counseling.

BIBLIOGRAPHY

1. Clark GR, Crowe P, Muszynska D, et al. Development of a diagnostic genetic test for simplex and autosomal recessive retinitis pigmentosa. Ophthalmology. 2010;117:2169-77.e3.
2. Telander DG, de Beus A, Small KW. (2013). Retinitis pigmentosa. [online] Available from www.emedicine.com/oph/TOPIC704.HTM. [Accessed September, 2013].

3A53. RETROLENTAL FIBROPLASIA (RLF; RETINOPATHY OF PREMATURITY)

General

Bilateral disease seen primarily in premature infants with immature retinal vessels; excessive use of oxygen is responsible for the majority of cases, but disease is seen despite oxygen restrictions or even when no oxygen supplementation is used; known factors that correlate with degrees of retinopathy of prematurity are low birth weight, short gestational age, length of time with supplemental oxygen, length of time on a mechanical ventilator; role of excessive light in newborn nurseries also has been proposed.

Ocular

Anterior or posterior synechiae; neovascularization of iris; pallor of optic disk; dragged disk; attenuated vessels; retinal detachment; dilation of veins; retinal folds; retinal hemorrhage; retrolental mass; vascular tortuosity; vasoconstriction of retina; retinal pigmentary changes; vitreous haze; vitreous traction; vitreous hemorrhages; cataract; glaucoma; leukocoria; myopia; shallow anterior chamber; opaque retrolental membrane; ciliary body drawn anteriorly; ciliary process around dilated pupil; absent pupillary reflexes; keratoconus; associated strabismus; amblyopia.

Clinical

Low birth weight; prematurity.

Laboratory

Diagnosis is made by clinical findings.

Treatment

Cryotherapy and laser surgery can be effective. Vitrectomy may be necessary.

BIBLIOGRAPHY

1. Bashour M, Menassa J, Gerontis CC. (2013). Retinopathy of prematurity. [online] Available from www.emedicine.com/oph/TOPIC413.HTM. [Accessed February, 2013].
2. Moshfeghi DM, Berrocal AM. Retinopathy of prematurity in the time of bevacizumab: incorporating the BEAT-ROP results into clinical practice. Ophthalmology. 2011;118(7):1227-8.
3. Wu WC, Yeh PT, Chen SN, et al. Effects and complications of bevacizumab use in patients with retinopathy of prematurity: a multicenter study in Taiwan. Ophthalmology. 2011;118(1):176-83.
4. Wheeler DT, Dobson V, Chiang MF, et al. Retinopathy of prematurity in infants weighing less than 500 grams at birth enrolled in the early treatment for retinopathy of prematurity study. Ophthalmology. 2011;118(6):1145-51.

3A54. RIEGER SYNDROME (AXENFELD-RIEGER SYNDROME; DYSGENESIS MESODERMALIS CORNEAE ET IRIDES; DYSGENESIS MESOSTROMALIS; AXENFELD POSTERIOR EMBRYOTOXON-JUVENILE GLAUCOMA)

General

Autosomal dominant; neural crest abnormality; 50% of patients develop glaucoma.

Ocular

Microphthalmia; congenital glaucoma; iris hypoplasia; deformed and acentric pupil; anterior synechiae; aniridia; microcornea; corneal opacities in Descemet's membrane parallel to the limbus; dislocated lens; optic atrophy; cataract; strabismus; ptosis; hypertelorism; keratoconus; posterior embryotoxon; broad iris processes to embryotoxon; iris stromal hypoplasia; corectopia; polycoria; secondary glaucoma.

Clinical

Face wide; hypodontia; underdeveloped maxilla; teeth deformities; myotonic dystrophy; facial anomalies: maxillary hypoplasia, protrusion of the lower lip, broad, flat nose; dental anomalies include absent teeth, pig-like incisors and decreased crown size; hypospadias.

Laboratory

Diagnosis is made by clinical findings.

Treatment/ocular

Congenital glaucoma can be treated with beta-blockers, prostaglandin analogs and carbonic anhydrase inhibitors. Surgery such as goniotomy or trabeculectomy can be used if IOP is not controlled.

BIBLIOGRAPHY

1. Eagle RC. Congenital, developmental and degenerative disorders of the iris and ciliary body. In: Albert DM, Jakobiec FA (Eds). Albert & Jakobiec's Principles and Practice of Ophthalmology: Clinical Practice, 3rd edition. Philadelphia, PA: WB Saunders; 1994. pp. 367-87.
2. Montes JG, Montes JC. Syndrome de Rieger, anomalie de axenfeld con glaucoma Juvenil familiar. Arch Soc Ophth Hisp Am. 1967;27:93.
3. Rieger H. Beitrage zur Kenntnis seltener Missbildungen der Iris. Graefes Arch Clin Esp Ophthalmol. 1935;133:602.
4. Wesley RK, Baker JD, Golnick AL. Rieger's syndrome: (oligodontia and primary mesodermal dysgenesis of the iris) clinical features and report of an isolated case. J Pediatr Ophthalmol Strabismus. 1978;15(2):67-70.

3A55. TOURETTE SYNDROME (GILLES DE LA TOURETTE SYNDROME; BRISSAUD II SYNDROME; CAPROLALIA GENERALIZED TIC; GUINON MYOSPASIA IMPULSIVA)

General

Etiology unknown; occurs at ages 7–8 years; emotional trauma is frequent precipitating factor; disturbed parent-child relationship frequently encountered.

Ocular

Blepharospasm; oculogyric deviations; dystonic neck movements.

Clinical

Chorea; caprolalia; echolalia tic; blinking and facial twitching.

Laboratory

No laboratory test is available.

Treatment

Alpha 2-adrenergic agonists and D2 dopamine medications are used to suppress tics.

BIBLIOGRAPHY

1. Hawley JS. (2012). Pediatric Tourette syndrome. [online] Available from www.emedicine.com/med/TOPIC3107. HTM. [Accessed September, 2013].

⊟ 4A. BERARDINELLI-SEIP SYNDROME (CONGENITAL GENERALIZED LIPODYSTROPHY)

General

Autosomal recessive; disorder of the hypothalamus.

Ocular

Punctate corneal infiltrations (lipodystrophia corneae).

Clinical

Advanced bone age; dilation of the third ventricle and basal cistern; frequent elevation of growth hormone; severe lipid levels; enlarged liver; diabetes mellitus; hyperpigmentation of axillae and chest wall; phlebomegaly.

Laboratory

Radiographic features include advanced skeletal age, bone cysts, and dilated cerebral ventricles and basal cisterns on pneumoencephalography.

Treatment

Leptin, an adipocyte hormone, which may improve insulin resistance, hyperglycemia, dyslipidemia, and hepatic steatosis may be useful. Surgical intervention may be helpful for patients with deformities.

⊟ BIBLIOGRAPHY

1. Janniger CK, Jagar C. (2012). Dermatologic manifestations of generalized lipodystrophy. [online] Available from www.emedicine.com/derm/TOPIC688.HTM. [Accessed September, 2013].

⊟ 4B. BRITTLE CORNEA SYNDROME (BRITTLE CORNEA, BLUE SCLERA AND RED HAIR SYNDROME; BLUE SCLERA SYNDROME)

General

Autosomal recessive; rare.

Ocular

Spontaneous perforation of cornea (brittle cornea); blue sclera; acute hydrops; microcornea; sclerocornea; cornea plana; keratoconus; keratoglobus.

Clinical

Red hair; associated with Ehlers-Danlos syndrome, osteogenesis imperfecta and Marfan's syndrome.

Laboratory

Diagnosis is made by clinical findings.

Treatment

Surgical correction of deformities, physiotherapy and the use of orthotic support and devices to assist mobility were the primary means of treatment for osteogenesis imperfecta. With the more recent understanding of the molecular mechanisms of the disease, medical treatment to increase bone mass and strength are gaining popularity.

⊟ BIBLIOGRAPHY

1. Ramachandran M, Achan P, Jones DHA, et al. (2012). Osteogenesis imperfecta. [online] Available from www.emedicine.com/orthoped/TOPIC530.HTM. [Accessed January, 2013].

⊟ 4C. CATARACT, MICROCORNEA SYNDROME

General

Autosomal dominant; prominent in Sicilian families.

Ocular

Cataracts; microcornea; myopia.

Clinical

None.

Laboratory

Diagnosis is made by clinical findings.

Treatment

Cataract surgery if vision decreases.

BIBLIOGRAPHY

1. McKusick VA. Mendelian Inheritance in Man; A Catalog of Human Genes and Genetic Disorders, 12th edition. Baltimore, USA: The Johns Hopkins University Press; 1998.
2. Hamosh A, Scott AF, Amberger J, et al. Online Mendelian Inheritance in Man (OMIM), a knowledge base of human genes and genetic disorders. Nucleic Acids Res. 2002;30(1):52-5.
3. Mollica F, Li Volti S, Tomarchio S, et al. Autosomal dominant cataract and microcornea associated with myopia in a Sicilian family. Clin Genet. 1985;28(1):42-6.
4. Polomeno RC, Cummings C. Autosomal dominant cataracts and microcornea. Can J Ophthalmol. 1979;14(4):227-9.

4D. COLOBOMATOUS, MICROPHTHALMIA AND MICROCORNEA SYNDROME

General

Autosomal dominant pattern of inheritance with complete penetrance.

Ocular

Bilateral inferonasal coloboma; axial enlargement; myopia; iridocorneal angle abnormalities; elevated IOP.

Clinical

None.

Laboratory

Diagnosis is made by clinical findings.

Treatment

See glaucoma.

BIBLIOGRAPHY

1. Toker E, Elcioglu N, Ozcan E, et al. Colobomatous macrophthalmia with microcornea syndrome: report of a new pedigree. Am J Med Genet. 2003;121A(1):25-30.

4E. CATARACT, CONGENITAL OR JUVENILE (CATARACT, JUVENILE, HUTTERITE TYPE)

General

Autosomal recessive; seen most frequently in the people of Japanese origin; autosomal dominant inheritance also has been reported.

Ocular

Retinitis pigmentosa; Usher syndrome (retinitis pigmentosa and congenital deafness); congenital cataract of the "i" phenotype; microphthalmos; keratoconus.

Clinical

Congenital deafness; galactokinase deficiency; epimerase deficiency.

Laboratory

Diagnosis is made by clinical findings.

Treatment

- *Cataract*: Change in glasses can sometimes improve a patient's visual function temporarily; however the most common treatment is cataract surgery.
- *Retinitis pigmentosa*: Vitamin A 15,000 IU/day is thought to slow the decline of retinal function; dark sunglasses for outdoor use; surgery for cataract; genetic counseling.

BIBLIOGRAPHY

1. McKusick VA. Mendelian Inheritance in Man; A Catalog of Human Genes and Genetic Disorders, 12th edition. Baltimore, USA: The Johns Hopkins University Press; 1998.

⊟ 4F. CONGENITAL CLOUDING OF THE CORNEA

General

Glaucoma is one of the common reasons for this condition. Other metabolic, genetic, idiopathic and developmental conditions can result in congenital clouding of the cornea.

Clinical

Fryns syndrome, Goldenhar-Gorlin syndrome, birth trauma, Peters' anomaly.

Ocular

Sclerocornea, dermoid tumors, congenital endothelial dystrophy. Rare cases include cornea plana, cornea keloids and congenital hereditary stromal dystrophy.

Laboratory

No laboratory findings for corneal clouding unless it is due to mucopolysaccharides. In that case, laboratory testing activity in leukocytes may be warranted.

Treatment

Treatment is primarily surgical. For patients with bilateral corneal opacity, PK is recommended.

⊟ BIBLIOGRAPHY

1. Scheinfeld NS, Freilich BD, Freilich J. (2012). Congenital clouding of the cornea. [online] Available from emedicine.medscape.com/article/1197148-overview. [Accessed September, 2013].

⊟ 4G. SPINOCEREBELLAR DEGENERATION AND CORNEAL DYSTROPHY (CORNEAL CEREBELLAR SYNDROME; CORNEAL DYSTROPHY WITH SPINOCEREBELLAR DEGENERATION)

General

Autosomal recessive; consanguineous parents.

Ocular

Corneal opacification; thickened Descemet membrane; degeneration of pannus; congenital cataracts; myopia; tilted optic disks.

Clinical

Mental retardation; progressive cerebellar abnormalities with variable dorsal column lesions; upper motor neuron involvement; histologic muscle abnormalities.

Laboratory

Diagnosis is made via slit-lamp examination.

Treatment

Treatment is based on the severity of the corneal decomposition. Hyperosmotic drops and ointments are used when corneal edema with corneal failure is present. Bandage contact lenses are used only as a temporary measure.

⊟ BIBLIOGRAPHY

1. Der Kaloustian VM, Jarudi NI, Khoury MJ, et al. Familial spinocerebellar degeneration with corneal dystrophy. Am J Med Genet. 1985;20:325-39.
2. McKusick VA. Mendelian Inheritance in Man; A Catalog of Human Genes and Genetic Disorders, 12th edition. Baltimore, USA: The Johns Hopkins University Press; 1998.
3. Online Mendelian Inheritance in Man, OMIM. McKusick-Nathans Institute for Genetic Medicine, Johns Hopkins University and National Center for Biotechnology Information, National Library of Medicine, February 12, 2007. Available from www.ncbi.nlm.nih.gov/omim. [Accessed September, 2013].
4. Mousa AR, Al-Din AS, Al-Nassar KE, et al. Autosomally inherited recessive spastic ataxia, macular dystrophy, congenital cataracts, myopia and vertically oval temporally tilted discs: report of a Bedouin family-a new syndrome. J Neurol Sci. 1986;76:105-21.

4H. CORNEA PLANA

General

Autosomal dominant; may be inherited as autosomal ominant or recessive.

Ocular

Hyperopia; hazy corneal limbus; opacities in corneal parenchyma and marked arcus; posterior embryotoxon; iris and lens abnormalities.

Clinical

Associated with epidermolysis bullosa dystrophica.

Laboratory

Clinical.

Treatment

Medical treatment includes the use of hyperosmotic drops, non-steroidal and steroid eye drops. Corneal transplant may be necessary.

BIBLIOGRAPHY

1. Duane TD. Clinical Ophthalmology. Philadelphia: JB Lippincott; 1987.
2. Hemady RK, Blum S, Sylvia BM, et al. Duplication of the lens, hourglass cornea, and cornea plana. Arch Ophthalmol. 1993;111:303.
3. McKusick VA. Mendelian Inheritance in Man; A Catalog of Human Genes and Genetic Disorders, 12th edition. Baltimore, USA: The Johns Hopkins University Press; 1998.

4I. DOWN SYNDROME (MONGOLISM; TRISOMY G; TRISOMY 21 SYNDROME; MONGOLOID IDIOCY)

General

Trisomy of chromosome 21.

Ocular

Hypertelorism; epicanthus; blepharitis; ectropion; nystagmus; esotropia; high myopia (30%); hyperopia; color blindness; yellow spots on the iris; hypoplasia of the iris; blepharoconjunctivitis; lens opacities (50%); keratoconus (may be acute); corneal hydrops; corneal ectasia; corneal edema; leukoma; lateral displacement of canaliculi and puncta; megaloblepharon; euryblepharon; decreased accommodation; Leber congenital amaurosis.

Clinical

Mental retardation; skeletal abnormalities; overextension of joints; deformed and low-set ears; short fifth finger; transverse palmar crease; fissured tongue; heart anomalies.

Laboratory

Amniocentesis during second trimester to check mothers who have low α-fetoprotein serum values, prenatal echography, craniofacial X-ray to check features and echocardiography.

Treatment

Primary care provider should coordinate the multisystemic evaluation. Awareness of systemic and ocular findings is essential for managing patients.

BIBLIOGRAPHY

1. Izquierdo NJ, Townsend W. (2011). Ophthalmologic manifestations of Down syndrome. [online] Available from www.emedicine.com/oph/TOPIC522.HTM. [Accessed August, 2013].

4J. FRANCOIS (2) DYSTROPHY (FRANCOIS-EVENS SYNDROME; SPECKLED CORNEAL DYSTROPHY)

General

Etiology unknown; congenital; nonprogressive; autosomal dominant, but sporadic cases have been reported.

Ocular

Corneal dystrophy characterized by minute punctate opacities found in all layers of the cornea; varies in size, form, and degree of opacity but is identical in both eyes; anterior limiting membrane is always intact.

Laboratory

Diagnosis is made by clinical findings

Treatment

Treatment is primarily surgical. Treatment of amblyopia and optical therapy can be helpful.

BIBLIOGRAPHY

1. Bron AJ. The corneal dystrophies. Curr Opin Ophthalmol. 1990;1:333.
2. Francois J. Heredity in Ophthalmology. St. Louis: CV Mosby; 1961.
3. Magalini SI, Scrascia E. Dictionary of Medical Syndromes, 2nd edition. Philadelphia: JB Lippincott; 1981.

4M. MEGALOCORNEA (CORNEA HAVING A HORIZONTAL DIAMETER OF MORE THAN 14 MM)

1. Aarskog syndrome (faciodigitogenital syndrome)
†2. Autosomal dominant or recessive trait
3. Congenital glaucoma (rare)
4. Craniosynostosis
5. Down syndrome
†6. Facial hemiatrophy
†7. Isolated
8. Marchesani syndrome (brachymorphia with spherophakia)
9. Marfan syndrome(arachnodactyly dysrophia mesodermalis congenita)
10. MMMM (megalocornea, macrocephaly, mental and motor retardation) syndrome
11. Mucopolysaccharidoses I-S (Scheie syndrome)
12. Neuhauser syndrome (megalocornea-mental retardation syndrome)
13. Oculocerebrorenal syndrome (Lowe syndrome)
14. Oculodental syndrome (Peter syndrome)
15. Osteogenesis imperfecta (van der Hoeve syndrome)
16. Oxycephaly (dysostosis craniofacial dyostosis)
17. Pierre Robin syndrome (micrognathia-glossoptosis syndrome)
18. Posterior embryotoxon (Rieger syndrome)
19. Rubella syndrome (Gregg syndrome)
†21. Sex-linked recessive trait
23. Sturge-Weber syndrome (meningocutaneous syndrome)

BIBLIOGRAPHY

1. Arffa RC. Grayson's Diseases of the Cornea, 3rd edition. St. Louis: Mosby-Year Book; 1991.
2. Frydman M, Berkenstadt M, Raas-Rothschild A, et al. Megalocornea, macrocephaly, mental and motor retardation (MMMM). Clin Genet. 1990;38:149-54.

†Indicates a general entry and therefore has not been described in detail in the text

4M1. AARSKOG SYNDROME (FACIAL-DIGITAL-GENITAL SYNDROME)

General

X-linked recessive; males fully affected; females exhibit partial features; normal birth weight and length.

Ocular

Telecanthus; hypertelorism; unilateral or bilateral blepharoptosis; strabismus; hyperopic astigmatism; large cornea.

Clinical

Short stature; triangular facies; deformity of hands and feet; anomalies of external genitalia; inguinal hernia; protruding umbilicus; abnormal cervical vertebrae; cryptorchidism.

Treatment

Primary goal is to prevent the development of a severe deformity rather.

Laboratory

Full and detailed physical examination; a radiologic evaluation is essential. Standard posteroanterior and lateral views are used for the initial evaluation.

BIBLIOGRAPHY

1. Letts RM, Jawadi AH. (2012). Congenital spinal deformity. [online] Available from www.emedicine.com/orthoped/TOPIC618.HTM. [Accessed September, 2013].

🖶 4M3. CONGENITAL AND INFANTILE CATARACTS

General

Rare, congenital opacity of lens.

Clinical

None.

Ocular

Microcornea, megalocornea, iris coloboma, aniridia, zonular dehiscence, strabismus, photophobia, sensory nystagmus, cataracts.

Laboratory

Diagnosis is made by clinical findings.

Treatment

Amblyopia therapy may be necessary in unilateral cataracts. Cataract surgical intervention is the usual therapy of choice.

🖶 BIBLIOGRAPHY

1. Bashour M, Menassa J, Gerontis CC. (2012). Congenital cataract. [online] Available from www.emedicine.com/oph/TOPIC45.HTM. [Accessed September, 2013].

🖶 4M4. CRANIOSYNOSTOSIS-MENTAL RETARDATION-CLEFTING SYNDROME

General

Autosomal recessive.

Ocular

Choroidal coloboma.

Clinical

Craniosynostosis; mental retardation; seizures; dysplastic kidneys; bat ears; cleft lip and palate; beaked nose; small posterior fontanel.

Laboratory

Serial radiographs, CT, MRI.

Treatment

Surgical treatment involves cranial expansion procedures.

🖶 BIBLIOGRAPHY

1. Jane JA, McKisic MS. (2012). Surgery for craniosynostosis. [online] Available from www.emedicine.com/med/TOPIC2897.HTM. [Accessed September, 2013].

🖶 4M5. DOWN SYNDROME (MONGOLISM; TRISOMY G; TRISOMY 21 SYNDROME; MONGOLOID IDIOCY)

General

Trisomy of chromosome 21.

Ocular

Hypertelorism; epicanthus; blepharitis; ectropion; nystagmus; esotropia; high myopia (30%); hyperopia; color blindness; yellow spots on the iris; hypoplasia of the iris; blepharoconjunctivitis; lens opacities (50%); keratoconus (may be acute); corneal hydrops; corneal ectasia; corneal edema; leukoma; lateral displacement of canaliculi and puncta; megaloblepharon; euryblepharon; decreased accommodation; Leber congenital amaurosis.

Clinical

Mental retardation; skeletal abnormalities; overextension of joints; deformed and low-set ears; short fifth finger; transverse palmar crease; fissured tongue; heart anomalies.

Laboratory

Amniocentesis during second trimester to check mothers who have low α-fetoprotein serum values, prenatal echography, craniofacial X-ray to check features and echocardiography.

Treatment

Primary care provider should coordinate the multisystemic evaluation. Awareness of systemic and ocular findings is essential for managing patients.

BIBLIOGRAPHY

1. Izquierdo NJ, Townsend W. (2011). Ophthalmologic manifestations of Down syndrome. [online] Available from www.emedicine.com/oph/TOPIC522.HTM. [Accessed August, 2013].

4M8. MARCHESANI SYNDROME (WEILL-MARCHESANI SYNDROME; INVERTED MARFAN SYNDROME; BRACHYMORPHY WITH SPHEROPHAKIA; DYSTROPHIA MESODERMALIS CONGENITA HYPERPLASTICA)

General

Pattern of inheritance uncertain; manifest at age of 9 months to 13 years.

Ocular

Lenticular myopia; secondary glaucoma (rare), caused by luxation of the lens; iridodonesis; ectopia lentis; spherophakia; optic atrophy; megalocornea; corneal opacity; acute pupillary block glaucoma.

Clinical

Brachydactyly; reduced growth; athletic build with abundant subcutaneous tissue; short neck and large thorax; short and clumsy hands and feet; decreased joint flexibility; hearing defects; inheritable connective tissue disorder, usually inherited as an autosomal recessive.

Laboratory

X-ray detects delayed carpal ossification.

Treatment/Glaucoma

Beta-blockers, carbonic anhydrase inhibitors and prostaglandin analogs. Surgery may be needed if IOP is uncontrolled.

BIBLIOGRAPHY

1. Hamosh A, Scott AF, Amberger J, et al. Online Mendelian Inheritance in Man, (OMIM), a knowledgebase of human genes and genetic disorders. Nucleic Acids Res. 2002;30(1):52-5
2. McKusick-Nathans Institute for Genetic Medicine, Johns Hopkins University and National Center for Biotechnology Information, National Library of Medicine, February 12, 2007. Available from www.ncbi.nlm.nih.gov/omim. [Accessed September, 2013].
3. Jensen AD, Cross HE, Paton Det al. Ocular complications in the Weill-Marchesani syndrome. Am J Ophthalmol. 1974; 77(2):261-9.
4. Marchesani O. Brachydactylie und Angeborene Kugellinse als Systemerkrankung. Klin Monatsbl Augenheilkd. 1939; 103:392.
5. McKusick VA. Mendelian Inheritance in Man; A Catalog of Human Genes and Genetic Disorders, 12th edition. Baltimore: The Johns Hopkins University Press; 1998.
6. Roy FH, Fraunfelder FT Fraunfelder FW. Roy and Fraunfelder's Current Ocular Therapy, 6th edition. Philadelphia: WB Saunders; 2008.
7. Willi M, Kut L, Cotlier E, et al. Pupillary-block glaucoma in the Marchesani syndrome. Arch Ophthalmol 1973; 90(6): 504-8.
8. Young ID, Fielder AR, Casey TA, et al. Weill-Marchesani syndrome in mother and son. Clin Genet. 1986;30(6):475-80.

4M9. MARFAN SYNDROME (DOLICHOSTENOMELIA; ARACHNODACTYLY; HYPERCHONDROPLASIA; DYSTROPHIA MESODERMALIS CONGENITA)

General

Hypoplastic form of dystrophia mesodermalis congenita; autosomal dominant; affects both sexes. It has been demonstrated that an abnormality of the gene coding for the connective tissue protein fibrillin is responsible for chronic Marfan syndrome.

Ocular

Exotropia; nystagmus; paralysis of accommodation; myopia (axial or lenticular); iridodonesis; miosis; persistent pupillary membrane; blue sclera; spherophakia; lens dislocation; cataract; megalocornea; retinal detachment (less frequently); pigmentary retinopathy; colobomata of macula, iris, optic nerve, and uveal tract (less frequently); keratoconus; central retinal artery occlusion; rhegmatogenous retinal detachment; syringoma.

Clinical

Arachnodactyly; skeletal anomalies; asymmetric thorax; dolichocephaly and high-arched palate; dissecting aneurysm; mitral valve prolapse; prominent ears; kyphoscoliosis; pectus excavatum; flat feet; hammer toes; pulmonary and kidney defects.

Laboratory

Genetic testing, molecular studies.

Treatment

- *Keratoconus*: Spectacle correction, hard contacts, avoid eye rubbing. If hydrops occur, discontinue contact lens, use sodium chloride (NaCl) drops and ointment, patching, and short course of steroids. As disease advances, PK, deep anterior lamellar keratoplasty intacs with laser grooves or collagen stabilization of cornea.
- *Cataract*: Change in glasses can sometimes improve a patient's visual function temporarily; however the most common treatment is cataract surgery.
- *Glaucoma*: Glaucoma medication should be the first plan of action. If medication is unsuccessful, a filtering surgical procedure with or without antimetabolites may be beneficial.
- *Strabismus*: Equalized vision with correct refractive error; surgery may be helpful in patient with diplopia.

BIBLIOGRAPHY

1. Chen H. (2011). Genetics of Marfan syndrome. [online] Available from www.emedicine.com/ped/TOPIC1372. HTM. [Accessed September, 2013].

4M10. MMMM SYNDROME (NEUHAUSER SYNDROME; MEGALOCORNEA, MACROCEPHALY, MENTAL AND MOTOR RETARDATION)

General

Rare.

Ocular

Megalocornea.

Clinical

Mental retardation; hearing loss; sensorineural complications; hypoplasia; corpus callosum; macrocephaly.

Laboratory/Ocular

Gonioscopy, A-scan ultrasound biometry.

Treatment

Spectacles; glaucoma or cataract surgery if necessary.

BIBLIOGRAPHY

1. Tominaga N, Kamimura N, Matsumoto T, et al. A case of megalocornea mental retardation syndrome complicated with bilateral sensorineural hearing loss. Pediat Int. 1999;41:392-4.
2. Tonaki H. Megalcornea-mental retardation syndrome. Turk J Pediatr. 2002;44:274-7.

4M11. SCHEIE SYNDROME (MUCOPOLYSACCHARIDOSIS IS; MPS IS; MPS V; MUCOPOLYSACCHARIDOSIS V)

General

Autosomal recessive; chondroitin sulfate B excreted in excess in the urine; formerly MPS V (*see* Hurler Syndrome; Hunter Syndrome; Sanfilippo-Good Syndrome; Morquio Syndrome; Maroteaux-Lamy Syndrome). Both sexes affected; deficiency of a-L-iduronidase; increased urinary dermatan and heparan sulfate; fibrous long-spacing collagen on histopathologic examination; least severe form of MPS.

Ocular

Night blindness; fields may show general constriction; ring scotoma; diffuse corneal haze to marked corneal clouding (progressive); bushy eyebrows; coarse eyelashes; optic atrophy; anisocoria; cataracts; proptosis; acid mucopolysaccharide deposits in the iris and sclera; tapetoretinal degeneration; glaucoma.

Clinical

Normal intelligence; broad facies; thickened joints; aortic valvular disease; psychosis; claw hand; carpal tunnel syndrome; excessive body hair; progressive juxta-articular cystic lesions.

Laboratory

Thin layer chromatography and radiography.

Treatment

Enzyme replacement therapy—patients with joint contractures may need surgery. Corneal transplant may be necessary if vision problems are severe.

⊟ BIBLIOGRAPHY

1. Banikazemi M. (2012). Genetics of mucopolysaccharidosis Type I. [online] Available from www.emedicine.com/ped/TOPIC2052.HTM. [Accessed September, 2013].

⊟ 4M12. NEUHAUSER SYNDROME (MEGALOCORNEA, MACROCEPHALY, MENTAL AND MOTOR RETARDATION)

General

Rare.

Ocular

Megalocornea.

Clinical

Mental retardation; hearing loss; sensorineural complications; hypoplasia; corpus callosum; macrocephaly.

Laboratory/Ocular

Gonioscopy, A-scan ultrasound biometry.

Treatment

Spectacles; glaucoma or cataract surgery if necessary.

⊟ BIBLIOGRAPHY

1. Tominaga N, Kamimura N, Matsumoto T, et al. A case of megalocornea mental retardation syndrome complicated with bilateral sensorineural hearing loss. Pediat Int. 1999;41:392-4.
2. Tonaki H. Megalcornea-mental retardation syndrome. Turk J Pediatr. 2002;44:274-7.

⊟ 4M13. LOWE SYNDROME (OCULO-CEREBRO-RENAL SYNDROME)

General

Essential enzyme or protein abnormality is unknown; sex-linked recessive trait (male incidence only); onset in early infancy.

Ocular

Nystagmus; congenital glaucoma; miotic pupils; no pupillary reaction; ectropion uveae; malformation of the anterior chamber angle and of the iris; Schlemm's canal may be absent with imperfect angle cleavage; blue sclera; cloudy cornea; cataracts; megalocornea; corneal dystrophy; buphthalmos; microphthalmos; microphakia; mydriasis; strabismus; lens punctate cortical opacities.

Clinical

Mental, psychomotor, and growth retardation; aminoaciduria; albuminuria; glycosuria; renal tubular acidosis; rickets; osteomalacia; muscular hypotony; hyporeflexia; hyperactivity with bizarre choreoathetoid movements and screaming.

Laboratory

Urine-aminoaciduria, proteinuria, calciuria, phosphaturia; serum-elevated acid phosphate; imaging studies—brain MRI—mild ventriculomegaly (one-third cases); ocular ultrasound—if dense cataract, rule out mass or retinal detachment posterior.

Treatment

Monitor and treat for glaucoma. If glaucoma develops, IOP lowering agents must be used. Often, these patients require surgical intervention with goniotomy, trabeculotomy, or a drainage filtration device. Congenital cataracts should be removed, ideally in the first 6 weeks of life, to optimize the visual potential.

⊟ BIBLIOGRAPHY

1. Alcorn DM. (2012). Oculocerebrorenal syndrome. [online] Available from www.emedicine.com/oph/TOPIC516.HTM. [Accessed September, 2013].

⊟ 4M14. OCULODENTAL SYNDROME (PETERS SYNDROME; RUTHERFORD SYNDROME)

General

Similar to Rieger syndrome and Meyer-Schwickerath-Weyer syndrome; Peters syndrome inherited as autosomal recessive with defect of corneogenetic mesoderm characterized by incomplete separation of lens vesicle, causing central opacities of cornea, shallow anterior chamber, synechiae, and remnants of pupillary membrane; anterior pole cataract; Rutherford syndrome inherited as autosomal dominant; exhibits iris and dental anomalies and mental retardation.

Ocular

High myopia; corneoscleral staphyloma; aniridia; macrocornea; opacities of the corneal margin; ectopia lentis with deposits of pigment; macular pigmentation; large excavation of optic nerve with atrophy.

Clinical

Oligodontia; microdontia; hypoplasia of enamel; abnormal tooth positions; hypertrophy of gums; failure of tooth eruption.

Treatment

See oral health specialist.

⊟ BIBLIOGRAPHY

1. Houston IB. Rutherford's syndrome. A familial oculo-dental disorder and electrophysiological study. Acta Paediatr Scand. 1966;55:233-8.
2. McKusick VA. Mendelian Inheritance in Man; A Catalog of Human Genes and Genetic Disorders, 12th edition. Baltimore: The Johns Hopkins University Press; 1998.

⊟ 4M15. VAN DER HOEVE SYNDROME (OSTEOGENESIS IMPERFECTA; OSTEOPSATHYROSIS; EKMAN SYNDROME; LOBSTEIN SYNDROME; SPURWAY SYNDROME; VROLIK SYNDROME; EDDOWES SYNDROME; BRITTLE BONE DISEASE) GLAUCOMA

General

Autosomal dominant.

Ocular

Glaucoma; blue sclera; keratoconus; cataract; optic nerve atrophy; retinopathy; retinal detachment.

Clinical

Brittle bones; deafness; hyperflexibility of ligaments; dental defects; developmental delay.

Laboratory

Deoxyribonucleic acid blood test, analysis of type I, III and V collagens synthesized by fibroblast, prenatal sonography.

Treatment

Synthetic analogs of pyrophosphate, cyclic intravenous pamidronate, growth hormone.

⊟ BIBLIOGRAPHY

1. Ramachandran M, Achan P, Jones DH, et al. (2012). Osteogenesis imperfecta. [online] Available from www.emedicine.com/orthoped/TOPIC530.HTM. [Accessed February, 2013].

4M16. CROUZON SYNDROME (DYSOSTOSIS CRANIOFACIALIS; OXYCEPHALY; CRANIOFACIAL DYSOSTOSIS; PARROT-HEAD SYNDROME; MÖBIUS-CROUZON SYNDROME; HEREDITARY CRANIOFACIAL DYSOSTOSIS)

General

Autosomal dominant; manifestations present at birth.

Ocular

Bilateral exophthalmos; hypertelorism (wide interpupillary distance); obliquity of palpebral fissures with outer canthus slanting downward; nystagmus; exotropia; upper field defects due to pressure upon the optic nerve on its lower part; bluish sclera; exposure keratitis in extreme exophthalmos; cataract; papilledema; secondary optic atrophy; corneal dystrophy; ptosis; strabismus; keratoconus.

Clinical

Prognathism; maxillary hypoplasia with short upper lip; synostosis of coronal and lambda sutures; parrot-beaked nose (psittachosrhina); widening temporal fossae; headaches.

Laboratory

Skull, spine, and hand radiography is usually necessary to confirm the diagnosis.

Treatment

Neurosurgical procedure is recommended in cases of intracranial hypertension leading to further optic atrophy.

BIBLIOGRAPHY

1. Chen H. (2013). Genetics of Crouzon syndrome. [online] Available from www.emedicine.com/ped/TOPIC511.HTM. [Accessed September, 2013].

4M17. PIERRE-ROBIN SYNDROME (ROBIN SYNDROME; MICROGNATHIA-GLOSSOPTOSIS SYNDROME)

General

Etiology unknown; manifestations at birth; pathogenesis based on arrested fetal development; history of intrauterine disturbance in early pregnancy (25% of cases); also increased incidence in offspring of mother's age 35 years or older; pathogenesis is thought to be incomplete development of the first brachial arch, which forms the maxilla and mandible.

Ocular

Microphthalmos; proptosis; ptosis; high myopia; glaucoma; cataract (rare); retinal disinsertion; megalocornea; iris atrophy; blue sclera; esotropia; conjunctivitis; distichiasis; vitreoretinal degeneration; retinal detachments.

Clinical

Micrognathia; cleft palate; glossoptosis; cyanosis; facial expression bird-like with flat base of nose and high-arched deformed palate with or without cleft; difficulty in breathing.

Laboratory

Diagnosis is made by clinical findings.

Treatment

Multidisciplinary approach is required to manage the complex features involved in the care of these children and their families.

BIBLIOGRAPHY

1. Tewfik TL, Trinh N, Teebi AS. (2012). Pierre Robin syndrome. [online] Available from www.emedicine.com/ent/TOPIC150.HTM. [Accessed September, 2013].

⊟ 4M18. RIEGER SYNDROME (AXENFELD-RIEGER SYNDROME; DYSGENESIS MESODERMALIS CORNEAE ET IRIDES; DYSGENESIS MESOSTROMALIS; AXENFELD POSTERIOR EMBRYOTOXON-JUVENILE GLAUCOMA)

General

Autosomal dominant; neural crest abnormality; 50% of patients develop glaucoma.

Ocular

Microphthalmia; congenital glaucoma; iris hypoplasia; deformed and acentric pupil; anterior synechiae; aniridia; microcornea; corneal opacities in Descemet's membrane parallel to the limbus; dislocated lens; optic atrophy; cataract; strabismus; ptosis; hypertelorism; keratoconus; posterior embryotoxon; broad iris processes to embryotoxon; iris stromal hypoplasia; corectopia; polycoria; secondary glaucoma.

Clinical

Face wide; hypodontia; underdeveloped maxilla; teeth deformities; myotonic dystrophy; facial anomalies: maxillary hypoplasia, protrusion of the lower lip, broad, flat nose; dental anomalies include absent teeth, pig-like incisors and decreased crown size; hypospadias.

Laboratory

Diagnosis is made by clinical findings.

Treatment/Ocular

Congenital glaucoma can be treated with beta-blockers, prostaglandin analogs and carbonic anhydrase inhibitors. Surgery such as goniotomy or trabeculectomy can be used if IOP is not controlled.

⊟ BIBLIOGRAPHY

1. Eagle RC. Congenital, developmental and degenerative disorders of the iris and ciliary body. In: Albert DM, Jakobiec FA (Eds). Albert & Jakobiec's Principles and Practice of Ophthalmology: Clinical Practice, 3rd edition. Philadelphia, PA: WB Saunders; 1994. pp. 367-87.
2. Montes JG, Montes JC. Syndrome de Rieger, anomalie de axenfeld con glaucoma Juvenil familiar. Arch Soc Ophth Hisp Am. 1967;27:93.
3. Rieger H. Beitrage zur Kenntnis seltener Missbildungen der Iris. Graefes Arch Clin Esp Ophthalmol. 1935;133:602.
4. Wesley RK, Baker JD, Golnick AL. Rieger's syndrome: (oligodontia and primary mesodermal dysgenesis of the iris) clinical features and report of an isolated case. J Pediatr Ophthalmol Strabismus. 1978;15:67-70.

⊟ 4M19. RUBELLA SYNDROME (CONGENITAL RUBELLA SYNDROME; GERMAN MEASLES; GREGG SYNDROME)

General

Rubella infection of the mother during first trimester of pregnancy; ocular disease is the most commonly found abnormality in patients with congenital rubella syndrome (75%), multiorgan disease is common (greater than 75%); no significant association has been found between gestational age and time of maternal infection and incidence of individual ocular conditions.

Ocular

Nystagmus; glaucoma; corneal haziness; cataracts; retinal pigmentary changes; appearance and central distribution of lesions are quite distinguishable from retinitis pigmentosa; retinopathy is not progressive and has little, if any, effect on vision; waxy atrophy of optic disk; conjunctivitis; megalocornea or microcornea; buphthalmos; microphthalmos; uveitis; iris atrophy; spherophakia; strabismus.

Clinical

Low-birth weight; diarrhea; pneumonia; urinary infection; hearing loss; heart disease; hepatosplenomegaly; mental retardation; inguinal hernias; ataxia; cardiac abnormalities.

Laboratory

Diagnosis is made by clinical findings. If in doubt, a rising titer of immunoglobulin M will indicate a recent infection.

Treatment

Treatment for rubella of the eye centers on glaucoma and cataract.

🗗 BIBLIOGRAPHY

1. Lombardo PC. (2011). Dermatologic Manifestations of Rubella. [online] Available from www.emedicine.com/derm/TOPIC380.HTM. [Accessed September, 2013].

🗗 4M23. STURGE-WEBER SYNDROME (MENINGOCUTANEOUS SYNDROME; VASCULAR ENCEPHALOTRIGEMINAL SYNDROME; NEURO-OCULOCUTANEOUS ANGIOMATOSIS; ENCEPHALOFACIAL ANGIOMATOSIS; ENCEPHALOTRIGEMINAL SYNDROME)

General

Trisomy 22 or partial trisomy inheritance. Variations include Jahnke syndrome (neuro-oculocutaneous angiomatosis without glaucoma), Schirmer syndrome (oculocutaneous angiomatosis with early glaucoma), Lawfordsyndrome (oculocutaneous angiomatosis with late glaucoma and no increase in volume of globe) and Mille syndrome (oculocutaneous syndrome with choroidal angioma but no glaucoma).

Ocular

Unilateral hydrophthalmos; secondary glaucoma (late) conjunctival angiomata (telangiectases); iris decoloration; nevoid marks or vascular dilation of the episclera; glioma; serous retinal detachment; choroidal angiomata; deep anterior chamber angle; port-wine stain of eyelids; buphthalmos; optic nerve cupping; anisometropia; hemianopsia; increased corneal diameter; enophthalmos; exophthalmos; optic atrophy; choroidal hemangioma; anterior chamber angle vascularization.

Clinical

Vascular port-wine nevus (face, scalp, limbs, trunk, leptomeninges); acromegaly; facial hemihypertrophy; intracranial angiomas; convulsion; mental retardation; obesity; limb atrophy.

Laboratory

Neuroimaging studies and the clinical examination have been the procedures of choice to establish the diagnosis.

Treatment

Anticonvulsants for seizure control, symptomatic and prophylactic therapy for headache and glaucoma treatment to reduce the IOP.

🗗 BIBLIOGRAPHY

1. Del Monte MA, Taravella M. (2012). Sturge-Weber syndrome. [online] Available from www.emedicine.com/oph/TOPIC348.HTM. [Accessed January, 2013].
2. Takeoka M, Riviello JJ. (2010). Pediatric Sturge-Weber syndrome. [online] Available from www.emedicine.com/neuro/TOPIC356.HTM. [Accessed January, 2013].

🗗 4N. MICROCORNEA (CORNEA WITH A HORIZONTAL DIAMETER OF LESS THAN 10 MM)

1. Associated ocular findings
   A. Aniridia and subluxated lenses
   B. Axenfeld syndrome (posterior embryotoxon)
   C. Colobomatous microphthalmia
   D. Congenital glaucoma
   †E. Corectopia and macular hypoplasia
   F. Hyperopia
   G. Meckel syndrome (dysencephala splanchnocystica syndrome)
   †H. Nanophthalmos
   I. Narrow-angle glaucoma
   J. Sclerocornea
2. Aberfeld syndrome (congenital blepharophimosis associated with generalized myopathy)

†3. Autosomal recessive or dominant trait

4. Carpenter syndrome (acrocephalopolysyndactyly II)
5. Cataract microcornea syndrome
6. Chromosome partial deletion (long-arm) syndrome
7. Ehlers-Danlos syndrome (fibrodysplasia elastica generalisata)
8. Gansslen syndrome (familial hemolytic icterus)
9. Hallermann-Streiff syndrome (dyscephalic mandibulooculofacial syndrome)
10. Hemifacial microsomia syndrome (Francois Haustrate syndrome)
12. Hutchinson-Gilford syndrome (progeria)
13. Laurence-Moon-Bardet-Biedl syndrome (retinitis pigmentosa-polydactylyadiposogenital syndrome)
14. Lenz microphthalmia syndrome
15. Little syndrome (nail patella syndrome)
16. Marchesani syndrome (mesodermal dysmorphodystrophy)
17. Marfan syndrome (arachnodactyly dystrophica mesodermalis congenita)
18. Meckel syndrome (dysencephalia splanchnocystica syndrome)
19. Meyer-Schwickerath-Weyers syndrome (oculodentodigital dysplasia)
20. Microcornea, glaucoma, absent frontal sinuses
21. Micro syndrome
22. Rieger syndrome (hypodontia and iris dysgenesis)
23. Ring chromosome
24. Roberts pseudothalidomide syndrome
25. Rubella syndrome (Gregg syndrome)
26. Sabin-Feldman syndrome
27. Schwartz syndrome (glaucoma associated with retinal detachment)
28. Smith-Magenis syndrome
29. Triploidy
30. Trisomy 13 (D trisomy, Patau syndrome)
31. Waardenburg syndrome (interoculoiridodermatoauditive dysplasia)

🗗 BIBLIOGRAPHY

1. Mandal AK, Singh AP, Rao L, et al. Roberts pseudothalidomide syndrome. Arch Ophthalmol. 2000;118:1462-3.
2. Mollica F, Li Volti S, Tomarchio S, et al. Autosomal dominant cataract and microcornea associated with myopia in a Sicilian family. Clin Genet. 1985;28:42-6.
3. Ranchod TM, Quiram PA, Hathaway N, et al. Microcornea, posterior megalolenticonus persistent fetal vasculature and coloboma. Ophthalmology. 2010;117:1843-7.
4. Roy FH. Ocular Syndromes and Systemic Diseases, 6th edition. New Delhi: Jaypee Brothers Medical Publishers; 2013.
5. Warburg M, Sjö O, Fledelius HC, et al. Autosomal recessive microcephaly, microcornea, congenital cataract, mental retardation, optic atrophy, and hypogenitalism. Arch Dis Child. 1993;147:1309-12.

†Indicates a general entry and therefore has not been described in detail in the text

🗗 4N1A. ANIRIDIA (CONGENITAL ANIRIDIA, HEREDITARY ANIRIDIA)

General

Hereditary, recessive (two-thirds of cases), can be dominant, sporadic or traumatic; absence of the iris; rare; usually bilateral unless due to trauma.

Ocular

Absence of iris; subluxed lens; iridodialysis; cataract; glaucoma; corneal scarring, vascularization, and edema; iris colobomata; round eccentric pupils; keratoconus.

Clinical

Cerebellar ataxia; mental retardation; Wilms' tumor (WT).

Laboratory

Chromosomal deletion, cytogenic analysis, submicroscopic deletions of WT gene with FISH technique, PCR genotyping halotypes across paired box gene 6 (PAX6)-WT1 region provides evidence of a chromosomal deletion.

Treatment

Systemic or topical glaucoma therapy.

🗗 BIBLIOGRAPHY

1. François J, Coucke D, Coppieters R. Aniridia-Wilms' tumor syndrome. Ophthalmologica. 1977;174(1):35-9.

2. Johns KJ, O'Day DM. Posterior chamber intraocular lenses after extracapsular cataract extraction in patients with aniridia. Ophthalmology. 1991;98(11):1698-702.
3. Kremer I, Rajpal RK, Rapuano CJ, et al. Results of penetrating keratoplasty in aniridia. Am J Ophthalmol. 1993;115(3): 317-20.
4. Magalini SI, Scrascia E. Dictionary of Medical Syndromes, 2nd edition. Philadelphia, PA: JB Lippincott; 1981.
5. Mintz-Hittner HA, Ferrell RE, Lyons LA, et al. Criteria to detect minimal expressivity within families with autosomal dominant aniridia. Am J Ophthalmol. 1992;114(6):700-7.
6. Nelson LB, Spaeth GL, Nowinski TS, et al. Aniridia. A review. Surv Ophthalmol. 1984;28(6):621-42.
7. Skeens HM, Brooks BP, Holland EJ. Congenital aniridia variant: minimally abnormal irides with severe limbal stem cell deficiency. Ophthalmology. 2011;118(7):1260-4.

⊟ 4N1A. DISLOCATION OF THE LENS

General

Ectopia lentis, occurs when the lens is not in its normal position.

Clinical

Marfan syndrome, Weill-Marchesani syndrome, sulfite-oxidase deficiency.

Laboratory

Diagnosis is made by clinical findings.

Treatment

Careful phacoemulsification; topical steroids should be given to control ocular inflammation.

⊟ BIBLIOGRAPHY

1. Eifrig CW. (2011). Ectopia lentis. [online] Available from www.emedicine.com/oph/TOPIC55.HTM. [Accessed September, 2013].

⊟ 4N1B. AXENFELD-RIEGER SYNDROME (POSTERIOR EMBRYOTOXON; AXENFELD SYNDROME)

General

Dominant inheritance; occasionally sporadic; variable in expression.

Ocular

Posterior embryotoxon: ring-like opacity of cornea; long trabecula; prominent Schwalbe line; iris adhesions to Schwalbe line and cornea with large abnormal iris processes or broad sheets of tissues of varying size and location; anterior layer of iris may appear hypoplastic; ectopia of the pupil not uncommon; polycoria occurs; ring-like opacity of the deep corneal layers extending several millimeters from the limbus in continuity with the sclera; keratoconus.

Laboratory

Patients may need workup for associated systemic abnormalities.

Treatment

Patients may need workup for associated systemic abnormalities, so referring to a pediatrician or an internist is important.

⊟ BIBLIOGRAPHY

1. Dersu II. (2012). Secondary congenital glaucoma. [online] Available from www.emedicine.com/oph/TOPIC141.HTM. [Accessed September, 2013].

⊟ 4N1C. COLOBOMATOUS, MICROPHTHALMIA AND MICROCORNEA SYNDROME

General

Autosomal dominant pattern of inheritance with complete penetrance.

Ocular

Bilateral inferonasal coloboma; axial enlargement; myopia; iridocorneal angle abnormalities; elevated IOP.

Clinical

None.

Laboratory

Diagnosis is made by clinical findings.

Treatment

See glaucoma.

⊟ BIBLIOGRAPHY

1. Toker E, Elcioglu N, Ozcan E, et al. Colobomatous macrophthalmia with microcornea syndrome: report of a new pedigree. Am J Med Genet. 2003;121A(1):25-30.

⊟ 4N1D. GLAUCOMA, CONGENITAL

General

Autosomal recessive; occurs more frequently in males; can occur isolated or associated with other systemic or ocular malformations (dysgenesis of iris, angle and peripheral cornea).

Ocular

Buphthalmos; corneal haze; glaucoma; epiphora.

Clinical

None.

Laboratory

Tonometry, corneal measurements, gonioscopy, and ophthalmoscopy should be performed in the operating room and carefully documented. IOPs recorded under general anesthesia are usually lower than those obtained in the office because of the effects of the anesthetic agents.

Treatment

Primary congenital glaucoma almost always is managed surgically; both goniotomy and trabeculotomy may be useful. When multiple goniotomies and/or trabeculotomies fail, the surgeon usually resorts to a filtering procedure.

⊟ BIBLIOGRAPHY

1. Ben-Zion I, Tomkins O, Moore DB, et al. Surgical results in the management of advanced primary congenital glaucoma in a rural pediatric population. Ophthalmology. 2011;118:231-5.
2. Bowman RJ, Dickerson M, Mwende J, et al. Outcomes of goniotomy for primary congential glaucoma in east Africa. Ophthalmology. 2011;118:236-40.
3. Cibis GW, Urban RC, Dahl AA. (2013). Primary congenital glaucoma. [online] Available from www.emedicine.com/oph/TOPIC138.HTM. [Accessed September, 2013].

⊟ 4N1F. HYPEROPIA, HIGH

General

Defect in eyesight in which the focal point falls behind the retina, resulting in farsightedness; autosomal recessive; eye shorter than normal.

Ocular

Farsightedness.

Clinical

None.

Laboratory

Diagnosis is made by clinical findings.

Treatment

Glasses, contact lens, conductive keratoplasty, laser-assisted in situ keratomileusis (LASIK) and phakic intraocular-lens (IOL).

BIBLIOGRAPHY

1. Roque MR, Roque BL, Limbonsiong R, et al. (2013). Conductive keratoplasty hyperopia and presbyopia. [online] Available from www.emedicine.com/oph/TOPIC736.HTM. [Accessed September, 2013].

4N1G. MECKEL SYNDROME (DYSENCEPHALIA SPLANCHNOCYSTIC SYNDROME; GRUBER SYNDROME)

General

Autosomal recessive; ocular manifestations are similar to those of trisomy 13–15 syndrome.

Ocular

Cryptophthalmos; clinical anophthalmos; microphthalmos; mongoloid slant of lid fissures; sclerocornea; microcornea; partial aniridia; cataract; retinal dysplasia; posterior staphyloma; optic nerve hypoplasia.

Clinical

Sloping forehead; posterior encephalocele; short neck; polydactyly and syndactyly (hands and feet); polycystic kidneys; cryptorchidism; cleft lip and palate; CNS abnormalities, including the Dandy-Walker malformation.

Laboratory

Chromosome analysis, MRI.

Treatment

Cardiac surgery may be warranted.

BIBLIOGRAPHY

1. Jayakar PB, Spiliopoulos M, Jayakar A. (2011). Meckel-Gruber syndrome. [online] Available from www.emedicine.com/ped/TOPIC1390.HTM. [Accessed September, 2013].

4N1I. PRIMARY ANGLE-CLOSURE GLAUCOMA (PRIMARY CLOSED ANGLE GLAUCOMA)

General

Obstruction of aqueous humor outflow forms the anterior chamber which results from closure of the angle by the peripheral root of the iris.

Clinical

Pain, nausea.

Ocular

Flare in the anterior chamber, conjunctival chemosis, hyperemia, corneal epithelial edema, folds in Descemet's membrane, peripheral anterior synechiae, increased IOP, visual field defect.

Laboratory

Diagnosis is made by clinical findings.

Treatment

Systemic hyperosmotic agents, topical pilocarpine every 5 minutes, laser iridotomy and if IOP does not respond, filtering surgery may be necessary.

BIBLIOGRAPHY

1. Noecker RJ, Kahook MY. (2011). Glaucoma, angle closure, acute. [online] Available from www.emedicine.com/oph/TOPIC255.HTM. [Accessed September, 2013].
2. Tham CC, Ritch R. (2012). Glaucoma, angle closure, chronic. [online] Available from www.emedicine.com/oph/TOPIC122.HTM. [Accessed September, 2013].

🗗 4N1J. SCLEROCORNEA

General

Autosomal dominant; feature of cornea plana.

Ocular

Malformation of cornea; indistinct limits of cornea and sclera.

Clinical

It is found in a patient with monosomy 21; may be found in association with hypertelorism, syndactyly, ambiguous genitalia and epidermolysis bullosa dystrophica.

Laboratory

Diagnosis is made by clinical findings.

Treatment

Check for elevated IOP. Medical treatment includes the use of hyperosmotic drops, nonsteroidal and steroidal eye drops. Corneal transplant may be necessary.

🗗 BIBLIOGRAPHY

1. Bloch N. [The different types of sclerocornea, their hereditary modes and concomitant congenital malformations]. J Genet Hum. 1965;14(2):133-72.
2. Doane JF, Sajjadi H, Richardson WP. Bilateral penetrating keratoplasty for sclerocornea in an infant with monosomy 21. Case report and review of the literature. Cornea. 1994;13(5):454-8.
3. Martínez-Frías ML, Bermejo E, Sánchez Otero T, et al. Sclerocornea, hypertelorism, syndactyly, and ambiguous genitalia. Am J Med Genet. 1994;49(2):195-7.
4. McKusick VA. Mendelian Inheritance in Man; A Catalog of Human Genes and Genetic Disorders, 12th edition. Baltimore, USA: The Johns Hopkins University Press; 1998.
5. Hamosh A, Scott AF, Amberger J, et al. Online Mendelian Inheritance in Man (OMIM), a knowledge base of human genes and genetic disorders. Nucleic Acids Res. 2002;30(1):52-5.
6. Sharkey JA, Kervick GN, Jackson AJ, et al. Cornea plana and sclerocornea in association with recessive epidermolysis bullosa dystrophica. Case report. Cornea. 1992;11(1): 83-5.

🗗 4N2. ABERFELD SYNDROME (SCHWARTZ-JAMPEL SYNDROME; CONGENITAL BLEPHAROPHIMOSIS ASSOCIATED WITH GENERALIZED MYOPATHY SYNDROME; OCULAR AND FACIAL ABNORMALITIES SYNDROME)

General

Etiology is not known; autosomal recessive inheritance, although there are reports of dominant inheritance; progressive disorder.

Ocular

Blepharophimosis; exotropia; myopia; congenital cataracts; microcornea.

Clinical

Myopathy; bone deformities; arachnodactyly; dwarfism; hypoplastic facial bones; hypertrichosis; kyphoscoliosis.

Laboratory

Physicians might consider referring suspected cases to genetic clinics that have affiliations with groups actively research so that genetic studies can be performed. Muscle biopsy findings are consistent with a myopathy.

Treatment

The goal is to reduce the abnormal muscle activity that causes stiffness. Botulinum toxin therapy may be considered for the treatment of blepharospasm. However, if ptosis is present this is contraindicated. Some medications that have been found useful in myotonic disorders include the anticonvulsants and the antiarrhythmics.

🗗 BIBLIOGRAPHY

1. Ault J, Berman SA, Dinnerstein E. (2012). Schwartz-Jampel syndrome. [online] Available from www.emedicine.com/neuro/TOPIC337.HTM. [Accessed September, 2013].

🗗 4N4. CARPENTER SYNDROME (ACROCEPHALOPOLYSYNDACTYLY TYPE II)

General

Hereditary; transmitted as an autosomal recessive trait; severe form of Apert syndrome; normal intelligence has been reported with this syndrome; polysyndactyly is not an absolute requirement for this diagnosis.

Ocular

Lateral displacement of inner canthus; epicanthal folds; microcornea; corneal opacities.

Clinical

Acrocephalopolysyndactyly; brachydactyly; peculiar facies; obesity; mental retardation; hypogonadism; generalized aminoaciduria; cryptorchidism; hypogenitalism.

Laboratory

Skull radiography, cranial CT.

Treatment

Carefully monitoring for signs and symptoms of elevated intracranial pressure is important. Surgery typically is indicated for increased intracranial pressure or for cosmetic reasons.

🗗 BIBLIOGRAPHY

1. Sheth RD, Ranalli N, Aldana P, et al. (2012). Pediatric craniosynostosis. [online] Available from www.emedicine.com/neuro/TOPIC80.HTM. [Accessed September, 2013].

🗗 4N5. CATARACT, MICROCORNEA SYNDROME

General

Autosomal dominant; prominent in Sicilian families.

Ocular

Cataracts; microcornea; myopia.

Clinical

None.

Laboratory

Diagnosis is made by clinical findings.

Treatment

Cataract surgery if vision decreases.

🗗 BIBLIOGRAPHY

1. McKusick VA. Mendelian Inheritance in Man; A Catalog of Human Genes and Genetic Disorders, 12th edition. Baltimore, USA: The Johns Hopkins University Press; 1998.
2. Hamosh A, Scott AF, Amberger J, et al. Online Mendelian Inheritance in Man (OMIM), a knowledgebase of human genes and genetic disorders. Nucleic Acids Res. 2002;30(1):52-5.
3. Mollica F, Li Volti S, Tomarchio S, et al. Autosomal dominant cataract and microcornea associated with myopia in a Sicilian family. Clin Genet. 1985;28(1):42-6.
4. Polomeno RC, Cummings C. Autosomal dominant cataracts and microcornea. Can J Ophthalmol. 1979;14(4):227-9.
5. Salmon JF, Wallis CE, Murray AD. Variable expressivity of autosomal dominant microcornea with cataract. Arch Ophthalmol. 1988;106(4):505-10.

🗗 4N6. CHROMOSOME 18 PARTIAL DELETION (LONG-ARM) SYNDROME [MONOSOMY 18 PARTIAL (LONG-ARM) SYNDROME; DE GROUCHY SYNDROME]

General

Deletion of approximately one-half of the long arm of chromosome 18.

Ocular

Hypertelorism; epicanthal folds; narrow palpebral fissure; nystagmus (horizontal); strabismus; myopia; astigmatism;

glaucoma; oval pupils; microcornea; posterior staphyloma; oblique disk; optic nerve staphyloma; optic nerve atrophy; microphthalmia; corneal opacities; iris hypoplasia; corectopia.

Clinical

Dwarfism; mental retardation; microcephaly; midface dysplasia; prominent antihelix and antitragus; congenital cardiac disease; abnormal, spindle-shaped fingers; genital defects.

Laboratory

Clinical.

Treatment

- *Glaucoma*: Glaucoma medication should be the first plan of action. If medication is unsuccessful, a filtering surgical procedure with or without antimetabotites may be beneficial.

- *Strabismus*: Equalized vision with correct refractive error; surgery may be helpful in patient with diplopia.

BIBLIOGRAPHY

1. de Grouchy J, Royer P, Salmon C, et al. Deletion Partielle des Bras Longs du Chromosome 18. Pathol Biol (France). 1964;12:579.
2. Ginsberg J, Perrin EV, Sueoka WT. Ocular manifestations in trisomy 18. Am J Ophthalmol. 1968;66:59.
3. Izquierdo NJ, Maumenee IH, Traboulsi EI. Anterior segment malformations in 18q- (de Grouchy) syndrome. Ophthalmic Pediatr Genet. 1993;14:91-4.
4. Levenson JE, Crandall BF, Sparkes RS. Partial deletion syndromes of chromosome 18. Ann Ophthalmol. 1971;3:756.
5. Mollica F, Li Volti S, Tomarchio S, et al. Autosomal dominant cataract and microcornea associated with myopia in a Sicilian family. Clin Genet. 1985;28:42-6.
6. Polomeno RC, Cummings C. Autosomal dominant cataracts and microcornea. Can J Ophthalmol. 1979;14:227-9.

4N7. EHLERS-DANLOS SYNDROME (FIBRODYSPLASIA ELASTICA GENERALISATA; CUTIS HYPERELASTICA; MEEKEREN-EHLERS-DANLOS SYNDROME; INDIAN RUBBER MAN SYNDROME; CUTIS LAXA)

General

Present at birth; autosomal dominant; two groups: cutaneous and articular; syndrome is one of the three primary disorders of elastic tissue [other two disorders are pseudoxanthoma elasticum (Grönblad-Strandberg syndrome) and senile elastosis]; inherited disorder of collagen biosynthesis.

Ocular

Hyperelasticity of palpebral skin; easy eversion of upper lid; ptosis; epicanthal folds; hypotony of extraocular muscles; strabismus; microcornea; thinning of cornea with keratoconus; thinning of sclera (blue sclera); subluxation of lens; angioid streaks; chorioretinal hemorrhages; retinitis proliferans with secondary detachment; macular degeneration; myopia; ruptured globe after minor trauma; limbus-to-limbus corneal thinning; acute hydrops; cornea plana; keratoglobus.

Clinical

Cutaneous manifestations include thin, atrophic, fragile skin, cutaneous hyperelasticity and pseudomolluscoid tumors; articular manifestations include excessive articular laxity and luxations; hypermobile joints.

Laboratory

Biochemical studies can detect alterations in collagen molecules in cultured skin fibroblasts. Molecular (DNA)-based testing is available. Diagnosis may by urinary analyte assay and clinical examination is the most common.

Treatment

Ascorbic acid therapy, in the event of skin lacerations seriously consider alternatives to sutures, including adhesive strips and wound glues, monitor for cardiac conditions and scoliosis.

BIBLIOGRAPHY

1. Steiner RD. (2011). Genetics of Ehlers-Danlos syndrome. [online] Available from www.emedicine.com/ped/TOPIC654.HTM. [Accessed September, 2013].

🗗 4N8. GANSSLEN SYNDROME (FAMILIAL HEMOLYTIC ICTERUS; HEMATOLOGIC-METABOLIC BONE DISORDER)

General

Autosomal dominant inheritance; occurs mainly in Caucasians.

Ocular

Hypertelorism; microphthalmos; epicanthus; narrowing of palpebral fissure; lid hemorrhages; myopia; dyschromatopsia; hypochromic heterochromia; scleral icterus; conjunctival hemorrhages; retinal pallor and edema in advanced stages; dilated retinal arteries and veins; round retinal hemorrhages in deeper retinal layers; retinal exudates and macular star.

Clinical

Splenomegaly; hemolytic crises; dental deformities; brachydactyly; polydactyly; congenital hip luxation; oxycephaly; deformities of the outer ear and otosclerosis.

Laboratory

Indirect Coomb's test and direct antibody test results are positive in the mother and affected newborn; serial maternal antibody titers are monitored until a critical titer of 1:32, which indicates that a high risk of fetal hydrops.

Treatment

Early exchange transfusion with type-O Rh-negative fresh RBCs with intensive phototherapy is usually required.

🗗 BIBLIOGRAPHY

1. Ganser SJ. Uber Einen Eigenarrigen Hysterischen Dammerzustand. Arch Psychiatr Nervenkrankh. 1898;30:633.
2. Magalini SI, Scrascia E. Dictionary of Medical Syndromes, 2nd edition. Philadelphia: JB Lippincott; 1981.

🗗 4N9. HALLERMANN-STREIFF SYNDROME [DYSCEPHALIC-MANDIBULO-OCULO-FACIAL SYNDROME; OCULO-MANDIBULO-DYSCEPHALY; ULLRICH-FREMERY-DOHNA SYNDROME; FRANCOIS DYSCEPHALIC SYNDROME; MANDIBULO-OCULO-FACIAL DYSCEPHALY SYNDROME; FRANCOIS-HALLERMANN-STREIFF SYNDROME; HALLERMANN-STREIFF-FRANCOIS SYNDROME; AUDRY I SYNDROME; DOHNA SYNDROME; FRANCOIS SYNDROME (1); DYSCEPHALY-TEETH ABNORMALITY-DWARFISM; DYSCEPHALIA OCULOMANDIBULARIS-HYPOTRICHOSIS; MANDIBULO-OCULAR DYSCEPHALIA HYPOTRICHOSIS; FREMERY-DOHNA SYNDROME; OCULO-MANDIBULO-FACIAL DYSCEPHALY]

General

Rare; familial occurrence and consanguinity; males and females are equally affected.

Ocular

Microphthalmos (bilateral); proptosis; nystagmus; strabismus; cataracts; bilateral optic atrophy; coloboma of optic disk, choroid, and iris; keratoglobus; microcornea; antimongoloid slant; iris atrophy; uveitis; blue sclera; persistent pupillary membrane; secondary glaucoma.

Clinical

Malformations of skull (brachycephaly), facial skeleton and jaws; erupted teeth at birth; diminished hair growth; hyperextensibility of joints; short stature; skin atrophy; mental deficiency; predisposition to upper airway compromise; obstructive sleep apnea.

Laboratory

Diagnosis is made by clinical findings.

Treatment

- *Cataract*: Change in glasses can sometimes improve a patient's visual function temporarily; however the most common treatment is cataract surgery.
- *Strabismus*: Equalized vision with correct refractive error; surgery may be helpful in patients with diplopia.
- *Uveitis*: Topical steroids and cycloplegic medication should be the initial treatment of choice. Oral steroids should be given if not responsive to topical steroids, immunosuppressants if bilateral disease that does not respond to oral steroids, periocular steroids for unilateral or posterior uveitis. Vitrectomy can be used for severe vitreous opacification. Cryotherapy and laser photocoagulation may be used for localized pars plana exudates.
- *Glaucoma*: Glaucoma medication should be the first plan of action. If medication is unsuccessful, a filtering surgical procedure with or without antimetabolites may be beneficial.

BIBLIOGRAPHY

1. François J, Victoria-Troncoso V. François' dyscephalic syndrome and skin manifestations. Ophthalmologica. 1981;183(2):63-7.
2. Roy FH, Fraunfelder FW, Fraunfelder FT. Roy and Fraunfelder's Current Ocular Therapy, 6th edition. Philadelphia, PA: WB Saunders; 2008.
3. Hallermann W. Vogelgesicht und Cataracta Congenita. Klin Monatsbl Augenheilkd. 1948;113:315-8.
4. Ronen S, Rozenmann Y, Isaacson M, et al. The early management of baby with Hallermann-Streiff-Francois syndrome. J Pediatr Ophthalmol Strabismus. 1979;16(2):119-21.
5. Spaepen A, Schrander-Stumpel C, Fryns JP, et al. Hallermann-Streiff syndrome: clinical and psychological findings in children. Nosologic overlap with oculodentodigital dysplasia? Am J Med Genet. 1991;41(4):517-20.
6. Streiff EB. Dysmorphic Mandibulo-faciale (Tete d'Oiseau) et Alterations Oculaires. Ophthalmologica. 1950;120(1-2): 79-83.

4N10. HEMIFACIAL MICROSOMIA SYNDROME (UNILATERAL FACIAL AGENESIS; OTOMANDIBULAR DYSOSTOSIS; FRANCOIS-HAUSTRATE SYNDROME)

General

No inheritance pattern; left side of face seems to be more frequently involved; facial asymmetry usually most obvious finding; both sexes affected; alteration of intrauterine environment is possible cause.

Ocular

Microphthalmos; congenital cystic ophthalmia; enophthalmos; strabismus; cataract; colobomata of iris, choroid, and retina.

Clinical

Microtia; macrostomia; failure of development of mandibular ramus and condyle; external auditory meatus may be absent; single or numerous ear tags; hypoplasia of facial muscles unilaterally; pulmonary agenesis (ipsilateral side); associated with Goldenhar syndrome.

Laboratory

X-ray, CT and MRI.

Treatment

Silastic implants remain one of the most common materials used for malar and submalar augmentation.

BIBLIOGRAPHY

1. Francois J, Haustrate L. Anomalies Colobomateuses du Globe Oculaire et Syndrome du Premier arc. Ann Ocul. 1954;187:340.
2. Geeraets WJ. Ocular Syndromes, 3rd edition. Philadelphia: Lea & Febiger; 1976.
3. Kobrynski L, Chitayat D, Zahed L, et al. Trisomy 22 and facioauriculovertebral (Goldenhar) sequence. Am J Med Genet. 1993;46:68-71.
4. Magalini SI, Scrascia E. Dictionary of Medical Syndromes, 2nd edition. Philadelphia: JB Lippincott; 1981.

4N12. HUTCHINSON-GILFORD SYNDROME (PROGERIA)

General

Inheritance unknown; belongs to group of ectodermal dysplasias (*see* Werner Syndrome-Progeria of Adults); elevated hyaluronic acid of unknown etiology, likely sporadic dominant mutation.

Ocular

Microphthalmia; hypotrichosis; microcornea; cataract.

Clinical

Appearance of "old age" in children; short stature to dwarfism; dyscephaly; atrophy of skin and subcutaneous adipose tissue; aplasia of maxilla; oligodontia; arteriosclerosis (premature); progeria.

Laboratory

Radiography findings usually manifest within the 1st or 2nd year of life and most commonly involve the skull, thorax, long bones, and phalanges.

Treatment

No effective therapy is available. Careful monitoring and referral to the proper specialists is important.

BIBLIOGRAPHY

1. Shah KN. (2013). Hutchinson-Gilford progeria. [online] Available from www.emedicine.com/derm/TOPIC731. HTM. [Accessed September, 2013].

4N13. LAURENCE-MOON-BARDET-BIEDL SYNDROME (BARDET-BIEDL SYNDROME; RETINITIS PIGMENTOSA-POLYDACTYLY-ADIPOSOGENITAL SYNDROME)

General

Recessive, autosomal dominant, and recessive sex-linked gene; male preponderance; onset in childhood; cases of Laurence-Moon-Bardet-Biedl belong to the group of heredoataxias.

Ocular

Ptosis; epicanthus; nystagmus; strabismus; night blindness; myopia; hypermetropia; iris coloboma; RP "bone corpuscles"; macular degeneration; attenuation of retinal vessels; choroidal atrophy; optic nerve atrophy; cataract; microphthalmia; keratoconus.

Clinical

Obesity (Fröhlich type); hypogenitalism; reduced intelligence and mental retardation; turricephaly; shortness of stature; atresia ani; genu valgum; congenital heart disease; polydactyly; body hair scant or absent; pseudogynecomastia.

Laboratory

Chromosomal analysis is recommended to confirm chromosomal sex and to evaluate for associated genetic syndromes.

Treatment

Consultation by pediatric endocrinologist and pediatric urologist is usually necessary.

BIBLIOGRAPHY

1. Telander DG, de Beus A, Small KW. (2012). Retinitis pigmentosa. [online] Available from www.emedicine.com/oph/TOPIC704.HTM. [Accessed September, 2013].

⊟ 4N14. LENZ MICROPHTHALMIA SYNDROME

General

X-linked recessive; female carriers.

Ocular

Microphthalmia; microcornea; ocular coloboma; colobomatous microphthalmia.

Clinical

Skeletal abnormalities of vertebral column, clavicles, and limbs; severe renal dysgenesis and hydroureters; dental anomalies; hypospadias and bilateral cryptorchidism; severe speech impairment; shortness of stature; long, cylindrical, and thin thorax; sloping shoulders; flat feet.

Laboratory

Diagnosis is made by clinical findings.

Treatment

None—ocular.

⊟ BIBLIOGRAPHY

1. Antoniades K, Tzouvelekis G, Doudou A, et al. A sporadic case of Lenz microphthalmia syndrome. Ann Ophthalmol. 1993;25:342-5.
2. Herrmann J, Optiz JM. The Lenz microphthalmia syndrome. Birth Defects. 1969;5:138-48.

⊟ 4N15. LITTLE SYNDROME (NAIL-PATELLA SYNDROME; HEREDITARY OSTEO-ONYCHO-DYSPLASIA; HOOD SYNDROME)

General

Inherited as autosomal dominant; affects males and females equally.

Ocular

Hypertelorism; ptosis; epicanthus; microcornea; keratoconus; sclerocornea; cataract; microphakia; light pigmentation of iris root with dark pigmented "clover-leaf" spots, referred to as the Lester line, not seen in all cases.

Clinical

Absent or hypoplastic patella; hypoplastic or dislocated head of radius; exostosis of skull bones; bilateral horns of iliac crests; longitudinal ridging of fingernails; glomerulonephritis; renal involvement; bilateral antecubital pterygia; arthrogryposis; disorder has been mapped to the long arm of chromosome 9; sensorineural hearing loss.

Laboratory

Conduct urinalysis, along with a microscopic analysis, to check for proteinuria and hematuria. Radiography findings reveal iliac horns. MRI to identify abnormal muscle insertions; renal biopsy.

Treatment

Renal dialysis and transplantation are necessary.

⊟ BIBLIOGRAPHY

1. Hoover-Fong J, McIntosh I, Sweeney E. (2012). Genetics of nail-patella syndrome. [online] Available from www.emedicine.com/ped/TOPIC1546.HTM. [Accessed September, 2013].

⊟ 4N16. MARCHESANI SYNDROME (WEILL-MARCHESANI SYNDROME; INVERTED MARFAN SYNDROME; BRACHYMORPHY WITH SPHEROPHAKIA; DYSTROPHIA MESODERMALIS CONGENITA HYPERPLASTICA)

General

Pattern of inheritance uncertain; manifest at age of 9 months to 13 years.

Ocular

Lenticular myopia; secondary glaucoma (rare), caused by luxation of the lens; iridodonesis; ectopia lentis;

spherophakia; optic atrophy; megalocornea; corneal opacity; acute pupillary block glaucoma.

Clinical

Brachydactyly; reduced growth; athletic build with abundant subcutaneous tissue; short neck and large thorax; short and clumsy hands and feet; decreased joint flexibility; hearing defects; inheritable connective tissue disorder, usually inherited as an autosomal recessive.

Laboratory

X-ray detects delayed carpal ossification.

Treatment/Glaucoma

Beta-blockers, carbonic anhydrase inhibitors and prostaglandin analogs. Surgery may be needed if IOP is uncontrolled.

⧉ BIBLIOGRAPHY

1. Hamosh A, Scott AF, Amberger J, et al. Online Mendelian Inheritance in Man, (OMIM), a knowledgebase of human genes and genetic disorders. Nucleic Acids Res. 2002;30(1):52-5
2. McKusick-Nathans Institute for Genetic Medicine, Johns Hopkins University and National Center for Biotechnology Information, National Library of Medicine, February 12, 2007. Available from www.ncbi.nlm.nih.gov/omim. [Accessed September, 2013].
3. Jensen AD, Cross HE, Paton Det al. Ocular complications in the Weill-Marchesani syndrome. Am J Ophthalmol. 1974; 77(2):261-9.
4. Marchesani O. Brachydactylie und Angeborene Kugellinse als Systemerkrankung. Klin Monatsbl Augenheilkd. 1939; 103:392.
5. McKusick VA. Mendelian Inheritance in Man; A Catalog of Human Genes and Genetic Disorders, 12th edition. Baltimore: The Johns Hopkins University Press; 1998.
6. Roy FH, Fraunfelder FT Fraunfelder FW. Roy and Fraunfelder's Current Ocular Therapy, 6th edition. Philadelphia: WB Saunders; 2008.
7. Willi M, Kut L, Cotlier E, et al. Pupillary-block glaucoma in the Marchesani syndrome. Arch Ophthalmol. 1973;90(6): 504-8.
8. Young ID, Fielder AR, Casey TA, et al. Weill-Marchesani syndrome in mother and son. Clin Genet. 1986;30(6): 475-80.

⧉ 4N17. MARFAN SYNDROME (DOLICHOSTENOMELIA; ARACHNODACTYLY; HYPERCHONDROPLASIA; DYSTROPHIA MESODERMALIS CONGENITA)

General

Hypoplastic form of dystrophia mesodermalis congenita; autosomal dominant; affects both sexes. It has been demonstrated that an abnormality of the gene coding for the connective tissue protein fibrillin is responsible for chronic Marfan syndrome.

Ocular

Exotropia; nystagmus; paralysis of accommodation; myopia (axial or lenticular); iridodonesis; miosis; persistent pupillary membrane; blue sclera; spherophakia; lens dislocation; cataract; megalocornea; retinal detachment (less frequently); pigmentary retinopathy; colobomata of macula, iris, optic nerve, and uveal tract (less frequently); keratoconus; central retinal artery occlusion; rhegmatogenous retinal detachment; syringoma.

Clinical

Arachnodactyly; skeletal anomalies; asymmetric thorax; dolichocephaly and high-arched palate; dissecting aneurysm; mitral valve prolapse; prominent ears; kyphoscoliosis; pectus excavatum; flat feet; hammer toes; pulmonary and kidney defects.

Laboratory

Genetic testing, molecular studies.

Treatment

- *Keratoconus*: Spectacle correction, hard contacts, avoid eye rubbing. If hydrops occur, discontinue contact lens, use NaCl drops and ointment, patching, and short course of steroids. As disease advances, PK, deep anterior lamellar keratoplasty intacs with laser grooves or collagen stabilization of cornea.

- *Cataract*: Change in glasses can sometimes improve a patient's visual function temporarily; however the most common treatment is cataract surgery.
- *Glaucoma*: Glaucoma medication should be the first plan of action. If medication is unsuccessful, a filtering surgical procedure with or without antimetabolites may be beneficial.

- *Strabismus*: Equalized vision with correct refractive error; surgery may be helpful in patient with diplopia.

BIBLIOGRAPHY

1. Chen H. (2011). Genetics of Marfan syndrome. [online] Available from www.emedicine.com/ped/TOPIC1372. HTM. [Accessed September, 2013].

4N18. MECKEL SYNDROME (DYSENCEPHALIA SPLANCHNOCYSTIC SYNDROME; GRUBER SYNDROME)

General

Autosomal recessive; ocular manifestations are similar to those of trisomy 13–15 syndrome.

Ocular

Cryptophthalmos; clinical anophthalmos; microphthalmos; mongoloid slant of lid fissures; sclerocornea; microcornea; partial aniridia; cataract; retinal dysplasia; posterior staphyloma; optic nerve hypoplasia.

Clinical

Sloping forehead; posterior encephalocele; short neck; polydactyly and syndactyly (hands and feet); polycystic kidneys; cryptorchidism; cleft lip and palate; CNS abnormalities, including the Dandy-Walker malformation.

Laboratory

Chromosome analysis, MRI.

Treatment

Cardiac surgery may be warranted.

BIBLIOGRAPHY

1. Jayakar PB, Spiliopoulos M, Jayakar A. (2011). Meckel-Gruber syndrome. [online] Available from www.emedicine.com/ped/TOPIC1390.HTM. [Accessed September, 2013].

4N19. MEYER-SCHWICKERATH-WEYERS SYNDROME (MICROPHTHALMOS SYNDROME; OCULODENTODIGITAL DYSPLASIA)

General

Etiology unknown; two types recognized: (I) dysplasia oculodentodigitalis and (II) dyscraniopygophalangie; type I is characterized by microphthalmia with possible iris pathology and glaucoma, oligodontia and brown pigmentation of teeth, camptodactyly, and possible absence of middle phalanx of second to fifth toes; type II consists of severe microphthalmos to anophthalmos, polydactyly, and developmental anomalies of nose and oral cavity; both sexes affected; present from birth; abnormal cerebral white matter.

Ocular

Microphthalmos; hypotrichosis; glaucoma; iris anomalies (eccentric pupil; changes in normal iris texture; remnants of pupillary membrane along iris margins); microcornea; hypertelorism; myopia; hyperopia; keratoconus.

Clinical

Thin, small nose with anteverted nostrils and hypoplastic alae; syndactyly; camptodactyly (fourth and fifth fingers); anomalies of middle phalanx of fifth finger and toe; hypoplastic teeth; wide mandible; alveolar ridge; sparse hair growth; visceral malformations.

Laboratory

Diagnosis is made by clinical findings.

Treatment

- *Glaucoma*: Glaucoma medication should be the first plan of action. If medication is unsuccessful, a filtering surgical procedure with or without antimetabotites may be beneficial.
- *Keratoconus*: Spectacle correction, hard contacts, avoid eye rubbing. If hydrops occur, discontinue contact lens, use NaCl drops and ointment, patching, and short course of steroids. As disease advances, PK, deep anterior lamellar keratoplasty intacs with laser grooves or collagen stabilization of cornea.

BIBLIOGRAPHY

1. Geeraets WK. Ocular Syndromes, 3rd edition. Philadelphia: Lea & Febiger; 1976.
2. Gutmann DH, Zackai EH, McDonald-McGinn DM, et al. Oculodentodigital dysplasia syndrome associated with abnormal cerebral white matter. Am J Med Genet. 1991; 41:18-20.
3. McKusick VA. Mendelian Inheritance in Man; A Catalog of Human Genes and Genetic Disorders, 12th edition. Baltimore: The Johns Hopkins University Press; 1998.

4N20. MORGAGNI SYNDROME (HYPEROSTOSIS FRONTALIS INTERNA SYNDROME; INTRACRANIAL EXOSTOSIS; METABOLIC CRANIOPATHY)

General

Dominant inheritance; onset around age 45 years; occurs almost exclusively in females.

Ocular

Cataract; optic nerve injury within the optic canal by bony protrusions, with resulting blindness.

Clinical

Hyperostosis frontalis interna; obesity (mainly trunk and proximal portions of limbs); hirsutism; menstrual disorders; hypertension; arteriosclerosis; headache; hypertrichosis; no case of male-to-male transmission is known; hyperprolactinemia.

Laboratory

CT scan of orbit.

Treatment

Cataract—change in glasses can sometimes improve a patient's visual function temporarily; however the most common treatment is cataract surgery.

BIBLIOGRAPHY

1. Falconer MA, Pierard BE. Failing vision caused by a bony spike compressing the optic nerve within the optic canal. Report of two cases associated with Morgagni's syndrome benefited by operation. Br J Ophthalmol. 1950;34:265.
2. Geeraets WK. Ocular Syndromes, 3rd edition. Philadelphia: Lea & Febiger; 1976.
3. McKusick VA. Mendelian Inheritance in Man; A Catalog of Human Genes and Genetic Disorders, 12th edition. Baltimore: The Johns Hopkins University Press; 1998.
4. Morgagni GB. De Sedibus et Causis Morborum Peranatomen Indagatis Libri Quinque (2 volumes). Venetiis: Typog. Remondiniana, 1761. Alexander B, English translation, 3 volumes. London, 1769. Select Med Classics. 1940;4:640.
5. Online Mendelian Inheritance in Man, OMIM. McKusick-Nathans Institute for Genetic Medicine, Johns Hopkins University and National Center for Biotechnology Information, National Library of Medicine, February 12, 2007. Available from www.ncbi.nlm.nih.gov/omim. [Accessed September, 2013].
6. Pawlikowski M, Komorowski J. Hyperostosis frontalis, galactorrhea, hyperprolactinemia, and Morgani-Stewart-Morel syndrome [Letter]. Lancet. 1983;1:474.

4N21. MICRO SYNDROME

General

Autosomal recessive microcephaly and microcornea; Muslim Pakistani inheritance; present at birth; consanguinity; autosomal recessive.

Ocular

Microcornea; congenital cataract; retinal dystrophy; optic nerve atrophy; ptosis; microphakia; microphthalmos; nuclear cataract; atonic pupils.

Clinical

Severe mental retardation; hypothalamic hypogenitalism; hypoplasia of the corpus callosum; short stature; cortical visual impairment; microcephaly; developmental delay.

Laboratory/Congenital Cataracts

Dilated examination, TORCH titers and venereal disease reaserch laboratory test.

Treatment/Congenital Cataracts

Cataract surgery is the treatment of choice.

BIBLIOGRAPHY

1. Ainsworth JR, Morton JE, Good P, et al. Micro syndrome in Muslim Pakistan children. Ophthalmology. 2001;108: 491-7.
2. Mégarbané A, Choueiri R, Bleik J, et al. Microcephaly, microphthalmia, congenital cataract, optic atrophy, short stature, hypotonia. Severe psychomotor retardation, and cerebral malformations: a second family with micro syndrome or a new syndrome? J Med Genet. 1999;36: 637-40.
3. Rodriguez C, Rufo M, Gomez de Terreros I. A second family with micro syndrome. Clin Dysmorphol. 1999;8:241-5.
4. Warburg M, Sjö O, Fledelius HC, et al. Autosomal recessive microcephaly, microcornea, congenital cataract, mental retardation, optic atrophy, and hypogenitalism: micro syndrome. Am J Dis Child. 1993;147:1309-12.

4N22. RIEGER SYNDROME (AXENFELD-RIEGER SYNDROME; DYSGENESIS MESODERMALIS CORNEAE ET IRIDES; DYSGENESIS MESOSTROMALIS; AXENFELD POSTERIOR EMBRYOTOXON-JUVENILE GLAUCOMA)

General

Autosomal dominant; neural crest abnormality; 50% of patients develop glaucoma.

Ocular

Microphthalmia; congenital glaucoma; iris hypoplasia; deformed and acentric pupil; anterior synechiae; aniridia; microcornea; corneal opacities in Descemet's membrane parallel to the limbus; dislocated lens; optic atrophy; cataract; strabismus; ptosis; hypertelorism; keratoconus; posterior embryotoxon; broad iris processes to embryotoxon; iris stromal hypoplasia; corectopia; polycoria; secondary glaucoma.

Clinical

Face wide; hypodontia; underdeveloped maxilla; teeth deformities; myotonic dystrophy; facial anomalies: maxillary hypoplasia, protrusion of the lower lip, broad, flat nose; dental anomalies include absent teeth, pig-like incisors and decreased crown size; hypospadias.

Laboratory

Diagnosis is made by clinical findings.

Treatment/Ocular

Congenital glaucoma can be treated with beta-blockers, prostaglandin analogs and carbonic anhydrase inhibitors. Surgery such as goniotomy or trabeculectomy can be used if IOP is not controlled.

BIBLIOGRAPHY

1. Eagle RC. Congenital, developmental and degenerative disorders of the iris and ciliary body. In: Albert DM, Jakobiec FA (Eds). Albert & Jakobiec's Principles and Practice of Ophthalmology: Clinical Practice, 3rd edition. Philadelphia, PA: WB Saunders; 1994. pp. 367-87.

2. Montes JG, Montes JC. Syndrome de Rieger, anomalie de axenfeld con glaucoma Juvenil familiar. Arch Soc Ophth Hisp Am. 1967;27:93.
3. Rieger H. Beitrage zur Kenntnis seltener Missbildungen der Iris. Graefes Arch Clin Esp Ophthalmol. 1935;133:602.
4. Wesley RK, Baker JD, Golnick AL. Rieger's syndrome: (oligodontia and primary mesodermal dysgenesis of the iris) clinical features and report of an isolated case. J Pediatr Ophthalmol Strabismus. 1978;15(2):67-70.

4N23. RING CHROMOSOME 6 (ANIRIDIA, CONGENITAL GLAUCOMA, AND HYDROCEPHALUS)

General

Rare disorder associated with various congenital anomalies; autosomal dominant with recessive sporadically reported.

Ocular

Microphthalmia; aniridia; congenital uveal ectropion; Rieger anomaly; congenital glaucoma; corneal clouding; prominent Schwalbe's line with attached iris strands; hypopigmented fundi; hypoplasia of iris stroma; strabismus; ptosis; nystagmus; megalocornea; iris coloboma; optic atrophy; hypertelorism; antimongoloid slant of palpebral fissures; ectopic pupils; angle anomalies; posterior embryotoxon; microcornea; colobomatous.

Clinical

Hydrocephalus; agenesis of corpus callosum; congenital heart defects; mental retardation; low-set malformed ears; broad nasal bridge; micrognathia; short neck; hand anomalies; high-arched palate; widely spaced nipples; deformity of feet; respiratory distress syndrome; hyperbilirubinemia; hypocalcemia; anemia; seizure; bulging anterior fontanel.

Laboratory

Diagnosis is made by clinical findings.

Treatment

Ptosis: If visual acuity is affected, most cases require surgical correction and there are several procedures that may be used including levator resection, repair or advancement and Fasanella-Servat procedure.

BIBLIOGRAPHY

1. Bateman JB. Chromosomal anomalies and the eye. In: Wright KW (Ed). Pediatric Ophthalmology and Strabismus. St Louis: Mosby; 1995. p. 595.
2. Chitayat D, Hahm SY, Iqbal MA, et al. Ring chromosome 6: report of a patient and literature review. Am J Med Genet. 1987;26(1):145-51.
3. DeLuise VP, Anderson DR. Primary infantile glaucoma (congenital glaucoma). Surv Ophthalmol. 1983;28(1):1-19.
4. Levin H, Ritch R, Barathur R, et al. Aniridia, congenital glaucoma, and hydrocephalus in a male infant with ring chromosome 6. Am J Med Genet. 1986;25(2):281-7.

4N24. ROBERTS PSEUDOTHALIDOMIDE SYNDROME (GLAUCOMA)

General

Rare autosomal recessive disorder characterized by prenatal and postnatal growth retardation, limb defects, and craniofacial anomalies.

Ocular

Cataracts; glaucoma; microcornea; corneal clouding.

Clinical

Patients usually do not survive past 1 month; patients often are mentally retarded.

Laboratory

Clinical.

Treatment

- *Cataract*: Change in glasses can sometimes improve a patient's visual function temporarily; however the most common treatment is cataract surgery.
- *Glaucoma*: Glaucoma medication should be the first plan of action. If medication is unsuccessful, a filtering surgical procedure with or without antimetabotites may be beneficial.

⊟ BIBLIOGRAPHY

1. Holden KR, Jabs EW, Sponseller PD. Roberts pseudothalidomide syndrome and normal intelligence: approaches to diagnosis and management. Dev Med Child Neurol. 1992;34:534-9.
2. Otano L, Matayoshi T, Gadow EC. Roberts syndrome: first-trimester prenatal diagnosis. Prenat Diagn. 1996;16:770-1.

⊟ 4N25. RUBELLA SYNDROME (CONGENITAL RUBELLA SYNDROME; GERMAN MEASLES; GREGG SYNDROME)

General

Rubella infection of the mother during first trimester of pregnancy; ocular disease is the most commonly found abnormality in patients with congenital rubella syndrome (75%), multiorgan disease is common (greater than 75%); no significant association has been found between gestational age and time of maternal infection and incidence of individual ocular conditions.

Ocular

Nystagmus; glaucoma; corneal haziness; cataracts; retinal pigmentary changes; appearance and central distribution of lesions are quite distinguishable from retinitis pigmentosa; retinopathy is not progressive and has little, if any, effect on vision; waxy atrophy of optic disk; conjunctivitis; megalocornea or microcornea; buphthalmos; microphthalmos; uveitis; iris atrophy; spherophakia; strabismus.

Clinical

Low-birth weight; diarrhea; pneumonia; urinary infection; hearing loss; heart disease; hepatosplenomegaly; mental retardation; inguinal hernias; ataxia; cardiac abnormalities.

Laboratory

Diagnosis is made by clinical findings. If in doubt, a rising titer of immunoglobulin M will indicate a recent infection.

Treatment

Treatment for rubella of the eye centers on glaucoma and cataract.

⊟ BIBLIOGRAPHY

1. Lombardo PC. (2011). Dermatologic manifestations of rubella. [online] Available from www.emedicine.com/derm/TOPIC380.HTM. [Accessed September, 2013].

⊟ 4N26. SABIN-FELDMAN SYNDROME (CHORIORETINITIS)

General

Etiology unknown; similar to toxoplasmosis; results of toxoplasma dye and complement fixation tests are negative; onset in early infancy.

Ocular

Microphthalmia; strabismus; fixed pupils; posterior lenticonus; microcornea; chorioretinitis or atrophic degenerative chorioretinal changes; optic atrophy.

Clinical

Cerebral calcifications (infrequent); convulsions (frequent); microcephaly; hydrocephalus.

Treatment

Lens extraction with irrigation-aspiration.

Laboratory

Clinical.

⊟ BIBLIOGRAPHY

1. Geeraets WJ. Ocular Syndromes, 3rd edition. Philadelphia: Lea & Febiger; 1976.
2. Sabin AB, Feldman HA. Chorioretinopathy associated with other evidence of cerebral damage in childhood: a syndrome of unknown etiology separable from congenital toxoplasmosis. J Pediatr. 1949;35:296.

⊟ 4N27. SCHWARTZ SYNDROME (RETINAL DETACHMENT)

General

Glaucoma associated with retinal detachment; caused by inflammation of trabecula or pigment granules obstructing outflow; photoreceptor outer segments identified in the aqueous humor of patients with this syndrome are thought to play a role in the elevation of IOP.

Ocular

Secondary open-angle glaucoma; retinal detachment; uveitis; myopia; blepharophimosis; long eyelashes; microcornea.

Clinical

Small stature; myotonia; expressionless facies; joint limitation in hips; dystrophy of epiphyseal cartilage, vertical shortness of vertebrae, short neck; low hairline.

Laboratory

Blood test, muscle biopsy, electromyography (EMG) and nerve conduction studies.

Treatment

Botulinum toxin type A is used to treat problems such as blepharospasm, blepharophimosis and ptosis; surgery may also be necessary.

⊟ BIBLIOGRAPHY

1. Ault J, Berman SA, Dinnerstein E. (2012). Schwartz-Jampel syndrome. [online] Available from www.emedicine.com/neuro/TOPIC337.HTM. [Accessed September, 2013].

⊟ 4N28. SMITH-MAGENIS SYNDROME

General

Mental retardation, physical dysmorphia, and behavior abnormalities due to a deletion at chromosome l7pl1.2.

Ocular

High myopia; retinal detachment; iris anomalies (absent collarette, nasal corectopia, stromal dysplasia); microcornea; strabismus; iris nodules called Wolfflin-Kruckmann spots.

Clinical

Wolfflin-Kruckmann spots may be confused with Brushfield spots, which are seen only in Down syndrome patients.

Laboratory

DNA analysis of the *FraX* promoter region should be ordered. Karyotype at the 500 band level and FISH probes should also be ordered. Brain MRI, head CT scan and skeletal film.

Treatment

No treatment is available for Smith-Magenis syndrome (SMS).

⊟ BIBLIOGRAPHY

1. Finucane BM, Jaeger ER, Kurtz MB, et al. Eye abnormalities in the Smith-Magenis contiguous gene deletion syndrome. Am J Med Genet. 1993;45:443-6.
2. Barnicoat AJ, Moller HU, Palmer RW, et al. An unusual presentation of Smith-Magenis syndrome with iris dysgenesis. Clin Dysmorphol. 1996;5:153-6.

⊟ 4N29. TRIPLOIDY SYNDROME (IRIS COLOBOMA)

General

Extra set of chromosomes due to diandry or digyny; still-birth or early neonatal death.

Ocular

Iris coloboma; microphthalmia; hypertelorism.

Clinical

Large placenta; prenatal growth deficits; large fontanels; syndactyly; heart defects; cleft lip; genital, brain, ear, and kidney malformations; meningomyelocele; micrognathia.

Laboratory/ocular

Diagnosis is made by clinical findings.

Treatment

None.

⊟ BIBLIOGRAPHY

1. Arvidsson CG, Hamberg H, Johnsson H, et al. A boy with complete triploidy and unusually long survival. Acta Paediatr Scand. 1986;75:507-10.
2. Crane JP, Beaver HA, Cheung SW. Antenatal ultrasound findings in fetal triploidy syndrome. J Ultrasound Med. 1985;4:519-24.
3. Kaufman MH. New insights into triploidy and tetraploidy, from an analysis of model systems for these conditions. Hum Reprod. 1991;6:8-16.
4. Magalim SI, Scrascia E. Dictionary of Medical Syndromes, 2nd edition. Philadelphia: JB Lippincott; 1981.
5. O'Brien WF, Knuppel RA, Kousseff B, et al. Elevated maternal serum alpha-fetoprotein in triploidy. Obstet Gynecol. 1988;71:994-5.
6. Rubenstein JB, Swayne LC, Dise CA, et al. Placental changes in fetal triploidy syndrome. J Ultrasound Med. 1986;5:545-50.
7. Strobel SL, Brandt JT. Abnormal hematologic features in a live-born female with triploidy. Arch Pathol Lab Med. 1985;109:775-7.
8. Walker S, Andrews J, Gregson NM, et al. Three further cases of triploidy in man surviving to birth. J Med Genet. 1973;10:135-41.

⊟ 4N30. TRISOMY 13 SYNDROME (TRISOMY D1 SYNDROME, PATAU SYNDROME, REESE SYNDROME) IRIS COLOBOMA

General

Extra chromosome in the D group; fatal in the first few months of life; trisomy 13–15 resembles trisomy D1.

Ocular

Anophthalmia; microphthalmia; iris coloboma; cataracts; retinal dysplasia; optic nerve coloboma; optic atrophy; iris dyplasia; calcified lens; retinal detachment; optic nerve hypoplasia; orbital cysts.

Clinical

Apneic spells; developmental deficiency of the nervous system; seizures (minor motor); deafness; cleft lip and palate; hemangiomata; horizontal palmar creases; hyperconvex fingernails; interventricular septal defects; renal abnormalities; cardiovascular changes; respiratory involvement; gastrointestinal disease; urogenital involvement; cerebral hypoplasia with hydrocephalus; mental retardation.

Laboratory

Immediate conventional cytogenetic test. Ultrasonography for any anomaly. Trisomy 13 is best identified through cytogenetic study of amniotic fluid.

Treatment

Surgical care is usually withheld for the first few months of life.

⊟ BIBLIOGRAPHY

1. Best RG, Gregg AR. (2012). Patau syndrome. [online] Available from www.emedicine.com/ped/TOPIC1745.HTM. [Accessed August, 2013].

🗗 4N31. WAARDENBURG SYNDROME (VAN DER HOEVE-HALBERSTAM-WAARDENBURG SYNDROME; WAARDENBURG-KLEIN SYNDROME; EMBRYONIC FIXATION SYNDROME; INTEROCULO-IRIDODERMATO-AUDITIVE DYSPLASIA; PIEBALDISM) HYPERTELORISM

General

Irregular dominant inheritance; developmental fault in neural crest with absence of the organ of Corti, aplasia of the spiral ganglion, and pigmentary changes; no sex preference; onset at birth.

Ocular

Hyperplasia of the medial portions of the eyebrows; hypertelorism; blepharophimosis; strabismus; heterochromia iridis; aniridia; microcornea; cornea plana; microphakia; abnormal fundus pigmentation; hypoplasia of optic nerve; synophrys; poliosis; hypopigmentation and hypoplasia of retina and choroid; epicanthus; lateral displacement of inferior puncta; lenticonus; underdevelopment of orbital bones; lateral displacement of inner canthi; hypopigmented iris.

Clinical

Congenital deafness; unilateral deafness or deaf-mutism; broad and high nasal root with absent nasofrontal angle; albinotic hair strain (unilateral); faint patches of skin pigmentation; pituitary tumor; nasal atresia; white forelock.

Laboratory

Molecular testing and audiology.

Treatment

Genetic counseling, audiology and otolaryngology management.

🗗 BIBLIOGRAPHY

1. Geeraets WJ. Ocular Syndromes, 3rd edition. Philadelphia: Lea & Febiger; 1976.
2. Jensen J, Rousing H. Dysplasia of the cochlea in a case of Wildervanck's syndrome. Adv Otorhinolaryngol. 1974;21:32.
3. Kôse G, Ozkan H, Ozdamar F, et al. Cholelithiasis in cervico-oculo-acoustic (Wildervanck's) syndrome. Acta Paediatr. 1993;82:890-1.
4. Schwartz RA, Bawle EV, Jozwiak S. (2013). Genetics of Waardenburg syndrome. [online] Available from www.emedicine.com/ped/TOPIC2422.HTM. [Accessed September, 2013].
5. Wildervanck LS. A cervico-oculo-acoustic-nerve syndrome. Ned Tijdschr Geneeskd. 1960;104:2600.

🗗 4O. MIDAS SYNDROME (MICROPHTHALMIA, DERMAL APLASIA AND SCLEROCORNEA)

General

X-linked phenotype; male—lethal trait.

Ocular

Bilateral microphthalmia; sclerocornea; blepharophimosis.

Clinical

Dermal aplasia; microcephaly; cardiomyopathy; ventricular fibrillation; congenital heart defect.

Laboratory/sclerocornea

No laboratory findings needed.

Treatment/Sclerocornea

Surgical care; PK is recommended.

🗗 BIBLIOGRAPHY

1. Cape CJ, Zaidman GW, Beck AD, et al. Phenotypic variation in ophthalmic manifestations of MIDAS syndrome (microphthalmia, dermal aplasia, and sclerocornea). Arch Ophthalmol. 2004;122(7):1070-4.
2. Happle R, Daniëls O, Koopman RJ. MIDAS syndrome (microphthalmia, dermal aplasia, and sclerocornea): an X-linked phenotype distinct from Goltz syndrome. Am J Med Genet. 1993;47(5):710-3.

⊟ 4P. MMMM SYNDROME (NEUHAUSER SYNDROME; MEGALOCORNEA, MACROCEPHALY, MENTAL AND MOTOR RETARDATION)

General

Rare.

Ocular

Megalocornea.

Clinical

Mental retardation; hearing loss; sensorineural complications; hypoplasia; corpus callosum; macrocephaly.

Laboratory/Ocular

Gonioscopy, A-scan ultrasound biometry.

Treatment

Spectacles; glaucoma or cataract surgery if necessary.

⊟ BIBLIOGRAPHY

1. Tominaga N, Kamimura N, Matsumoto T, et al. A case of megalocornea mental retardation syndrome complicated with bilateral sensorineural hearing loss. Pediat Int. 1999;41:392-4.
2. Tonaki H. Megalcornea-mental retardation syndrome. Turk J Pediatr. 2002;44:274-7.

⊟ 4Q. MYOTONIC DYSTROPHY SYNDROME (MYOTONIA ATROPHICA SYNDROME; DYSTROPHIA MYOTONICA; CURSCHMANN-STEINERT SYNDROME)

General

Rare autosomal dominant disease; onset at the age of 20 years; condition is worsened by administration of neostigmine (Prostigmin); associated with an unstable DNA sequence composed of varying numbers of CTG triplet repeats (which allows a specific molecular test for this disorder).

Ocular

Mild ptosis (occasionally); myotonic cataract with small, dot-like subcapsular cortical opacities during early stage, with polychromatic properties on biomicroscopic examination; corneal epithelial dystrophy; loss of corneal sensitivity; tapetoretinal degeneration; macular red spot; macular degeneration; chorioretinitis; pilomatrixomas; ocular hypotony; pattern pigmentary changes; abnormal saccades.

Clinical

Progressive muscular atrophy with selection of certain muscles (mainly sternocleidomastoid, temporalis, dorsiflexor muscles of the ankle, anterior oblique); myotonia; bland facial expression; speech disturbance due to involvement of vocal cords and palatal muscles; dysphagia; endocrine disturbances.

Laboratory

Diagnosis is made by clinical findings.

Treatment

- *Ptosis*: If visual acuity is affected, most cases require surgical correction and there are several procedures that may be used including levator resection, repair or advancement and Fasanella-Servat procedure.
- *Cataract*: Change in glasses can sometimes improve a patient's visual function temporarily; however, the most common treatment is cataract surgery.
- *Corneal dystrophy*: Mild cases—can be observed and soft contact lenses are helpful; PK may be necessary; graft recurrences are treated by superficial keratectomy, PTK or repeat PK.

- *Macular degeneration*: No treatment is available for non-neovascular age-related macular degeneration (AMD). Preventative therapy includes no smoking, control of hypertension, cholesterol, and blood sugar, exercise and vitamins. Neovascular AMD treatment consists of laser, avastin and lucentis.

BIBLIOGRAPHY

1. Brooke NM, Cwik VE. Myotonic dystrophy. In: Bradley WG (Ed). Neurology in Clinical Practice: Principles of Diagnosis and Management, 2nd edition. Boston, USA: Butterworth-Heinemann; 1995. pp. 2020-2.
2. Gjertsen IK, Sandvig KU, Eide N, et al. Recurrence of secondary opacification and development of a dense posterior vitreous membrane in patients with myotonic dystrophy. J Cataract Refract Surg. 2003;29(1):213-6.
3. Kimizuka Y, Kiyosawa M, Tamai M, et al. Retinal changes in myotonic dystrophy. Clinical and follow-up evaluation. Retina. 1993;13(2):129-35.
4. Koca MR, Horn F, Korth M. Alterations of saccadic eye movements in myotonic dystrophy. Graefes Arch Clin Exp Ophthalmol. 1992;230(5):437-41.
5. Kuwabara T, Lessell S. Electron microscopic study of extraocular muscles in myotonic dystrophy. Am J Ophthalmol. 1976;82(2):303-9.
6. Mausolf FA, Burns CA, Burian HM. Morphologic and functional retinal changes in myotonic dystrophy unrelated to quinine therapy. Am J Ophthalmol. 1972;74(6):1141-3.
7. Meyer E, Navon D, Auslender L, et al. Myotonic dystrophy: pathological study of the eyes. Ophthalmologica. 1980;181(3-4):215-20.
8. Reardon W, MacMillan JC, Myring J, et al. Cataract and myotonic dystrophy: the role of molecular diagnosis. Br J Ophthalmol. 1993;77(9):579-83.
9. Rosa N, Lanza M, Borrelli M, et al. Low intraocular pressure resulting from ciliary body detachment in patients with myotonic dystrophy. Ophthalmology. 2011;118(2):260-4.

4R. MULTIPLE ENDOCRINE NEOPLASIA 2B OR 3 (MEN 2B OR 3)

General

Autosomal dominant inheritance; multiple endocrine neoplasia (MEN) type 3 has been separated from MEN2 because of low incidence of associated parathyroid disease in these cases; poor prognosis; several different point mutations in the RET protooncogene on chromosome 10 have been associated with the MEN type 2 syndromes.

Ocular

Prominent corneal nerves in clear stroma; diffuse, nodular thickening of eyelids; nasal displacement of lacrimal puncta; rostral displacement of eyelashes; eversion of eyelids; subconjunctival neuromas; thickened conjunctival nerves; decreased tear formation; prominent eyebrows; impaired pupillary dilation; thickened iris nerves; increased IOP (rare); localized orbital neurofibromas (orbit, conjunctiva); lesions of the tongue resembling neuromas.

Clinical

May be present at birth or develop later; 50% show complete syndrome of multiple neuromas (lips, tongue, eyelids), bumpy lips, pheochromocytoma, and medullary carcinoma; others exhibit variable combinations of the preceding, without the pheochromocytoma; diarrhea; Marfanoid habitus.

Laboratory

Genetic screening, biochemical screening, CT scanning or MRI.

Treatment

Surgery is the treatment of choice. Hormone replacement therapy after total thyroidectomy.

BIBLIOGRAPHY

1. Richards ML, Carter SM, Gross SJ. (2012). Type 2 multiple endocrine neoplasia. [online] Available from www.emedicine.com/med/TOPIC1520.HTM. [Accessed September, 2013].

🗗 4S. RING DERMOID SYNDROME (AMBLYOPIA)

General

Autosomal dominant; usually bilateral.

Ocular

Dermoid choristoma; conjunctival plaques of keratinization; corneal lipid deposition; irregular corneal astigmatism; amblyopia; concomitant strabismus.

Laboratory

Diagnosis is made by clinical findings.

Treatment

Strabismus—equalized vision with correct refractive error. Surgery may be helpful in patient with diplopia.

🗗 BIBLIOGRAPHY

1. Henkind P, Marinoff G, Manas A, et al. Bilateral corneal dermoids. Am J Ophthalmol. 1973;76(6):972-7.
2. Mattos J, Contreras F, O'Donnell FE, et al. Ring dermoid syndrome. A new syndrome of autosomal dominantly inherited, bilateral, annular limbal dermoids with corneal and conjunctival extension. Arch Ophthalmol. 1980;98(6):1059-61.
3. McKusick VA. Mendelian Inheritance in Man; A Catalog of Human Genes and Genetic Disorders, 12th edition. Baltimore: The Johns Hopkins University Press; 1998.
4. McKusick-Nathans Institute for Genetic Medicine, Johns Hopkins University and National Center for Biotechnology Information, National Library of Medicine (2007). Online Mendelian Inheritance in Man®, (OMIM®). [online] Available from www.ncbi.nlm.nih.gov/omim. [Accessed September, 2013].
5. Oakman JH, Lambert SR, Grossniklaus HE, et al. Corneal dermoid: case report and review of classification. J Pediatr Ophthalmol Strabismus. 1993;30(6):388-91.

🗗 4T. SCLEROCORNEA

General

Autosomal dominant; feature of cornea plana.

Ocular

Malformation of cornea; indistinct limits of cornea and sclera.

Clinical

It is found in a patient with monosomy 21; may be found in association with hypertelorism, syndactyly, ambiguous genitalia and epidermolysis bullosa dystrophica.

Laboratory

Diagnosis is made by clinical findings.

Treatment

Check for elevated IOP. Medical treatment includes the use of hyperosmotic drops, nonsteroidal and steroidal eye drops. Corneal transplant may be necessary.

🗗 BIBLIOGRAPHY

1. Bloch N. [The different types of sclerocornea, their hereditary modes and concomitant congenital malformations]. J Genet Hum. 1965;14(2):133-72.
2. Doane JF, Sajjadi H, Richardson WP. Bilateral penetrating keratoplasty for sclerocornea in an infant with monosomy 21. Case report and review of the literature. Cornea. 1994;13(5):454-8.
3. Martínez-Frías ML, Bermejo E, Sánchez Otero T, et al. Sclerocornea, hypertelorism, syndactyly, and ambiguous genitalia. Am J Med Genet. 1994;49(2):195-7.
4. McKusick VA. Mendelian Inheritance in Man; A Catalog of Human Genes and Genetic Disorders, 12th edition. Baltimore, USA: The Johns Hopkins University Press; 1998.
5. Hamosh A, Scott AF, Amberger J, et al. Online Mendelian Inheritance in Man (OMIM), a knowledge base of human genes and genetic disorders. Nucleic Acids Res. 2002;30(1):52-5.
6. Sharkey JA, Kervick GN, Jackson AJ, et al. Cornea plana and sclerocornea in association with recessive epidermolysis bullosa dystrophica. Case report. Cornea. 1992;11(1):83-5.

4U. SENTER SYNDROME (KERATITIS-ICHTHYOSIS-DEAFNESS SYNDROME; KID SYNDROME; ICHTHYOSIFORM ERYTHRODERMA, CORNEAL INVOLVEMENT, AND DEAFNESS (KERATITIS)

General

Autosomal recessive.

Ocular

Corneal involvement.

Clinical

Ichthyosiform erythroderma; deafness; hepatomegaly; hepatic cirrhosis; glycogen storage; short stature; mental retardation; hepatitis.

Laboratory

Diagnosis is made by clinical findings.

Treatment

Steroids or antibiotics may be useful.

BIBLIOGRAPHY

1. McKusick VA. Mendelian Inheritance in Man: A Catalog of Human Genes and Genetic Disorders, 12th edition. Baltimore, USA: The Johns Hopkins University Press; 1998.
2. Hamosh A, Scott AF, Amberger J, et al. Online Mendelian Inheritance in Man (OMIM), a knowledge base of human genes and genetic disorders. Nucleic Acids Res. 2002;30(1):52-5.
3. Senter TP, Jones KL, Sakati N, et al. Atypical ichthyosiform erythroderma and congenital neurosensory deafness a distinct syndrome. J Pediatr. 1978;92(1):68-72.
4. Wilson GN, Squires RH, Weinberg AG. Keratitis, hepatitis, ichthyosis, and deafness: report and review of KID syndrome. Am J Med Genet. 1991;40(3):255-9.

4V. SNAIL TRACKS OF CORNEA

This condition involves irregular, discontinuous grayish white streaks or patches, usually orientated horizontally and obliquely on the corneal endothelium.
1. Corneal buttons preserved in corneal storage medium
2. Following ocular surgery
3. Ocular trauma

BIBLIOGRAPHY

1. Alfonso E, Tucker GS, Batlle JF, et al. Snailtracks of the corneal endothelium. Ophthalmology. 1986;99:344-9.

4W. WEYERS SYNDROME (2) (WEYERS IV SYNDROME; LRIDODENTAL DYSPLASIA; DENTOIRIDEAL DYSPLASIA; DYSGENESIS IRIDODENTALIS; DYSGENESIS MESODERMALIS CORNEAE ET IRIDES WITH DIGODONTIA) CORNEAL OPACITY

General

Present from birth; hereditary; etiology unknown.

Ocular

Dysplasia; small perforation of iris; pupillary synechiae; microphthalmia; corneal opacity.

Clinical

Dwarfism; myotonic dystrophy; microdontia; oligodontia; hypoplasia of dental enamel.

Laboratory

Clinical.

Treatment

None.

BIBLIOGRAPHY

1. Magalini SI, Scrascia E. Dictionary of Medical Syndromes, 2nd edition. Philadelphia: JB Lippincott; 1981. p. 864.

2. Weyers H. Dysgenesis Irido-dentalis. Ein Neues Syndrome mit obweichdendem Chromosomalen Geschlecht bei Weiblichen Merkmalträgern. Presented at the Meeting of Deutsche Gessellschaft fuer Kinderheilkunde, Kassel, Germany: 1960.

4X. WHIPPLE DISEASE (INTESTINAL LIPODYSTROPHY) PAPILLEDEMA

General

Multisystem disorder; prominent in males; onset between 4th decade and 7th decade; etiology is unknown.

Ocular

Ophthalmoplegia (vertical gaze involved more than horizontal gaze); papilledema; intraocular inflammation; vitreous opacities; bilateral panuveitis; small, round grayish retinal lesions; chemosis; supranuclear ophthalmoplegia; myoclonic ocular jerks; pendular nystagmus.

Clinical

Pneumonia; pleurisy; tonsillitis; sinusitis; cystitis; arthritis; fever; leukocytosis; diarrhea; malabsorption; death; dyspnea; weight loss; lymphadenopathy; polyserositis; gray pigmentation of skin; dementia; facial jerks; rhythmic movement of the mouth, jaw, and extremities.

Laboratory

The following test may be useful to screen for the presence of malabsorption but they are not specific for the disease: Sudan strain of stool, serum carotene, serum albumin, prothrombin time and CT scan.

Treatment

Antibiotic therapy.

BIBLIOGRAPHY

1. Roberts IM. (2011). Whipple disease. [online] Available from www.emedicine.com/med/TOPIC2409.HTM. [Accessed September, 2013].

5. KERATITIS

5A. ACTINOMYCOSIS

General

Gram-positive *Actinomyces israelii*.

Ocular

Hypopyon; conjunctivitis; keratitis; corneal ulcer; proptosis; uveitis; dacryocystitis; yellow nodules on conjunctiva and eyelids; occlusion of nasolacrimal canaliculi; canaliculitis; orbital abscess; endophthalmitis (rare).

Clinical

Chronic inflammatory induration and sinus formation.

Laboratory

Canalicular discharge may be sent for Gram stain/Giemsa stain, cultures and sensitivities (i.e. blood agar, Sabouraud, anaerobic) and special stains (i.e. calcofluor white stain).

Treatment

Penicillins and cephalosporins are useful. Subconjunctival penicillin coadministered with systemic iodides and topical sulfacetamide or penicillin can be used.

BIBLIOGRAPHY

1. Roque MR, Roque BL, Foster CS. (2012). Actinomycosis in ophthalmology. [online] Available from www.emedicine.com/oph/TOPIC491.HTM. [Accessed September, 2013].

⊟ 5B. CORNEAL ULCER (BACTERIAL CORNEAL ULCERS, BACTERIAL KERATITIS)

General

Rapid progression with corneal destruction within 48 hours. Predisposing factors include contact lens wearers, trauma, contaminated ocular medications.

Clinical

None.

Ocular

Corneal ulceration, stromal abscess formation and anterior segment inflammation.

Laboratory

Chocolate agar plate, Gram's stain, blood agar plate, brain-heart infusion broth, meat-glucose broth, Giemsa stain, Sabouraud's dextrose agar (fungus).

Treatment

Fluoroquinolone.

⊟ BIBLIOGRAPHY

1. Murillo-Lopez FH. (2012). Bacterial keratitis. [online] Available from www.emedicine.com/oph/TOPIC98.HTM. [Accessed September, 2013].

⊟ 5C. CENTRAL STERILE CORNEAL ULCERATION

General

Either infectious or sterile, this inflammatory condition is associated with the disruption of the epithelial layer involving the stroma.

Clinical

Herpes simplex virus, herpes zoster virus, Sjögren syndrome, facial palsy, vitamin A deficiency, Wegener's granulomatosis, rheumatoid arthritis (RA).

Ocular

Corneal scarring, neovascularization, blindness, and corneal perforation. Herpes, contact lens use, lagophthalmos, sicca.

Treatment

It is important to first exclude infectious etiologies. Antibiotics, preservative-free (PF) artificial tears; for chemical burs prednisone is useful; oral tetracycline can be used in combination of topical tetracycline.

Laboratory

Corneal smears and cultures, corneal scraping, complete workup to rule out infectious or systemic inflammatory disease.

⊟ BIBLIOGRAPHY

1. Farooqui SZ, Foster CS, Ma JJ. (2011). Central sterile corneal ulceration. [online] Available from emedicine.medscape.com/article/1196936-overview. [Accessed September, 2013].

⊟ 5D. CORNEAL OPACITY-DIFFUSE

†1. Acromesomelic dysplasia
†*2. Birth trauma
3. Cockayne syndrome
†*4. Congenital hereditary endothelial dystrophy
†5. Congenital hereditary stromal dystrophy
6. Cystinosis
†7. Fabry syndrome
8. Fetal rubella effects
9. GM gangliosidosis type 1
10. Hurler syndrome
†11. Infection
12. Maroteaux-Lamy syndrome
13. Morquio syndrome
14. Mucolipidosis III
15. Mucolipidosis IV
16. Multiple sulfatase deficiency

17. MPS VII
18. Pachyonychia congenita syndrome
19. Pena-Shokeir type II syndrome [cerebrooculofacial-skeletal (COFS) syndrome]
20. Rutherford syndrome
21. Scheie syndrome
*22. Sclerocornea
23. Seip syndrome
24. Sialidosis, Goldberg type

†25. Trisomy syndrome
†26. 18q syndrome

BIBLIOGRAPHY

1. Isenberg SJ. The Eye in Infancy. Chicago: Year Book Medical; 1989.

†Indicates a general entry and therefore has not been described in detail in the text

5D3. COCKAYNE SYNDROME (DWARFISM WITH RETINAL ATROPHY AND DEAFNESS; MICKEY MOUSE SYNDROME)

General

Autosomal recessive; onset in second year of life; wide spectrum of symptoms and severity of the disease suggest that biochemical and genetic heterogeneity exist.

Ocular

Enophthalmos; cataracts; pigmentary degeneration of retina; optic atrophy; band keratopathy; exotropia; nystagmus; absence of foveal reflex; corneal dystrophy; corneal perforation; anhidrosis; exposure keratitis; decreased blinking.

Clinical

Dwarfism (nanism) with disproportionately long limbs, large hands, and large feet; kyphosis; deformed limbs; thickened skull; intracranial calcifications; mental retardation; prognathism; deafness (often partial); precociously senile appearance; sensitivity to sunlight, with skin pigmentation and scarring; dental caries.

Laboratory

Brain CT scan may reveal calcifications and cortical atrophy.

Treatment

Photoprotection with sunscreens and clothing are useful. Cochlear implantation can help minimize the effects of auditory impairment.

BIBLIOGRAPHY

1. Imaeda S. (2012). Cockayne syndrome. [online] Available from www.emedicine.com/derm/TOPIC717.HTM. [Accessed September, 2013]

5D6. LIGNAC-FANCONI SYNDROME (FANCONI-LIGNAC SYNDROME; CYSTINOSIS SYNDROME; CYSTINE STORAGE-AMINOACIDURIA-DWARFISM SYNDROME; RENAL RICKETS; NEPHROPATHIC CYSTINOSIS)

General

Autosomal recessively inherited storage disorder in which nonprotein cystine accumulates within cellular lysosomes; occurs primarily in children; prognosis in children with renal tubular insufficiency and dwarfism poor, with survival past age 10 years rare without renal transplant.

Ocular

Cystine crystals located in conjunctiva, cornea, sclera, iris, ciliary body, lens, and perhaps choroid; general clouding of cornea caused by dense deposition of cystine crystals; pupillary block glaucoma; photophobia; band keratopathy; posterior synechiae with thickened stroma of iris; decreased visual function; patchy retinopathy; visual field constriction.

Clinical

Fanconi syndrome with rickets; dwarfism; glomerular dystrophy; renal failure; oral motor dysfunction.

Laboratory

The diagnosis is made based on tests that document the excessive loss of substances in the urine (e.g. amino acids, glucose, phosphate, bicarbonate) in the absence of high plasma concentrations.

Treatment

Replacement of substances lost in the urine. Liver transplantation is sometimes necessary.

BIBLIOGRAPHY

1. Fathallah-Shaykh S, Spitzer A. (2013). Fanconi syndrome. [online] Available from www.emedicine.com/ped/TOPIC756.HTM. [Accessed September, 2013].

5D8. RUBELLA SYNDROME (CONGENITAL RUBELLA SYNDROME; GERMAN MEASLES; GREGG SYNDROME)

General

Rubella infection of the mother during first trimester of pregnancy; ocular disease is the most commonly found abnormality in patients with congenital rubella syndrome (75%), multiorgan disease is common (greater than 75%); no significant association has been found between gestational age and time of maternal infection and incidence of individual ocular conditions.

Ocular

Nystagmus; glaucoma; corneal haziness; cataracts; retinal pigmentary changes; appearance and central distribution of lesions are quite distinguishable from retinitis pigmentosa; retinopathy is not progressive and has little, if any, effect on vision; waxy atrophy of optic disk; conjunctivitis; megalocornea or microcornea; buphthalmos; microphthalmos; uveitis; iris atrophy; spherophakia; strabismus.

Clinical

Low-birth weight; diarrhea; pneumonia; urinary infection; hearing loss; heart disease; hepatosplenomegaly; mental retardation; inguinal hernias; ataxia; cardiac abnormalities.

Laboratory

Diagnosis is made by clinical findings. If in doubt, a rising titer of immunoglobulin M will indicate a recent infection.

Treatment

Treatment for rubella of the eye centers on glaucoma and cataract.

BIBLIOGRAPHY

1. Lombardo PC. (2011). Dermatologic manifestations of rubella. [online] Available from www.emedicine.com/derm/TOPIC380.HTM. [Accessed September, 2013].

5D9. GANGLIOSIDOSIS GMI TYPE 1 [GENERALIZED GANGLIOSIDOSIS (INFANTILE); NORMAN-LANDING SYNDROME; PSEUDO-HURLER LIPOIDOSIS]

General

Absence of A, B, and C isoenzymes of β-galactosidase visceral tissue and mucopolysaccharides in visceral tissues; both sexes affected; autosomal recessive; onset from birth; death from age 6 months to 2 years; defect has been localized to chromosome 3 (3p12-3p13).

Ocular

Macular cherry-red spots; optic disk pallor; nystagmus; esotropia; corneal clouding; retinal artery tortuosity and narrowing; retinitis pigmentosa; macular cherry-red spot found in 50% of patients with this disorder.

Clinical

Cerebral degeneration combined with visceromegaly and skeletal dysplasia; mental and motor retardation; seizures; deafness; spastic quadriplegia; feeding difficulties; recurrent bronchopneumonia; broad nose; frontal bossing; prominent maxilla; hepatosplenomegaly.

Laboratory

Diagnosis is dependent upon demonstration of specific enzymatic deficiency in peripheral blood leukocytes or cultured fibroblasts.

Treatment

Treatment primarily is directed at symptomatic relief.

BIBLIOGRAPHY

1. Ierardi-Curto L. (2013). Lipid storage disorders. [online] Available from www.emedicine.com/ped/TOPIC1310. HTM. [Accessed September, 2013].

5D10. HURLER SYNDROME (PFAUNDLER-HURLER SYNDROME; GARGOYLISM; DYSOSTOSIS MULTIPLEX; MPS IH SYNDROME; SYSTEMIC MUCOPOLYSACCHARIDOSIS TYPE IH; MUCOPOLYSACCHARIDOSIS IH)

General

Autosomal recessive inheritance; in addition to corneal opacities and enlargement of the head at birth, other symptoms become apparent at the end of the 1st year; death occurs usually before 20 years; gross excess of chondroitin sulfate band, heparitin sulfate in the urine (*see* Hunter Syndrome; Sanfilippo-Good Syndrome; Morquio-Brailsford Syndrome; Scheie Syndrome; Maroteaux-Lamy Syndrome). Jensen suggested that the pathogenesis of the various mucopolysaccharidoses is the same but that the variations in the defective enzymes cause the different types; most common mucopolysaccharidosis (MPS), decreased iduronidase.

Ocular

Proptosis; hypertelorism; thick, enlarged lids; esotropia; diffuse haziness of the cornea at birth progressive to milky opacity; retinal pigmentary changes may exist; macular edema and absence of foveal reflex; optic atrophy; megalocornea; bushy eyebrows; coarse eyelashes; mucopolysaccharide deposits of iris, lens, and sclera; enlarged optic foramen; retinal detachment; anisocoria; buphthalmos; nystagmus; secondary open-angle glaucoma; progressive retinopathy with vascular narrowing; hyperpigmentation of the fundus; bone spicule; papilledema.

Clinical

Dorsolumbar kyphosis; head deformities with depressed nose bridge; short cervical spine; short limbs; macroglossia; enlarged liver and spleen; short stature; facial dysmorphism; progressive psychomotor retardation.

Laboratory

Blood smears-abnormal cytoplasmic inclusions in lymphocytes; urine: increased excretion of dermatan sulfate and heparin sulfate.

Treatment

- *Macular edema*: Use of corticosteroids, carbonic anhydrase inhibitors and NSAIDs are the mainstay of treatment. If traditional therapy is not effective, intraocular injections of Avastin® may be helpful. In cases that have vitreous strand tugging against the macula, pars plana vitrectomy may be necessary.
- *Retinal detachment*: Scleral buckle, pneumatic retinopexy and vitrectomy may be used to close all the breaks.
- *Glaucoma*: Glaucoma medication should be the first plan of action. If medication is unsuccessful, a filtering surgical procedure with or without antimetabolites may be beneficial.
- *Papilledema*: Underlying cause should be determined and treated. Systemic acetazolamide is the medical therapy of choice.

BIBLIOGRAPHY

1. Banikazemi M. (2012). Genetics of mucopolysaccharidosis type I. [online] Available from www.emedicine.com/ped/TOPIC1031.HTM. [Accessed July, 2013].

5D12. MAROTEAUX-LAMY SYNDROME (SYSTEMIC MUCOPOLYSACCHARIDOSIS TYPE VI; MPS VI SYNDROME; MUCOPOLYSACCHARIDOSIS VI)

General

Onset in infancy; etiology unknown; autosomal recessive; excessive urinary excretion of chondroitin sulfate B; lysosomal storage disease; deficiency of the enzyme arylsulfatase B; multiple clinical phenotypes.

Ocular

Corneal haziness and opacities; pupillary membrane remnants.

Clinical

Skeleton deformities; restriction of articular movements; dyspnea; heart murmur; hearing impairment.

Laboratory

Urine-excessive glycosaminoglycan—dermatan sulfate or chondroitin sulfate B.

Treatment

Enzyme replacement, bone marrow transplant and stem cell therapy is in the experimental stage.

BIBLIOGRAPHY

1. Roy FH, Fraunfelder FT, Fraunfelder FW. Roy and Fraunfelder's Current Ocular Therapy, 6th edition. Philadelphia, PA: WB Saunders; 2008.
2. Kenyon KR, Topping TM, Green WR, et al. Ocular pathology of the Maroteaux-Lamy syndrome (systemic mucopolysaccharidosis type VI). Histologic and ultrastructural report of two cases. Am J Ophthalmol. 1972;73(5):718-41.
3. Matalon R, Arbogast B, Dorfman A. Deficiency of chondroitin sulfate N-acetylgalactosamine 4-sulfate sulfatase in Maroteaux-Lamy syndrome. Biochem Biophys Res Commun. 1974;61(4):1450-7.
4. Quigley HA, Kenyon KR. Ultrastructural and histochemical studies of a newly recognized form of systemic mucopolysaccharidosis. (Maroteaux-Lamy syndrome, mild phenotype). Am J Ophthalmol. 1974;77(6):809-18.
5. Voskoboeva E, Isbrandt D, von Figura K, et al. Four novel mutant alleles of the arylsulfatase B gene in two patients with intermediate form of mucopolysaccharidosis VI (Maroteaux-Lamy syndrome). Hum Genet. 1994;93(3):259-64.

5D13. MORQUIO SYNDROME (MORQUIO-BRAILSFORD SYNDROME; BRAILSFORD-MORQUIO DYSTROPHY; FAMILIAL OSSEOUS DYSTROPHY; KERATOSULFATURIA; MPS IV; MUCOPOLYSACCHARIDOSIS IV; SPONDYLOEPIPHYSEAL DYSPLASIA; OSTEOCHONDRODYSTROPHIA DEFORMANS; INFANTILE HEREDITARY CHONDRODYSPLASIA; HEREDITARY POLY TOPIC ENCHONDRAL DYSOSTOSIS; HEREDITARY OSTEOCHONDRODYSTROPHY; ECCENTRO-OSTEOCHONDRODYSPLASIA; DYSOSTOSIS ENCHONDRALIS META-EPIPHYSARIA; MORQUIO-ULLRICH SYNDROME; ATYPICAL CHONDRODYSTROPHY; CHONDRODYSTROPHIA TARDA; CHONDRO-OSTEODYSTROPHY)

General

Autosomal recessive dystrophy of cartilage and bone; slight predilection for males; apparent between ages 4 and 10 years; excess production of keratosulfate (*see* Hurler Syndrome; Hunter Syndrome; Sanfilippo-Good Syndrome; Scheie Syndrome; Maroteaux-Lamy Syndrome); autosomal recessive; abnormal N-acetylgalactosamine-G-sulfate sulfatase.

Ocular

Enophthalmos; ptosis; excessive tear secretion; ocular hypotony; miosis; occasionally hazy cornea; bushy eyebrows; optic nerve atrophy; moderate-to-late corneal clouding.

Clinical

Dwarfism; skeletal deformities (progressive); delayed ossification of epiphyses; decreased muscle tone; deafness; weak extremities; waddling gait; coarse broad mouth; spaced teeth; aortic regurgitation; normal intelligence.

Laboratory

Blood-Reilly's granules in leukocytes; X-ray—flat vertebrae and odontoid hypoplasia.

Treatment

Treatment is limited to supportive care.

BIBLIOGRAPHY

1. Bittar T, Washington ER. (2012). Mucopolysaccharidosis. [online] Available from www.emedicine.com/orthoped/TOPIC203.HTM. [Accessed September, 2013].

5D14. ML III (PSEUDO-HURLER POLYDYSTROPHY; MUCOLIPIDOSIS III)

General

Autosomal recessive disorder, almost indistinguishable biochemically from mucolipidosis II; decreased levels of N-acetylglucosamine phosphotransferase.

Ocular

Increased corneal thickness; wrinkled maculopathy; granular pigmentary changes of fundus; papilledema; hyperopic astigmatism; corneal opacities; retinal vascular tortuosity; visual field defects.

Clinical

Joint stiffness; coarse facial feature; short stature; aortic valve disease; arm and hand deformities; self-mutilation of the distal phalanges; carpal tunnel syndrome.

Laboratory

Clinical.

Treatment

- *Corneal opacities*: Medical treatment includes the use of hyperosmotic drops, nonsteroidal and steroid eye drops. Corneal transplant may be necessary.
- *Papilledema*: Underlying cause should be determined and treated. Systemic acetazolamide is the medical therapy of choice.

BIBLIOGRAPHY

1. Duane TD. Clinical Ophthalmology. Philadelphia: JB Lippincott; 1987.
2. Zammarchi E, Savelli A, Donati MA, et al. Self-mutilation in a patient with mucolipidosis III. Pediatr Neurol. 1994;11:68-70.

5D15. ML IV (MUCOLIPIDOSIS IV; BERMAN SYNDROME)

General

Storage disease in which corneal clouding is an early sign with no evidence of systemic involvement until age of 1 year; autosomal recessive; cases seen in Ashkenazi Jews; abnormal neuraminidase.

Ocular

Corneal clouding; corneal opacities; epithelial edema; retinal atrophy; pale optic nerve; diffuse corneal clouding present at birth or in early infancy.

Clinical

Progressive psychomotor retardation; skeletal dysplasia; facial anomalies.

Laboratory

Clinical.

Treatment

- *Corneal opacities*: Medical treatment includes the use of hyperosmotic drops, nonsteroidal and steroid eye drops. Corneal transplant may be necessary.

BIBLIOGRAPHY

1. Roy H. (2013). Xanthelasma. [online] Available from www.emedicine.com/oph/TOPIC610.HTM. [Accessed September, 2013].

5D16. ARYLSULFATASE A DEFICIENCY (METACHROMATIC LEUKODYSTROPHY; SULFATIDE LIPOIDOSIS SYNDROME; GREENFIELD DISEASE; SCHOLZ SYNDROME; SCHOLZ-BIELSCHOWSKY-HENNEBERG SYNDROME; VAN BOGAERT-NYSSEN DISEASE; VAN BOGAERT-NYSSEN-PEIFFER DISEASE; FAMILIAL PROGRESSIVE CEREBRAL SCLEROSIS; INFANTILE PROGRESSIVE CEREBRAL SCLEROSIS; INFANTILE METACHROMATIC LEUKODYSTROPHY; LEUKODYSTROPHIA CEREBRI PROGRESSIVA METACHROMATICA DIFFUSA; OPTICOCHLEODENTATE DEGENERATION)

General

Accumulation of sulfatide caused by deficient activity of arylsulfatase A; autosomal recessive; familial form of metachromatic leukodystrophy; Greenfield disease (late infantile form); van Bogaert-Nyssen-Peiffer syndrome (adult form); affects central and peripheral nervous systems by demyelination and by accumulation of metachromatic material.

Ocular

Visual loss in association with optic atrophy; strabismus; macular cherry-red spot; corneal opacification; oculomotor disorders (nystagmus, strabismus); optic nerve and retinal demyelination.

Clinical

Motor and mental deterioration with spasticity; paralysis; seizures; dementia; death in early childhood, although attenuated and adult forms of the disease occur; schizophrenia; temporo-occipital demyelination; unreactive to visual and auditory stimuli; adult form: moodiness, withdrawal, megalomania, hallucinations, violent reactions, and dementia.

Laboratory

Arylsulfatase A enzyme activity may be decreased in leukocytes or in cultured skin fibroblasts. Brain MRI may identify white matter lesions and atrophy.

Treatment

There is no effective treatment to reverse the deterioration and loss of function. Bone marrow or cord blood transplantation may be useful in individuals with asymptomatic late infantile and early juvenile forms of the disease.

BIBLIOGRAPHY

1. Ikeda AK, Moore T, Steiner RD. (2012). Metachromatic leukodystrophy. [online] Available from www.emedicine.com/ped/TOPIC2893.HTM. [Accessed September, 2013].

5D17. BETA-GLUCURONIDASE DEFICIENCY (MUCOPOLYSACCHARIDOSIS VII; MPS VII)

General

Autosomal recessive disorder associated with enzyme deficiency of β-glucuronidase; disorder combines clinical and biochemical features of the Morquio and Sanfilippo syndromes.

Ocular

Clouding of the cornea.

Clinical

Dwarfism; hepatosplenomegaly; skeletal deformity; mental retardation; hernias; unusual facies; delayed psychomotor development; frequent symptomatic pulmonary infections.

Laboratory

Urine-elevated glycosaminoglycans and oligosaccharides; blood-vacuoles in lymphocytes and fibroblasts. Metachromatic granular inclusions (Alder bodies) in leukocytes.

Treatment

No treatment is available for the underlying disorder, and care must be supportive.

BIBLIOGRAPHY

1. Banikazemi M, Varma S. (2011). Genetics of mucopolysaccharidosis type VII. [online] Available from www.emedicine.com/ped/TOPIC858.HTM. [Accessed September, 2013].

⊞ 5D18. JADASSOHN-LEWANDOWSKY SYNDROME (PACHYONYCHIA CONGENITA)

General

Autosomal dominant inheritance; three variants: type I has symmetric keratoses of hands and feet and follicular keratosis of body; type II same as type I, plus leukokeratosis; type III same as type I with corneal changes; gene for this disorder has been found to be closely linked to the keratin gene cluster on 17q12-q21; disorder usually develops in early infancy.

Ocular

Dyskeratosis of the cornea; bilateral cataract.

Clinical

Keratosis and hyperhidrosis of palms and soles, whereas the remaining skin is usually rather dry; bullous lesions may occur with secondary infections, mainly during warm seasons; leukokeratosis of oral mucosa (mainly tongue); follicular keratosis; congenital pachyonychia (nails not only may be thickened but also may be frequently inflamed and lost with aggravation at sites of regrowth); hoarse voice; epidermoid cysts; oral leukokeratosis.

Laboratory

Electron microscopy can be performed by using plantar or palmar skin samples. Electron microscopy shows thickened and clumped intermediate filaments, as well as enlarged keratohyaline granules.

Treatment

The thickened nail plate can be softened by using 20% salicylic acid ointment or 20–40% urea and 10% salicylic acid in an emulsifying ointment with occlusive dressings. The affected nails can be removed under local or general anesthesia; however, unless the nail matrix is partially removed, nails regrow.

⊞ BIBLIOGRAPHY

1. George SJ. (2012). Pachyonychia congenital. [online] Available from www.emedicine.com/derm/TOPIC812.HTM. [Accessed September, 2013].

⊞ 5D19. CEREBRO-OCULO-FACIO-SKELETAL SYNDROME (COFS SYNDROME)

General

Inherited as autosomal recessive disorder; death within the first 3 years of life; feeding difficulties secondary to incoordination of the swallowing mechanism.

Ocular

Microphthalmia; blepharophimosis; cataracts.

Clinical

Microcephaly; hypotonia; prominent nasal root; large ear pinnae; flexion contractures at elbows and knees; camptodactylia; osteoporosis; kyphosis; scoliosis; congenital muscular dystrophy.

Laboratory

Clinical.

Treatment

Change in glasses can sometimes improve a patient's visual function temporarily; however the most common treatment is cataract surgery.

⊞ BIBLIOGRAPHY

1. Geeraets WJ. Ocular Syndromes, 3rd edition. Philadelphia: Lea & Febiger; 1976.
2. Gershoni-Baruch R, Ludatscher RM, Lichtig C, et al. Cerebrooculo-facio-skeletal syndrome: further delineation. Am J Med Genet. 1991;41:74-7.

3. Lowry RB, MacLean R, McLean DM, et al. Cataracts, microcephaly, kyphosis and limited joint movement in two siblings. A new syndrome. J Pediatr. 1971;79:282.
4. McKusick VA. Mendelian Inheritance in Man; A Catalog of Human Genes and Genetic Disorders, 12th edition. Baltimore: The Johns Hopkins University Press; 1998.
5. Online Mendelian Inheritance in Man, OMIM. McKusick-Nathans Institute for Genetic Medicine, Johns Hopkins University and National Center for Biotechnology Information, National Library of Medicine, February 12, 2007. Available from www.ncbi.nlm.nih.gov/omim. [Accessed September, 2013].
6. Pena SD, Shokeir MK. Autosomal recessive cerebro-oculo-facio-skeletal (COFS) syndrome. Clin Genet. 1974;5:285.

5D20. OCULODENTAL SYNDROME (PETERS SYNDROME; RUTHERFORD SYNDROME)

General

Similar to Rieger syndrome and Meyer-Schwickerath-Weyer syndrome; Peters syndrome inherited as autosomal recessive with defect of corneogenetic mesoderm characterized by incomplete separation of lens vesicle, causing central opacities of cornea, shallow anterior chamber, synechiae, and remnants of pupillary membrane; anterior pole cataract; Rutherford syndrome inherited as autosomal dominant; exhibits iris and dental anomalies and mental retardation.

Ocular

High myopia; corneoscleral staphyloma; aniridia; macrocornea; opacities of the corneal margin; ectopia lentis with deposits of pigment; macular pigmentation; large excavation of optic nerve with atrophy.

Clinical

Oligodontia; microdontia; hypoplasia of enamel; abnormal tooth positions; hypertrophy of gums; failure of tooth eruption.

Treatment

See oral health specialist.

BIBLIOGRAPHY

1. Houston IB. Rutherford's syndrome. A familial oculo-dental disorder and electrophysiological study. Acta Paediatr Scand. 1966;55:233-8.
2. McKusick VA. Mendelian Inheritance in Man; A Catalog of Human Genes and Genetic Disorders, 12th edition. Baltimore: The Johns Hopkins University Press; 1998.

5D21. SCHEIE SYNDROME (MUCOPOLYSACCHARIDOSIS IS; MPS IS; MPS V; MUCOPOLYSACCHARIDOSIS V

General

Autosomal recessive; chondroitin sulfate B excreted in excess in the urine; formerly MPS V (*see* Hurler Syndrome; Hunter Syndrome; Sanfilippo-Good Syndrome; Morquio Syndrome; Maroteaux-Lamy Syndrome). Both sexes affected; deficiency of a-L-iduronidase; increased urinary dermatan and heparan sulfate; fibrous long-spacing collagen on histopathologic examination; least severe form of MPS.

Ocular

Night blindness; fields may show general constriction; ring scotoma; diffuse corneal haze to marked corneal clouding (progressive); bushy eyebrows; coarse eyelashes; optic atrophy; anisocoria; cataracts; proptosis; acid mucopolysaccharide deposits in the iris and sclera; tapetoretinal degeneration; glaucoma.

Clinical

Normal intelligence; broad facies; thickened joints; aortic valvular disease; psychosis; claw hand; carpal tunnel syndrome; excessive body hair; progressive juxta-articular cystic lesions.

Laboratory

Thin layer chromatography and radiography.

Treatment

Enzyme replacement therapy—patients with joint contractures may need surgery. Corneal transplant may be necessary if vision problems are severe.

🗗 BIBLIOGRAPHY

1. Banikazemi M. (2012). Genetics of mucopolysaccharidosis type I. [online] Available from www.emedicine.com/ped/TOPIC2052.HTM. [Accessed September, 2013].

🗗 5D22. SCLEROCORNEA

General

Autosomal dominant; feature of cornea plana.

Ocular

Malformation of cornea; indistinct limits of cornea and sclera.

Clinical

It is found in a patient with monosomy 21; may be found in association with hypertelorism, syndactyly, ambiguous genitalia and epidermolysis bullosa dystrophica.

Laboratory

Diagnosis is made by clinical findings.

Treatment

Check for elevated IOP. Medical treatment includes the use of hyperosmotic drops, nonsteroidal and steroidal eye drops. Corneal transplant may be necessary.

🗗 BIBLIOGRAPHY

1. Bloch N. [The different types of sclerocornea, their hereditary modes and concomitant congenital malformations]. J Genet Hum. 1965;14(2):133-72.
2. Doane JF, Sajjadi H, Richardson WP. Bilateral penetrating keratoplasty for sclerocornea in an infant with monosomy 21. Case report and review of the literature. Cornea. 1994;13(5):454-8.

🗗 5D23. BERARDINELLI-SEIP SYNDROME (CONGENITAL GENERALIZED LIPODYSTROPHY)

General

Autosomal recessive; disorder of the hypothalamus.

Ocular

Punctate corneal infiltrations (lipodystrophia corneae).

Clinical

Advanced bone age; dilation of the third ventricle and basal cistern; frequent elevation of growth hormone; severe lipid levels; enlarged liver; diabetes mellitus; hyperpigmentation of axillae and chest wall; phlebomegaly.

Laboratory

Radiographic features include advanced skeletal age, bone cysts, and dilated cerebral ventricles and basal cisterns on pneumoencephalography.

Treatment

Leptin, an adipocyte hormone, which may improve insulin resistance, hyperglycemia, dyslipidemia, and hepatic steatosis may be useful. Surgical intervention may be helpful for patients with deformities.

🗗 BIBLIOGRAPHY

1. Janniger CK, Jagar C. (2012). Dermatologic manifestations of generalized lipodystrophy. [online] Available from www.emedicine.com/derm/TOPIC688.HTM. [Accessed September, 2013].

5D24. GOLDBERG DISEASE

General

Unclassified syndrome with features of mucopolysaccharidoses, sphingolipidoses, and mucolipidoses; deficiency of neuraminidase; located in chromosome 20q 13.1.

Ocular

Macular cherry-red spot; corneal clouding; cerebromacular degeneration.

Clinical

Dwarfism; Gargoyle facies; mental retardation; seizures; hearing disorder.

Laboratory

Diagnosis is made by clinical findings.

Treatment

For patients with bilateral and visually disabling corneal opacity, PK is recommended.

BIBLIOGRAPHY

1. Scheinfeld NS, Freilich BD, Freilich J. (2013). Congenital clouding of the cornea. [online] Available from www.emedicine.com/oph/TOPIC771.HTM. [Accessed September, 2013].
2. Banikazemi M. (2012). Genetics of mucopolysaccharidosis type I. [online] Available from www.emedicine.com/ped/TOPIC2052.HTM. [Accessed September, 2013].

5E. CORNEAL OPACITY-LOCALIZED, CONGENITAL

1. Acromegaloid changes, cutis verticis gyrata, and corneal leukoma
†2. Aniridia
†3. Autosomal dominant colomba
4. Cataract microcornea syndrome
†*5. Dermoid limbal, central, and ring
6. Fetal alcohol syndrome
7. Fetal rubella effects
†8. Fetal transfusion syndrome
†9. Fucosidosis
†10. Group 13-trisomy phenotype
11. Keratoconus posticus circumscriptus
12. Meesman syndrome
13. Peters anomaly and short stature
14. Pillay syndrome(ophthalmomandibulomelic dysplasia)
15. Radial aplasia, anterior chamber cleavage syndrome
16. Richner-Hanhart syndrome
17. Rieger syndrome
†18. Trisomy syndrome
19. Waardenburg syndrome
†20. Wedge-shaped stromal opacity
†21. 4p syndrome
22. 11q syndrome
23. 18q syndrome

BIBLIOGRAPHY

1. Isenberg SJ. The Eye in Infancy. Chicago: Year Book Medical; 1989.
2. Roy FH. Ocular Syndromes and Systemic Diseases, 4th edition. New Delhi: Jaypee Brothers Medical Publishers; 2013.

†Indicates a general entry and therefore has not been described in detail in the text

5E1. ACL SYNDROME (ACROMEGALOID, CUTIS VERTICIS GYRATA, CORNEAL LEUKOMA SYNDROME)

General

Autosomal dominant; rare; three features include (1) cutis verticis, (2) associated with acromegaly and (3) corneal leukoma; onset by age of 1 year.

Ocular

Bilateral corneal leukoma; keratitis.

Clinical

Unusually tall; large hands, feet, and chin; skin of hands very soft; skin of scalp lies in folds; frontal bosses; ear calcification; pituitary tumors; abnormal dermal ridge patterns; enlargement of supraorbital arch of frontal bone.

Laboratory

aCL antibodies react primarily to membrane phospho-lipids, such as cardiolipin and phosphatidylserine. Of the three known isotypes of aCL (i.e. IgG, IgM, IgA). IgG correlates most strongly with thrombotic events.

Treatment

For patients with bilateral and visually disabling corneal opacity, PK is recommended.

BIBLIOGRAPHY

1. Belilos E, Carsons S. (2012). Antiphospholipid syndrome. [online] Available from www.emedicine.com/med/TOP-IC2923.HTM. [Accessed September, 2013].
2. Scheinfeld NS, Freilich BD, Freilich J. (2013). Congenital clouding of the cornea. [online] Available from www.emedicine.com/oph/TOPIC771.HTM. [Accessed September, 2013].

5E4. CATARACT, MICROCORNEA SYNDROME

General

Autosomal dominant; prominent in Sicilian families.

Ocular

Cataracts; microcornea; myopia.

Clinical

None.

Laboratory

Diagnosis is made by clinical findings.

Treatment

Cataract surgery if vision decreases.

BIBLIOGRAPHY

1. McKusick VA. Mendelian Inheritance in Man; A Catalog of Human Genes and Genetic Disorders, 12th edition. Baltimore, USA: The Johns Hopkins University Press; 1998.
2. Hamosh A, Scott AF, Amberger J, et al. Online Mendelian Inheritance in Man (OMIM), a knowledge base of human genes and genetic disorders. Nucleic Acids Res. 2002;30(1):52-5.
3. Mollica F, Li Volti S, Tomarchio S, et al. Autosomal dominant cataract and microcornea associated with myopia in a Sicilian family. Clin Genet. 1985;28(1):42-6.
4. Polomeno RC, Cummings C. Autosomal dominant cataracts and microcornea. Can J Ophthalmol. 1979;14(4):227-9.

5E6. FETAL ALCOHOL SYNDROME

General

Dysgenesis in children born to alcoholic mothers; both sexes affected; onset from birth.

Ocular

Antimongoloid slant of lid fissures; lateral displacement of inner canthi; ptosis; epicanthi; strabismus; myopia; optic nerve hypoplasia; diffuse corneal clouding; iridocorneal abnormalities with central corneal edema; lens opacification; motility disorders.

Clinical

Growth retardation; delayed development (physical and intellectual); maxillary hypoplasia; micrognathia; large, low-set ears; abnormal motor function; irritability; microcephaly; cerebral nervous system dysfunctions; abnormal philtrum; flattened nasal bridge; cardiovascular defects; thin upper lip.

Laboratory

If suspected, consult a subspecialist (e.g. geneticist, developmentalist) to confirm the diagnosis.

Treatment

Treat for associated birth defects and intervention for potential cognitive and behavioral abnormalities. Vitrectomy may be necessary.

BIBLIOGRAPHY

1. Vaux KK, Chambers C. (2012). Fetal alcohol syndrome. [online] Available from www.emedicine.com/ped/TOP-IC767.HTM. [Accessed September, 2013].

5E7. RUBELLA SYNDROME (CONGENITAL RUBELLA SYNDROME; GERMAN MEASLES; GREGG SYNDROME)

General

Rubella infection of the mother during first trimester of pregnancy; ocular disease is the most commonly found abnormality in patients with congenital rubella syndrome (75%), multiorgan disease is common (greater than 75%); no significant association has been found between gestational age and time of maternal infection and incidence of individual ocular conditions.

Ocular

Nystagmus; glaucoma; corneal haziness; cataracts; retinal pigmentary changes; appearance and central distribution of lesions are quite distinguishable from retinitis pigmentosa; retinopathy is not progressive and has little, if any, effect on vision; waxy atrophy of optic disk; conjunctivitis; megalocornea or microcornea; buphthalmos; microphthalmos; uveitis; iris atrophy; spherophakia; strabismus.

Clinical

Low-birth weight; diarrhea; pneumonia; urinary infection; hearing loss; heart disease; hepatosplenomegaly; mental retardation; inguinal hernias; ataxia; cardiac abnormalities.

Laboratory

Diagnosis is made by clinical findings. If in doubt, a rising titer of immunoglobulin M will indicate a recent infection.

Treatment

Treatment for rubella of the eye centers on glaucoma and cataract.

BIBLIOGRAPHY

1. Lombardo PC. (2011). Dermatologic manifestations of rubella. [online] Available from www.emedicine.com/derm/TOPIC380.HTM. [Accessed September, 2013].

5E11. KERATOCONUS POSTICUS CIRCUMSCRIPTUS (KPC; KPC WITH ASSOCIATED MALFORMATIONS)

General

Autosomal recessive; rare; abnormality in corneal curvature centrally localized on its posterior surface in association with opacification of the overlying stroma; may be an anterior chamber cleavage defect with failure of normal separation of the lens and iris from the cornea.

Ocular

Corneal opacities; retinal coloboma; ptosis; hyperopia; iridocorneal adhesions; hypertelorism.

Clinical

Cleft lip; cleft palate; neck webbing; short stature; mental retardation; inguinal hernia; undescended testes; tight heel cords; vertebral anomalies; delayed bone age; double ureters; cone-shaped epiphyses; stubby limbs and digits; limitation of extension and supination of the elbows; brachydactyly; fifth finger clinodactyly; frequent urinary tract infections; prominent nose; mild maxillary hypoplasia; low posterior hairline; short, broad feet with bilateral pes cavus; bilateral ureteric reflux.

Laboratory

Corneal topography.

Treatment

Rigid CLs are the mainstay of treatment, intrastromal corneal rings (Intacs) have shown some success and corneal graft is sometimes necessary.

BIBLIOGRAPHY

1. McKusick VA. Mendelian Inheritance in Man; A Catalog of Human Genes and Genetic Disorders, 12th edition. Baltimore: The Johns Hopkins University Press; 1998.
2. Online Mendelian Inheritance in Man, OMIM. McKusick-Nathans Institute for Genetic Medicine, Johns Hopkins University and National Center for Biotechnology Information, National Library of Medicine, February 12, 2007. Available from www.ncbi.nlm.nih.gov/omim. [Accessed September, 2013].
3. Young ID, Macrae WG, Hughes HE, et al. Keratoconus posticus circumscriptus, cleft lip and palate, genitourinary abnormalities, short stature, and mental retardation in sibs. J Med Genet. 1982;19:332-6.

5E12. CORNEAL DYSTROPHY, MEESMANN EPITHELIAL (MEESMANN EPITHELIAL DYSTROPHY OF CORNEA)

General

Autosomal dominant; rare; onset 1st year of life; possible that a disturbance of the cytoplasmic ground substance results in cellular homogenization with cyst formation.

Ocular

Myriads of fine punctate opacities in epithelium and Bowman membrane of cornea; thickening of the epithelial basement membrane of cornea; keratoconus.

Clinical

None.

Laboratory

Diagnosis is made by clinical findings.

Treatment

Usually not treatment. Bandage contact lens can be used to reduce discomfort and reduce visual loss.

BIBLIOGRAPHY

1. Tremblay M, Dubé I. Meesmann's corneal dystrophy: ultrastructural features. Can J Ophthalmol. 1982;17:24-8.
2. Fine BS, Yanoff M, Pitts E, et al. Meesmann's epithelial dystrophy of cornea. Am J Ophthalmol. 1977;83:633-42.
3. McKusick VA. Mendelian Inheritance in Man: A Catalog of Human Genes and Genetic Disorders, 12th edition. Baltimore: The Johns Hopkins University Press; 1998.

5E13. PETERS ANOMALY

General

Autosomal recessive; may be morphologic entity with several eye syndromes, including Rieger syndrome, Mietens syndrome and fetal alcohol syndrome; may be due to a developmental field defect, a contiguous gene syndrome, or a defective homeotic gene controlling development of the eye and other body structures.

Ocular

Corneal opacification; lenticulocorneal adherence; iris adhesions; glaucoma; cataract; narrow lid fissures; colobomatous microphthalmia; persistent hyperplastic primary vitreous; retinal detachment; iris nodules.

Clinical

Short-limbed dwarfism; broad face; thin upper lip; hypoplastic columella; hypospadias; cleft lip and palate; craniofacial abnormalities; congenital heart disease; horseshoe kidney; polycystic kidneys; Wilms' tumor; mental retardation; external ear anomalies; camptodactyly.

Laboratory

Diagnosis is made by clinical findings.

Treatment

Glaucoma therapy, peripheral optical iridectomy, filtration surgery, cryoablation, or a tube shunt may be necessary if medications do not control the pressure. Corneal transplantation may be necessary if visual acuity is decreased.

BIBLIOGRAPHY

1. Giri G. (2012). Peters anomaly. [online] Available from www.emedicine.com/oph/TOPIC112.HTM. [Accessed September, 2013].

🔁 5E14. PILLAY SYNDROME (OPHTHALMOMANDIBULOMELIC DYSPLASIA)

General

Autosomal dominant; both sexes affected.

Ocular

Corneal opacities.

Clinical

Temporomandibular fusion; obtuse mandibular angle; short forearms.

Laboratory

Diagnosis is made by clinical findings.

Treatment

Check for elevated IOP. Medical treatment includes the use of hyperosmotic drops, non-steroidal and steroid eye drops. Corneal transplant may be necessary.

🔁 BIBLIOGRAPHY

1. Magalini SI, Scrascia E. Dictionary of Medical Syndromes, 2nd edition. Philadelphia: Lippincott; 1981.
2. Pillay VK. Ophthalmomandibulomelic dysplasia. An hereditary syndrome. J Bone Joint Surg. 1964;46:858-62.

🔁 5E15. ANTERIOR CHAMBER CLEAVAGE SYNDROME (REESE-ELLSWORTH SYNDROME; PETERS-PLUS SYNDROME)

General

Abnormalities in the embryologic development of the anterior chamber due to failure of normal migration of mesodermal cells across the anterior segment of the eye or failure of later differentiation of the mesodermal elements; various conditions described as congenital: central anterior synechiae, persistent mesenchymal tissue in the chamber angle, posterior embryotoxon, congenital corneal hyaline membrane, posterior marginal dysplasia, prominent Schwalbe's line, mesodermal dysgenesis, and internal corneal ulcer seem all to fall in this same category of the anterior chamber cleavage syndrome; condition is present at birth; about 80% are bilateral; autosomal dominant inheritance; may be associated with congenital sensory neuropathy and ichthyosis.

Ocular

Increased IOP; adhesions between the iris and cornea; persistence of mesenchymal tissue in the chamber angle; usually shallow anterior chamber; iris coloboma and hypoplasia; prominent Schwalbe's ring; contiguous hyaloid membrane; corneal opacities of various density with or without edema, usually at the site of iris adhesion; anterior pole cataract; remains of hyaloid artery.

Clinical

Dental anomalies; mental retardation; cleft palate; syndactyly; craniofacial dysostosis; myotonic dystrophy.

Laboratory

Diagnosis is made by clinical findings.

Treatment

- *Glaucoma*: Glaucoma medication should be the first plan of action. If medication is unsuccessful, a filtering surgical procedure with or without antimetabolites may be beneficial.
- *Cataract*: Change in glasses can sometimes improve a patient's visual function temporarily; however, the most common treatment is cataract surgery.

🔁 BIBLIOGRAPHY

1. Giri G. (2012). Peters Anomaly. [online] Available from www.emedicine.com/oph/TOPIC112.HTM. [Accessed September, 2013].

5E16. HANHART SYNDROME (RICHNER SYNDROME; RECESSIVE KERATOSIS PALMOPLANTARIS; PSEUDOHERPETIC KERATITIS; RICHNER-HANHART SYNDROME; TYROSINEMIA II; TYROSINOSIS; PSEUDODENDRITIC KERATITIS)

General

Autosomal recessive; consanguinity.

Ocular

Excess tearing; photophobia; dendritic lesions of the cornea with corneal sensitivity not affected; keratitis; papillary hypertrophy of conjunctiva; corneal haze; neovascularization of cornea; cataract; nystagmus.

Clinical

Dyskeratosis palmoplantaris; diffuse keratosis; dystrophy of nails; hypotrichosis; mental retardation (usually pronounced); sensorineural hearing loss.

Laboratory

Serum-plasma tyrosine 16–62 mg/dL; urine-tyrosinuria and tyrosyluria; liver biopsy—decreased cytoplasmic tyrosine aminotransferase (cTAT) activity.

Treatment

Topical keratolytics, topical retinoids, potent topical steroids with or without keratolytics in dermatoses with an inflammatory component.

BIBLIOGRAPHY

1. Lee RA, Yassaee M, Bowe WP, et al. (2011). Keratosis Palmaris et Plantaris. [online] www.emedicine.com/derm/TOPIC589.HTM. [Accessed September, 2013].

5E17. RIEGER SYNDROME (AXENFELD-RIEGER SYNDROME; DYSGENESIS MESODERMALIS CORNEAE ET IRIDES; DYSGENESIS MESOSTROMALIS; AXENFELD POSTERIOR EMBRYOTOXON-JUVENILE GLAUCOMA)

General

Autosomal dominant; neural crest abnormality; 50% of patients develop glaucoma.

Ocular

Microphthalmia; congenital glaucoma; iris hypoplasia; deformed and acentric pupil; anterior synechiae; aniridia; microcornea; corneal opacities in Descemet's membrane parallel to the limbus; dislocated lens; optic atrophy; cataract; strabismus; ptosis; hypertelorism; keratoconus; posterior embryotoxon; broad iris processes to embryotoxon; iris stromal hypoplasia; corectopia; polycoria; secondary glaucoma.

Clinical

Face wide; hypodontia; underdeveloped maxilla; teeth deformities; myotonic dystrophy; facial anomalies: maxillary hypoplasia, protrusion of the lower lip, broad, flat nose; dental anomalies include absent teeth, pig-like incisors and decreased crown size; hypospadias.

Laboratory

Diagnosis is made by clinical findings.

Treatment/Ocular

Congenital glaucoma can be treated with beta-blockers, prostaglandin analogs and carbonic anhydrase inhibitors. Surgery such as goniotomy or trabeculectomy can be used if IOP is not controlled.

BIBLIOGRAPHY

1. Eagle RC. Congenital, developmental and degenerative disorders of the iris and ciliary body. In: Albert DM, Jakobiec FA (Eds). Albert & Jakobiec's Principles and Practice of Ophthalmology: Clinical Practice, 3rd edition. Philadelphia, PA: WB Saunders; 1994. pp. 367-87.
2. Montes JG, Montes JC. Syndrome de Rieger, anomalie de axenfeld con glaucoma Juvenil familiar. Arch Soc Ophth Hisp Am. 1967;27:93.
3. Rieger H. Beitrage zur Kenntnis seltener Missbildungen der Iris. Graefes Arch Clin Esp Ophthalmol. 1935;133:602.
4. Wesley RK, Baker JD, Golnick AL. Rieger's syndrome: (oligodontia and primary mesodermal dysgenesis of the iris) clinical features and report of an isolated case. J Pediatr Ophthalmol Strabismus. 1978;15(2):67-70.

5E19. WAARDENBURG SYNDROME (VAN DER HOEVE-HALBERSTAM-WAARDENBURG SYNDROME; WAARDENBURG-KLEIN SYNDROME; EMBRYONIC FIXATION SYNDROME; INTEROCULO-IRIDODERMATO-AUDITIVE DYSPLASIA; PIEBALDISM) HYPERTELORISM

General

Irregular dominant inheritance; developmental fault in neural crest with absence of the organ of Corti, aplasia of the spiral ganglion, and pigmentary changes; no sex preference; onset at birth.

Ocular

Hyperplasia of the medial portions of the eyebrows; hypertelorism; blepharophimosis; strabismus; heterochromia iridis; aniridia; microcornea; cornea plana; microphakia; abnormal fundus pigmentation; hypoplasia of optic nerve; synophrys; poliosis; hypopigmentation and hypoplasia of retina and choroid; epicanthus; lateral displacement of inferior puncta; lenticonus; underdevelopment of orbital bones; lateral displacement of inner canthi; hypopigmented iris.

Clinical

Congenital deafness; unilateral deafness or deaf-mutism; broad and high nasal root with absent nasofrontal angle; albinotic hair strain (unilateral); faint patches of skin pigmentation; pituitary tumor; nasal atresia; white forelock.

Laboratory

Molecular testing and audiology.

Treatment

Genetic counseling, audiology and otolaryngology management.

BIBLIOGRAPHY

1. Schwartz RA, Bawle EV, Jozwiak S. (2013). Genetics of Waardenburg syndrome. [online] Available from www.emedicine.com/ped/TOPIC2422.HTM. [Accessed September, 2013].

5E22. 11Q- SYNDROME

General

Chromosome 11 deletion syndrome.

Ocular

Telecanthus/hypertelorism; rarely, congenital glaucoma, cyclopia.

Clinical

Psychomotor retardation, trigonocephaly, broad depressed nasal bridge, micrognathia, low-set abnormal ears, cardiac anomalies, hand and foot anomalies, renal agenesis, anal atresia, supratentorial white matter abnormality on CT or MRI; microphallus; holoprosencephaly; female preponderance.

Laboratory

Clinical.

Treatment

See congenital glaucoma.

BIBLIOGRAPHY

1. Helmuth RA, Weaver DD, Wills ER. Holoprosencephaly, ear abnormalities, congenital heart defect, and microphallus in a patient with 11q- mosaicism. Am J Med Genet. 1989;32:178-81.
2. Ishida Y, Watanabe N, Ishihara Y, et al. The 11q- syndrome with mosaic partial deletion of 11q. Acta Paediatr Jpn. 1992;34:592-6.
3. Leegte B, Kerstjens-Frederikse WS, Deelstra K, et al. 11q-syndrome: three cases and a review of the literature. Genet Couns. 1999;10:305-13.

🖶 5E23. 18Q- SYNDROME (18Q DELETION SYNDROME)

General

Chromosome 18q deletion syndrome.

Ocular

Macular "fibrosis"; optic disk abnormalities with tractional retinal detachment, retinal degeneration, and tilting of the optic disk.

Clinical

Microcephaly; short stature; hypotonia; hypothyroidism; diabetes mellitus; short neck; sensorineural hearing loss; sensorimotor axonal neuropathy; mild-to-moderate mental retardation; chronic arthritis; seizures.

Laboratory

Clinical.

Treatment

Retinal detachment: Scleral buckle, pneumatic retinopexy and vitrectomy may be used to close all the breaks.

🖶 BIBLIOGRAPHY

1. Gordon MF, Bressman S, Brin MF, et al. Dystonia in a patient with deletion of 18q. Mov Disord. 1995;10:496-9.
2. Hansen US, Herline T. Chronic arthritis in a boy with 18q-syndrome. J Rheumatol. 1994;21:1958-9.

🖶 5F. SANDS OF THE SAHARA SYNDROME (DIFFUSE LAMELLAR KERATITIS)

General

Interface inflammation after LASIK.

Ocular

Interface inflammation after LASIK is a rare but potential sight-threatening complication; syndrome presents 1–5 days after LASIK; affected patients often complain of decreased or cloudy vision, foreign body sensation and photophobia; symptoms may be mild or severe; cause of the interface debris is unknown, but microkeratome material is implicated.

Laboratory

Diagnosis is made by clinical findings.

Treatment

Increments in strength and frequency of topical steroids and discontinuing NSAIDs.

🖶 BIBLIOGRAPHY

1. Kaufman SC, Maitchouk DY, Chiou AG, et al. Interface inflammation after laser in situ keratomileusis. Sands of the Sahara syndrome. J Cataract Refract surg. 1998;24(12):1589-93.
2. Smith RJ, Maloney RK. Diffuse lamellar keratitis. A new syndrome in lamellar refractive surgery. Ophthalmology. 1998;105(9):1721-6.

🖶 5G. FILAMENTARY KERATITIS

General

Etiology unknown.

Clinical

None.

Ocular

Fine filaments develop on front surface of cornea. Move with lid movement.

Laboratory

Diagnosis is made by clinical findings.

Treatment

Debridement of filaments with forceps or cotton-tipped applicator, NaCl drops and ointment, soft contact lens and punctal occlusion.

BIBLIOGRAPHY

1. Roy FH, Fraunfelder FW, Fraunfelder FT. Roy and Fraunfelder's Current Ocular Therapy, 6th edition. London; Elsevier; 2008.

5H. FUNGAL KERATITIS

General

It can occur following trauma or in immunosuppressed individuals.

Clinical

None.

Ocular

Central or pericentral corneal ulcer, photophobia, pain.

Laboratory

- *Corneal smear*: Giemsa stain, potassium hydroxide (KOH) or Gomori's methenamine-silver stain.
- *Culture*: Sabouraud's dextrose agar, brain-heart infusion broth.

Treatment

- *Yeast*: Amphotericin hourly while awake for 48 hours then every 2 hours.
- *Fungal*: Natamycin 5% every hour for 48 hours, then every 2 hours. Excisional keratoplasty may be necessary.

BIBLIOGRAPHY

1. Shi W, Wang T, Xie L, et al. Risk factors, clinical features, and outcomes of recurrent fungal keratitis after corneal transplantation. Ophthalmology. 2010;117(5):890-6.
2. Singh D, Verma A. (2012). Fungal keratitis. [online] Available from www.emedicine.com/oph/TOPIC99.HTM. [Accessed September, 2013].

5I. HLA-B27 SYNDROMES

General

Human leukocyte antigen system is the major histocompatibility complex (MHC) found on chromosome 6; associated with inflammatory disease.

Ocular

Uveitis; Reiter's syndrome; keratitis; band keratopathy; iris bombe; pigment dispersion; papillary miosis; iris nodules; cystoid macular edema (CME); disk edema; pars plana exudates; choroiditis.

Clinical

Ankylosing spondylitis; arthritis; inflammatory bowel disease; psoriatic arthritis.

Laboratory

Careful history and physical examination usually helps in distinguishing between the uveitic entities associated with systemic disease and HLA-B27 from those that are not associated with HLA-B27.

Treatment

Topical or systemic corticosteroids and topical cycloplegics are useful. Periocular corticosteroid injections are extremely useful in acute, recalcitrant or noncompliant cases, particularly when posterior segment involvement occurs. Immunosuppressive therapy may be necessary in refractory cases or in those patients with corticosteroid-induced side effects. The primary goal is to eliminate all cells, thereby minimizing complications including cataracts, CME, hypotony or glaucoma.

BIBLIOGRAPHY

1. Di Lorenzo AL. (2011). HLA-B27 syndromes. [online] Available from www.emedicine.com/oph/TOPIC721.HTM. [Accessed September, 2013].

5J. INTERSTITIAL KERATITIS

General

Nonsuppurative inflammation characterized by cellular infiltrates, usually caused by syphilis but can be secondary to bacterial, viral, parasitic and autoimmune causes.

Clinical

Syphilis; tuberculosis; leprosy; Lyme disease; *Acathamoeba; Leishmania*; Epstein-Barr; mumps; Cogan's syndrome.

Ocular

Decreased vision; photophobia; tearing; blepharospasm; dense, white stromal necrosis of the cornea.

Laboratory

Diagnosis is made by clinical findings; serologic testing is done to determine the cause.

Treatment

Treat the underlying disorder.

Ocular

Topical corticosteroids; if permanent corneal opacity occurs corneal transplant may be necessary.

BIBLIOGRAPHY

1. Majmudar PA. (2011). Interstitial keratitis overview of interstitial keratitis. [online] Available from emedicine.medscape.com/article/1194376-overview. [Accessed September, 2013].

5K. KERATITIS FUGAX HEREDITARIA

General

Autosomal dominant; onset from the age of 4–12 years; characterized by acute attacks of keratitis.

Ocular

Keratitis; corneal opacities.

Clinical

None.

Laboratory

Diagnosis is made by clinical findings.

Treatment

Initiate broad-spectrum antibiotics with the following: tobramycin every hour alternating with fortified cefazolin (50 mg/mL) one drop every hour. If the corneal ulcer is small, peripheral and no impending perforation is present, intensive monotherapy with fluoroquinolones is an alternative treatment.

BIBLIOGRAPHY

1. Mills TJ, Mills LD. (2011). Corneal ulceration and ulcerative keratitis in emergency medicine. [online] Available from www.emedicine.com/emerg/TOPIC115.HTM. [Accessed September, 2013].

5L. SENTER SYNDROME (KERATITIS-ICHTHYOSIS-DEAFNESS SYNDROME; KID SYNDROME; ICHTHYOSIFORM ERYTHRODERMA, CORNEAL INVOLVEMENT, AND DEAFNESS (KERATITIS)

General

Autosomal recessive.

Ocular

Corneal involvement.

Clinical

Ichthyosiform erythroderma; deafness; hepatomegaly; hepatic cirrhosis; glycogen storage; short stature; mental retardation; hepatitis.

Laboratory

Diagnosis is made by clinical findings.

Treatment

Steroids or antibiotics may be useful.

BIBLIOGRAPHY

1. McKusick VA. Mendelian Inheritance in Man: A Catalog of Human Genes and Genetic Disorders, 12th edition. Baltimore, USA: The Johns Hopkins University Press; 1998.

5M. DIMMER SYNDROME (KERATITIS NUMMULARIS)

General

Onset after minor ocular trauma.

Ocular

Photophobia; ocular pain; excessive lacrimation; discoid infiltration of superficial layers of cornea without adjacent conjunctivitis.

Laboratory

None.

Treatment

Keratitis: Local treatment is used for prevention and reduction of corneal damage. Systemic therapy is used for controlling the underlying disease. Tissue adhesives may be necessary for impending perforation. Keratectomy, conjunctival resection, amniotic membrane transplantation and keratoplasty may be necessary.

BIBLIOGRAPHY

1. Dimmer F. Weber Eine der Keratitis Nurmnularis. Mahestehende Hirnhutentzuendung Augenheilkd. 1905;13:621-35.
2. Magalini SI, Scrascia E. Dictionary of Medical Syndromes, 2nd edition. Philadelphia, PA: Lippincott Williams and Wilkins; 1981.

5O. EPITHELIAL EROSION SYNDROME (METAHERPETIC KERATITIS; KAUFMAN SYNDROME; FRANCESCHETTI DYSTROPHY; POSTTRAUMATIC KERATITIS)

General

It is most likely caused by herpes simplex virus; previous corneal trauma or autosomal dominant.

Ocular

Recurrent erosions of the corneal epithelium, usually seen within weeks or months after herpes simplex infection of the cornea; "loose" epithelium is removed from the underlying Bowman's membrane mechanically by lid blinking; defects are irregular in shape and stain positively with fluorescein dye; underlying corneal stroma usually shows some edema; pain upon opening eyes in morning.

Clinical

Mild fever; occasionally herpetic skin lesions.

Laboratory

Diagnosis is made by clinical findings.

Treatment

Goal of therapy is regenerating or repairing the epithelial basement membrane to restore the adhesion between the epithelium and the anterior stroma, topical lubrication therapy, bandage soft contact lenses, debridement of the epithelium and basement membrane or anterior stromal micropuncture may be useful.

BIBLIOGRAPHY

1. Verma A, Ehrenhaus MP. (2012). Recurrent corneal erosion. [online] Available from www.emedicine.com/oph/TOPIC113.HTM. [Accessed September, 2013].

5P. MOOREN'S ULCER (CHRONIC SERPIGINOUS ULCER OF THE CORNEA, ULCUS)

General

Chronic and progressive disorder of cornea.

Clinical

None.

Ocular

Ulcerative keratitis.

Laboratory

Diagnosis is made by clinical findings.

Treatment

- *Topical*: Cycloplegic agents, steroids, antibiotic drops. Bandage contact lens and cyanoacrylate glue over perforation may be useful.
- *Surgical*: Conjunctival recession/resection, conjunctival excision and superficial lamellar keratectomy.
- *Systemic*: If hepatitis C virus (HCV) is detected, treat with interferon alpha and Roferon-A if chronic HCV is detected; if no chronic HCV is detected, an immunosuppressive specialist should be involved.

BIBLIOGRAPHY

1. Murillo-Lopez FH. (2012). Corneal ulcer. [online] Available from www.emedicine.com/oph/TOPIC249.HTM. [Accessed September, 2013].

5Q. NEUROPARALYTIC KERATITIS (NEUTROPIC KERATITIS, TRIGEMINIAL NEUROPATHIC KERATOPATHY)

General

Numbness of the cornea from injury of trigeminal nerve. Causes include surgery of trigeminal neuralgias, surgery of acoustic neuroma and herpes zoster ophthalmicus and Riley-Day syndrome.

Clinical

None.

Ocular

Abnormalities of the tear film and cornea, punctate keratopathy, epithelial detachment, stromal lysis.

Laboratory

Diagnosis is made by clinical findings.

Treatment

- *Stage 1:* Punctate keratopathy is treated with intermittent patching. Oral tetracyclines and discontinuing contact lens may be helpful.
- *Stage 2:* Epithelial detachment—atropine, Blenderm or temporary tarsorrhaphy. Botulinum toxin into levator palpebrae superioris.
- *Stage 3:* Closure of lid—atropine and botulinum toxin and antibiotics and systemic antibiotic. Permanent tarsorrhaphy.

BIBLIOGRAPHY

1. Graham RH, Hendrix MA. (2012). Neurotrophic keratopathy. [online] Available from www.emedicine.com/oph/TOPIC106.HTM. [Accessed September, 2013].

5R. COGAN (1) SYNDROME (NONSYPHILITIC INTERSTITIAL KERATITIS)

General

Cause unknown; perhaps a generalized hypersensitivity reaction; most frequently affects young adults; unclear etiology; several studies suggest an autoimmunomediated process, possibly a vasculitis.

Ocular

Blepharospasm; lacrimation; congested conjunctival vessels; little or no reaction in anterior chamber but ciliary injection present; interstitial keratitis (unilateral or bilateral); granular-type infiltrates; patchy distribution in deeper stroma; later vascularization; conjunctivitis; corneal opacity; uveitis; nystagmus.

Clinical

Vestibuloauditory symptoms (similar to Ménière syndrome); nausea; vomiting; vertigo; tinnitus (abrupt onset); rapidly progressive deafness; loss of equilibration (*see* Ménière syndrome); aortic insufficiency; sensorineural testing; lacunar infarcts.

Laboratory

Leukocytosis in 75%, neutrophilia in 50%, mild eosinophilia in 17%, relative lymphopenia in 25%, anemia in 33%, thrombocytosis in 30% and ESR of greater than 20 in 75%.

Treatment

Corticosteroids and antibiotics are useful. Corneal transplantation may be necessary for corneal opacity.

BIBLIOGRAPHY

1. Majmudar PA. (2011). Interstitial keratitis overview of interstitial keratitis. [online] Available from www.emedicine.com/oph/TOPIC101.HTM. [Accessed September, 2013].

5S. PANNUS (SUPERFICIAL VASCULAR INVASION CONFINED TO A SEGMENT OF THE CORNEA OR EXTENDING AROUND THE ENTIRE LIMBUS)

*1. Acne rosacea
†*2. Allergic marginal infiltration
*3. Anoxic contact lens overwear syndrome
4. Ariboflavinosis keratopathy
*5. Contact lens usage
6. Deerfly fever (tularemia)
7. Degenerative-blind degenerative eyes; often associated with bullous keratopathy
8. Dermatitis herpetiformis (Duhring-Brocq disease)
†9. Drugs including the following:
- Benoxinate
- Benzalkonium
- Butacaine
- Chlorhexidine
- Cocaine
- Dibucaine
- Dyclonine
- F3T
- Ibuprofen
- Idoxuridine
- IDU
- Iodine solution
- Oxyphenbutazone
- Phenacaine
- Phenylbutazone
- Piperocaine
- Proparacaine
- Silicone
- Tetracaine
- Thimerosal
- Trifluridine
- Urokinase
- Vidarabine
10. Fuchs corneal dystrophy (degenerative pannus)
†11. Glaucoma (degenerative pannus)
12. *Haemophilus influenzae*
13. Histiocytosis X (Hand-Schüller-Christian syndrome)
14. Hypoparathyroidism
15. Inclusion conjunctivitis in infants and adults (micropannus, chlamydia)
16. Keratoconjunctivitis sicca

* Indicates most frequent

17. Leishmaniasis
†18. Leprosy (Hansen disease)
†19. Linear nevus sebaceous of Jadassohn
†20. Lyell disease (toxic epidermal necrolysis or scalded skin syndrome)
†21. Lymphopathia venereum
†22. Molluscum contagiosum
†23. Ocular cicatricial pemphigoid
†24. Onchocerciasis (river blindness)
†25. Papilloma (wart)
†26. Pellagra (avitaminosis B12)
†27. Pemphigus foliaceus (Cazenave disease)
†28. Phlyctenular keratoconjunctivitis
†29. Siemens disease (keratosis follicularis spinulosa decalvans)
†*30. Staphylococcal keratoconjunctivitis (micropannus)
†31. Stevens-Johnson syndrome (mucocutaneous ocular syndrome)
†*32. Superior limbic keratoconjunctivitis (micropannus)
†33. Terrien disease (senile marginal atrophy)

†34. Trachoma
†35. Tuberculosis
†36. Vaccinia
†37. Vernal conjunctivitis (micropannus)
†38. Vitamin B12 deficiency (Addison pernicious anemia syndrome)

BIBLIOGRAPHY

1. Arffa RC. Grayson's Diseases of the Cornea, 3rd edition. St. Louis: Mosby-Year Book; 1991.
2. Dixon WS, Bron AJ. Fluorescein angiographic demonstration of corneal vascularization in contact lens wearers. Am J Ophthalmol. 1973;75:1010-5.
3. Fraunfelder FT, Fraunfelder FW. Drug-induced ocular side effects. Woburn, MA: Butterworth-Heinemann; 2001.
4. Roy FH. Ocular Syndromes and Systemic Diseases, 4th edition. Philadelphia: Lippincott Williams & Wilkins; 2007.

---

†Indicates a general entry and therefore has not been described in detail in the text

5S1. ACNE ROSACEA (ACNE ERYTHEMATOSA; OCULAR ROSACEA)

General

Etiology unknown; usually occurs in women 30–50 years of age; pathogenetic mechanism remains unclear.

Ocular

Conjunctivitis; corneal neovascularization (wedge-shaped); keratitis; meibomianitis; blepharitis; recurrent chalazion; conjunctival hyperemia; superficial punctate keratopathy; corneal vascularization, thinning, perforation, and scarring; episcleritis; scleritis; iritis; nodular conjunctivitis.

Clinical

Symmetrical erythema; papules; pustules; telangiectasia; sebaceous gland hypertrophy of the forehead, malar eminences, and nose.

Laboratory

Diagnosis is made by clinical findings.

Treatment

Systemic antibiotics are useful in most cases.

BIBLIOGRAPHY

1. Banasikowaska AK, Singh S. (2012). Rosacea. [online] Available from www.emedicine.com/derm/TOPIC377.HTM. [Accessed July, 2013].

5S3. ANOXIC OVERWEAR SYNDROME

General

It is caused by a reduction in oxygen supply due to continuously worn hydrogel lenses; allergic or toxic reactions to preservatives used in the cleaning process.

Ocular

Refractive error changes; endothelial cell changes; physical trauma to the anterior surface of the cornea; corneal neovascularization; giant papillary conjunctivitis; contact lens deposits; acute red eye syndrome.

Laboratory

Diagnosis is made by clinical findings.

Treatment

Observation; topical steroid drops; reduce time one individual uses contact lens; corneal laser photocoagulation.

◫ BIBLIOGRAPHY

1. Binder PS. The physiologic effects of extended wear soft contact lenses. Ophthalmology. 1980;87:745-9.
2. Sarver MD, Baggett DA, Harris MG, et al. Corneal edema with hydrogel lenses and eye closure: effect of oxygen transmissibility. Am J Optom Physiol Opt. 1981;58:386-92.

◫ 5S4. AVITAMINOSIS B2 (ARIBOFLAVINOSIS; PELLAGRA)

General

Niacin deficiency.

Ocular

Conjunctivitis; corneal vascularization; keratitis; pupillary dilation; optic atrophy; optic neuritis; cataract; blepharitis; central scotoma; marked photophobia.

Clinical

Occasional cranial nerve palsies; dermatitis; glossitis; gastrointestinal and nervous system dysfunction; mental deterioration; diarrhea; stomatitis.

Laboratory

Therapeutic response to niacin in a patient with the typical symptoms and signs of pellagra establishes the diagnosis.

Treatment

Niacin taken orally is usually effective in reversing the clinical manifestations.

◫ BIBLIOGRAPHY

1. Rabinowitz SS, Feygina V, Reddy S, et al. (2012). Pediatric pellagra. [online] Available from www.emedicine.com/ped/TOPIC1755.HTM. [Accessed September, 2013].

◫ 5S5. NEOVASCULARIZATION, CORNEAL CONTACT LENS RELATED

General

Pathologic state in which new blood vessels extending in the corneal stroma from trauma, inflammation, infection, toxic insults secondary to contact lens usage.

Clinical

None.

Ocular

Vessel ingrowth into the cornea, ocular irritation.

Laboratory

Diagnosis is made by clinical findings.

Treatment

Observation, eliminate cause, topical steroid drops, reduced time for an individual using contact lens, corneal laser photocoagulation.

◫ BIBLIOGRAPHY

1. Weissman BA, Yeung KK. (2011). Neovascularization, corneal, CL-related. [online] Available from emedicine.medscape.com/article/1195886-overview. [Accessed September, 2013].

5S6. DEERFLY FEVER (FRANCIS DISEASE; RABBIT FEVER; TULAREMIA; DEERFLY TULAREMIA)

General

Acute infectious disease caused by *Francisella (Pasteurella) tularensis.*

Ocular

Chemosis; conjunctivitis; corneal ulcer; endophthalmitis; dacryocystitis; optic atrophy; iris prolapse; chalazion; corneal opacity; pannus.

Clinical

Local ulcerative lesion; suppuration of regional lymph nodes; fever; prostration; myalgia; severe headache; pneumonia.

Laboratory

Diagnosis is usually based on serology results. Tularemia tube agglutination testing is the most commonly used serological test.

Treatment

Systemic antibiotics.

BIBLIOGRAPHY

1. Cleveland KO, Gelfand M, Raugi GJ. (2013). Tularemia. [online] Available from www.emedicine.com/med/TOPIC2326.HTM. [Accessed September, 2013].

5S7. CORNEAL EDEMA (BULLOUS KERATOPATHY, EPITHELIAL EDEMA, STROMAL EDEMA)

General

It may be caused by endothelial dysfunction, corneal hypoxia and elevated IOP.

Clinical

None.

Ocular

Swelling of cornea, loss of vision, pain.

Laboratory

Diagnosis is made by clinical findings.

Treatment

Control IOP, hypertonic salt solution or ointment, soft contact lens, anterior stromal puncture or conjunctival flap, PTK, hair dryer held at arm's length and posterior lamellar keratoplasty.

BIBLIOGRAPHY

1. Taravella M, Walker M. (2012). Postoperative corneal edema. [online] Available from www.emedicine.com/oph/TOPIC64.HTM. [Accessed September, 2013].

5S8. DERMATITIS HERPETIFORMIS (DUHRING-BROCQ DISEASE)

General

Malignant; atypical; does not respond well to sulfone or sulfapyridine therapy; uncommon; autoimmune blistering dermatosis; pruritic eruption involving the scalp, buttocks, lower back, and extensor surface of arms; autoantibody is generally of immunoglobulin A class causing deposition at the dermal-epidermal junction.

Ocular

Bullae of conjunctiva, skin, and mucous membranes; blisters are intraepithelial (acantholysis) and usually do not leave scars; epithelium desquamates in patches; corneal and conjunctival vascularization; symblepharon; cataract.

Clinical

Vesicles; erythema; pruritus; burning; eruption classically involves extensor surface of the knees, elbows, buttocks, sacrum, scapula, and scalp.

Laboratory

Diagnosis is made by clinical findings and skin biopsy.

Treatment

Dapsone and sulfapyridine are the primary medications used for therapy. Avoidance of gluten is also helpful.

BIBLIOGRAPHY

1. Miller JL, Zaman SA. (2013). Dermatitis herpetiformis. [online] Available from www.emedicine.com/derm/TOPIC95.HTM. [Accessed September, 2013].

5S10. FUCHS' CORNEAL DYSTROPHY (FUCHS' ENDOTHELIAL DYSTROPHY OF THE CORNEA, COMBINED DYSTROPHY OF FUCHS', ENDOTHELIAL DYSTROPHY OF THE CORNEA, EPITHELIAL DYSTROPHY OF FUCHS', FUCHS' EPITHELIAL-ENDOTHELIAL DYSTROPHY)

General

Bilateral, slowly progressive, primary corneal disease, which results in vision loss due to corneal edema. Autosomal dominant and usually not clinically evident until the 4th or 5th decade of life.

Clinical

None.

Ocular

Central corneal guttae; gray, thickened appearance of Descemet's membrane; stromal edema; subepithelial edema; decreased visual acuity.

Laboratory

Diagnosis is made by clinical findings. The characteristics include endothelium producing an abnormal, banded, posterior layer of Descemet's membrane with characteristics of central guttae excrescences which are a hallmark of this disease.

Treatment

Early intervention includes NaCl 5% solution or ointment and the use of a hair dryer on low heat setting for tear film evaporation and corneal deturgescence. Surgical intervention includes corneal transplantation, EK, DLEK and DSEK.

BIBLIOGRAPHY

1. Singh D, Mittal V. (2012). Fuchs endothelial dystrophy. [online] Available from www.emedicine.com/oph/TOPIC91.HTM. [Accessed September, 2013].

5S12. HAEMOPHILUS INFLUENZAE

General

Gram-negative rod.

Ocular

Conjunctivitis; cellulitis; tenonitis; uveitis; vitreous opacity; pannus; corneal opacity.

Clinical

Pharyngitis; epiglottitis; laryngotracheitis; pneumonia; bronchitis; otitis media; meningitis; cellulitis; septic arthritis; sinusitis.

Laboratory

Gram-negative coccobacillus with eight biotypes and six serotypes. Gram stain and culture.

Treatment

Antibiotics are the mainstay of treatment. Invasive and serious infections are best treated with an intravenous third-generation cephalosporin until antibiotic sensitivities are available.

🗗 BIBLIOGRAPHY

1. Devarajan VR. (2012). Haemophilus influenzae infections. [online] Available from www.emedicine.com/med/TOPIC936.HTM. [Accessed September, 2013].

🗗 5S13. HISTIOCYTOSIS X (HAND-SCHULLER-CHRISTIAN SYNDROME; LIPOID GRANULOMA; XANTHOMATOUS GRANULOMA SYNDROME; SCHULLER-CHRISTIAN-HAND SYNDROME; LETTERER-SIWE SYNDROME; ACUTE HISTIOCYTOSIS X; EOSINOPHILIC GRANULOMA; RETICULOENDOTHELIOSIS SYNDROME)

General

The term histiocytosis X has been proposed to include Letterer-Siwe disease, Hand-Schuller-Christian disease, and eosinophilic granuloma of bone; there are sufficient grounds to treat Hand-Schuller-Christian and Letterer-Siwe together as different phases of the same disease process; eosinophilic granuloma most likely represents a reaction pattern, sharing some histologic features with the first two but nonetheless carrying a more benign prognosis; Letterer-Siwe disease is referred to as acute differentiated histiocytosis; Hand-Schuller-Christian disease is referred to as subacute differentiated or chronic differentiated histiocytosis; Letterer-Siwe etiology is unknown, onset is in infancy and early childhood, and prognosis is generally poor; Hand-Schuller-Christian etiology is unknown, onset is in childhood, male preponderance is 2:1, and prognosis is chronic with remissions; eosinophil may play a contributory pathophysiologic role.

Ocular

Exophthalmos; ocular pulsations; orbital roof defects; xanthelasma; blepharitis; internal ophthalmoplegia; nystagmus; retinal hemorrhages; papilledema; optic atrophy; uveitis; hypopyon; pannus; bullous keratopathy; corneal ulcer; hypochromic heterochromia; retinal detachment; cataract; scleritis.

Clinical

Hepatosplenomegaly; lymphadenopathy; skin lesions with papular eruptions; ecchymosis; purpura; bone lesions; anemia; fatigue; anorexia; fever; xanthoma of the skin; diabetes insipidus; skull defects; lung fibrosis; cardiac insufficiency.

Laboratory

Diagnosis is made by clinical findings.

Treatment

Treatment is a combination of radiation and chemotherapy.

🗗 BIBLIOGRAPHY

1. Christian HA. Defects in membranous bones, exophthalmos and diabetes insipidus, Volume 1. New York: Paul B. Hoeber; 1919. p. 390.
2. Duane TD. Clinical Ophthalmology. Philadelphia: JB Lippincott; 1987.
3. Roy FH, Fraunfelder FW, Fraunfelder FT. Roy and Fraunfelder's Current Ocular Therapy, 6th edition. Philadelphia: WB Saunders; 2008.
4. Hand A. Polyuria and tuberculosis. Arch Pediatr. 1893;10:673.
5. Mittelman D, Apple DJ, Goldberg MF. Ocular involvement in Letterer-Siwe disease. Am J Ophthalmol. 1973;75:261-5.
6. Pearlstone AD, Flom L. Letterer-Siwe's disease. J Pediatr Ophthalmol. 1970;77:103-5.
7. Petersen RA, Kuwabara T. Ocular manifestations of familial lymphohistiocytosis. Arch Ophthalmol. 1968;79:413.
8. Trocme SD, Aldave AJ. The eye and the eosinophil. Surv Ophthalmol. 1994;39:241-52.

⊟ 5S14. HYPOPARATHYROIDISM

General

Deficient secretion of PTH.

Ocular

Keratitis; blepharospasm; ptosis; cataract; madarosis; optic neuritis; papilledema; conjunctivitis; myopia; ocular colobomata.

Clinical

Decreased blood calcium; increased serum phosphate; tetany; muscle cramps; stridor; carpopedal spasms; convulsions; lethargy; personality changes; mental retardation; intracranial calcification; choreoathetosis; hemiballismus; renal agenesis.

Laboratory

Diagnosis made rests on the functional capacity of the adrenal cortex to synthesize cortisol. This is accomplished primarily by use of the rapid ACTH stimulation test (Cortrosyn, cosyntropin, or Synacthen).

Treatment

Endocrinologist should be consulted for the acute care and chronic care.

⊟ BIBLIOGRAPHY

1. Gonzalez-Campoy JM. (2012). Hypoparathyroidism. [online] Available from www.emedicine.com/med/TOPIC1131.HTM. [Accessed September, 2013].

⊟ 5S15. CHLAMYDIA (INCLUSION CONJUNCTIVITIS; PARATRACHOMA)

General

Organism that infects the epithelium of mucoid surfaces; sexually transmitted; major cause of non-gonococcal urethritis in men and cervicitis in women; major cause of neonatal ophthalmia; *Chlamydia trachomatis* is an intracellular bacterium lacking respiratory enzymes that has an affinity for mucosal epithelium; serotypes A through C have been epidemiologically associated with trachoma; serotypes E through K have been associated with genital infection and keratoconjunctivitis in sexually active adults and neonates; other serotypes have been associated with lymphogranuloma venereum and Reiter syndrome.

Ocular

Follicular conjunctivitis; corneal opacities; keratitis; corneal ulcer; lid edema; uveitis.

Clinical

Pneumonia; gastrointestinal disturbances; genital discharge.

Laboratory

Giemsa stain, cell culture—time intensive, direct fluorescent monoclonal antibiotics to stain smears.

Treatment

Three to six weeks of oral tetracycline (500 mg qid), oral doxycycline (100 mg bid), or oral erythromycin stearate (500 mg qid). Simultaneous treatment of all sexual partners is important to prevent reinfection.

⊟ BIBLIOGRAPHY

1. Bashour M. (2012) Ophthalmologic manifestations of chlamydia. [online] Available from www.emedicine.com/oph/TOPIC494.HTM. [Accessed September, 2013].

5S16. KERATOCONJUNCTIVITIS SICCA AND SJÖGREN'S SYNDROME

General

Autoimmune disease, seen more frequently in females.

Clinical

Xerostomia (dry mouth), dry nasal and genital mucosa.

Ocular

Severe dry eyes, corneal ulceration, corneal perforation, corneal scarring and vascularization.

Laboratory

Biopsy of lip and lachrymal gland positive, anti-nuclear antibody rheumatoid factor (RF) and anti-ro (Sjögren's specific A) and anti-La (Sjögren specific B). Elevated IgG level positive—predication for positive biopsy.

Treatment

Severe cases—immunosuppressive agents such as cyclosporin A and corticosteroids. Frequent application of tear substitutes, steroids, punctal plugs, bandage contacts and partial tarsorrhaphy.

BIBLIOGRAPHY

1. Foster CS, Yuksel E, Anzaar F, et al. (2013). Dry eye syndrome. [online] Available from www.emedicine.com/oph/TOPIC597.HTM. [Accessed September, 2013].

5S17. LEISHMANIASIS

General

It is caused by protozoa *Leishmania*.

Ocular

Conjunctivitis; ulcerative keratitis; ulcerating granulomatous lid lesions; lid edema; interstitial keratitis; subacute focal retinitis; retinal hemorrhage; iridocyclitis; unilateral chronic granulomatous blepharitis.

Clinical

Lesions in spleen, liver, and large intestine; fever; leukopenia; cutaneous lesions on the face.

Laboratory

Diagnosis of leishmaniasis has been confirmed by isolating, visualizing, and culturing the parasite from infected tissue. Over recent years, significant advances in PCR techniques have allowed for the highly sensitive and rapid diagnosis of specific *Leishmania* species.

Treatment

Sodium stibogluconate, amphotericin B (AmBisome) and pentamidine, dapsone, ketoconazole and fluconazole are drugs used for treatment. Which drug is best suited is dependent on what part of the world the patient is in.

BIBLIOGRAPHY

1. Stark CG. (2013). Leishmaniasis. [online] Available from www.emedicine.com/med/TOPIC1275.HTM. [Accessed September, 2013].

5T. TERRIEN DISEASE (TERRIEN MARGINAL DEGENERATION; GUTTER DYSTROPHY; PERIPHERAL FURROW KERATITIS; SENILE MARGINAL ATROPHY)

General

Rare; no known cause; 75% of patients are males from the age 10–70 years.

Ocular

Usually bilateral; may be asymmetrical; peripheral, fine, yellow-white, punctate stromal opacities associated with mild, superficial corneal vascularization; progressive thinning leads to peripheral gutter formation; decrease in visual acuity; loss of Bowman membrane and anterior stromal lamella with partial replacement of these tissues by a vascularized connective tissue; fatty deposits; thin stroma; thickness changes in Descemet's membrane; regular recurring attacks of pain and inflammation; keratoconus; reported association with Terrien's marginal degeneration.

Clinical

None.

Laboratory

Diagnosis is made by clinical findings.

Treatment/Ocular

Mild cases can be observed and soft contact lenses are helpful; PK may be necessary; graft recurrences are treated by superficial keratectomy, PTK or repeat PK.

BIBLIOGRAPHY

1. Ashenhurst M, Slomovic A. Corneal hydrops in Terrien's marginal degeneration: an unusual complication. Can J Ophthalmol. 1987;22(6):328-30.
2. Austin P, Brown SI. Inflammatory Terrien's marginal corneal disease. Am J Ophthalmol. 1981;92(2):189-92.
3. Friedlaender MH. Allergy and Immunology of the Eye, Illustrated edition. Hagerstown, MD: Harper & Row; 1979. p. 190.
4. Kremer I. Terrien's marginal degeneration associated with vernal conjunctivitis. Am J Ophthalmol. 1991;111(4):517-8.
5. Lopez JS, Price FW, Whitcup SM, et al. Immunohistochemistry of Terrien's and Mooren's corneal degeneration. Arch Ophthalmol. 1991;109(7):988-92.

5U. PERIPHERAL ULCERATIVE KERATITIS

General

Ulceration in the peripheral cornea; relatively uncommon; may be presenting characteristics of a systemic disease.

Clinical

Connective and vasculitic disease; herpes simplex, varicella; human immunodeficiency virus (HIV); syphilis; hepatitis; bacillary dysentery; *Salmonella*.

Ocular

Pain; foreign body sensation; tearing; photophobia; decreased visual acuity.

Laboratory

Testing should be focused on the suspected systemic disease.

Treatment

Local treatment is used for prevention and reduction of corneal damage. Systemic therapy is used for controlling the underlying disease. Tissue adhesives may be necessary for impending perforation. Keratectomy, conjunctival resection, amniotic membrane transplantation and keratoplasty may be necessary.

BIBLIOGRAPHY

1. Yu EN, Foster CS. (2012). Peripheral ulcerative keratitis. [online] Available from emedicine.medscape.com/article/1195980-overview. [Accessed September, 2013].

5V. PISK (PRESSURE INDUCED INTRALAMELLAR STROMAL KERATITIS)

General

It is associated with LASIK postoperative patients.

Ocular

Elevated IOP; ocular discomfort; blurred vision; stromal keratitis.

Clinical

None.

Laboratory

Diagnosis is made by clinical findings.

Treatment

Topical glaucoma therapy, nonsteroidal anti-inflammatory agents.

BIBLIOGRAPHY

1. Belin MW, Hannush SB, Yau CW, et al. Elevated intraocular pressure-induced interlamellar stromal keratitis. Ophthalmology. 2002;109(10):1929-33.
2. Caceres V. Post-LASIK IOP measurements may help detect PISK. EyeWorld. 2005;72-3.

5W. HANHART SYNDROME (RICHNER SYNDROME; RECESSIVE KERATOSIS PALMOPLANTARIS; PSEUDOHERPETIC KERATITIS; RICHNER-HANHART SYNDROME; TYROSINEMIA II; TYROSINOSIS; PSEUDODENDRITIC KERATITIS)

General

Autosomal recessive; consanguinity.

Ocular

Excess tearing; photophobia; dendritic lesions of the cornea with corneal sensitivity not affected; keratitis; papillary hypertrophy of conjunctiva; corneal haze; neovascularization of cornea; cataract; nystagmus.

Clinical

Dyskeratosis palmoplantaris; diffuse keratosis; dystrophy of nails; hypotrichosis; mental retardation (usually pronounced); sensorineural hearing loss.

Laboratory

- *Serum*: Plasma tyrosine 16–62 mg/dL
- *Urine*: Tyrosinuria and tyrosylvria
- *Liver biopsy*: Decreased cytoplasmic tyrosine aminotransferase (cTAT) activity.

Treatment

Topical keratolytics, topical retinoids, potent topical steroids with or without keratolytics in dermatosis with an inflammatory component.

BIBLIOGRAPHY

1. Lee RA, Yassaee M, Bowe WP, et al. (2011). Keratosis palmaris et plantaris. [online] Available from www.emedicine.com/derm/TOPIC589.HTM. [Accessed September, 2013].

5X. RELAPSING FEVER (RECURRENT FEVER)

General

Acute infectious disease caused by *Borrelia* transmitted by lice; characterized by recurrent bouts of fever separated by relatively asymptomatic periods; there is an endemic form of rheumatic fever transmitted by tick vectors and spirochetes of the genus *Borrelia*.

Ocular

Extraocular muscle paralysis; uveitis; interstitial keratitis; hypopyon; conjunctivitis; optic nerve atrophy; subconjunctival and retinal hemorrhages; ptosis; mydriasis; retinal venous occlusion.

Clinical

Toxemia and febrile paroxysms are separated by afebrile periods.

Laboratory

Diagnosis is confirmed by bone marrow aspirates, cerebrospinal fluids or spirochetes in peripheral smears.

Treatment

The drugs of choice include doxycycline, penicillin G, chloramphenicol or erythromycin.

BIBLIOGRAPHY

1. Akhter K, Dorsainvil PA, Cunha BA. (2012). Relapsing fever. [online] Available from www.emedicine.com/med/TOPIC1999.HTM. [Accessed September, 2013].

🖭 5Y. ROCKY MOUNTAIN SPOTTED FEVER

General

Acute systemic disease caused by *Rickettsia rickettsii* transmitted by a wood tick or dog tick.

Ocular

Conjunctivitis; optic atrophy; cotton-wool spots; scotoma; uveitis; optic neuritis; paralysis of accommodation; paralysis of extraocular muscles; retinal vascular occlusion; vitreal opacity; hypopyon; anterior uveitis with fibrin clots.

Clinical

Fever; chills; headache; muscle aches; rash.

Laboratory

Early diagnosis depends on clinical and epidemiological grounds. PCR has high sensitivity and specificity.

Treatment

Intravenous tetracycline and chloramphenicol should be started as soon as possible. Oral doxycycline, tetracycline and chloramphenicol may be considered but only if patient is not acutely ill.

🖭 BIBLIOGRAPHY

1. Cunha BA, O'Brien MS. (2011). Rocky mountain spotted fever. [online] Available from www.emedicine.com/oph/TOPIC503.HTM. [Accessed September, 2013].

🖭 5Z. SANDWICH INFECTIOUS KERATITIS SYNDROME (SIK SYNDROME)

General

Bacterial and fungal organisms infiltration of the interface between donor and host corneas following DLEK, DALK, DSAEK and anterior lamellar keratoplasty (ALK).

Clinical

None.

Ocular

Infectious infiltrates in the interface of the cornea which are white, small, irregular or circular.

Laboratory

Careful slit-lamp examination is essential and any interface infiltrate should be monitored closely. Cultures are difficult to get because the infection is intracorneal.

Treatment

Intensive antibiotic treatment regimen is necessary, if fungal infection is identified and the use of antifungal agents is recommended. If medical treatment fails, a therapeutic penetrating keratoplasty (TPK) may be necessary.

🖭 BIBLIOGRAPHY

1. John T, Park T. New techniques, new corneal complication. Sandwich infectious keratitis, or SIK syndrome, can be difficult to diagnose and manage. Rev Ophthalmol. 2009;16:3.
2. John T. Selective tissue corneal transplantation: a great step forward in global visual restoration. Expert Rev Ophthalmol. 2006;1(1):5-8.

🖭 5SAA. SUPERIOR LIMBIC KERATOCONJUNCTIVITIS (THEODORES SUPERIOR LIMBIC KERATOCONJUNCTIVITIS, SLK)

General

Corneal disease affecting the superior limbus.

Clinical

None.

Ocular

Hyperemia, thickened upper bulbar conjunctiva in a "corridor-like" distribution, fine papillary inflammation of superior palpebral conjunctival, punctate erosion over the superior and perilimbal cornea and superior filamentary keratopathy.

Laboratory

Giemsa-stained scraping of upper conjunctiva demonstrates keratinized cells.

Treatment

Topical lubricants and mast cells stabilizers, punctal plugs, silver nitrate treatment on upper tarsal and bulbar conjunctiva, bandage contact lens, brief focal applications of thermal cautery and recession of involved superior bulbar conjunctiva.

BIBLIOGRAPHY

1. Oakman JH. (2011). Superior limbic keratoconjunctivitis. [online] Available from www.emedicine.com/oph/TOPIC103.HTM. [Accessed September, 2013].

5SBB. PERIPHERAL ULCERATIVE KERATITIS

General

Ulceration in the peripheral cornea; relatively uncommon; may be presenting characteristics of a systemic disease.

Clinical

Connective and vasculitic disease; herpes simplex, varicella; HIV; syphilis; hepatitis; bacillary dysentery; *Salmonella*.

Ocular

Pain; foreign body sensation; tearing; photophobia; decreased visual acuity.

Laboratory

Testing should be focused on the suspected systemic disease.

Treatment

Local treatment is used for prevention and reduction of corneal damage. Systemic therapy is used for controlling the underlying disease. Tissue adhesives may be necessary for impending perforation. Keratectomy, conjunctival resection, amniotic membrane transplantation and keratoplasty may be necessary.

BIBLIOGRAPHY

1. Yu EN, Foster CS. (2012). Peripheral ulcerative keratitis. [online] Available from emedicine.medscape.com/article/1195980-overview. [Accessed September, 2013].

5SCC. ULTRAVIOLET KERATITIS

General

Radiation injury, ultraviolet (UV) absorbed by cornea, most commonly from welder's equipment but sun tanning beds, flood lamps, lightning and electric sparks can also be the cause.

Ocular

Foreign body sensation; irritation; pain; photophobia; reduced visual acuity; tearing and blepharospasm.

Laboratory

Slit-lamp examination with fluorescein uptake and straining along with history.

Treatment

Topical cycloplegic drops and antibiotic ointment; pressure patch is the traditional therapy. Some physicians feel that a pressure patch delays re-epithelialization and opt for cycloplegics and antibiotics only.

BIBLIOGRAPHY

1. Brozen R, Fromm C. (2011). Ultraviolet keratitis. [online] Available from emedicine.medscape.com/article/799025-overview. [Accessed September, 2013].

5SDD. VERNAL KERATOCONJUNCTIVITIS (ATOPIC KERATOCONJUNCTIVITIS, ALLERGIC CONJUNCTIVITIS, GIANT PAPILLARY CONJUNCTIVITIS)

General

Bilateral, chronic, severe allergy, more frequent in young males and during the spring time.

Clinical

Atopy present in half of the cases.

Ocular

Giant papillae conjunctivitis.

Laboratory

Diagnosis is made by clinical findings.

Treatment

Ocular lubricants, nonsteroidal anti-inflammatory and steroidal drops, oral nonsteroidal anti-inflammatory or steroids; supratarsal steroids; surgical excision, cryotherapy and beta irradiation of papillae.

BIBLIOGRAPHY

1. Ventocilla M, Bloomenstein MR, Majmudar PA. (2012). Allergic conjunctivitis. [online] Available from www.emedicine.com/oph/TOPIC85.HTM. [Accessed September, 2013].

6. TRAUMA

6A. CORNEAL ABRASIONS, CONTUSIONS, LACERATIONS AND PERFORATIONS

General

Loss of corneal epithelium from direct or indirect injury.

Clinical

None.

Ocular

Photophobia, tearing, eye pain, foreign body sensation, corneal abrasion, laceration or perforation.

Laboratory

Diagnosis is made by clinical findings.

Treatment

Topical antibiotic and cycloplegic agents, pain medication, pressure patching and bandage contact lens.

BIBLIOGRAPHY

1. Giri G. (2012). Corneoscleral laceration. [online] Available from www.emedicine.com/oph/TOPIC108.HTM. [Accessed September, 2013].Clinical: None
2. Verma A, Khan FH. (2011). Corneal abrasion. [online] Available from www.emedicine.com/oph/TOPIC247.HTM. [Accessed September, 2013].

6B. COGAN (1) SYNDROME (NONSYPHILITIC INTERSTITIAL KERATITIS)

General

Cause unknown; perhaps a generalized hypersensitivity reaction; most frequently affects young adults; unclear etiology; several studies suggest an autoimmunomediated process, possibly a vasculitis.

Ocular

Blepharospasm; lacrimation; congested conjunctival vessels; little or no reaction in anterior chamber but ciliary injection present; interstitial keratitis (unilateral or bilateral); granular-type infiltrates; patchy distribution in deeper stroma; later vascularization; conjunctivitis; corneal opacity; uveitis; nystagmus.

Clinical

Vestibuloauditory symptoms (similar to Ménière syndrome); nausea; vomiting; vertigo; tinnitus (abrupt onset); rapidly progressive deafness; loss of equilibration (*see* Ménière syndrome); aortic insufficiency; sensorineural testing; lacunar infarcts.

Laboratory

Leukocytosis in 75%, neutrophilia in 50%, mild eosinophilia in 17%, relative lymphopenia in 25%, anemia in 33%, thrombocytosis in 30% and ESR of greater than 20 in 75%.

Treatment

Corticosteroids and antibiotics are useful. Corneal transplantation may be necessary for corneal opacity.

⊟ BIBLIOGRAPHY

1. Majmudar PA. (2011). Interstitial keratitis overview of interstitial keratitis. [online] Available from www.emedicine.com/oph/TOPIC101.HTM. [Accessed September, 2013].

⊟ 6C. CORNEAL EDEMA (BULLOUS KERATOPATHY, EPITHELIAL EDEMA, STROMAL EDEMA)

General

It may be caused by endothelial dysfunction, corneal hypoxia and elevated IOP.

Clinical

None.

Ocular

Swelling of cornea, loss of vision, pain.

Laboratory

Diagnosis is made by clinical findings.

Treatment

Control IOP, hypertonic salt solution or ointment, soft contact lens, anterior stromal puncture or conjunctival flap, PTK, hair dryer held at arm's length and posterior lamellar keratoplasty.

⊟ BIBLIOGRAPHY

1. Taravella M, Walker M. (2012). Postoperative corneal edema. [online] Available from www.emedicine.com/oph/TOPIC64.HTM. [Accessed September, 2013].

⊟ 6D. CORNEAL EDEMA, POSTOPERATIVE

General

Irreversible corneal edemas are used as a complication of cataract surgery; it occur infrequently following cataract surgery; it occurs more frequently with anterior chamber IOL than posterior IOLs. There is an increased incidence in patients with Fuchs' corneal dystrophy. Older individuals with less endothelial reserve are more prone.

Clinical

None.

Ocular

Stromal and intercellular epithelial edema; bullous keratopathy; corneal dystrophy; poor vision; cornea guttata; discomfort.

Laboratory

Specular microscopy; endothelial layer photos; ultrasound pachymetry and optical pachymetry.

Treatment

Hypertonic agents such as Muro 128; bandage contact lenses may be useful for discomfort; corneal transplant and management of the intraocular lens may be necessary.

⊟ BIBLIOGRAPHY

1. Taravella M, Walker M. (2012). Postoperative corneal edema. [online] Available from emedicine.medscape.com/article/1193218-overview. [Accessed September, 2013].

⎘ 6E. DESCEMET MEMBRANE FOLDS

General

Descemet membrani is position between the stroma and the endothelial cell layer. Any conditon that may cause inflammation to the cornea or the anterior chamber can result in descemet membrane folds.

Clinical

Diagnosis is made by clinical findings.

Ocular

Corneal edema and anterior chamber inflammation. Ocular infections, inflammation after surgery, retained lens fragments, retinal detachment, endophthalmitis, trauma or injury, such as blunt trauma or chemical injury.

Treatment

Treat inflammation using steroidal, nonsteroidal, and osmotic agents. Surgical care via PK is available.

Laboratory

B-scan if the view of the posterior pole is obscured. Gonioscopy is performed to reveal lens fragments in the anterior chamber.

⎘ BIBLIOGRAPHY

1. Graham RH, Shuler MF. (2012). Descemet membrane folds. [online] Available from emedicine.medscape.com/article/1196103-overview. [Accessed September, 2013].

⎘ 6F. CORNEAL FOREIGN BODY

General

Foreign body lodged in the corneal epithelium usually metal, glass or organic material; may be superficial or embedded. It is seen in males more frequently than females secondary to their activities.

Clinical

None.

Ocular

Pain, photophobia, tearing, conjunctival and ciliary injection; epithelial defect; corneal edema; rust ring with metallic injury.

Laboratory

Slit-lamp examination; Seidel test; and if intraocular involvement is suspected, B-scan, orbital CT scan and ultrasound biomicroscopy.

Treatment

Removal with a sterile spud or needle under topical anesthesia; if a rust ring remains, a rust ring drill may be used. The patient is treated with antibiotics, cycloplegics and a pressure patch or bandage contact lens.

⎘ BIBLIOGRAPHY

1. Bashour M. (2012). Corneal foreign body treatment and management. [online] Available from emedicine.medscape.com/article/1195581-treatment. [Accessed September, 2013].

⎘ 6G. CORNEAL GRAFT REJECTION OR FAILURE

General

Five-year failure rate for grafts is approximately 35%, mostly due to rejection; immunologic response of the host to the donor corneal tissue; more frequent in individuals under the age of 60 years.

Clinical

None.

Ocular

Decreased visual acuity, redness, irritation, photophobia; epithelial, stromal and endothelial edema.

Laboratory

Diagnosis is made by clinical findings.

Treatment

Topical corticosteroids used aggressively; subconjunctival injections of corticosteroids; systemic corticosteroids.

IOP must be monitored and if the pressure becomes elevated, glaucoma medication will be necessary.

BIBLIOGRAPHY

1. Jacobs J, Taravella M. (2012). Corneal graft rejection. [online] Available from emedicine.medscape.com/article/1193505-overview. [Accessed September, 2013].

6H. HERPES SIMPLEX

General

Large, complex DNA virus.

Ocular

Conjunctivitis; keratitis; iridocyclitis; corneal ulcer; uveitis; hyphema; hypopyon; iris atrophy; cataract; scleritis; dacryoadenitis; blepharitis; acute retinal necrosis.

Clinical

Recurrent skin vesicles on lids, perioral area, nose and genitalia; meningitis, encephalitis.

Laboratory

Viral cultures.

Treatment

Antiviral therapy, topical or oral, is an effective treatment of epithelial herpes infection.

BIBLIOGRAPHY

1. Wang JC, Ritterband DC. (2012). Ophthalmologic manifestations of herpes simplex keratitis. [online] Available from www.emedicine.com/oph/TOPIC100.HTM. [Accessed September, 2013].

6I. CORNEAL MELT POSTOPERATIVE

General

Corneal melt may be associated with infectious, inflammatory or trophic causes. Two of the most common causes of corneal melt are: herpes simplex virus and retained lenticular material.

Ocular

Postoperative corneal melt can occur with almost all ocular operations. Some of the major surgeries include: pterygium surgery, refractive surgery, epikeratophakia, keratomileusis, keratoplasty, glaucoma surgeries, trabeculectomy, vitreous surgery, cataract, and rectus muscle surgery (rare).

Clinical

Sjögren syndrome, RA, lupus.

Treatment

Ocular and systemic treatments are recommended for such disorder.

Laboratory

Diagnosis is made by clinical findings.

BIBLIOGRAPHY

1. Verma A. (2011). Postoperative corneal melt. [online] Available from emedicine.medscape.com/article/1193347-overview. [Accessed September, 2013].

⊟ 6J. CORNEAL MUCOUS PLAQUES

General

Abnormal collections of a mixture of mucus, epithelial cells and proteinaceous and lipoidal material adhering to cornea.

Clinical

None.

Ocular

Corneal mucous plaque.

Laboratory

Diagnosis is made by clinical findings.

Treatment

Lubricants for dry eyes, cyclosporine A, steroids and non-steroidal anti-inflammatory agents may also be necessary.

⊟ BIBLIOGRAPHY

1. Graham RH. (2012). Corneal mucous plaques. [online] Available from www.emedicine.com/oph/TOPIC682.HTM. [Accessed September, 2013].

⊟ 6K. MYOPIA, INTRACORNEAL RINGS

General

The intrastromal corneal ring is a device designed to correct mild-to-moderate myopia by flattening the anterior curvature of the cornea.

Clinical

None.

Ocular

Inability to *see* well as distance; side effects of the surgery may include increased IOP, overcorrection, decrease corneal sensation, decrease in contrast sensitivity.

Laboratory

Refractive history including contact lens wear, keratometry, uncorrected and best corrected vision, slit-lamp examination, tonometry, manifest and cycloplegic refraction, dilated fundus examination.

Treatment

Glasses or contact lens can be used to correct myopia. If patient is unhappy with glasses or contact lens, intracorneal rings can be considered.

⊟ BIBLIOGRAPHY

1. Roque MR, Roque BL, Limbonsiong R, et al. (2012). Intracorneal rings myopia. [online] Available from emedicine.medscape.com/article/1221441-overview. [Accessed September, 2013].

⊟ 6L. NEOVASCULARIZATION, CORNEAL CONTACT LENS RELATED

General

Pathologic state in which new blood vessels extending in the corneal stroma from trauma, inflammation, infection, toxic insults secondary to contact lens usage.

Clinical

None.

Ocular

Vessel ingrowth into the cornea, ocular irritation.

Laboratory

Diagnosis is made by clinical findings.

Treatment

Observation, eliminate cause, topical steroid drops, reduced time for an individual using contact lens, corneal laser photocoagulation.

BIBLIOGRAPHY

1. Weissman BA, Yeung KK. (2011). Neovascularization, corneal, CL-related. [online] Available from emedicine.medscape.com/article/1195886-overview. [Accessed September, 2013].

6M. MUCOUS MEMBRANE PEMPHIGOID

General

Immune-mediated disease characterized by autoantibodies to the basement membrane zone at the subepithelial junction of the mucous membranes.

Ocular

Progressive cicatrizing conjunctivitis; symblepharon; corneal clouding.

Clinical

Nasal and oral mucosa cicatrization; trachea and esophagus cicatrization.

Laboratory

Diagnosis is made by clinical findings.

Treatment

No topical agent is effective. Systemic corticosteroids can control the progression of the disease. Surgeries include marginal rotation of the eyelid, mucous membrane grafting, retractor placation and fornix reconstruction.

BIBLIOGRAPHY

1. Foster CS, Hamam R, Letko E. (2011). Ophthalmologic manifestations of cicatricial pemphigoid. [online] Available from www.emedicine.com/oph/TOPIC83.HTM. [Accessed September, 2013].

6N. ULTRAVIOLET KERATITIS

General

Radiation injury, UV absorbed by cornea, most commonly from welder's equipment but sun tanning beds, flood lamps, lightning and electric sparks can also be the cause.

Ocular

Foreign body sensation; irritation; pain; photophobia; reduced visual acuity; tearing and blepharospasm.

Laboratory

Slit-lamp examination with fluorescein uptake and straining along with history.

Treatment

Topical cycloplegic drops and antibiotic ointment; pressure patch is the traditional therapy. Some physicians feel that a pressure patch delays re-epithelialization and opt for cycloplegics and antibiotics only.

BIBLIOGRAPHY

1. Brozen R, Fromm C. (2011). Ultraviolet keratitis. [online] Available from emedicine.medscape.com/article/799025-overview. [Accessed September, 2013].

CHAPTER
21

Extraocular Muscles

⊟ 1A. PARALYSIS OF SIXTH NERVE (ABDUCENS PALSY)

This type of paralysis produces palsy of the lateral rectus (LR) muscle with esotropia increasing when the eye is moved laterally. The course of the sixth nerve makes it more vulnerable to injury than other cranial nerves.

1. *Intracerebral*
   A. Foville syndrome (Foville peduncular syndrome)
   B. Gaucher disease (cerebroside lipidosis)
   C. Hydrocephalus
   †D. Inflammatory lesions such as meningoencephalitis, cerebellitis and abscess
   †E. Lateral ventricular cyst
   F. Leukemia
   G. Millard-Gubler syndrome (abducens-facial hemiplegia alternans)
   H. *Mycoplasma pneumoniae*
   †I. Nuclear aplasia—autosomal dominant
   J. Platybasia (cerebellomedullary malformation syndrome)
   †K. Spontaneous subdural hematoma
   L. Thrombosis or aneurysm of nutrient vessels to sixth nucleus-basilar artery
   M. Tumors—intracranial, pontine glioma, or metastatic tumor from breast, thyroid glands, or nasopharynx
      1. Primary
         a. Gliomas such as astrocytomas, ependymomas and medulloblastomas
         b. Other primary tumors, including meningiomas, pinealomas, craniopharyngiomas and hemangiomas
      †2. Metastatic lesions such as those from the nasopharynx, rhabdomyosarcoma (RMS) and neuroblastomas

   N. Wernicke encephalopathy-thiamine deficiency in alcoholics with sixth nerve palsy, paresis of horizontal conjugate gaze, nystagmus, ataxia and Korsakoff psychosis

2. *Intracranial*
   A. Carotid artery aneurysm (foramen lacerum syndrome)
   B. Cerebellopontine angle tumor such as acoustic neuroma, producing unilateral deafness, facial paralysis, diplopia and papilledema
   C. Chickenpox
   D. Coccidioidomycosis
   †E. Congenital absence of sixth nerve
   †F. Cushing syndrome II (angle tumor syndrome)
   G. Dandy-Walker syndrome (atresia of the foramen Magendie)
   H. Diphtheria
   I. Gradenigo syndrome—osteitis of petrous tip of pyramid following homolateral mastoid or middle ear infection; facial pain (fifth nerve involvement)
   J. Greig syndrome (ocular hypertelorism syndrome)
   K. Hydrophobia (rabies)
   L. Hydrocephalus (decreased intracranial pressure)
   †M. Increased intracranial pressure
   N. Malaria
   †O. Massive pituitary adenoma
   P. Measles
   Q. Meningitis
   R. Möbius syndrome (congenital paralysis of sixth and seventh nerves)
   S. Neuritis because of diseases such as diabetes mellitus, herpes zoster, poliomyelitis, lead or arsenic poisoning, multiple sclerosis (MS), syphilis, brucellosis

T. Ophthalmoplegic migraine syndrome

†U. Osteosarcoma

V. Passow syndrome (status dysraphicus syndrome)

W. Pseudotumor cerebri (Symonds syndrome)

X. Raymond syndrome (pontine syndrome)

Y. Relapsing polychondritis

†Z. Skeletal dysplasia (mental retardation, abducens palsy)-X-linked

†AA. Skull fractures—usually crush injury

†BB. Spontaneous dissection of the internal carotid artery

†CC. Subdural hematoma

DD. Trichinellosis

†EE. Tumor extension as chordoma

†FF. Vascular lesions, because of congenital aneurysm, arteriovenous fistulas, diabetes, hypertension

†GG. Water-soluble contrast myelography

3. *Lesions affecting exit of sixth nerve from cranial cavity*

A. Cavernous sinus syndrome (Foix syndrome)

†B. Le Fort I maxillary osteotomy

†C. Optic nerve sheath fenestration

D. Orbital apex lesion

†E. Percutaneous thermal ablation of trigeminal nerve rootlet

F. Sphenocavernous syndrome

G. Sphenopalatine fossa lesion—loss of tearing and paresis of second division of fifth nerve, most frequently because of malignant tumor

H. Superior orbital fissure syndrome

I. Tolosa-Hunt syndrome (painful ophthalmoplegia)

†J. Transient in newborns

4. *Other*

A. Cluster headache

B. Cretinism (hypothyroid goiter)

C. Duane syndrome (retraction syndrome)

D. Engelmann syndrome (hereditary multiple diaphyseal sclerosis)

†E. Following lumbar puncture (LP), lumbar anesthesia, or Pantopaque injection for myelography

F. Kahler disease (multiple myeloma)

G. Lupus erythematosus (Kaposi-Libman-Sacks syndrome)

H. Myasthenia gravis

†I. Optic nerve sheath fenestration (rare)

J. Preeclampsia

K. Sarcoidosis

†L. Secondary to immunization or viral illness

†M. Toxic substances such as arsenic, carbon tetrachloride, dichloroacetylene, dilantin, gold salts, isoniazid, nitrofuran, thalidomide, trichloroethylene, furaltadone (Altafur), lithium

---

†Indicates a general entry and therefore has not been described in detail in the text

Treatment

- Truly isolated cases often are benign. They can be followed with a serial examination, at least every 6 weeks, over a 6-month period to note decreasing symptoms (diplopia) and resolution of the paretic LR (increasing motility).

- Children with sixth nerve palsy who are in the amblyopic age group can be treated with an alternating patching to decrease their chances of developing any amblyopia in the paretic eye. Additionally, prescribing the full amount of hyperopic correction helps to decrease the esodeviation by relaxing the child's accommodative effort.

- Adult patients and those children beyond the amblyopic age can be patched or have their lenses "fogged" with clear tape or nail polish to reduce their diplopia. Fresnel prisms also can be prescribed as an alternative.

- Older patients in whom giant cell arteritis is a consideration should start the standard treatment with prednisone or intravenous methylprednisolone as soon as possible.

⊟ BIBLIOGRAPHY

1. Ehrenhaus MP, Hajee ME, Roy H. (2012). Abducens nerve palsy. [online] Available from www.emedicine.com/oph/TOPIC158.HTM. [Accessed September, 2013].

2. Lee CH, Hammel JM. (2013). Temporal arteritis in emergency medicine. [online] Available from www.emedicine.com/emerg/TOPIC568.HTM. [Accessed September, 2013].

3. Goodwin J. (2012). Oculomotor nerve palsy. [online] Available from www.emedicine.com/oph/TOPIC183.HTM. [Accessed September, 2013].

4. Lee AG, Berlie CL, Costello F. (2012). Ophthalmologic manifestations of multiple sclerosis. [online] Available from www.emedicine.com/oph/TOPIC179.HTM. [Accessed September, 2013].

5. Lopez JI, Bechtel KA, Rothrock JF. (2013). Pediatric headache. [online] Available from www.emedicine.com/emerg/TOPIC382.HTM. [Accessed September, 2013].

6. Nelson SL. (2013). Hydrocephalus. [online] Available from www.emedicine.com/neuro/TOPIC161.HTM. [Accessed September, 2013].

7. Bardorf CM, Stavern GV, Garcia-Valenzuela E. (2013). Horner syndrome. [online] Available from www.emedicine.com/oph/TOPIC336.HTM. [Accessed September, 2013].

8. Bennett NJ, Domachowske J, Abuhammour W. (2013). Pediatric rocky mountain spotted fever. [online] Available from www.emedicine.com/ped/TOPIC2709.HTM. [Accessed September, 2013].

9. Lewis RA. (2013). Chronic inflammatory demyelinating polyradiculoneuropathy. [online] Available from www.emedicine.com/neuro/TOPIC467.HTM. [Accessed September, 2013].

10. Robertson WC, Chawla J. (2012). Pediatric idiopathic intracranial hypertension. [online] Available from www.emedicine.com/neuro/TOPIC537.HTM. [Accessed September, 2013].

⊟ 1.1A. FOVILLE SYNDROME (FOVILLE PEDUNCULAR SYNDROME)

General

Pontine area tumor, hemorrhage, tuberculoma, MS, or unilateral obstruction of paramedian branches may cause clinical manifestations.

Ocular

Paralysis of cranial nerve VI; paralysis of conjugate movement to the side of the lesion; abduction or horizontal gaze deficit.

Clinical

Peripheral facial palsy; contralateral hemiplegia; headache; ipsilateral: facial weakness, loss of taste, facial analgesia, Homer syndrome and deafness.

Laboratory

Computed tomography (CT) and magnetic resonance imaging (MRI).

Treatment

See neurologist.

⊟ BIBLIOGRAPHY

1. Bedi HK, Devpura JC, Bomb BS. Clinical tuberculoma of pons presenting as Foville's syndrome. J Indian Med Assoc. 1973;61(4):184-5.
2. Foville AL. Note sur une Paralysie Peu Connue des Certains Muscles de l'Oeil, et Sa Liaison avec Quelques Points de l'Anatomie et la Physiologic de la Protuberance Annulaire. Bull Soc Anat (Paris). 1858;33:393.
3. Geeraets WJ. Ocular Syndromes, 3rd edition. Philadelphia, USA: Lea & Febiger; 1976.
4. Newman NJ. Third, fourth, and sixth nerve lesions and the cavernous sinus. In: Albert DM, Jakobiec FA, Miller JW, Azar DT, Blodi BA (Eds). Albert & Jakobiec's Principles and Practice of Ophthalmology, 3rd edition. Philadelphia, USA: WB Saunders; 1994. p. 2458.

⊟ 1.1B. GAUCHER SYNDROME (GLUCOCEREBROSIDE STORAGE DISEASE; GLUCOSYL CERAMIDE LIPIDOSIS; CEREBROSIDE LIPIDOSIS)

General

Storage of glucocerebroside in the reticuloendothelial system; autosomal recessive; occurs frequently in Jewish families; onset at any age; onset usually sudden in the infantile form; disease belongs to group of lipid storage disturbances such as ganglioside (Tay-Sachs), sphingomyelin (Niemann-Pick) and ceramide trihexoside (Fabry) (*see* Tay-Sachs syndrome; Niemann-Pick syndrome; Fabry syndrome); caused by glucosylceramide β-glucosidase (glucocerebrosidase) deficiency; psychomotor deterioration apparent before age of 6 months.

Ocular

Strabismus; brown-yellowish, wedge-shaped pinguecula; corneal clouding; oculomotor paralysis; gaze palsies.

Clinical

Infantile form: generalized hypertonia, opisthotonus, dysphagia, vomiting, laryngeal spasm, dyspnea; chronic form: hepatosplenomegaly, lymphadenopathy, mild-to-moderate anemia, yellowish-brown patchy skin pigmentation.

Laboratory

Infiltration by cells with "onion-peel" cytoplasm, called Gaucher cells, is caused by a lipid storage disorder (i.e. glucosylceramide lipidosis). Gaucher cells clog or infiltrate the bone marrow, spleen and liver.

Treatment

Treat the underlying disease and provide supportive measures for symptomatic patients. Treat anemia with packed red blood cell transfusions.

⊟ BIBLIOGRAPHY

1. Besa EC. (2013). Myelophthisic anemia. [online] Available from www.emedicine.com/med/TOPIC1562.HTM. [Accessed September, 2013].

⊟ 1.1C. EXTREME HYDROCEPHALUS SYNDROME (KLEEBLATTSCHÄDEL SYNDROME; CLOVERLEAF SKULL SYNDROME; HYDROCEPHALUS; CHONDRODYSTROPHICUS CONGENITA)

General

Secondary obstruction of cerebrospinal fluid (CSF) circulation caused by some primary disease such as maternal rubella, rhesus (Rh) incompatibility, or hydramnion; Arnold-Chiari syndrome has similar associated findings; almost all affected children are born dead.

Ocular

Exophthalmos with downward placement and downward rotation of the globes; propulsion of globes; upper lid retraction and lower lids covering almost half of the downwardly rotated cornea; nystagmus; strabismus; exposure keratitis; optic nerve atrophy.

Clinical

Extreme hydrocephalus; low-set ears; thin and spastic extremities with digital anomalies; convulsions; spina bifida.

Laboratory

CT, MRI, ultrasound through the anterior fontanelle.

Treatment

Surgical treatment is the preferred therapeutic option and shunts are performed in the majority of patients.

⊟ BIBLIOGRAPHY

1. Nelson SL (2013). Hydrocephalus. [online] Available from www.emedicine.com/neuro/TOPIC161.HTM. [Accessed September, 2013].

⊟ 1.1F. LEUKEMIA

General

Acute or chronic blood disorder.

Ocular

Engorgement of conjunctival vessels; papillary hypertrophy; aggregations of tumor cells in conjunctiva, choroid and orbit; secondary glaucoma; retinal venous engorgement and tortuosity with pronounced constrictions; retinal hemorrhages; retinal detachment; cotton-wool spots; macular edema; papilledema; optic atrophy; optic neuritis; paralysis of extraocular muscles; hypopyon; vitreous opacities; retinal sea fans; perilimbal subconjunctival infiltrates; corneal leukemic infiltration (rare); shallow serous retinal detachments; hyphema; iris neovascularization; central retinal vein occlusion; vitreous infiltrates.

Clinical

Frequent involvement of central nervous system (CNS); intracranial hemorrhage; thrombocytopenia; rising white cell count.

Laboratory

Complete blood count (CBC) and differential, bone marrow aspiration, immunophenotyping, chromosomal analysis.

Treatment

Chemotherapy with or without radiotherapy.

⊟ BIBLIOGRAPHY

1. Wu L, Evans T, Martinez J. (2012). Leukemias. [online] Available from www.emedicine.com/oph/TOPIC489.HTM. [Accessed September, 2013].

⊡ 1.1G. MILLARD-GUBLER SYNDROME (ABDUCENS-FACIAL HEMIPLEGIA ALTERNANS)

General

Vascular, infectious, or tumorous lesion at the base of the pons affecting the nuclei of the sixth and seventh nerves and fibers of the pyramidal tract; demyelinating disease.

Ocular

Diplopia; esotropia; paralysis external rectus muscle (often bilateral); in unilateral cases, there is deviation of eyes to side opposite lesion and inability to move them toward side of lesion; abduction of eye prevented by destruction of sixth nerve nucleus; opposite eye cannot be voluntarily adducted but can converge and move in this position by rotatory and caloric stimulation.

Clinical

Ipsilateral facial paralysis; contralateral hemiplegia of arm and leg from involvement of pyramidal tract.

Laboratory/Diplopia

None.

Treatment/Diplopia

Occluding one eye, Fresnel prism, anticholinergic agent and cortisteroids may be needed in the treatment of myasthenia gravis.

⊡ BIBLIOGRAPHY

1. Geeraets WJ. Ocular Syndromes, 3rd edition. Philadelphia, USA: Lea & Febiger; 1976.
2. Gubler A. De l'Hemiplegie Alterne Envisagee Comme Signe de Lesion de la Protuberance Annulaire et Comme Preuve de la Decussation des Nerfs Faciaux. Gaz Hebd Med Chir. 1856;3:749,789,811.
3. Minderhoud JM. Diagnostic significance of symptomatology in brain stem ischaemic infarction. Eur Neurol. 1971;5(6):343-53.
4. Newman NJ. Third, fourth and sixth nerve lesions and the cavernous sinus. In: Albert DM, Jakobiec FA, Miller JW, Azar DT, Blodi BA (Eds). Albert & Jakobiec's Principles and Practice of Ophthalmology, 3rd edition. Philadelphia, USA: WB Saunders; 1994. p. 2458.

⊡ 1.1H. PNEUMOCOCCAL INFECTIONS (STREPTOCOCCUS PNEUMONIAE INFECTIONS)

General

Gram-positive diplococcus *Streptococcus pneumoniae;* some strains are encapsulated while others are not; ocular infections usually are caused by the encapsulated strains; conjunctivitis and corneal scarring produced in an animal model have been attributed to a hemolytic cytolytic exopeptidase.

Ocular

Hypopyon; conjunctivitis; keratitis; corneal ulcer; endophthalmitis; dacryocystitis; uveitis; orbital cellulitis; secondary glaucoma; ophthalmia neonatorum.

Clinical

Upper respiratory infection; chills; sharp pain in hemithorax; cough with sputum production; fever; headache; gastrointestinal symptoms.

Laboratory

Gram stain demonstrates Gram-positive cocci in pairs. The unattached end of each coccus is slightly pointed outward.

Treatment

Impetigo, oral antibiotics and topical antibiotic ointment; preseptal cellulitis, oral antibiotics; orbital cellulitis, need team of infectious disease specialist, otolaryngologist and ophthalmologist to develop plan of therapy; dacryocystitis, oral and topical antibiotics, dacryocystorhinostomy may be necessary; conjunctivitis, topical antibiotic; keratitis, topical antibiotics; poststreptococcal reactive arthritis can occur with uveitis, topical steroids and cycloplegics; endophthalmitis, prompt and aggressive therapy with topical, intravitreal and sometimes systemic antibiotics and pars plana vitrectomy; post-refractive surgery keratitis, flap raised, cultured and treated. Occasionally the flap should be amputated.

⊡ BIBLIOGRAPHY

1. Muench DF, Rajnik M. (2013). Pneumococcal infections. [online] Available from www.emedicine.com/med/TOPIC1848.HTM. [Accessed September, 2013].

1.1J. ARNOLD-CHIARI SYNDROME (PLATYBASIA SYNDROME; CEREBELLOMEDULLARY MALFORMATION SYNDROME; BASILAR IMPRESSIONS)

General

Malformation of the hindbrain; developmental deformity of the occipital bone and upper cervical spine; recognized in children or adults; clinical picture may be indistinguishable from that of Dandy-Walker syndrome in infants.

Ocular

Horizontal, vertical and rotary forms of nystagmus; vertical nystagmus in both upgaze and downgaze is most common; papilledema; esotropia; Duane's retraction syndrome (association); oscillopsia.

Clinical

Hydrocephalus; cerebellar ataxia; bilateral pyramidal tract signs.

Laboratory

CT scans are used most commonly for the diagnosis of hydrocephalus and for the evaluation of suspected shunt malfunction.

Treatment

Early recognition and treatment is important because of the potential life-threatening symptoms. Early surgical intervention, especially in infants may prevent irreversible changes and death.

BIBLIOGRAPHY

1. Incesu L, Khosla A, Aiello MR. (2011). Imaging in Chiari II malformation. [online] Available from www.emedicine.com/radio/TOPIC150.HTM. [Accessed September, 2013].

1.1L. VERTEBRAL BASILAR ARTERY SYNDROME (INTRANUCLEAR OPHTHALMOPLEGIA)

General

"Whiplash" injury with hyperextension of the neck followed by rapid forward movement of the head or osteoarthritis of the cervical spine, cervical ribs (*see* craniocervical syndrome).

Ocular

Nystagmus (postural); internuclear ophthalmoplegia; visual deterioration; visual hallucinations may be associated with a decrease in consciousness; homonymous hemianopsia (bilateral); contralateral hemianopic visual field defect.

Clinical

Severe, throbbing occipital headache associated with neck pain; vertigo from ischemia of the internal auditory artery, from the temporoparietal cortex or from ischemia in the lateral tegmentum of the pons; nausea and vomiting; ataxia; hemiparesis; quadriplegia; dysarthria; dysphagia; deafness; dyslexia; atonia; confusion; coma; tremor.

Laboratory/Ocular

Diagnosis is made by clinical findings.

Treatment

Nystagmus: Seesaw—visual field to consider neoplastic or vascular etiologies. Upbeat nystagmus—may indicate MS, cerebellar degeneration, tumors or infarcts. Treatment is directed toward identification and resolution of underlying cause. Downbeat nystagmus—affects the cerebellum or craniocervical junction including Arnold-Chiari malformation, MS, trauma, tumor, infarction and many toxic metabolic entities. MRI may indicate a surgically correctable lesion. "Periodic alternating nystagmus" is continuous horizontal nystagmus from stroke, tumor, MS, trauma, infection, drug intoxication. It can occur from cataract, vitreous hemorrhage or optic atrophy.

BIBLIOGRAPHY

1. Caplan LR. Posterior cerebral artery syndrome. In: Vinken PJ, Bruyn GW, Klawans HL (Eds). Handbook of Clinical Neurology, Vascular Diseases (part I, vol. 53). Amsterdam: Elsevier Science; 1988.
2. Caplan LR. "Top of the basilar" syndrome. Neurology. 1980;30:72-9.
3. Hoyt WF. Transient bilateral blurring of vision: considerations of an episodic ischemic symptom of vertebral-basilar insufficiency. Arch Ophthalmol. 1963;70:746.
4. Millikan CH, Siekert RG. Studies in cerebrovascular disease: I. the syndrome of intermittent insufficiency of the basilar arterial system. Proc Staff Meet Mayo Clin. 1955;30:61-8.

🗗 1.1M1. CRANIOPHARYNGIOMA

General

Benign congenital tumors arising from epithelial remnants of Rathke pouch; most common nonglial intracranial tumors in childhood; second most common sellar-parasellar tumor primarily in children or young adults; 35% of cases occur in patients over age of 40 years.

Ocular

Paresis of third or sixth nerve; optic nerve atrophy; optic neuritis; papilledema; dilation of pupil; diplopia; hemianopsia; nystagmus; scotoma; visual field defects; visual loss.

Clinical

Hydrocephalus; infantilism; diabetes insipidus; abnormal sexual development; headaches; acute aseptic meningitis.

Laboratory

Cranial CT and MRI are the current imaging standards.

Treatment

Although controversial, aggressive surgical treatment to attempt gross total resection is sometimes considered. Second option is planned limited surgery followed by radiotherapy.

🗗 BIBLIOGRAPHY

1. Bobustuc GC, Groves MD, Fuller GN, et al. (2012). Craniopharyngioma. [online] Available from www.emedicine.com/neuro/TOPIC584.HTM. [Accessed September, 2013].

🗗 1.1M1. HEMANGIOMA

General

It can occur throughout the body, but particularly in the head; primary intraosseous orbital hemangiomas is rare; capillary hemangioma of the orbit and eyelids generally is unilateral.

Ocular

Hemangiomas of lids or orbit; ptosis; strabismus; amblyopia; proptosis; optic atrophy; hypermetropia; cavernous hemangiomas are the most common benign orbital tumors of adults.

Clinical

Ipsilateral hemangiomas of the brain and meninges.

Laboratory

Neuroimaging can be of great assistance in making the diagnosis.

Treatment

Most of these lesions regress on their own; there is no need to intervention. If spontaneous regression does not occur corticosteroids, in various formulations, may be considered. Topical application of timolol has been useful in some cases.

🗗 BIBLIOGRAPHY

1. Karmel M. Topical timolol for capillary hemangioma. Eyenet. 2010.
2. Seiff S, Zwick OM, DeAngelis DD, et al. (2011). Capillary hemangioma. [online] Available from www.emedicine.com/oph/TOPIC691.HTM. [Accessed September, 2013].

1.1N. WERNICKE SYNDROME I (SUPERIOR HEMORRHAGIC POLIOENCEPHALO-PATHIC SYNDROME; HEMORRHAGIC POLIOENCEPHALITIS SUPERIOR SYNDROME; ENCEPHALITIS HEMORRHAGICA SUPERIORIS; AVITAMINOSIS B; THIAMINE DEFICIENCY; BERIBERI; GAYET-WERNICKE SYNDROME; WERNICKE-KORSAKOFF SYNDROME) PTOSIS

General

Lack of vitamin B or thiamine; focal vascular lesions in the gray matter around third and fourth ventricles and Sylvian aqueduct; alcoholics (adults); beriberi of all ages.

Ocular

Ptosis; acute bilateral nuclear ophthalmoplegia; complete ophthalmoplegia; retinal hemorrhages; optic atrophy; optic neuritis; conjunctivitis; blepharitis; nutritional amblyopia; central scotoma; papilledema; nystagmus; absolute pupillary paralysis or Argyll Robertson pupils; accommodative palsy.

Clinical

Early prostration; lethargy; irritability; stupor; delirium; mental disturbances to Korsakoff psychosis; ataxia; tremors; peripheral neuritis; anorexia; vomiting; insomnia; perspiration; tachycardia; hallucinations; retrograde amnesia; apathy; anxiety; fear; defective concentration; cardiomyopathy.

Laboratory

Electrolyte studies, serum thiamine levels, CBC. Evaluation of hypoxemia, hypercarbia, acidosis, or alkalosis. Serum/urine toxin drug screen and liver enzymes.

Treatment

Parenteral thiamine is the treatment of choice.

BIBLIOGRAPHY

1. Xiong GL, Kenedi CA. (2013). Wernicke-Korsakoff syndrome. [online] Available from www.emedicine.com/med/TOPIC2405.HTM. [Accessed September, 2013].

1.2A. FORAMEN LACERUM SYNDROME (ANEURYSM OF INTERNAL CAROTID ARTERY SYNDROME)

General

Most commonly caused by congenital aneurysm involving the intradural portion of the carotid artery.

Ocular

Periorbital pain; ptosis; oculomotor paralysis with ptosis, diplopia, and internal ophthalmoplegia; cranial nerves IV and VI may be involved; homonymous hemianopia (occasionally); loss of pupillary reflexes for light and accommodation; papilledema; optic atrophy.

Clinical

Meningism; mental disturbances; unilateral frontal or orbital headache; migraine attacks.

Laboratory

CT, MRI, angiography, magnetic resonance angiography (MRA).

Treatment

Endovascular balloon occlusion.

BIBLIOGRAPHY

1. Dailey EJ, Holloway JA, Murto RE, et al. Evaluation of ocular signs and symptoms in cerebral aneurysms. Arch Ophthalmol. 1964;71:463-74.
2. Geeraets WJ. Ocular syndromes, 3rd edition. Philadelphia: Lea & Febiger; 1976.
3. Misra M, Mohanty AB, Rath S. Giant aneurysm of internal carotid artery presenting features of retrobulbar neuritis. Indian J Ophthalmol. 1991;39:28-9.

1.2B. CUSHING (2) SYNDROME (ANGLE TUMOR SYNDROME; CEREBELLOPONTINE ANGLE SYNDROME; PONTOCEREBELLAR ANGLE TUMOR SYNDROME; ACOUSTIC NEUROMA SYNDROME)

General

Tumor involving cranial nerves V, VI, VII and VIII, and brainstem; occurs between ages of 30 years and 45 years.

Ocular

Paresis orbicularis muscle (VII); paresis external rectus muscle (VI); mixed nystagmus with head tilt; palsies of extraocular muscles are accounted for by increased intracranial pressure if the aqueduct of Sylvius is closed by the growing tumor; decreased corneal reflex V (homolateral and early sign); bilateral papilledema (increased intracranial pressure).

Clinical

Deafness (homolateral); labyrinth function disturbed or lost; tinnitus; hyperesthesia of the face; homolateral facial nerve paresis (total paralysis rare); hoarseness; difficulties in swallowing; unilateral limb ataxia; gait ataxia; nuchal headache; emesis; facial pain, numbness and paresis; progressive unilateral hearing loss.

Laboratory

The diagnostic test for acoustic tumors is gadolinium-enhanced MRI.

Treatment

Surgical excision of the tumor, arresting tumor growth using stereotactic radiation therapy, careful serial observation.

BIBLIOGRAPHY

1. Kutz JW, Roland PS, Isaacson B. (2012). Acoustic neuroma. [online] Available from www.emedicine.com/ent/TOPIC239.HTM. [Accessed September, 2013].

1.2C. CHICKENPOX (VARICELLA)

General

Acute exanthematous disease; highly contagious; children between ages of 2 and 8 years.

Ocular

Conjunctival ulcer; corneal ulcer; descemetocele; corneal opacity; keratitis; paresis of third, fourth and sixth nerves; optic neuritis; papilledema; retinitis; hemorrhagic retinopathy; uveitis; cataract; paralytic mydriasis; phthisis bulbi; unifocal choroiditis; dendritic keratitis; acute retinal necrosis [in a patient with acquired immunodeficiency syndrome (AIDS)]; disciform keratitis.

Clinical

Fever; malaise; rash; pruritus.

Laboratory

Diagnosis is made by clinical findings.

Treatment

Isolation oral antihistamines, such as diphenhydramine and hydroxyzine, are used for severe pruritus and acetaminophen is recommended for use for the reduction of fever.

BIBLIOGRAPHY

1. Bechtel KA, Chatterjee A, Lichenstein R, et al. (2013). Pediatric chickenpox. [online] Available from www.emedicine.com/emerg/TOPIC367.HTM. [Accessed September, 2013].

🖥 1.2D. COCCIDIOIDOMYCOSIS (VALLEY FEVER, SAN JOAQUIN FEVER)

General

It is caused by fungus *Coccidioides immitis*.

Ocular

Conjunctivitis; choroiditis; uveitis; retinal hemorrhages; vitreal opacity; vitreal floaters; episcleritis; hypopyon; granulomatous lesion of optic nerve head; paralysis of sixth cranial nerve; secondary glaucoma; papilledema; mutton fat keratitic precipitates; necrotizing granulomatous conjunctivitis; iridocyclitis.

Clinical

Mild respiratory illness; cavity lung lesion.

Laboratory

Routine culture media, IgM antibody for acute, IgG antibody for present or past infection.

Treatment

Systemic fluconazole or amphotericin B is the treatment of choice. Ocular treatment includes topical amphotericin B and use of steroids sparingly.

🖥 BIBLIOGRAPHY

1. Hospenthal DR, Thompson GR, Oppenheimer AP, et al. (2013). Coccidioidomycosis. [online] Available from www.emedicine.com/ped/TOPIC423.HTM. [Accessed September, 2013].

🖥 1.2G. DANDY-WALKER SYNDROME (ATRESIA OF THE FORAMEN OF MAGENDIE)

General

Manifested in infants; malformation and stenosis of the foramina of Luschka and Magendie; dilation of fourth ventricle.

Ocular

Ptosis; sixth nerve paralysis; papilledema.

Clinical

Hydrocephalus (varies in severity) with enlargement of the skull and thinning of the bone predominantly in occipital region; loss of tendon reflexes; basilar impression; scoliosis; hydromelia.

Laboratory

CT, MRI, ultrasound and angiography.

Treatment

Shunt to treat associated hydrocephalus.

🖥 BIBLIOGRAPHY

1. Incesu L, Khosla A. (2013). Imaging in Dandy-Walker malformation. [online] Available from www.emedicine.com/radio/TOPIC206.HTM. [Accessed September, 2013].

🖥 1.2H. DIPHTHERIA

General

Acute infectious disease caused by *Corynebacterium diphtheriae*; severity is dependent upon the amount of exotoxin absorbed prior to initiation of specific therapy.

Ocular

Conjunctivitis; xerophthalmia; keratitis; corneal ulcer; blepharitis; cellulitis of lid; meibomianitis; ptosis; dacryocystitis; cataract; central retinal artery occlusion; optic neuritis; accommodative spasm or paralysis; convergence paralysis; divergence paralysis; paralysis of third, fourth, or sixth nerve; paralysis of accommodation (in children); ocular motor nerve paresis; choroiditis; cranial neuropathies involving the trigeminal, vagus, and hypoglossal cranial nerves; myocarditis.

Clinical

Local inflammatory lesion, with effect on heart, kidneys and nervous system.

Laboratory

Gram-positive rods commonly affect children younger than 10 years.

Treatment

Systemic treatment involves use of diphtheria antitoxin and antibiotics. Ocular treatment includes diphtheria antitoxin and high titer y-globulin preparation. Topical penicillin G ointment helps to eradicate the bacilli.

BIBLIOGRAPHY

1. Demirci CS, Abuhammour W. (2013). Pediatric diphtheria. [online] Available from www.emedicine.com/ped/TOPIC596.HTM. [Accessed September, 2013].

1.2I. GRADENIGO SYNDROME (TEMPORAL SYNDROME; LANNOIS-GRADENIGO SYNDROME)

General

It is caused by extradural abscess of the petrous portion of the temporal bone; good prognosis.

Ocular

Ipsilateral paralysis (cranial nerve VI); transient involvement of cranial nerves III and IV occasionally present; severe pain in area of ophthalmic branch (cranial nerve V); photophobia; lacrimation; reduced corneal sensitivity; optic nerve involvement occasionally present.

Clinical

Inner ear infection with deafness; mastoiditis; facial paresis possible; temperature may be elevated; meningeal signs possible; can occur rarely as a complication of otitis media.

Laboratory

CT and MRI.

Treatment

See otolaryngologist.

BIBLIOGRAPHY

1. De Graaf J, Cats H, de Jager AE, et al. Gradenigo's syndrome: a rare complication of otitis media. Clin Neurol Neurosurg. 1988;90(3):237-9.
2. Gradenigro G. A special syndrome of endocranial otitic complications. Ann Otol Rhinol Laryngol. 1904;13:637.
3. Joffe WS. Clinical nerve disease. Int Ophthalmol Clin. 1967;7(4):823-38.

1.2J. GREIG SYNDROME (OCULAR HYPERTELORISM SYNDROME; HYPERTELORISM; PRIMARY EMBRYONIC HYPERTELORISM; HYPERTELORISM OCULARIS)

General

Condition is rare; sporadic or hereditary; autosomal dominant or sex linked; if not associated with mental deficiency, then adequate mental and physical development is found.

Ocular

Hypertelorism (wide spacing of orbits); enophthalmos; epicanthus; deformities of eyelids and brows; defects of the palpebral fissure; bilateral sixth nerve paralysis; esotropia; astigmatism; optic atrophy by tension on the optic nerve; strabismus.

Clinical

Skull may show mild malformations, including bitemporal eminences and decreased anteroposterior diameter; harelip; high-arched palate; cleft palate; broad and flat nasal root; mental impairment.

Laboratory

Diagnosis is made by clinical findings.

Treatment

Minor degrees of deformity (referred to as telecanthus) can be corrected by removing a small amount of bone in the midline. A limited frontal craniotomy is performed in the midline osteotomy.

BIBLIOGRAPHY

1. Jackson IT, Malhotra G. (2012). Congenital syndromes. [online] Available from www.emedicine.com/plastic/TOPIC183.HTM. [Accessed September, 2013].

1.2K. HYDROPHOBIA (LYSSA; RABIES)

General

Acute viral zoonosis of the CNS.

Ocular

Lid retraction; widening of palpebral fissure; retinal hemorrhages; mydriasis; paralysis of third, fourth, fifth, or seventh nerve; bilateral optic neuritis; branch retinal artery occlusion; vaccine-induced autoimmune demyelinative optic neuritis.

Clinical

Fever; headache; nausea; numbness; tingling; acute sensitiveness to sound and light; laryngeal and pharyngeal spasms; increased muscle tonus; convulsions; delirium; coma; death.

Laboratory

Saliva can be tested by virus isolation or reverse transcription followed by polymerase chain reaction (PCR). Suspected infections animal should be quarantined for 10 days.

Treatment

Before the onset of symptoms, both passive and active immunizations are effective for preventing progression to full-blown rabies. In exposures to high-risk species, initiate treatment immediately pending laboratory examination of the animal, if it is caught.

BIBLIOGRAPHY

1. Gompf SG, Pham TM, Somboonwit C, et al. (2013). Rabies. [online] Available from www.emedicine.com/med/TOPIC1374.HTM. [Accessed September, 2013].

1.2L. EXTREME HYDROCEPHALUS SYNDROME (KLEEBLATTSCHÄDEL SYNDROME; CLOVERLEAF SKULL SYNDROME; HYDROCEPHALUS; CHONDRODYSTROPHICUS CONGENITA)

General

Secondary obstruction of CSF circulation caused by some primary disease such as maternal rubella, Rh incompatibility, or hydramnion; Arnold-Chiari syndrome has similar associated findings; almost all affected children are born dead.

Ocular

Exophthalmos with downward placement and downward rotation of the globes; propulsion of globes; upper lid retraction and lower lids covering almost half of the downwardly rotated cornea; nystagmus; strabismus; exposure keratitis; optic nerve atrophy.

Clinical

Extreme hydrocephalus; low-set ears; thin and spastic extremities with digital anomalies; convulsions; spina bifida.

Laboratory

CT, MRI, ultrasound through the anterior fontanel.

Treatment

Surgical treatment is the preferred therapeutic option and shunts are performed in the majority of patients.

BIBLIOGRAPHY

1. Nelson SL, Murro AM, Talavera F, et al. (2013). Hydrocephalus. [online] Available from www.emedicine.com/neuro/TOPIC161.HTM. [Accessed September, 2013].

⊟ 1.2N. MALARIA

General

It is caused by *Plasmodium* which is transmitted by mosquito bite, blood transfusion, or contaminated needles and syringes.

Ocular

Proliferative retinitis; vascular embolism; keratitis; ocular herpes simplex; blepharitis; optic atrophy; papilledema; papillitis; optic neuritis; anisocoria; Argyll Robertson pupil; vitreal hemorrhages and opacity; cataract; myopia; strabismus; uveitis; scleral icterus; scotoma; lagophthalmos; ptosis; subconjunctival hemorrhages; paralysis of third, fourth, or sixth nerve; epibulbar hemorrhage involving the conjunctiva, episclera, tendinous insertion of the medial rectus.

Clinical

Fever; anemia; splenomegaly; death.

Laboratory

Blood smear.

Treatment

Consult infectious disease specialist.

⊟ BIBLIOGRAPHY

1. Perez-Jorge EV, Herchline TE. (2013). Malaria. [online] Available from www.emedicine.com/med/TOPIC1385.HTM. [Accessed September, 2013].

⊟ 1.2P. MEASLES (MORBILLI; RUBEOLA)

General

Acute, extremely communicable disease that affects young school-aged children; caused by paramyxovirus.

Ocular

Hypopyon; uveitis; conjunctivitis; Koplik (Hirschberg) spots of conjunctiva; keratitis; corneal ulcer; cellulitis of lid; dacryocystitis; congenital cataract; optic atrophy; optic neuritis; strabismus; pigmentary retinopathy; iris prolapse; hemianopsia; secondary glaucoma; central retinal artery occlusion; orbital cellulitis; accommodative spasm; paralysis of sixth nerve; keratoconus.

Clinical

Maculopapular rash; fever.

Laboratory

Diagnosis is made by clinical findings.

Treatment

Good hydration.

⊟ BIBLIOGRAPHY

1. Chen SS, Fennelly G. (2013). Measles. [online] Available from www.emedicine.com/derm/TOPIC259.HTM. [Accessed September, 2013].

⊟ 1.2Q. MENINGOCOCCEMIA (NEISSERIA MENINGITIDES; MENINGITIS)

General

Systemic bacterial infection caused by *Neisseria meningitides*; can be present chronically in patients with immune deficiencies including deficient complement levels.

Ocular

Photophobia; conjunctivitis; chemosis; keratitis; uveitis; panophthalmitis; retinal endophlebitis; macular edema; papillitis; optic neuritis; paresis of sixth or seventh nerve; nystagmus; miosis; hippus; cortical blindness; papilledema (rare); conjunctival petechiae; strabismus.

Clinical

Meningitis; fever; malaise; joint pain; splenic enlargement.

Laboratory

Cultures from blood, spinal fluid, or joint fluid.

Treatment

Treat with antibiotics promptly.

🗗 BIBLIOGRAPHY

1. Javid MH, Ahmed SH. (2013). Meningococcemia. [online] Available from www.emedicine.com/med/TOPIC1445.HTM. [Accessed September, 2013].

🗗 1.2R. MÖBIUS II SYNDROME (CONGENITAL FACIAL DIPLEGIA; CONGENITAL PARALYSIS OF THE SIXTH AND SEVENTH NERVES; CONGENITAL OCULOFACIAL PARALYSIS; VON GRAEFES SYNDROME)

General

Congenital; possibly failure of development of facial nerve cells or primary defect of muscles deriving from first two brachial arches or both; recovery in a few weeks or non-progressive permanent paralysis of face; asymmetrical; if incomplete, usually spares lower face and platysma.

Ocular

Proptosis; ptosis; weakness of abductor muscles; normal convergence; limitation to internal rotation in lateral movements; esotropia.

Clinical

Facial diplegia; deafness; loss of vestibular responses; webbed fingers or toes; clubfoot.

Laboratory

Diagnosis is made by clinical findings.

Treatment

Ptosis: If visual acuity is affected most cases require surgical correction and there are several procedures that may be used including levator resection, repair or advancement and Fasanella-Servat.

🗗 BIBLIOGRAPHY

1. Abbott RL, Metz HS, Weber AA. Saccadic velocity studies in Möbius syndrome. Ann Ophthalmol. 1978;10:619-23.
2. Fenichel GM. Congenital facial asymmetry (aplasia of facial muscles). In: Fenichel GM (ed). Clinical pediatric neurology, 2nd edition. Philadelphia: WB Saunders; 1993. pp. 341-2.
3. Kawai M, Momoi T, Fujii T, et al. The syndrome of Möbius sequence, peripheral neuropathy, and hypogonadotropic hypogonadism. Am J Med Genet. 1990;37:578-82.
4. Menkes JH, Kenneth T. Möbius syndrome. In: Menkes JH (ed). Textbook of child neurology, 5th edition. Baltimore: Williams & Wilkins; 1995. pp. 309-10.
5. Merz M, Wójtowicz S. The Möbius syndrome. Report of electromyographic examinations in two cases. Am J Ophthalmol. 1967;63(4):837-40.
6. Möbius PJ. über angeborene doppelseitige Abducens-Facialislahmung. Munch Med Wochenschr. 1888;35:91-108.
7. Pucket CL, Beg SA. Facial reanimation in Möbius syndrome. South Med J. 1978;71(12):1498-501.

🗗 1.2S. DIABETES MELLITUS

General

Complex disorder of carbohydrate, lipid and protein metabolism characterized by hyperglycemia and a relative or total lack of insulin. Development is influenced by both genetic and environmental factors. Most commonly occurs in middle or late life (type II) and is seen most commonly in the obese. Diabetes can occur in the 1st or 2nd decade of life (type I) and usually involves the lack of insulin production by the pancreas and the need for insulin therapy.

Clinical

Atherosclerosis, nephropathy, neuropathy, polyuria, polydipsia, polyphagia, obesity, elevated plasma glucose and elevated A1C.

Ocular

Diabetic retinopathy, vitreous hemorrhage, macular edema, cataract, glaucoma, asteroid hyalosis, extraocular muscle paralysis, rubeosis iridis, corneal hypesthesia, optic nerve atrophy; papillopathy.

Laboratory

Diagnosis made by fasting plasma glucose of greater than 126 mg/dL and 2-hour post-glucose load (75 g) plasma glucose of greater than 200 mg/dL and confirmed by repeat test.

Treatment

Goals include elimination of symptoms, by reduction of blood sugar and blood pressure. Smoking cessation, aspirin therapy, weight loss, exercise, diabetic diet as well as oral medication and/or insulin are all used in the treatment of diabetes. Diabetic retinopathy is most successfully treated with retinal photocoagulation. Pars plana vitrectomy is sometimes necessary to remove vitreous hemorrhage. Other ocular problems caused by diabetes such as cataracts and glaucoma are treated in traditional methods.

BIBLIOGRAPHY

1. Khardori R. (2013). Type 2 diabetes mellitus. [online] Available from www.emedicine.medscape.com/article/117853-overview. [Accessed September, 2013].

1.2S. HERPES ZOSTER

General

Caused by varicella zoster virus; about 75% of cases occur in persons over age of 45 years; condition is more frequent with advancing age and in patients who are immunocompromised by drugs or disease; in particular, an increasing number of patients with herpes zoster ophthalmicus are immunosuppressed.

Ocular

Conjunctivitis; keratitis; recurrent corneal ulcer; neuralgia; zoster rash of eyelids; uveitis; iris atrophy; scleritis; cataract; optic neuritis; paralysis of third nerve; proptosis; paralysis of lids; orbital apex syndrome; retinitis; neurotrophic keratitis; acute retinal necrosis; progressive outer retinal necrosis; ocular motor nerve pareses; tonic pupil; encephalitis; vasculitis.

Clinical

Local lesions involving the posterior or root ganglia; nerve damage; tissue scarring.

Laboratory

Diagnosed mostly on the basis of the characteristic pain and appearance of the dermatomal rashes.

Treatment

Antiviral agents, systemic corticosteroids, antidepressants and adequate pain control. Immunocompetent adults aged 60 years or older, benefit from receipt of the herpes zoster vaccine and have a lower incidence of herpes zoster.

BIBLIOGRAPHY

1. Ghaznawi N, Virdi A, Dayan A, et al. Herpes Zoster Ophthalmicus: Comparison of disease in patients 60 years and older versus younger than 60 years. Ophthalmology. 2011;118:2242-50.
2. Tseng HF, Smith N, Harpaz R, et al. Herpes zoster vaccine in older adults and the risk of subsequent herpes zoster disease. JAMA. 2011;305(2):160-6.

1.2S. POLIOMYELITIS (INFANTILE PARALYSIS)

General

Acute viral infection characterized by varying degrees of neuronal injury, with special localization in the anterior horns and motor nuclei of the brainstem.

Ocular

Diplopia; nystagmus; paralysis of third, fourth, and sixth nerves; paresis of seventh nerve; papilledema; visual agnosia; Homer's syndrome; pupillary paralysis; optic neuritis;

ophthalmoparesis; transient visual loss; internuclear ophthalmoplegia; papillary disturbances, spasm of near reflex.

Clinical

Flaccid paralysis of many muscle groups; death from asphyxia and involvement of vital centers in the brainstem.

Laboratory

Obtain specimens from the CSF, stool and throat for viral cultures.

Treatment

No antivirals are effective against polioviruses. The treatment of poliomyelitis is mainly supportive and will involve physical therapist and rehabilitation therapist, pulmonologist, neurologist, immunologist and infectious diseases specialist.

BIBLIOGRAPHY

1. Estrada B. (2012). Pediatric poliomyelitis. [online] Available from www.emedicine.com/ped/TOPIC1843.HTM. [Accessed September, 2013].

1.2S. DISSEMINATED SCLEROSIS (MULTIPLE SCLEROSIS)

General

Disseminated demyelination affecting white matter of the brain, spinal cord, and optic nerves; etiology unknown.

Ocular

Nystagmus; ptosis; myokymia; optic atrophy; papillitis; optic neuritis; anisocoria; Argyll Robertson pupil; Marcus Gunn pupil; hippus, decreased or absent papillary reaction to light; periphlebitis; visual field defects; gaze palsy; paralysis of third or sixth nerve; uveitis; oscillopsia; Uhthoff symptom (reduction of visual acuity with exercise or ocular hyperthermia); pars planitis; retinal venous sheathing; retinitis; granulomatous uveitis.

Clinical

Incoordination; paresthesia; spasticity; tic douloureux; urinary frequency and infections; progressive disability; paralysis; death.

Laboratory

MRI, CSF positive for oligoclonal band, albumin and IgG index; brainstem auditory evoked response (BAER) and somato-sensory evoked potentials (SEP).

Treatment

Patients with MS may require multiple consultations to rule out other causes for their symptoms. Drugs such as immunodulator, immunosuppressors, anti-Parkinson agent, CNS stimulants are all used in the management of the disease.

BIBLIOGRAPHY

1. Luzzio C, Dangond F. (2013). Multiple sclerosis. [online] Available from www.emedicine.com/neuro/topic228.htm. [Accessed September, 2013].

1.2S. ACQUIRED LUES (SYPHILIS; ACQUIRED SYPHILIS; LUES VENEREA; MALUM VENEREUM)

General

Causative agent, *Treponema pallidum,* usually transmitted sexually.

Ocular

Conjunctival chancroid; conjunctivitis; keratitis; blepharitis; ptosis; iris atrophy; hippus; dacryocystitis; optic nerve atrophy; optic neuritis; periostitis; episcleritis; scleritis; nystagmus; uveitis; vitreous hemorrhages; paralysis of sixth nerve; papilledema; retinal hemorrhages; retinitis proliferans; oculogyric crisis; neuroretinitis; papilledema (associated with aseptic meningitis); diffuse or multifocal chorioretinitis; vertical supranuclear gaze palsy; Benedikt syndrome.

Clinical

Primary lesion associated with regional lymphadenopathy; secondary bacteremic stage associated with generalized mucocutaneous lesions; tertiary stage characterized by destructive mucocutaneous, musculoskeletal, or parenchymal lesions, aortitis, or CNS disease; syphilis and human immunodeficiency virus (HIV) infection often coexist in the same patient who experiences a higher incidence and greater severity of neurologic and ocular manifestations; a significant percentage of patients infected with HIV-I and *T. pallidum* become seronegative to syphilis testing.

Laboratory

Serologic nontreponemal tests include Venereal Disease Research Laboratory (VDRL) and rapid plasma reagin (RPR).

Treatment

The goals are to reduce morbidity and to prevent complications. Penicillin is the antibiotic of choice for treating syphilis. Ocular syphilis should be treated the same as patients with neurosyphilis.

BIBLIOGRAPHY

1. Majmudar PA. (2011). Interstitial Keratitis Overview of Interstitial Keratitis. [online] Available from www.emedicine.com/oph/TOPIC453.HTM. [Accessed September, 2013].
2. Euerle B, Chandrasekar PH, Diaz MM, et al. (2012). Syphilis. [online] Available from www.emedicine.com/med/TOPIC2224.HTM. [Accessed September, 2013].

1.2S. BANG DISEASE (BRUCELLOSIS; MALTA FEVER; MEDITERRANEAN FEVER; PIG BREEDER DISEASE; GIBRALTAR FEVER; UNDULANT FEVER)

General

Transmitted to man from animals or animal products containing bacteria of the genus Brucella; human infection results from ingestion of infected animal tissue and milk products or through skin wounds directly bathed in freshly killed animal tissues.

Ocular

Conjunctivitis; punctate keratitis; optic neuritis; swollen optic nerves; chorioretinitis; extraocular muscle palsies; phlyctenules; dacryoadenitis; papilledema; episcleritis; macular edema; phthisis bulbi; uveitis; vitreous opacities; changes in intraocular pressure (IOP; early decrease or late increase).

Clinical

Fever; icterus; weakness; sweats; general malaise; mammary abscess.

Laboratory

Increasing serum agglutination test.

Treatment

The goal of medical therapy is to prevent complications and relapses. Multidrug antimicrobial regimens are the mainstay of therapy. Ocular treatment includes topical steroids and cycloplegics for uveitis.

BIBLIOGRAPHY

1. Al-Nassir W. (2011). Brucellosis. [online] Available from www.emedicine.com/med/TOPIC248.HTM. [Accessed September, 2013].

1.2T. OPHTHALMOPLEGIC MIGRAINE SYNDROME

General

Symptoms produced by ipsilateral herniation of hippocampal gyrus of temporal lobe through incisura tentorii; dependent upon unilateral cerebral edema due to vascular or vasomotor phenomena, intracranial aneurysm, or tumor; incidence may be greater in women with the initial attack in the 1st decade of life; pathogenesis is unclear, but it is likely secondary to ischemia of the ocular motor nerve.

Ocular

Severe unilateral supraorbital pain; ptosis; transitory partial or complete homolateral oculomotor paralysis; fourth or sixth nerve occasionally involved; retinal hemorrhages; papilledema (may be bilateral); moderate to severe headache with partial to complete cranial nerve III paresis including the pupil; more than one ocular nerve may be affected.

Clinical

Migraine headache, not present in all instances; dizziness; diminution in sense of smell; hypalgesia contralateral side of face; nausea/vomiting may be present; recurrent sinus arrest.

Laboratory

Clinical.

Treatment

Ptosis: If visual acuity is affected, most cases require surgical correction and there are several procedures that may be used including levator resection, repair or advancement and Fasanella-Servat.

⊟ BIBLIOGRAPHY

1. Bazak I, Margulis T, Shnaider H, et al. Ophthalmoplegic migraine and recurrent sinus arrest. J Neurol Neurosurg Psychiatry. 1991;54:935.
2. Ehlers H. On pathogenesis of ophthalmoplegic migraine. Acta Psychiatr Neurol (Scand). 1928;3:219.
3. Geeraets WJ. Ocular Syndromes, 3rd edition. Philadelphia: Lea & Febiger; 1976.
4. Gulkilik G, Cagatay H, Oba E, et al. Ophthalmoplegic migraine associated with recurrent isolated ptosis. Ann Ophthal. 2010;41:206-12.
5. Raskin NH. Migraine and other headaches. In: Rowland LP (Ed). Merritt's Textbook of Neurology, 9th edition. Baltimore: Williams & Wilkins; 1995. pp. 837-45.
6. Stommel EW, Ward TN, Harris RD. Ophthalmoplegic migraine or Tolosa-Hunt syndrome? Headache. 1994;34:177.
7. Van Pelt W, Andermann F. On the early onset of ophthalmologic migraine. Am J Dis Child. 1964;107:628.
8. Vijayan N. Ophthalmoplegic migraine: ischemic or compressive neuropathy? Headache. 1980;20:300-4.

⊟ 1.2V. PASSOW SYNDROME (BREMER STATUS DYSRAPHICUS; STATUS DYSRAPHICUS SYNDROME; SYRINGOMYELIA; SYRINGOBULBIA)

General

Congenital nonclosure of the neural tube; familial occurrence or may be sporadic; insidious onset in 2nd to 3rd decade of life.

Ocular

Enophthalmos; ptosis; rotatory nystagmus; heterochromia iridis; anterior uveitis; corneal anesthesia; neuroparalytic keratitis; paralysis of third, fifth, sixth, and seventh cranial nerves; Horner syndrome; anisocoria; papilledema; optic atrophy; zonular cataract (*see* Horner Syndrome).

Clinical

Anesthesia over area of first division of trigeminal nerve; facial hemiatrophy; facial nerve paralysis; muscular weakness; cervical ribs; kyphoscoliosis; spina bifida; unilateral numbness of fingers; loss of deep reflexes; insensitivity to pain and temperature in affected areas; neurogenic bladder.

Laboratory

MRI, CT.

Treatment

Suboccipital and cervical decompression, laminectomy and syringotomy, shunts, fourth ventriculostomy, terminal ventriculostomy and neuroendoscopic surgery may be considered.

⊟ BIBLIOGRAPHY

1. Al-Shatoury HA, Galhom AA, Wagner FC. (2012). Syringomyelia. [online] Available from emedicine.medscape.com/article/1151685-overview. [Accessed September, 2013].

1.2W. SYMONDS SYNDROME (OTITIC HYDROCEPHALUS SYNDROME; SEROUS MENINGITIS SYNDROME; BENIGN INTRACRANIAL HYPERTENSION; PSEUDOTUMOR CEREBRI)

General

Children and adolescents; protracted course; increased CSF, but without increase in protein or cells.

Ocular

Sixth nerve palsy, ipsilateral side with otitis media; retinal hemorrhages and exudates; moderate-to-marked papilledema followed by secondary optic atrophy; unilateral or bilateral swelling of the optic nerve head have been reported; cranial nerve third and fourth involvement; bilateral retinal vein occlusion.

Clinical

Greatly increased pressure of spinal fluid, often greater than 300 mm Hg, without increased cells or protein; intermittent headaches; otitis media; chronic renal failure; chronic myeloid leukemia.

Laboratory

Imaging studies such as MRI to rule out tumors of brain and spinal cord and LP.

Treatment

Carbonic anhydrase inhibitors such as acetazolamide and furosemide are useful.

BIBLIOGRAPHY

1. Chang D, Nagamoto G, Smith WE. Benign intracranial hypertension and chronic renal failure. Cleve Clin J Med. 1992;59(4):419-22.
2. Chari C, Rao NS. Benign intracranial hypertension-its unusual manifestations. Headache. 1991;31(9):599-600.
3. Chern S, Magargal LE, Brav SS. Bilateral central retinal vein occlusion as an initial manifestation of pseudotumor cerebri. Ann Ophthalmol. 1991;23(2):54-7.
4. Roy FH, Fraunfelder FW, Fraunfelder FT. Roy and Fraunfelder's Current Ocular Therapy, 6th edition. Philadelphia, PA: WB Saunders; 2008.
5. Venable HP. Pseudo-tumor cerebri. J Natl Med Assoc. 1970;62(6):435-40.
6. Venable HP. Pseudo-tumor cerebri: further studies. J Natl Med Assoc. 1973;65(3):194-7.

1.2X. RAYMOND SYNDROME [RAYMOND-CESTAN SYNDROME; CESTAN (2) SYNDROME; PONTINE SYNDROME; DISASSOCIATION OF LATERAL GAZE SYNDROME]

General

Lesion involving the pyramidal tracts as they traverse the pons; posterior longitudinal bundle and medial lemniscus may be involved; tumor and vascular thromboses are common causes; can be caused iatrogenically after neurosurgical procedures.

Ocular

Ipsilateral abducens palsy; paralysis of lateral conjugate gaze.

Clinical

Contralateral hemiplegia; anesthesia of the face, limbs, and trunk.

Laboratory

CT scan of head.

Treatment

Tape or base-out prism on one eye glass may be useful. Botulinum toxin type A into the antagonist medial recturs muscle; if no improvement after 6–12 months, recess/resect of medial and LR.

BIBLIOGRAPHY

1. Isobe I, Fujita T, Yoshida K, et al. Rare case of Raymond-Cestan syndrome. Naika. 1970;26:388-92.
2. Raymond F, Cestan R. Trois Observations de Paralysie des Mouvements Associes des Globes Oculaires. Rev Neural (Paris). 1901;9:70-7.
3. Seyer H, Honegger J, Schott W, et al. Raymond's syndrome following petrosal sinus sampling. Acta Neurachir. 1994;131:157-9.

1.2Y. RELAPSING POLYCHONDRITIS (JAKSCH WARTENHOST SYNDROME; MEYENBURG-ALTHERZ-VEHLINGER SYNDROME; VON MEYENBERG II SYNDROME)

General

Episodic, yet generally progressive; onset usually in middle life; possibly caused by lysosomal labilizing factor of endogenous or exogenous toxic nature or immunologic reactions; possible association with Reiter's syndrome.

Ocular

Conjunctivitis; corneal ulcer; exophthalmos; panophthalmitis; phthisis bulbi; proptosis; optic neuritis; papilledema; retinal detachment; blue sclera; episcleritis; scleromalacia; vitreous opacity; cataracts; nystagmus; retinal artery thrombosis; keratoconjunctivitis sicca; secondary glaucoma; scotoma; uveitis; paresis of third or sixth nerve; conjunctival mass (salmon patch); chorioretinitis.

Clinical

Destruction of cartilage and eventual replacement with connective tissue; polyarthritis; chondritis; tracheal collapse; bronchial collapse; anemia; liver dysfunction; death; malaise; fever; dyspnea; changes in pitch of voice; hearing impairment; vertigo; deformed ears; aortic valve insufficiency.

Laboratory

No specific serologic markers.

Treatment

No therapy.

BIBLIOGRAPHY

1. Compton N, Buckner JH, Harp KI, et al. (2012). Polychondritis. [online] Available from emedicine.medscape.com/article/331475-overview. [Accessed September, 2013].

1.2DD. TRICHINELLOSIS (TRICHINOSIS)

General

Parasite *Trichinella* enters the body by ingestion of infected meat (usually poorly cooked pork).

Ocular

Conjunctivitis; splinter hemorrhages of conjunctiva; paralysis of sixth nerve; exophthalmos; proptosis; uveitis; optic neuritis; papilledema; retinal hemorrhages; dyschromatopsia; scotoma; secondary glaucoma; encysted parasites in the extraocular muscles.

Clinical

Fever; urticaria; respiratory symptoms; muscle pain; myalgias and severe proximal muscle weakness; impaired coordination.

Laboratory

Leukocytosis and eosinophilia elevated serum levels of lactic dehydrogenase, aldolase and creatine phosphokinase (50% cases).

Treatment

Mebendazole orally is the treatment of choice. In severe cases, prednisone may be used in conjunction with antihelminthic agent.

BIBLIOGRAPHY

1. Arnold LK. (2012). Trichinellosis/Trichinosis. [online] Available from www.emedicine.com/emerg/TOPIC612.HTM. [Accessed September, 2013].

🗗 1.3A. FOIX SYNDROME (CAVERNOUS SINUS SYNDROME; HYPOPHYSEAL-SPHENOIDAL SYNDROME; CAVERNOUS SINUS NEURALGIA SYNDROME; GODTFREDSEN SYNDROME; CAVERNOUS SINUS-NASOPHARYNGEAL TUMOR SYNDROME; CAVERNOUS SINUS THROMBOSIS)

General

Causes include tumor of lateral sinus wall or sphenoid bone, intracranial aneurysm, cavernous and lateral sinus thrombosis, or lesions; multiple myeloma; may result from infarctions or cancer or be idiopathic.

Ocular

Proptosis; severe ocular and periorbital pain; lid edema; paresis or paralysis of cranial nerves III, IV, V, and VI; corneal anesthesia; optic atrophy.

Clinical

Postauricular edema; trigeminal neuralgia; deviation of the tongue toward paralyzed side; patients usually have prominent manifestations of sepsis and paranasal sinus; local skin infections are the most common cause.

Laboratory

CT, MRI.

Treatment

Radiotherapy, anticoagulation, high-dose antibiotic therapy.

🗗 BIBLIOGRAPHY

1. Kattah JC, Pula JH. (2012). Cavernous sinus syndromes. [online] Available from www.emedicine.com/neuro/topic572.htm. [Accessed September, 2013].

🗗 1.3D. ORBITAL FRACTURE, APEX

General

It affects the most posterior portion of the pyramidal-shaped orbit, positioned at the craniofacial junction. Usually associated with blunt or penetrating trauma to the face or skull.

Clinical

Intracranial or facial trauma.

Ocular

Visual loss; optic neuropathy; optic nerve sheath hematoma; optic nerve impingement; optic nerve compression; retrobulbar hemorrhage; extraocular muscle nerve palsy; diplopia; afferent pupil defect; periocular ecchymosis; proptosis.

Laboratory

CT scan is most appropriate to make diagnosis.

Treatment

In cases that involve decreased vision and optic nerve injury, medical or surgical nerve decompression should be considered. Corticosteroids should be the initial treatment and if it is not effective, surgical intervention is necessary.

🗗 BIBLIOGRAPHY

1. Patel B, Taylor SF. (2012). Apex orbital fracture. [online] Available from emedicine.medscape.com/article/1218196-overview. [Accessed September, 2013].

⊟ 1.3F. SPHENOCAVERNOUS SYNDROME

General

Lesion in the cavernous sinus; similar to the superior orbital fissure syndrome (Rochon-Duvigneaud syndrome) and orbital apex syndrome (*see* Rochon-Duvigneaud syndrome).

Ocular

Proptosis; edema; paresis of cranial nerves III, IV and VI (paralysis of the abducens nerve precedes paralysis of the oculomotor nerve, because the abducens is situated between the internal carotid artery and the cavernous sinus wall); conjunctival edema.

Laboratory

CT and MRI.

Clinical

Paresis of the first (sometimes second and third) division of cranial nerve V; sinusitis.

Treatment

- *Proptosis*: Ocular lubricants are beneficial for controlling the corneal exposure.
- *Paresis of cranial nerves III*: Prism therapy, surgical—muscle surgery on the affected muscle, occlusion of the involved eye to relieve diplopia.

⊟ BIBLIOGRAPHY

1. Geeraets WJ. Ocular Syndromes, 3rd edition. Philadelphia, PA: Lea & Febiger; 1976. p. 404.
2. Jefferson G. Concerning injuries, aneurysms and tumours involving the cavernous sinus. Trans Ophthalmol Soc UK. 1953;73:117.
3. Sekhar LN, Linskey ME, Sen CN, et al. Surgical management of lesions within the cavernous sinus. Clin Neurosurg. 1991;37:440-89.
4. Watson NJ, Dick AD, Hutchinson CH. A case of sinusitis presenting with spheno-cavernous syndrome: discussion of the differential diagnosis. Scott Med J. 1991;36(6):179-80.

⊟ 1.3G. SLUDER SYNDROME (SPHENOPALATINE GANGLION NEURALGIA SYNDROME; LOWER FACIAL NEURALGIA SYNDROME)

General

Irritation of the sphenopalatine ganglion; attacks of pain last from minutes to days (*see* Charlin syndrome).

Ocular

Severe orbital pain; increased lacrimation during episodes of pain.

Clinical

Unilateral facial pain, mainly root of nose, orbit, and mastoid area; episodes of headaches; nasal congestion.

Laboratory

Clinical.

Treatment

Identify pain and treat.

⊟ BIBLIOGRAPHY

1. Geeraets WJ. Ocular Syndromes, 3rd edition. Philadelphia: Lea & Febiger; 1976.
2. Miller NR (Ed). Walsh and Hoyt's Clinical Neuro-Ophthalmology (Volume II), 4th edition. Baltimore: Williams & Wilkins; 1982.
3. Seltzer AP. Facial pain. J Natl Med Assoc. 1971;63:354.
4. Sluder G. The role of sphenopalatine (Meckel's) ganglion in nasal headaches. NY Med J. 1908;87:989.

⧉ 1.3H. ROCHON-DUVIGNEAUD SYNDROME (SUPERIOR ORBITAL FISSURE SYNDROME) OPTIC ATROPHY

General

Inflammatory, traumatic, tumor, or vascular lesions such as meningioma of the sphenoid, carotid aneurysm, and arachnoiditis; infections originating in the maxillary sinus.

Ocular

Mild exophthalmos; lid edema; partial or complete ophthalmoplegia (III, IV and VI); decreased corneal sensitivity; papilledema; optic atrophy.

Clinical

Decreased sensitivity in area of nasociliary, lacrimal, frontal, and ophthalmic nerve distribution; may result from a metastatic tumor.

Laboratory

CBC count, erythrocyte sedimentation rate (ESR), thyroid function test, fluorescent treponemal antibody (FTA), antinuclear antibody (ANA), lupus erythematosus (LE) preparation, antineutrophil cytoplasmic antibody (ANCA), serum protein electrophoresis, Lyme titer, angiotensin-converting enzyme (ACE) level and HIV titer are helpful. CSF, anti-GQ1b antibodies, and MRI of the brain and the orbits.

Treatment

Corticosteroids are the treatment of choice.

⧉ BIBLIOGRAPHY

1. Falcone F, Lazow SK, Berger JR, et al. Superior orbital fissure syndrome. Secondary to infected dentigerous cyst of the maxillary sinus. NY State Dental J. 1994;60:62-4.
2. Hedstrom J, Parsons J, Maloney PL, et al. Superior orbital fissure syndrome: report of a case. J Oral Surg. 1974; 32: 198-201.
3. Phanthumchinda K, Hemachuda T. Superior orbital fissure syndrome as a presenting symptom in hepatocellular carcinoma. J Med Assoc Thailand. 1992;75:62-5.
4. Rochon-Duvigneaud A. Quelques Cas de Paralysie de Tous les Nerfs Orbitaires (Ophtalmoplegie Totale avec Amaurose et Anesthesie dans le Domaine de l'Ophtalmique d'Origine Syphilitique). Arch Ophthalmol. 1896;16:746.

⧉ 1.3I. TOLOSA-HUNT SYNDROME (PAINFUL OPHTHALMOPLEGIA)

General

Symptoms last from days to weeks; attacks recur at intervals of months or years; inflammatory lesion of cavernous sinus; onset most frequent in fifth decade of life; recurrent Tolosa-Hunt syndrome has been observed in some patients.

Ocular

Steadily "growing" retro-orbital pain; ptosis; involvement of cranial nerves III, IV, VI, and first division of V; scintillating scotomata; sluggish pupil reaction to light; corneal sensitivity diminished; optic neuritis.

Clinical

Inflammatory lesions of cavernous sinus.

Laboratory

MRI with axial and coronal views of brain, typically showing thickening and enhancement of involved cavernous sinus. Cerebral angiography is done to rule out aneurysm. Blood count, ESR, ANA, ANCA and ACE levels may be abnormal.

Treatment

Corticosteroids is often used to treat the chronic granulomatous inflammation of the cavernous sinus.

⧉ BIBLIOGRAPHY

1. Taylor DC. (2012). Tolosa-Hunt syndrome. [online] Available from www.emedicine.com/neuro/TOPIC373.HTM. [Accessed September, 2013].

1.4A. RAEDER SYNDROME (PARATRIGEMINAL PARALYSIS; HORTON HEADACHE; HISTAMINE CEPHALALGIA; CILIARY NEURALGIA; CLUSTER HEADACHE; PERIODIC MIGRAINOUS NEURALGIA)

General

Interruption of sympathetic fibers about the carotid artery and involvement of the fifth nerve; meningioma and aneurysm of the internal carotid artery are the most frequent causes; prominent in males; possible pathogenetic mechanism of this condition is an ischemic injury of the gasserian ganglion.

Ocular

Mild enophthalmos; mild ptosis (unilateral); epiphora; scotoma possible; hypotonia; unilateral miosis; increased tear secretion; periocular pain; Homer syndrome.

Clinical

Facial pain; occasionally weakness of the jaw muscles; headaches (V-region); hypertension; associated inflammatory processes are not infrequent.

Laboratory

Brain scan to rule out meningioma and basilar artery aneurysm.

Treatment

Oxygen inhalation and sumatriptan subcutaneous is useful in acute attacks.

BIBLIOGRAPHY

1. Bardorf CM, van Stavern G, Garcia-Valenzuela E. (2012). Horner syndrome. [online] Available from www.emedicine.com/oph/TOPIC336.HTM. [Accessed September, 2013].

1.4B. CRETINISM (HYPOTHYROID GOITER; HYPOTHYROIDISM; JUVENILE HYPOTHYROIDISM; MYXEDEMA)

General

Deficient thyroid function.

Ocular

Blepharitis; ptosis; enophthalmos; temporal madarosis; decreased tear secretion; glaucoma; proptosis; optic atrophy; optic neuritis; blue dot cataract; conjunctivitis; scleritis; optic disk hemorrhage and arcuate scotoma associated with glaucoma.

Clinical

Myxedema; larynx and tongue swollen; hoarse speech; dry, yellowish skin; slow pulse; mental retardation; infertility; pericardial effusion; cardiac enlargement; physical development retarded.

Laboratory

Clinical.

Treatment

- *Blepharitis*: Oral tetracyclines, omega-3 fatty acids, flax seed oil or fish oil. Ocular therapy include eyelid scrubs, warm compresses, bacitracin ointment to lid margins, topical cyclosporine A and preservative free lubricants.
- *Ptosis*: If visual acuity is affected, most cases require surgical correction and there are several procedures that may be used including levator resection, repair or advancement and Fasanella-Servat.
- *Glaucoma*: Glaucoma medication should be the first plan of action. If medication is unsuccessful, a filtering surgical procedure with or without antimetabotites may be beneficial.
- *Cataract*: Change in glasses can sometimes improve a patient's visual function temporarily; however the most common treatment is cataract surgery.

BIBLIOGRAPHY

1. Daniel MS, Postellon DC. (2013). Congenital hypothyroidism. [online] Available from www.emedicine.com/ped/TOPIC501.HTM. [Accessed September, 2013].

1.4C. DUANE SYNDROME (RETRACTION SYNDROME; STILLING SYNDROME; TURK-STILLING SYNDROME)

General

Autosomal dominant; more frequent in females; manifestations in infancy; was thought to be secondary to fibrosis of the LR muscle or abnormal check ligaments; now established to be due to congenital aberrant innervation affecting third and seventh cranial nerves.

Ocular

Narrowing of palpebral fissure on adduction, widening on abduction; primary global retraction; deficiency of medial and lateral recti motility; limitation of abduction in affected eye usually is complete; retraction of the globe with attempted adduction varies from 1 mm to 10 mm; convergence insufficiency; heterochromia irides; left eye is more frequently involved.

Clinical

Associated Klippel-Feil syndrome; malformation of face, ears and teeth.

Laboratory

Diagnosis is made by clinical findings.

Treatment

Indications for surgery include anomalous head position, strabismus in primary gaze, significant upshoot or downshoot in adduction and cosmetically significant palpebral fissure. Duane retraction syndrome type 1 (DRS-1) (absent abduction, esotropia in primary position and head turn toward the affected side to fuse) medial rectus recession of the affected eye; DRS with exotropia—recess LR of involved side. Retraction of the globe—recess medial and LR of involved eye. Upshoots and downshoots—recess the LR.

BIBLIOGRAPHY

1. Verma A. (2011). Duane syndrome. [online] Available from www.emedicine.com/oph/TOPIC326.HTM. [Accessed September, 2013].

1.4D. ENGELMANN SYNDROME [OSTEOPATHIA HYPEROSTOTICA (SCLEROTICANS) MULTIPLEX INFANTILIS; DIAPHYSEAL DYSPLASIA; CAMURATI-ENGELMANN DISEASE; HEREDITARY MULTIPLE DIAPHYSEAL SCLEROSIS; JUVENILE PAGET DISEASE]

General

Etiology unknown; progressive resorption and deposits of bone with thickening of periosteum and changes of cortex as evident by diagnostic X-ray studies in the intermediate portion of the long bones.

Ocular

Exophthalmos; hypertelorism (secondary); ptosis; lagophthalmos; LR palsy; convergence insufficiency; epiphora; cataract; tortuous retinal vessels; papilledema; optic atrophy.

Clinical

Pain in extremities; poorly developed musculature; waddling gait; delayed ambulation; scaly skin; delayed dentition; deafness; hypogonadism; pain in both legs; aching in the forearms; episodic temporofrontal and occipital headache.

Laboratory

Clinical.

Treatment

- *Exophthalmos*: Reversing the problem which is causing the exophthalmos is the treatment of choice and will minimize the ocular complications. Ocular lubricants are beneficial for control of the corneal exposure.
- *Ptosis*: If visual acuity is affected, most cases require surgical correction and there are several procedures that may be used including levator resection, repair or advancement and Fasanella-Servat.

- *Cataract*: Change in glasses can sometimes improve a patient's visual function temporarily; however the most common treatment is cataract surgery.
- *Papilledema*: Underlying cause should be determined and treated. Systemic acetazolamide is the medical therapy of choice.

BIBLIOGRAPHY

1. Brodrick JD. Luxation of the globe in Engelmann's disease. Am J Ophthalmol. 1977;83:870-3.
2. De Vits A, Keymeulen B, Bossuyt A, et al. Progressive diaphyseal dysplasia (Camurati-Engelmann's disease). Improvement of clinical signs and of bone scintigraphy during pregnancy. Clin Nucl Med. 1994;19:104-7.
3. Engelmann G. Ein Fall von Osteopathia Hyperostotica (Scleroticans) Infantilis. Fortschr Geb Roentgen Strahl. 1929;39:1101.
4. Morse PH, Walsh FB, McCormick JR. Ocular findings in hereditary diaphyseal dysplasia (Engelmann's disease). Am J Ophthalmol. 1969;68:100.
5. Roy FH, Fraunfelder FW, Fraunfelder FT. Roy and Fraunfelder's Current Ocular Therapy, 6th edition. Philadelphia: WB Saunders; 2007.

1.4F. KAHLER DISEASE (MYELOMATOSIS; MULTIPLE MYELOMA)

General

Disseminated malignancy of plasma cells located predominantly in the bone marrow.

Ocular

Tumor of orbit common, with proptosis or displacement of globe; conjunctival sledging and segmentation; crystalline deposits of cornea and conjunctiva; cotton-wool spots; retrobulbar neuritis; occlusion of central retinal artery and vein; palsy of sixth nerve; vitreous hemorrhage; dilated veins and hemorrhages; retinal microaneurysms; choroidal detachment; amaurosis fugax; myeloma infiltrates in orbit, iris, choroid, retina, sclera, and optic nerve; corneal opacities; ciliary body cysts; iritis; glaucoma; subluxation of lens; papilledema; corneal edema; cavernous sinus syndrome; bilateral superficial punctate keratitis; central retinal vein occlusion; crystalline keratopathy in a vortex distribution; spontaneous endocapsular hematoma.

Clinical

Bone pain; fractures; dehydration; hypercalcemia; hyperuricemia; proteinuria; inclination to infection; hyperviscosity.

Laboratory

Comprehensive metabolic panel to assess a patient's total protein, albumin and globulin, blood urea nitrogen (BUN), creatinine, and uric acid, MRI scan, bone marrow aspirate and biopsy.

Treatment

Bone marrow transplantation and radiation may be beneficial. Patients often benefit from the expertise of an orthopedic surgeon versed in oncologic management because prophylactic fixation of impending pathologic fractures is occasionally warranted.

BIBLIOGRAPHY

1. Seiter K, Shah D. (2013). Multiple myeloma. [online] Available from www.emedicine.com/med/TOPIC1521.HTM. [Accessed September, 2013].

1.4G. DISSEMINATED LUPUS ERYTHEMATOSUS (SYSTEMIC LUPUS ERYTHEMATOSUS; LUPUS ERYTHEMATOSUS; KAPOSI-LIBMAN-SACK SYNDROME, SLE)

General

Possible etiology includes viral infections and genetic predisposition; immunologic abnormalities.

Ocular

Keratitis; keratoconjunctivitis sicca; corneal ulcer; optic nerve atrophy; optic neuritis; papilledema; arteritis; central retinal vein occlusion; retinal detachment; microaneurysm; scleritis; uveitis; ptosis; conjunctivitis; paralysis of third nerve; homonymous hemianopsia; multifocal microinfarcts; mydriasis; nystagmus; proptosis; orbital myositis; pseudoretinitis pigmentosa; photophobia.

Clinical

Polyarthritis; morning stiffness; fever; malaise; fatigue; polyserositis; renal disease; CNS disease; anemia; leukopenia; maculopapular rash in a "butterfly" distribution over malar region; alopecia.

Laboratory

Antibodies to double-stranded DNA or the Smith (Sm) antigen or a false-positive serology test for syphilis; positive ANA test that is caused by a medication.

Treatment

Fever, rash, musculoskeletal, and serositis manifestations respond to hydroxychloroquine and nonsteroidal anti-inflammatory drugs (NSAIDs). Low-to-moderate dose steroids are necessary for acute flares. CNS involvement and renal disease constitute more serious disease and often require high-dose steroids and other immunosuppression agents. Diffuse proliferative lupus nephritis has been treated with cyclophosphamide induction therapy.

BIBLIOGRAPHY

1. Bartles CM, Muller D. (2012). Systemic erythematosus lupus. [online] Available from www.emedicine.com/med/TOPIC2228.HTM. [Accessed September, 2013].

1.4H. ERB-GOLDFLAM SYNDROME (ERB II SYNDROME; HOPPE-GOLDFLAM DISEASE; PSEUDOPARALYTIC SYNDROME; MYASTHENIA GRAVIS)

General

Occurs at any age; more frequent between ages 20 and 40 years; more females affected than males; progressive; spontaneous; symptoms improve or resolve with rest in early stages of disease (*see* myasthenia gravis, neonatal or infantile); caused by autoantibodies against the acetylcholine receptor at the neuromuscular junction, leading to abnormal fatigability and weakness of skeletal muscle.

Ocular

Transient diplopia; ptosis of upper eyelids.

Clinical

Excessive fatigability of musculature; symptoms appear and increase as day progresses; expressionless face; sagging jaw; difficulty in chewing and talking; nasal regurgitation.

Laboratory

Ice test—crushed ice in surgical glove over ptotic eyelid for 2 minutes and watch for brief elevation of eyelid; Tensilon test and prostigmin test may result in the elevation of ptotic eyelid or improved strabismus in individuals with myasthenia gravis.

Treatment

Adrenal corticosteroids are frequently used. In some cases, mycophenolate mofetil, cyclosporine and cyclophosphamide may be useful. Patching one eye or using prisms may be helpful.

BIBLIOGRAPHY

1. Erb W. Zur Casuistick der Bulbaren La hmungen. Arch Psychiatr Vervenkr. 1879;9:325-50.
2. Roy FH, Fraunfelder FT, Fraunfelder FW. Roy and Fraunfelder's Current Ocular Therapy, 6th edition. London, UK: Elsevier; 2008.
3. Goldflam S. Vebereinen Scheinbar Keilbaren Bulbarparalytischem Symptom Complex mit Betheiligung der Extremitaten. Dtsch Z Nerven. 1983;4:312-52.
4. Kim JH, Hwang JM, Hwang YS, et al. Childhood ocular myasthenia gravis. Ophthalmology. 2003;110(7):1458-62.
5. Lepore FE, Sanborn GE, Slevin JT. Pupillary dysfunction in myasthenia gravis. Ann Neurol. 1979;6(1):29-33.
6. Sommer N, Melms A, Weller M, et al. Ocular myasthenia gravis. A critical review of clinical and pathophysiological aspects. Doc Ophthalmol. 1993;84(4):309-33.

1.4J. ECLAMPSIA AND PREECLAMPSIA (TOXEMIA OF PREGNANCY; PREECLAMPSIA)

General

Disorders of cells in glomeruli of kidneys that occur during gestation or shortly after delivery.

Ocular

Cortical blindness; nystagmus; mydriasis; absolute pupillary paralysis; ptosis; choroidal detachment; retinal detachment; cotton wool exudates; optic atrophy; retinal hemorrhages; petechial hemorrhages and focal edema in the occipital cortex.

Clinical

Hypertension; edema; proteinuria; convulsions; coma; death; cardiac failure; weight gain.

Laboratory

CT of head, MRI, cerebral angiography, laboratory studies—CBC count, platelet count, 24-hour urine for protein/creatinine, electrolytes, liver function tests, aspartate aminotransferase, uric acid, serum glucose

Treatment

Eclamptic convulsions are life-threatening emergencies and require the proper treatment to decrease maternal morbidity and mortality. Deliver immediately by cesarean delivery, depending on the maternal and fetal condition.

BIBLIOGRAPHY

1. Ross MG. (2012). Eclampsia. [online] Available from www.emedicine.com/med/TOPIC633.HTM. [Accessed September, 2013].

1.4K. SCHAUMANN SYNDROME (BESNIER-BOECK-SCHAUMANN SYNDROME; BOECK SARCOID; SARCOIDOSIS)

General

Etiology unknown; theories include tuberculosis, hypersensitivity to pine pollen, virus infection; affects blacks most often; chronic course with spontaneous remissions (*see* Heerfordt's syndrome); hilar or paratracheal nodes with erythema nodosum; onset most often in middle and old age; ocular involvement in 20–25% of all cases.

Ocular

Orbital granulomatous mass; bony defects; cutaneous and subcutaneous nodules; myogenic palsy; lacrimal gland adenopathy; decreased tear formation; secondary glaucoma; granulomatous uveitis with iris nodules, cells and flare; mutton fat keratic precipitates; keratitis sicca; vitreous floaters; band-shaped keratitis; complicated cataract; inflammatory retinal exudates; "candle wax drippings"; optic nerve atrophy; neuritis; eyelid nodules; ocular nerve enlargement (granuloma).

Clinical

Lymphadenopathy; hilar nodes; fatigue; cystic, punched-out or reticulated changes in small bones (mainly, hands and feet); muscle wasting; contractures; weakness in legs and arms.

Laboratory

Chest X-ray, CT scan, and MRI of the brain.

Treatment

Glucocorticoids are the treatment of choice.

BIBLIOGRAPHY

1. Sharma GD. (2011). Pediatric sarcoidosis. [online] Available from www.emedicine.com/ped/TOPIC2043.HTM. [Accessed September, 2013].

🖰 1B. MILLARD-GUBLER SYNDROME (ABDUCENS-FACIAL HEMIPLEGIA ALTERNANS)

General

Vascular, infectious or tumorous lesion at the base of the pons affecting the nuclei of the sixth and seventh nerves and fibers of the pyramidal tract; demyelinating disease.

Ocular

Diplopia; esotropia; paralysis of external rectus muscle (often bilateral); in unilateral cases, there is deviation of eyes to sides opposite lesion and inability to move them toward the side of lesion; abduction of eye is prevented by destruction of sixth nerve nucleus; opposite eye cannot be voluntarily adducted but can converge and move in this position by rotatory and caloric stimulation.

Clinical

Ipsilateral facial paralysis; contralateral hemiplegia of arm and leg from involvement of pyramidal tract.

Laboratory/Diplopia

None.

Treatment/Diplopia

Occluding one eye, Fresnel prism, anticholinergic agent, and corticosteroids may be needed in the treatment of myasthenia gravis.

🖰 BIBLIOGRAPHY

1. Geeraets WJ. Ocular Syndromes, 3rd edition. Philadelphia, PA: Lea & Febiger; 1976.
2. Gubler A. De l'Hémiplegie alterne envisagée comme signe de lésion de la protubérance annulaire et comme preuve de la décussation des nerfs faciaux. Gaz Hebd Med Chir. 1856;3:749,789,811.
3. Minderhoud JM. Diagnostic significance of symptomatology in brain stem ischemic infarction. Eur Neurol. 1971;5(6):343-53.
4. Newman NJ. Third, fourth and sixth nerve lesions and the cavernous sinus. In: Albert DM, Jakobiec FA (Eds). Albert & Jakobiec's Principles and Practice of Ophthalmology: Clinical Practice, 5th edition. Philadelphia, PA: WB Saunders; 1994. pp. 245-51.

🖰 2A. ACCOMMODATIVE ESOTROPIA

General

Hereditary, onset between the age of 6 months and 5 years.

Clinical

None.

Ocular

Uncorrected hyperopia with insufficient fusional divergence. The hyperopia averages 5 diopters. The esotropia has equal distance and near.

Laboratory

Diagnosis is made by clinical findings.

Treatment

Amblyopia therapy; spectacle correction—full cycloplegia refraction if esotropia has same distance and near; greater near than distant esotropia—bifocals up to +3.50 diopters set high at mid-pupil; gradually reduce the power to maintain fusion, contact lens if patient is capable; ectothiophate iodine is used to reduce use of spectacles and if residual esotropia after full correction is observed, consider strabismus surgery.

🖰 BIBLIOGRAPHY

1. Noyes C, Gupta RR. (2012). Accommodative esotropia. [online] Available from www.emedicine.com/oph/TOPIC554.HTM. [Accessed September, 2013].

2B. ACQUIRED NONACCOMMODATIVE ESOTROPIA

General

Convergent deviation with onset after the age of 6 months, unaffected by accommodation.

Clinical

None.

Ocular

Esotropia is same in all fields of gaze, amblyopia.

Laboratory

Diagnosis is made by clinical findings.

Treatment

Amblyopia therapy, eyeglasses if significant refractive error; orthoptics; unilateral surgery—recess medial rectus and resect LR or bilateral surgery—recess both medial rectus.

BIBLIOGRAPHY

1. Pascotto A, Fioretto M, Saccà SC, et al. (2012). Acquired esotropia. [online] Available from www.emedicine.com/oph/TOPIC327.HTM. [Accessed September, 2013].

2C. A ESOTROPIA SYNDROME

General

Esotropia greater looking up by 15 prism diopters than looking down; an overaction of superior oblique muscles or underaction of inferior rectus muscles; fusion may be obtained by chin elevation; mongoloid (upward) slant of lid fissures; may be accommodative, nonaccommodative or paralytic esotropia components.

Laboratory

Diagnosis is made by clinical findings.

Treatment

Recess the medial rectus bilaterally with a half tendon up-shift. If unilateral surgery is performed, recess medial rectus with upshift and resect the LR with a half tendon downshift. With significant oblique overaction, recess the medial rectus bilaterally or recess the medial rectus and resect the LR unilaterally for esotropia in primary position; weaken the superior oblique bilaterally if 25 diopters from up to down.

BIBLIOGRAPHY

1. Beyer-Machule C, von Noorden GK. Atlas of Ophthalmic Surgery: Lids, Orbits, Extraocular Muscles. New York, USA: Thieme Publishing Group; 1985.
2. Hwang J, Wright KW. Strabismus syndromes. In: Wright KW (Ed). Pediatric Ophthalmology and Strabismus. St. Louis: Mosby; 1995. p. 223.
3. Roy FH. Practical management of eye problems: glaucoma, strabismus, visual fields. Philadelphia: Lea & Febiger; 1975. pp. 32-134.

2D. AXENFELD-SCHURENBERG SYNDROME (CYCLIC OCULOMOTOR PARALYSIS)

General

Congenital manifestation; frequently unilateral.

Ocular

Cyclic oculomotor paralysis (paralysis alternating with spasm); during periods of paralysis, lid exhibits ptosis and affected eye is abducted; during spasm, lid is raised, deviation of affected eye is either inward or outward, and pupil is fixed and contracted.

Laboratory

Diagnosis is made by clinical findings.

Treatment

Prism therapy; surgical—muscle surgery on the affected muscle, and occlusion at the involved eye to relief diplopia.

BIBLIOGRAPHY

1. Axenfeld T, Schurenberg L. Beitrage zur Kenntnis der Ange-borenen Beweglichkeitsdefekte des Auges. Klin Monastbl Augenheilkd. 1901;39:64.

2. Hamed LM. Oculomotor palsy with cyclic spasm. In: Margo CE, Mames R, Hamed LM (Eds). Diagnostic Problems in Clinical Ophthalmology, illustrated edition. Philadelphia, PA: WB Saunders; 1994. p. 712.
3. Levy MR. Cyclic oculomotor paralysis with optic atrophy. Am J Ophthalmol. 1968;65(5):766-9.
4. Purvin V. Oculomotor palsy in children. In: Margo CE, Mames R, Hamed LM (Eds). Diagnostic Problems in Clinical Ophthalmology, illustrated edition. Philadelphia, PA: WB Saunders; 1994. pp. 682-3.

2E. COGAN (2) SYNDROME (OCULOMOTOR APRAXIA SYNDROME; WIEACKER SYNDROME)

General

X-linked; oculomotor apraxia and muscle atrophy; prevalent in males; corpus callosum can be hypoplastic.

Ocular

Rapid and frequent blinking; conjugate palsy; congenital oculomotor apraxia with patient unable to move eyes voluntarily to one side but with otherwise normal ocular movements; patient fixes objects by head tilt and turning, which causes further ocular deviation via the vestibular reflex; compensation for this overshoot is accomplished by some jerky eye movements with final fixation possible and gradual return of the head to the primary position; may be associated with abnormal electroretinographic responses.

Clinical

Slow progression, predominantly distal muscle atrophy; congenital contracture of feet; dyspraxia of face and tongue muscles; mild mental retardation.

Laboratory

Diagnosis is made by clinical findings.

Treatment

None.

BIBLIOGRAPHY

1. Borchert MS, Sadun AA, Sommers JD, et al. Congenital oculo motor apraxia. Findings with magnetic resonance imaging. J Clin Neuroophthalmol. 1987;7(2):104-7.
2. Cogan DG. A type of congenital ocular motor apraxia presenting jerky head movement. Trans Am Acad Ophthalmol Otolaryngol. 1952;56(6):853-62.
3. Magni R, Spadea L, Pece A, et al. Electroretinographic findings in congenital oculomotor apraxia (Cogan's syndrome). Doc Ophthalmol. 1994;86(3):259-66.
4. Vassella F, Lütschg J, Mumenthaler M. Cogan's congenital ocular motor apraxia in two successive generations. Dev Med Child Neurol. 1972;14(6):788-96.

2F. CONGENITAL ESOTROPIA (INFANTILE ESOTROPIA)

General

Inward turning of the eye which is manifested by 6 months of age.

Clinical

None.

Ocular

Esotropia, amblyopia, coloboma, hypoplasia, retinoblastoma.

Laboratory

Diagnosis is made by clinical findings.

Treatment

Correct refractive error, amblyopia therapy, medial rectus recession and/or LR resection in one or both eyes.

BIBLIOGRAPHY

1. Ocampo VV, Foster CS. (2012). Infantile esotropia. [online] Available from www.emedicine.com/oph/TOPIC328.HTM. [Accessed September, 2013].

2G. ESOTROPIA: HIGH ACCOMMODATIVE CONVERGENCE TO ACCOMMODATION RATIO

General

The ratio of accommodative convergence [(AC) to accommodation (A) (AC/A)] is a measure of responsiveness of convergence for each diopter of accommodation; onset is from the age of 1–7 years.

Clinical

None.

Ocular

Esotropia, accommodation is greater at near than distance.

Laboratory

Diagnosis is made by clinical findings.

Treatment

Goal—achievement of alignment distance and nearby use of single vision lens—full prescription.

BIBLIOGRAPHY

1. Noyes C, Gupta RR. (2012). Esotropia with high AC/A ratio. [online] Available from www.emedicine.com/oph/TOPIC557.HTM. [Accessed September, 2013].

2H. MARCUS GUNN SYNDROME (JAW-WINKING SYNDROME; CONGENITAL TRIGEMINOOCULOMOTOR SYNKINESIS)

General

Familial occurrence is rare, although dominant inheritance has been reported; symptoms caused by abnormal connections between external pterygoid muscle and levator palpebrae, with supranuclear or supranuclear-nuclear involvement (*see* Marin Amat syndrome).

Ocular

Unilateral congenital ptosis in more than 90% of cases; 10% have spontaneous onset, usually in older persons; lid elevates rapidly when mouth is opened or mandible is moved to one or the other side; left eye seems to be more frequently affected than right eye; high incidences of strabismus (36%); amblyopia (34%); bilateral jaw-winking; decreased abduction.

Clinical

Stimulation of ipsilateral pterygoid with chewing, opening mouth, sucking or contralateral jaw thrusts.

Laboratory

Diagnosis is made by clinical findings.

Treatment

Treat amblyopia, if mild ptosis and for mild jaw-winking, consider Muller's muscle conjunctival resection; severe jaw-winking, release levator and perform a frontalis sling usually bilaterally; unilateral ptosis mild jaw-winking, consider levator relapse and advanced frontalis muscle to the superior tarsus.

BIBLIOGRAPHY

1. Blaydon SM. (2011). Marcus Gunn jaw-winking syndrome. [online] Available from www.emedicine.com/oph/TOPIC608.HTM. [Accessed September, 2013].

2I. PARALYSIS OF THIRD NERVE (OCULOMOTOR NERVE)

This type of paralysis includes ptosis, an inability to rotate the eye upward or inward, a dilated unreactive pupil (iridoplegia), and paralysis of accommodation (cycloplegia).

1. *Intracerebral*
   A. Lesion of red nucleus (Benedikt syndrome): Homolateral oculomotor paralysis with contralateral intention tremor.

B. Myasthenia gravis and mesencephalic cavernous angioma.

C. Nuclear types: Pareses of a single or a few extraocular muscles supplied by the oculomotor nerve in one or both eyes; there may or may not be pupillary disturbances (mydriasis, sluggish pupillary reaction) and paresis of accommodation; in tumors within or near the midbrain (pinealomas), there is a combination of isolated muscle pareses with vertical gaze palsy, possibly a disturbance of convergence, and nystagmus retractorius (Parinaud syndrome, Sylvian aqueduct syndrome); includes Axenfeld-Schurenberg syndrome (cyclic oculomotor paralysis), Bruns syndrome (postural change syndrome), Claude syndrome (inferior nucleus ruber syndrome), congenital vertical retraction syndrome, and Nothnagel syndrome (ophthalmoplegia-cerebellar ataxia syndrome).

D. Occlusion of basilar artery: Due to emboli especially but also to hemorrhage or aneurysm.

E. Recurrent third nerve palsy secondary to vascular spasm of migraine.

F. Syndrome of cerebral peduncle (Weber syndrome): Homolateral oculomotor paralysis and cross-hemiplegia.

†G. Tumors.

2. *Intracranial*

A. Amebic dysentery

†B. Aneurysm rupture at base of brain: Third nerve paralysis, pain around the face (fifth nerve), and headache

C. Botulism

D. Chickenpox

E. Craniopharyngioma

F. Dengue fever

G. Devic syndrome (optical myelitis)

H. Diphtheria

I. Encephalitis, acute

†J. Hepatic failure

†K. Hepatitis

L. Influenza

M. Lockjaw (tetanus)

†N. Lymphoma

O. Malaria

P. Measles immunization

Q. Meningococcal meningitis

R. Multiple sclerosis (disseminated sclerosis)

S. Ophthalmic migraine

T. Periarteritis nodosa

U. Poliomyelitis

V. Polyneuritis because of toxins such as alcohol, lead, arsenic, and carbon monoxide; dinitrophenol or carbon disulfide poisoning; or diabetes mellitus, herpes zoster, or mumps

W. Rabies

X. Relapsing polychondritis

Y. Smallpox vaccination

†Z. Subdural hematoma

AA. Syphilis (acquired lues)

BB. Temporal arteritis syndrome (Hutchinson-Horton-Magrath-Brown syndrome)

CC. Tuberculosis

3. *Lesions affecting exit from cranial cavity*

A. Cavernous sinus syndrome: Paralysis of third, fourth, and sixth nerves with proptosis

   1. Aneurysm (arteriovenous fistula syndrome): Pupil involved
   2. Carotid-cavernous fistula
   †3. Cavernous sinus thrombosis
   †4. Extension from lateral sinus thrombosis
   †5. Extension of nasopharyngeal tumor
   †6. Pituitary adenoma: Lateral extension
   7. Tolosa-Hunt syndrome (painful ophthalmoplegia)

B. Superior orbital fissure syndrome: Same as for cavernous sinus syndrome except exophthalmos is less likely to occur and optic nerve involvement and miotic pupil are more likely

   1. Aneurysm of internal carotid artery syndrome (foramen lacerum syndrome): Pupil involved
   †2. Occlusion of superior ophthalmic vein
   †3. Skull fractures or hemorrhage
   4. Sphenoid sinus suppuration (sphenocavernous syndrome)
   5. Temporal syndrome (Gradenigo syndrome)
   6. Tumors, such as sphenoid ridge meningioma (Rochon-Duvigneaud syndrome), nasopharyngeal tumor, metastatic carcinoma, RMS, chordoma, and sarcoma

†C. Orbital apex: Involvement of third, fourth, sixth, and first division of fifth cranial nerves and optic nerve proptosis is common.

4. *Other*

A. Alber-Schonberg syndrome (marble bone disease, osteopetrosis)

†B. Associated with aspirin poisoning

†C. Congenital
D. Hodgkin disease
E. Lupus erythematosus (Kaposi-Libman-Sacks syndrome)
F. Myasthenia gravis (masquerade)
G. Passow syndrome (status dysraphicus syndrome)
H. Porphyria cutanea tarda (PCT)
I. Sarcoid (Schaumann syndrome)

Treatment

- Third cranial nerve palsy from ischemia in the nerve trunk is believed to result from insufficiency of the vasa nervosa or small vessels that supply the nerve.
- Third cranial nerve palsy is most frequent in persons older than age 60 years and in those with prominent or long-standing atherosclerotic risk factors, such as diabetes or hypertension.
  - The key finding in these patients is relative sparing of the pupillary sphincter with complete or near-complete palsy of the extraocular muscles innervated by the third cranial nerve, including levator palpebrae.
  - Ironically, these patients may have very severe pain in the eye or orbit ipsilateral to the involved nerve. The pathogenesis of this pain is not understood, but it is common in patients with medial palsy and does not in itself suggest aneurysm as the cause.
- Medical management is actually watchful waiting, since there is no direct medical treatment that alters the course of the disease. Fortunately, nearly all patients undergo spontaneous remission of the palsy, usually within 6–8 weeks.
  - Treatment during the symptomatic interval is directed at alleviating symptoms, mainly pain and diplopia.
  - Nonsteroidal anti-inflammatory drugs are the first-line treatment of choice for the pain. Diplopia is not a problem when ptosis occludes the involved eye.
  - When diplopia is from large-angle divergence of the visual axes, patching one eye is the only practical short-term solution. When the angle of deviation is smaller, fusion in primary position often can be achieved using horizontal or vertical prism or both.

- Since the condition is expected to resolve spontaneously within a few weeks, most physicians would prescribe the prism as Fresnel paste on.
- Patients who do not recover from third cranial nerve palsy after 6–12 months may become candidates for eye muscle resection or recession to treat persistent and stable-angle diplopia. Some of these patients also may require some form of lid-lift surgery for persistent ptosis that restricts vision or is cosmetically unacceptable to the patient.

BIBLIOGRAPHY

1. Goodwin J. (2012). Oculomotor nerve palsy. [online] Available from www.emedicine.com/oph/TOPIC183.HTM. [Accessed September, 2013].
2. Eggenberger ER. (2012). Anisocoria. [online] Available from www.emedicine.com/oph/TOPIC160.HTM. [Accessed September, 2013].
3. Lee AG, Berlie CL, Costello F. (2012). Ophthalmologic manifestations of multiple sclerosis. [online] Available from www.emedicine.com/oph/TOPIC179.HTM. [Accessed September, 2013].
4. Patel B, Taylor SF. (2012). Apex Orbital Fracture. [online] Available from emedicine.medscape.com/article/1218196-overview. [Accessed September, 2013].
5. Wessels IF. (2013). Diplopia. [online] Available from www.emedicine.com/oph/TOPIC191.HTM. [Accessed September, 2013].
6. Lopez JI, Bechtel KA, Rothrock JF. (2013). Pediatric headache. [online] Available from emedicine.medscape.com/article/2110861-overview. [Accessed September, 2013].
7. Cohen AJ, Mercandetti M. (2011). Adult ptosis. [online] Available from www.emedicine.com/oph/TOPIC201.HTM. [Accessed September, 2013].
8. Jonathan L Brisman. (2012). Neurosurgery for cerebral aneurysm. [online] Availble from www.emedicine.com/med/TOPIC3468.HTM. [Accessed September, 2013].
9. Cruz-Flores S, Muengtaweepongsa S. (2012). Basilar artery thrombosis. [online] Availble from www.emedicine.com/neuro/TOPIC407.HTM. [Accessed September, 2013].
10. Verma A. (2012). Duane syndrome. [online] Available from www.emedicine.com/oph/TOPIC326.HTM. [Accessed September, 2013].
11. Suh DW. (2012). Congenital ptosis. [online] Available from emedicine.medscape.com/article/1212815-overview. [Accessed September, 2013].

†Indicates a general entry and therefore has not been described in detail in the text

21.1A. BENEDIKT SYNDROME (TEGMENTAL SYNDROME)

General

Lesion of the inferior nucleus tuber with obstruction of the third nerve; arteriosclerotic occlusion of branches of the basilar artery, trauma and hemorrhages in the midbrain, and neoplasm most common causes.

Ocular

Homolateral paralysis of cranial nerve III (oculomotor); involves associated movements of convergence, elevation, and depression of the eyes; loss of reflex to light and accommodation, diplopia.

Clinical

Unilateral hyperkinesis; contralateral hemiparesis, coarse tremor of upper extremity (greatly increased during movement), hemihypoesthesia, and absent deep sensibility; ipsilateral ataxia. There is at least one reported case of an HIV-positive patient with Benedikt syndrome who had elevated toxoplasma IgG titers.

Laboratory

CT, MRI, transcranial Doppler.

Treatment

Ocular: Patients who do not recover from third cranial nerve palsy after 6–12 months may become candidates for eye muscle resection or recession to treat persistent and stable-angle diplopia.

BIBLIOGRAPHY

1. Kaye V, Brandstate ME. (2011). Vertebrobasilar stroke overview of vertebrobasilar stroke. [online] Available from www.emedicine.com/pmr/TOPIC143.HTM. [Accessed September, 2013].
2. Goodwin J. (2012). Oculomotor nerve palsy. [online] Available from www.emedicine.com/oph/TOPIC183.HTM. [Accessed September, 2013].

21.1B. ERB-GOLDFLAM SYNDROME (ERB II SYNDROME; HOPPE-GOLDFLAM DISEASE; PSEUDOPARALYTIC SYNDROME; MYASTHENIA GRAVIS)

General

Occurs at any age; more frequent between ages 20–40 years; more females affected than males; progressive; spontaneous; symptoms improve or resolve with rest in early stages of disease (*see* myasthenia gravis, neonatal or infantile); caused by autoantibodies against the acetylcholine receptor at the neuromuscular junction, leading to abnormal fatigability and weakness of skeletal muscle.

Ocular

Transient diplopia; ptosis of upper eyelids.

Clinical

Excessive fatigability of musculature; symptoms appear and increase as day progresses; expressionless face; sagging jaw; difficulty in chewing and talking; nasal regurgitation.

Laboratory

Ice test—crushed ice in surgical glove over ptotic eyelid for 2 minutes and watch for brief elevation of eyelid; Tensilon test and prostigmin test may result in the elevation of ptotic eyelid or improved strabismus in individuals with myasthenia gravis.

Treatment

Adrenal corticosteroids are frequently used. In some cases, mycophenolate mofetil, cyclosporine and cyclophosphamide may be useful. Patching one eye or using prisms may be helpful.

BIBLIOGRAPHY

1. Erb W. Zur Casuistick der Bulbaren La hmungen. Arch Psychiatr Vervenkr. 1879;9:325-50.
2. Roy FH, Fraunfelder FT, Fraunfelder FW. Roy and Fraunfelder's Current Ocular Therapy, 6th edition. London, UK: Elsevier; 2008.
3. Goldflam S. Vebereinen Scheinbar Keilbaren Bulbarparalytischem Symptom Complex mit Betheiligung der Extremitaten. Dtsch Z Nerven. 1983;4:312-52.
4. Kim JH, Hwang JM, Hwang YS, et al. Childhood ocular myasthenia gravis. Ophthalmology. 2003;110(7):1458-62.
5. Lepore FE, Sanborn GE, Slevin JT. Pupillary dysfunction in myasthenia gravis. Ann Neurol. 1979;6(1):29-33.
6. Sommer N, Melms A, Weller M, et al. Ocular myasthenia gravis. A critical review of clinical and pathophysiological aspects. Doc Ophthalmol. 1993;84(4):309-33.

21.1C. PARINAUD OCULOGLANDULAR SYNDROME (PARINAUD CONJUNCTIVA-ADENITIS SYNDROME; CATSCRATCH OCULOGLANDULAR SYNDROME; CATSCRATCH DISEASE; BARTONELLA HENSELAE)

General

Most frequently seen in children; incubation time 7–10 days; caused by small pleomorphic Gram-negative bacillus; good prognosis; affects both sexes; about 90% of patients with this condition have serologic evidence of infection by *Rochalimaea henselae*.

Ocular

Conjunctivitis; retrotarsal conjunctival granulations; formation of granulomata in anterior segment about 3 mm high and 2–6 mm in diameter; inferior fornix usually affected; ulceration common; neuroretinitis; optic neuritis.

Clinical

Tender, red papule at the site of a cat scratch; regional preauricular and cervical lymphadenitis (often only one gland involved); irregular fever for 4–5 days and malaise; fever; parotid gland swelling.

Laboratory

Histopathology of biopsied lymph node of Warthin-Starry silver stain.

Treatment

Symptomatic treatment includes warm compresses, analgesics and antipyretics. Aspiration of lymph node if distention causes pain. Antibiotics may be necessary in severe cases.

BIBLIOGRAPHY

1. Nervi SJ. (2011). Catscratch disease. [online]. Available from www.emedicine.com/med/TOPIC304.HTM. [Accessed November, 2012].
2. Chi SL, Stinnett S, Eggenberger E, et al. Clinical characteristics in 53 patients with cat scratch optic neuropathy. Ophthalmology. 2012;119:183-7.

21.1C. KOERBER-SALUS-ELSCHNIG SYNDROME (SYLVIAN AQUEDUCT SYNDROME; NYSTAGMUS RETRACTORIUS SYNDROME)

General

It is caused by tumor or inflammation in the region of aqueduct of Sylvius, third and fourth ventricle, or corpora quadrigemina.

Ocular

Lid retraction may be associated with midbrain lesions above the posterior commissure; paresis of vertical gaze; tonic spasm of convergence on attempted upward gaze; clonic convergence movements or convergence nystagmus; vertical nystagmus on gaze up or down; nystagmus retractorius with spasmodic retraction of the eyes when an attempt is made to move them in any direction; occasional extraocular muscle paresis.

Clinical

Headaches; dizziness; hypertension; possible hemiparesis; ataxia; hemitremor; Babinski's sign.

Laboratory

CT, MRI.

Treatment

- *Lid retraction:* Identify systemic abnormalities as thyroid; 6 month stabilizing before eyelid surgery.
- *Local:* Ocular lubrication (drops or ointment). Botulinum toxin type A may also be useful.

BIBLIOGRAPHY

1. Elschnig A. Nystagmus Retractorius, ein Cerebrales Herd-symptom. Med Klin. 1913;9:8.
2. Geeraets WJ. Ocular Syndromes, 3rd edition. Philadelphia, PA: Lea & Febiger; 1976.

2I.1C. AXENFELD-SCHURENBERG SYNDROME (CYCLIC OCULOMOTOR PARALYSIS)

General

Congenital manifestation; frequently unilateral.

Ocular

Cyclic oculomotor paralysis (paralysis alternating with spasm); during periods of paralysis, lid exhibits ptosis and affected eye is abducted; during spasm, lid is raised, deviation of affected eye is either inward or outward, and pupil is fixed and contracted.

Laboratory

Diagnosis is made by clinical findings.

Treatment

Prism therapy; surgical—muscle surgery on the affected muscle, and occlusion at the involved eye to relief diplopia.

BIBLIOGRAPHY

1. Axenfeld T, Schurenberg L. Beitrage zur Kenntnis der Angeborenen Beweglichkeitsdefekte des Auges. Klin Monastbl Augenheilkd. 1901;39:64.
2. Hamed LM. Oculomotor palsy with cyclic spasm. In: Margo CE, Mames R, Hamed LM (Eds). Diagnostic Problems in Clinical Ophthalmology, illustrated edition. Philadelphia, PA: WB Saunders; 1994. p. 712.
3. Levy MR. Cyclic oculomotor paralysis with optic atrophy. Am J Ophthalmol. 1968;65(5):766-9.
4. Purvin V. Oculomotor palsy in children. In: Margo CE, Mames R, Hamed LM (Eds). Diagnostic Problems in Clinical Ophthalmology, illustrated edition. Philadelphia, PA: WB Saunders; 1994. pp. 682-3.

2I.1C. BRUNS SYNDROME (POSTURAL CHANGE SYNDROME)

General

It is caused by tumors of the third, fourth, or lateral ventricle or by lesions of the midline in the brain.

Ocular

Partial ophthalmoplegia (third nerve paralysis) and gaze paralysis; oculomotor paresis associated with postural change of head or body; amaurosis or transient blindness; flashes of light.

Clinical

Severe paroxysmal headache; nausea and vomiting; vertigo; irregular respiration; apnea; syncope; tachycardia; free-floating cysts within the fourth ventricle may produce intermittent foramen obstruction and Bruns syndrome; Kramer reported a patient with a free-floating cysticercus cyst with this condition.

Laboratory

CT scan of head.

Treatment

Consultation with a neurologist.

BIBLIOGRAPHY

1. Geeraets WJ Ocular syndromes, 3rd edition. Philadelphia; Lea & Febiger;1976.
2. Bruns O. Neuropathologische Demonstrationen. Neurol Centralbl. 1902;21:561.

2I.1C. CLAUDE SYNDROME (INFERIOR NUCLEUS RUBER SYNDROME; RUBRO-SPINAL-CEREBELLAR-PEDUNCLE SYNDROME)

General

Paramedian mesencephalic lesion starting in midbrain; often occlusion of terminal branches of the paramedian arteries supplying the inferior portion of the nucleus ruber.

Ocular

Paralysis of ipsilateral oculomotor and trochlear nerves (III, IV).

Clinical

It may be associated with motor hemiplegia.

Laboratory

Diagnosis is made by clinical findings.

Treatment

Prisms may be useful for small deviations. Botulinum toxin may also be useful. For deviation greater than 15 prism diopters, strabismus surgery may be required.

BIBLIOGRAPHY

1. Claude H. Inferior nucleus ruber syndrome. Rev Neurol. 1912; 1:311.
2. Cremieux G, Serratrice G. A case of retraction nystagmus associated with Claude's syndrome. Mars Med (Fre). 1972;109:635.
3. Gaymard B, Saudeau D, de Toffol B, et al. Two mesencephalic lacunar infarcts presenting as Claude's syndrome and pure motor hemiparesis. Eur Neurol. 1991;31:152-5.
4. Geeraets WJ. Ocular Syndromes, 3rd edition. Philadelphia, PA: Lea & Febiger; 1976.

21.1C. NOTHNAGEL SYNDROME (OPHTHALMOPLEGIA-CEREBELLAR ATAXIA SYNDROME)

General

Lesion of superior cerebellar peduncle, red nucleus and emerging oculomotor fibers such as pineal tumor, or tumor or vascular disturbance in corpora quadrigemina or vermis cerebelli (*see* Bruns syndrome).

Ocular

Oculomotor paresis; gaze paralysis most frequently upward, combined with some degree of internal or external ophthalmoplegia.

Clinical

Cerebellar ataxia; poor upper extremity movements; neoplasia; infarction; midbrain lesion.

Laboratory

CT and MRI of brain.

Treatment

See neurologist.

BIBLIOGRAPHY

1. Magalini SI, Scrascia E. Dictionary of Medical Syndromes, 2nd edition. Philadelphia, PA: Lippincott Williams and Wilkins; 1981.
2. Nothnagel H. Topische Diagnostik Der Gehirnkrankheiten. Berlin: Nabu Press; 2010. p. 220.

21.1D. VERTEBRAL BASILAR ARTERY SYNDROME (INTRANUCLEAR OPHTHALMOPLEGIA)

General

"Whiplash" injury with hyperextension of the neck followed by rapid forward movement of the head or osteoarthritis of the cervical spine, cervical ribs (*see* Cranio-cervical syndrome).

Ocular

Nystagmus (postural); internuclear ophthalmoplegia; visual deterioration; visual hallucinations may be associated with a decrease in consciousness; homonymous hemianopsia (bilateral); contralateral hemianopic visual field defect.

Clinical

Severe, throbbing occipital headache associated with neck pain; vertigo from ischemia of the internal auditory artery, from the temporoparietal cortex or from ischemia in the lateral tegmentum of the pons; nausea and vomiting; ataxia; hemiparesis; quadriplegia; dysarthria; dysphagia; deafness; dyslexia; atonia; confusion; coma; tremor.

Laboratory/Ocular

Diagnosis is made by clinical findings.

Treatment

- *Seesaw nystagmus*: Visual field to consider neoplastic or vascular etiologies.
- *Upbeat nystagmus*: May indicate MS, cerbellar degeneration, tumors or infarcts. Treatment is directed toward identification and resolution of underlying cause.
- *Downbeat nystagmus*: Affects the cerebellum or craniocervical junction including Arnold-Chiari malformation, MS, trauma, tumor, infarction and many toxic metabolic entities. MRI may indicate a surgically correctable lesion. Periodic alternating nystagmus is continous horizontal nystagmus from stroke, tumor, MS, trauma, infection, drug intoxication. Can occur from cataract, vitreous hemorrhage or optic atrophy.

BIBLIOGRAPHY

1. Caplan LR. Posterior cerebral artery syndrome. In: Vinken PJ, Bruyn GW; Klawans HL (Eds). Handbook of Clinical Neurology, Vascular Diseases. Amsterdam: Elsevier Science; 1988.
2. Caplan LR. "Top of the basilar" syndrome. Neurology. 1980;30:72.
3. Hoyt WF. Transient bilateral blurring of vision: considerations of an episodic ischemic symptom of vertebral-basilar insufficiency. Arch Ophthalmol. 1963;70:746.
4. Millikan CH, Siekert RG. Studies in cerebrovascular disease: I. the syndrome of intermittent insufficiency of the basilar arterial system. Proc Mayo Clin. 1965;30:61.

21.1E. MIGRAINE (VASCULAR HEADACHE)

General

Recurrent attacks of pain in the head; usually unilateral; often familial.

Ocular

Abnormal visual sensations; scotoma generally restricted to one-half of the visual field; complete blindness; unilateral transient visual loss; photopsia; branch retinal artery occlusions; anisocoria.

Clinical

Nausea; vomiting; anorexia; sensory, motor, and mood disturbances; fluid imbalance; headache.

Laboratory

Investigation studies; rule out comorbid disease, exclude other causes of headaches such as structural and/or metabolic; neurological examination; LP followed by CT scan or MRI.

Treatment

Treatment is based on the severity of the case.

BIBLIOGRAPHY

1. Chawla J, Blanda M, Braswell R, et al. (2011). Migraine headache. [online] Available from www.emedicine.com/neuro/TOPIC218.HTM. [Accessed September, 2013].

21.1F. WEBER SYNDROME (WEBER-DUBLER SYNDROME; CEREBELLAR PEDUNCLE SYNDROME; ALTERNATING OCULOMOTOR PARALYSIS; VENTRAL MEDIAL MIDBRAIN SYNDROME) PTOSIS

General

Lesion of the peduncle (crus), pons or medulla, which interrupts the third nerve before it emerges from the peduncle and interrupts fibers in the pyramidal tract above the level of the third nuclei; hemorrhage and thrombosis; tumor of the pituitary region, extending posteriorly; also may result in secondary to cerebrovascular disease.

Ocular

Ptosis; homolateral third nerve palsy (usually complete); fixed, dilated pupil.

Clinical

Contralateral hemiplegia; contralateral paralysis of face and tongue (supranuclear type).

Laboratory

Diagnosis is made by clinical findings.

Treatment

Ptosis: If visual acuity is affected, most cases require surgical correction and there are several procedures that may be used including levator resection, repair or advancement and Fasanella-Servat.

BIBLIOGRAPHY

1. Kistler JP, Ropper AH, Martin JB. Cerebrovascular diseases. In: Isselbacher KJ, Braunwald E, Wilson JD, Martin JB, Fauci A, Kasper DL (Eds). Harrison's Principles of Internal Medicine, 13th edition. New York: McGraw-Hill; 1994. pp. 2242-3.
2. Miller NR (Ed). Walsh and Hoyt's Clinical Neuro-Ophthalmology, 44th edition. Baltimore, USA: Williams & Wilkins; 1995. pp. 238-44.
3. Newman NJ. Third, fourth and sixth-nerve lesions and the cavernous sinus. In: Albert DM, Jakobiec FA (Eds). Albert & Jakobiec's Principles and Practice of Ophthalmology: Clinical Practice, 5th edition. Philadelphia, PA: WB Saunders; 1994. pp. 245-51.
4. Weber H. A contribution to the pathology of the crura cerebri. Med Chir Trans. 1863;46:121-40.1.
5. Wolf BS, Newman CM, Khilnani MT. The posterior inferior cerebellar artery on vertebral angiography. Am J Roentgenol Radium Ther Nucl Med. 1962;87:322-37.

21.2A. AMEBIASIS (AMEBIC DYSENTERY, ENTAMOEBA HISTOLYTICA)

General

It is caused by *Entamoeba histolytica*; *E. histolytica* cysts in stools are diagnostic.

Ocular

Conjunctivitis; iridocyclitis; hypopyon; central choroiditis; retinal hemorrhages; retinal perivasculitis; macular edema; corneal ulceration; granulomatous and nongranulomatous uveitis; vitreous hemorrhage.

Clinical

Chronic dysentery; abscesses of liver and brain; toxic megacolon.

Laboratory

Enzyme immunoassay (EIA) is the best test for making the specific diagnosis of *E. histolytica*.

Treatment

Metronidazole is considered the drug of choice for symptomatic, invasive disease. Asymptomatic intestinal infection may be treated with iodoquinol, paromomycin, or diloxanide furoate.

BIBLIOGRAPHY

1. Lacasse A, Cleveland KO, Cantey JR, et al. Amebiasis. [online] Availble from www.emedicine.com/ped/TOPIC80.HTM. [Accessed September, 2013].

21.2C. BOTULISM

General

It is caused by a toxin-producing strain of *Clostridium botulinum*; it occurs primarily after the ingestion of contaminated food; the organism can produce a neurotoxin, the effect of which can be life threatening.

Ocular

Absent optokinetic nystagmus, absent vertical gaze; marked limitation of horizontal gaze; ptosis; diplopia; decreased tear secretion; mydriasis; paralysis of accommodation; nystagmus; optic atrophy; optic neuritis; extraocular muscle paresis.

Clinical

Dizziness; severe respiratory impairment; gastrointestinal disturbances; dysphagia; dysarthria; postural hypotension.

Laboratory

Toxin assay for early diagnosis, whereas later cases are more likely to yield a positive specimen culture.

Treatment

Antitoxin appears to be the only effective medication. Supportive care such as ventilation and parenteral nutrition are necessary for the duration of the paralytic illness.

BIBLIOGRAPHY

1. Patel B, Taylor SF. (2012). Ophthalmologic manifestations of botulism. [online] Available from www.emedicine.com/oph/TOPIC493.HTM. [Accessed September, 2013].

21.2D. CHICKENPOX (VARICELLA)

General

Acute exanthematous disease; highly contagious; children ages between 2 and 8 years.

Ocular

Conjunctival ulcer; corneal ulcer; descemetocele; corneal opacity; keratitis; paresis of third, fourth, and sixth nerves; optic neuritis; papilledema; retinitis; hemorrhagic retinopathy; uveitis; cataract; paralytic mydriasis; phthisis bulbi; unifocal choroiditis; dendritic keratitis; acute retinal necrosis (in a patient with AIDS); disciform keratitis.

Clinical

Fever; malaise; rash; pruritus.

Laboratory

Diagnosis is made by clinical findings.

Treatment

Isolation oral antihistamines, such as diphenhydramine and hydroxyzine, are used for severe pruritus and acetaminophen is recommended for use for the reduction of fever.

BIBLIOGRAPHY

1. Bechtel KA. (2011). Pediatric chickenpox. [online] Available from www.emedicine.com/emerg/TOPIC367.HTM. [Accessed September, 2013].

21.2E. CRANIOPHARYNGIOMA

General

Benign congenital tumors arising from epithelial remnants of Rathke's pouch; most common non-glial intracranial tumors in childhood; second most common sellar-parasellar tumor primarily in children or young adults; 35% of cases occur in patients over age of 40 years.

Ocular

Paresis of third or sixth nerve; optic nerve atrophy; optic neuritis; papilledema; dilation of pupil; diplopia; hemianopia; nystagmus; scotoma; visual field defects; visual loss.

Clinical

Hydrocephalus; infantilism; diabetes insipidus; abnormal sexual development; headaches; acute aseptic meningitis.

Laboratory

Cranial CT and MRI are the current imaging standards.

Treatment

Although controversial, aggressive surgical treatment to attempt gross total resection is sometimes considered. Second option is planned limited surgery followed by radiotherapy.

BIBLIOGRAPHY

1. Bobustuc GC, Groves MD, Fuller GN, et al. (2012). Craniopharyngioma. [online] Available from www.emedicine.com/neuro/TOPIC584.HTM. [Accessed September, 2013].

21.2F. DENGUE FEVER

General

Endemic over the tropics and subtropics; caused by four distinct serogroups of dengue viruses, types 1–4, Group B arboviruses; transmitted solely by mosquitoes of the genus *Aedes*.

Ocular

Lid edema; conjunctivitis; ocular and retrobulbar pain accentuated by ocular movement; dacryoadenitis; keratitis; corneal ulcer; iritis; retinal or vitreous hemorrhages; ocular motor paresis; optic atrophy.

Clinical

Hemorrhagic fever, severe headache; backache; joint pain; rigors; insomnia; anorexia; loss of taste; epistaxis; rashes; maculopapular rash; myalgia; human infection with four serotypes of dengue virus causing two diseases: classic dengue fever and dengue hemorrhagic fever (50% mortality).

Laboratory

Basic metabolic panel, liver function test, coagulation studies, chest X-ray, serial ultrasonography.

Treatment

A self-limited illness, and only supportive care is required. Acetaminophen may be used to treat patients with symptomatic fever. Dengue hemorrhagic fever warrant closer observation. Rehydration with intravenous fluids, plasma expander, transfusion and shock therapy may be necessary.

BIBLIOGRAPHY

1. Shepherd SM, Hinfey PB, Shoff WH. (2012). Dengue. [online] Available from www.emedicine.com/med/TOPIC528.HTM. [Accessed September, 2013].

21.2G. DEVIC SYNDROME (OPHTHALMOENCEPHALOMYELOPATHY; OPTIC MYELITIS; NEUROMYELITIS OPTICA)

General

Etiology unknown; frequent between the ages of 20 years and 50 years; mortality rate up to 50%; associated with chickenpox.

Ocular

Ptosis is rare; ocular muscle palsy (rare); abducens and oculomotor palsy; paralysis of conjugate gaze; blindness; onset usually very sudden in one eye, followed soon by blindness in the other eye; miosis; bilateral optic neuritis (unilateral involvement is rare); optic atrophy; pupillary dysfunction.

Clinical

Prodromal signs: headache; sore throat; fever and malaise; ascending myelitis with resulting pain, which may be severe; numbness; weakness; paralysis.

Laboratory

Diagnosis is made by clinical findings.

Treatment

Steroids orally or intravenously may be useful.

BIBLIOGRAPHY

1. Schatz MP, Carter JE. (2011). Childhood optic neuritis. [online] Available from www.emedicine.com/oph/TOPIC343.HTM. [Accessed September, 2013].

🔲 21.2H. DIPHTHERIA

General

Acute infectious disease caused by *C. diphtheriae*; severity is dependent upon the amount of exotoxin absorbed prior to initiation of specific therapy.

Ocular

Conjunctivitis; xerophthalmia; keratitis; corneal ulcer; blepharitis; cellulitis of lid; meibomianitis; ptosis; dacryocystitis; cataract; central retinal artery occlusion; optic neuritis; accommodative spasm or paralysis; convergence paralysis; divergence paralysis; paralysis of third, fourth, or sixth nerve; paralysis of accommodation (in children); ocular motor nerve paresis; choroiditis; cranial neuropathies involving the trigeminal, vagus, and hypoglossal cranial nerves; myocarditis.

Clinical

Local inflammatory lesion, with effect on heart, kidneys, and nervous system.

Laboratory

Gram-positive rods commonly affect children younger than 10 years.

Treatment

Systemic treatment involves use of diphtheria antitoxin and antibiotics. Ocular treatment includes diphtheria antitoxin and high titer y-globulin preparation. Topical penicillin-G ointment helps to eradicate the bacilli.

🔲 BIBLIOGRAPHY

1. Demirci CS. (2011). Pediatric diphtheria. [online] Available from www.emedicine.com/ped/TOPIC596.HTM. [Accessed September, 2013].

🔲 21.2I. ENCEPHALITIS, ACUTE

General

In approximately 0.1–0.2% of patients having rubeola (measles), an acute encephalitis is seen within 1 week after the onset of the rash; a case of immunosuppressive encephalitis can present with focal seizures leading to progressive obtundation.

Ocular

Papillitis; optic atrophy; ocular motor palsies; nystagmus; optic neuritis or neuroretinitis.

Clinical

Rise in temperature; drowsiness; irritability; meningismus; vomiting and headache; stupor; convulsions; coma.

Laboratory

Perform head CT, with and without contrast agent, before LP to search for evidence of elevated intracerebral pressure. MRI is useful. Viral serology.

Treatment

Evaluate and treat for shock or hypotension, treat systemic complications, acyclovir.

🔲 BIBLIOGRAPHY

1. Howes DS, Lazoff M. (2013). Encephalitis. [online] Available from www.emedicine.com/emerg/TOPIC163.HTM. [Accessed September, 2013].

🔲 21.2L. INFLUENZA

Ocular

Conjunctivitis; subconjunctival hemorrhages; keratitis; tenonitis; ptosis; cellulitis of orbit and lid; dacryocystitis; retinal hemorrhage; cataract; episcleritis; hypopyon; optic neuritis; uveitis; panophthalmitis; vitreal hemorrhage; paralysis of third or fourth nerve; uveitis following vaccination for influenza.

Clinical

Headache; fever; malaise; muscular aching; substernal soreness; nasal stuffiness; nausea.

Laboratory

The criterion standard for diagnosing influenza A and B is a viral culture of nasal-pharyngeal samples, throat samples, or both.

Treatment

Prevention is the most effective therapy. Two new drugs have been marketed recently for treatment of influenza A and B. These are the neuraminidase inhibitors, oseltamivir and zanamivir.

BIBLIOGRAPHY

1. Derlet RW. (2012). Influenza. [online] Available from www.emedicine.com/med/TOPIC1170.HTM. [Accessed September, 2013].

21.2M. LOCKJAW (TETANUS)

General

Acute infectious disease affecting nervous system; causative agent is *Clostridium tetani*; bacteria enters body through a puncture wound, abrasion, cut, or burn.

Ocular

Chemosis; keratitis; nystagmus; uveitis; corneal ulcer; cellulitis of orbit; hypopyon; panophthalmitis; pupil paralysis; pseudoptosis; blepharospasm; paralysis of third or seventh nerve; may occur following perforating ocular injuries.

Clinical

Severe muscle spasms; dysphagia; trismus; facial palsy; muscle stiffness; irritability.

Laboratory

Gram-positive spore-forming bacteria, laboratory studies are of little value.

Treatment

Passive immunization with human tetanus immune globulin shortens the course of tetanus and may lessen its severity. Benzodiazepines have emerged as the mainstay of symptomatic therapy for tetanus.

BIBLIOGRAPHY

1. Hinfey PB. (2012). Tetanus. [online] Available from www.emedicine.com/med/TOPIC2254.HTM. [Accessed September, 2013].

21.2O. MALARIA

General

It is caused by *Plasmodium*, which is transmitted by mosquito bite, blood transfusion, or contaminated needles and syringes.

Ocular

Proliferative retinitis; vascular embolism; keratitis; ocular herpes simplex; blepharitis; optic atrophy; papilledema; papillitis; optic neuritis; anisocoria; Argyll Robertson pupil; vitreal hemorrhages and opacity; cataract; myopia; strabismus; uveitis; scleral icterus; scotoma; lagophthalmos; ptosis; subconjunctival hemorrhages; paralysis of third, fourth, or sixth nerve; epibulbar hemorrhage involving the conjunctiva, episclera, tendinous insertion of the medial rectus.

Clinical

Fever; anemia; splenomegaly; death.

Laboratory

Blood smear.

Treatment

Consult infectious disease specialist.

BIBLIOGRAPHY

1. Perez-Jorge EV, Herchline TE. (2013). Malaria. [online] Available from www.emedicine.com/med/TOPIC1385.HTM. [Accessed September, 2013].

⊟ 2I.2P. MEASLES (MORBILLI; RUBEOLA)

General

Acute, extremely communicable disease that affects young school-aged children; caused by paramyxovirus.

Ocular

Hypopyon; uveitis; conjunctivitis; Koplik (Hirschberg) spots of conjunctiva; keratitis; corneal ulcer; cellulitis of lid; dacryocystitis; congenital cataract; optic atrophy; optic neuritis; strabismus; pigmentary retinopathy; iris prolapse; hemianopsia; secondary glaucoma; central retinal artery occlusion; orbital cellulitis; accommodative spasm; paralysis of sixth nerve; keratoconus.

Clinical

Maculopapular rash; fever.

Laboratory

Diagnosis is made by clinical findings.

Treatment

Good hydration.

⊟ BIBLIOGRAPHY

1. Chen SS. (2011). Measles. [online] Available from www.emedicine.com/derm/TOPIC259.HTM. [Accessed September, 2013].

⊟ 2I.2Q. MENINGOCOCCEMIA (NEISSERIA MENINGITIDES; MENINGITIS)

General

Systemic bacterial infection caused by *N. meningitides*; can be present chronically in patients with immune deficiencies including deficient complement levels.

Ocular

Photophobia; conjunctivitis; chemosis; keratitis; uveitis; panophthalmitis; retinal endophlebitis; macular edema; papillitis; optic neuritis; paresis of sixth or seventh nerve; nystagmus; miosis; hippus; cortical blindness; papilledema (rare); conjunctival petechiae; strabismus.

Clinical

Meningitis; fever; malaise; joint pain; splenic enlargement.

Laboratory

Cultures from blood, spinal fluid, or joint fluid.

Treatment

Treat with antibiotics promptly.

⊟ BIBLIOGRAPHY

1. Javid MH, Ahmed SH. (2012). Meningococcemia. [online] Available from www.emedicine.com/med/TOPIC1445.HTM. [Accessed September, 2013].

⊟ 2I.2R. DISSEMINATED SCLEROSIS (MULTIPLE SCLEROSIS)

General

Disseminated demyelination affecting white matter of the brain, spinal cord, and optic nerves; etiology is unknown.

Ocular

Nystagmus; ptosis; myokymia; optic atrophy; papillitis; optic neuritis; anisocoria; Argyll Robertson pupil; Marcus Gunn pupil; hippus, decreased or absent papillary reaction to light; periphlebitis; visual field defects; gaze palsy; paralysis of third or sixth nerve; uveitis; oscillopsia; Uhthoff symptom (reduction of visual acuity with exercise or ocular hyperthermia); pars planitis; retinal venous sheathing; retinitis; granulomatous uveitis.

Clinical

Incoordination; paresthesia; spasticity; tic douloureux; urinary frequency and infections; progressive disability; paralysis; death.

Laboratory

MRI, CSF positive for oligoclonal band, albumin and immunoglobulin G (IgG) index; BAER and somatosensory-evoked potentials (SEP).

Treatment

Patients with MS may require multiple consultations to rule out other causes for their symptoms. Drugs such as immunomodulators, immunosuppressors, antiparkinson agents, CNS stimulants are all used in the management of the disease.

BIBLIOGRAPHY

1. Luzzio C, Dangond F. (2012). Multiple sclerosis. [online] Available from www.emedicine.com/neuro/topic228.htm. [Accessed September, 2013].

21.2S. OPHTHALMOPLEGIC MIGRAINE SYNDROME

General

Symptoms produced by ipsilateral herniation of hippocampal gyrus of temporal lobe through incisura tentorii; dependent upon unilateral cerebral edema due to vascular or vasomotor phenomena, intracranial aneurysm, or tumor; incidence may be greater in women with the initial attack in the 1st decade of life; pathogenesis is unclear, but it is likely secondary to ischemia of the ocular motor nerve.

Ocular

Severe unilateral supraorbital pain; ptosis; transitory partial or complete homolateral oculomotor paralysis; fourth or sixth nerve occasionally involved; retinal hemorrhages; papilledema (may be bilateral); moderate to severe headache with partial to complete cranial nerve III paresis including the pupil; more than one ocular nerve may be affected.

Clinical

Migraine headache, not present in all instances; dizziness; diminution in sense of smell; hypalgesia contralateral side of face; nausea/vomiting may be present; recurrent sinus arrest.

Laboratory

Clinical.

Treatment

Ptosis: If visual acuity is affected, most cases require surgical correction and there are several procedures that may be used including levator resection, repair or advancement and Fasanella-Servat.

BIBLIOGRAPHY

1. Bazak I, Margulis T, Shnaider H, et al. Ophthalmoplegic migraine and recurrent sinus arrest. J Neurol Neurosurg Psychiatry. 1991;54:935.
2. Ehlers H. On pathogenesis of ophthalmoplegic migraine. Acta Psychiatr Neurol (Scand). 1928;3:219.
3. Geeraets WJ. Ocular Syndromes, 3rd edition. Philadelphia: Lea & Febiger; 1976.
4. Gulkilik G, Cagatay H, Oba E, et al. Ophthalmoplegic migraine associated with recurrent isolated ptosis. Ann Ophthal. 2010;41:206-12.
5. Raskin NH. Migraine and other headaches. In: Rowland LP (Ed). Merritt's Textbook of Neurology, 9th edition. Baltimore: Williams & Wilkins; 1995. pp. 837-45.
6. Stommel EW, Ward TN, Harris RD. Ophthalmoplegic migraine or Tolosa-Hunt syndrome? Headache. 1994;34:177.
7. Van Pelt W, Andermann F. On the early onset of ophthalmologic migraine. Am J Dis Child. 1964;107:628.
8. Vijayan N. Ophthalmoplegic migraine: ischemic or compressive neuropathy? Headache. 1980;20:300-4.

⊟ 21.2T KUSSMAUL DISEASE (KUSSMAUL-MAIER DISEASE; NECROTIZING ANGIITIS; PAN)

General

Progressive process of vascular inflammation and necrosis, manifested by numerous nodules along the course of small and medium-sized arteries; lesions are segmental in distribution, have a predilection for bifurcation and involve all but the pulmonary arteries; arteries in gastrointestinal tract, kidneys, and muscles are particularly affected; affects primarily males between ages 20 years and 50 years.

Ocular

Retinal detachment; cotton-wool patches; polyarteritis nodosa lesion of arteries; pseudoretinitis pigmentosa; conjunctivitis; corneal ulcer; tenonitis; ptosis; exophthalmos; uveitis; optic atrophy; cataract; scleritis; paralysis of extraocular muscles; neuroretinitis; macular star; peripheral ulcerative keratitis; retinal vasculitis; pseudotumor of the orbit; central retinal artery occlusion.

Clinical

Fever; myalgia; hypertension; gastrointestinal disorders; neuropathy; respiratory infection; weight loss; anginal pain; hemiplegia; convulsion; acute brain syndrome; skin lesions; diffuse erythema; purpura; urticaria; gangrene; tachycardia; pericarditis; aortitis; painful facial swelling; diplopia.

Laboratory

Diagnosis is made by clinical findings.

Treatment

- *Retinal detachment*: Scleral buckle, pneumatic retinopexy and vitrectomy may be used to close all the breaks.
- *Corneal ulcer*: Corneal cultures may be taken and treatment is initiated. Treatment includes a broad spectrum of antibiotics and cycloplegic drops.
- *Uveitis*: Topical steroids and cycloplegic medication should be the initial treatment of choice. Oral steroids if not responsive to topical steroids, immunosuppressants if bilateral disease that does not respond to oral steroids, periocular steroids for unilateral or posterior uveitis. Vitrectomy can be used for severe vitreous opacification. Cryotherapy and laser photocoagulation may be used for localized pars plana exudates.

⊟ BIBLIOGRAPHY

1. Akova YA, Jabbur NS, Foster CS. Ocular presentation of polyarteritis nodosa. Clinical course and management with steroid and cytotoxic therapy. Ophthalmology. 1993;100(12):1775-81.
2. Kussmaul A, Maier R. Ueber Eine Bisher Nicht Beschriebene Eigenthumliche Artenener Krankung (Periarteritis Nodosa), die Mit Morbus Brightii und Rapid Fortschreitender Allgemeiner Muskellahumung Einhergeht. Dtsch Arch Klin Med. 1866;1:484-518.
3. Matsuda A, Chin S, Ohashi T. A case of neuroretinitis associated with long-standing polyarteritis nodosa. Ophthalmologica. 1994;208(3):168-71.
4. Roy FH, Fraunfelder FW, Fraunfelder FT. Roy and Fraunfelder's Current Ocular Therapy, 6th edition. Philadelphia: WB, Saunders; 2008.
5. Solomon SM, Solomon JH. Bilateral central retinal artery occlusions in polyarteritis nodosa. Ann Ophthalmol. 1978; 10(5):567-9.

⊟ 21.2U. POLIOMYELITIS (INFANTILE PARALYSIS)

General

Acute viral infection characterized by varying degrees of neuronal injury, with special localization in the anterior horns and motor nuclei of the brainstem.

Ocular

Diplopia; nystagmus; paralysis of third, fourth, and sixth nerves; paresis of seventh nerve; papilledema; visual agnosia; Homer syndrome; pupillary paralysis; optic neuritis; ophthalmoparesis; transient visual loss; internuclear ophthalmoplegia; papillary disturbances, spasm of near reflex.

Clinical

Flaccid paralysis of many muscle groups; death from asphyxia and involvement of vital centers in the brainstem.

Laboratory

Obtain specimens from the CSF, stool, and throat for viral cultures.

Treatment

No antivirals are effective against polioviruses. The treatment of poliomyelitis is mainly supportive and will involve physical therapist and rehabilitation therapist, pulmonologist, neurologist, immunologist and infectious diseases specialist.

⊟ BIBLIOGRAPHY

1. Estrada B. (2012). Pediatric poliomyelitis. [online] Available from www.emedicine.com/ped/TOPIC1843.HTM. [Accessed September, 2013].

⊟ 21.2V. ALCOHOLISM

General

Classified into three groups; (1) symptoms of mental disease, (2) physiologic poison, or (3) result of social drinking; addiction compounds other health disorders.

Ocular

Congestion of conjunctiva; amblyopia; diplopia; night blindness; nystagmus; cataracts; paralysis of accommodation; paralysis of extraocular muscles; esophoria for distance fixation; acute visual loss; cotton-wool spots; cherry-red spot (associated with pancreatitis).

Clinical

Tremors; seizures; delirium; alcoholic hepatitis; cirrhosis; gastritis; pancreatitis; cancer of mouth and esophagus; peripheral neuropathy; organic brain disease; hypertension; cardiomyopathy; hypoglycemia; anemia; hyperuricemia; susceptibility to infections; skeletal myopathies.

Treatment

Address the issue, strongly encourage alcoholic anonymous (AA) and encourage family members to contact Al-Anon and Alateen.

⊟ BIBLIOGRAPHY

1. Thompson W, Lande RG, Kalapatapu RK. (2013). Alcoholism. [online] Available from www.emedicine.com/med/TOPIC98.HTM. [Accessed September, 2013].

⊟ 21.2V. HERPES ZOSTER

General

Caused by varicella zoster virus; about 75% of cases occur in persons over age of 45 years; condition is more frequent with advancing age and in patients who are immunocompromised by drugs or disease; in particular, an increasing number of patients with herpes zoster ophthalmicus are immunosuppressed.

Ocular

Conjunctivitis; keratitis; recurrent corneal ulcer; neuralgia; zoster rash of eyelids; uveitis; iris atrophy; scleritis; cataract; optic neuritis; paralysis of third nerve; proptosis; paralysis of lids; orbital apex syndrome; retinitis; neurotrophic keratitis; acute retinal necrosis; progressive outer retinal necrosis; ocular motor nerve pareses; tonic pupil; encephalitis; vasculitis.

Clinical

Local lesions involving the posterior or root ganglia; nerve damage; tissue scarring.

Laboratory

Diagnosed mostly on the basis of the characteristic pain and appearance of the dermatomal rashes.

Treatment

Antiviral agents, systemic corticosteroids, antidepressants, and adequate pain control. Immunocompetent adults aged 60 years or older, benefit from receipt of the herpes zoster vaccine and have a lower incidence of herpes zoster.

BIBLIOGRAPHY

1. Diaz MM, Foster CS, Walton RC, et al. (2011). Herpes zoster ophthalmicus. [online] Available from www.emedicine.com/oph/TOPIC257.HTM. [Accessed September, 2013].
2. Ghaznawi N, Virdi A, Dayan A, et al. Herpes zoster ophthalmicus: comparison of disease in patients 60 years and older versus younger than 60 years. Ophthalmology. 2011;118(11):2242-50.
3. Ho J, Xirasagar S, Lin H. Increased risk of a cancer diagnosis after herpes zoster ophthalmicus: a nationwide population-based study. Ophthalmology. 2011;118(6):1076-81.
4. Tseng HF, Smith N, Harpaz R, et al. Herpes zoster vaccine in older adults and the risk of subsequent herpes zoster disease. JAMA. 2011;305(2):160-6.

21.2V. MUMPS

General

Viral infection.

Ocular

Conjunctivitis; keratitis; corneal ulcer; tenonitis; exophthalmos; microphthalmos; optic atrophy; optic neuritis; papillitis; scleritis; uveitis; cortical blindness; congenital punctal occlusion; paralysis of extraocular muscles; dacryoadenitis; iritis; paralysis of accommodation; internal and external ophthalmoparesis.

Clinical

Affects the parotid glands, but infection of other glandular tissue occurs, including the lacrimal gland and testicles; encephalitis; meningitis.

Laboratory

Mumps virus by acute serologic studies.

Treatment

Generous hydration and alimentation, analgesics for headaches. No antiviral agent is available.

BIBLIOGRAPHY

1. Defendi GL. (2012). Mumps. [online] Available from www.emedicine.com/ped/TOPIC1503.HTM. [Accessed September, 2013].

21.2W. HYDROPHOBIA (LYSSA; RABIES)

General

Acute viral zoonosis of the CNS.

Ocular

Lid retraction; widening of palpebral fissure; retinal hemorrhages; mydriasis; paralysis of third, fourth, fifth, or seventh nerve; bilateral optic neuritis; branch retinal artery occlusion; vaccine-induced autoimmune demyelinative optic neuritis.

Clinical

Fever; headache; nausea; numbness; tingling; acute sensitiveness to sound and light; laryngeal and pharyngeal spasms; increased muscle tonus; convulsions; delirium; coma; death.

Laboratory

Saliva can be tested by virus isolation or reverse transcription followed by PCR. Suspected infectious animal should be quarantined for 10 days.

Treatment

Before the onset of symptoms, both passive and active immunizations are effective for preventing progression to full-blown rabies. In exposures to high-risk species, initiate treatment immediately pending laboratory examination of the animal, if it is caught.

BIBLIOGRAPHY

1. Gompf SG. (2011). Rabies. [online] Available from www.emedicine.com/med/TOPIC1374.HTM. [Accessed September, 2013].

21.2X. RELAPSING POLYCHONDRITIS (JAKSCH WARTENHOST SYNDROME; MEYENBURG-ALTHERZ-VEHLINGER SYNDROME; VON MEYENBERG II SYNDROME)

General

Episodic, yet generally progressive; onset usually in middle life; possibly caused by lysosomal labilizing factor of endogenous or exogenous toxic nature or immunologic reactions; possible association with Reiter's syndrome.

Ocular

Conjunctivitis; corneal ulcer; exophthalmos; panophthalmitis; phthisis bulbi; proptosis; optic neuritis; papilledema; retinal detachment; blue sclera; episcleritis; scleromalacia; vitreous opacity; cataracts; nystagmus; retinal artery thrombosis; keratoconjunctivitis sicca; secondary glaucoma; scotoma; uveitis; paresis of third or sixth nerve; conjunctival mass (salmon patch); chorioretinitis.

Clinical

Destruction of cartilage and eventual replacement with connective tissue; polyarthritis; chondritis; tracheal collapse; bronchial collapse; anemia; liver dysfunction; death; malaise; fever; dyspnea; changes in pitch of voice; hearing impairment; vertigo; deformed ears; aortic valve insufficiency.

Laboratory

No specific serologic markers.

Treatment

No therapy.

BIBLIOGRAPHY

1. Compton N, Buckner JH, Harp KI, et al. (2012). Polychondritis. [online] Available from emedicine.medscape.com/article/331475-overview. [Accessed September, 2013].

21.2Y. SMALLPOX (VARIOLA)

General

Highly contagious cutaneous disease caused by viral infection.

Ocular

Conjunctivitis; keratitis; corneal ulcer; hypopyon; endophthalmitis; congenital corneal clouding; albinotic spots on iris; choroiditis; vitreous opacities; papillitis; extraocular muscle palsies; entropion; dacryocystitis; chorioretinitis; optic neuritis; and vesicles of the eyelid; preauricular adenopathy; eyelid ulcerating pustules; several conditions predispose to the spread of vaccinia, including eczema, hypogammaglobulinemia, steroid therapy, and AIDS.

Clinical

Fever, headache, and vomiting prior to appearance of the rash on the face, upper trunk, and down to the extremities.

Laboratory

Brick-shaped virions viewed with electron microscopy examination, virus culture from live cells, or DNA analysis using PCR and smallpox skin specimen should be collected.

Treatment

No known treatment is effective.

BIBLIOGRAPHY

1. Hussain AN, Hussain F, Alam M, et al. (2011). Smallpox. [online] Available from www.emedicine.com/med/TOPIC3545.HTM. [Accessed September, 2013].

⊟ 21.2AA. ACQUIRED LUES (SYPHILIS; ACQUIRED SYPHILIS; LUES VENEREA; MALUM VENEREUM)

General

Causative agent, *T. pallidum*, usually transmitted sexually.

Ocular

Conjunctival chancroid; conjunctivitis; keratitis; blepharitis; ptosis; iris atrophy; hippus; dacryocystitis; optic nerve atrophy; optic neuritis; periostitis; episcleritis; scleritis; nystagmus; uveitis; vitreous hemorrhages; paralysis of sixth nerve; papilledema; retinal hemorrhages; retinitis proliferans; oculogyric crisis; neuroretinitis; papilledema (associated with aseptic meningitis); diffuse or multifocal chorioretinitis; vertical supranuclear gaze palsy; Benedikt syndrome.

Clinical

Primary lesion associated with regional lymphadenopathy; secondary bacteremic stage associated with generalized mucocutaneous lesions; tertiary stage characterized by destructive mucocutaneous, musculoskeletal, or parenchymal lesions, aortitis, or CNS disease; syphilis and HIV infection often coexist in the same patient who experiences a higher incidence and greater severity of neurologic and ocular manifestations; a significant percentage of patients infected with HIV-I and *T. pallidum* become seronegative to syphilis testing.

Laboratory

Serologic nontreponemal tests include VDRL and RPR.

Treatment

The goals are to reduce morbidity and to prevent complications. Penicillin is the antibiotic of choice for treating syphilis. Ocular syphilis should be treated the same as patients with neurosyphilis.

⊟ BIBLIOGRAPHY

1. Euerle B, Chandrasekar PH, Diaz MM, et al. (2012). Syphilis. [online] Available from www.emedicine.com/med/TOPIC2224.HTM. [Accessed September, 2013].
2. Majmudar PA. (2011). Interstitial keratitis overview of interstitial keratitis. [online] Available from www.emedicine.com/oph/TOPIC453.HTM. [Accessed September, 2013].

⊟ 21.2BB. TEMPORAL ARTERITIS SYNDROME (CRANIAL ARTERITIS SYNDROME; GIANT CELL ARTERITIS; HUTCHINSON-HORTON-MAGATH-BROWN SYNDROME)

General

Etiology unknown; mainly females; mainly Whites; ages 55–80 years; temporal artery shows inflammatory thickening; arteritis of the vessels supplying the optic nerve.

Ocular

Transient ptosis; partial or complete loss of vision on the affected side; retinal detachment; exudates and hemorrhages; narrowing of retinal vessels; obstruction of the central retinal artery; optic atrophy; ischemic optic neuropathy; acute decreased IOP; corneal hypesthesia; palsies of extraocular muscles; hemorrhagic glaucoma; diplopia; hemorrhages on or around the disk.

Clinical

Throbbing headache; hyperalgesia of the scalp; malaise; anorexia; weakness; weight loss; fever; nodular pulmonary nodules; cough; otitis with deafness.

Laboratory

Elevated ESR greater than 50 mm/hour, positive temporal artery biopsy.

Treatment

Systemic corticosteroids are the therapy of choice.

⊟ BIBLIOGRAPHY

1. Allen AW, Biega T, Varma MK. (2012). Temporal arteritis imaging. [online] Available from www.emedicine.com/radio/TOPIC675.HTM. [Accessed September, 2013].
2. Walvick MD, Walvick MP. Giant cell arteritis: laboratory predictors of a positive temporal artery biopsy. Ophthalmology. 2011;118(6):1201-4.

21.2CC. TUBERCULOSIS

General

Communicable disease caused by the acid-fast bacillus *Mycobacterium tuberculosis.*

Ocular

Conjunctivitis; subconjunctival nodules (tuberculomas); keratitis; pannus; corneal ulcer; blepharitis; cellulitis; meibomianitis; uveitis; dacryocystitis; chronic orbital cellulitis; retinitis; scleritis; scleral perforation; hypopyon; vitreous hemorrhages; optic neuritis; optic atrophy; tuberculous panophthalmitis; choroidal tubercles; intraorbital extraocular lesions.

Clinical

Pulmonary infection; pyuria; hematuria; epididymitis; dysuria; flank pain; distorted calyces; productive cough.

Laboratory

Acid-fast bacillus culture of body fluids including vitreous and aqueous. PCR is 89% positive for pulmonary infection.

Treatment

A course of chemotherapy (isoniazid, rifampin, pyrazinamide and ethambutol or streptomycin) for a period of 6 months is the recommended therapy.

BIBLIOGRAPHY

1. Collins JK. Handbook of Clinical Ophthalmology. New York: Masson; 1982.
2. DeVoe AG, Locatcher-Khorazo D. The external manifestations of ocular tuberculosis. Trans Am Ophthalmol Soc. 1964;62:203-12.
3. D'Souza P, Garg R, Dhaliwal RS, et al. Orbital tuberculosis. Int Ophthalmol. 1994;18:149-52.
4. Gupta V, Gupta A, Arora S, et al. Presumed tubercular serpiginous like choroiditis. Ophthalmology. 2003;110:1744-9.
5. Patkar S, Singhania BK, Agrawal A. Intraorbital extraocular tuberculosis: a report of three cases. Surg Neurol. 1994; 42:320-1.
6. Roy, FH, Fraunfelder FW, Fraunfelder FT. Roy and Fraunfelder's Current Ocular Therapy, 6th editon. Philadelphia: WB Saunders; 2008.
7. Tejada P, Mendez MJ, Negreira S. Choroidal tubercles with tuberculous meningitis. Int Ophthalmol. 1994;18:115-8.

21.3A. CAROTID ARTERY SYNDROME (CAVERNOUS SINUS FISTULA SYNDROME; RED-EYED SHUNT SYNDROME)

General

Seventy-five percent of cases caused by trauma; others occur spontaneously or are congenital; fistula from carotid artery to cavernous sinus.

Ocular

Progressive, pulsating exophthalmos; distended pulsating superior orbital vein; venous congestion of lids; variable ophthalmoplegia, depending on involvement of cranial nerves III to VI; secondary glaucoma; congestion of conjunctiva with chemosis; corneal ulcerations; eversion of the lower lid; loss of corneal sensation; retinal edema; engorgement of retinal veins; papilledema; optic atrophy; ocular bruit that may be subjective and/or objective; diplopia; visual decrease; choroidal folds; dilated superior ophthalmic vein.

Clinical

Severe unilateral headache; buzzing noise.

Laboratory

Orbital ultrasonography, CT, six-vessel cranial digital subtraction angiography—characterization of the arterial supply and venous drainage of fistula.

Treatment

Use of intraocular lowering agent and topical lubrication is the ocular treatment of choice.

⛬ BIBLIOGRAPHY

1. Dailey EJ, Holloway JA, Murto RE, et al. Evaluation of ocular signs and symptoms in cerebral aneurysms. Arch Ophthalmol. 1964;71:463-74.
2. Duane TD. Clinical Ophthalmology. Philadelphia: JB Lippincott; 1987.
3. Flaharty PM, Lieb WE, Sergott RC, et al. Color Doppler imaging. A new noninvasive technique to diagnose and monitor carotid cavernous sinus fistulas. Arch Ophthalmol. 1991;109:522-6.
4. Gonshor LG, Kline LB. Choroidal folds and dural cavernous sinus fistula. Arch Ophthalmol. 1991;109:1065-6.
5. Phelps CD, Thompson HS, Ossoinig KC. The diagnosis and prognosis of atypical carotid cavernous fistula. Am J Ophthalmol. 1982;93:423-36.
6. Roy FH, Fraunfelder FW, Fraunfelder FT. Roy and Fraunfelder's Current Ocular Therapy, 6th edition. Philadelphia: WB Saunders; 2008.
7. Travers B. A case of aneurysm by anastomosis in the orbit, cured by ligation of common carotid artery. Med Chir Trans. 1917;2:1-420.

⛬ 21.3A1. ARTERIOVENOUS FISTULA (ARTERIOVENOUS ANEURYSM; ARTERIOVENOUS ANGIOMA; ARTERIOVENOUS MALFORMATION; CIRSOID ANEURYSM; RACEMOSE HEMANGIOMA; VARICOSE ANEURYSM)

General

Abnormal communications between arteries and veins that allow arterial blood to enter the vein directly without traversing a capillary network; may be congenital or secondary to penetrating trauma or blunt trauma.

Ocular

Uveitis; chemosis and neovascularization of conjunctiva; bullous keratopathy; eyelid edema; ptosis; exophthalmos; iris atrophy; papilledema; retinal hemorrhages; cataract; paresis of third or sixth nerves; glaucoma; upper lid tumor; total choroidal detachment; leaking retinal macroaneurysms; central retinal vein occlusion; iris neovascularization.

Clinical

Cerebral hemorrhage; death; substernal pain; dyspnea; varicose veins.

Laboratory

Orbital ultrasonography, CT and six-vessel cranial digital subtraction angiography.

Treatment

Obtain emergent neurosurgical consultation for definitive treatment.

⛬ BIBLIOGRAPHY

1. Zebian RC, Kazzi AA. (2013). Emergent management of subarachnoid hemorrhage. [online] Available from www.emedicine.com/emerg/topic559.htm. [Accessed September, 2013].

⛬ 21.3A2. CAROTID ARTERY SYNDROME (CAVERNOUS SINUS FISTULA SYNDROME; RED-EYED SHUNT SYNDROME)

General

Seventy-five percent of cases caused by trauma; others occur spontaneously or are congenital; fistula from carotid artery to cavernous sinus.

Ocular

Progressive, pulsating exophthalmos; distended pulsating superior orbital vein; venous congestion of lids; variable ophthalmoplegia, depending on involvement of cranial nerves III to VI; secondary glaucoma; congestion of conjunctiva with chemosis; corneal ulcerations; eversion of the lower lid; loss of corneal sensation; retinal edema; engorgement of retinal veins; papilledema; optic atrophy; ocular bruit that may be subjective and/or objective; diplopia; visual decrease; choroidal folds; dilated superior ophthalmic vein.

Clinical

Severe unilateral headache; buzzing noise.

Laboratory

Orbital ultrasonography, CT, six-vessel cranial digital subtraction angiography—characterization of the arterial supply and venous drainage of fistula.

Treatment

Use of intraocular lowering agent and topical lubrication is the ocular treatment of choice.

🖬 BIBLIOGRAPHY

1. Dailey EJ, Holloway JA, Murto RE, et al. Evaluation of ocular signs and symptoms in cerebral aneurysms. Arch Ophthalmol. 1964;71:463-74.
2. Duane TD. Clinical Ophthalmology. Philadelphia: JB Lippincott; 1987.
3. Flaharty PM, Lieb WE, Sergott RC, et al. Color Doppler imaging. A new noninvasive technique to diagnose and monitor carotid cavernous sinus fistulas. Arch Ophthalmol. 1991;109:522-6.
4. Gonshor LG, Kline LB. Choroidal folds and dural cavernous sinus fistula. Arch Ophthalmol. 1991;109:1065-6.
5. Phelps CD, Thompson HS, Ossoinig KC. The diagnosis and prognosis of atypical carotid cavernous fistula. Am J Ophthalmol. 1982;93:423-36.
6. Roy FH, Fraunfelder FW, Fraunfelder FT. Roy and Fraunfelder Current Ocular Therapy, 6th edition. Philadelphia: WB Saunders; 2008.
7. Travers B. A case of aneurysm by anastomosis in the orbit, cured by ligation of common carotid artery. Med Chir Trans. 1917;2:1-420.

🖬 21.3A7. TOLOSA-HUNT SYNDROME (PAINFUL OPHTHALMOPLEGIA)

General

Symptoms last from days to weeks; attacks recur at intervals of months or years; inflammatory lesion of cavernous sinus; onset most frequent in 5th decade of life; recurrent Tolosa-Hunt syndrome has been observed in some patients.

Ocular

Steadily "growing" retro-orbital pain; ptosis; involvement of cranial nerves III, IV, VI and first division of V; scintillating scotoma; sluggish pupil reaction to light; corneal sensitivity diminished; optic neuritis.

Clinical

Inflammatory lesions of cavernous sinus.

Laboratory

MRI with axial and coronal views of brain, typically showing thickening and enhancement of involved cavernous sinus. Cerebral angiography is done to rule out aneurysm. Blood count, ESR, ANA, ANCA and ACE levels may be abnormal.

Treatment

Corticosteroids is often used to treat the chronic granulomatous inflammation of the cavernous sinus.

🖬 BIBLIOGRAPHY

1. Taylor DC. (2012). Tolosa-Hunt syndrome. [online] Available from www.emedicine.com/neuro/TOPIC373.HTM. [Accessed September, 2013].

🖬 21.3B. ROCHON-DUVIGNEAUD SYNDROME (SUPERIOR ORBITAL FISSURE SYNDROME) OPTIC ATROPHY

General

Inflammatory, traumatic, tumor, or vascular lesions such as meningioma of the sphenoid, carotid aneurysm, and arachnoiditis; infections originating in the maxillary sinus.

Ocular

Mild exophthalmos; lid edema; partial or complete ophthalmoplegia (III, IV and VI); decreased corneal sensitivity; papilledema; optic atrophy.

Clinical

Decreased sensitivity in area of nasociliary, lacrimal, frontal, and ophthalmic nerve distribution; may result from a metastatic tumor.

Laboratory

CBC count, ESR, thyroid function test, FTA, ANA, LE preparation, ANCA, serum protein electrophoresis, Lyme titer, ACE level and HIV titer are helpful. CSF, anti-GQ1b antibodies, and MRI of the brain and the orbits.

Treatment

Corticosteroids are the treatment of choice.

BIBLIOGRAPHY

1. Falcone F, Lazow SK, Berger JR, et al. Superior orbital fissure syndrome. Secondary to infected dentigerous cyst of the maxillary sinus. NY State Dental J. 1994;60:62-4.
2. Hedstrom J, Parsons J, Maloney PL, et al. Superior orbital fissure syndrome: report of a case. J Oral Surg. 1974; 32:198-201.
3. Phanthumchinda K, Hemachuda T. Superior orbital fissure syndrome as a presenting symptom in hepatocellular carcinoma. J Med Assoc Thailand. 1992;75:62-5.
4. Rochon-Duvigneaud A. Quelques Cas de Paralysie de Tous les Nerfs Orbitaires (Ophtalmoplegie Totale avec Amaurose et Anesthesie dans le Domaine de l'Ophtalmique d'Origine Syphilitique). Arch Ophthalmol. 1896;16:746.

21.3B1. FORAMEN LACERUM SYNDROME (ANEURYSM OF INTERNAL CAROTID ARTERY SYNDROME)

General

Most commonly caused by congenital aneurysm involving the intradural portion of the carotid artery.

Ocular

Periorbital pain; ptosis; oculomotor paralysis with ptosis, diplopia, and internal ophthalmoplegia; cranial nerves IV and VI may be involved; homonymous hemianopia (occasionally); loss of pupillary reflexes for light and accommodation; papilledema; optic atrophy.

Clinical

Meningism; mental disturbances; unilateral frontal or orbital headache; migraine attacks.

Laboratory

CT, MRI, angiography, MRA.

Treatment

Endovascular balloon occlusion.

BIBLIOGRAPHY

1. Dailey EJ, Holloway JA, Murto RE, et al. Evaluation of ocular signs and symptoms in cerebral aneurysms. Arch Ophthalmol. 1964;71:463-74.
2. Geeraets WJ. Ocular syndromes, 3rd edition. Philadelphia: Lea & Febiger; 1976.
3. Misra M, Mohanty AB, Rath S. Giant aneurysm of internal carotid artery presenting features of retrobulbar neuritis. Indian J Ophthalmol. 1991;39:28-9.

21.3B4. SPHENOCAVERNOUS SYNDROME

General

Lesion in the cavernous sinus; similar to the superior orbital fissure syndrome (Rochon-Duvigneaud syndrome) and orbital apex syndrome (*see* Rochon-Duvigneaud syndrome).

Ocular

Proptosis; edema; paresis of cranial nerves III, IV and VI (paralysis of the abducens nerve precedes paralysis of the oculomotor nerve, because the abducens is situated between the internal carotid artery and the cavernous sinus wall); conjunctival edema.

Laboratory

CT and MRI.

Clinical

Paresis of the first (sometimes second and third) division of cranial nerve V; sinusitis.

Treatment

- *Proptosis*: Ocular lubricants are beneficial for controlling the corneal exposure.
- *Paresis of cranial nerves III*: Prism therapy, surgical—muscle surgery on the affected muscle, occlusion of the involved eye to relieve diplopia.

BIBLIOGRAPHY

1. Geeraets WJ. Ocular Syndromes, 3rd edition. Philadelphia, PA: Lea & Febiger; 1976. p. 404.
2. Jefferson G. Concerning injuries, aneurysms and tumours involving the cavernous sinus. Trans Ophthalmol Soc UK. 1953;73:117.

3. Sekhar LN, Linskey ME, Sen CN, et al. Surgical management of lesions within the cavernous sinus. Clin Neurosurg. 1991;37:440-89.

4. Watson NJ, Dick AD, Hutchinson CH. A case of sinusitis presenting with spheno-cavernous syndrome: discussion of the differential diagnosis. Scott Med J. 1991;36(6):179-80.

21.3B5. GRADENIGO SYNDROME (TEMPORAL SYNDROME; LANNOIS-GRADENIGO SYNDROME)

General

It is caused by extradural abscess of the petrous portion of the temporal bone; good prognosis.

Ocular

Ipsilateral paralysis (cranial nerve VI); transient involvement of cranial nerves III and IV occasionally present; severe pain in area of ophthalmic branch (cranial nerve V); photophobia; lacrimation; reduced corneal sensitivity; optic nerve involvement occasionally present.

Clinical

Inner ear infection with deafness; mastoiditis; facial paresis possible; temperature may be elevated; meningeal signs possible; can occur rarely as a complication of otitis media.

Laboratory

CT and MRI.

Treatment

See otolaryngologist.

BIBLIOGRAPHY

1. De Graaf J, Cats H, de Jager AE, et al. Gradenigo's syndrome: a rare complication of otitis media. Clin Neurol Neurosurg. 1988;90(3):237-9.
2. Gradenigro G. A special syndrome of endocranial otitic complications. Ann Otol Rhinol Laryngol. 1904;13:637.
3. Joffe WS. Clinical nerve disease. Int Ophthalmol Clin. 1967;7(4):823-38.

21.3B6. ROCHON-DUVIGNEAUD SYNDROME (SUPERIOR ORBITAL FISSURE SYNDROME) OPTIC ATROPHY

General

Inflammatory, traumatic, tumor, or vascular lesions such as meningioma of the sphenoid, carotid aneurysm, and arachnoiditis; infections originating in the maxillary sinus.

Ocular

Mild exophthalmos; lid edema; partial or complete ophthalmoplegia (III, IV and VI); decreased corneal sensitivity; papilledema; optic atrophy.

Clinical

Decreased sensitivity in area of nasociliary, lacrimal, frontal, and ophthalmic nerve distribution; may result from a metastatic tumor.

Laboratory

CBC count, ESR, thyroid function test, FTA, ANA, LE preparation, ANCA, serum protein electrophoresis, Lyme titer, ACE level and HIV titer are helpful. CSF, anti-GQ1b antibodies, and MRI of the brain and the orbits.

Treatment

Corticosteroids are the treatment of choice.

BIBLIOGRAPHY

1. Falcone F, Lazow SK, Berger JR, et al. Superior orbital fissure syndrome. Secondary to infected dentigerous cyst of the maxillary sinus. NY State Dental J. 1994;60:62-4.
2. Hedstrom J, Parsons J, Maloney PL, et al. Superior orbital fissure syndrome: report of a case. J Oral Surg. 1974; 32:198-201.
3. Phanthumchinda K, Hemachuda T. Superior orbital fissure syndrome as a presenting symptom in hepatocellular carcinoma. J Med Assoc Thailand. 1992;75:62-5.
4. Rochon-Duvigneaud A. Quelques Cas de Paralysie de Tous les Nerfs Orbitaires (Ophtalmoplegie Totale avec Amaurose et Anesthesie dans le Domaine de l'Ophtalmique d'Origine Syphilitique). Arch Ophthalmol. 1896;16:746.

🗗 21.4A. ALBERS-SCHONBERG DISEASE (MARBLE BONE DISEASE; OSTEOSCLEROSIS FRAGILIS GENERALISATA; OSTEOPETROSIS; OSTEOPOIKILOSIS; OSTEOSCLEROSIS CONGENITA DIFFUSA)

General

Simple recessive inheritance, also dominant transmission; benign form is asymptomatic in about 50% of cases and known under the synonym Henck-Assmann syndrome; prognosis is poor for malignant form, with death usually in infancy.

Ocular

Oculomotor paralysis; cranial nerve VII palsy; optic atrophy; ptosis; exophthalmos; papilledema; nystagmus; anisocoria; congenital cataracts; hypertelorism; visual loss in infancy; nasolacrimal duct obstruction; keratoconus.

Clinical

Cartilage and bone thickening; multiple fractures; hyperchromic anemia; osteomyelitis; severe forms: jaundice, hepatosplenomegaly, skeleton sclerosis, lymphadenopathy, and hydrocephalus in infants; mild forms: nerve compression, fractures, and milder form of anemia; pancytopenia from marrow obliteration; low serum calcium; elevated phosphorus.

Laboratory

Radiologic features are usually diagnostic. Patients usually have generalized osteosclerosis. Bones may be uniformly sclerotic, but alternating sclerotic and lucent bands may be noted in iliac wings and near ends of long bones. The bones might be club-like or appear like a bone within bone.

Treatment

- *Infantile therapy*: Vitamin D appears to help by stimulating dormant osteoclasts and thus stimulate bone resorption. Large doses of calcitriol, along with restricted calcium intake, sometimes improve osteopetrosis dramatically.
- *Adult therapy*: No specific medical treatment exists for the adult type.

🗗 BIBLIOGRAPHY

1. Blank R, Bhargava A. (2012). Osteopetrosis. [online] Available from www.emedicine.com/med/TOPIC1692.HTM. [Accessed September, 2013].

🗗 21.4D. HODGKIN DISEASE

General

Hodgkin disease begins in the lymph nodes and usually spreads in a predictable fashion along contiguous chains of nodes; etiology may be viral; prevalent in males.

Ocular

Keratitis; uveitis; cataract; retinal hemorrhages; vasculitis; Horner syndrome; cortical blindness; papilledema; paralysis of oculomotor nerve; episcleritis; visual field defects; infiltration of choroid, conjunctiva, lacrimal gland, and orbit; papillitis; retrobulbar neuritis; opsoclonus-myoclonus; keratitis sicca; infiltrative optic neuropathy; association with Vogt-Koyanagi-Harada syndrome; bilateral serous detachments of the macula.

Clinical

Painless cervical, axillary, or inguinal lymph node swelling; fever; weight loss; anemia; generalized pruritus.

Laboratory

Biopsy of lymph glands is diagnostic.

Treatment

The goal of therapy is to induce a complete remission with radiation therapy, chemotherapy or bone marrow transplantation.

🗗 BIBLIOGRAPHY

1. Lash BW, Dessain SK, Argiris A. (2012). Hodgkin Lymphoma. [online] Available from www.emedicine.com/med/TOPIC1022.HTM. [Accessed September, 2013].

⊟ 21.4E. DISSEMINATED LUPUS ERYTHEMATOSUS (SYSTEMIC LUPUS ERYTHEMATOSUS; LUPUS ERYTHEMATOSUS; KAPOSI-LIBMAN-SACK SYNDROME, SLE)

General

Possible etiology includes viral infections and genetic predisposition; immunologic abnormalities.

Ocular

Keratitis; keratoconjunctivitis sicca; corneal ulcer; optic nerve atrophy; optic neuritis; papilledema; arteritis; central retinal vein occlusion; retinal detachment; microaneurysm; scleritis; uveitis; ptosis; conjunctivitis; paralysis of third nerve; homonymous hemianopsia; multifocal microinfarcts; mydriasis; nystagmus; proptosis; orbital myositis; pseudoretinitis pigmentosa; photophobia.

Clinical

Polyarthritis; morning stiffness; fever; malaise; fatigue; polyserositis; renal disease; CNS disease; anemia; leukopenia; maculopapular rash in a "butterfly" distribution over malar region; alopecia.

Laboratory

Antibodies to double-stranded DNA or the Smith (Sm) antigen or a false-positive serology test for syphilis; positive ANA test that is caused by a medication.

Treatment

Fever, rash, musculoskeletal, and serositis manifestations respond to hydroxychloroquine and NSAIDs. Low-to-moderate dose steroids are necessary for acute flares. CNS involvement and renal disease constitute more serious disease and often require high-dose steroids and other immunosuppression agents. Diffuse proliferative lupus nephritis has been treated with cyclophosphamide induction therapy.

⊟ BIBLIOGRAPHY

1. Bartles CM, Muller D. (2012). Systemic erythematosus lupus. [online] Available from www.emedicine.com/med/TOPIC2228.HTM. [Accessed September, 2013].

⊟ 21.4F. ERB-GOLDFLAM SYNDROME (ERB II SYNDROME; HOPPE-GOLDFLAM DISEASE; PSEUDOPARALYTIC SYNDROME; MYASTHENIA GRAVIS)

General

Occurs at any age; more frequent between ages 20 and 40 years; more females affected than males; progressive; spontaneous; symptoms improve or resolve with rest in early stages of disease (*see* myasthenia gravis, neonatal or infantile); caused by autoantibodies against the acetylcholine receptor at the neuromuscular junction, leading to abnormal fatigability and weakness of skeletal muscle.

Ocular

Transient diplopia; ptosis of upper eyelids.

Clinical

Excessive fatigability of musculature; symptoms appear and increase as day progresses; expressionless face; sagging jaw; difficulty in chewing and talking; nasal regurgitation.

Laboratory

Ice test—crushed ice in surgical glove over ptotic eyelid for 2 minutes and watch for brief elevation of eyelid; Tensilon test and prostigmin test may result in the elevation of ptotic eyelid or improved strabismus in individuals with myasthenia gravis.

Treatment

Adrenal corticosteroids are frequently used. In some cases, mycophenolate mofetil, cyclosporine and cyclophosphamide may be useful. Patching one eye or using prisms may be helpful.

⊟ BIBLIOGRAPHY

1. Erb W. Zur Casuistick der Bulbaren La hmungen. Arch Psychiatr Vervenkr. 1879;9:325-50.
2. Roy FH, Fraunfelder FT, Fraunfelder FW. Roy and Fraunfelder's Current Ocular Therapy, 6th edition. London, UK: Elsevier; 2008.
3. Goldflam S. Vebereinen Scheinbar Keilbaren Bulbarparalytischem Symptom Complex mit Betheiligung der Extremitaten. Dtsch Z Nerven. 1983;4:312-52.
4. Kim JH, Hwang JM, Hwang YS, et al. Childhood ocular myasthenia gravis. Ophthalmology. 2003;110(7):1458-62.
5. Lepore FE, Sanborn GE, Slevin JT. Pupillary dysfunction in myasthenia gravis. Ann Neurol. 1979;6(1):29-33.
6. Sommer N, Melms A, Weller M, et al. Ocular myasthenia gravis. A critical review of clinical and pathophysiological aspects. Doc Ophthalmol. 1993;84(4):309-33.

🗗 21.4G. PASSOW SYNDROME (BREMER STATUS DYSRAPHICUS; STATUS DYSRAPHICUS SYNDROME; SYRINGOMYELIA; SYRINGOBULBIA)

General

Congenital nonclosure of the neural tube; familial occurrence or may be sporadic; insidious onset in 2nd to 3rd decade of life.

Ocular

Enophthalmos; ptosis; rotatory nystagmus; heterochromia iridis; anterior uveitis; corneal anesthesia; neuroparalytic keratitis; paralysis of third, fifth, sixth, and seventh cranial nerves; Horner syndrome; anisocoria; papilledema; optic atrophy; zonular cataract (*see* Horner Syndrome).

Clinical

Anesthesia over area of first division of trigeminal nerve; facial hemiatrophy; facial nerve paralysis; muscular weakness; cervical ribs; kyphoscoliosis; spina bifida; unilateral numbness of fingers; loss of deep reflexes; insensitivity to pain and temperature in affected areas; neurogenic bladder.

Laboratory

MRI, CT.

Treatment

Suboccipital and cervical decompression, laminectomy and syringotomy, shunts, fourth ventriculostomy, terminal ventriculostomy and neuroendoscopic surgery may be considered.

🗗 BIBLIOGRAPHY

1. Al-Shatoury HA, Galhom AA, Wagner FC. (2012). Syringomyelia. [online] Available from emedicine.medscape.com/article/1151685-overview. [Accessed September, 2013].

🗗 21.4H. PORPHYRIA CUTANEA TARDA

General

Disorder of porphyria metabolism; highest incidence in Bantu population; both sexes affected; onset between ages 40 and 60 years; insidious onset; autosomal dominant; light-sensitive dermatitis in later adult life; associated with excretion of large amounts of uroporphyrin in urine.

Ocular

Synophrys; keratitis; palsies of third and seventh cranial nerves; scleromalacia perforans; optic atrophy; retinal hemorrhages and cotton-wool spots; macular edema; pinguecula; pterygium; brownish pigmentation in conjunctiva and lid margin.

Clinical

Cutaneous manifestations are solar hypersensitivity, vesiculobullous lesions, ulcerations, severe scarring, and hypertrichosis; erythrodontia.

Laboratory

Urinary porphyrin levels are abnormally high, with several hundred to several thousand micrograms excreted in a 24-hour period. Direct immunofluorescence examination can help differentiate PCT from immunobullous diseases with dermoepidermal junction cleavage (epidermolysis bullosa acquisita, lupus erythematosus) in which the perivascular immunoglobulin deposition found in PCT is not observed.

Treatment

Sunlight avoidance, therapeutic phlebotomy to reduce iron stores, chelation with desferrioxamine; iron-rich foods should be consumed in moderation.

🗗 BIBLIOGRAPHY

1. Poh-Fitzpatrick MB. (2012). Porphyria cutanea tarda. [online] Available from www.emedicine.com/derm/TOPIC344.HTM. [Accessed September, 2013].

21.41. SCHAUMANN SYNDROME (BESNIER-BOECK-SCHAUMANN SYNDROME; BOECK SARCOID; SARCOIDOSIS)

General

Etiology unknown; theories include tuberculosis, hypersensitivity to pine pollen, virus infection; affects blacks most often; chronic course with spontaneous remissions (*see* Heerfordt's syndrome); hilar or paratracheal nodes with erythema nodosum; onset most often in middle and old age; ocular involvement in 20–25% of all cases.

Ocular

Orbital granulomatous mass; bony defects; cutaneous and subcutaneous nodules; myogenic palsy; lacrimal gland adenopathy; decreased tear formation; secondary glaucoma; granulomatous uveitis with iris nodules, cells and flare; mutton fat keratic precipitates; keratitis sicca; vitreous floaters; band-shaped keratitis; complicated cataract; inflammatory retinal exudates; "candle wax drippings"; optic nerve atrophy; neuritis; eyelid nodules; ocular nerve enlargement (granuloma).

Clinical

Lymphadenopathy; hilar nodes; fatigue; cystic, punched-out or reticulated changes in small bones (mainly, hands and feet); muscle wasting; contractures; weakness in legs and arms.

Laboratory

Chest X-ray, CT scan, and MRI of the brain.

Treatment

Glucocorticoids are the treatment of choice.

BIBLIOGRAPHY

1. Sharma GD. (2011). Pediatric sarcoidosis. [online] Available from www.emedicine.com/ped/TOPIC2043.HTM. [Accessed September, 2013].

2J. V ESOTROPIA SYNDROME

General

Esotropia is greater looking down by 15 prism diopters than looking up; may have underaction of superior oblique or overaction of inferior oblique; antimongoloid (downward) slant of lid fissures; may have accommodative, nonaccommodative or paralytic esotropia components.

Clinical

Fusion is obtained by chin depression.

Laboratory

Diagnosis is made by clinical findings.

Treatment

Recess the medial rectus bilaterally with a half tendon downward. If unilateral surgery is performed, recess medial rectus with downshift and resect the LR with a half tendon upshift. With significant oblique overaction, recess the medial rectus bilaterally or recess the medial rectus and resect the LR unilaterally for esotropia in primary position; weaken the superior oblique bilaterally if 25 diopters from up to down.

BIBLIOGRAPHY

1. Thacker N, Rosenbaum AL, Velez FG. (2012). V-pattern esotropia and exotropia. [online] Available from www.emedicine.com/oph/TOPIC561.HTM. [Accessed September, 2013].

⊟ 2K. WEBER SYNDROME (WEBER-DUBLER SYNDROME; CEREBELLAR PEDUNCLE SYNDROME; ALTERNATING OCULOMOTOR PARALYSIS; VENTRAL MEDIAL MIDBRAIN SYNDROME) PTOSIS

General

Lesion of the peduncle (crus), pons or medulla, which interrupts the third nerve before it emerges from the peduncle and interrupts fibers in the pyramidal tract above the level of the third nuclei; hemorrhage and thrombosis; tumor of the pituitary region, extending posteriorly; also may result in secondary to cerebrovascular disease.

Ocular

Ptosis; homolateral third nerve palsy (usually complete); fixed, dilated pupil.

Clinical

Contralateral hemiplegia; contralateral paralysis of face and tongue (supranuclear type).

Laboratory

Diagnosis is made by clinical findings.

Treatment

Ptosis: If visual acuity is affected, most cases require surgical correction and there are several procedures that may be used including levator resection, repair or advancement and Fasanella-Servat.

⊟ BIBLIOGRAPHY

1. Kistler JP, Ropper AH, Martin JB. Cerebrovascular diseases. In: Isselbacher KJ, Braunwald E, Wilson JD, Martin JB, Fauci A, Kasper DL (Eds). Harrison's Principles of Internal Medicine, 13th edition. New York: McGraw-Hill; 1994. pp. 2242-3.
2. Miller NR (Ed). Walsh and Hoyt's Clinical Neuro-Ophthalmology, 44th edition. Baltimore, USA: Williams & Wilkins; 1995. pp. 238-44.
3. Newman NJ. Third, fourth and sixth-nerve lesions and the cavernous sinus. In: Albert DM, Jakobiec FA (Eds). Albert & Jakobiec's Principles and Practice of Ophthalmology: Clinical Practice, 5th edition. Philadelphia, PA: WB Saunders; 1994. pp. 245-51.
4. Weber H. A contribution to the pathology of the crura cerebri. Med Chir Trans. 1863;46:121-40.1.
5. Wolf BS, Newman CM, Khilnani MT. The posterior inferior cerebellar artery on vertebral angiography. Am J Roentgenol Radium Ther Nucl Med. 1962;87:322-37.

⊟ 3. SIXTH NERVE

⊟ 3A. ACQUIRED EXOTROPIA

General

Exodeviation is characterized by visual axes that form a divergent angle. Intermittent exotropia, sensory exotropia and exotropia with neurologic causes are all types of acquired exotropia. More common in Middle East, Africa and Asia.

Clinical

Neurological issues.

Ocular

Exophoria, intermittent exotropia, diplopia, bitemporal suppression, asthenopia and closing of one eye in bright light, amblyopia.

Laboratory

Diagnosis is made by clinical findings.

Treatment

Nonsurgical treatment involves correction of refractive error, occlusion therapy for amblyopia, orthoptics and Botox® injections. Treatment of neurologic defect is also important. Surgery is only considered when the patient has poor control of the deviation, diplopia and severe asthenopia.

⊟ BIBLIOGRAPHY

1. Thacker N, Velez FG, Rosenbaum AL. (2012). Acquired exotropia. [online] Available from emedicine.medscape.com/article/1199004-overview. [Accessed September, 2013].

⊟ 3B. A EXOTROPIA SYNDROME

General

Exotropia is greater looking down by 15 prism diopters than looking up; mongoloid (upward) slant of lid fissures; alternating sursumduction and associated vertical divergence; overaction of superior oblique muscles or underaction of inferior oblique or inferior rectus muscles; fusion is obtained by chin depression.

Laboratory

Diagnosis is made by clinical findings.

Treatment

Recess the LR with downshift. If unilateral surgery is performed, recess the LR with downshift and resect the medial rectus with upshift. With oblique dysfunction, recess the rectus bilateral and weaken the superior oblique bilaterally.

⊟ BIBLIOGRAPHY

1. Hardesty HH. Superior oblique tenotomy. Arch Ophthalmol. 1972;88(2):181-4.
2. Hwang J, Wright KW. Strabismus syndromes. In: Wright KW (Ed). Pediatric Ophthalmology and Strabismus. St. Louis: Mosby; 1995. p. 223.
3. Roy FH. Practical Management of Eye Problems: Glaucoma, Strabismus, Visual Fields, illustrated edition. Philadelphia, PA: Lea & Febiger; 1975. pp. 144-5.

⊟ 3C. BASIC AND INTERMITTENT EXOTROPIA

General

Divergent misalignment of visual axis.

Clinical

None.

Ocular

Exotropias are more frequent with visual field defects and craniofacial syndromes, amblyopia.

Laboratory

Diagnosis is made by clinical findings.

Treatment

Minus lenses, prisms, orthoptic exercises and occlusion. Surgical—recession of LR or resection of medial rectus.

⊟ BIBLIOGRAPHY

1. Thacker N, Velez FG, Rosenbaum AL. (2012). Acquired exotropia. [online] Available from www.emedicine.com/oph/TOPIC329.HTM. [Accessed September, 2013].
2. Bashour M, Gerontis CC. (2012). Congenital exotropia. [online] Available from www.emedicine.com/oph/TOPIC330.HTM. [Accessed September, 2013].

⊟ 3D. V EXOTROPIA SYNDROME

General

Exotropia greater looking up by 15 diopters than looking down; underaction of superior oblique or overaction of inferior oblique muscles; antimongoloid (downward) slant of lid fissures.

Clinical

Fusion is obtained by chin elevation.

Laboratory

Diagnosis is made by clinical findings.

Treatment

Recess the LR with upshift. If unilateral surgery is performed, recess the LR with upshift and resect the medial rectus with downshift. With oblique dysfunction, recess the rectus bilateral and weaken the superior oblique bilaterally.

⊟ BIBLIOGRAPHY

1. Thacker N, Rosenbaum AL, Velez FG. (2012). V-pattern esotropia and exotropia. [online] Available from www.emedicine.com/oph/TOPIC561.HTM. [Accessed September, 2013].

4. FOURTH NERVE

4A. BROWN SYNDROME (SUPERIOR OBLIQUE TENDON SHEATH SYNDROME)

General

Etiology unknown; affects both sexes; present from birth; may be congenital or acquired (secondary to trauma, orbital surgery, or injections, or following delivery).

Ocular

Bilateral ptosis with associated backward head tilt; widening of palpebral fissure with attempted upward gaze; ocular movements show failure in the direction of superior oblique action; may be associated with underaction of the inferior oblique; adduction or abduction restricted or completely abolished; choroidal coloboma.

Laboratory

Diagnosis is made by clinical findings.

Treatment

Once systemic disease is excluded, patients' inflammation can be treated with anti-inflammatory medication. Oral ibuprofen is a good first-line choice. Local steroid injections in the area of the trochlea and oral corticosteroids can be used for inflammation. Once the inflammatory disease process is controlled, patients with inflammatory Brown syndrome may show spontaneous resolution. Congenital Brown syndrome is unlikely to improve spontaneously; therefore, surgery is important to consider as an option.

BIBLIOGRAPHY

1. Wright KW, Salvador MG. (2012). Brown syndrome. [online] Available from www.emedicine.com/oph/TOPIC552.HTM. [Accessed September, 2013].
2. Suh DW, Oystreck DT, Hunter DG. Long-term results of an intraoperative adjustable superior oblique tendon suture spacer using nonabsorbable suture for Brown Syndrome. Ophthalmology. 2008;115(10):1800-4.

4B. CANINE TOOTH SYNDROME (CLASS VII SUPERIOR OBLIQUE PALSY)

General

It is caused by trauma to the trochlear area, producing a "double Brown syndrome"; secondary to strengthening the superior oblique along with a residual superior oblique palsy, or a combination of local trauma to the trochlea causing restriction to upgaze along with closed head trauma producing a fourth nerve palsy.

Ocular

Underaction of the superior oblique and the inferior oblique on the same side.

Clinical

None.

Laboratory

Diagnosis is made by clinical findings.

Treatment

- *Class I*: The greatest vertical deviation in the field of action of inferior oblique—weakened inferior oblique.
- *Class II*: The greatest vertical deviation in the field of action of the underacting superior oblique—superior oblique strengthening.
- *Class III*: An equal vertical deviation of inferior oblique and superior oblique—either inferior oblique or superior oblique surgery.

BIBLIOGRAPHY

1. Ellis FD, Helveston EM. Superior oblique palsy: diagnosis and classification. Int Ophthalmol Clin. 1976;16(3): 127-35.
2. Roy FH, Fraunfelder FW, Fraunfelder FT. Roy and Fraunfelder's Current Ocular Therapy, 6th edition. Philadelphia, PA: WB Saunders; 2008.

4C. CONGENITAL EPIBLEPHARON INFERIOR OBLIQUE INSUFFICIENCY SYNDROME

General

Prognosis is good with treatment; present in infancy; inversion of lash line occurs with epiblepharon, and is exaggerated by the inferior oblique insufficiency.

Ocular

Narrow interpupillary distance; some ocular prominence; epicanthus; epiblepharon exaggerated in downward gaze; spastic entropion with retroflexion of the eyelashes; epiblepharon becomes less pronounced with growth and development; usually bilateral but in some cases asymmetrical; inferior oblique insufficiency usually unilateral; persistent unilateral keratoconjunctival irritation by the inverted cilia; lacrimation due to conjunctival and corneal irritation.

Clinical

Chubby cheeks (occasionally).

Laboratory

Diagnosis is made by clinical findings.

Treatment

None.

BIBLIOGRAPHY

1. Duke-Elder WS (Ed). System of Ophthalmology, 2nd edition. St Louis: CV Mosby; 1976. pp. 167-84.
2. Swan KC. The syndrome of congenital epiblepharon and inferior oblique insufficiency. Am J Ophthalmol. 1955; 39(4):130-6.

4E. PROXIMAL AND DISTAL CLICK SYNDROME OF THE SUPERIOR OBLIQUE TENDON (SIMULATED SUPERIOR OBLIQUE TENDON SYNDROME)

General

Produced by quick head movements; caused by adhesions (secondary to trauma and inflammation) or frontal sinus surgery; proximal click adhesions in front to trochlea; distal click adhesions behind trochlea; associated with Brown syndrome.

Ocular

Decreased elevation in adduction; downshoot of the affected eye on adduction; overaction of the tethered inferior oblique after cutting superior oblique tendon; widening of palpebral fissure on adduction; diplopia.

Clinical

Rheumatoid arthritis.

Laboratory

Diagnosis is made by clinical findings.

Treatment

Superior oblique split tendon lengthening technique, tenotomy and superior oblique recession may be useful procedures.

BIBLIOGRAPHY

1. Brown HW. True and simulated superior oblique tendon sheath syndromes. Doc Ophthalmol. 1973;34(1):123-36.
2. Pittke EC. The proximal and distal click syndrome of the superior oblique tendon. Graefes Arch Clin Exp Ophthalmol. 1987;225(1):28-32.

🗗 4F. SUPERIOR OBLIQUE MYOKYMIA

General

Twitching of superior oblique; rare; occurs in adults; frequently chronic.

Clinical

None.

Ocular

Oscillopsia (microtremor, twitching and vertical and/or torsional diplopia).

Laboratory

MRI to identify vascular compression.

Treatment

Systemic—tegretol, topical—betaxolol, surgical—weaken the affected superior oblique and ipsilateral inferior oblique.

🗗 BIBLIOGRAPHY

1. Roy FH, Fraunfelder FW, Fraunfelder FT. Roy and Fraunfelder's Current Ocular Therapy, 6th edition. London, UK: Elsevier; 2008.

🗗 4H. TROCHLEAR NERVE PALSY (FOURTH NERVE PALSY)

General

Paralysis of the fourth cranial nerve which can be congenital or acquired. Etiology is obscure for congenital disease. Head trauma, diabetes, atherosclerosis, tumor, aneurysm, MS and hypertension are causes for acquired disease.

Clinical

History of head trauma, diabetes, tumor, aneurysm, MS, hypotension, atherosclerosis.

Ocular

Vertical diplopia, head tilt, superior oblique muscle depression, which causes abduction of the globe and intorts, V-pattern esotropia, torticollis.

Laboratory

Diagnosis is made by clinical findings.

Treatment

Prisms may be useful for small deviations. Botulinum toxin may also be useful. For deviation greater than 15 prism diopters, strabismus surgery may be required.

🗗 BIBLIOGRAPHY

1. Sheik ZA, Hutcheson KA. (2012). Trochlear nerve palsy. [online] Available from emedicine.medscape.com/article/1200187-overview. [Accessed September, 2013].

🗗 5. NYSTAGMUS

🗗 5A. BLOCKED NYSTAGMUS SYNDROME (NYSTAGMUS BLOCKAGE SYNDROME; NYSTAGMUS COMPENSATION SYNDROME)

General

Von Noorden documented this syndrome with electrooculographic recordings.

Ocular

Bilateral or monocular convergence where the adducted eye(s) cannot be abducted to the midline; if monocular, it may alternate; esotropia increases with prolonged fixation; head turn; nystagmus.

Clinical

None.

Laboratory

Clinical—electrooculographic recordings.

Treatment

- *Strabismus*: Equalized vision with correct refractive error; surgery may be helpful in patient with diplopia.
- *Nystagmus*:
  - *Seesaw*: Visual field to consider neoplastic or vascular etiologies.
  - *Upbeat*: May indicate MS, cerbellar degeneration, tumors or infarcts. Treatment is directed towards identification and resolution of underlying cause.
  - *Downbeat*: Affects the cerebellum or craniocervical junction including Arnold-Chiari malformation, MS, trauma, tumor, infarction and many toxic metabolic entities. MRI may indicate a surgically correctable lesion. Periodic alternating nystagmus is continuous horizontal nystagmus from stroke, tumor, MS, trauma, infection, drug intoxication. Can occur from cataract, vitreous hemorrhage or optic atrophy.

BIBLIOGRAPHY

1. Bardorf CM, Stavern GV, Garcia-Valenzuela E. (2012). Acquired nystagmus. [online] Available from www.emedicine.com/oph/TOPIC339.HTM. [Accessed September, 2013].

5B. CATARACT, MICROPHTHALMIA AND NYSTAGMUS

General

Autosomal recessive.

Ocular

Miosis; cataract; nystagmus; microphthalmia.

Clinical

None.

Laboratory

Diagnosis is made by clinical findings.

Treatment

Cataract surgery if vision decreases.

BIBLIOGRAPHY

1. McKusick VA. Mendelian Inheritance in Man: A Catalog of Human Genes and Genetic Disorders, 12th edition. Baltimore, USA: The Johns Hopkins University Press; 1998.
2. Hamosh A, Scott AF, Amberger J, et al. Online Mendelian Inheritance in Man (OMIM), a knowledge base of human genes and genetic disorders. Nucleic Acids Res. 2002;30(1):52-5.
3. Temtamy SA, Shalash BA. Genetic heterogeneity of the syndrome: microphthalmia with congenital cataract. Birth Defects Orig Artic Ser. 1974;10(4):292-3.
4. Zeiter HJ. Congenital microphthalmos: A pedigree of four affected siblings and an additional report of forty four sporadic cases. Am J Ophthalmol. 1963;55:910-22.

5C. EPIPHYSEAL DYSPLASIA, MICROCEPHALY, AND NYSTAGMUS

General

Autosomal recessive.

Ocular

Nystagmus; retinitis pigmentosa.

Clinical

Epiphyseal dysplasia; microcephaly; short stature.

Laboratory

Diagnosis is made by clinical findings.

Treatment

Retinitis pigmentosa: Vitamin A 15,000 IU/day is thought to slow the decline of retinal function, dark sunglasses for outdoor use, surgery for cataract, genetic counseling.

BIBLIOGRAPHY

1. Parikh S, Batra P, Do TT. (2012). Diastrophic dysplasia. [online] Available from www.emedicine.com/orthoped/TOPIC632.HTM. [Accessed September, 2013].
2. Temtamy SA, Shalach BA. Genetic heterogeneity of the syndrome: microphthalmos with congenital cataract. Birth Defects. 1974;10:292-3.
3. Zeiter HJ. Congenital microphthalmos: a pedigree of 4 affected siblings and an additional report of 44 sporadic cases. Am J Ophthalmol. 1963;55:910-22.

5D. HENNEBERT SYNDROME (LUETIC-OTITIC-NYSTAGMUS SYNDROME)

General

It is caused by congenital syphilis; manifestations in childhood; when a fistula in the labyrinth exists, compression of the external auditory meatus will produce nystagmus of a wide amplitude (diagnostic of fistula).

Ocular

Spontaneous nystagmus when the column of air in the auditory canal is compressed; interstitial keratitis; disseminated syphilitic chorioretinitis may be present.

Clinical

Vertigo; fistula in the labyrinth; deafness; other clinical manifestations of congenital syphilis may be present such as "saddle" nose and Hutchinson teeth.

Laboratory

Serologic testing is commonly used to confirm diagnosis of syphilis.

Treatment

Penicillin remains the treatment of choice.

BIBLIOGRAPHY

1. Waseem M, Aslam M. (2011). Pediatric syphilis. [online] Available from www.emedicine.com/ped/TOPIC2193.HTM. [Accessed September, 2013].

5E. KARSCH-NEUGEBAUER SYNDROME (NYSTAGMUS-SPLIT HAND SYNDROME)

General

Autosomal dominant.

Ocular

Horizontal nystagmus; strabismus; cataract; fundus changes.

Clinical

Split hand and split foot deformities; monodactylous hands.

Laboratory

Diagnosis is made by clinical findings.

Treatment

Baclofen has been effective in treating the periodic alternating nystagmus. Retrobulbar or intramuscular injection of Botox® has been demonstrated to abolish nystagmus temporarily. Strabismus surgery is used in patients with certain forms of nystagmus with varying degrees of success.

BIBLIOGRAPHY

1. Karsch J. Erbliche Augenmissbildung in Verbendung mit Spalthand Und-Fuss. Z Augenheikunde. 1936;89:274-9.
2. McKusick VA. Mendelian Inheritance in Man: A Catalog of Human Genes and Genetic Disorders, 12th edition. Baltimore, USA: The Johns Hopkins University Press; 1998.
3. Hamosh A, Scott AF, Amberger J, et al. Online Mendelian Inheritance in Man (OMIM), a knowledge base of human genes and genetic disorders. Nucleic Acids Res. 2002;30(1):52-5.
4. Neugebauer H. Splathand Und-Fuss mit Familiaerer Besonderheit. Z Orthop. 1962;95:500-6.

5F. KOERBER-SALUS-ELSCHNIG SYNDROME (SYLVIAN AQUEDUCT SYNDROME; NYSTAGMUS RETRACTORIUS SYNDROME)

General

It is caused by tumor or inflammation in the region of aqueduct of Sylvius, third and fourth ventricle, or corpora quadrigemina.

Ocular

Lid retraction may be associated with midbrain lesions above the posterior commissure; paresis of vertical gaze; tonic spasm of convergence on attempted upward gaze; clonic convergence movements or convergence nystagmus; vertical nystagmus on gaze up or down; nystagmus retractorius with spasmodic retraction of the eyes when an attempt is made to move them in any direction; occasional extraocular muscle paresis.

Clinical

Headaches; dizziness; hypertension; possible hemiparesis; ataxia; hemitremor; Babinski's sign.

Laboratory

CT, MRI.

Treatment

- *Lid retraction*: Identify systemic abnormalities as thyroid; treat: 6 month stabilizing before eyelid surgery.
- *Local*: Ocular lubrication (drops or ointment). Botulinum toxin type A may also be useful.

BIBLIOGRAPHY

1. Elschnig A. Nystagmus Retractorius, ein Cerebrales Herdsymptom. Med Klin. 1913;9:8.
2. Geeraets WJ. Ocular Syndromes, 3rd edition. Philadelphia, PA: Lea & Febiger; 1976.

5G. LENOBLE-AUBINEAU SYNDROME (NYSTAGMUS-MYOCLONIA SYNDROME)

General

Familial; pathogenesis is not known; prevalent in males; manifest during first years of life; X-linked dominant inheritance has been reported in one family.

Ocular

Congenital nystagmus associated with fasciculations of muscles spontaneously elicited by mechanical stimulation or cold.

Clinical

Tremors of head and limbs; myoclonic movements of extremities and trunk; hypospadias; abnormalities of teeth; facial asymmetry; localized edema.

Laboratory

Diagnosis is made by clinical findings.

Treatment

Baclofen, gabapentin, retrobulbar injection of Botox® may be useful for nystagmus.

BIBLIOGRAPHY

1. Lenoble E, Aubineau E. Nystagmus-Myoclonia Syndrome: Une Variete Nouvelle de Myoclonie Congenitale Pouvant Etre Hereditaire et Familiale A Nystagmus Constant. Rev Med (Paris). 1906;26:471.
2. Magalini SI, Scrascia E. Dictionary of Medical Syndromes, 2nd edition. Philadelphia, PA: Lippincott Williams and Wilkins; 1981.
3. McKusick VA. Mendelian Inheritance in Man: A Catalog of Human Genes and Genetic Disorders, 12th edition. Baltimore, USA: The Johns Hopkins University Press; 1998.
4. Hamosh A, Scott AF, Amberger J, et al. Online Mendelian Inheritance in Man (OMIM), a knowledgebase of human genes and genetic disorders. Nucleic Acids Res. 2002;30(1):52-5.

5H. NYSTAGMUS

General

A repetitive involuntary eye movement that often indicates an underlying ocular or neurologic disorder.

Ocular

Oscillopsia, vertical and/or torsional diplopia, superior oblique myokymia.

Clinical

Vertigo.

Laboratory

Diagnosis is made by clinical findings.

Treatment

- *Nystagmus*:
  - *Seesaw*: Visual field to consider neoplastic or vascular etiologies.

- *Upbeat*: It may indicate MS, cerebellar degeneration, tumors or infarcts. Treatment is directed toward the identification and resolution of underlying cause.
- *Downbeat*: It affects the cerebellum or craniocervical junction including Arnold-Chiari malformation, MS, trauma, tumor, infarction and many toxic metabolic entities. MRI may indicate a surgically correctable lesion. Periodic alternating nystagmus is continuous horizontal nystagmus from stroke, tumor, MS, trauma, infection and drug intoxication. It can occur from cataract, vitreous hemorrhage or optic atrophy.

BIBLIOGRAPHY

1. Bardorf CM, Stavern GV, Garcia-Valenzuela E. (2012). Acquired nystagmus. [online] Available from www.emedicine.com/oph/TOPIC339.HTM. [Accessed September, 2013].
2. Curtis T, Wheeler DT. (2012). Congenital nystagmus. [online] Available from www.emedicine.com/oph/TOPIC688.HTM. [Accessed September, 2013].

5I. NYSTAGMUS COMPENSATION SYNDROME

General

Congenital [*see* Ethan syndrome, primary; Ethan syndrome, secondary; nystagmus blockage syndrome (NBS)].

Ocular

Esotropia; amblyopia; onset may be preceded by manifesting nystagmus; abnormal head posture toward the adducted fixing eye; nystagmus reduced or absent, with the fixing eye adducted.

Clinical

Abnormal head position.

Laboratory

Diagnosis is made by clinical findings.

Treatment

Strabismus: Equalized vision with correct refractive error; surgery may be helpful in patients with diplopia.

BIBLIOGRAPHY

1. Frank JW. Diagnostic signs in the nystagmus compensation syndrome. J Pediatr Ophthalmol Strabismus. 1979;16(5):317-20.
2. von Noorden GK. The nystagmus compensation (blockage) syndrome. Am J Ophthalmol. 1976;82(2):283-90.

5J. NYSTAGMUS, CONGENITAL (CONGENITAL IDIOPATHIC NYSTAGMUS)

General

Autosomal dominant; pattern of inheritance in congenital nystagmus, whether of the "motor" or "sensory" type, may be autosomal dominant, recessive or sex-linked.

Ocular

Vertical and horizontal nystagmus; this nystagmus occasionally is vertical or torsional; in addition, periodic alternating, downbeat and seesaw nystagmus may be present at birth; normal electroretinogram.

Clinical

None.

Laboratory

Diagnosis is made by clinical findings.

Treatment

Baclofen, gabapentin, retrobulbar injection of Botox®.

🗗 BIBLIOGRAPHY

1. Curtis T, Wheeler DT. (2012). Congenital nystagmus. [online] Available from www.emedicine.com/oph/TOPIC688.HTM. [Accessed September, 2013].

🗗 5K. NYSTAGMUS, PRIMARY HEREDITARY (CONGENITAL NYSTAGMUS)

General

Autosomal recessive, sex-linked or irregular dominant; may be associated with albinism.

Ocular

Horizontal nystagmus; myopia.

Clinical

Head spasms; carpopedal spasms (Trousseau sign); Chvostek sign.

Laboratory

Diagnosis is made by clinical findings.

Treatment

- *Nystagmus*:
  - *Seesaw*: Visual field to consider neoplastic or vascular etiologies.
  - *Upbeat*: It may indicate MS, cerebellar degeneration, tumors or infarcts. Treatment is directed toward the identification and resolution of underlying cause.
  - *Downbeat*: It affects the cerebellum or craniocervical junction including Arnold-Chiari malformation, MS, trauma, tumor, infarction and many toxic metabolic entities. MRI may indicate a surgically correctable lesion. Periodic alternating nystagmus is continuous horizontal nystagmus from stroke, tumor, MS, trauma, infection and drug intoxication. It can occur from cataract, vitreous hemorrhage or optic atrophy.

🗗 BIBLIOGRAPHY

1. Curtis T, Wheeler DT. (2012). Congenital nystagmus. [online] Available from www.emedicine.com/oph/TOPIC688.HTM. [Accessed September, 2013].
2. Allen M. Primary hereditary nystagmus: case study with genealogy. J Hered. 1942;33:454-6.
3. Gutmann DH, Brooks ML, Emanuel BS, et al. Congenital nystagmus in a (40, XX/45, X) mosaic woman from a family with X-linked congenital nystagmus. Am J Med Genet. 1991;39(2):167-9.
4. Lavin PJ. Congenital nystagmus. In: Bradley WG (Ed). Neurology in Clinical Practice, 2nd edition. Boston, USA: Butterworth-Heinemann; 1995. p. 200.
5. McKusick VA. Mendelian Inheritance in Man: A Catalog of Human Genes and Genetic Disorders, 12th edition. Baltimore, USA: The Johns Hopkins University Press; 1998.
6. Hamosh A, Scott AF, Amberger J, et al. Online Mendelian Inheritance in Man (OMIM), a knowledgebase of human genes and genetic disorders. Nucleic Acids Res. 2002;30(1):52-5.
7. Stromberg A, Pavan-Langston D. Extraocular muscles, strabismus, and nystagmus. In: Pavan-Langston D (Ed). Nystagmus: Manual of Ocular Diagnosis and Therapy, 4th edition. Boston, USA: Little, Brown and Company; 1995. pp. 333-6.

🗗 5L. NYSTAGMUS, VOLUNTARY

General

Autosomal dominant; usually it is purely horizontal, but it may be vertical or torsional.

Ocular

Voluntary rapid to-and-fro synchronous movements of eyes.

Clinical

Simultaneous head tremor has been associated with this condition.

Laboratory

Diagnosis is made by clinical findings.

Treatment

None—ocular.

⊟ BIBLIOGRAPHY

1. Keyes MJ. Voluntary nystagmus in two generations. Arch Neurol. 1973;29(1):63-4.
2. Lee J, Gresty M. A case of "voluntary nystagmus" and head tremor. J Neurol Neurosurg Psychiatry. 1993;56(12):1321-2.
3. McKusick VA. Mendelian Inheritance in Man: A Catalog of Human Genes and Genetic Disorders, 12th edition. Baltimore, USA: The Johns Hopkins University Press; 1998.
4. Hamosh A, Scott AF, Amberger J, et al. Online Mendelian Inheritance in Man (OMIM), a knowledge base of human genes and genetic disorders. Nucleic Acids Res. 2002;30(1):52-5.
5. Miller NR (Ed). Walsh and Hoyt's Clinical Neuro-Ophthalmology, 4th edition. Baltimore, USA: Williams & Wilkins; 1985. p. 45-54.

⊟ 6. OPHTHALMOPLEGIA

⊟ 6A. ACUTE OPHTHALMOPLEGIA (ACUTE ONSET OF EXTRAOCULAR MUSCLE PALSY)

1. Infranuclear
   A. Aneurysm of internal carotid artery or circle of Willis
   †B. Trauma
      1. Orbital fracture
      2. Orbital hematoma
   C. Orbital cellulitis secondary to acute paranasal sinusitis including mucormycosis in a diabetic
   D. Ophthalmoplegic migraine
   E. Myasthenia gravis
   †F. Orbital pseudotumor
   G. Orbital tumors
      †1. Lymphoma
      †2. Metastatic
      3. Rhabdomyosarcoma
   H. Occlusion of ophthalmic artery
2. *Nuclear*
   A. Acute and subacute infections
      1. Infectious encephalitis
         a. Viral encephalitis
            †i. Anterior poliomyelitis
            †ii. Encephalitis lethargica and other epidemic viral encephalitides
            iii. Fisher syndrome (ophthalmoplegia, ataxia, areflexia)
            iv. Rabies
            v. Vaccinal encephalitis
            vi. Varicella, variola, measles, mumps, influenza, infectious mononucleosis
            vii. Zoster

b. Organismal encephalitic infections
   i. Typhoid
   ii. Scarlet fever
   iii. Whooping cough
   †iv. Gas gangrene
   †v. Septicemia
   vi. Pneumonia
   vii. Typhus
   viii. Malaria
c. Acute CNS diseases
   †i. Acute demyelinating diseases-acute encephalomyelitis, acute MS disseminated.
   ii. Neuritic infections
      †a. Polyradiculoneuritis
      †b. Epidemic paralyzing vertigo
      c. Acute infectious (rheumatic) polyneuritis
      †d. Interstitial neuritis-meningitis, cranial sinusitis, petrositis, nasal sinusitis, orbital periostitis, orbital abscess
   iii. Widespread infections
      †a. Meningovascular syphilis
      b. Mucormycosis (AIDS)
      c. Tuberculosis
      d. Torula and cryptococcosis
   iv. Toxic conditions
      a. Diphtheria
      b. Tetanus
      c. Botulism
   v. Allergic conditions

a. Sarcoidosis syndrome (Schaumann syndrome)

†b. Recurrent multiple cranial nerve palsies

B. Metabolic diseases

1. Deficiency diseases

a. Thiamine deficiency (Wernicke- Korsakoff syndrome)

†b. Nicotinic acid deficiency: Pellagra

†c. Ascorbic acid deficiency: Scurvy

2. Diabetes

3. Anemias

a. Primary anemia: Leukemia

†b. Secondary anemia (loss of blood)

†4. Exophthalmic ophthalmoplegia

5. Porphyria

†C. Poisoning such as lead, carbon monoxide, snake poisons, wasp stings, ergot, sulfuric acid, phosphorus, triorthoceresylphosphate, and dichloroacetylene

†D. Drugs, include the following:

- Acebutolol
- Acetohexamide
- Acetophenazine
- Adrenal cortex injection
- Alcohol
- Aldosterone
- Allobarbital
- Amitriptyline
- Amobarbital
- Amodiaquine
- Atenolol
- Amoxapine
- Amphotericin B
- Aprobarbital
- Aspirin
- Auranofin
- Aurothioglucose
- Aurothioglycanide
- Barbital
- Beclomethasone
- Betamethasone
- Botulin A toxin
- Bupivacaine
- Butabarbital
- Butalbital
- Butallylonal
- Butaperazine
- Butethal
- Calcitriol
- Carbamazepine
- Carisoprodol
- Carphenazine
- Chloral hydrate
- Chlorambucil
- Chlordiazepoxide
- Chloroform
- Chloroprocaine
- Chloroquine
- Chlorpromazine
- Chlorpropamide
- Cisplatin
- Clomipramine
- Clonazepam
- Clorazepate
- Colchicine
- Cortisone
- Cyclobarbital
- Cyclopentobarbital
- Cytarabine
- Desipramine
- Desoxycorticosterone
- Dexamethasone
- Dextrothyroxine
- Diazepam
- Dibucaine
- Diethazine
- Digitalis
- Digitoxin
- Dimethyl tubocurarine iodide
- Diphenhydramine
- Diphenylhydantoin
- Diphtheria and tetanus toxoids (adsorbed)
- Diphtheria and tetanus toxoids and pertussis
- Diphtheria toxoid (adsorbed)
- Disulfiram
- Doxepin
- DPT vaccine
- Ergocalciferol
- Ethambutol
- Ethopropazine
- Etidocaine
- Fludrocortisone
- Fluphenazine
- Fluprednisolone
- Flurazepam
- Glyburide

- Gold Au 198
- Gold sodium thiomalate
- Gold sodium thiosulfate
- Griseofulvin
- Halazepam
- Heptabarbital
- Hexachlorophene
- Hexethal
- Hexobarbital
- Hydrocortisone
- Hydroxychloroquine
- Imipramine
- Indomethacin
- Influenza virus vaccine
- Insulin
- Iodide and iodine solutions and compounds
- Iophendylate
- Isoniazid
- Ketoprofen
- Labetalol
- Levodopa
- Levothyroxine
- Lidocaine
- Liothyronine
- Liotrix
- Lorazepam
- Measles and rubella virus vaccine (live)
- Measles virus vaccine
- Measles, mumps, and rubella virus vaccine
- Mephenesin
- Mephobarbital
- Mepivacaine
- Meprobamate
- Mesoridazine
- Metharbital
- Methdilazine
- Methitural
- Methohexital
- Methotrexate
- Methotrimeprazine
- Methoxiflurane
- Methyl alcohol
- Methyldopa
- Methylene blue
- Methylprednisolone
- Metoclopramide
- Metocurine iodide
- Metoprolol
- Metrizamide
- Midazolam
- Mumps virus vaccine (live)
- Nadolol
- Nalidixic acid
- Naproxen
- Nitrazepam
- Nitrofurantoin
- Nortriptyline
- Oral contraceptives
- Oxazepam
- Oxyphenbutazone
- Paramethadione
- Paramethasone
- Pentobarbital
- Periciazine
- Perphenazine
- Phenytoin
- Phenobarbital
- Phenylbutazone
- Pindolol
- Piperacetazine
- Piperazine
- Piperocaine
- Poliovirus vaccine
- Prazepam
- Prednisolone
- Prednisone
- Prilocaine
- Primidone
- Probarbital
- Procaine
- Prochlorperazine
- Promazine
- Promethazine
- Propiomazine
- Propoxycaine
- Proprandol
- Protriptyline
- Quinacrine
- Radioactive iodides
- Rubella and mumps virus vaccine (live)
- Rubella virus vaccine (live)
- Secobarbital
- Sodium salicylate
- Succinylcholine
- Talbutal
- Temazepam
- Tetracaine

- Thiamylal
- Thiethylperazine
- Thiopental
- Thiopropazate
- Thioproperazine
- Thioridazine
- Thyroglobulin
- Thyroid trifluoperazine
- Tolazamide
- Tolbutamide
- Triamcinolone
- Trichloroethylene
- Triflupromazine
- Trimeprazine
- Trimethadione
- Trimipramine
- Tubocurarine
- Vaccine (adsorbed)
- Vinbarbital
- Vinblastine
- Vincristine
- Vitamin A
- Vitamin D
- Vitamin D_2
- Vitamin D_3

†E. Neoplasms and cysts

†F. Trauma affecting the midbrain, base of the skull, and orbit

G. Vascular lesions as arteriosclerosis, hemorrhage and thrombosis in the midbrain, subarachnoid, hemorrhage, aneurysms, congenitally dilated arteries, giant-cell arteritis

†H. Idiopathic: Etiologic basis undetermined.

BIBLIOGRAPHY

1. Fraunfelder FT, Fraunfelder FW. Drug-induced ocular side effects. Woburn, MA: Butterworth-Heinemann; 2001.
2. Pacifici L, Passarelli F, Papa G, et al. Acute third cranial nerve ophthalmoplegia: possible pathogenesis from alpha-II-interferon treatment. Ital J Neurol Sci. 1993;14:579-80.
3. Roy FH. Ocular Syndromes and Systemic Diseases, 6th edition. New Delhi: Jaypee Brothers Medical Publishers; 2013.

†Indicates a general entry and therefore has not been described in detail in the text

6A1B1. INTERNAL ORBITAL FRACTURES (BLOWOUT FRACTURE)

General

Trauma that involves the walls of the orbit leaving the bony rim intact.

Clinical

Tripod fracture of the zygoma.

Ocular

Proptosis, enophthalmos, diplopia.

Laboratory

Computed tomography.

Treatment

The transconjunctival approach with lateral canthotomy and cantholysis is preferred to expose the orbital floor, nasal approach to further expose the medial wall.

BIBLIOGRAPHY

1. Cohen AJ, Mercandetti M. (2012). Orbital floor fractures (blowout). [online] Available from www.emedicine.com/plastic/TOPIC485.HTM. [Accessed September, 2013].

6A1C. ORBITAL CELLULITIS AND ABSCESS

General

Potentially life threatening; requires prompt evaluation and treatment.

Clinical

Sinusitis, ear infection, diabetes, dental disease.

Ocular

Orbital pain, proptosis, diplopia, decreased ocular motility, eyelid swelling and erythema, vision loss.

Laboratory

Diagnosis is made by clinical findings.

Treatment

Intravenous and oral antibiotic.

⊟ BIBLIOGRAPHY

1. Harrington JN. (2012). Orbital cellulitis. [online] Available from www.emedicine.com/oph/TOPIC205.HTM. [Accessed September, 2013].

⊟ 6A1D. OPHTHALMOPLEGIC MIGRAINE SYNDROME

General

Symptoms produced by ipsilateral herniation of hippocampal gyrus of temporal lobe through incisura tentorii; dependent upon unilateral cerebral edema due to vascular or vasomotor phenomena, intracranial aneurysm, or tumor; incidence may be greater in women with the initial attack in the 1st decade of life; pathogenesis is unclear, but it is likely secondary to ischemia of the ocular motor nerve.

Ocular

Severe unilateral supraorbital pain; ptosis; transitory partial or complete homolateral oculomotor paralysis; fourth or sixth nerve occasionally involved; retinal hemorrhages; papilledema (may be bilateral); moderate to severe headache with partial to complete cranial nerve III paresis including the pupil; more than one ocular nerve may be affected.

Clinical

Migraine headache, not present in all instances; dizziness; diminution in sense of smell; hypalgesia contralateral side of face; nausea/vomiting may be present; recurrent sinus arrest.

Laboratory

Clinical.

Treatment

Ptosis: If visual acuity is affected, most cases require surgical correction and there are several procedures that may be used including levator resection, repair or advancement and Fasanella-Servat.

⊟ BIBLIOGRAPHY

1. Bazak I, Margulis T, Shnaider H, et al. Ophthalmoplegic migraine and recurrent sinus arrest. J Neurol Neurosurg Psychiatry. 1991;54:935.
2. Ehlers H. On pathogenesis of ophthalmoplegic migraine. Acta Psychiatr Neurol (Scand). 1928;3:219.
3. Geeraets WJ. Ocular Syndromes, 3rd edition. Philadelphia: Lea & Febiger; 1976.
4. Gulkilik G, Cagatay H, Oba E, et al. Ophthalmoplegic migraine associated with recurrent isolated ptosis. Ann Ophthal. 2010;41:206-12.
5. Raskin NH. Migraine and other headaches. In: Rowland LP (Ed). Merritt's Textbook of Neurology, 9th edition. Baltimore: Williams & Wilkins; 1995. pp. 837-45.
6. Stommel EW, Ward TN, Harris RD. Ophthalmoplegic migraine or Tolosa-Hunt syndrome? Headache. 1994;34:177.
7. Van Pelt W, Andermann F. On the early onset of ophthalmologic migraine. Am J Dis Child. 1964;107:628.
8. Vijayan N. Ophthalmoplegic migraine: ischemic or compressive neuropathy? Headache. 1980;20:300-4.

⊟ 6A1E. ERB-GOLDFLAM SYNDROME (ERB II SYNDROME; HOPPE-GOLDFLAM DISEASE; PSEUDOPARALYTIC SYNDROME; MYASTHENIA GRAVIS)

General

Occurs at any age; more frequent between ages 20 and 40 years; more females affected than males; progressive; spontaneous; symptoms improve or resolve with rest in early stages of disease (*see* myasthenia gravis, neonatal or infantile); caused by autoantibodies against the acetylcholine receptor at the neuromuscular junction, leading to abnormal fatigability and weakness of skeletal muscle.

Ocular

Transient diplopia; ptosis of upper eyelids.

Clinical

Excessive fatigability of musculature; symptoms appear and increase as day progresses; expressionless face; sagging jaw; difficulty in chewing and talking; nasal regurgitation.

Laboratory

Ice test—crushed ice in surgical glove over ptotic eyelid for 2 minutes and watch for brief elevation of eyelid; Tensilon test and prostigmin test may result in the elevation of ptotic eyelid or improved strabismus in individuals with myasthenia gravis.

Treatment

Adrenal corticosteroids are frequently used. In some cases, mycophenolate mofetil, cyclosporine and cyclophosphamide may be useful. Patching one eye or using prisms may be helpful.

BIBLIOGRAPHY

1. Erb W. Zur Casuistick der Bulbaren La hmungen. Arch Psychiatr Vervenkr. 1879;9:325-50.
2. Roy FH, Fraunfelder FT, Fraunfelder FW. Roy and Fraunfelder's Current Ocular Therapy, 6th edition. London, UK: Elsevier; 2008.
3. Goldflam S. Vebereinen Scheinbar Keilbaren Bulbarparalytischem Symptom Complex mit Betheiligung der Extremitaten. Dtsch Z Nerven. 1983;4:312-52.
4. Kim JH, Hwang JM, Hwang YS, et al. Childhood ocular myasthenia gravis. Ophthalmology. 2003;110(7):1458-62.
5. Lepore FE, Sanborn GE, Slevin JT. Pupillary dysfunction in myasthenia gravis. Ann Neurol. 1979;6(1):29-33.
6. Sommer N, Melms A, Weller M, et al. Ocular myasthenia gravis. A critical review of clinical and pathophysiological aspects. Doc Ophthalmol. 1993;84(4):309-33.

6A1G3. RHABDOMYOSARCOMA (CORNEAL EDEMA)

General

Most common malignant orbital neoplasm of childhood; usually occurs before age 10 years; more commonly seen in males; rarely may develop in adults; shows evidence of striated muscle differentiation; has been divided into three histopathologic types: (1) embryonal, (2) alveolar and (3) pleomorphic.

Ocular

Choroidal folds; corneal edema; exposure keratitis; RMS of orbit or extraocular muscles; decreased motility; proptosis; papilledema; orbital edema; enlarged optic foramen; erosion of bony walls of orbit; pupil irregularity; epiphora; glaucoma; visual loss; nasolacrimal duct obstruction; conjunctival mass.

Clinical

Metastasis to the lymph system, bone marrow and lungs; headaches.

Laboratory

Liver, renal and cytogenetic testing; CT and bone scanning; MRI, ultrasonography and echocardiography.

Treatment

Chemotherapy radiation and surgically removing the tumor are used to treat patients with RMS.

BIBLIOGRAPHY

1. Cripe TP. (2011). Pediatric Rhabdomyosarcoma. [online] Available from www.emedicine.com/ped/TOPIC2005.HTM. [Accessed September, 2013].

6A1H. RETINAL ARTERY OCCLUSION

General

This condition involves a sudden, painless visual loss.

Clinical

Temporal arteritis, jaw claudication, scalp tenderness.

Ocular

Ophthalmoscopic examination, a diffuse retinal pallor and a cherry-red spot in macula are noted.

Laboratory

To determine etiology; CBC to evaluate blood disorders, ESR, blood cultures, carotid ultrasound imaging, fluorescein angiogram.

Treatment

Intraocular pressure lowering medications, carbogen therapy, hyperbaric oxygen. Vitrectomy may be necessary.

BIBLIOGRAPHY

1. Graham RH, Ebrahim SA. (2012). Central retinal artery occlusion. [online] Available from www.emedicine.com/oph/TOPIC387.HTM. [Accessed September, 2013].

🗗 6A2.A1AIII. FISHER SYNDROME (OPHTHALMOPLEGIA ATAXIA AREFLEXIA SYNDROME; MILLER-FISHER SYNDROME)

General

Acute idiopathic polyneuritis; prognosis good; complete recovery over several weeks (variant of Guillain-Barré syndrome; *see* Guillain-Barré syndrome).

Ocular

Moderate ptosis; complete external and almost complete internal ophthalmoplegia; diplopia; sluggish pupil reaction to light; may present without total ophthalmoplegia.

Clinical

Dizziness; severe ataxia; loss of tendon reflexes; chest pains; difficulties in chewing; diminished or absent sense of vibration; upper respiratory tract infection preceding this syndrome.

Laboratory

Diagnosis usually is made on clinical grounds. Laboratory studies are useful to rule out other diagnoses.

Treatment

Monitored closely for changes in blood pressure, heart rate and other arrhythmias. Temporary pacing may be required for patients with second-degree and third-degree heart block.

🗗 BIBLIOGRAPHY

1. Fisher M. An unusual variant of acute idiopathic polyneuritis (syndrome of ophthalmoplegia, ataxia and areflexia). N Engl J Med. 1956;255(2):57-65.
2. Igarashi Y, Takeda M, Maekawa H, et al. Fisher's syndrome without total ophthalmoplegia. Ophthalmologica. 1992;205(3):163-7.
3. Swick HM. Pseudointernuclear ophthalmoplegia in acute idiopathic polyneuritis (Fisher's syndrome). Am J Ophthalmol. 1974;77(5):725-8.

🗗 6A2.A1AIV. HYDROPHOBIA (LYSSA; RABIES)

General

Acute viral zoonosis of the CNS.

Ocular

Lid retraction; widening of palpebral fissure; retinal hemorrhages; mydriasis; paralysis of third, fourth, fifth, or seventh nerve; bilateral optic neuritis; branch retinal artery occlusion; vaccine-induced autoimmune demyelinative optic neuritis.

Clinical

Fever; headache; nausea; numbness; tingling; acute sensitiveness to sound and light; laryngeal and pharyngeal spasms; increased muscle tonus; convulsions; delirium; coma; death.

Laboratory

Saliva can be tested by virus isolation or reverse transcription followed by PCR. Suspected infections animal should be quarantined for 10 days.

Treatment

Before the onset of symptoms, both passive and active immunizations are effective for preventing progression to full-blown rabies. In exposures to high-risk species, initiate treatment immediately pending laboratory examination of the animal, if it is caught.

🗗 BIBLIOGRAPHY

1. Gompf SG, Pham TM, Somboonwit C, et al. (2013). Rabies. [online] Available from www.emedicine.com/med/TOPIC1374.HTM. [Accessed September, 2013].

🗗 6A2.A1AVI. CHICKENPOX (VARICELLA)

General

Acute exanthematous disease; highly contagious; children between ages of 2 and 8 years.

Ocular

Conjunctival ulcer; corneal ulcer; descemetocele; corneal opacity; keratitis; paresis of third, fourth and sixth nerves; optic neuritis; papilledema; retinitis; hemorrhagic retinopathy; uveitis; cataract; paralytic mydriasis; phthisis bulbi; unifocal choroiditis; dendritic keratitis; acute retinal necrosis (in a patient with AIDS); disciform keratitis.

Clinical

Fever; malaise; rash; pruritus.

Laboratory

Diagnosis is made by clinical findings.

Treatment

Isolation oral antihistamines, such as diphenhydramine and hydroxyzine, are used for severe pruritus and acetaminophen is recommended for use for the reduction of fever.

🗗 BIBLIOGRAPHY

1. Bechtel KA, Chatterjee A, Lichenstein R, et al. (2013). Pediatric chickenpox. [online] Available from www.emedicine.com/emerg/TOPIC367.HTM. [Accessed September, 2013].

🗗 6A2.A1AVI. SMALLPOX (VARIOLA)

General

Highly contagious cutaneous disease caused by viral infection.

Ocular

Conjunctivitis; keratitis; corneal ulcer; hypopyon; endophthalmitis; congenital corneal clouding; albinotic spots on iris; choroiditis; vitreous opacities; papillitis; extraocular muscle palsies; entropion; dacryocystitis; chorioretinitis; optic neuritis; and vesicles of the eyelid; preauricular adenopathy; eyelid ulcerating pustules; several conditions predispose to the spread of vaccinia, including eczema, hypogammaglobulinemia, steroid therapy, and AIDS.

Clinical

Fever, headache, and vomiting prior to appearance of the rash on the face, upper trunk, and down to the extremities.

Laboratory

Brick-shaped virions viewed with electron microscopy examination, virus culture from live cells, or DNA analysis using PCR and smallpox skin specimen should be collected.

Treatment

No known treatment is effective.

🗗 BIBLIOGRAPHY

1. Hussain AN, Hussain F, Alam M, et al. (2011). Smallpox. [online] Available from www.emedicine.com/med/TOPIC3545.HTM. [Accessed September, 2013].

🗗 6A2.A1AVI. MEASLES (MORBILLI; RUBEOLA)

General

Acute, extremely communicable disease that affects young school-aged children; caused by paramyxovirus.

Ocular

Hypopyon; uveitis; conjunctivitis; Koplik (Hirschberg) spots of conjunctiva; keratitis; corneal ulcer; cellulitis of lid; dacryocystitis; congenital cataract; optic atrophy; optic neuritis; strabismus; pigmentary retinopathy; iris prolapse; hemianopsia; secondary glaucoma; central retinal artery occlusion; orbital cellulitis; accommodative spasm; paralysis of sixth nerve; keratoconus.

Clinical

Maculopapular rash; fever.

Laboratory

Diagnosis is made by clinical findings.

Treatment

Good hydration.

🖶 BIBLIOGRAPHY

1. Chen SS, Fennelly G. (2013). Measles. [online] Available from www.emedicine.com/derm/TOPIC259.HTM. [Accessed September, 2013].

🖶 6A2.A1AVI. MUMPS

General

Viral infection.

Ocular

Conjunctivitis; keratitis; corneal ulcer; tenonitis; exophthalmos; microphthalmos; optic atrophy; optic neuritis; papillitis; scleritis; uveitis; cortical blindness; congenital punctal occlusion; paralysis of extraocular muscles; dacryoadenitis; iritis; paralysis of accommodation; internal and external ophthalmoparesis.

Clinical

Affects the parotid glands, but infection of other glandular tissue occurs, including the lacrimal gland and testicles; encephalitis; meningitis.

Laboratory

Mumps virus by acute serologic studies.

Treatment

Generous hydration and alimentation, analgesics for headaches. No antiviral agent is available.

🖶 BIBLIOGRAPHY

1. Defendi GL. (2012). Mumps. [online] Available from www.emedicine.com/ped/TOPIC1503.HTM. [Accessed September, 2013].

🖶 6A2.A1AVI. INFLUENZA

General

Viral infection; fever, muscle ache.

Ocular

Conjunctivitis; subconjunctival hemorrhages; keratitis; tenonitis; ptosis; cellulitis of orbit and lid; dacryocystitis; retinal hemorrhage; cataract; episcleritis; hypopyon; optic neuritis; uveitis; panophthalmitis; vitreal hemorrhage; paralysis of third or fourth nerve; uveitis following vaccination for influenza.

Clinical

Headache; fever; malaise; muscular aching; substernal soreness; nasal stuffiness; nausea.

Laboratory

The standard criterion for diagnosing influenza A and B is a viral culture of nasal-pharyngeal samples, throat samples, or both.

Treatment

Prevention is the most effective therapy. Two new drugs have been marketed recently for treatment of influenza A and B. These are the neuraminidase inhibitors, oseltamivir and zanamivir.

🖶 BIBLIOGRAPHY

1. Derlet RW. (2012). Influenza. [online] Available from www.emedicine.com/med/TOPIC1170.HTM. [Accessed September, 2013].

⊟ 6A2.A1AVII. HERPES ZOSTER

General

It is caused by varicella zoster virus; about 75% of cases occur in persons over age of 45 years; condition is more frequent with advancing age and in patients who are immunocompromised by drugs or disease; in particular, an increasing number of patients with herpes zoster ophthalmicus are immunosuppressed.

Ocular

Conjunctivitis; keratitis; recurrent corneal ulcer; neuralgia; zoster rash of eyelids; uveitis; iris atrophy; scleritis; cataract; optic neuritis; paralysis of third nerve; proptosis; paralysis of lids; orbital apex syndrome; retinitis; neurotrophic keratitis; acute retinal necrosis; progressive outer retinal necrosis; ocular motor nerve pareses; tonic pupil; encephalitis; vasculitis.

Clinical

Local lesions involving the posterior or root ganglia; nerve damage; tissue scarring.

Laboratory

Diagnosed mostly on the basis of the characteristic pain and appearance of the dermatomal rashes.

Treatment

Antiviral agents, systemic corticosteroids, antidepressants and adequate pain control. Immunocompetent adults aged 60 years or older, benefit from receipt of the herpes zoster vaccine and have a lower incidence of herpes zoster.

⊟ BIBLIOGRAPHY

1. Ghaznawi N, Virdi A, Dayan A, et al. Herpes Zoster Ophthalmicus: Comparison of disease in patients 60 years and older versus younger than 60 years. Ophthalmology. 2011;118:2242-50.
2. Tseng HF, Smith N, Harpaz R, et al. Herpes zoster vaccine in older adults and the risk of subsequent herpes zoster disease. JAMA. 2011;305:160-6.

⊟ 6A2.A1BI. ABDOMINAL TYPHUS (ENTERIC FEVER; TYPHOID FEVER)

General

Causative agent, *Salmonella typhi*.

Ocular

Conjunctivitis; chemosis; corneal ulcer; tenonitis; paralysis of extraocular muscles; endophthalmitis; panophthalmitis; optic neuritis; retinal detachment; central scotoma; central retinal artery emboli; iritis with or without hypopyon; choroiditis; retinal hemorrhages; bilateral optic neuritis; abnormal ocular motility (likely secondary to thrombotic infarcts affecting the ocular motor nerve nuclei, fascicles, brainstem, or cerebral hemispheres).

Clinical

Fever; headache; bradycardia; splenomegaly; maculopapular rash; leukopenia; encephalitis. Salmonella may produce an illness characterized by fever and bacteremia without any other manifestations of enterocolitis or enteric fever, which is particularly common in patients with AIDS.

Laboratory

Gram-negative bacillus isolation from blood culture (50–70% of cases). Positive stool culture is less frequent.

Treatment

Early detection, antibiotic therapy and adequate fluids, electrolytes, and nutrition reduce the rate of complications and reduce the case-fatality rate.

⊟ BIBLIOGRAPHY

1. Brusch JL. (2011). Typhoid fever. [online] Available from www.emedicine.com/med/TOPIC2331.HTM. [Accessed September, 2013].

🖳 6A2.A1BII. STREPTOCOCCUS (SCARLET FEVER)

General

Gram-positive bacteria that can invade any tissue.

Ocular

Conjunctivitis; corneal ulcer; blepharitis; scarlatinal rash of lid; erysipelas dermatitis of lid; gangrene of lid; endophthalmitis; proptosis; dacryocystitis; optic neuritis; orbital cellulitis; uveitis; hypopyon; secondary glaucoma; paralysis of extraocular muscles; infectious crystalline keratopathy; scleritis.

Clinical

Pharyngitis; impetigo; scarlet fever; pneumonia; bacteremia; rheumatic fever; glomerulonephritis.

Laboratory

Gram-positive cocci growing in pairs or chains. Throat culture and sensitivity are useful.

Treatment

Penicillin is the drug of choice.

🖳 BIBLIOGRAPHY

1. Zabawski EJ. (2011). Scarlet Fever. [online] Available from www.emedicine.com/emerg/TOPIC518.HTM. [Accessed September, 2013].

🖳 6A2.A1BIII. PERTUSSIS (WHOOPING COUGH)

General

Causative agent is *Haemophilus pertussis (Bordetella pertussis)*; not all patients who develop pertussis encephalopathy are children.

Ocular

Conjunctivitis; severe cortical blindness; papilledema; choroiditis; retinal ischemia; ocular muscle palsies; hemorrhages of eyelids, conjunctiva, orbit, anterior chamber, and retina; chronic papilledema; optic neuritis; retinal and vitreous hemorrhages, and even intracranial and subarachnoid hemorrhage associated with increased intrathoracic and intra–abdominal pressures during coughing.

Clinical

Respiratory tract infection; nasal discharge; cough ending with a loud crowing; inspiratory noise (the whoop); thick mucoid sputum; soreness over trachea; ulcer of glottis; vomiting; tetany; encephalopathy; cortical blindness.

Laboratory

The standard criterion for diagnosis of pertussis is isolation of B pertussis in culture.

Treatment

The goals of therapy include limiting the number of paroxysms, observing the severity of cough, providing assistance when necessary, and maximizing nutrition, rest, and recovery. Antimicrobial agents help to prevent the spread of the infection.

🖳 BIBLIOGRAPHY

1. Bocka JJ, McNeil BK, Aronoff SC. (2013). Pertussis. [online] Available from www.emedicine.com/ped/TOPIC1778.HTM. [Accessed September, 2013].

6A2.A1BVI. PNEUMOCOCCAL INFECTIONS (STREPTOCOCCUS PNEUMONIAE INFECTIONS)

General

Gram-positive diplococcus *S. pneumoniae*; some strains are encapsulated while others are not; ocular infections usually are caused by the encapsulated strains; conjunctivitis and corneal scarring produced in an animal model have been attributed to a hemolytic cytolytic exopeptidase.

Ocular

Hypopyon; conjunctivitis; keratitis; corneal ulcer; endophthalmitis; dacryocystitis; uveitis; orbital cellulitis; secondary glaucoma; ophthalmia neonatorum.

Clinical

Upper respiratory infection; chills; sharp pain in hemithorax; cough with sputum production; fever; headache; gastrointestinal symptoms.

Laboratory

Gram stain demonstrates Gram-positive cocci in pairs. The unattached end of each cocci is slightly pointed outward.

Treatment

Impetigo, oral antibiotics and topical antibiotic ointment; preseptal cellulitis, oral antibiotics; orbital cellulitis, need team of infectious disease specialist, otolaryngologist and ophthalmologist to develop plan of therapy; dacryocystitis, oral and topical antibiotics, dacryocystorhinostomy may be necessary; conjunctivitis, topical antibiotic; keratitis, topical antibiotics; poststreptococcal reactive arthritis can occur with uveitis, topical steroids and cycloplegics; endophthalmitis, prompt and aggressive therapy with topical, intravitreal and sometimes systemic antibiotics and pars plana vitrectomy; post-refractive surgery keratitis, flap raised, cultured and treated. Occasionally the flap should be amputated.

BIBLIOGRAPHY

1. Muench DF. (2012). Pneumococcal infections. [online] Available from www.emedicine.com/med/TOPIC1848.HTM. [Accessed September, 2013].

6A2.A1BVII. JAPANESE RIVER FEVER (MITE-BORNE TYPHUS; RURAL TYPHUS; SCRUB TYPHUS; TROPICAL TYPHUS; TSUTSUGAMUSHI DISEASE; TYPHUS)

General

Acute febrile illness by *Rickettsia tsutsugamushi* transmitted by the larval form of a mite.

Ocular

Keratitis; uveitis; paracentral scotoma; vitreous opacity; nystagmus; retinal hemorrhages; exudates; edema.

Clinical

Chills; fever; malaise; headache; lymphadenopathy; generalized aching.

Laboratory

The confirmatory tests are the indirect immunoperoxidase test and the immunofluorescent assay. An infection is confirmed by a four-fold increase in antibody titers between acute and convalescent serum specimens.

Treatment

Treatment must be initiated early in the course of the disease, based on presumptive diagnosis, to reduce morbidity and mortality. Doxycycline and chloramphenicol are both effective.

BIBLIOGRAPHY

1. Cennimo DJ, Dieudonne A. (2013). Scrub Typhus. [online] Available from emedicine.medscape.com/article/971797-overview. [Accessed September, 2013].

⊟ 6A2.A1BVIII. MALARIA

General

Caused by Plasmodium, which is transmitted by mosquito bite, blood transfusion, or contaminated needles and syringes.

Ocular

Proliferative retinitis; vascular embolism; keratitis; ocular herpes simplex; blepharitis; optic atrophy; papilledema; papillitis; optic neuritis; anisocoria; Argyll Robertson pupil; vitreal hemorrhages and opacity; cataract; myopia; strabismus; uveitis; scleral icterus; scotoma; lagophthalmos; ptosis; subconjunctival hemorrhages; paralysis of third, fourth, or sixth nerve; epibulbar hemorrhage involving the conjunctiva, episclera, tendinous insertion of the medial rectus.

Clinical

Fever; anemia; splenomegaly; death.

Laboratory

Blood smear.

Treatment

Consult infectious disease specialist.

⊟ BIBLIOGRAPHY

1. Perez-Jorge EV, Herchline TE. (2013). Malaria. [online] Available from www.emedicine.com/med/TOPIC1385. HTM. [Accessed September, 2013].

⊟ 6A2.A1CIIC. GUILLAIN-BARRÉ SYNDROME (LANDRY PARALYSIS; ACUTE INFECTIOUS NEURITIS; ACUTE POLYRADICULITIS; ACUTE FEBRILE POLYNEURITIS; ACUTE IDIOPATHIC POLYNEURITIS; INFLAMMATORY POLYRADICULONEUROPATHY; LANDRY-GUILLAIN-BARRÉ-STROHL SYNDROME; POSTINFECTIOUS POLYNEURITIS)

General

Etiology unknown; occurs from age 16–50 years.

Ocular

Facial nerve paralysis with paralytic ectropion of the lower eyelid; mild-to-complete external ophthalmoplegia; optic neuritis; papilledema; ptosis; anisocoria; nystagmus; dyschromatopsia; scotoma; bilateral tonic pupils.

Clinical

Polyneuritis involving facial peripheral motor nerves and spinal cord; facial diplegia; bladder incontinence; variable degrees of paralysis, usually beginning in lower extremities; tendon reflexes absent; involvement of respiratory muscles possible; paresthesia (symmetrical).

Laboratory

Cytomegalovirus (CMV), Epstein-Barr virus and human immunodeficiency (HIV) have been most closely associated with this condition.

Treatment

Plasma exchange have shown to be beneficial. Corneal exposure is treated with topical therapy or lateral tarsorrhaphies if warranted.

⊟ BIBLIOGRAPHY

1. Andary MT, Oleszek JL, Cha-Kim A. (2012). Guillain-Barre Syndrome. [online] Available from www.emedicine.com/pmr/TOPIC48.HTM. [Accessed September, 2013].

6A2.A1CIIIB. ACQUIRED IMMUNODEFICIENCY SYNDROME (AIDS; ACQUIRED CELLULAR IMMUNODEFICIENCY; ACQUIRED IMMUNODEFICIENCY)

General

Acquired breakdown of the immune system followed by disease that takes advantage of the body's collapsed defenses; acquired by shared drug needles or sexual intercourse; occurs most frequently in homosexually active men (75%), intravenous drug abusers (13%), and Haitian immigrants (6%).

Ocular

Retinal cotton-wool spots; CMV retinitis; retinal periphlebitis; conjunctival Kaposi sarcoma; necrotizing retinitis; retinal hemorrhages; conjunctivitis sicca; orbital Burkitt lymphoma; peripheral retinochoroiditis; vitreitis; fungal corneal ulcer; hypopyon; acute glaucoma; third nerve palsy; anterior uveitis; atypical retinitis; orbital pseudotumor; herpes zoster ophthalmicus; herpes simplex keratitis; bacterial keratitis; molluscum contagiosum; CMV retinitis; toxoplasma retinitis; acute retinal necrosis; HIV retinitis; syphilitic retinitis; *Pneumocystis carinii* choroiditis; fungal and bacterial endophthalmitis; fungal choroiditis; conjunctival microvasculopathy; keratitis sicca; subconjunctival hemorrhage.

Clinical

Because of lowered immunity, one third develops Kaposi sarcoma; pneumonia caused by *P. carinii*; death.

Laboratory

Enzyme-linked immunosorbent assay (ELISA) test is used for screening other tests are used to evaluate false-positive and false-negative test results.

Treatment

Medical consultations are required for systemic treatment. The treatment of CMV retinitis can include drugs such as ganciclovir, valganciclovir, fomivirsen, foscarnet and cidofovir. All of these drugs have specific adverse effects and complicate the decision to use for treatment.

BIBLIOGRAPHY
1. Dubin J. (2011). Rapid testing for HIV. [online] Available from www.emedicine.com/emerg/TOPIC253.HTM. [Accessed September, 2013].

6A2.A1CIIIC. TUBERCULOSIS

General

Communicable disease caused by the acid-fast bacillus *M. tuberculosis*.

Ocular

Conjunctivitis; subconjunctival nodules (tuberculomas); keratitis; pannus; corneal ulcer; blepharitis; cellulitis; meibomianitis; uveitis; dacryocystitis; chronic orbital cellulitis; retinitis; scleritis; scleral perforation; hypopyon; vitreous hemorrhages; optic neuritis; optic atrophy; tuberculous panophthalmitis; choroidal tubercles; intraorbital extraocular lesions.

Clinical

Pulmonary infection; pyuria; hematuria; epididymitis; dysuria; flank pain; distorted calyces; productive cough.

Laboratory

Acid-fast bacillus culture of body fluids including vitreous and aqueous. PCR is 89% positive for pulmonary infection.

Treatment

A course of chemotherapy (isoniazid, rifampin, pyrazinamide and ethambutol or streptomycin) for a period of 6 months is the recommended therapy.

BIBLIOGRAPHY
1. Collins JK. Handbook of Clinical Ophthalmology. New York: Masson; 1982.
2. DeVoe AG, Locatcher-Khorazo D. The external manifestations of ocular tuberculosis. Trans Am Ophthalmol Soc. 1964;62:203-12.
3. D'Souza P, Garg R, Dhaliwal RS, et al. Orbital tuberculosis. Int Ophthalmol. 1994; 18:149-52.
4. Gupta V, Gupta A, Arora S, et al. Presumed tubercular serpiginous like choroiditis. Ophthalmology. 2003;110:1744-9.
5. Patkar S, Singhania BK, Agrawal A. Intraorbital extraocular tuberculosis: a report of three cases. Surg Neurol 1994; 42:320-1.
6. Roy FH, Fraunfelder FW, Fraunfelder FT. Roy and Fraunfelder's Current Ocular Therapy, 6th editon. Philadelphia: WB Saunders; 2008.
7. Tejada P, Mendez MJ, Negreira S. Choroidal tubercles with tuberculous meningitis. Int Ophthalmol. 1994;18:115-8.

⊟ 6A2.A1CIIID. CRYPTOCOCCOSIS (TORULOSIS)

General

A pulmonary infection caused by *Cryptococcus neoformans*, a saprophyte found in weathered pigeon droppings, soil, and unpasteurized cow's milk; infection acquired through respiratory system and usually manifests as meningoencephalitis; higher incidence in patients with AIDS.

Ocular

Blurred or poor vision; diplopia; uveitis; papilledema; retinal detachment; retinal hemorrhage and exudates; secondary glaucoma; vitreous reaction; retinitis; proptosis; a mass over the optic nerve head; disease process can be bilateral or unilateral; cranial nerve VI palsy; visual loss; conjunctivitis.

Clinical

Severe headache; dizziness; ataxia; vomiting; tinnitus; memory disturbances; Jacksonian convulsions; fever usually is absent; occurs frequently in patients with leukemia or lymphoma.

Laboratory

The diagnosis is based on skin biopsy findings evaluated after fungal staining and culture.

Treatment

The goal of pharmacotherapy is either to terminate the infection when possible or to control the infection and to reduce morbidity when cure is not possible.

⊟ BIBLIOGRAPHY

1. King JW, DeWitt ML. (2013). Cryptococcosis. [online] Available from www.emedicine.com/med/TOPIC482.HTM. [Accessed September, 2013].

⊟ 6A2.A1CIVA. DIPHTHERIA

General

Acute infectious disease caused by *C. diphtheriae*; severity is dependent upon the amount of exotoxin absorbed prior to initiation of specific therapy.

Ocular

Conjunctivitis; xerophthalmia; keratitis; corneal ulcer; blepharitis; cellulitis of lid; meibomianitis; ptosis; dacryocystitis; cataract; central retinal artery occlusion; optic neuritis; accommodative spasm or paralysis; convergence paralysis; divergence paralysis; paralysis of third, fourth, or sixth nerve; paralysis of accommodation (in children); ocular motor nerve paresis; choroiditis; cranial neuropathies involving the trigeminal, vagus, and hypoglossal cranial nerves; myocarditis.

Clinical

Local inflammatory lesion, with effect on heart, kidneys and nervous system.

Laboratory

Gram-positive rods commonly affect children younger than 10 years.

Treatment

Systemic treatment involves use of diphtheria antitoxin and antibiotics. Ocular treatment includes diphtheria antitoxin and high titer y-globulin preparation. Topical penicillin G ointment helps to eradicate the bacilli.

⊟ BIBLIOGRAPHY

1. Demirci CS, Abuhammour W. (2013). Pediatric diphtheria. [online] Available from www.emedicine.com/ped/TOPIC596.HTM. [Accessed September, 2013].

6A2.A1CIVB. LOCKJAW (TETANUS)

General

Acute infectious disease affecting nervous system; causative agent is *Clostridium tetani;* bacteria enters body through a puncture wound, abrasion, cut, or burn.

Ocular

Chemosis; keratitis; nystagmus; uveitis; corneal ulcer; cellulitis of orbit; hypopyon; panophthalmitis; pupil paralysis; pseudoptosis; blepharospasm; paralysis of third or seventh nerve; may occur following perforating ocular injuries.

Clinical

Severe muscle spasms; dysphagia; trismus; facial palsy; muscle stiffness; irritability.

Laboratory

Gram-positive spore-forming bacteria, laboratory studies are of little value.

Treatment

Passive immunization with human tetanus immune globulin shortens the course of tetanus and may lessen its severity. Benzodiazepines have emerged as the mainstay of symptomatic therapy for tetanus.

BIBLIOGRAPHY

1. Hinfey PB. (2012). Tetanus. [online] Available from www.emedicine.com/med/TOPIC2254.HTM. [Accessed September, 2013].

6A2.A1CIVC. BOTULISM

General

It is caused by a toxin-producing strain of *C. botulinum;* it occurs primarily after the ingestion of contaminated food; the organism can produce a neurotoxin, the effect of which can be life threatening.

Ocular

Absent optokinetic nystagmus, absent vertical gaze; marked limitation of horizontal gaze; ptosis; diplopia; decreased tear secretion; mydriasis; paralysis of accommodation; nystagmus; optic atrophy; optic neuritis; extraocular muscle paresis.

Clinical

Dizziness; severe respiratory impairment; gastrointestinal disturbances; dysphagia; dysarthria; postural hypotension.

Laboratory

Toxin assay for early diagnosis, whereas later cases are more likely to yield a positive specimen culture.

Treatment

Antitoxin appears to be the only effective medication. Supportive care such as ventilation and parenteral nutrition are necessary for the duration of the paralytic illness.

BIBLIOGRAPHY

1. Patel B, Taylor SF. (2012). Ophthalmologic manifestations of botulism. [online] Available from www.emedicine.com/oph/TOPIC493.HTM. [Accessed September, 2013].

6A2.A1CVA. SCHAUMANN SYNDROME (BESNIER-BOECK-SCHAUMANN SYNDROME; BOECK SARCOID; SARCOIDOSIS)

General

Etiology unknown; theories include tuberculosis, hypersensitivity to pine pollen, virus infection; affects blacks most often; chronic course with spontaneous remissions (*see* Heerfordt's syndrome); hilar or paratracheal nodes with erythema nodosum; onset most often in middle and old age; ocular involvement in 20–25% of all cases.

Ocular

Orbital granulomatous mass; bony defects; cutaneous and subcutaneous nodules; myogenic palsy; lacrimal gland adenopathy; decreased tear formation; secondary glaucoma; granulomatous uveitis with iris nodules, cells and flare; mutton fat keratic precipitates; keratitis sicca; vitreous floaters; band-shaped keratitis; complicated cataract;

inflammatory retinal exudates; "candle wax drippings"; optic nerve atrophy; neuritis; eyelid nodules; ocular nerve enlargement (granuloma).

Clinical

Lymphadenopathy; hilar nodes; fatigue; cystic, punched-out or reticulated changes in small bones (mainly, hands and feet); muscle wasting; contractures; weakness in legs and arms.

Laboratory

Chest X-ray, CT scan, and MRI of the brain.

Treatment

Glucocorticoids are the treatment of choice.

🖅 BIBLIOGRAPHY

1. Sharma GD. (2011). Pediatric sarcoidosis. [online] Available from www.emedicine.com/ped/TOPIC2043.HTM. [Accessed September, 2013].

🖅 6A.2B1A. WERNICKE SYNDROME I (SUPERIOR HEMORRHAGIC POLIOENCEPHA-LOPATHIC SYNDROME; HEMORRHAGIC POLIOENCEPHALITIS SUPERIOR SYNDROME; ENCEPHALITIS HEMORRHAGICA SUPERIORIS; AVITAMINOSIS B; THIAMINE DEFICIENCY; BERIBERI; GAYET-WERNICKE SYNDROME; WERNICKE-KORSAKOFF SYNDROME) PTOSIS

General

Lack of vitamin B or thiamine; focal vascular lesions in the gray matter around third and fourth ventricles and Sylvian aqueduct; alcoholics (adults); beriberi of all ages.

Ocular

Ptosis; acute bilateral nuclear ophthalmoplegia; complete ophthalmoplegia; retinal hemorrhages; optic atrophy; optic neuritis; conjunctivitis; blepharitis; nutritional amblyopia; central scotoma; papilledema; nystagmus; absolute pupillary paralysis or Argyll Robertson pupils; accommodative palsy.

Clinical

Early prostration; lethargy; irritability; stupor; delirium; mental disturbances to Korsakoff psychosis; ataxia; tremors; peripheral neuritis; anorexia; vomiting; insomnia; perspiration; tachycardia; hallucinations; retrograde amnesia; apathy; anxiety; fear; defective concentration; cardiomyopathy.

Laboratory

Electrolyte studies, serum thiamine levels, CBC. Evaluation of hypoxemia, hypercarbia, acidosis, or alkalosis. Serum/urine toxin drug screen and liver enzymes.

Treatment

Parenteral thiamine is the treatment of choice.

🖅 BIBLIOGRAPHY

1. Xiong GL, Kenedi CA. (2013). Wernicke-Korsakoff syndrome. [online] Available from www.emedicine.com/med/TOPIC2405.HTM. [Accessed September, 2013].

🖅 6A.2B2. DIABETES MELLITUS

General

Complex disorder of carbohydrate, lipid and protein metabolism characterized by hyperglycemia and a relative or total lack of insulin. Development is influenced by both genetic and environmental factors. Most commonly occurs in middle or late life (type II) and is seen most commonly in the obese. Diabetes can occur in the 1st or 2nd decade of life (type I) and usually involves the lack of insulin production by the pancreas and the need for insulin therapy.

Clinical

Atherosclerosis; nephropathy; neuropathy; polyuria; polydipsia; polyphagia; obesity; elevated plasma glucose and elevated glycated hemoglobin (A1C).

Ocular

Diabetic retinopathy; vitreous hemorrhage; macular edema; cataract; glaucoma; asteroid hyalosis; extraocular muscle paralysis; rubeosis iridis; corneal hypesthesia; optic nerve atrophy; papillopathy.

Laboratory

Diagnosis made by fasting plasma glucose of greater than 126 mg/dL and 2 hours post glucose load (75 g) plasma glucose of greater than 200 mg/dL and confirmed by repeat test.

Treatment

Goals include elimination of symptoms, by reduction of blood sugar and blood pressure. Smoking cessation, aspirin therapy, weight loss, exercise, diabetic diet as well as oral medication and/or insulin are all used in the treatment of diabetes. Diabetic retinopathy is most successfully treated with retinal photocoagulation. Pars plana vitrectomy is sometimes necessary to remove vitreous hemorrhage. Other ocular problems caused by diabetes such as cataracts and glaucoma are treated in traditional methods.

BIBLIOGRAPHY

1. Khardori R. (2012). Type 2 diabetes mellitus. [online] Available from emedicine.medscape.com/article/117853-overview. [Accessed September, 2013].

6A.2B3A. LEUKEMIA

General

Acute or chronic blood disorder.

Ocular

Engorgement of conjunctival vessels; papillary hypertrophy; aggregations of tumor cells in conjunctiva, choroid and orbit; secondary glaucoma; retinal venous engorgement and tortuosity with pronounced constrictions; retinal hemorrhages; retinal detachment; cotton-wool spots; macular edema; papilledema; optic atrophy; optic neuritis; paralysis of extraocular muscles; hypopyon; vitreous opacities; retinal sea fans; perilimbal subconjunctival infiltrates; corneal leukemic infiltration (rare); shallow serous retinal detachments; hyphema; iris neovascularization; central retinal vein occlusion; vitreous infiltrates.

Clinical

Frequent involvement of CNS; intracranial hemorrhage; thrombocytopenia; rising white cell count.

Laboratory

Complete blood count and differential, bone marrow aspiration, immunophenotyping, chromosomal analysis.

Treatment

Chemotherapy with or without radiotherapy.

BIBLIOGRAPHY

1. Wu L, Evans T, Martinez J. (2012). Leukemias. [online] Available from www.emedicine.com/oph/TOPIC489.HTM. [Accessed September, 2013].

6A.2B5 PORPHYRIA CUTANEA TARDA

General

Disorder of porphyria metabolism; highest incidence in Bantu population; both sexes affected; onset between ages 40 and 60 years; insidious onset; autosomal dominant; light-sensitive dermatitis in later adult life; associated with excretion of large amounts of uroporphyrin in urine.

Ocular

Synophrys; keratitis; palsies of third and seventh cranial nerves; scleromalacia perforans; optic atrophy; retinal hemorrhages and cotton-wool spots; macular edema; pinguecula; pterygium; brownish pigmentation in conjunctiva and lid margin.

Clinical

Cutaneous manifestations are solar hypersensitivity, vesiculobullous lesions, ulcerations, severe scarring, and hypertrichosis; erythrodontia.

Laboratory

Urinary porphyrin levels are abnormally high, with several hundred to several thousand micrograms excreted in a 24-hour period. Direct immunofluorescence examination can help differentiate PCT from immunobullous diseases with dermoepidermal junction cleavage (epidermolysis bullosa acquisita, lupus erythematosus) in which the perivascular immunoglobulin deposition found in PCT is not observed.

Treatment

Sunlight avoidance, therapeutic phlebotomy to reduce iron stores, chelation with desferrioxamine; iron-rich foods should be consumed in moderation.

BIBLIOGRAPHY

1. Poh-Fitzpatrick MB. (2012). Porphyria cutanea tarda. [online] Available from www.emedicine.com/derm/TOPIC344.HTM. [Accessed September, 2013].

6A.2G TEMPORAL ARTERITIS SYNDROME (CRANIAL ARTERITIS SYNDROME; GIANT CELL ARTERITIS; HUTCHINSON-HORTON-MAGATH-BROWN SYNDROME)

General

Etiology unknown; mainly females; mainly Whites; ages 55–80 years; temporal artery shows inflammatory thickening; arteritis of the vessels supplying the optic nerve.

Ocular

Transient ptosis; partial or complete loss of vision on the affected side; retinal detachment; exudates and hemorrhages; narrowing of retinal vessels; obstruction of the central retinal artery; optic atrophy; ischemic optic neuropathy; acute decreased IOP; corneal hypesthesia; palsies of extraocular muscles; hemorrhagic glaucoma; diplopia; hemorrhages on or around the disk.

Clinical

Throbbing headache; hyperalgesia of the scalp; malaise; anorexia; weakness; weight loss; fever; nodular pulmonary nodules; cough; otitis with deafness.

Laboratory

Elevated ESR greater than 50 mm/hour, positive temporal artery biopsy.

Treatment

Systemic corticosteroids are the therapy of choice.

BIBLIOGRAPHY

1. Allen AW, Biega T, Varma MK. (2012). Temporal arteritis imaging. [online] Available from www.emedicine.com/radio/TOPIC675.HTM. [Accessed September, 2013].
2. Walvick MD, Walvick MP. Giant cell arteritis: laboratory predictors of a positive temporal artery biopsy. Ophthalmology. 2011;118(6):1201-4.

6B. BIELSCHOWSKY-LUTZ-COGAN SYNDROME (INTERNUCLEAR OPHTHALMOPLEGIA)

General

Lesion in the medial longitudinal fasciculus; anterior internuclear ophthalmoplegia consists of paresis of convergence with paresis of homolateral medial rectus muscle during lateral gaze toward opposite side of the lesion; in the posterior internuclear ophthalmoplegia, convergence is not affected, while the homolateral medial rectus muscle is paralytic on lateral gaze; the most common cause in young patients include a demyelinating process such as MS, whereas an ischemic process is more common in the elderly; other reported causes of brainstem infarction associated with internuclear ophthalmoplegia include sickle cell trait, periarteritis nodosa, Wernicke encephalopathy, "crack" cocaine smoking.

Ocular

Unilateral or bilateral palsy of the medial rectus muscle during conjugate lateral gaze but with or without normal function of this muscle during convergence, depending on the type of internuclear ophthalmoplegia; dissociated nystagmus in the maximal abducted contralateral eye.

Laboratory

CT and MRI.

Treatment

Intravenous (IV) and oral steroids may be beneficial.

⊟ BIBLIOGRAPHY

1. Lee AG, Berlie CL, Costello F. (2012). Ophthalmologic manifestations of multiple sclerosis. [online] Available from www.emedicine.com/oph/TOPIC179.HTM. [Accessed September, 2013].
2. Luzzio C, Dangond F. (2012). Multiple sclerosis. [online] Available from www.emedicine.com/emerg/TOPIC321.HTM. [Accessed September, 2013].

⊟ 6C. BILATERAL COMPLETE OPHTHALMOPLEGIA (BILATERAL PALSY OF OCULAR MUSCLES, PTOSIS, WITH PUPIL AND ACCOMMODATION INVOLVEMENT)

[†]1. Arteriosclerotic hemorrhage and occlusion
2. Cerebellopontine angle tumors (Cushing syndrome II)
3. Encephalitis, acute
4. Fisher syndrome (ophthalmoplegia-ataxia areflexia syndrome)
5. Giant-cell arteritis (Hutchinson-Horton-Magath-Brown syndrome)
6. Kiloh-Nevin syndrome (ocular myeomyopathy)
[†]7. Midbrain tumors
8. Multiple sclerosis (rare)
9. Mucormycosis
10. OHAHA syndrome (ophthalmoplegia, hypotonia, ataxia hypacusis, athetosis)
[†]11. Orbital abscess
12. Parinaud syndrome (conjunctiva-adenitis syndrome)
[†]13. Retrobulbar block complication
14. Rochon-Duvigneaud syndrome (superior orbital fissure syndrome)
15. Rollet syndrome (orbital apex-sphenoidal syndrome)
16. Syphilis (acquired lues)
[†]17. Trauma
18. Wernicke encephalopathies (thiamine deficiency)
19. Whipple disease (intestinal lipodystrophy)

⊟ BIBLIOGRAPHY

1. McKusick VA. Mendelian Inheritance in Man, 12th edition. Baltimore: Johns Hopkins Hospital Press; 1998.
2. Roy FH, Fraunfelder FT, Fraunfelder FW: Roy and Fraunfelder's Current Ocular Therapy, 6th edition. Philadelphia: WB Saunders; 2008.
3. Sergott RC, Glaser JS, Berger LJ. Simultaneous, bilateral diabetic ophthalmoplegia. Ophthalmology. 1984;91:18-22.

[†]Indicates a general entry and therefore has not been described in detail in the text

---

⊟ 6C2. CUSHING (2) SYNDROME (ANGLE TUMOR SYNDROME; CEREBELLOPONTINE ANGLE SYNDROME; PONTOCEREBELLAR ANGLE TUMOR SYNDROME; ACOUSTIC NEUROMA SYNDROME)

General

Tumor involving cranial nerves V, VI, VII, and VIII and brainstem; occurs between ages 30 and 45 years.

Ocular

Paresis orbicularis muscle (VII); paresis external rectus muscle (VI); mixed nystagmus with head tilt; palsies of extraocular muscles are accounted for by increased intracranial pressure if the aqueduct of Sylvius is closed by the growing tumor; decreased corneal reflex V (homolateral and early sign); bilateral papilledema (increased intracranial pressure).

Clinical

Deafness (homolateral); labyrinth function disturbed or lost; tinnitus; hyperesthesia of the face; homolateral facial nerve paresis (total paralysis rare); hoarseness; difficulties in swallowing; unilateral limb ataxia; gait ataxia; nuchal headache; emesis; facial pain, numbness and paresis; progressive unilateral hearing loss.

Laboratory

The diagnostic test for acoustic tumors is gadolinium-enhanced MRI.

Treatment

Surgical excision of the tumor; arresting tumor growth using stereotactic radiation therapy; careful serial observation.

BIBLIOGRAPHY

1. Kutz JW, Roland PS, Isaacson B. (2012). Acoustic neuroma. [online] Available from www.emedicine.com/ent/TOPIC239.HTM. [Accessed September, 2013].

6C3. ENCEPHALITIS, ACUTE

General

In approximately 0.1–0.2% of patients having rubeola (measles), an acute encephalitis is seen within 1 week after the onset of the rash; a case of immunosuppressive encephalitis can present with focal seizures leading to progressive obtundation.

Ocular

Papillitis; optic atrophy; ocular motor palsies; nystagmus; optic neuritis or neuroretinitis.

Clinical

Rise in temperature; drowsiness; irritability; meningismus; vomiting and headache; stupor; convulsions; coma.

Laboratory

Perform head CT, with and without contrast agent, before LP to search for evidence of elevated intracerebral pressure MRI is useful, viral serology.

Treatment

Evaluate and treat for shock or hypotension, treat systemic complications, acyclovir.

BIBLIOGRAPHY

1. Howes DS, Lazoff M. (2013). Encephalitis. [online] Available from www.emedicine.com/emerg/TOPIC163.HTM. [Accessed September, 2013].

6C4. FISHER SYNDROME (OPHTHALMOPLEGIA ATAXIA AREFLEXIA SYNDROME; MILLER-FISHER SYNDROME)

General

Acute idiopathic polyneuritis; prognosis good; complete recovery over several weeks (variant of Guillain-Barré syndrome; *see* Guillain-Barré syndrome).

Ocular

Moderate ptosis; complete external and almost complete internal ophthalmoplegia; diplopia; sluggish pupil reaction to light; may present without total ophthalmoplegia.

Clinical

Dizziness; severe ataxia; loss of tendon reflexes; chest pains; difficulties in chewing; diminished or absent sense of vibration; upper respiratory tract infection preceding this syndrome.

Laboratory

Diagnosis usually is made on clinical grounds. Laboratory studies are useful to rule out other diagnoses.

Treatment

Monitored closely for changes in blood pressure, heart rate and other arrhythmias. Temporary pacing may be required for patients with second-degree and third-degree heart block.

BIBLIOGRAPHY

1. Fisher M. An unusual variant of acute idiopathic polyneuritis (syndrome of ophthalmoplegia, ataxia and areflexia). N Engl J Med. 1956;255(2):57-65.
2. Igarashi Y, Takeda M, Maekawa H, et al. Fisher's syndrome without total ophthalmoplegia. Ophthalmologica. 1992;205(3):163-7.
3. Swick HM. Pseudointernuclear ophthalmoplegia in acute idiopathic polyneuritis (Fisher's syndrome). Am J Ophthalmol. 1974;77(5):725-8.

6C5. TEMPORAL ARTERITIS SYNDROME (CRANIAL ARTERITIS SYNDROME; GIANT CELL ARTERITIS; HUTCHINSON-HORTON-MAGATH-BROWN SYNDROME)

General

Etiology unknown; mainly females; mainly Whites; ages 55–80 years; temporal artery shows inflammatory thickening; arteritis of the vessels supplying the optic nerve.

Ocular

Transient ptosis; partial or complete loss of vision on the affected side; retinal detachment; exudates and hemorrhages; narrowing of retinal vessels; obstruction of the central retinal artery; optic atrophy; ischemic optic neuropathy; acute decreased IOP; corneal hypesthesia; palsies of extraocular muscles; hemorrhagic glaucoma; diplopia; hemorrhages on or around the disk.

Clinical

Throbbing headache; hyperalgesia of the scalp; malaise; anorexia; weakness; weight loss; fever; nodular pulmonary nodules; cough; otitis with deafness.

Laboratory

Elevated ESR greater than 50 mm/hour, positive temporal artery biopsy.

Treatment

Systemic corticosteroids are the therapy of choice.

BIBLIOGRAPHY

1. Allen AW, Biega T, Varma MK. (2012). Temporal arteritis imaging. [online] Available from www.emedicine.com/radio/TOPIC675.HTM. [Accessed September, 2013].
2. Walvick MD, Walvick MP. Giant cell arteritis: laboratory predictors of a positive temporal artery biopsy. Ophthalmology. 2011;118(6):1201-4.

6C6. KILOH-NEVIN SYNDROME (MUSCULAR DYSTROPHY OF EXTERNAL OCULAR MUSCLES; OCULAR MYOPATHY)

General

Etiology unknown; autosomal dominant.

Ocular

Ptosis; orbicularis muscle weakness; ocular myopathy; diplopia progressing to bilateral myopathic ophthalmoplegia; may be associated with pigmentary retinopathy and heart block (*see* Kearns-Sayre syndrome).

Clinical

Progressive muscular dystrophy in which facial muscles may be involved; occasionally, hereditary ataxia; pain; myokymia.

Laboratory

Diagnosis is made by clinical findings.

Treatment

Topical keratolytics, systemic and topical retinoids, potent topical steroids.

BIBLIOGRAPHY

1. Duszowa J, Koraszewska-Matuszewska B, Niebrój TK. The Kiloh-Nevin syndrome. Klin Oczna. 1974;44:805-7.
2. Kiloh LG, Nevin S. Progressive dystrophy of the external ocular muscles. Brain. 1951;74:115.

6C8. DISSEMINATED SCLEROSIS (MULTIPLE SCLEROSIS)

General

Disseminated demyelination affecting white matter of the brain, spinal cord, and optic nerves; etiology unknown.

Ocular

Nystagmus; ptosis; myokymia; optic atrophy; papillitis; optic neuritis; anisocoria; Argyll Robertson pupil; Marcus Gunn pupil; hippus, decreased or absent papillary reaction to light; periphlebitis; visual field defects; gaze palsy; paralysis of third or sixth nerve; uveitis; oscillopsia; Uhthoff symptom (reduction of visual acuity with exercise or ocular hyperthermia); pars planitis; retinal venous sheathing; retinitis; granulomatous uveitis.

Clinical

Incoordination; paresthesia; spasticity; tic douloureux; urinary frequency and infections; progressive disability; paralysis; death.

Laboratory

MRI, CSF positive for oligoclonal band, albumin and IgG index; BAER and SEP.

Treatment

Patients with MS may require multiple consultations to rule out other causes for their symptoms. Drugs such as immunodulator, immunosuppressors, anti-Parkinson agent, CNS stimulants are all used in the management of the disease.

BIBLIOGRAPHY

1. Luzzio C, Dangond F. (2013). Multiple Sclerosis. [online] Available from www.emedicine.com/neuro/topic228.htm. [Accessed September, 2013].

6C9. MUCORMYCOSIS (PHYCOMYCOSIS)

General

Acute, often fatal infection caused by saprophytic fungi; associated with diabetes mellitus and ketoacidosis.

Ocular

Corneal ulcer; striate keratopathy; ptosis; panophthalmitis; proptosis; cellulitis of orbit; immobile pupil; retinitis; optic neuritis; paralysis of extraocular muscles; central retinal artery thrombosis.

Clinical

Epistaxis; nasal discharge; facial pain; facial palsies; anhidrosis; cranial nerve or peripheral motor and sensory nerve deficits may occur.

Laboratory

Tissue biopsy and culture of paranasal sinuses demonstrate the presence of the fungi, which appear as broad, irregular, nonseptate, branching hyphae on Hematoxylin and Eosin (H & E) stain.

Treatment

Amphotericin B.

BIBLIOGRAPHY

1. Crum-Cianflone NF. (2011). Mucormycosis. [online] Available from www.emedicine.com/oph/TOPIC225.HTM. [Accessed September, 2013].

6C10. OHAHA SYNDROME (OPHTHALMOPLEGIA, HYPOTONIA, ATAXIA, HYPOACUSIS, ATHETOSIS)

General

Ophthalmoplegia, hypotonia, ataxia, hypoacusis, athetosis (OHAHA) are distinguishing symptoms; sudden onset of deafness at an age after patient has learned to speak.

Ocular

Kernicterus; strabismus; nystagmus; ocular migraine; ophthalmoplegia; vascular spasm in branches of the ophthalmic artery; intact convergence.

Clinical

Hemiplegia; athetosis; choreoathetosis; tremor; hypoxia; corticospinal tract disease; diabetes mellitus; ataxia; medulloblastoma; asynergia; dysdiadochokinesis; Holmes rebound phenomenon; acute cerebellar lesion; dysmetria; dysarthria; Fox syndrome; vascular occlusion; congenital athetosis.

Laboratory

Diagnosis is made by clinical findings.

Treatment

- *Strabismus*: Equalized vision with correct refractive error; surgery may be helpful in patients with diplopia.
- *Local*: Ocular lubrication (drops or ointments) may be useful for exposure.

BIBLIOGRAPHY

1. Kallio AK, Jauhiainen T. A new syndrome of ophthalmoplegia, hypoacusis, ataxia, hypotonia, and athetosis (OHAHA). Adv Audiol. 1985;3:84-90.
2. McKusick VA. Mendelian Inheritance in Man; A Catalog of Human Genes and Genetic Disorders, 12th edition. Baltimore, USA: The Johns Hopkins University Press; 1998.
3. Hamosh A, Scott AF, Amberger J, et al. Online Mendelian Inheritance in Man (OMIM), a knowledgebase of human genes and genetic disorders. Nucleic Acids Res. 2002;30(1):52-5.
4. Woody RC, Blaw ME. Ophthalmoplegic migraine in infancy. Clin Pediatr (Phila). 1986;25(2):82-4.

6C12. PARINAUD OCULOGLANDULAR SYNDROME (PARINAUD CONJUNCTIVA-ADENITIS SYNDROME; CATSCRATCH OCULOGLANDULAR SYNDROME; CATSCRATCH DISEASE; BARTONELLA HENSELAE)

General

Most frequently seen in children; incubation time 7–10 days; caused by small pleomorphic Gram-negative bacillus; good prognosis; affects both sexes; about 90% of patients with this condition have serologic evidence of infection by *R. henselae*.

Ocular

Conjunctivitis; retrotarsal conjunctival granulations; formation of granulomata in anterior segment about 3 mm high and 2–6 mm in diameter; inferior fornix usually affected; ulceration common; neuroretinitis; optic neuritis.

Clinical

Tender, red papule at the site of a cat scratch; regional preauricular and cervical lymphadenitis (often only one gland involved); irregular fever for 4–5 days and malaise; fever; parotid gland swelling.

Laboratory

Histopathology of biopsied lymph node of Warthin-Starry silver stain.

Treatment

Symptomatic treatment includes warm compresses, analgesics and antipyretics. Aspiration of lymph node if distention causes pain. Antibiotics may be necessary in severe cases.

BIBLIOGRAPHY

1. Nervi SJ. (2011). Catscratch Disease. [online]. Available from www.emedicine.com/med/TOPIC304.HTM. [Accessed November, 2012].
2. Chi SL, Stinnett S, Eggenberger E, et al. Clinical characteristics in 53 patients with cat scratch optic neuropathy. Ophthalmology. 2012;119:183-7.

6C14. ROCHON-DUVIGNEAUD SYNDROME (SUPERIOR ORBITAL FISSURE SYNDROME) OPTIC ATROPHY

General

Inflammatory, traumatic, tumor, or vascular lesions such as meningioma of the sphenoid, carotid aneurysm, and arachnoiditis; infections originating in the maxillary sinus.

Ocular

Mild exophthalmos; lid edema; partial or complete ophthalmoplegia (III, IV and VI); decreased corneal sensitivity; papilledema; optic atrophy.

Clinical

Decreased sensitivity in area of nasociliary, lacrimal, frontal, and ophthalmic nerve distribution; may result from a metastatic tumor.

Laboratory

CBC count, ESR, thyroid function test, FTA, ANA, LE preparation, ANCA, serum protein electrophoresis, Lyme titer, ACE level and HIV titer are helpful. CSF, anti-GQ1b antibodies, and MRI of the brain and the orbits.

Treatment

Corticosteroids are the treatment of choice.

BIBLIOGRAPHY

1. Falcone F, Lazow SK, Berger JR, et al. Superior orbital fissure syndrome. Secondary to infected dentigerous cyst of the maxillary sinus. NY State Dental J. 1994;60:62-4.
2. Hedstrom J, Parsons J, Maloney PL, et al. Superior orbital fissure syndrome: report of a case. J Oral Surg. 1974;32: 198-201.
3. Phanthumchinda K, Hemachuda T. Superior orbital fissure syndrome as a presenting symptom in hepatocellular carcinoma. J Med Assoc Thailand. 1992;75:62-5.
4. Rochon-Duvigneaud A. Quelques Cas de Paralysie de Tous les Nerfs Orbitaires (Ophtalmoplegie Totale avec Amaurose et Anesthesie dans le Domaine de l'Ophtalmique d'Origine Syphilitique). Arch Ophthalmol. 1896;16:746.

6C15. ROLLET SYNDROME (ORBITAL APEX-SPHENOIDAL SYNDROME) OPTIC NEURITIS

General

Lesion in the apex of the orbit (neoplastic, hemorrhagic, or inflammatory) involving the third, fourth, and sixth cranial nerves, the ophthalmic branch of the fifth sympathetic fibers when they pass through the sphenoidal fissure, and the optic nerve; manifestations vary greatly with extent of lesion; pain is frequent early sign; orbital fissure syndrome and sphenocavernous syndrome are similar; sudden onset.

Ocular

Exophthalmos; ptosis; hyperesthesia or anesthesia of the upper lid; ophthalmoplegia (partial or complete); wide pupil with loss of reaction on accommodation; neuralgic pain in the region of the ophthalmic branch of cranial nerve V; anesthesia of the cornea; papilledema; optic neuritis; optic atrophy; diplopia; herpes zoster ophthalmicus.

Clinical

Hyperesthesia or anesthesia of the forehead; inflammation of cavernous sinuses; meningoencephalitis.

Laboratory

Diagnosis is made by clinical findings.

Treatment

Exophthalmos: Reversing the problem which is causing the exophthalmos is the treatment of choice and will minimize the ocular complications. Ocular lubricants are beneficial for control of the corneal exposure.

BIBLIOGRAPHY

1. Bourke RD, Pyle J. Herpes zoster ophthalmicus and the orbital apex syndrome. Aust N Z J Ophthalmol. 1994;22:77-80.

🖰 6C16. ACQUIRED LUES (SYPHILIS; ACQUIRED SYPHILIS; LUES VENEREA; MALUM VENEREUM)

General

Causative agent, *T. pallidum*, usually transmitted sexually.

Ocular

Conjunctival chancroid; conjunctivitis; keratitis; blepharitis; ptosis; iris atrophy; hippus; dacryocystitis; optic nerve atrophy; optic neuritis; periostitis; episcleritis; scleritis; nystagmus; uveitis; vitreous hemorrhages; paralysis of sixth nerve; papilledema; retinal hemorrhages; retinitis proliferans; oculogyric crisis; neuroretinitis; papilledema (associated with aseptic meningitis); diffuse or multifocal chorioretinitis; vertical supranuclear gaze palsy; Benedikt syndrome.

Clinical

Primary lesion associated with regional lymphadenopathy; secondary bacteremic stage associated with generalized mucocutaneous lesions; tertiary stage characterized by destructive mucocutaneous, musculoskeletal, or parenchymal lesions, aortitis, or CNS disease; syphilis and HIV infection often coexist in the same patient who experiences a higher incidence and greater severity of neurologic and ocular manifestations; a significant percentage of patients infected with HIV-I and *T. pallidum* become seronegative to syphilis testing.

Laboratory

Serologic nontreponemal tests include VDRL and RPR.

Treatment

The goals are to reduce morbidity and to prevent complications. Penicillin is the antibiotic of choice for treating syphilis. Ocular syphilis should be treated the same as patients with neurosyphilis.

🖰 BIBLIOGRAPHY

1. Euerle B, Chandrasekar PH, Diaz MM, et al. (2012). Syphilis. [online] Available from www.emedicine.com/med/TOPIC2224.HTM. [Accessed September, 2013].
2. Majmudar PA. (2011). Interstitial keratitis overview of interstitial keratitis. [online] Available from www.emedicine.com/oph/TOPIC453.HTM. [Accessed September, 2013].

🖰 6C18. WERNICKE SYNDROME I (SUPERIOR HEMORRHAGIC POLIOENCEPHALO-PATHIC SYNDROME; HEMORRHAGIC POLIOENCEPHALITIS SUPERIOR SYNDROME; ENCEPHALITIS HEMORRHAGICA SUPERIORIS; AVITAMINOSIS B; THIAMINE DEFICIENCY; BERIBERI; GAYET-WERNICKE SYNDROME; WERNICKE-KORSAKOFF SYNDROME) PTOSIS

General

Lack of vitamin B or thiamine; focal vascular lesions in the gray matter around third and fourth ventricles and Sylvian aqueduct; alcoholics (adults); beriberi of all ages.

Ocular

Ptosis; acute bilateral nuclear ophthalmoplegia; complete ophthalmoplegia; retinal hemorrhages; optic atrophy; optic neuritis; conjunctivitis; blepharitis; nutritional amblyopia; central scotoma; papilledema; nystagmus; absolute pupillary paralysis or Argyll Robertson pupils; accommodative palsy.

Clinical

Early prostration; lethargy; irritability; stupor; delirium; mental disturbances to Korsakoff psychosis; ataxia; tremors; peripheral neuritis; anorexia; vomiting; insomnia; perspiration; tachycardia; hallucinations; retrograde amnesia; apathy; anxiety; fear; defective concentration; cardiomyopathy.

Laboratory

Electrolyte studies, serum thiamine levels, CBC. Evaluation of hypoxemia, hypercarbia, acidosis, or alkalosis. Serum/urine toxin drug screen and liver enzymes.

Treatment

Parenteral thiamine is the treatment of choice.

🖰 BIBLIOGRAPHY

1. Xiong GL, Kenedi CA. (2013). Wernicke-Korsakoff syndrome. [online] Available from www.emedicine.com/med/TOPIC2405.HTM. [Accessed September, 2013].

🗗 6C19. WHIPPLE DISEASE (INTESTINAL LIPODYSTROPHY) PAPILLEDEMA

General

Multisystem disorder; prominent in males; onset between 4th decade and 7th decade; etiology is unknown.

Ocular

Ophthalmoplegia (vertical gaze involved more than horizontal gaze); papilledema; intraocular inflammation; vitreous opacities; bilateral panuveitis; small, round grayish retinal lesions; chemosis; supranuclear ophthalmoplegia; myoclonic ocular jerks; pendular nystagmus.

Clinical

Pneumonia; pleurisy; tonsillitis; sinusitis; cystitis; arthritis; fever; leukocytosis; diarrhea; malabsorption; death; dyspnea; weight loss; lymphadenopathy; polyserositis; gray pigmentation of skin; dementia; facial jerks; rhythmic movement of the mouth, jaw, and extremities.

Laboratory

The following test may be useful to screen for the presence of malabsorption but they are not specific for the disease: Sudan strain of stool, serum carotene, serum albumin, prothrombin time and CT scan.

Treatment

Antibiotic therapy.

🗗 BIBLIOGRAPHY

1. Roberts IM. (2011). Whipple disease. [online] Available from www.emedicine.com/med/TOPIC2409.HTM. [Accessed September, 2013].

🗗 6D. INTERNAL ORBITAL FRACTURES (BLOWOUT FRACTURE)

General

Trauma that involves the walls of the orbit leaving the bony rim intact.

Clinical

Tripod fracture of the zygoma.

Ocular

Proptosis, enophthalmos, diplopia.

Laboratory

Computed tomography.

Treatment

The transconjunctival approach with lateral canthotomy and cantholysis is preferred to expose the orbital floor, nasal approach to further expose the medial wall.

🗗 BIBLIOGRAPHY

1. Cohen AJ, Mercandetti M. (2012). Orbital floor fractures (blowout). [online] Available from www.emedicine.com/plastic/TOPIC485.HTM. [Accessed September, 2013].

🗗 6E. CEREBELLAR ATAXIA, INFANTILE, WITH PROGRESSIVE EXTERNAL OPHTHALMOPLEGIA

General

Autosomal recessive; neurologic lesion.

Ocular

Paralysis of all extraocular muscles; ptosis; retinal degeneration; blindness.

Clinical

Spinocerebellar degeneration; ataxia.

Laboratory

None.

Treatment

None.

⊟ BIBLIOGRAPHY

1. Jampel RS, Okazaki H, Bernstein H. Ophthalmoplegia and retinal degeneration associated with spinocerebellar ataxia. Arch Ophthalmol. 1961;66(2):247-59.

2. McKusick VA. Mendelian Inheritance in Man: A Catalog of Human Genes and Genetic Disorders, 12th edition. Baltimore, USA: The Johns Hopkins University Press; 1998.

⊟ 6F. CHRONIC OPHTHALMOPLEGIA (CPEO) SLOW ONSET OF EXTRAOCULAR MUSCLE PALSY

1. Degenerative conditions
   †A. Amyotrophic lateral sclerosis-progressive bulbar palsy
   B. Chronic progressive external ophthalmoplegia (CPEO)
   C. Hereditary ataxias-Friedreich ataxia, Sanger-Brown ataxia
   D. Progressive supranuclear palsy
   E. Syringomyelia (syringobulbia)
   F. Thyroid myopathy (Graves disease)
2. Infective conditions
   †A. Diffuse sclerosis
   B. Disseminated sclerosis (MS)
   C. Syphilis

Treatment

- Several small studies have shown evidence of clinical improvement in patients treated with CoQ10.
- For ptosis, adhesive tape and lid crutches can be used to assist patients with advanced CPEO.
- Bell phenomenon is absent in many patients with CPEO; therefore, ptosis surgery often is contraindicated.

Because a silicone sling is reversible, it could be a possibility for some patients.

- Patients with oculopharyngeal dystrophy who experience severe dysphagia may be treated with cricopharyngeal myotomy, but a gastrostomy tube often is more practical.
- Strabismus surgery can be helpful in carefully selected patients if diplopia occurs and the patient has had a stable deviation for several months.

⊟ BIBLIOGRAPHY

1. Roy H. (2013). Chronic progressive external ophthalmoplegia. [online] Available from www.emedicine.com/oph/TOPIC510.HTM. [Accessed September, 2013].
2. Basu AP, Posner E, McFarland R, et al. (2012). Kearns-Sayre Syndrome. [online] Available from www.emedicine.com/ped/TOPIC2763.HTM. [Accessed September, 2013].
3. Sripathi N. (2012). Facioscapulohumeral dystrophy. [online] Available from www.emedicine.com/neuro/TOPIC133.HTM. [Accessed September, 2013].

---

†Indicates a general entry and therefore has not been described in detail in the text

⊟ 6F1B. OPHTHALMOPLEGIA, PROGRESSIVE EXTERNAL

General

Autosomal recessive; progressive limitation of ocular motility with clinical sparing of pupillary function; underlying pathogenesis is secondary to a mitochondrial cytopathy; appearance of ragged-red fibers in the abnormal muscles is primarily caused by mitochondrial accumulations beneath the plasma membrane and between the myofibrils.

Ocular

Oculopharyngeal muscular dystrophy; retinitis pigmentosa; progressive external ophthalmoplegia; some patients show only ptosis and ophthalmoplegia; most patients have multisystem involvement.

Clinical

Heart block; ataxia.

Laboratory

Thyroid studies, acetylcholine receptor antibody. MRI, CT and ultrasound may show enlarged extraocular muscles.

Treatment

If ptosis is present lid crutches may be helpful or ptosis surgery. Strabismus surgery may be helpful in patients with diplopia.

BIBLIOGRAPHY

1. Roy H. (2011). Chronic progressive external ophthalmoplegia. [online] Available from www.emedicine.com/oph/TOPIC510.HTM. [Accessed September, 2013].

6F1C. FRIEDREICH ATAXIA (SPINOCEREBELLAR ATAXIA)

General

Etiology unknown, either autosomal recessive or dominant; progressive; incapacitating by the age of 20 years; death from secondary diseases or cardiac failure; prevalent in males.

Ocular

Nystagmus; optic atrophy; there is a form of Friedreich ataxia (FA) associated with congenital glaucoma.

Clinical

Kyphoscoliosis; tremor; dysmetria; asynergia; slow ataxic speech; paresthesias; Babinski sign; headache; retarded growth; mental retardation; polyuria; polydipsia; deformity of feet (onset in first year of life); clumsy gait and difficult to turn arms, head and trunk; deafness.

Laboratory

MRI is the study of choice in the evaluation of the atrophic changes.

Treatment

Results of treating ataxia in FA have generally been disappointing. No therapeutic measures are known to alter the natural history of the neurological disease.

BIBLIOGRAPHY

1. Chawla J. (2012). Friedreich ataxia. [online] Available from www.emedicine.com/neuro/TOPIC139.HTM. [Accessed September, 2013].

6F1C. BROWN-MARIE SYNDROME (BROWN-MARIE ATAXIC SYNDROME; SANGER BROWN SYNDROME; HEREDITARY ATAXIA SYNDROME; MARIE HEREDITARY ATAXIA)

General

Cause unknown; simple recessive inheritance, although irregular dominant transmission has been observed.

Ocular

Nystagmus; strabismus; ophthalmoplegia; anisocoria; Argyll Robertson pupil; retinitis pigmentosa; optic nerve atrophy; retrobulbar optic neuritis.

Clinical

Hereditary ataxia; choreiform movements; athetosis; pyramidal tract paresis; speech difficulties; hyperreflexia.

Laboratory

CT and MRI.

Treatment

Treatment is directed to symptoms. Pharmocologic therapy has provided only minimal benefits.

BIBLIOGRAPHY

1. Azevedo CJ, Berman SA. (2012). Olivopontocerebellar Atrophy. [online] Available from www.emedicine.com/neuro/TOPIC282.HTM. [Accessed September, 2013].

6F1D. STEELE-RICHARDSON-OLSZEWSKI SYNDROME (PROGRESSIVE SUPRANUCLEAR PALSY)

General

Nerve cell degeneration centered in the brainstem; resemblance to Lhermitte pyramidopallidal syndrome and to Jakob disease with dementia and rigidity; onset in the 6th decade of life; prominent in males.

Ocular

Supranuclear ophthalmoplegia affecting chiefly vertical gaze, especially downward.

Clinical

Pseudobulbar palsy; dysarthria; dystonic rigidity of neck and upper trunk; axial rigidity; bradykinesia; pyramidal signs; parkinsonism; frontal lobe-type dementia.

Laboratory

No specific laboratory or imaging findings.

Treatment

No medication is effective and only few patients respond to dopaminergic or anticholineric drugs.

BIBLIOGRAPHY

1. Eggenberger ER, Clark D. (2013). Progressive supranuclear palsy. [online] Available from www.emedicine.com/neuro/TOPIC328.HTM. [Accessed September, 2013].

6F1E. PASSOW SYNDROME (BREMER STATUS DYSRAPHICUS; STATUS DYSRAPHICUS SYNDROME; SYRINGOMYELIA; SYRINGOBULBIA)

General

Congenital nonclosure of the neural tube; familial occurrence or may be sporadic; insidious onset in 2nd to 3rd decade of life.

Ocular

Enophthalmos; ptosis; rotatory nystagmus; heterochromia iridis; anterior uveitis; corneal anesthesia; neuroparalytic keratitis; paralysis of third, fifth, sixth, and seventh cranial nerves; Horner syndrome; anisocoria; papilledema; optic atrophy; zonular cataract (*see* Horner Syndrome).

Clinical

Anesthesia over area of first division of trigeminal nerve; facial hemiatrophy; facial nerve paralysis; muscular weakness; cervical ribs; kyphoscoliosis; spina bifida; unilateral numbness of fingers; loss of deep reflexes; insensitivity to pain and temperature in affected areas; neurogenic bladder.

Laboratory

MRI, CT.

Treatment

Suboccipital and cervical decompression, laminectomy and syringotomy, shunts, fourth ventriculostomy, terminal ventriculostomy and neuroendoscopic surgery may be considered.

BIBLIOGRAPHY

1. Al-Shatoury HA, Galhom AA, Wagner FC. (2012). Syringomyelia. [online] Available from emedicine.medscape.com/article/1151685-overview. [Accessed September, 2013].

6F1F. BASEDOW SYNDROME (GRAVES DISEASE; HYPERTHYROIDISM; THYROTOXICOSIS; EXOPHTHALMIC GOITER; PARRY DISEASE)

General

Diffuse toxic goiter; inherited as a simple autosomal recessive; penetrance greater in females; however, dominant mode of inheritance and variable penetrance are possible; uncommon in either sex before the age of 15 years.

Ocular

Exophthalmos; swelling of eyelids and discoloration of upper eyelids; lid lag (von Graefe's sign); globe lag (Koeber's sign); lid trembling on gentle closure (Rosenbach's sign); reduced blinking (Stellwag's sign); retraction of upper lid; difficulty in everting upper lid (Gifford's sign); convergence weakness (Möbius's sign); impaired fixation on extreme lateral gaze (Suker's sign); possible external ophthalmoplegia (Ballet's sign); Dalrymple's sign (staring appearance); tearing; photophobia; epiphora; prolapse of lacrimal gland; neuroretinal edema; tortuous vessels; papilledema and papillitis; anisocoria; keratitis; increased IOP on upgaze; decreased visual acuity; enlargement of the extraocular muscles; increased volume of the extraorbital fat; superior rectus muscle enlargement; decreased venous outflow.

Clinical

Tachycardia; anxiety; insomnia; loss of weight; hyperhidrosis; restlessness; myocarditis (toxic); atrial fibrillation.

Laboratory

Visual field testing, forced duction testing for restrictive myopathy, CT, MRI, T4 and thyroid-stimulating hormone, thyroid-stimulating immunoglobulins.

Treatment

There is no immediate treatment; the disease is self-limited but prolonged course over 1 or more years. 5% of patients may require surgical intervention which could be orbital decompression, strabismus surgery, lid-lengthening surgery or blepharoplasty.

BIBLIOGRAPHY

1. Ing E. (2012). Thyroid-associated orbitopathy. [online] Available from www.emedicine.com/oph/TOPIC237.HTM. [Accessed September, 2013].
2. Regensburg NI, Wiersinga WM, Berendschot TT, et al. Do subtypes of Graves' orbitopathy exist? Ophthalmology. 2011;118:191-6.

6F2B. DISSEMINATED SCLEROSIS (MULTIPLE SCLEROSIS)

General

Disseminated demyelination affecting white matter of the brain, spinal cord, and optic nerves; etiology unknown.

Ocular

Nystagmus; ptosis; myokymia; optic atrophy; papillitis; optic neuritis; anisocoria; Argyll Robertson pupil; Marcus Gunn pupil; hippus, decreased or absent papillary reaction to light; periphlebitis; visual field defects; gaze palsy; paralysis of third or sixth nerve; uveitis; oscillopsia; Uhthoff symptom (reduction of visual acuity with exercise or ocular hyperthermia); pars planitis; retinal venous sheathing; retinitis; granulomatous uveitis.

Clinical

Incoordination; paresthesia; spasticity; tic douloureux; urinary frequency and infections; progressive disability; paralysis; death.

Laboratory

MRI, CSF positive for oligoclonal band, albumin and IgG index; BAER and SEP.

Treatment

Patients with MS may require multiple consultations to rule out other causes for their symptoms. Drugs such as immunodulator, immunosuppressors, anti-Parkinson agent, CNS stimulants are all used in the management of the disease.

BIBLIOGRAPHY

1. Luzzio C, Dangond F. (2013). Multiple sclerosis. [online] Available from www.emedicine.com/neuro/topic228.htm. [Accessed September, 2013].

6F2C. ACQUIRED LUES (SYPHILIS; ACQUIRED SYPHILIS; LUES VENEREA; MALUM VENEREUM)

General

Causative agent, *T. pallidum*, usually transmitted sexually.

Ocular

Conjunctival chancroid; conjunctivitis; keratitis; blepharitis; ptosis; iris atrophy; hippus; dacryocystitis; optic nerve atrophy; optic neuritis; periostitis; episcleritis; scleritis; nystagmus; uveitis; vitreous hemorrhages; paralysis of sixth nerve; papilledema; retinal hemorrhages; retinitis proliferans; oculogyric crisis; neuroretinitis; papilledema (associated with aseptic meningitis); diffuse or multifocal chorioretinitis; vertical supranuclear gaze palsy; Benedikt syndrome.

Clinical

Primary lesion associated with regional lymphadenopathy; secondary bacteremic stage associated with generalized mucocutaneous lesions; tertiary stage characterized by destructive mucocutaneous, musculoskeletal, or parenchymal lesions, aortitis, or CNS disease; syphilis and HIV infection often coexist in the same patient who experiences a higher incidence and greater severity of neurologic and ocular manifestations; a significant percentage of patients infected with HIV-I and *T. pallidum* become seronegative to syphilis testing.

Laboratory

Serologic nontreponemal tests include VDRL and RPR.

Treatment

The goals are to reduce morbidity and to prevent complications. Penicillin is the antibiotic of choice for treating syphilis. Ocular syphilis should be treated the same as patients with neurosyphilis.

BIBLIOGRAPHY

1. Euerle B, Chandrasekar PH, Diaz MM, et al. (2012). Syphilis. [online] Available from www.emedicine.com/med/TOPIC2224.HTM. [Accessed September, 2013].
2. Majmudar PA. (2011). Interstitial keratitis overview of interstitial keratitis. [online] Available from www.emedicine.com/oph/TOPIC453.HTM. [Accessed September, 2013].

6G. CHRONIC PROGRESSIVE EXTERNAL OPHTHALMOPLEGIA (CPEO; OPHTHALMOPLEGIA PLUS)

General

A general term covering many conditions; onset at any age; familial history; conditions associated with CPEO include myotonic dystrophy, Kearns-Sayre syndrome and oculopharyngeal dystrophy; disorders that rarely cause external ophthalmoplegia include congenital disorders (abetalipoproteinemia, Refsum disease, extraocular fibrosis syndrome, Möbius syndrome), progressive supranuclear palsy, endocrine exophthalmos, myasthenia gravis and MS; now considered to be a mitochondrial cytopathy with varied clinical presentation; four distinct disorders of ophthalmic importance are: (1) CPEO or Kearns-Sayre syndrome, (2) myoclonus epilepsy with ragged-red fibers (MERRF), (3) mitochondrial encephalopathy, lactic acidosis and stroke-like episodes (MELAS) and (4) Leber optic neuropathy.

Ocular

Exposure keratopathy; filamentary keratitis; keratoconjunctivitis sicca; corneal scarring; esotropia; exotropia; gaze paralysis; ptosis; levator paralysis; cataract; optic atrophy; diplopia; tapetoretinal degeneration; constriction of visual field; retinitis pigmentosa.

Clinical

Weakness; weight loss; myopathic or Hutchinson facies; cardiac abnormalities; CNS abnormalities.

Laboratory

No specific test; diagnosis is based on the clinical evidence.

Treatment

A complex disorder requiring the involvement of physicians from various specialties, including neurology, cardiology, ophthalmology and endocrinology.

⬚ BIBLIOGRAPHY

1. Roy H. (2011). Chronic progressive external ophthalmoplegia. [online] Available from www.emedicine.com/oph/TOPIC510.HTM. [Accessed September, 2013].

⬚ 6H. DOMINANT OPTIC ATROPHY SYNDROME (DOMINANT OPTIC ATROPHY, DEAFNESS, PTOSIS, OPHTHALMOPLEGIA, DYSTAXIA, AND MYOPATHY)

General

Autosomal dominant disorder; ptosis, ophthalmoplegia, dystaxia, and nonspecific myopathy occur in midlife; optic atrophy and hearing loss occur in early life; autosomal dominant inheritance.

Ocular

Ptosis; ophthalmoplegia; progressive optic atrophy; abnormal electroretinography; diplopia; ocular myopathy; nystagmus; focal temporal excavation of optic disk; dyschromatopsia (blue-yellow); myopia; temporal pallor of the optic nerve.

Clinical

Sensorineural hearing loss; myopathy; dystaxia.

Laboratory

Diagnosis is made by clinical findings.

Treatment

Oral steroids and sometimes IV steroids are necessary.

⬚ BIBLIOGRAPHY

1. Del Porto G, Vingolo EM, Steindl K, et al. Clinical heterogeneity of dominant optic atrophy: the contribution of visual function investigations to diagnosis. Graefes Arch Clin Exp Ophthalmol. 1994;232(12):717-27.
2. Eliott D, Traboulsi EI, Maumenee IH. Visual prognosis in autosomal dominant optic atrophy (Kjer type). Am J Ophthalmol. 1993;115(3):360-7.

⬚ 6I. EXTERNAL OPHTHALMOPLEGIA (PARALYSIS OF OCULAR MUSCLES INCLUDING PTOSIS WITH SPARING OF PUPIL AND ACCOMMODATION)

†1. Abiotrophy-specific for one particular tissue, bilateral, symmetric
2. Amyloidosis (Lubarsch-Pick syndrome)
3. Aneurysm of internal carotid artery (foramen lacerum syndrome)
4. Bassen-Kornzweig syndrome (familial hypolipoproteinemia)
5. Bee sting
6. Chronic progressive external ophthalmoplegia
†7. Congenital and familial
8. Diabetes mellitus (Willis disease)
9. Diphtheria
10. Epidemic encephalitis
11. Friedreich ataxia
12. Garcin syndrome (Schmincke tumor unilateral cranial paralysis)
13. Graves disease (hyperthyroidism)
14. Jacod syndrome (petrosphenoidal space syndrome)
15. Kearns-Sayre syndrome (ophthalmoplegic retinal degeneration syndrome)
16. Mumps
17. Myasthenia gravis (Erb-Goldflam syndrome)
18. Myotonic dystrophy (Curschmann-Steinert syndrome)
†19. Myositis

20. Nevus sebaceous of Jadassohn
21. Nothnagel syndrome (ophthalmoplegia-cerebellar ataxia syndrome)
22. Oculopharyngeal syndrome (progressive muscular dystrophy with ptosis and dysphagia)
23. Olivopontocerebellar atrophy III (with retinal degeneration)-dominant
24. Ophthalmoplegia, progressive external, and scoliosis (horizontal gaze paralysis, familial)-recessive
25. Pernicious anemia
26. Polyradiculoneuronitis (Guillain-Barré and Fisher syndromes)
27. Progressive facial hemiatrophy (Parry-Romberg syndrome)
†28. Pseudotumor (orbital)
29. Refsum syndrome (heredopathia atactica polyneuritiformis syndrome)
30. Scleroderma (progressive systemic sclerosis)
31. Shy-Drager syndrome (orthostatic hypotension syndrome)
32. Shy-Gonatas syndrome (accumulation of lipids in muscles simulates gargoylism)

†33. Statin drugs
34. Tick paralysis (Lyme disease, Rocky Mountain spotted fever)
†35. Vincristine: May have fifth and seventh nerve and peripheral neuropathies
36. Wernicke encephalopathies (beriberi, thiamine deficiency)

BIBLIOGRAPHY

1. Fassati A, Bordoni A, Amboni P, et al. Chronic progressive external ophthalmoplegia: a correlative study of quantitative molecular data and histochemical and biochemical profile. J Neurol Sci. 1994;123:140-6.
2. Fraunfelder FW, Richards AB. Diplopia, Blepharoptosis and Ophthalmoplegia and 3-Hydroxy-3 Methyl-Glutaryl-CoA Reductase Inhibitor Use. Ophthalmology. 2008;115:2282-5.
3. McKusick VA. Mendelian Inheritance in Man, 12th editiion. Baltimore: Johns Hopkins University Press; 1998.
4. Roy FH. Ocular Syndromes and Systemic Diseases, 6th edition. New Dehli: Jaypee Brothers Medical Publishers; 2013.

†Indicates a general entry and therefore has not been described in detail in the text

61.2. LUBARSCH-PICK SYNDROME (PRIMARY AMYLOIDOSIS; IDIOPATHIC AMYLOIDOSIS; AMYLOIDOSIS)

General

Rare condition of unknown etiology; inherited as a dominant trait, with male preponderance; characterized by amyloid accumulation in muscles and in gastrointestinal and genitourinary tracts.

Ocular

Internal and external ophthalmoplegia; diminished lacrimation; amyloid deposits in conjunctival, episcleral, and ciliary vessels; vitreous opacities; amyloid deposits in the corneal stroma; retinal hemorrhages and perivascular exudates; paralysis of extraocular muscles; pseudopodia lentis; strabismus fixus convergens; keratoconus.

Clinical

Peripheral neuropathy (extremities); heart failure; defective hepatic and renal functions with hepatosplenomegaly; waxy skin lesions; muscular weakness (progressive); multiple myeloma; hoarseness; chronic gastrointestinal symptoms.

Laboratory

Biopsy-staining with Congo red demonstrates apple-green birefringence under polarized light; distinctive fibrillar ultrastructure.

Treatment

Deoxydoxorubicin had demonstrated some clinical benefit.

BIBLIOGRAPHY

1. Biswas J, Badrinath SS, Rao NA. Primary nonfamilial amyloidosis of the vitreous. A light microscopic and ultrastructural study. Retina. 1992;12(3):251-3.
2. Goebel HH, Friedman AH. Extraocular muscle involvement in idiopathic primary amyloidosis. Am J Ophthalmol. 1971;71(5):1121-7.

61.3. FORAMEN LACERUM SYNDROME (ANEURYSM OF INTERNAL CAROTID ARTERY SYNDROME)

General

Most commonly caused by congenital aneurysm involving the intradural portion of the carotid artery.

Ocular

Periorbital pain; ptosis; oculomotor paralysis with ptosis, diplopia, and internal ophthalmoplegia; cranial nerves IV and VI may be involved; homonymous hemianopia (occasionally); loss of pupillary reflexes for light and accommodation; papilledema; optic atrophy.

Clinical

Meningism; mental disturbances; unilateral frontal or orbital headache; migraine attacks.

Laboratory

CT, MRI, angiography, MRA.

Treatment

Endovascular balloon occlusion.

BIBLIOGRAPHY

1. Dailey EJ, Holloway JA, Murto RE, et al. Evaluation of ocular signs and symptoms in cerebral aneurysms. Arch Ophthalmol. 1964;71:463-74.
2. Geeraets WJ. Ocular syndromes, 3rd edition. Philadelphia: Lea & Febiger; 1976.
3. Misra M, Mohanty AB, Rath S. Giant aneurysm of internal carotid artery presenting features of retrobulbar neuritis. Indian J Ophthalmol. 1991;39:28-9.

61.4. BASSEN-KORNZWEIG SYNDROME (ABETALIPOPROTEINEMIA; ACANTHOCYTOSIS; FAMILIAL HYPOLIPOPROTEINEMIA)

General

Inability to absorb and transport lipids; predominant in males; autosomal recessive inheritance; acanthocytosis, a peculiar burr cell malformation of the red blood cells; the basic defect is thought to be an inability to synthesize the apolipoprotein B peptide of low-density and very-low-density lipoproteins.

Ocular

Ptosis (may be present); nystagmus; progressive external ophthalmoplegia; retinitis pigmentosa (usually atypical); retinopathy develops with age after 10–14 years; optic atrophy occasionally; epicanthal folds; cataract; optic nerve pallor; hypopigmentation of retina; macular degeneration; dyschromatopsia.

Clinical

Steatorrhea; hypocholesterolemia; neurologic disorder with ataxia (similar to Friedreich ataxia); areflexia; Babinski sign; muscle weakness (facial, lingual; proximal and distal); slurred speech; lordosis; kyphosis.

Laboratory

Most patients will exhibit acanthocytosis on peripheral blood smear.

Treatment

Medical care is symptomatic and supportive.

BIBLIOGRAPHY

1. Gross KV, Lorenzo N. (2012). Neuroacanthocytosis syndromes. [online] Available from www.emedicine.com/neuro/TOPIC502.HTM. [Accessed September, 2013].

🗔 61.5. BEE STING OF THE EYE (BEE STING OF THE CORNEA)

General

Occurs when the toothed lancet of the stinging apparatus penetrates the cornea.

Ocular

Conjunctival hemorrhage, chemosis, and hyperemia; corneal abscess; keratitis; lid edema; iris depigmentation; iridoplegia; iritis; lacrimation; apoplectic visual loss; acute disk swelling secondary to acute demyelination.

Clinical

Laryngeal edema; anaphylaxis; death; localized tissue edema; fever.

Laboratory

Diagnosis usually is confirmed by patient's history.

Treatment

Remove foreign body from the eye.

🗔 BIBLIOGRAPHY

1. Vankawala HH, de Moor C, Park R. (2012). Hymenoptera stings. [online] Available from www.emedicine.com/emerg/TOPIC55.HTM. [Accessed September, 2013].

🗔 61.6. CHRONIC PROGRESSIVE EXTERNAL OPHTHALMOPLEGIA (CPEO; OPHTHALMOPLEGIA PLUS)

General

A general term covering many conditions; onset at any age; familial history; conditions associated with CPEO include myotonic dystrophy, Kearns-Sayre syndrome and oculopharyngeal dystrophy; disorders that rarely cause external ophthalmoplegia include congenital disorders (abetalipoproteinemia, Refsum disease, extraocular fibrosis syndrome, Möbius syndrome), progressive supranuclear palsy, endocrine exophthalmos, myasthenia gravis and MS; now considered to be a mitochondrial cytopathy with varied clinical presentation; four distinct disorders of ophthalmic importance are: (1) CPEO or Kearns-Sayre syndrome, (2) MERRF, (3) MELAS and (4) Leber optic neuropathy.

Ocular

Exposure keratopathy; filamentary keratitis; keratoconjunctivitis sicca; corneal scarring; esotropia; exotropia; gaze paralysis; ptosis; levator paralysis; cataract; optic atrophy; diplopia; tapetoretinal degeneration; constriction of visual field; retinitis pigmentosa.

Clinical

Weakness; weight loss; myopathic or Hutchinson facies; cardiac abnormalities; CNS abnormalities.

Laboratory

No specific test; diagnosis is based on the clinical evidence.

Treatment

A complex disorder requiring the involvement of physicians from various specialties, including neurology, cardiology, ophthalmology and endocrinology.

🗔 BIBLIOGRAPHY

1. Roy H. (2011). Chronic progressive external ophthalmoplegia. [online] Available from www.emedicine.com/oph/TOPIC510.HTM. [Accessed September, 2013].

🗔 61.8. DIABETES MELLITUS

General

Complex disorder of carbohydrate, lipid and protein metabolism characterized by hyperglycemia and a relative or total lack of insulin. Development is influenced by both genetic and environmental factors. Most commonly occurs in middle or late life (type II) and is seen most commonly in the obese. Diabetes can occur in the 1st or 2nd decade of life (type I) and usually involves the lack of insulin production by the pancreas and the need for insulin therapy.

Clinical

Atherosclerosis, nephropathy, neuropathy, polyuria, polydipsia, polyphagia, obesity, elevated plasma glucose and elevated A1C.

Ocular

Diabetic retinopathy, vitreous hemorrhage, macular edema, cataract, glaucoma, asteroid hyalosis, extraocular muscle paralysis, rubeosis iridis, corneal hypesthesia, optic nerve atrophy; papillopathy.

Laboratory

Diagnosis made by fasting plasma glucose of greater than 126 mg/dL and 2-hour post-glucose load (75 g) plasma glucose of greater than 200 mg/dL and confirmed by repeat test.

Treatment

Goals include elimination of symptoms, by reduction of blood sugar and blood pressure. Smoking cessation, aspirin therapy, weight loss, exercise, diabetic diet as well as oral medication and/or insulin are all used in the treatment of diabetes. Diabetic retinopathy is most successfully treated with retinal photocoagulation. Pars plana vitrectomy is sometimes necessary to remove vitreous hemorrhage. Other ocular problems caused by diabetes such as cataracts and glaucoma are treated in traditional methods.

BIBLIOGRAPHY

1. Khardori R. (2013). Type 2 diabetes mellitus. [online] Available from www.emedicine.medscape.com/article/117853-overview. [Accessed September, 2013].

61.9. DIPHTHERIA

General

Acute infectious disease caused by *C. diphtheriae*; severity is dependent upon the amount of exotoxin absorbed prior to initiation of specific therapy.

Ocular

Conjunctivitis; xerophthalmia; keratitis; corneal ulcer; blepharitis; cellulitis of lid; meibomianitis; ptosis; dacryocystitis; cataract; central retinal artery occlusion; optic neuritis; accommodative spasm or paralysis; convergence paralysis; divergence paralysis; paralysis of third, fourth, or sixth nerve; paralysis of accommodation (in children); ocular motor nerve paresis; choroiditis; cranial neuropathies involving the trigeminal, vagus, and hypoglossal cranial nerves; myocarditis.

Clinical

Local inflammatory lesion, with effect on heart, kidneys and nervous system.

Laboratory

Gram-positive rods commonly affect children younger than 10 years.

Treatment

Systemic treatment involves use of diphtheria antitoxin and antibiotics. Ocular treatment includes diphtheria antitoxin and high titer y-globulin preparation. Topical penicillin G ointment helps to eradicate the bacilli.

BIBLIOGRAPHY

1. Demirci CS, Abuhammour W. (2013). Pediatric diphtheria. [online] Available from www.emedicine.com/ped/TOPIC596.HTM. [Accessed September, 2013].

61.10. ENCEPHALITIS, ACUTE

General

In approximately 0.1–0.2% of patients having rubeola (measles), an acute encephalitis is seen within 1 week after the onset of the rash; a case of immunosuppressive encephalitis can present with focal seizures leading to progressive obtundation.

Ocular

Papillitis; optic atrophy; ocular motor palsies; nystagmus; optic neuritis or neuroretinitis.

Clinical

Rise in temperature; drowsiness; irritability; meningismus; vomiting and headache; stupor; convulsions; coma.

Laboratory

Perform head CT, with and without contrast agent, before LP to search for evidence of elevated intracerebral pressure. MRI is useful. Viral serology.

Treatment

Evaluate and treat for shock or hypotension, treat systemic complications, acyclovir.

⊟ BIBLIOGRAPHY

1. Howes DS, Lazoff M. (2013). Encephalitis. [online] Available from www.emedicine.com/emerg/TOPIC163.HTM. [Accessed September, 2013].

⊟ 6I.11. FRIEDREICH ATAXIA (SPINOCEREBELLAR ATAXIA)

General

Etiology unknown, either autosomal recessive or dominant; progressive; incapacitating by the age of 20 years; death from secondary diseases or cardiac failure; prevalent in males.

Ocular

Nystagmus; optic atrophy; there is a form of Friedreich ataxia (FA) associated with congenital glaucoma.

Clinical

Kyphoscoliosis; tremor; dysmetria; asynergia; slow ataxic speech; paresthesias; Babinski sign; headache; retarded growth; mental retardation; polyuria; polydipsia; deformity of feet (onset in 1st year of life); clumsy gait and difficult to turn arms, head and trunk; deafness.

Laboratory

MRI is the study of choice in the evaluation of the atrophic changes.

Treatment

Results of treating ataxia in FA have generally been disappointing. No therapeutic measures are known to alter the natural history of the neurological disease.

⊟ BIBLIOGRAPHY

1. Chawla J. (2012). Friedreich ataxia. [online] Available from www.emedicine.com/neuro/TOPIC139.HTM. [Accessed September, 2013].

⊟ 6I.12. GARCIN SYNDROME (HALF-BASE SYNDROME; SCHMINCKE TUMOR-UNILATERAL CRANIAL PARALYSIS)

General

Causes include tumors of nasopharynx, rapidly progressing growth of a sarcoma of base of skull, meningitis, and cranial polyneuritis; cranial nerves VIII to XII are most frequently involved.

Ocular

Ptosis (unilateral); unilateral external ophthalmoplegia; papilledema.

Clinical

Difficulties in swallowing; impairment of speech; hearing defect; respiratory difficulties; sensory disturbances; hoarseness.

Laboratory

MRI with gadolinium and fat suppression is the radiologic modality of choice; transnasal biopsy of nasopharyngeal mass.

Treatment

Radiation therapy is the primary mode of management of nasopharyngeal carcinoma.

⊟ BIBLIOGRAPHY

1. Bruce JN, Fetell MR. Tumors of the skull and cranial nerves. In: Rowland LP (Ed). Merritt's Textbook of Neurology, 9th edition. Baltimore: Williams & Wilkins; 1995. pp. 320-9.

61.13. BASEDOW SYNDROME (GRAVES DISEASE; HYPERTHYROIDISM; THYROTOXICOSIS; EXOPHTHALMIC GOITER; PARRY DISEASE)

General

Diffuse toxic goiter; inherited as a simple autosomal recessive; penetrance greater in females; however, dominant mode of inheritance and variable penetrance are possible; uncommon in either sex before the age of 15 years.

Ocular

Exophthalmos; swelling of eyelids and discoloration of upper eyelids; lid lag (von Graefe's sign); globe lag (Koeber's sign); lid trembling on gentle closure (Rosenbach's sign); reduced blinking (Stellwag's sign); retraction of upper lid; difficulty in everting upper lid (Gifford's sign); convergence weakness (Möbius's sign); impaired fixation on extreme lateral gaze (Suker's sign); possible external ophthalmoplegia (Ballet's sign); Dalrymple's sign (staring appearance); tearing; photophobia; epiphora; prolapse of lacrimal gland; neuroretinal edema; tortuous vessels; papilledema and papillitis; anisocoria; keratitis; increased IOP on upgaze; decreased visual acuity; enlargement of the extraocular muscles; increased volume of the extraorbital fat; superior rectus muscle enlargement; decreased venous outflow.

Clinical

Tachycardia; anxiety; insomnia; loss of weight; hyperhidrosis; restlessness; myocarditis (toxic); atrial fibrillation.

Laboratory

Visual field testing, forced duction testing for restrictive myopathy, CT, MRI, T4 and thyroid-stimulating hormone, thyroid-stimulating immunoglobulins.

Treatment

There is no immediate treatment; the disease is self-limited but prolonged course over 1 or more years. Five percent of patients may require surgical intervention which could be orbital decompression, strabismus surgery, lid-lengthening surgery or blepharoplasty.

BIBLIOGRAPHY

1. Ing E. (2012). Thyroid-associated orbitopathy. [online] Available from www.emedicine.com/oph/TOPIC237.HTM. [Accessed September, 2013].
2. Regensburg NI, Wiersinga WM, Berendschot TT, et al. Do subtypes of Graves' orbitopathy exist? Ophthalmology. 2011;118:191-6.

61.14. JACOD SYNDROME (NEGRI-JACOD SYNDROME; PETROSPHENOIDAL SPACE SYNDROME)

General

Lesion involving cranial nerves II to VI; most frequently a malignant nasopharyngeal tumor originating in lateropharyngeal area.

Ocular

Ophthalmoplegia; unilateral blindness; trigeminal neuralgia (ophthalmic branch); descending optic atrophy if cranial nerve II is involved; amaurosis fugax.

Clinical

Trigeminal neuralgia (at the beginning the first and second divisions of nerve V are involved; later the third division is affected as well); unilateral or bilateral enlargement of cervical lymph nodes (30%); deafness; palatal muscle paralysis.

Laboratory

MRI with gadolinium and fat suppression is the radiologic modality of choice. Transnasal biopsy of nasopharyngeal mass may also be necessary.

Treatment

External beam radiation therapy is the primary mode of management; chemotherapeutic approaches have been devised to improve the response rates.

BIBLIOGRAPHY

1. Lin H, Fee WH. (2012). Malignant nasopharyngeal tumors. [online] Available from www.emedicine.com/ent/TOPIC269.HTM. [Accessed September, 2013].

61.15. KEARNS-SAYRE SYNDROME (OPHTHALMOPLEGIA PLUS SYNDROME; KEARNS-SHY SYNDROME; KEARNS DISEASE)

General

Etiology unknown; sporadic (nonhereditary); onset before age of 20 years; external ophthalmoplegia; complete heart block.

Ocular

Pigmentary degeneration of retina; progressive external ophthalmoplegia; corneal decompensation; optic neuritis.

Clinical

Abnormal mitochondria with paracrystalline inclusion in muscle cell; heart block; limb weakness; hyperglycemic acidotic coma; death; cerebellar dysfunction.

Laboratory

Best means of achieving definitive diagnosis is via analysis of a muscle biopsy specimen, with quantification of the level of deletion using Southern blot analysis.

Treatment

No disease-modifying therapy exists for Kearns-Sayre syndrome but symptoms can be treated traditionally.

BIBLIOGRAPHY

1. Basu AP, Posner E, McFarland R. (2012). Kearns-Sayre syndrome. [online] Available from www.emedicine.com/ped/TOPIC2763.HTM. [Accessed September, 2013].

61.16. MUMPS

General

Viral infection.

Ocular

Conjunctivitis; keratitis; corneal ulcer; tenonitis; exophthalmos; microphthalmos; optic atrophy; optic neuritis; papillitis; scleritis; uveitis; cortical blindness; congenital punctal occlusion; paralysis of extraocular muscles; dacryoadenitis; iritis; paralysis of accommodation; internal and external ophthalmoparesis.

Clinical

Affects the parotid glands, but infection of other glandular tissue occurs, including the lacrimal gland and testicles; encephalitis; meningitis.

Laboratory

Mumps virus by acute serologic studies.

Treatment

Generous hydration and alimentation, analgesics for headaches. No antiviral agent is available.

BIBLIOGRAPHY

1. Defendi GL. (2012). Mumps. [online] Available from www.emedicine.com/ped/TOPIC1503.HTM. [Accessed September, 2013].

61.17. ERB-GOLDFLAM SYNDROME (ERB II SYNDROME; HOPPE-GOLDFLAM DISEASE; PSEUDOPARALYTIC SYNDROME; MYASTHENIA GRAVIS)

General

Occurs at any age; more frequent between ages 20 and 40 years; more females affected than males; progressive; spontaneous; symptoms improve or resolve with rest in early stages of disease (*see* myasthenia gravis, neonatal or infantile); caused by autoantibodies against the acetylcholine receptor at the neuromuscular junction, leading to abnormal fatigability and weakness of skeletal muscle.

Ocular

Transient diplopia; ptosis of upper eyelids.

Clinical

Excessive fatigability of musculature; symptoms appear and increase as day progresses; expressionless face; sagging jaw; difficulty in chewing and talking; nasal regurgitation.

Laboratory

Ice test—crushed ice in surgical glove over ptotic eyelid for 2 minutes and watch for brief elevation of eyelid; Tensilon test and prostigmin test may result in the elevation of ptotic eyelid or improved strabismus in individuals with myasthenia gravis.

Treatment

Adrenal corticosteroids are frequently used. In some cases, mycophenolate mofetil, cyclosporine and cyclophosphamide may be useful. Patching one eye or using prisms may be helpful.

🗗 BIBLIOGRAPHY

1. Erb W. Zur Casuistick der Bulbaren La hmungen. Arch Psychiatr Vervenkr. 1879;9:325-50.

🗗 6I.18. MYOTONIC DYSTROPHY SYNDROME (MYOTONIA ATROPHICA SYNDROME; DYSTROPHIA MYOTONICA; CURSCHMANN-STEINERT SYNDROME)

General

Rare autosomal dominant disease; onset at about age 20 years; condition is worsened by administration of neostigmine (Prostigmin); associated with an unstable DNA sequence composed of varying numbers of CTG triplet repeats (which allows a specific molecular test for this disorder).

Ocular

Mild ptosis (occasionally); myotonic cataract with small, dot-like subcapsular cortical opacities during early stage, with polychromatic properties on biomicroscopic examination; corneal epithelial dystrophy; loss of corneal sensitivity; tapetoretinal degeneration; macular red spot; macular degeneration; chorioretinitis; pilomatrixomas; ocular hypotony; pattern pigmentary changes; abnormal saccades.

Clinical

Progressive muscular atrophy with selection of certain muscles (mainly stern-ocleidomastoid, temporalis, dorsiflexor muscles of the ankle, anterior oblique); myotonia; bland facial expression; speech disturbance due to involvement of vocal cords and palatal muscles; dysphagia; endocrine disturbances.

Laboratory

Clinical.

Treatment

- *Ptosis*: If visual acuity is affected most cases require surgical correction and there are several procedures that may be used including levator resection, repair or advancement and Fasanella-Servat.
- *Cataract*: Change in glasses can sometimes improve a patient's visual function temporarily; however the most common treatment is cataract surgery.
- *Corneal dystrophy*: Mild cases can be observed and soft contact lenses are helpful, penetrating keratoplasty may be necessary, graft recurrences treated by superficial keratectomy, phototherapeutic keratectomy or repeat penetrating keratoplasty.
- *Macular degeneration*: No treatment available for non-neovascular AMD. Preventative therapy includes no smoking, control of hypertension, cholesterol, and blood sugar, exercise and vitamins. Neovascular AMD treatment consists of laser, Avastin and Lucentis.

🗗 BIBLIOGRAPHY

1. Brooke NM, Cwik VE. Myotonic dystrophy. In: Bradley WG, Daroff RB, Fenichel GM, Jankovic J (Eds). Neurology in Clinical Practice, 2nd edition. Boston: Butterworth-Heinemann; 1995. pp. 2020-2.
2. Gjertsen IK, Sandvig KU, Eide N, et al. Recurrence of secondary opacification and development of a dense posterior vitreous membrane in patients with myotonic dystrophy. J Cataract Refract Surg. 2003;29:213-6.
3. Goldflam S. Vebereinen Scheinbar Keilbaren Bulbarparalytischem Symptom Complex mit Betheiligung der Extremitaten. Dtsch Z Nerven. 1983;4:312-52.
4. Kim JH, Hwang JM, Hwang YS, et al. Chilhood ocular myasthenia gravis. Ophthalmology. 2003;110:1458-62.
5. Kimizuka Y, Kiyosawa M, Tamai M, et al. Retinal changes in myotonic dystrophy. Clinical and follow-up evaluation. Retina. 1993;13:129-35.
6. Koca MR, Horn F, Korth M. Alterations of saccadic eye movements in myotonic dystrophy. Graefes Arch Clin Exp Ophthalmol. 1992;230:437-41.
7. Kuwabara T, Lessell S. Electron microscopic study of extraocular muscles in myotonic dystrophy. Am J Ophthalmol. 1976;82:303-39.
8. Lepore FE. Pupillary dysfunction in myasthenia gravis. Ann Neurol. 1979;6:29-33.

9.   Mausolf FA, Burns CA, Burian HM. Morphologic and functional retinal changes in myotonic dystrophy unrelated to quinine therapy. Am J Ophthalmol. 1972;74:1141-3.

10. Meyer E, Navon D, Auslender L, et al. Myotonic dystrophy: pathological study of the eyes. Ophthalmologica. 1980;181:215-20.

11. Reardon W, MacMillan JC, Myring J, et al. Cataract and myotonic dystrophy: the role of molecular diagnosis. Br J Ophthalmol. 1993;77:579-83.

12. Rosa N, Lanza M, Borrelli M, et al. Low intraocular pressure resulting from ciliary body detachment in patients with myotonic dystrophy. Ophthalmology. 2011;118:260-4.

13. Roy FH, Fraunfelder FT, Fraunfelder FW. Roy and Fraunfelder's Current Ocular Therapy, 6th edition. London: Elsevier; 2008.

14. Sommer N, Melms A, Weller M, et al. Ocular myasthenia gravis. A critical review of clinical and pathophysiological aspects. Doc Ophthalmol. 1993;84:309-33.

🖶 61.20. LINEAR NEVUS SEBACEUS OF JADASSOHN (NEVUS SEBACEUS OF JADASSOHN; JADASSOHN-TYPE ANETODERMA; ORGANOID NEVUS SYNDROME; SEBACEUS NEVUS SYNDROME)

General

Skin nevus caused by failure of separation of skin appendages from adjacent epithelium during the 3rd month of gestation.

Ocular

Proptosis; epibulbar lipodermoids; colobomata of eyelids, iris, and choroid; antimongoloid fissures; ocular motor palsies; nystagmus; teratomas of orbit and aberrant lacrimal glands; corneal vascularization; vision defects; conjunctival dermolipomas; choristomas of conjunctiva, sclera; corneal vascularization/opacification; colobomas of uvea, retina, optic disk, and lids; optic nerve hypoplasia; microphthalmia; anophthalmia; hemangioma of the sclera/conjunctiva.

Clinical

Circumscribed lesions of the face and scalp with excessively large sebaceous glands; papillomatous epidermal hyperplasia; seizures; skeletal abnormalities, particularly in skull; failure to thrive; convulsion; mental retardation.

Laboratory

Epidermis shows papillomatous hyperplasia. In the dermis, the numbers of mature sebaceous glands are increased. Ectopic apocrine glands are often found in the deep dermis beneath sebaceous glands.

Treatment

Photodynamic therapy with topical aminolevulinic acid. Full-thickness skin excision is usually required, and topical destruction.

🖶 BIBLIOGRAPHY

1.   Al Hammadi A, Lebwohl MG. (2012). Nevus Sebaceus. [online] Available from www.emedicine.com/derm/TOPIC296.HTM. [Accessed September, 2013].

🖶 61.21. NOTHNAGEL SYNDROME (OPHTHALMOPLEGIA-CEREBELLAR ATAXIA SYNDROME)

General

Lesion of superior cerebellar peduncle, red nucleus and emerging oculomotor fibers such as pineal tumor, or tumor or vascular disturbance in corpora quadrigemina or vermis cerebelli (*see* Bruns syndrome).

Ocular

Oculomotor paresis; gaze paralysis most frequently upward, combined with some degree of internal or external ophthalmoplegia.

Clinical

Cerebellar ataxia; poor upper extremity movements; neoplasia; infarction; midbrain lesion.

Laboratory

CT and MRI of brain.

Treatment

See neurologist.

BIBLIOGRAPHY

1. Magalini SI, Scrascia E. Dictionary of Medical Syndromes, 2nd edition. Philadelphia, PA: Lippincott Williams and Wilkins; 1981.

2. Nothnagel H. Topische Diagnostik Der Gehirnkrankheiten. Berlin: Nabu Press; 2010. p. 220.

61.22. OCULOPHARYNGEAL SYNDROME (PROGRESSIVE MUSCULAR DYSTROPHY WITH PTOSIS AND DYSPHAGIA; OCULOPHARYNGEAL MUSCULAR DYSTROPHY)

General

Etiology unknown; autosomal dominant inheritance; no CNS pathology; muscles of pharynx, hypopharynx, and proximal third of esophagus involved with myopathy; onset late in life; progressive hereditary myopathy in which the levator palpebrae and pharyngeal muscles are selectively involved; progressive usually symmetrical blepharoptosis with or without dysphagia appears in the 5th decade.

Ocular

Ptosis.

Clinical

Dysphagia; occasionally weakness of facial muscles.

Laboratory/Ocular

Diagnosis is made by clinical findings.

Treatment

Ptosis: If visual acuity is affected, most cases require surgical correction and there are several procedures that may be used including levator resection, repair or advancement and Fasanella-Servat.

BIBLIOGRAPHY

1. Codère F. Oculopharyngeal muscular dystrophy. Can J Ophthalmol. 1993;28(1):1-2.
2. Duranceau A, Forand MD, Fauteux JP. Surgery in oculopharyngeal muscular dystrophy. Am J Surg. 1980;139(1):33-9.
3. Jordan DR, Addison DJ. Surgical results and pathological findings in the oculopharyngeal dystrophy syndrome. Can J Ophthalmol. 1993;28(1):15-8.
4. Molgat YM, Rodrigue D. Correction of blepharoptosis in oculopharyngeal muscular dystrophy: review of 91 cases. Can J Ophthalmol. 1993;28(1):11-4.
5. Murphy SF, Drachman DB. The oculopharyngeal syndrome. JAMA. 1968;203(12):1003-8.
6. Taylor EW. Progressive vagus-glossopharyngeal paralysis with ptosis: contribution to a group of family diseases. J Nerv Ment Dis. 1915;42(3):129-39.

61.23. OLIVOPONTOCEREBELLAR ATROPHY III (OPCA III; OPCA WITH RETINAL DEGENERATION)

General

Autosomal dominant; neurologic lesion; dominant with variable penetration.

Ocular

Retinopathy variable: peripheral, macular and circumpapillary; retinal degeneration; blindness; external ophthalmoplegia; variable electroretinogram function.

Clinical

Ataxia.

Laboratory

Anti-Purkinje cell antibodies, MRI.

Treatment

Treatment is directed to symptoms.

BIBLIOGRAPHY

1. Azevedo CJ, Berman SA. (2012). Olivopontocerebellar atrophy. [online] Available from www.emedicine.com/neuro/TOPIC282.HTM. [Accessed September, 2013].

🖶 61.24. PROGRESSIVE EXTERNAL OPHTHALMOPLEGIA AND SCOLIOSIS

General

Rare; isolated muscle dystrophic involvement of extraocular muscles; onset in childhood or early adulthood; slowly progressive.

Ocular

Horizontal gaze paralysis; pendular nystagmus; ptosis; orbicularis oculi weakness.

Clinical

Scoliosis; facial myokymia; contracture of facial muscles.

Laboratory

Diagnosis is made by clinical findings.

Treatment

- *Nystagmus*:
  - *Seesaw*: Visual field to consider neoplastic or vascular etiologies.
  - *Upbeat*: It may indicate MS, cerebellar degeneration, tumors or infarcts. Treatment is directed toward the identification and resolution of underlying cause.
  - *Downbeat*: It affects the cerebellum or craniocervical junction including Arnold-Chiari malformation, MS, trauma, tumor, infarction and many toxic metabolic entities. MRI may indicate a surgically correctable lesion. Periodic alternating nystagmus is continuous horizontal nystagmus from stroke, tumor, MS, trauma, infection and drug intoxication. It can occur from cataract, vitreous hemorrhage or optic atrophy.
  - *Ptosis*: If visual acuity is affected, most cases require surgical correction and there are several procedures that may be used including levator resection, repair or advancement and Fasanella-Servat.

🖶 BIBLIOGRAPHY

1. Roddi R, Riggio E, Gilbert PM, et al. Clinical evaluation of techniques used in the surgical treatment of progressive hemifacial atrophy. J Craniomaxillofac Surg. 1994;22(1):23-32.
2. Moore MH, Wong KS, Proudman TW, et al. Progressive hemifacial atrophy (Romberg's disease): skeletal involvement and treatment. Br J Plast Surg. 1993;46(1):39-44.

🖶 61.25. ADDISON PERNICIOUS ANEMIA SYNDROME (PERNICIOUS ANEMIA SYNDROME; VITAMIN B12 DEFICIENCY ANEMIA; MACROCYTIC ANEMIA; BIERMER SYNDROME)

General

Autosomal dominant; female preponderance; onset between ages 30 and 50 years; lack of intrinsic factor normally produced in the fundus of stomach and important for absorption of vitamin B12 in the intestinal tract; infrequent ocular involvement.

Ocular

Central scotoma, centrocecal scotomata, and field contractions in a few cases; retinal hemorrhages (round with white center) at the posterior pole; both retina and disk may have a whitish, hazy appearance; optic neuritis (ischemic); optic atrophy; palsies of extraocular muscles; ocular hypotony; cataract; bilateral, slowly progressive optic neuropathy, unclear etiology.

Clinical

Megaloblastic anemia (chronic and progressive); hypochlorhydria; glossitis; stomatitis; constipation or diarrhea; paresthesias and numbness; incoordination; ataxia; sphincter malfunction.

Laboratory

The peripheral blood usually shows a macrocytic anemia with a mild leukopenia and thrombocytopenia.

Treatment

The cause of the failure to absorb cobalamin (Cbl) should be determined. Vitamin B12 is available as either cyanocobalamin or hydroxocobalamin and each are useful in the treatment of vitamin B_{12} deficiency.

🖶 BIBLIOGRAPHY

1. Schick P, Conrad ME. (2013). Pernicious anemia. [online] Available from www.emedicine.com/med/TOPIC1799.HTM. [Accessed September, 2013].

61.26. GUILLAIN-BARRÉ SYNDROME (LANDRY PARALYSIS; ACUTE INFECTIOUS NEURITIS; ACUTE POLYRADICULITIS; ACUTE FEBRILE POLYNEURITIS; ACUTE IDIO-PATHIC POLYNEURITIS; INFLAMMATORY POLYRADICULONEUROPATHY; LANDRY-GUILLAIN-BARRÉ-STROHL SYNDROME; POSTINFECTIOUS POLYNEURITIS)

General

Etiology unknown; occurs from age 16–50 years.

Ocular

Facial nerve paralysis with paralytic ectropion of the lower eyelid; mild-to-complete external ophthalmoplegia; optic neuritis; papilledema; ptosis; anisocoria; nystagmus; dyschromatopsia; scotoma; bilateral tonic pupils.

Clinical

Polyneuritis involving facial peripheral motor nerves and spinal cord; facial diplegia; bladder incontinence; variable degrees of paralysis, usually beginning in lower extremities; tendon reflexes absent; involvement of respiratory muscles possible; paresthesia (symmetrical).

Laboratory

Cytomegalovirus, Epstein-Barr virus and HIV have been most closely associated with this condition.

Treatment

Plasma exchange have shown to be beneficial. Corneal exposure is treated with topical therapy or lateral tarsorrhaphies if warranted.

BIBLIOGRAPHY

1. Andary MT, Oleszek JL, Cha-Kim A. (2012). Guillain-Barrè Syndrome. [online] Available from www.emedicine.com/pmr/TOPIC48.HTM. [Accessed September, 2013].

61.26. FISHER SYNDROME (OPHTHALMOPLEGIA ATAXIA AREFLEXIA SYNDROME; MILLER-FISHER SYNDROME)

General

Acute idiopathic polyneuritis; prognosis good; complete recovery over several weeks (variant of Guillain-Barré syndrome; *see* Guillain-Barré syndrome).

Ocular

Moderate ptosis; complete external and almost complete internal ophthalmoplegia; diplopia; sluggish pupil reaction to light; may present without total ophthalmoplegia.

Clinical

Dizziness; severe ataxia; loss of tendon reflexes; chest pains; difficulties in chewing; diminished or absent sense of vibration; upper respiratory tract infection preceding this syndrome.

Laboratory

Diagnosis usually is made on clinical grounds. Laboratory studies are useful to rule out other diagnoses.

Treatment

Monitored closely for changes in blood pressure, heart rate and other arrhythmias. Temporary pacing may be required for patients with second-degree and third-degree heart block.

BIBLIOGRAPHY

1. Fisher M. An unusual variant of acute idiopathic polyneuritis (syndrome of ophthalmoplegia, ataxia and areflexia). N Engl J Med. 1956;255(2):57-65.
2. Igarashi Y, Takeda M, Maekawa H, et al. Fisher's syndrome without total ophthalmoplegia. Ophthalmologica. 1992;205(3):163-7.
3. Swick HM. Pseudointernuclear ophthalmoplegia in acute idiopathic polyneuritis (Fisher's syndrome). Am J Ophthalmol. 1974;77(5):725-8.

🔲 61.27. ROMBERG SYNDROME (PARRY-ROMBERG SYNDROME; PROGRESSIVE HEMIFACIAL ATROPHY; PROGRESSIVE FACIAL HEMIATROPHY; FACIAL HEMIATROPHY) ENOPHTHALMUS

General

Autosomal dominant; irritation in the peripheral trophic sympathetic system; onset in the 2nd decade; both sexes affected.

Ocular

Enophthalmos; outer canthus lowered; absence of nasal portion of eyebrow; ptosis; paresis of ocular muscles; miosis; iritis; iridocyclitis; heterochromia iridis; keratitis; neuroparalytic keratitis; cataracts; choroiditis; Fuchs' heterochromic cyclitis; retinal vascular abnormalities; association with Coats syndrome and exudative stellate neuroretinopathy; scleral melting.

Clinical

Atrophy of soft tissue on one side of the face, including tongue; trigeminal neuralgia and/or paresthesia; alopecia and poliosis not uncommon.

Laboratory/Ocular

Neuroimaging, CT scan of the orbits, MRI and bone scans.

Treatment/Ocular

Chemotherapy, ionizing radiation or immunosuppressive treatments.

🔲 BIBLIOGRAPHY

1. Aracena T, Roca FP, Barragan M. Progressive hemifacial atrophy (Parry-Romberg syndrome): report of two cases. Ann Ophthalmol. 1979;11:953-8.
2. Gass JD, Harbin TS, Del Piero EJ. Exudative stellate neuroretinopathy and Coats' syndrome in patients with progressive hemifacial atrophy. Eur J Ophthalmol. 1991;1:2-10.
3. Hoang-Xuan T, Foster CS, Jakobiec FA, et al. Romberg's progressive hemifacial atrophy: an association with scleral melting. Cornea. 1991;10:361-6.
4. La Hey E, Baarsma GS. Fuchs' heterochromic cyclitis and retinal vascular abnormalities in progressive hemifacial atrophy. Eye. 1993;7:426-8.
5. Parry CH. Collections from Unpublished Papers, Volume I. London: Underwood; 1825.
6. Romberg MH. Trophoneurosen. Klin Ergebn. Berlin: A. Forster; 1846.

🔲 61.29. REFSUM SYNDROME (HEREDOPATHIA ATACTICA POLYNEURITIFORMIS SYNDROME; PHYTANIC ACID OXIDASE DEFICIENCY; PHYTANIC ACID STORAGE DISEASE; REFSUM-THIEBAUT SYNDROME)

General

Autosomal recessive; disorder of lipid metabolism; interstitial hypertrophic polyneuropathy; delamination of myelin sheaths; onset usually between ages 4 and 7 years; caused by deficiency of phytanic acid hydroxylase.

Ocular

Progressive external ophthalmoplegia; night blindness; visual field constriction; pupillary abnormalities; corneal opacities; retinal degeneration beginning in macula; atypical RP; cataracts.

Clinical

Spinocerebellar ataxia; deafness (progressive); polyneuritis-like effect on limbs; CNS degeneration; ichthyosis; sensory changes; wasting of extremities; complete heart block; relapses and remissions in adolescence; normal intelligence.

Laboratory

Check phytanic acid in serum.

Treatment

Dietary restriction of phytanic acid, plasma exchange.

🔲 BIBLIOGRAPHY

1. Zalewska A, Schwartz RA. (2011). Refsum disease. [online] Available from www.emedicine.com/derm/TOPIC705.HTM. [Accessed September, 2013].

🗗 61.30. PROGRESSIVE SYSTEMIC SCLEROSIS (SCLERODERMA; SYSTEMIC SCLERODERMA)

General

Chronic connective tissue disease of unknown etiology; chronic and usually progressive disorder; typical onset is 3rd-5th decade; ratio of women to men is 4:1; primary sites of pathology are the arterioles and capillaries of affected organs.

Ocular

Marginal corneal ulcers; shortened fornices of the conjunctiva; ptosis; cotton-wool patches of retina; papilledema; retinal hemorrhages; cicatrization of conjunctiva and cornea; blepharitis; blepharospasm; thready, tenacious yellow-white conjunctival discharge; hypertrophy of lacrimal gland; episcleritis; ocular myositis; Sjögren syndrome; uveitis; vitreous haze; keratitis sicca; decreased corneal sensation; iritis; ischemic choroidopathy; iris sectorial atrophy; blepharophimosis; heterochromia; keratoconus; central retinal vein occlusion; branch retinal vein occlusion.

Clinical

Vascular insufficiency; Raynaud's phenomenon; malaise; weight loss; stiffness; fever; polyarticular arthritis; diffuse edema of the hands; calcinosis; esophageal involvement; sclerodactyly; telangiectasis; esophageal stricture; renal failure; diffuse interstitial fibrosis.

Laboratory

No specific test establishes diagnosis. Hypergammaglobulinemia—50% of cases ANA increased in 40–70% cases.

Treatment

Skin thickening can be treated with D-penicillamine and other experimental drugs. Pruritus can be treated with moisturizers and histamine. Raynaud's phenomenon can be treated with calcium channel blockers. Renal crisis episodes are best prevented and treated with the aggressive use of ACE inhibitors. Myositis may be treated cautiously with steroids.

🗗 BIBLIOGRAPHY

1. Jimenez SA, Cronin PM, Koenig AS, et al. (2012). Scleroderma. [online] Available from www.emedicine.com/med/TOPIC2076.HTM. [Accessed September, 2013].

🗗 61.31. SHY-DRAGER SYNDROME (ORTHOSTATIC HYPOTENSION SYNDROME; SHY-MEGEE-DRAGER SYNDROME)

General

Etiology unknown; gradual onset; adults; progressive degeneration of the nervous system.

Ocular

External ophthalmoplegia; iris atrophy; ocular sympathetic and parasympathetic insufficiency (alternating Homer syndrome, cholinergic supersensitivity, decreased lacrimation, and corneal hypesthesia).

Clinical

Orthostatic hypotension; rigidity; tremor; adiadochokinesia; wasting of muscles; mental retardation; impotence; dysphagia; bilateral vocal cord paralysis; neurogenic bladder; anhidrosis; extremity weakness and paresthesias; dizziness; abnormal postural balance.

Laboratory

No laboratory studies are indicated.

Treatment

No effective systemic therapy is known.

🗗 BIBLIOGRAPHY

1. Dalvi AI, Rauschkolb PK, Berman SA. (2012). Striatonigral degeneration. [online] Available from www.emedicine.com/neuro/TOPIC354.HTM. [Accessed September, 2013].

⊞ 61.32. SHY-GONATAS SYNDROME

General

Unknown etiology; similar to Hunter and Refsum syndromes; accumulation of lipids in muscles simulates gargoylism; present from birth.

Ocular

Mild proptosis; hypertelorism; ptosis; external ophthalmoplegia (progressive); concentric visual field constriction; keratopathy with possible corneal ulcer; lattice-like white opacities in the area of Bowman membrane; retinal pigmentary degeneration (atypical retinitis pigmentosa) with difficulties with night vision.

Clinical

Weakness of extremities (proximal); myopathy and neuropathy; cerebellar ataxia.

Laboratory

Clinical.

Treatment

- *Ptosis*: If visual acuity is affected, most cases require surgical correction and there are several procedures that may be used including levator resection, repair or advancement and Fasanella-Servat.
- *Corneal ulcer*: Corneal cultures may be taken and treatment initiated. Treatment includes a broad spectrum of antibiotics and cycloplegic drops.

⊞ BIBLIOGRAPHY

1. Geeraets WJ. Ocular Syndromes, 3rd edition. Philadelphia: Lea & Febiger; 1976.
2. Gonatas NK. A generalized disorder of nervous system, skeletal muscle and heart resembling Refsum's disease and Hurler's syndrome. II. Ultrastructure. Am J Med. 1967;42:169.
3. Shy GM, Silberberg DH, Appel SH, et al. A generalized disorder of nervous system, skeletal muscle and heart resembling Refsum's disease and Hurler's syndrome. I. Clinical, pathologic and biochemical characteristics. Am J Med. 1967;42:163.

⊞ 61.34. LYME DISEASE

General

It is caused by tick bite; symptoms resolve after treatment.

Ocular

Keratitis may occur up to 5 years after the first episode; diplopia; photophobia; ischemic optic neuropathy; iritis; panophthalmitis; conjunctivitis; exudative retinal detachment; choroiditis; vitreitis; multiple cranial nerve palsies; association with acute, posterior, multifocal, placoid, pigment epitheliopathy; branch retinal artery occlusion.

Clinical

Arthritis; increased intracranial pressure; effusion of knees; swelling of wrists.

Laboratory

Immunofluorescent assay (IFA) and ELISA.

Treatment

Oral antibiotics for 2–3 weeks: tetracycline 500 mg four times a day, doxycycline 100 mg two times a day, phenoxymethyl penicillin 500 mg four times a day, or amoxicillin 500 mg three to four times a day.

⊞ BIBLIOGRAPHY

1. Zaidman GW. (2011). Ophthalmic Aspects of Lyme Disease Overview of Lyme Disease. [online] Available from www.emedicine.com/oph/TOPIC262.HTM. [Accessed September, 2013].

61.34. ROCKY MOUNTAIN SPOTTED FEVER

General

Acute systemic disease caused by *Rickettsia rickettsii* transmitted by a wood tick or dog tick.

Ocular

Conjunctivitis; optic atrophy; cotton-wool spots; scotoma; uveitis; optic neuritis; paralysis of accommodation; paralysis of extraocular muscles; retinal vascular occlusion; vitreal opacity; hypopyon; anterior uveitis with fibrin clots.

Clinical

Fever; chills; headache; muscle aches; rash.

Laboratory

Early diagnosis depends on clinical and epidemiological grounds. PCR has high sensitivity and specificity.

Treatment

Intravenous tetracycline and chloramphenicol should be started as soon as possible. Oral doxycycline, tetracycline and chloramphenicol may be considered but only if patient is not acutely ill.

BIBLIOGRAPHY

1. Cunha BA, O'Brien MS. (2011). Rocky mountain spotted fever. [online] Available from www.emedicine.com/oph/TOPIC503.HTM. [Accessed September, 2013].

61.36. WERNICKE SYNDROME I (SUPERIOR HEMORRHAGIC POLIOENCEPHALO-PATHIC SYNDROME; HEMORRHAGIC POLIOENCEPHALITIS SUPERIOR SYNDROME; ENCEPHALITIS HEMORRHAGICA SUPERIORIS; AVITAMINOSIS B; THIAMINE DEFICIENCY; BERIBERI; GAYET-WERNICKE SYNDROME; WERNICKE-KORSAKOFF SYNDROME) PTOSIS

General

Lack of vitamin B or thiamine; focal vascular lesions in the gray matter around third and fourth ventricles and Sylvian aqueduct; alcoholics (adults); beriberi of all ages.

Ocular

Ptosis; acute bilateral nuclear ophthalmoplegia; complete ophthalmoplegia; retinal hemorrhages; optic atrophy; optic neuritis; conjunctivitis; blepharitis; nutritional amblyopia; central scotoma; papilledema; nystagmus; absolute pupillary paralysis or Argyll Robertson pupils; accommodative palsy.

Clinical

Early prostration; lethargy; irritability; stupor; delirium; mental disturbances to Korsakoff psychosis; ataxia; tremors; peripheral neuritis; anorexia; vomiting; insomnia; perspiration; tachycardia; hallucinations; retrograde amnesia; apathy; anxiety; fear; defective concentration; cardiomyopathy.

Laboratory

Electrolyte studies, serum thiamine levels, CBC. Evaluation of hypoxemia, hypercarbia, acidosis, or alkalosis. Serum/urine toxin drug screen and liver enzymes.

Treatment

Parenteral thiamine is the treatment of choice.

BIBLIOGRAPHY

1. Xiong GL, Kenedi CA. (2013). Wernicke-Korsakoff syndrome. [online] Available from www.emedicine.com/med/TOPIC2405.HTM. [Accessed September, 2013].

6J. FISHER SYNDROME (OPHTHALMOPLEGIA ATAXIA AREFLEXIA SYNDROME; MILLER-FISHER SYNDROME)

General

Acute idiopathic polyneuritis; prognosis good; complete recovery over several weeks (variant of Guillain-Barré syndrome; *see* Guillain-Barré syndrome).

Ocular

Moderate ptosis; complete external and almost complete internal ophthalmoplegia; diplopia; sluggish pupil reaction to light; may present without total ophthalmoplegia.

Clinical

Dizziness; severe ataxia; loss of tendon reflexes; chest pains; difficulties in chewing; diminished or absent sense of vibration; upper respiratory tract infection preceding this syndrome.

Laboratory

Diagnosis usually is made on clinical grounds. Laboratory studies are useful to rule out other diagnoses.

Treatment

Monitored closely for changes in blood pressure, heart rate and other arrhythmias. Temporary pacing may be required for patients with second-degree and third-degree heart block.

BIBLIOGRAPHY

1. Fisher M. An unusual variant of acute idiopathic polyneuritis (syndrome of ophthalmoplegia, ataxia and areflexia). N Engl J Med. 1956;255(2):57-65.
2. Igarashi Y, Takeda M, Maekawa H, et al. Fisher's syndrome without total ophthalmoplegia. Ophthalmologica. 1992;205(3):163-7.
3. Swick HM. Pseudointernuclear ophthalmoplegia in acute idiopathic polyneuritis (Fisher's syndrome). Am J Ophthalmol. 1974;77(5):725-8.

6K. INTERNUCLEAR OPHTHALMOPLEGIA

This condition comprises paralysis of the medial rectus muscles on attempted conjugate lateral gaze without other evidence of third nerve paralysis due to involvement of medial longitudinal fasciculus. Jerk nystagmus of abducting eye and vertical nystagmus, usually on upward gaze, may be present.

1. *Bilateral*
   A. Arnold-Chiari malformation (cerebellomedullary malformation syndrome)
   †B. "Crack" cocaine
   C. Fabry disease (glycosphingolipid lipidosis)
   †D. Inflammation, such as upper respiratory infection
   †E. Midbrain infarction
   *F. Multiple sclerosis (disseminated sclerosis)
   G. Myasthenia gravis (Erb-Goldflam syndrome)
   †H. Occlusive vascular disease
   I. Oculocerebellar tegmental syndrome
   †J. Pontine hematoma

   K. Syphilis (acquired lues)
   L. Temporal arteritis
   M. Vertebral basilar artery syndrome (whiplash injury)
   N. Webino syndrome (wall-eyed exotropia bilateral internuclear ophthalmoplegia)
   O. Wernicke encephalopathy
2. *Unilateral*
   A. Bielschowsky-Lutz-Cogan syndrome (internuclear ophthalmoplegia)
   B. Cryptococcosis (torulosis)
   C. Multiple sclerosis (disseminated sclerosis)
   D. Myasthenia gravis (Erb-Goldflam syndrome)
   E. Neuro-Behçet Disease
   †F. Tumors of the brainstem
   †*G. Vascular lesion-infarct of small branch of basilar artery

*Indicates most frequent
†Indicates a general entry and therefore has not been described in detail in the text

BIBLIOGRAPHY

1. Kaye V, Brandstate ME. (2011). Vertebrobasilar Stroke Overview of Vertebrobasilar Stroke. [online] Available from www.emedicine.com/pmr/TOPIC143.HTM. [Accessed September, 2013].

2. Landolfi J, Venkataramana A. (2013). Brainstem Gliomas. [online] Available from www.emedicine.com/neuro/TOPIC40.HTM. [Accessed September, 2013].
3. Lee AG, Berlie CL, Costello F. (2012). Ophthalmologic manifestations of multiple sclerosis. [online] Available from www.emedicine.com/oph/TOPIC179.HTM. [Accessed September, 2013].
4. Papamitsakis NI. (2013). Lacunar Syndrome. [online] Available from www.emedicine.com/neuro/TOPIC695.HTM. [Accessed September, 2013].
5. Ramachandran TS. (2013). Tuberculous Meningitis. [online] Available from www.emedicine.com/neuro/TOPIC385.HTM. [Accessed September, 2013].
6. Rust RS. (2012). Diffuse Sclerosis. [online] Available from www.emedicine.com/neuro/TOPIC92.HTM. [Accessed September, 2013].
7. Roque MR, Roque BL, Miserocchi E, et al. (2013). Ophthalmologic manifestations of giant cell arteritis. [online] Available from www.emedicine.com/oph/TOPIC254.HTM. [Accessed September, 2013].

6K.1A. ARNOLD-CHIARI SYNDROME (PLATYBASIA SYNDROME; CEREBELLOMEDULLARY MALFORMATION SYNDROME; BASILAR IMPRESSIONS)

General

Malformation of the hindbrain; developmental deformity of the occipital bone and upper cervical spine; recognized in children or adults; clinical picture may be indistinguishable from that of Dandy-Walker syndrome in infants.

Ocular

Horizontal, vertical, and rotary forms of nystagmus; vertical nystagmus in both upgaze and downgaze is most common; papilledema; esotropia; Duane retraction syndrome (association); oscillopsia.

Clinical

Hydrocephalus; cerebellar ataxia; bilateral pyramidal tract signs.

Laboratory

CT scans are used most commonly for the diagnosis of hydrocephalus and for the evaluation of suspected shunt malfunction.

Treatment

Early recognition and treatment is important because of the potential life-threatening symptoms. Early surgical intervention, especially in infants may prevent irreversible changes and death.

BIBLIOGRAPHY

1. Incesu L, Khosla A, Aiello MR. (2011). Imaging in Chiari II malformation. [online] Available from www.emedicine.com/radio/TOPIC150.HTM. [Accessed September, 2013].

6K.1C. FABRY DISEASE (ANGIOKERATOMA CORPORIS DIFFUSUM SYNDROME; DIFFUSE ANGIOKERATOSIS; FABRY-ANDERSON SYNDROME; GLYCOSPHINGOLIPID LIPIDOSIS; GLYCOSPHINGOLIPIDOSIS)

General

Lipoid storage disorder; X-linked recessive inheritance; lack of α-galactosidase A enzyme.

Ocular

Swelling of eyelids; varicosities of palpebral and bulbar conjunctiva; corneal dystrophy; corneal opacities; increased tortuosity of retinal vessels and aneurysmal dilatations; cornea verticillata; cataract; central retinal artery occlusion; internuclear paralysis of extraocular muscles; papilledema; tortuosity and caliber irregularity of conjunctival vessels; characteristic cream-colored whorl-like opacity in deep part of corneal epithelium; posterior cataract; occasional edema of optic disk and retina.

Clinical

Angiokeratoma of the skin with small, grouped papular lesions mainly over the scrotum, thighs, buttocks, sacral area, umbilical area, and lips; elevated blood pressure; disturbance in sweat secretion; pain in arms and legs; enlarged heart; albuminuria.

Laboratory

Reduced α-galactosidase A level in plasma; elevated trihexosyl ceramide levels in urine and plasma.

Treatment

Primarily surgical and is usually a corneal transplant. After surgery, treatment of amblyopia and optical therapy can be helpful.

BIBLIOGRAPHY

1. Banikazemi M, Desnick RJ, Astrin KH. (2012). Genetics of Fabry disease. [online] Available from www.emedicine.com/ped/TOPIC2888.HTM. [Accessed September, 2013].

6K.1F. DISSEMINATED SCLEROSIS (MULTIPLE SCLEROSIS)

General

Disseminated demyelination affecting white matter of the brain, spinal cord, and optic nerves; etiology unknown.

Ocular

Nystagmus; ptosis; myokymia; optic atrophy; papillitis; optic neuritis; anisocoria; Argyll Robertson pupil; Marcus Gunn pupil; hippus, decreased or absent papillary reaction to light; periphlebitis; visual field defects; gaze palsy; paralysis of third or sixth nerve; uveitis; oscillopsia; Uhthoff symptom (reduction of visual acuity with exercise or ocular hyperthermia); pars planitis; retinal venous sheathing; retinitis; granulomatous uveitis.

Clinical

Incoordination; paresthesia; spasticity; tic douloureux; urinary frequency and infections; progressive disability; paralysis; death.

Laboratory

MRI, CSF positive for oligoclonal band, albumin and IgG index; BAER and SEP.

Treatment

Patients with MS may require multiple consultations to rule out other causes for their symptoms. Drugs such as immunodulator, immunosuppressors, anti-Parkinson agent, CNS stimulants are all used in the management of the disease.

BIBLIOGRAPHY

1. Luzzio C, Dangond F. (2013). Multiple Sclerosis. [online] Available from www.emedicine.com/neuro/topic228.htm. [Accessed September, 2013].

6K.1G. ERB-GOLDFLAM SYNDROME (ERB II SYNDROME; HOPPE-GOLDFLAM DISEASE; PSEUDOPARALYTIC SYNDROME; MYASTHENIA GRAVIS)

General

Occurs at any age; more frequent between ages 20 and 40 years; more females affected than males; progressive; spontaneous; symptoms improve or resolve with rest in early stages of disease (*see* myasthenia gravis, neonatal or infantile); caused by autoantibodies against the acetylcholine receptor at the neuromuscular junction, leading to abnormal fatigability and weakness of skeletal muscle.

Ocular

Transient diplopia; ptosis of upper eyelids.

Clinical

Excessive fatigability of musculature; symptoms appear and increase as day progresses; expressionless face; sagging jaw; difficulty in chewing and talking; nasal regurgitation.

Laboratory

Ice test—crushed ice in surgical glove over ptotic eyelid for 2 minutes and watch for brief elevation of eyelid; Tensilon test and prostigmin test may result in the elevation of ptotic eyelid or improved strabismus in individuals with myasthenia gravis.

Treatment

Adrenal corticosteroids are frequently used. In some cases, mycophenolate mofetil, cyclosporine and cyclophosphamide may be useful. Patching one eye or using prisms may be helpful.

☐ BIBLIOGRAPHY

1. Erb W. Zur Casuistick der Bulbaren La hmungen. Arch Psychiatr Vervenkr. 1879;9:325-50.
2. Roy FH, Fraunfelder FT, Fraunfelder FW. Roy and Fraunfelder's Current Ocular Therapy, 6th edition. London, UK: Elsevier; 2008.

☐ 6K.1I. OCULOCEREBELLAR TEGMENTAL SYNDROME

General

Vascular lesion of mesencephalon with softening in peduncular area.

Ocular

Paralysis of associated ocular movements (internuclear anterior ophthalmoplegia).

Clinical

Sudden onset of hemiplegia with rapid recovery; bilateral cerebellar syndrome.

Laboratory

Diagnosis is made by clinical findings.

Treatment

Treat vascular lesion.

☐ BIBLIOGRAPHY

1. Fournier A, Ducoulombier H, Cousin J, et al. [Oculo-cerebello-myoclonic syndrome and neuroblastoma]. J Sci Med Lille. 1972;90(5):189-97.
2. Rodriquez B, et al. A new type of peduncular syndrome: internuclear ophthalmoplegia and bilateral cerebellar syndrome from a tegmental lesion. Arch Urug Med. 1945;10:353; Am J Ophthalmol. 1946;29:511.

☐ 6K.1K. ACQUIRED LUES (SYPHILIS; ACQUIRED SYPHILIS; LUES VENEREA; MALUM VENEREUM)

General

Causative agent, *T. pallidum*, usually transmitted sexually.

Ocular

Conjunctival chancroid; conjunctivitis; keratitis; blepharitis; ptosis; iris atrophy; hippus; dacryocystitis; optic nerve atrophy; optic neuritis; periostitis; episcleritis; scleritis; nystagmus; uveitis; vitreous hemorrhages; paralysis of sixth nerve; papilledema; retinal hemorrhages; retinitis proliferans; oculogyric crisis; neuroretinitis; papilledema (associated with aseptic meningitis); diffuse or multifocal chorioretinitis; vertical supranuclear gaze palsy; Benedikt syndrome.

Clinical

Primary lesion associated with regional lymphadenopathy; secondary bacteremic stage associated with generalized mucocutaneous lesions; tertiary stage characterized by destructive mucocutaneous, musculoskeletal, or parenchymal lesions, aortitis, or CNS disease; syphilis and HIV infection often coexist in the same patient who experiences a higher incidence and greater severity of neurologic and ocular manifestations; a significant percentage of patients infected with HIV-I and *T. pallidum* become seronegative to syphilis testing.

Laboratory

Serologic nontreponemal tests include VDRL and RPR.

Treatment

The goals are to reduce morbidity and to prevent complications. Penicillin is the antibiotic of choice for treating syphilis. Ocular syphilis should be treated the same as patients with neurosyphilis.

☐ BIBLIOGRAPHY

1. Euerle B, Chandrasekar PH, Diaz MM, et al. (2012). Syphilis. [online] Available from www.emedicine.com/med/TOPIC2224.HTM. [Accessed September, 2013].
2. Majmudar PA. (2011). Interstitial keratitis overview of interstitial keratitis. [online] Available from www.emedicine.com/oph/TOPIC453.HTM. [Accessed September, 2013].

6K.1L. TEMPORAL ARTERITIS SYNDROME (CRANIAL ARTERITIS SYNDROME; GIANT CELL ARTERITIS; HUTCHINSON-HORTON-MAGATH-BROWN SYNDROME)

General

Etiology unknown; mainly females; mainly Whites; ages 55–80 years; temporal artery shows inflammatory thickening; arteritis of the vessels supplying the optic nerve.

Ocular

Transient ptosis; partial or complete loss of vision on the affected side; retinal detachment; exudates and hemorrhages; narrowing of retinal vessels; obstruction of the central retinal artery; optic atrophy; ischemic optic neuropathy; acute decreased IOP; corneal hypesthesia; palsies of extraocular muscles; hemorrhagic glaucoma; diplopia; hemorrhages on or around the disk.

Clinical

Throbbing headache; hyperalgesia of the scalp; malaise; anorexia; weakness; weight loss; fever; nodular pulmonary nodules; cough; otitis with deafness.

Laboratory

Elevated ESR greater than 50 mm/hour, positive temporal artery biopsy.

Treatment

Systemic corticosteroids are the therapy of choice.

BIBLIOGRAPHY

1. Allen AW, Biega T, Varma MK. (2012). Temporal arteritis imaging. [online] Available from www.emedicine.com/radio/TOPIC675.HTM. [Accessed September, 2013].
2. Walvick MD, Walvick MP. Giant cell arteritis: laboratory predictors of a positive temporal artery biopsy. Ophthalmology. 2011;118(6):1201-4.

6K.1M. CRANIOCERVICAL SYNDROME (WHIPLASH INJURY)

General

Disturbed accommodation is due to a central lesion rather than a peripheral lesion of the ciliary muscle; Horner syndrome observed where a palsy of the cervical sympathetics occurs (*see* Horner Syndrome).

Ocular

General ocular pain; enophthalmos; mild ptosis; reduced ability to accommodate; disturbance in ocular movements; primarily those extraocular muscles innervated by the oculomotor nerve are involved; convergence insufficiency; nystagmus (gaze direction and vestibular, central, peripheral, and mixed type); vestibular impairment in more than 50% of cases; asthenopia; fogging; double vision; miosis; mydriasis; retinal arteriolar pressure may show changes in systolic and diastolic pressure and be more pronounced than changes in the brachial blood pressure; decreased stereoacuity; vitreous detachment.

Clinical

Headache; vertigo; dizziness; neck and back pain.

Laboratory

Radiographs in the neutral, flexed, and extended positions, should be obtained and the degree of movement measured.

Treatment

Physical therapy, cervical fusion should be considered with great caution and only after aggressive nonsurgical care has failed; intra-articular facet joint injections and medial branch blocks.

BIBLIOGRAPHY

1. Windsor RE, Hankley D, Cone-Sullivan LA, et al. (2012). Cervical Facet Syndrome. [online] Available from www.emedicine.com/sports/TOPIC20.HTM. [Accessed September, 2013].

🗗 6K.1N. WEBINO SYNDROME (WALL-EYED BILATERAL INTERNUCLEAR OPHTHALMOPLEGIA)

General

Differential diagnosis includes demyelinating disease, arteriosclerotic cerebrovascular disease, trauma, Arnold-Chiari malformation, syphilis, periarteritis nodosa, glioma, cryptococcal meningitis and premature infants; usually represents midline involvement of oculomotor nucleus.

Ocular

Wall-eyed internuclear ophthalmoplegia (bilateral internuclear ophthalmoplegia with exotropia).

Clinical

Depends on cause; associated with MS in young patients.

Laboratory

Diagnosis is made by clinical findings.

Treatment

Evaluate internuclear ophthalmoplegia.

🗗 BIBLIOGRAPHY

1. Daroff RE, Hoyt WE. Supranuclear disorders of ocular control systems in man. In: Bach-Y-Rita P, Collins CC (Eds). The Control of Eye Movements. Orlando, FL: Academic Press; 1971. p. 223.
2. Lepore FE, Nissenblatt MJ. Bilateral internuclear ophthalmoplegia after intrathecal chemotherapy and cranial irradiation. Am J Ophthalmol. 1981;92(6):851-3.
3. Miller NR (Ed). Walsh and Hoyt's Clinical Neuro-Ophthalmology, 4th edition. Baltimore, USA: Williams & Wilkins; 1995. p. 4323.

🗗 6K.1O. WERNICKE SYNDROME I (SUPERIOR HEMORRHAGIC POLIOENCEPHALOPATHIC SYNDROME; HEMORRHAGIC POLIOENCEPHALITIS SUPERIOR SYNDROME; ENCEPHALITIS HEMORRHAGICA SUPERIORIS; AVITAMINOSIS B; THIAMINE DEFICIENCY; BERIBERI; GAYET-WERNICKE SYNDROME; WERNICKE-KORSAKOFF SYNDROME) PTOSIS

General

Lack of vitamin B or thiamine; focal vascular lesions in the gray matter around third and fourth ventricles and Sylvian aqueduct; alcoholics (adults); beriberi of all ages.

Ocular

Ptosis; acute bilateral nuclear ophthalmoplegia; complete ophthalmoplegia; retinal hemorrhages; optic atrophy; optic neuritis; conjunctivitis; blepharitis; nutritional amblyopia; central scotoma; papilledema; nystagmus; absolute pupillary paralysis or Argyll Robertson pupils; accommodative palsy.

Clinical

Early prostration; lethargy; irritability; stupor; delirium; mental disturbances to Korsakoff psychosis; ataxia; tremors; peripheral neuritis; anorexia; vomiting; insomnia; perspiration; tachycardia; hallucinations; retrograde amnesia; apathy; anxiety; fear; defective concentration; cardiomyopathy.

Laboratory

Electrolyte studies, serum thiamine levels, CBC. Evaluation of hypoxemia, hypercarbia, acidosis, or alkalosis. Serum/urine toxin drug screen and liver enzymes.

Treatment

Parenteral thiamine is the treatment of choice.

🗗 BIBLIOGRAPHY

1. Xiong GL, Kenedi CA. (2013). Wernicke-Korsakoff syndrome. [online] Available from www.emedicine.com/med/TOPIC2405.HTM. [Accessed September, 2013].

6K.2A. BIELSCHOWSKY-LUTZ-COGAN SYNDROME (INTERNUCLEAR OPHTHALMOPLEGIA)

General

Lesion in the medial longitudinal fasciculus; anterior internuclear ophthalmoplegia consists of paresis of convergence with paresis of homolateral medial rectus muscle during lateral gaze toward opposite side of the lesion; in the posterior internuclear ophthalmoplegia, convergence is not affected, while the homolateral medial rectus muscle is paralytic on lateral gaze; the most common cause in young patients include a demyelinating process such as MS, whereas an ischemic process is more common in the elderly; other reported causes of brainstem infarction associated with internuclear ophthalmoplegia include sickle cell trait, periarteritis nodosa, Wernicke encephalopathy, "crack" cocaine smoking.

Ocular

Unilateral or bilateral palsy of the medial rectus muscle during conjugate lateral gaze but with or without normal function of this muscle during convergence, depending on the type of internuclear ophthalmoplegia; dissociated nystagmus in the maximal abducted contralateral eye.

Laboratory

CT and MRI.

Treatment

Intravenous (IV) and oral steroids may be beneficial.

BIBLIOGRAPHY

1. Lee AG, Berlie CL, Costello F. (2012). Ophthalmologic manifestations of multiple sclerosis. [online] Available from www.emedicine.com/oph/TOPIC179.HTM. [Accessed September, 2013].
2. Luzzio C, Dangond F. (2012). Multiple sclerosis. [online] Available from www.emedicine.com/emerg/TOPIC321.HTM. [Accessed September, 2013].

6K.2B. CRYPTOCOCCOSIS (TORULOSIS)

General

A pulmonary infection caused by *Cryptococcus neoformans*, a saprophyte found in weathered pigeon droppings, soil, and unpasteurized cow's milk; infection acquired through respiratory system and usually manifests as meningoencephalitis; higher incidence in patients with AIDS.

Ocular

Blurred or poor vision; diplopia; uveitis; papilledema; retinal detachment; retinal hemorrhage and exudates; secondary glaucoma; vitreous reaction; retinitis; proptosis; a mass over the optic nerve head; disease process can be bilateral or unilateral; cranial nerve VI palsy; visual loss; conjunctivitis.

Clinical

Severe headache; dizziness; ataxia; vomiting; tinnitus; memory disturbances; Jacksonian convulsions; fever usually is absent; occurs frequently in patients with leukemia or lymphoma.

Laboratory

The diagnosis is based on skin biopsy findings evaluated after fungal staining and culture.

Treatment

The goal of pharmacotherapy is either to terminate the infection when possible or to control the infection and to reduce morbidity when cure is not possible.

BIBLIOGRAPHY

1. King JW, DeWitt ML. (2013). Cryptococcosis. [online] Available from www.emedicine.com/med/TOPIC482.HTM. [Accessed September, 2013].

⊟ 6K.2C. DISSEMINATED SCLEROSIS (MULTIPLE SCLEROSIS)

General

Disseminated demyelination affecting white matter of the brain, spinal cord, and optic nerves; etiology unknown.

Ocular

Nystagmus; ptosis; myokymia; optic atrophy; papillitis; optic neuritis; anisocoria; Argyll Robertson pupil; Marcus Gunn pupil; hippus, decreased or absent papillary reaction to light; periphlebitis; visual field defects; gaze palsy; paralysis of third or sixth nerve; uveitis; oscillopsia; Uhthoff symptom (reduction of visual acuity with exercise or ocular hyperthermia); pars planitis; retinal venous sheathing; retinitis; granulomatous uveitis.

Clinical

Incoordination; paresthesia; spasticity; tic douloureux; urinary frequency and infections; progressive disability; paralysis; death.

Laboratory

MRI, CSF positive for oligoclonal band, albumin and IgG index; BAER and SEP.

Treatment

Patients with MS may require multiple consultations to rule out other causes for their symptoms. Drugs such as immunodulator, immunosuppressors, anti-Parkinson agent, CNS stimulants are all used in the management of the disease.

⊟ BIBLIOGRAPHY

1. Luzzio C, Dangond F. (2013). Multiple sclerosis. [online] Available from www.emedicine.com/neuro/topic228.htm. [Accessed September, 2013].

⊟ 6K.2D. ERB-GOLDFLAM SYNDROME (ERB II SYNDROME; HOPPE-GOLDFLAM DISEASE; PSEUDOPARALYTIC SYNDROME; MYASTHENIA GRAVIS)

General

Occurs at any age; more frequent between ages 20 years and 40 years; more females affected than males; progressive; spontaneous; symptoms improve or resolve with rest in early stages of disease (*see* myasthenia gravis, neonatal or infantile); caused by autoantibodies against the acetylcholine receptor at the neuromuscular junction, leading to abnormal fatigability and weakness of skeletal muscle.

Ocular

Transient diplopia; ptosis of upper eyelids.

Clinical

Excessive fatigability of musculature; symptoms appear and increase as day progresses; expressionless face; sagging jaw; difficulty in chewing and talking; nasal regurgitation.

Laboratory

Ice test—crushed ice in surgical glove over ptotic eyelid for 2 minutes and watch for brief elevation of eyelid; Tensilon test and prostigmin test may result in the elevation of ptotic eyelid or improved strabismus in individuals with myasthenia gravis.

Treatment

Adrenal corticosteroids are frequently used. In some cases, mycophenolate mofetil, cyclosporine and cyclophosphamide may be useful. Patching one eye or using prisms may be helpful.

⊟ BIBLIOGRAPHY

1. Erb W. Zur Casuistick der Bulbaren La hmungen. Arch Psychiatr Vervenkr. 1879;9:325-50.
2. Roy FH, Fraunfelder FT, Fraunfelder FW. Roy and Fraunfelder's Current Ocular Therapy, 6th edition. London, UK: Elsevier; 2008.
3. Goldflam S. Vebereinen Scheinbar Keilbaren Bulbarparalytischem Symptom Complex mit Betheiligung der Extremitaten. Dtsch Z Nerven. 1983;4:312-52.
4. Kim JH, Hwang JM, Hwang YS, et al. Chilhood ocular myasthenia gravis. Ophthalmology. 2003;110:1458-62.
5. Lepore FE. Pupillary dysfunction in myasthenia gravis. Ann Neurol. 1979;6:29-33.
6. Sommer N, Melms A, Weller M, et al. Ocular myasthenia gravis. A critical review of Clinical and pathophysiological aspects. Doc Ophthalmol. 1993;84:309-33.

6K.2E. BEHÇET SYNDROME (DERMATO-STOMATO-OPHTHALMIC SYNDROME; OCULOBUCCOGENITAL SYNDROME; GILBERT SYNDROME)

General

Virus infection; occurs in adults; chronic disease; complete remission is rare; etiology is unknown.

Ocular

Muscle palsies (occasional); nystagmus (occasional); conjunctivitis; hypopyon; iritis; recurrent uveitis; keratoconjunctivitis sicca; keratitis; vitreous hemorrhages; thrombophlebitis retinal veins (occasional); retinal hemorrhages; optic neuritis (occasional); macular edema; optic nerve atrophy; retinitis; secondary glaucoma; retinal vasculitis; disk edema; panophthalmitis; optic neuropathy; skin lesions, posterior uveitis and systemic complications have been associated with loss of vision with this disorder; corneal immune ring opacity.

Clinical

Aphthous lesions of mucous membranes of the mouth and genitalia; cerebellar signs; convulsions; paraplegia; skin erythema (multiforme, bullosum); arthritis; urethritis; glossitis; recurrent fever.

Laboratory

Nonspecific human leukocyte antigen (HLA) B51 positive may help to support diagnosis.

Treatment

The goals of therapy are to suppress inflammation, to reduce the frequency and severity of recurrences, and to minimize involvement of the retina. To be effective, treatment must be started early. Extent of involvement and severity of disease determine the choice of medication. Treatment options include corticosteroids, cytotoxic agents, cyclosporine, and colchicine.

BIBLIOGRAPHY

1. Bashour M. (2012). Ophthalmologic manifestations of Behcet disease. [online] Available from www.emedicine.com/oph/TOPIC425.HTM. [Accessed September, 2013].

6L. IVIC SYNDROME (RADIAL RAY DEFECTS, HEARING IMPAIRMENT, INTERNAL OPHTHALMOPLEGIA, THROMBOCYTOPENIA)

General

Autosomal dominant; Institute Venezolano de Investigacionas Cientificas (IVIC); observed in 1800s from Canary islands in Venezuela; it has been observed in descendants of a family that migrated to Venezuela from the Canary islands.

Ocular

Strabismus; internal ophthalmoplegia.

Clinical

Malformed upper limb; short distal phalanx; hearing loss; thrombocytopenia; leukocytosis; imperforate anus; radial ray defect.

Laboratory

Diagnosis is made by clinical findings.

Treatment

Traditional surgery is done for esotropia or exotropia.

BIBLIOGRAPHY

1. Areas S, Penchaszadeh VB, Pinto-Cisternas J, et al. The IVIC syndrome: a new autosomal dominant complex pleiotropic syndrome with radial ray hypoplasia, hearing impairment, internal ophthalmoplegia, and thrombocytopenia. Am J Med Genet. 1980;6(1):25-59.
2. Czeizel A, Göblyös P, Kodaj I. IVIC syndrome: report of a third family. Am J Med Genet. 1989;33(2):282-3.
3. McKusick VA. Mendelian Inheritance in Man; A Catalog of Human Genes and Genetic Disorders, 12th edition. Baltimore, USA: The Johns Hopkins University Press; 1998.
4. Hamosh A, Scott AF, Amberger J, et al. Online Mendelian Inheritance in Man (OMIM), a knowledgebase of human genes and genetic disorders. Nucleic Acids Res. 2002;30(1):52-5.

🗗 6M. KEARNS-SAYRE SYNDROME (OPHTHALMOPLEGIA PLUS SYNDROME; KEARNS-SHY SYNDROME; KEARNS DISEASE)

General

Etiology unknown; sporadic (nonhereditary); onset before age of 20 years; external ophthalmoplegia; complete heart block.

Ocular

Pigmentary degeneration of retina; progressive external ophthalmoplegia; corneal decompensation; optic neuritis.

Clinical

Abnormal mitochondria with paracrystalline inclusion in muscle cell; heart block; limb weakness; hyperglycemic acidotic coma; death; cerebellar dysfunction.

Laboratory

Best means of achieving definitive diagnosis is via analysis of a muscle biopsy specimen, with quantification of the level of deletion using Southern blot analysis.

Treatment

No disease-modifying therapy exists for Kearns-Sayre syndrome but symptoms can be treated traditionally.

🗗 BIBLIOGRAPHY

1. Basu AP, Posner E, McFarland R. (2012). Kearns-Sayre syndrome. [online] Available from www.emedicine.com/ped/TOPIC2763.HTM. [Accessed September, 2013].

🗗 6N. MYOPIA-OPHTHALMOPLEGIA SYNDROME

General

Sex-linked; characteristics seen in males; carried by females.

Ocular

Ptosis; myopia; complete or partial ophthalmoplegia; abnormal pupil; progressive degeneration of retina and choroid.

Clinical

Patellar reflex absent; Achilles reflex absent; spina bifida; cardiac defects; absent deep tendon reflex in carriers only.

Laboratory

Clinical.

Treatment

- *Ptosis*: If visual acuity is affected, most cases require surgical correction and there are several procedures that may be used including levator resection, repair or advancement and Fasanella-Servat.
- *Ophthalmoplegia*: A complex disorder requiring the involvement of physicians from various specialties, including neurology, cardiology, ophthalmology, and endocrinology.

🗗 BIBLIOGRAPHY

1. McKusick VA. Mendelian Inheritance in Man; A Catalog of Human Genes and Genetic Disorders, 12th edition. Baltimore: The Johns Hopkins University Press; 1998.
2. Online Mendelian Inheritance in Man, OMIM. McKusick-Nathans Institute for Genetic Medicine, Johns Hopkins University and National Center for Biotechnology Information, National Library of Medicine, February 12, 2007. Available from www.ncbi.nlm.nih.gov/omim. [Accessed September, 2013].
3. Ortiz de Zarate JC. Recessive sex-linked inheritance of congenital external ophthalmoplegia and myopia coincident with other dysplasias. Br J Ophthalmol. 1966;50:606-7.

⊟ 6O. NOTHNAGEL SYNDROME (OPHTHALMOPLEGIA-CEREBELLAR ATAXIA SYNDROME)

General

Lesion of superior cerebellar peduncle, red nucleus and emerging oculomotor fibers such as pineal tumor, or tumor or vascular disturbance in corpora quadrigemina or vermis cerebelli (*see* Bruns syndrome).

Ocular

Oculomotor paresis; gaze paralysis most frequently upward, combined with some degree of internal or external ophthalmoplegia.

Clinical

Cerebellar ataxia; poor upper extremity movements; neoplasia; infarction; midbrain lesion.

Laboratory

CT and MRI of brain.

Treatment

See neurologist.

⊟ BIBLIOGRAPHY

1. Magalini SI, Scrascia E. Dictionary of Medical Syndromes, 2nd edition. Philadelphia, PA: Lippincott Williams and Wilkins; 1981.
2. Nothnagel H. Topische Diagnostik Der Gehirnkrankheiten. Berlin: Nabu Press; 2010. p. 220.

⊟ 6P. OHAHA SYNDROME (OPHTHALMOPLEGIA, HYPOTONIA, ATAXIA, HYPOACUSIS, ATHETOSIS)

General

Ophthalmoplegia, hypotonia, ataxia, hypoacusis, athetosis (OHAHA) are distinguishing symptoms; sudden onset of deafness at an age after patient has learned to speak.

Ocular

Kernicterus; strabismus; nystagmus; ocular migraine; ophthalmoplegia; vascular spasm in branches of the ophthalmic artery; intact convergence.

Clinical

Hemiplegia; athetosis; choreoathetosis; tremor; hypoxia; corticospinal tract disease; diabetes mellitus; ataxia; medulloblastoma; asynergia; dysdiadochokinesis; Holmes rebound phenomenon; acute cerebellar lesion; dysmetria; dysarthria; Fox syndrome; vascular occlusion; congenital athetosis.

Laboratory

Diagnosis is made by clinical findings.

Treatment

- *Strabismus*: Equalized vision with correct refractive error; surgery may be helpful in patients with diplopia.
- *Local*: Ocular lubrication (drops or ointments) may be useful for exposure.

⊟ BIBLIOGRAPHY

1. Kallio AK, Jauhiainen T. A new syndrome of ophthalmoplegia, hypoacusis, ataxia, hypotonia, and athetosis (OHAHA). Adv Audiol. 1985;3:84-90.
2. McKusick VA. Mendelian Inheritance in Man; A Catalog of Human Genes and Genetic Disorders, 12th edition. Baltimore, USA: The Johns Hopkins University Press; 1998.
3. Hamosh A, Scott AF, Amberger J, et al. Online Mendelian Inheritance in Man (OMIM), a knowledgebase of human genes and genetic disorders. Nucleic Acids Res. 2002;30(1):52-5.
4. Woody RC, Blaw ME. Ophthalmoplegic migraine in infancy. Clin Pediatr (Phila). 1986;25(2):82-4.

6Q. OPHTHALMOPLEGIA, FAMILIAL STATIC

General

Autosomal dominant; forms include internal, external and total ophthalmoplegia.

Ocular

Ptosis; almost completely fixed eyes; nystagmoid movements; unequal pupils; pupil paralysis.

Clinical

None.

Laboratory

Diagnosis is made by clinical findings.

Treatment

Ptosis: If visual acuity is affected, most cases require surgical correction and there are several procedures that may be used including levator resection, repair or advancement and Fasanella-Servat procedure.

BIBLIOGRAPHY

1. Lees F. Congenital, static familial ophthalmoplegia. J Neurol Neurosurg Psychiatry. 1960;23:46-51.

6R. PAINFUL OPHTHALMOPLEGIA (PALSY OF OCULAR MUSCLES WITH PAIN)

†1. Adenocarcinoma metastatic to the orbit
†2. Atypical facial neuralgia
3. Cavernous sinus syndrome (Foix syndrome)
†4. Collier sphenoidal palsy
†5. Diabetic ophthalmoplegia
†6. Intracavernous carotid aneurysm
†7. Myositis (orbital)
†8. Nasopharyngeal tumor
9. Ophthalmoplegic migraine
10. Orbital abscess (mucormycosis-diabetes, immunosuppressed, AIDS)
11. Orbital apex sphenoidal syndrome (Rollet syndrome)
†12. Orbital periostitis
13. Postherpetic neuralgia
†14. Pseudotumor of orbit
15. Superior orbital fissure syndrome (Rochon-Duvigneaud syndrome, including superior orbital fissuritis)
16. Temporal arteritis
17. Tic douloureux of the first trigeminal division
18. Tolosa-Hunt syndrome (inflammatory lesion of cavernous sinus)

BIBLIOGRAPHY

1. Mannor GE, Rose GE, Moseley IF, et al. Outcome of orbital myositis. Ophthalmology. 1997;104:409-14.
2. Roy FH, Fraunfelder FT, Fraunfelder FW. Roy and Fraunfelder's Current Ocular Therapy, 6th edition. Philadelphia: WB Saunders; 2008.
3. Sananman ML, Weintroub MI. Remitting ophthalmoplegia due to rhabdomyosarcoma. Arch Ophthalmol. 1971;86:459-61.

†Indicates a general entry and therefore has not been described in detail in the text

6R3. FOIX SYNDROME (CAVERNOUS SINUS SYNDROME; HYPOPHYSEAL-SPHENOIDAL SYNDROME; CAVERNOUS SINUS NEURALGIA SYNDROME; GODTFREDSEN SYNDROME; CAVERNOUS SINUS-NASOPHARYNGEAL TUMOR SYNDROME; CAVERNOUS SINUS THROMBOSIS)

General

Causes include tumor of lateral sinus wall or sphenoid bone, intracranial aneurysm, cavernous and lateral sinus thrombosis, or lesions; multiple myeloma; may result from infarctions or cancer or be idiopathic.

Ocular

Proptosis; severe ocular and periorbital pain; lid edema; paresis or paralysis of cranial nerves III, IV, V, and VI; corneal anesthesia; optic atrophy.

Clinical

Postauricular edema; trigeminal neuralgia; deviation of the tongue toward paralyzed side; patients usually have prominent manifestations of sepsis and paranasal sinus; local skin infections are the most common cause.

Laboratory

CT, MRI.

Treatment

Radiotherapy, anticoagulation, high-dose antibiotic therapy.

BIBLIOGRAPHY

1. Kattah JC, Pula JH. (2012). Cavernous sinus syndromes. [online] Available from www.emedicine.com/neuro/topic572.htm. [Accessed September, 2013].

6R9. OPHTHALMOPLEGIC MIGRAINE SYNDROME

General

Symptoms produced by ipsilateral herniation of hippocampal gyrus of temporal lobe through incisura tentorii; dependent upon unilateral cerebral edema due to vascular or vasomotor phenomena, intracranial aneurysm, or tumor; incidence may be greater in women with the initial attack in the 1st decade of life; pathogenesis is unclear, but it is likely secondary to ischemia of the ocular motor nerve.

Ocular

Severe unilateral supraorbital pain; ptosis; transitory partial or complete homolateral oculomotor paralysis; fourth or sixth nerve occasionally involved; retinal hemorrhages; papilledema (may be bilateral); moderate to severe headache with partial to complete cranial nerve III paresis including the pupil; more than one ocular nerve may be affected.

Clinical

Migraine headache, not present in all instances; dizziness; diminution in sense of smell; hypalgesia contralateral side of face; nausea/vomiting may be present; recurrent sinus arrest.

Laboratory

Clinical.

Treatment

Ptosis: If visual acuity is affected, most cases require surgical correction and there are several procedures that may be used including levator resection, repair or advancement and Fasanella-Servat.

BIBLIOGRAPHY

1. Bazak I, Margulis T, Shnaider H, et al. Ophthalmoplegic migraine and recurrent sinus arrest. J Neurol Neurosurg Psychiatry. 1991;54:935.
2. Ehlers H. On pathogenesis of ophthalmoplegic migraine. Acta Psychiatr Neurol (Scand). 1928;3:219.
3. Geeraets WJ. Ocular Syndromes, 3rd edition. Philadelphia: Lea & Febiger; 1976.
4. Gulkilik G, Cagatay H, Oba E, et al. Ophthalmoplegic migraine associated with recurrent isolated ptosis. Ann Ophthal. 2010;41:206-12.
5. Raskin NH. Migraine and other headaches. In: Rowland LP (Ed). Merritt's Textbook of Neurology, 9th edition. Baltimore: Williams & Wilkins; 1995. pp. 837-45.
6. Stommel EW, Ward TN, Harris RD. Ophthalmoplegic migraine or Tolosa-Hunt syndrome? Headache. 1994;34:177.
7. Van Pelt W, Andermann F. On the early onset of ophthalmologic migraine. Am J Dis Child. 1964;107:628.
8. Vijayan N. Ophthalmoplegic migraine: ischemic or compressive neuropathy? Headache. 1980;20:300-4.

6R10. MUCORMYCOSIS (PHYCOMYCOSIS)

General

Acute, often fatal infection caused by saprophytic fungi; associated with diabetes mellitus and ketoacidosis.

Ocular

Corneal ulcer; striate keratopathy; ptosis; panophthalmitis; proptosis; cellulitis of orbit; immobile pupil; retinitis; optic neuritis; paralysis of extraocular muscles; central retinal artery thrombosis.

Clinical

Epistaxis; nasal discharge; facial pain; facial palsies; anhidrosis; cranial nerve or peripheral motor and sensory nerve deficits may occur.

Laboratory

Tissue biopsy and culture of paranasal sinuses demonstrate the presence of the fungi, which appear as broad, irregular, nonseptate, branching hyphae on Hematoxylin and Eosin (H & E) stain.

Treatment

Amphotericin B.

BIBLIOGRAPHY

1. Crum-Cianflone NF. (2011). Mucormycosis. [online] Available from www.emedicine.com/oph/TOPIC225.HTM. [Accessed September, 2013].

6R10. ACQUIRED IMMUNODEFICIENCY SYNDROME (AIDS; ACQUIRED CELLULAR IMMUNODEFICIENCY; ACQUIRED IMMUNODEFICIENCY)

General

Acquired breakdown of the immune system followed by disease that takes advantage of the body's collapsed defenses; acquired by shared drug needles or sexual intercourse; occurs most frequently in homosexually active men (75%), intravenous drug abusers (13%), and Haitian immigrants (6%).

Ocular

Retinal cotton-wool spots; CMV retinitis; retinal periphlebitis; conjunctival Kaposi sarcoma; necrotizing retinitis; retinal hemorrhages; conjunctivitis sicca; orbital Burkitt lymphoma; peripheral retinochoroiditis; vitreitis; fungal corneal ulcer; hypopyon; acute glaucoma; third nerve palsy; anterior uveitis; atypical retinitis; orbital pseudotumor; herpes zoster ophthalmicus; herpes simplex keratitis; bacterial keratitis; molluscum contagiosum; CMV retinitis; toxoplasma retinitis; acute retinal necrosis; HIV retinitis; syphilitic retinitis; *P. carinii* choroiditis; fungal and bacterial endophthalmitis; fungal choroiditis; conjunctival microvasculopathy; keratitis sicca; subconjunctival hemorrhage.

Clinical

Because of lowered immunity, one third develops Kaposi sarcoma; pneumonia caused by *P. carinii*; death.

Laboratory

ELISA test is used for screening other tests are used to evaluate false-positive and false-negative test results.

Treatment

Medical consultations are required for systemic treatment. The treatment of CMV retinitis can include drugs such as ganciclovir, valganciclovir, fomivirsen, foscarnet and cidofovir. All of these drugs have specific adverse effects and complicate the decision to use for treatment.

BIBLIOGRAPHY

1. Dubin J. (2011). Rapid Testing for HIV. [online] Available from www.emedicine.com/emerg/TOPIC253.HTM. [Accessed September, 2013].

6R11. ROLLET SYNDROME (ORBITAL APEX-SPHENOIDAL SYNDROME) OPTIC NEURITIS

General

Lesion in the apex of the orbit (neoplastic, hemorrhagic, or inflammatory) involving the third, fourth, and sixth cranial nerves, the ophthalmic branch of the fifth sympathetic fibers when they pass through the sphenoidal fissure, and the optic nerve; manifestations vary greatly with extent of lesion; pain is frequent early sign; orbital fissure syndrome and sphenocavernous syndrome are similar; sudden onset.

Ocular

Exophthalmos; ptosis; hyperesthesia or anesthesia of the upper lid; ophthalmoplegia (partial or complete); wide pupil with loss of reaction on accommodation; neuralgic pain in the region of the ophthalmic branch of cranial nerve V; anesthesia of the cornea; papilledema; optic neuritis; optic atrophy; diplopia; herpes zoster ophthalmicus.

Clinical

Hyperesthesia or anesthesia of the forehead; inflammation of cavernous sinuses; meningoencephalitis.

Laboratory

Diagnosis is made by clinical findings.

Treatment

Exophthalmos: Reversing the problem which is causing the exophthalmos is the treatment of choice and will minimize the ocular complications. Ocular lubricants are beneficial for control of the corneal exposure.

BIBLIOGRAPHY

1. Bourke RD, Pyle J. Herpes zoster ophthalmicus and the orbital apex syndrome. Aust N Z J Ophthalmol. 1994;22: 77-80.
2. Goldberg RA, Hannani K, Toga AW. Microanatomy of the orbital apex. Computed tomography and microcryoplaning of soft and hard tissue. Ophthalmology. 1992;99:1447-52.

6R13. HUNT SYNDROME (RAMSAY-HUNT SYNDROME; GENICULATE NEURALGIA; HERPES ZOSTER AURICULARIS)

General

Herpes of the geniculate ganglion; course is prolonged; characterized by severe pain that frequently precedes skin and mucosal lesions and may persist for some time after lesions have disappeared; sulfuiduronate enzyme deficiency.

Ocular

Diminished lacrimation; absence of motor corneal reflex on affected side, whereas consensual reflex of noninvolved eye remains normal.

Clinical

Herpes zoster lesions of external ear and oral mucosa; severe pain in area of external auditory meatus and pinna; diminished hearing; tinnitus; vertigo, facial palsy; diminution or total loss of superficial and deep facial reflexes; zoster lesions may involve the scalp, face, and neck; hoarseness; absence of auricular lesions has been reported; progressive dementia; extensive frontal white matter change; myoclonus; ataxia; facial paralysis; tinnitus; hearing loss; hyperacusis; vertigo; dysgeusia; seizures; cerebellar ataxia; schizophrenia-like symptoms.

Laboratory

Diagnosed mostly on the basis of the characteristic pain and appearance of the dermatomal rashes.

Treatment

Antiviral agents, systemic corticosteroids, antidepressants, and adequate pain control.

BIBLIOGRAPHY

1. Adour KK. Otological complications of herpes zoster. Ann Neurol. 1994;35:S62-4.
2. Blackley B, Friedmann I, Wright I. Herpes zoster auris associated with facial nerve palsy and auditory nerve symptoms: a case report with histopathological findings. Acta Otolaryngol. 1967;63:533-50.
3. Collins JF. Handbook of Clinical Ophthalmology. New York: Masson; 1982.
4. Hori T, Mizukami K, Suzuki T, et al. Ramsay Hunt syndrome with mental disorder. Jpn J Psychiatry Neurol. 1991;45:873-7.
5. Hunt JR. On herpetic inflammations of the geniculate ganglion: a new syndrome and its complications. J Nerv Ment Dis N Y. 1907;34:73.
6. Kobayashi K, Morikawa K, Fukutani Y et al. Ramsay Hunt syndrome: progressive mental deterioration in association with unusual cerebral white matter change. Clin Neuropathol. 1994;13(2):88-96.
7. Shapiro BE, Slattery M, Pessin MS. Absence of auricular lesions in Ramsay Hunt syndrome. Neurology. 1994;44:773-4.

6R15. ROCHON-DUVIGNEAUD SYNDROME (SUPERIOR ORBITAL FISSURE SYNDROME) OPTIC ATROPHY

General

Inflammatory, traumatic, tumor, or vascular lesions such as meningioma of the sphenoid, carotid aneurysm, and arachnoiditis; infections originating in the maxillary sinus.

Ocular

Mild exophthalmos; lid edema; partial or complete ophthalmoplegia (III, IV and VI); decreased corneal sensitivity; papilledema; optic atrophy.

Clinical

Decreased sensitivity in area of nasociliary, lacrimal, frontal, and ophthalmic nerve distribution; may result from a metastatic tumor.

Laboratory

CBC count, ESR, thyroid function test, FTA, ANA, LE preparation, ANCA, serum protein electrophoresis, Lyme titer, ACE level and HIV titer are helpful. CSF, anti-GQ1b antibodies, and MRI of the brain and the orbits.

Treatment

Corticosteroids are the treatment of choice.

BIBLIOGRAPHY

1. Falcone F, Lazow SK, Berger JR, et al. Superior orbital fissure syndrome. Secondary to infected dentigerous cyst of the maxillary sinus. NY State Dental J. 1994;60:62-4.
2. Hedstrom J, Parsons J, Maloney PL, et al. Superior orbital fissure syndrome: report of a case. J Oral Surg. 1974; 32:198-201.
3. Phanthumchinda K, Hemachuda T. Superior orbital fissure syndrome as a presenting symptom in hepatocellular carcinoma. J Med Assoc Thailand. 1992;75:62-5.
4. Rochon-Duvigneaud A. Quelques Cas de Paralysie de Tous les Nerfs Orbitaires (Ophtalmoplegie Totale avec Amaurose et Anesthesie dans le Domaine de l'Ophtalmique d'Origine Syphilitique). Arch Ophthalmol. 1896;16:746.

6R16. TEMPORAL ARTERITIS SYNDROME (CRANIAL ARTERITIS SYNDROME; GIANT CELL ARTERITIS; HUTCHINSON-HORTON-MAGATH-BROWN SYNDROME)

General

Etiology unknown; mainly females; mainly Whites; ages 55–80 years; temporal artery shows inflammatory thickening; arteritis of the vessels supplying the optic nerve.

Ocular

Transient ptosis; partial or complete loss of vision on the affected side; retinal detachment; exudates and hemorrhages; narrowing of retinal vessels; obstruction of the central retinal artery; optic atrophy; ischemic optic neuropathy; acute decreased IOP; corneal hypesthesia; palsies of extraocular muscles; hemorrhagic glaucoma; diplopia; hemorrhages on or around the disk.

Clinical

Throbbing headache; hyperalgesia of the scalp; malaise; anorexia; weakness; weight loss; fever; nodular pulmonary nodules; cough; otitis with deafness.

Laboratory

Elevated ESR greater than 50 mm/hour, positive temporal artery biopsy.

Treatment

Systemic corticosteroids are the therapy of choice.

BIBLIOGRAPHY

1. Allen AW, Biega T, Varma MK. (2012). Temporal arteritis imaging. [online] Available from www.emedicine.com/radio/TOPIC675.HTM. [Accessed September, 2013].
2. Walvick MD, Walvick MP. Giant cell arteritis: laboratory predictors of a positive temporal artery biopsy. Ophthalmology. 2011;118(6):1201-4.

6R17. TIC DOULOUREUX (TRIGEMINAL NEURALGIA)

General

Brief, sharp, unilateral facial pain that usually occurs in the middle or lower face; occurs more often in females; occurs most frequently in persons over age 40 years; right side affected more than left side.

Ocular

Ipsilateral hyperemia with the pain of conjunctiva; periorbital pain; ipsilateral lacrimation during the pain; decreased corneal sensitivity; photophobia.

Clinical

Pain triggered by chewing, swallowing, laughing, brushing teeth, shaving, or combing hair; may be present with MS.

Laboratory

MRI and MRA will demonstrate structural compression of the trigeminal rootlet.

Treatment

Systemic medication such as carbamazepine and phenytoin are particularly useful.

BIBLIOGRAPHY

1. Huff JS. (2012). Trigeminal neuralgia in emergency medicine. [online] Available from www.emedicine.com/emerg/TOPIC617.HTM. [Accessed September, 2013].

6R18. TOLOSA-HUNT SYNDROME (PAINFUL OPHTHALMOPLEGIA)

General

Symptoms last from days to weeks; attacks recur at intervals of months or years; inflammatory lesion of cavernous sinus; onset most frequent in 5th decade of life; recurrent Tolosa-Hunt syndrome has been observed in some patients.

Ocular

Steadily "growing" retro-orbital pain; ptosis; involvement of cranial nerves III, IV, VI and first division of V; scintillating scotoma; sluggish pupil reaction to light; corneal sensitivity diminished; optic neuritis.

Clinical

Inflammatory lesions of cavernous sinus.

Laboratory

MRI with axial and coronal views of brain, typically showing thickening and enhancement of involved cavernous sinus. Cerebral angiography is done to rule out aneurysm. Blood count, ESR, ANA, ANCA and ACE levels may be abnormal.

Treatment

Corticosteroids is often used to treat the chronic granulomatous inflammation of the cavernous sinus.

BIBLIOGRAPHY

1. Taylor DC. (2012). Tolosa-Hunt syndrome. [online] Available from www.emedicine.com/neuro/TOPIC373.HTM. [Accessed September, 2013].

6S. OPHTHALMOPLEGIA, PROGRESSIVE EXTERNAL

General

Autosomal recessive; progressive limitation of ocular motility with clinical sparing of pupillary function; underlying pathogenesis is secondary to a mitochondrial cytopathy; appearance of ragged-red fibers in the abnormal muscles is primarily caused by mitochondrial accumulations beneath the plasma membrane and between the myofibrils.

Ocular

Oculopharyngeal muscular dystrophy; retinitis pigmentosa; progressive external ophthalmoplegia; some patients show only ptosis and ophthalmoplegia; most patients have multisystem involvement.

Clinical

Heart block; ataxia.

Laboratory

Thyroid studies, acetylcholine receptor antibody. MRI, CT and ultrasound may show enlarged extraocular muscles.

Treatment

If ptosis is present, lid crutches may be helpful or ptosis surgery. Strabismus surgery may be helpful in patients with diplopia.

BIBLIOGRAPHY

1. Roy H. (2011). Chronic progressive external ophthalmoplegia. [online] Available from www.emedicine.com/oph/TOPIC510.HTM. [Accessed September, 2013].

6T. OPHTHALMOPLEGIA, PROGRESSIVE EXTERNAL, WITH RAGGED RED FIBERS

General

Autosomal dominant.

Ocular

Progressive ophthalmoplegia.

Clinical

Ragged-red fibers in skeletal muscle from the extremities; subsarcolemmal clusters of mitochondria containing paracrystalline inclusions.

Laboratory

Thyroid studies, acetylcholine receptor antibody. MRI, CT and ultrasound may show enlarged extraocular muscles.

Treatment

If ptosis is present, lid crutches may be helpful or ptosis surgery. Strabismus surgery may be helpful in patients with diplopia.

BIBLIOGRAPHY

1. Roy H. (2011). Chronic progressive external ophthalmoplegia. [online] Available from www.emedicine.com/oph/TOPIC510.HTM. [Accessed September, 2013].

6U. OPHTHALMOPLEGIA, PROGRESSIVE EXTERNAL, WITH SCROTAL TONGUE AND MENTAL DEFICIENCY

General

Autosomal dominant.

Ocular

Progressive external ophthalmoplegia; progressive chorioretinal sclerosis; bilateral ptosis; convergence paresis; myopia; optic atrophy; retinitis pigmentosa.

Clinical

Bilateral facial weakness; lingua scrotalis; mental retardation; cerebellar ataxia; weakness and spasticity of the limbs.

Laboratory

Thyroid studies, acetylcholine receptor antibody. MRI, CT and ultrasound may show enlarged extraocular muscles.

Treatment

If ptosis is present, lid crutches may be helpful or ptosis surgery. Strabismus surgery may be helpful in patients with diplopia.

BIBLIOGRAPHY

1. Roy H. (2011). Chronic progressive external ophthalmoplegia. [online] Available from www.emedicine.com/oph/TOPIC510.HTM. [Accessed September, 2013].

6V. PROGRESSIVE EXTERNAL OPHTHALMOPLEGIA AND SCOLIOSIS

General

Rare; isolated muscle dystrophic involvement of extraocular muscles; onset in childhood or early adulthood; slowly progressive.

Ocular

Horizontal gaze paralysis; pendular nystagmus; ptosis; orbicularis oculi weakness.

Clinical

Scoliosis; facial myokymia; contracture of facial muscles.

Laboratory

Diagnosis is made by clinical findings.

Treatment

- *Nystagmus*:
  - Seesaw nystagmus: Visual field to consider neoplastic or vascular etiologies.
  - Upbeat nystagmus: It may indicate MS, cerebellar degeneration, tumors or infarcts. Treatment is directed toward the identification and resolution of underlying cause.
  - Downbeat nystagmus: It affects the cerebellum or craniocervical junction including Arnold-Chiari malformation, MS, trauma, tumor, infarction and many toxic metabolic entities. MRI may indicate a surgically correctable lesion. Periodic alternating nystagmus is continuous horizontal nystagmus from stroke, tumor, MS, trauma, infection and drug intoxication. It can occur from cataract, vitreous hemorrhage or optic atrophy.
- *Ptosis*: If visual acuity is affected, most cases require surgical correction and there are several procedures that may be used including levator resection, repair or advancement and Fasanella-Servat.

BIBLIOGRAPHY

1. Moore MH, Wong KS, Proudman TW, et al. Progressive hemifacial atrophy (Romberg's disease): skeletal involvement and treatment. Br J Plast Surg. 1993;46(1):39-44.
2. Roddi R, Riggio E, Gilbert PM, et al. Clinical evaluation of techniques used in the surgical treatment of progressive hemifacial atrophy. J Craniomaxillofac Surg. 1994;22(1):23-32.

6W. PSEUDOOPHTHALMOPLEGIA SYNDROME (ROTH-BIELSCHOWSKY SYNDROME)

General

Supranuclear lesion in the temporal lobe.

Ocular

Paralysis of lateral gaze in one direction; vestibular nystagmus in which the fast phase is absent on the ipsilateral side but the slow phase is present.

Clinical

Basal ganglia or tectal lesion.

Laboratory

Diagnosis is made by clinical findings.

Treatment

See neurologist.

BIBLIOGRAPHY

1. Bielschowsky A. Das Klinische Bild der Assoziierten Blicklahmung und Seine Bedeutung fur die Topische Diagnostik. Munchen Med Wochenschr. 1903;40:1666.
2. Cogan DG, Adams RD. Type of paralysis of conjugate gaze (ocular motor apraxia). AMA Arch Ophthalmol. 1953;50(4):434-42.
3. Geeraets WJ. Ocular Syndromes, 3rd edition. Philadelphia, PA: Lea & Febiger; 1976.
4. Roth WC. Demonstration von Kranken mit Ophthalmoplegie. Neurol Zentbl. 1901;20:921.

🗗 6X. TOLOSA-HUNT SYNDROME (PAINFUL OPHTHALMOPLEGIA)

General

Symptoms last from days to weeks; attacks recur at intervals of months or years; inflammatory lesion of cavernous sinus; onset most frequent in 5th decade of life; recurrent Tolosa-Hunt syndrome has been observed in some patients.

Ocular

Steadily "growing" retro-orbital pain; ptosis; involvement of cranial nerves III, IV, VI, and first division of V; scintillating scotomata; sluggish pupil reaction to light; corneal sensitivity diminished; optic neuritis.

Clinical

Inflammatory lesions of cavernous sinus.

Laboratory

MRI with axial and coronal views of brain, typically showing thickening and enhancement of involved cavernous sinus. Cerebral angiography is done to rule out aneurysm. Blood count, ESR, ANA, ANCA and ACE levels may be abnormal.

Treatment

Corticosteroids is often used to treat the chronic granulomatous inflammation of the cavernous sinus.

🗗 BIBLIOGRAPHY

1. Taylor DC. (2012). Tolosa-Hunt syndrome. [online] Available from www.emedicine.com/neuro/TOPIC373.HTM. [Accessed September, 2013].

🗗 6Y. WEBINO SYNDROME (WALL-EYED BILATERAL INTERNUCLEAR OPHTHALMOPLEGIA)

General

Differential diagnosis includes demyelinating disease, arteriosclerotic cerebrovascular disease, trauma, Arnold-Chiari malformation, syphilis, periarteritis nodosa, glioma, Cryptococcal meningitis and premature infants; usually represents midline involvement of oculomotor nucleus.

Ocular

Wall-eyed internuclear ophthalmoplegia (bilateral internuclear ophthalmoplegia with exotropia).

Clinical

Depends on cause; associated with MS in young patients.

Laboratory

Diagnosis is made by clinical findings.

Treatment

Evaluate internuclear ophthalmoplegia.

🗗 BIBLIOGRAPHY

1. Daroff RE, Hoyt WE. Supranuclear disorders of ocular control systems in man. In: Bach-Y-Rita P, Collins CC (Eds). The Control of Eye Movements. Orlando, FL: Academic Press; 1971. p. 223.
2. Lepore FE, Nissenblatt MJ. Bilateral internuclear ophthalmoplegia after intrathecal chemotherapy and cranial irradiation. Am J Ophthalmol. 1981;92(6):851-3.
3. Miller NR (Ed). Walsh and Hoyt's Clinical Neuro-Ophthalmology, 4th edition. Baltimore, USA: Williams & Wilkins; 1995. p. 4323.

🗗 7. CONGENITAL VERTICAL RETRACTION SYNDROME

General

Congenital.

Ocular

Aberrant regeneration of the oculomotor nerve; concurrent protective eyelid closure; congenital alterations in the extraocular muscle, its insertion and peripheral innervation; nystagmus retractorius; surgical or traumatic rearrangement of orbital structures may account for retraction.

Clinical

None.

Laboratory

Diagnosis is made by clinical findings.

Treatment

None.

BIBLIOGRAPHY

1. Khodadoust AA, von Noorden GK. Bilateral vertical retraction syndrome. A family study. Arch Ophthalmol. 1967;78(5):606-12.
2. Osher RH, Schatz NJ, Duane TD. Acquired orbital retraction syndrome. Arch Ophthalmol. 1980;98(10):1798-802.
3. Pesando P, Nuzzi G, Maraini G. Vertical retraction syndrome. Ophthalmologica. 1978;177(5):254-9.

8. DUANE SYNDROME (RETRACTION SYNDROME; STILLING SYNDROME; TURK-STILLING SYNDROME)

General

Autosomal dominant; more frequent in females; manifestations in infancy; was thought to be secondary to fibrosis of the LR muscle or abnormal check ligaments; now established to be due to congenital aberrant innervation affecting third and seventh cranial nerves.

Ocular

Narrowing of palpebral fissure on adduction, widening on abduction; primary global retraction; deficiency of medial and lateral recti motility; limitation of abduction in affected eye usually is complete; retraction of the globe with attempted adduction varies from 1 mm to 10 mm; convergence insufficiency; heterochromia irides; left eye is more frequently involved.

Clinical

Associated Klippel-Feil syndrome; malformation of face, ears and teeth.

Laboratory

Diagnosis is made by clinical findings.

Treatment

Indications for surgery include anomalous head position, strabismus in primary gaze, significant upshot or downshoot in adduction and cosmetically significant palpebral fissure. Duane retraction syndrome type 1 (DRS-1) (absent abduction, esotropia in primary position and head turn toward the affected side to fuse) medial rectus recession of the affected eye; DRS with exotropia—recess LR of involved side. Retraction of the globe—recess medial and lateral rectus of involved eye. Upshoots and downshoots—recess the LR.

BIBLIOGRAPHY

1. Verma A. (2011). Duane syndrome. [online] Available from www.emedicine.com/oph/TOPIC326.HTM. [Accessed September, 2013].

9. GENERAL FIBROSIS SYNDROME (CONGENITAL ENOPHTHALMOS WITH OCULAR MUSCLE FIBROSIS AND PTOSIS; CONGENITAL FIBROSIS OF THE INFERIOR RECTUS WITH PTOSIS; STRABISMUS FIXUS; VERTICAL RETRACTION SYNDROME (CONGENITAL FIBROSIS SYNDROME)

General

Present from birth; familial history; apparent autosomal dominant transmission; sex-linked recessive transmission is also reported.

Ocular

Ptosis; enophthalmos; disk hypoplasia; astigmatism; esotropia; exotropia; hypotropia; nystagmus; visual loss; positive forced duction test; it may be associated with

Marcus Gunn jaw-winking and synergistic divergence in attempted right gaze.

Clinical

None.

Laboratory

Neuroimaging is the most essential laboratory study.

Treatment

Surgically approximating normal orbital bone positions, before addressing soft tissue volume loss.

⧉ BIBLIOGRAPHY

1. Soparkar CN. (2012). Enophthalmos. [online] Available fromwww.emedicine.com/oph/TOPIC617.HTM.[Accessed September, 2013].

CHAPTER 22

Eyelids

1. DISORDERS

1A. ABERFELD SYNDROME (SCHWARTZ-JAMPEL SYNDROME; CONGENITAL BLEPHAROPHIMOSIS ASSOCIATED WITH GENERALIZED MYOPATHY SYNDROME; OCULAR AND FACIAL ABNORMALITIES SYNDROME)

General

Etiology is not known; autosomal recessive inheritance, although there are reports of dominant inheritance; progressive disorder.

Ocular

Blepharophimosis; exotropia; myopia; congenital cataracts; microcornea.

Clinical

Myopathy; bone deformities; arachnodactyly; dwarfism; hypoplastic facial bones; hypertrichosis; kyphoscoliosis.

Laboratory

Physicians might consider referring suspected cases to genetic clinics that have affiliations with groups actively research so that genetic studies can be performed. Muscle biopsy findings are consistent with a myopathy.

Treatment

The goal is to reduce the abnormal muscle activity that causes stiffness. Botulinum toxin therapy may be considered for the treatment of blepharospasm. However, if ptosis is present this is contraindicated. Some medications that have been found useful in myotonic disorders include the anticonvulsants and the antiarrhythmics.

BIBLIOGRAPHY

1. Ault J, Berman SA, Dinnerstein E. (2012). Schwartz-Jampel syndrome. [online] Available from www.emedicine.com/neuro/TOPIC337.HTM. [Accessed September, 2013].

1B. BELL'S PALSY (IDIOPATHIC FACIAL PARALYSIS)

General

Unilateral facial nerve paralysis of sudden onset and gradual recovery involving the nerve as it runs through the fallopian canal; etiology unknown; more common in adults.

Ocular

Corneal ulcer; paralysis of seventh nerve; ectropion; lagophthalmos; ptosis; epiphora; decreased visual acuity; diplopia; ocular irritation; exposure keratitis.

Clinical

Aching in the ear or mastoid; tingling or numbness of cheek or mouth; alteration of taste; hyperacusis; epiphora; facial weakness; most commonly and frequently affected cranial nerve with herpes zoster is the facial nerve.

Laboratory

It is not diagnosed by clinical findings.

Treatment

Most patients recover without treatment. If spontaneous recovery does not occur, the most widely accepted treatment is corticosteroids.

BIBLIOGRAPHY

1. Taylor DC, Khoromi S, Zachariah SB. (2012). Bell palsy. [online] Available from www.emedicine.com/neuro/TOPIC413.HTM. [Accessed September, 2013].

1C. BLEPHAROCHALASIS

General

Rare, with recurrent episodic painless periorbital edema.

Clinical

None.

Ocular

Skin of the lids is thin and baggy.

Laboratory

Diagnosis is made by clinical findings.

Treatment

Cold compress may be of some use. Surgical—excise the redundant skin, reposition the ectopic lacrimal gland and reconstruct lateral canthal tendon.

BIBLIOGRAPHY

1. Roy FH, Fraunfelder FW, Fraunfelder FT. Roy and Fraunfelder's Current Ocular Therapy, 6th edition. London, UK: Elsevier; 2008.

1D. BLEPHAROPHIMOSIS SYNDROME (SIMOSA SYNDROME)

General

Dominantly inherited tetrad of ptosis, epicanthus inversus, telecanthus and blepharophimosis.

Ocular

Scarred or contracted in the secondary blepharophimosis because of ocular pemphigus or trachoma; ectropion; epicanthus inversus; lacrimal puncta displacement; ptosis; telecanthus; optic nerve coloboma; angle dysgenesis; optic nerve hypoplasia; amblyopia; strabismus.

Clinical

Low-set ears; low nasal bridge.

Laboratory

Diagnosis is made by clinical findings.

Treatment

The ptosis is corrected by frontalis fixation at an early age. Canthoplasties may be performed to improve the blepharophimosis. The considerable epicanthus is usually best left until early adolescence, since the degree of this problem tends to diminish with time and the skin becomes easier to move.

BIBLIOGRAPHY

1. Bashour M. (2012). Ptosis blepharoplasty. [online] Available from www.emedicine.com/ent/TOPIC97.HTM. [Accessed September, 2013].

⊟ 1E. BLEPHAROPTOSIS, MYOPIA, ECTOPIA LENTIS

General

Autosomal dominant.

Ocular

Ptosis; high-grade myopia; ectopia lentis; displacement of crystalline lens of eye; connective tissue defect of sclera, zonules, and levator aponeurosis.

Clinical

None.

Laboratory

Diagnosis is made by clinical findings.

Treatment

Observation is only required in mild cases of congenital ptosis if no signs of amblyopia, strabismus, and abnormal head posture are present. Surgical correction may be necessary with more severe cases. Earlier intervention may be required if significant amblyopia or ocular torticollis is present.

⊟ BIBLIOGRAPHY

1. Suh DW. (2012). Congenital ptosis. [online] Available from www.emedicine.com/oph/TOPIC345.HTM. [Accessed September, 2013].

⊟ 1F. CHARGE ASSOCIATION (MULTIPLE CONGENITAL ANOMALIES SYNDROME; COLOBOMA, HEART DISEASE, ATRESIA, RETARDED GROWTH, GENITAL HYPOPLASIA, EAR MALFORMATION ASSOCIATION)

General

Syndrome consists of four of six major manifestations of ocular coloboma, heart disease, atresia, retarded growth and development, genital hypoplasia, and ear malformations with or without hearing loss.

Ocular

Blepharoptosis; iris coloboma; optic nerve coloboma; macular hypoplasia; lacrimal canalicular atresia; nasolacrimal duct obstruction.

Clinical

Microcephaly; brachycephaly; malformed ear; bilateral finger contractures; heart disease; genital hypoplasia; heart disease; choanal atresia; retarded growth; hearing loss; facial nerve palsies; mental retardation.

Laboratory

CHD7 mutation analysis is diagnostic in 58–71% of individuals who meet the clinical criteria, head computed tomography (CT) and magnetic resonance imaging (MRI), cranial ultrasound.

Treatment

Secure airway, stabilize the patient, exclude major life-threatening congenital anomalies and transfer the individual with coloboma of the eye, heart defects, atresia of the nasal choanae, retardation of growth and/or development, genital and/or urinary abnormalities, and ear abnormalities and deafness (CHARGE) syndrome to a specialist center with pediatric otolaryngologist and other subspecialty services.

⊟ BIBLIOGRAPHY

1. Tegay DH, Yedowitz JC. (2012). CHARGE syndrome. [online] Available from www.emedicine.com/ped/TOPIC367.HTM. [Accessed September, 2013].

🗗 1G. LID COLOBOMA

1. Amniogenic band syndrome (amniotic bands-Streeter anomaly)
2. Epidermal nevus syndrome
3. Fraser syndrome
4. Frontonasal dysplasia syndrome
5. Goldenhar syndrome (oculoauriculovertebral dysplasia)
6. Miller syndrome
7. Nager syndrome
8. Nevus sebaceous of Jadassohn (linear sebaceous nevus syndrome)
9. Palpebral coloboma-lipoma syndrome
†*10. Traumatic
11. Treacher Collins-Franceschetti syndrome (mandibulofacial dysostosis)

Treatment

Protecting the cornea is important in the treatment of lid coloboma.

🗗 BIBLIOGRAPHY

1. Bashour M. (2012). Eyelid Coloboma. [online] Available from www.emedicine.com/oph/TOPIC673.HTM. [Accessed September, 2013].

Indicates a general entry and therefore has not been described in detail in the text

🗗 1G1. AMNIOGENIC BAND SYNDROME (RING CONSTRICTION; STREETER DYSPLASIA)

General

It is caused by fetus swallowing one or more of the free-floating strands that result from amniotic rupture; the tension of these strands intraorally and extraorally produces secondary tears and deformations; no hereditary factor known.

Ocular

Upward slant of palpebral fissures; bilateral upper and lower lid colobomas; telecanthus; bilateral corneal opacities; microphthalmos; strabismus; hypertelorism; epibulbar choristoma; unilateral chorioretinal defects or lacuna (rare).

Clinical

Craniofacial and limb abnormalities.

Laboratory

Diagnosis is made by clinical findings.

Treatment

Equalized vision with correct refractive error; surgery may be helpful in patient with strabismus.

🗗 BIBLIOGRAPHY

1. Braude LS, Miller M, Cuttone J. Ocular abnormalities in the anmiogenic band syndrome. Br J Ophthalmol. 1981;65:299-303.
2. Hashemi K, Traboulsi EI, Chavis R, et al. Chorioretinal lacuna in the anmiotic band syndrome. J Pediatr Ophthalmol Strabismus. 1991;28:238-9.
3. Miller MT, Deutsch TA, Cronin C, et al. Amniotic bands as a cause of ocular anomalies. Am J Ophthalmol. 1987;104:270-9.
4. Murata T, Hashimoto S, Ishibashi T, et al. A case of anmiotic band syndrome with bilateral epibulbar choristoma. Br J Ophthalmol. 1992;76:685-7.
5. Streeter GL. Focal deficiencies in fetal tissues and their relation to intrauterine amputation. Contrib Embryol Carney Inst. 1930;22:1-44.

🗗 1G2. EPIDERMAL NEVUS SYNDROME (ICHTHYOSIS HYSTRIX)

General

One or a combination of the following epidermal nevi described as nevus unius lateris, ichthyosis hystrix, linear nevus sebaceous, or congenital acanthosis nigricans; autosomal dominant.

Ocular

Blepharoptosis and fibroma on bulbar conjunctiva; antimongoloid eyelid fissures; eyelid colobomata; horizontal and rotary nystagmus; esotropia; conjunctival tumors; corneal opacities; corectopia and colobomata of the iris.

Clinical

Somatic anomalies involving the skeletal and central nervous system (CNS); anomalies of bone formation; atrophy; ankylosis; vitamin D-resistant rickets; bone cysts; mental retardation; cortical atrophy; hydrocephalus; focal and grand mal epilepsy; cerebrovascular tumors; cortical blindness.

Laboratory

Histologic examination, electroencephalogram (EEG), MRI.

Treatment

Vitamin D analogs may work by inhibiting epidermal proliferation, promoting keratinocyte differentiation, and/or exerting immunosuppressive effects on lymphoid cells.

BIBLIOGRAPHY

1. Schwartz RA, Jozwiak S. (2013). Epidermal nevus syndrome. [online] Available from www.emedicine.com/derm/TOPIC732.HTM. [Accessed September, 2013].

1G3. CRYPTOPHTHALMIA SYNDROME (CRYPTOPHTHALMOS SYNDACTYLY SYNDROME; FRASER SYNDROME)

General

Autosomal recessive.

Ocular

Microphthalmia; epibulbar dermoid; cryptophthalmos; enophthalmia; eyebrows partially or completely missing; skin from forehead completely covers one or both eyes, but the globes can be palpated beneath the skin; in unilateral cases, the fellow eye may present lid coloboma; buphthalmos; conjunctival sac partially or totally obliterated; absence of trabeculae, Schlemm canal, and ciliary muscles; cornea is differentiated from the sclera; lens anomalies from complete absence to hypoplasia, dislocation, and calcification.

Clinical

Syndactyly (finger, toes) (about 40%); coloboma of alae nasi and nostrils; urogenital abnormalities, including pseudohermaphroditism and renal hypoplasia; abnormal, bizarre hairline; narrow external auditory meatus and malformation of ossicles; cleft lip and palate may occur; atresia or hypoplasia of larynx in some cases; hoarse voice; dysplastic pinna; meatal stenosis; glottic web and subglottic stenosis.

Laboratory

Antenatal ultrasonography; radiography of the abdomen; contrast enema; rectal biopsy.

Treatment

Management of the congenital defects.

BIBLIOGRAPHY

1 Rosen NG, Zitsman J, Aidlen JT. (2013). Atresia, Stenosis, and Other Obstruction of the Colon. [online] Available from www.emedicine.com/ped/TOPIC2928.HTM. [Accessed September, 2013].

1G4. FRONTONASAL DYSPLASIA SYNDROME (MEDIAN CLEFT FACE SYNDROME)

General

Congenital disorder without genetic background; condition may present a variety of facial malformations, depending on the stage of embryonic development at which interference occurs.

Ocular

Hypertelorism; anophthalmia or microphthalmia; significant refractive errors; strabismus; nystagmus; eyelid ptosis; optic nerve hypoplasia; optic nerve colobomas; cataract; corneal dermoid; inflammatory retinopathy.

Clinical

Broad nasal root may be associated with median nasal groove and cleft of nose and/or upper lip; cleft of ala nasi (unilateral or bilateral); V-shaped hair prolongation into forehead.

Laboratory

CT, MRI and physical examination.

Treatment

Reconstruction surgery may be warranted.

⊟ BIBLIOGRAPHY

1. Kinsey JA, Streeten BW. Ocular abnormalities in the medial cleft face syndrome. Am J Ophthalmol. 1977;83:261.
2. Roarty JD, Pron GE, Siegel-Bartelt J, et al. Ocular manifestations of frontonasal dysplasia. Plast Reconstr Surg. 1994;93:25-30.
3. Sedano HO, Cohen MM, Jirasek J, et al. Frontonasal dysplasia. J Pediatr. 1970;76:906-13.
4. Weaver D, Bellinger D. Bifid nose associated with midline cleft of the upper lip: case report. Arch Otolaryngol. 1946;44:480.

⊟ 1G5. GOLDENHAR SYNDROME (OCULO-AURICULO-VERTEBRAL DYSPLASIA; GOLDENHAR-GORLIN SYNDROME)

General

Most cases have been sporadic, but cases of autosomal dominant and recessive inheritance have been reported; male preponderance (60%); present at birth.

Ocular

Anophthalmia; colobomata of choroid, iris, and eyelid; antimongolian slant of lid fissure; epibulbar dermoid or lipodermoids of conjunctiva, cornea, and orbit; tilted optic disk; nerve hypoplasia; microphthalmia; macular heterotopia; tortuous retinal vessels.

Clinical

Frontal bulging of the skull; receding chin; malar hypoplasia; micrognathia and macrostomia; auricular appendices (single or multiple); multiple vertebral anomalies; preauricular fistulas; mental retardation.

Laboratory

Clinical.

Treatment

Dermoids: Surgery for function or cosmesis.

⊟ BIBLIOGRAPHY

1. Tewfik TL, Al-Noury KI. (2013). Manifestations of craniofacial syndromes. [online] Available from www.emedicine.com/ent/TOPIC319.HTM. [Accessed September, 2013].

⊟ 1G6. MILLER SYNDROME (POSTAXIAL ACROFACIAL DYSOSTOSIS; GENEE-WIEDEMANN SYNDROME)

General

Cause unknown; sporadic and familial cases known as Genee-Wiedemann syndrome.

Ocular

Ectropion.

Clinical

Malar hypoplasia; cleft palate and lip; postaxial limb deficiency; cup-shaped ears.

Laboratory

Diagnosis is made by clinical findings.

Treatment

- *Ectropion*: Topical ocular lubricants.
  - Congenital: Full-thickness skin graft with canthal tendon tightening.
  - Involutional: Tighten lid by resecting full-thickness wedge-medial spindle procedure for punctal eversion.

Paralytic may require a fascia lata sling procedure if does not resolve in 3–6 months.

BIBLIOGRAPHY

1. Chrzanowska KH, Fryns JP, Krajewska-Walasek M, et al. Phenotype variability in the Miller acrofacial dysostosis syndrome: report of two further patients. Clin Genet. 1989;35:157-60.

1G7. NAGER SYNDROME (NAGER ACROFACIAL DYOSTOSIS)

General

Rare congenital syndrome characterized by mandibulofacial dyostosis with associated radial defects.

Ocular

Downward slanting palpebral fissures; absent eyelashes in the medial third of the lower lids.

Clinical

Mandibular and malar hypoplasia; dysplastic ears with conductive deafness; variable degrees of palatal clefting; upper limb malformation (often bilateral hand deformities).

Laboratory

Clinical.

Treatment

None—ocular.

BIBLIOGRAPHY

1. Danziger I, Brodsky L, Perry R, et al. Nager's acrofacial dysostosis. Case report and review of the literature. Int J Pediatr Otorhinolaryngol. 1990;20:225-40.
2. Friedman RA, Wood E, Pransky SM, et al. Nager acrofacial dysostosis: management of a difficult airway. Int J Pediatr Otorhinolaryngol. 1996;35:69-72.
3. Pfeiffer RA, Stoess H. Acrofacial dysostosis (Nager syndrome): synopsis and report of a new case. Am J Med Genet. 1983;15:255-60.

1G8. LINEAR NEVUS SEBACEUS OF JADASSOHN (NEVUS SEBACEUS OF JADASSOHN; JADASSOHN-TYPE ANETODERMA; ORGANOID NEVUS SYNDROME; SEBACEUS NEVUS SYNDROME)

General

Skin nevus caused by failure of separation of skin appendages from adjacent epithelium during the 3rd month of gestation.

Ocular

Proptosis; epibulbar lipodermoids; colobomata of eyelids, iris, and choroid; antimongoloid fissures; ocular motor palsies; nystagmus; teratomas of orbit and aberrant lacrimal glands; corneal vascularization; vision defects; conjunctival dermolipomas; choristomas of conjunctiva, sclera; corneal vascularization/opacification; colobomas of uvea, retina, optic disk, and lids; optic nerve hypoplasia; microphthalmia; anophthalmia; hemangioma of the sclera/conjunctiva.

Clinical

Circumscribed lesions of the face and scalp with excessively large sebaceous glands; papillomatous epidermal hyperplasia; seizures; skeletal abnormalities, particularly in skull; failure to thrive; convulsion; mental retardation.

Laboratory

Epidermis shows papillomatous hyperplasia. In the dermis, the numbers of mature sebaceous glands are increased. Ectopic apocrine glands are often found in the deep dermis beneath sebaceous glands.

Treatment

Photodynamic therapy with topical aminolevulinic acid. Full-thickness skin excision is usually required, and topical destruction.

BIBLIOGRAPHY

1. Al Hammadi A, Lebwohl MG. (2012). Nevus sebaceous. [online] Available from www.emedicine.com/derm/TOPIC296.HTM. [Accessed September, 2013].

1G9. PALPEBRAL COLOBOMA-LIPOMA SYNDROME (NASOPALPEBRAL LIPOMA-COLOBOMA)

General

Autosomal dominant; described in a Venezuelan family.

Ocular

Coloboma of upper and lower lids at junction between their middle and inner thirds; fat deposits of both upper lids; malposition of lacrimal puncta; hypertelorism; telecanthus.

Clinical

Broad nasal bridge; fatty accumulations on nasal bridge and nasolabial area; maxillary hypoplasia.

Laboratory

Diagnosis is made by clinical findings.

Treatment

Corneal protection is the primary goal in the medical treatment of eyelid colobomas. The eyelid coloboma is large; immediate surgical closure is usually needed to prevent corneal compromise.

BIBLIOGRAPHY

1. Bashour M. (2012). Eyelid coloboma. [online] Available from www.emedicine.com/oph/TOPIC673.HTM. [Accessed September, 2013].

1G11. FRANCESCHETTI SYNDROME (FRANCESCHETTI-ZWAHLEN-KLEIN SYNDROME; TREACHER COLLINS SYNDROME; MANDIBULOFACIAL DYSOSTOSIS; MANDIBULOFACIAL SYNDROME; EYELID-MALAR-MANDIBLE SYNDROME; OCULOVERTEBRAL SYNDROME; BERRY SYNDROME; FRANCESCHETTI-ZWAHLEN SYNDROME; ZWAHLEN SYNDROME; BILATERAL FACIAL AGENESIS; BERRY-FRANCESCHETTI-KLEIN SYNDROME; FRANCESCHETTI-KLEIN SYNDROME; FRANCESCHETTI SYNDROME (II); TREACHER COLLINS-FRANCESCHETTI SYNDROME; WEYERS-THIER SYNDROME)

General

Irregular dominant inheritance; Weyers-Thier syndrome has similar features, except it is a unilateral variant; prevalent in Caucasians.

Ocular

Microphthalmia; oblique position of eyes with lateral downward slope of palpebral fissures; temporal lower lid coloboma; lack of cilia on middle third of lower lid; iris coloboma; underdeveloped orbicularis oculi muscle; cataract; optic disk hypoplasia.

Clinical

Fish-like face with sunken cheek bones, receding chin, and large, wide mouth; absent or malformed external ears with auricular appendages; high palate and possible harelip; hypoplastic zygomatic arch with absence of normal malar eminences; prolonged hairline on the cheek; deafness; micrognathia; glossoptosis; cleft palate.

Laboratory

Full craniofacial CT scan (axial and coronal slices from the top of the skull through the cervical spine), brain MRI.

Treatment

Operative repair is based upon the anatomic deformity and timing of correction is done according to physiologic need and development.

⊡ BIBLIOGRAPHY

1. Tolarova MM, Wong GB, Varma S. (2012). Mandibulofacial Dysostosis (Treacher Collins Syndrome). [online] Available from www.emedicine.com/ped/TOPIC1364.HTM. [Accessed September, 2013].

⊡ 1H. EYELID CONTUSIONS, LACERATIONS, AND AVULSIONS

General

Trauma to the eyelid, blowout fracture.

Clinical

None.

Ocular

Eyelid contusion, laceration or avulsion.

Laboratory

CT scan for orbital fracture, MRI for soft-tissue contrast.

Treatment

Oral and topical antibiotics, debridement of wound, repair of laceration with sutures, repair of canicular injury if laceration of canthus may require an oculoplastic surgeon.

⊡ BIBLIOGRAPHY

1. Ing E. (2012). Eyelid laceration. [online] Available from www.emedicine.com/oph/TOPIC219.HTM. [Accessed September, 2013].

⊡ 1I. DERMATOCHALASIS

General

Redundant and lax eyelid skin and muscle, commonly seen in the elderly; loss of elastic tissue and weakening of connective tissue are the causative factors; most frequently in the upper lid but can be seen in lower lid.

Clinical

Renal failure, trauma, cutis laxa, Ehlers-Danlos syndrome, amyloidosis, xanthelasma, thyroid abnormalities and genetics predispose individuals.

Ocular

Visual field loss, blepharitis, entropion, ectropion and trichiasis.

Laboratory

Diagnosis is made by clinical findings. Visual field testing can document field loss.

Treatment

Blepharoplasty is the treatment of choice. Lid hygiene and topical antibiotic may be necessary for blepharitis.

⊡ BIBLIOGRAPHY

1. Gilliland GD. (2012). Dermatochalasis. [online] Available from emedicine.medscape.com/article/1212294-overview. [Accessed September, 2013].

⊡ 1J. DOMINANT OPTIC ATROPHY SYNDROME (DOMINANT OPTIC ATROPHY, DEAFNESS, PTOSIS, OPHTHALMOPLEGIA, DYSTAXIA, AND MYOPATHY)

General

Autosomal dominant disorder; ptosis, ophthalmoplegia, dystaxia, and nonspecific myopathy occur in midlife; optic atrophy and hearing loss occur in early life; autosomal dominant inheritance.

Ocular

Ptosis; ophthalmoplegia; progressive optic atrophy; abnormal electroretinography; diplopia; ocular myopathy; nystagmus; focal temporal excavation of optic disk; dyschromatopsia (blue-yellow); myopia; temporal pallor of the optic nerve.

Clinical

Sensorineural hearing loss; myopathy; dystaxia.

Laboratory

Diagnosis is made by clinical findings.

Treatment

Oral steroids and sometimes, intravenous steroids are necessary.

BIBLIOGRAPHY

1. Del Porto G, Vingolo EM, Steindl K, et al. Clinical heterogeneity of dominant optic atrophy: the contribution of visual function investigations to diagnosis. Graefes Arch Clin Exp Ophthalmol. 1994;232(12):717-27.
2. Eliott D, Traboulsi EI, Maumenee IH. Visual prognosis in autosomal dominant optic atrophy (Kjer type). Am J Ophthalmol. 1993;115(3):360-7.

1K. DUCK-BILL LIPS AND PTOSIS

General

Autosomal dominant.

Ocular

Ptosis; strabismus; hypertelorism.

Clinical

Short philtrum; duck-bill lips; low-set ears; broad forehead; slightly anteverted nose and flat nasal bridge; slightly wide-spaced teeth and high-arched palate; slightly receding chin; slightly wide-set nipples; two phalanges in both fifth fingers; impaired speech.

Laboratory

Diagnosis is made by clinical findings.

Treatment

Observation in mild cases with no abnormal head position or amblyopia. More severe cases may require levator muscle resection, frontalis suspension procedure, Fasanella-Servat procedure, Müller muscle-conjunctival resection.

BIBLIOGRAPHY

1. Suh DW. (2012). Congenital ptosis. [online] Available from www.emedicine.com/oph/TOPIC345.HTM. [Accessed September, 2013].

1L. ECTROPION (LID MARGIN TURNED OUTWARD FROM THE EYEBALL)

1. *Congenital ectropion*
   A. With distichiasis
   †B. With tight septum; microblepharon
   C. With partial coloboma
   D. With mandibulofacial dysostosis (Franceschetti syndrome)
   †E. With megaloblepharon (euryblepharon)
   F. With microphthalmos or buphthalmos
   G. Cerebrooculofacioskeletal syndrome
   H. Down syndrome (mongolism)
   I. Hartnup syndrome (niacin deficiency)
   J. Lowe syndrome (oculocerebrorenal syndrome)
   K. Miller syndrome
   L. Milroy disease (oromandibular dystonia)
   M. Robinow syndrome
   N. Sjögren-Larsson syndrome (SLS)

2. *Acquired ectropion*
   A. Spastic ectropion
      1. Acute spastic ectropion
      2. Blepharophimosis syndrome
      †3. Chronic spastic ectropion becoming cicatricial ectropion
      †4. Hypothermal injury
      5. Myasthenia gravis-afternoon onset (Erb-Goldflam syndrome)
      6. Siemen syndrome (hereditary ectodermal dysplasia syndrome)
   B. Atonic ectropion
      1. Anophthalmic socket
      1. Bell palsy (Idiopathic facial paralysis)
      2. Guillain-Barré syndrome (acute infectious neuritis)

3. Paralytic ectropion-lagophthalmos, such as in seventh nerve palsy
4. Senile ectropion-tissue relaxation

C. Cicatricial ectropion
1. Amendola syndrome
2. Blastomycosis
3. Collodion baby syndrome (congenital ichthyosis)
†4. Chronic dermatitis
†5. Cutaneous T-cell
†6. Etretinate therapy
†7. Excessive skin excision
†8. Facial bums and scarring
†9. Hydroa vacciniforme
10. Kabuki makeup syndrome
11. Leprosy (Hansen disease)
12. Orbital fracture repair
13. Palmoplantar keratodermia
†14. Postblepharoplasty ectropion
15. Psoriasis (psoriasis vulgaris)
†16. Radiation
17. Sézary syndrome (malignant cutaneous reticulosis syndrome)
†18. Systemic fluorouracil
†19. Thermal bums
†20. Trauma
†21. Transformation from chronic spastic ectropion
22. Zinsser-Engman-Cole syndrome (dyskeratosis congenita with pigmentation)

D. Allergic ectropion: Anaphylactic, contact, and microbial (usually temporary)
1. Danbolt-Closs syndrome (acrodermatitis enteropathica)
2. Elschnig syndrome

E. Mechanical
1. Kaposi disease (multiple idiopathic hemorrhagic sarcoma)
2. Leiomyoma
†3. Lumps (chalazion, cysts, neurofibroma)

Treatment

Lubricating ointments are recomended when cornea is exposed. Surgery may also be an option.

BIBLIOGRAPHY

1. Ing E. (2012). Ectropion. [online] Available from www.emedicine.com/oph/TOPIC211.HTM. [Accessed September, 2013].

---

†Indicates a general entry and therefore has not been described in detail in the text

1L1A. DISTICHIASIS (DISTICHIASIS WITH CONGENITAL ANOMALIES OF THE HEART AND PERIPHERAL VASCULATURE)

General

Autosomal dominant.

Ocular

Double rows of eyelashes; congenital ectropion; absence of Meibomian glands; replacement of dense collagenous tissue of the tarsal plates by loose areolar tissue.

Clinical

Congenital heart defects; ventricular septal defects; stress-induced asystole; visible varicosities; chronic venous disease of the legs; sinus bradycardia.

Laboratory

Diagnosis is made by clinical findings.

Treatment

Symptomatic—therapeutic contact lenses as well as lubricating drops and ointments. Epilation with electrolysis cryosurgery, double freeze-thaw down to -20°F, lid splitting procedure.

BIBLIOGRAPHY

1. Rostami S. (2011). Distichiasis. [online] Available from www.emedicine.com/oph/TOPIC603.HTM. [Accessed September, 2013].

🗗 1L1C. EYELID COLOBOMA

General

Full-thickness lid defect generally in the junction of the medial and middle third of the upper lid; causes include trauma, surgical accident or a congenital defect. Most constant feature of Treacher-Collins syndrome.

Clinical

Treacher-Collins syndrome.

Ocular

Full-thickness lid defect; dry eye syndrome; corneal defects.

Laboratory

Diagnosis is made by clinical observation.

Treatment

Temporary treatment involves articial tears, ointment, bandage contact lens and bedtime patching until surgery can be performed. Surgical treatment usually involves direct closure.

🗗 BIBLIOGRAPHY

1. Bashour M. (2012). Eyelid coloboma. [online] Available from www.emedicine.com/oph/TOPIC673.HTM. [Accessed September, 2013].

🗗 1L1D. FRANCESCHETTI SYNDROME (FRANCESCHETTI-ZWAHLEN-KLEIN SYNDROME; TREACHER COLLINS SYNDROME; MANDIBULOFACIAL DYSOSTOSIS; MANDIBULOFACIAL SYNDROME; EYELID-MALAR-MANDIBLE SYNDROME; OCULOVERTEBRAL SYNDROME; BERRY SYNDROME; FRANCESCHETTI-ZWAHLEN SYNDROME; ZWAHLEN SYNDROME; BILATERAL FACIAL AGENESIS; BERRY-FRANCESCHETTI-KLEIN SYNDROME; FRANCESCHETTI-KLEIN SYNDROME; FRANCESCHETTI SYNDROME (II); TREACHER COLLINS-FRANCESCHETTI SYNDROME; WEYERS-THIER SYNDROME)

General

Irregular dominant inheritance; Weyers-Thier syndrome has similar features, except it is a unilateral variant; prevalent in Caucasians.

Ocular

Microphthalmia; oblique position of eyes with lateral downward slope of palpebral fissures; temporal lower lid coloboma; lack of cilia on middle third of lower lid; iris coloboma; underdeveloped orbicularis oculi muscle; cataract; optic disk hypoplasia.

Clinical

Fish-like face with sunken cheek bones, receding chin, and large, wide mouth; absent or malformed external ears with auricular appendages; high palate and possible harelip; hypoplastic zygomatic arch with absence of normal malar eminences; prolonged hairline on the cheek; deafness; micrognathia; glossoptosis; cleft palate.

Laboratory

Full craniofacial CT scan (axial and coronal slices from the top of the skull through the cervical spine), brain MRI.

Treatment

Operative repair is based upon the anatomic deformity and timing of correction is done according to physiologic need and development.

🗗 BIBLIOGRAPHY

1. Tolarova MM, Wong GB, Varma S. (2012). Mandibulofacial dysostosis (Treacher Collins Syndrome). [online] Available from www.emedicine.com/ped/TOPIC1364.HTM. [Accessed September, 2013].

1L1F. PEDIATRIC CONGENITAL GLAUCOMA (PRIMARY INFANTILE GLAUCOMA, BUPHTHALMOS)

General

Rare, found in infants who have aqueous outflow obstruction.

Clinical

None.

Ocular

Open angle glaucoma, photophobia, cloudy cornea, blepharospasm and lacrimation.

Laboratory

Diagnosis is made by clinical findings.

Treatment

Prompt surgical intervention for intraocular pressure (IOP) control which includes angle surgery, goniotomy and trabeculotomy, correction of ametropia, rigorours amblyopia treatment.

BIBLIOGRAPHY

1. Cibis GW, Urban RC, Dahl AA. (2013). Primary congenital glaucoma. [online] Available from www.emedicine.com/oph/TOPIC138.HTM. [Accessed September, 2013].

1L1G. CEREBRO-OCULO-FACIO-SKELETAL SYNDROME (COFS SYNDROME)

General

Inherited as autosomal recessive disorder; death within the first 3 years of life; feeding difficulties secondary to incoordination of the swallowing mechanism.

Ocular

Microphthalmia; blepharophimosis; cataracts.

Clinical

Microcephaly; hypotonia; prominent nasal root; large ear pinnae; flexion contractures at elbows and knees; camptodactylia; osteoporosis; kyphosis; scoliosis; congenital muscular dystrophy.

Laboratory

Clinical.

Treatment

Change in glasses can sometimes improve a patient's visual function temporarily; however the most common treatment is cataract surgery.

BIBLIOGRAPHY

1. Geeraets WJ. Ocular Syndromes, 3rd edition. Philadelphia: Lea & Febiger; 1976.
2. Gershoni-Baruch R, Ludatscher RM, Lichtig C, et al. Cerebrooculo-facio-skeletal syndrome: Further delineation. Am J Med Genet. 1991;41:74-7.
3. Lowry RB, MacLean R, McLean DM, et al. Cataracts, microcephaly, kyphosis and limited joint movement in two siblings. A new syndrome. J Pediatr. 1971;79:282-4.
4. McKusick VA. Mendelian Inheritance in Man; A Catalog of Human Genes and Genetic Disorders, 12th edition. Baltimore, USA: The Johns Hopkins University Press; 1998.
5. Online Mendelian Inheritance in Man, OMIM. McKusick-Nathans Institute for Genetic Medicine, Johns Hopkins University and National Center for Biotechnology Information, National Library of Medicine, February 12, 2007. Available from www.ncbi.nlm.nih.gov/omim. [Accessed September, 2013].
6. Pena SD, Shokeir MK. Autosomal recessive cerebrooculofacio-skeletal (COFS) syndrome. Clin Genet. 1974;5:285–93.

1L1H. DOWN SYNDROME (MONGOLISM; TRISOMY G; TRISOMY 21 SYNDROME; MONGOLOID IDIOCY)

General

Trisomy of chromosome 21.

Ocular

Hypertelorism; epicanthus; blepharitis; ectropion; nystagmus; esotropia; high myopia (30%); hyperopia; color blindness; yellow spots on the iris; hypoplasia of the iris; blepharoconjunctivitis; lens opacities (50%); keratoconus (may be acute); corneal hydrops; corneal ectasia; corneal edema; leukoma; lateral displacement of canaliculi and puncta; megaloblepharon; euryblepharon; decreased accommodation; Leber congenital amaurosis.

Clinical

Mental retardation; skeletal abnormalities; overextension of joints; deformed and low-set ears; short fifth finger; transverse palmar crease; fissured tongue; heart anomalies.

Laboratory

Amniocentesis during second trimester to check mothers who have low α-fetoprotein serum values, prenatal echography, craniofacial X-ray to check features and echocardiography.

Treatment

Primary care provider should coordinate the multisystemic evaluation. Awareness of systemic and ocular findings is essential for managing patients.

BIBLIOGRAPHY

1. Izquierdo NJ, Townsend W. (2011). Ophthalmologic manifestations of Down syndrome. [online] Available from www.emedicine.com/oph/TOPIC522.HTM. [Accessed August, 2013].

1L1I. HARTNUP SYNDROME (PELLAGRA-CEREBELLAR ATAXIA-RENAL AMINOACIDURIA SYNDROME; H DISEASE; NIACIN DEFICIENCY)

General

Recessive; inborn error in amino acid metabolism with abnormal metabolism of tryptophan; both sexes affected; present from infancy.

Ocular

Ectropion; symblepharon; nystagmus; scleral ulcers; corneal leukoma; photophobia; diplopia during attacks.

Clinical

Dermatitis (similar to pellagra) with skin eruptions; progressive mental retardation; cerebellar ataxia.

Laboratory

Therapeutic response to niacin in a patient with the typical symptoms and signs establishes the diagnosis.

Treatment

Oral therapy with nicotinamide or niacin usually is effective in reversing the clinical manifestations.

BIBLIOGRAPHY

1. Hegyi V, Schwartz RA. (2012). Dermatologic manifestations of pellagra. [online] Available from www.emedicine.com/derm/TOPIC621.HTM. [Accessed August, 2013].

1L1J. LOWE SYNDROME (OCULO-CEREBRO-RENAL SYNDROME)

General

Essential enzyme or protein abnormality is unknown; sex-linked recessive trait (male incidence only); onset in early infancy.

Ocular

Nystagmus; congenital glaucoma; miotic pupils; no pupillary reaction; ectropion uveae; malformation of the anterior chamber angle and of the iris; Schlemm's canal may be absent with imperfect angle cleavage; blue sclera; cloudy cornea; cataracts; megalocornea; corneal dystrophy; buphthalmos; microphthalmos; microphakia; mydriasis; strabismus; lens punctate cortical opacities.

Clinical

Mental, psychomotor, and growth retardation; aminoaciduria; albuminuria; glycosuria; renal tubular acidosis; rickets; osteomalacia; muscular hypotony; hyporeflexia; hyperactivity with bizarre choreoathetoid movements and screaming.

Laboratory

Urine-aminoaciduria, proteinuria, calciuria, phosphaturia; serum-elevated acid phosphate; imaging studies—brain MRI—mild ventriculomegaly (one-third cases); ocular ultrasound—if dense cataract, rule out mass or retinal detachment posterior.

Treatment

Monitor and treat for glaucoma. If glaucoma develops, IOP lowering agents must be used. Often, these patients require surgical intervention with goniotomy, trabeculotomy, or a drainage filtration device. Congenital cataracts should be removed, ideally in the first 6 weeks of life, to optimize the visual potential.

BIBLIOGRAPHY

1. Alcorn DM. (2012). Oculocerebrorenal syndrome. [online] Available from www.emedicine.com/oph/TOPIC516.HTM. [Accessed September, 2013].

1L1K. MILLER SYNDROME (POSTAXIAL ACROFACIAL DYSOSTOSIS; GENEE-WIEDEMANN SYNDROME)

General

Cause unknown; sporadic and familial cases known as Genee-Wiedemann syndrome.

Ocular

Ectropion.

Clinical

Malar hypoplasia; cleft palate and lip; postaxial limb deficiency; cup-shaped ears.

Laboratory

Diagnosis is made by clinical findings.

Treatment

- *Ectropion*: Topical ocular lubricants.
  - Congenital: Full-thickness skin graft with canthal tendon tightening.
  - Involutional: Tighten lid by resecting full-thickness wedge-medial spindle procedure for punctal eversion. Paralytic may require a fascia lata sling procedure if does not resolve in 3–6 months.

BIBLIOGRAPHY

1. Chrzanowska KH, Fryns JP, Krajewska-Walasek M, et al. Phenotype variability in the Miller acrofacial dysostosis syndrome: report of two further patients. Clin Genet. 1989;35:157-60.

⊟ 1L1L. NONNE-MILROY-MEIGE DISEASE (CHRONIC HEREDITARY LYMPHEDEMA; MILROY DISEASE; MEIGE DISEASE; MEIGE-MILROY SYNDROME; NONNE-MILROY SYNDROME; CHRONIC HEREDITARY EDEMA; CHRONIC HEREDITARY TROPHEDEMA; CHRONIC TROPHEDEMA; ELEPHANTIASIS CONGENITA HEREDITARIA; FAMILIAL HEREDITARY EDEMA; HEREDITARY EDEMA; IDIOPATHIC HEREDITARY LYMPHEDEMA; PSEUDOEDEMATOUS HYPODERMAL HYPERTROPHY; PSEUDOELEPHANTIASIS NEUROARTHRITICA; OROMANDIBULAR DYSTONIA; BLEPHAROSPASM-OROMANDIBULAR DYSTONIA; CONGENITAL TROPHEDEMA; TROPHOLYMPHEDEMA; TROPHONEUROSIS; ELEPHANTIASIS ARABUM CONGENITA)

General

Autosomal dominant; prevalent in females; two types: praecox at birth to 35 years and tarda after age 35 years.

Ocular

Lid and conjunctival edema; blepharoptosis; distichiasis; strabismus; buphthalmos; ectropion.

Clinical

Lymphedema; mandibulofacial dysostosis; unilateral or bilateral edema of ankle ascending to the knee and eventually above; rough, pigmented skin over swollen parts.

Laboratory

Clincal findings.

Treatment

Prevention of infection and control local complications.

⊟ BIBLIOGRAPHY

1. Rossy KM, Scheinfeld NS. (2013). Lymphedema. [online] Available from www.emedicine.com/med/TOPIC1482. HTM. [Accessed September, 2013].

⊟ 1L1M. ROBINOW-SILVERMAN-SMITH SYNDROME (ACHONDROPLASTIC DWARFISM; MESOMELIC DWARFISM; ROBINOW DWARFISM)

General

Autosomal dominant; both sexes affected; present from birth.

Ocular

Hypertelorism; epicanthal folds.

Clinical

Dwarfism; shortened forearms; bulging forehead; depressed nasal bridge; hypoplastic mandible; small, upturned nose; micrognathia; crowded teeth; penile hypoplasia.

Laboratory

Radiography, CT scan, MRI, and ultrasound.

Treatment

No specific treatment exists.

⊟ BIBLIOGRAPHY

1. Khan AN, Rahim R, MacDonald S. (2013). Achondroplasia imaging. [online] Available from www.emedicine.com/radio/TOPIC809.HTM. [Accessed September, 2013].

⊟ 1L1N. SJÖGREN-LARSSON SYNDROME (OLIGOPHRENIA ICHTHYOSIS SPASTIC DIPLEGIA SYNDROME)

General

Rare; autosomal recessive; consanguinity; loss of neurons and gliosis throughout gray matter; autosomal recessively inherited disorder characterized by the triad of congenital ichthyosis, spastic diplegia or tetraplegia, and mental retardation.

Ocular

Hypertelorism; ichthyosis of lid; chorioretinitis with macular and perimacular pigment degeneration or bright, glistening intraretinal dots; atypical retinitis pigmentosa; blepharitis; conjunctivitis; keratitis; tan/white areas of retinal pigment epithelium loss; maculopathy.

Clinical

Oligophrenia idiocy; ichthyosis (congenital); spastic disorders; epilepsy; speech defect.

Laboratory

Measurement of fatty aldehyde dehydrogenase (FALDH) or fatty alcohol: NAD^+ oxidoreductase on cultured skin fibroblast.

Treatment

Moisturizing creams and keratolytic agent such as alpha-hydroxyacid, salicylic acid, and urea. Standard anticonvulsant are used to treat recurrent seizures. Surgery procedures such as tendon lengthening, adduction release, dorsal root rhizotomy may help some patients with SLS.

⊟ BIBLIOGRAPHY

1. Rizzo WB. (2012). Genetics of Sjogren-Larsson syndrome. [online] Available from www.emedicine.com/ped/TOPIC2111.HTM. [Accessed September, 2013].
2. Rob L, Veen VD, Fuijkschot J, et al. Patients with Sjögren-Larsson syndrome lack macular pigment. Ophthalmology. 2010;117:966-71.

⊟ 1L2A1. ECTROPION

General

Outward turning of eyelid which can be congenital or acquired.

Clinical

Facial abnormalities.

Ocular

Eyelid turning outward, exposure keratopathy, ocular irritation or infection.

Laboratory

Diagnosis is made by clinical findings.

Treatment

- *Ectropion*: Topical ocular lubricants.
  - Congenital: Full thickness skin graft with canthal tendon tightening.
  - Involutional: Tighten the lid by resecting full-thickness wedge-medial spindle procedure for punctal eversion. Paralytic may require a fascia lata sling procedure if it does not resolve in 3–6 months.

⊟ BIBLIOGRAPHY

1. Ing E. (2012). Ectropion. [online] Available from www.emedicine.com/oph/TOPIC211.HTM. [Accessed September, 2013].

🗗 1L2A2. BLEPHAROPHIMOSIS SYNDROME (SIMOSA SYNDROME)

General

Dominantly inherited tetrad of ptosis, epicanthus inversus, telecanthus and blepharophimosis.

Ocular

Scarred or contracted in the secondary blepharophimosis because of ocular pemphigus or trachoma; ectropion; epicanthus inversus; lacrimal puncta displacement; ptosis; telecanthus; optic nerve coloboma; angle dysgenesis; optic nerve hypoplasia; amblyopia; strabismus.

Clinical

Low-set ears; low nasal bridge.

Laboratory

Diagnosis is made by clinical findings.

Treatment

The ptosis is corrected by frontalis fixation at an early age. Canthoplasties may be performed to improve the blepharophimosis. The considerable epicanthus is usually best left until early adolescence, since the degree of this problem tends to diminish with time and the skin becomes easier to move.

🗗 BIBLIOGRAPHY

1. Bashour M. (2012). Ptosis blepharoplasty. [online] Available from www.emedicine.com/ent/TOPIC97.HTM. [Accessed September, 2013].

🗗 1L2A5. ERB-GOLDFLAM SYNDROME (ERB II SYNDROME; HOPPE-GOLDFLAM DISEASE; PSEUDOPARALYTIC SYNDROME; MYASTHENIA GRAVIS)

General

Occurs at any age; more frequent between ages 20–40 years; more females affected than males; progressive; spontaneous; symptoms improve or resolve with rest in early stages of disease (*see* myasthenia gravis, neonatal or infantile); caused by autoantibodies against the acetylcholine receptor at the neuromuscular junction, leading to abnormal fatigability and weakness of skeletal muscle.

Ocular

Transient diplopia; ptosis of upper eyelids.

Clinical

Excessive fatigability of musculature; symptoms appear and increase as day progresses; expressionless face; sagging jaw; difficulty in chewing and talking; nasal regurgitation.

Laboratory

Ice test—crushed ice in surgical glove over ptotic eyelid for 2 minutes and watch for brief elevation of eyelid; Tensilon test and prostigmin test may result in the elevation of ptotic eyelid or improved strabismus in individuals with myasthenia gravis.

Treatment

Adrenal corticosteroids are frequently used. In some cases, mycophenolate mofetil, cyclosporine and cyclophosphamide may be useful. Patching one eye or using prisms may be helpful.

🗗 BIBLIOGRAPHY

1. Erb W. Zur Casuistick der Bulbaren La hmungen. Arch Psychiatr Vervenkr. 1879;9:325-50.
2. Roy FH, Fraunfelder FT, Fraunfelder FW. Roy and Fraunfelder's Current Ocular Therapy, 6th edition. London, UK: Elsevier; 2008.
3. Goldflam S. Vebereinen Scheinbar Keilbaren Bulbarparalytischem Symptom Complex mit Betheiligung der Extremitaten. Dtsch Z Nerven. 1983;4:312-52.
4. Kim JH, Hwang JM, Hwang YS, et al. Childhood ocular myasthenia gravis. Ophthalmology. 2003;110(7):1458-62.
5. Lepore FE, Sanborn GE, Slevin JT. Pupillary dysfunction in myasthenia gravis. Ann Neurol. 1979;6(1):29-33.
6. Sommer N, Melms A, Weller M, et al. Ocular myasthenia gravis. A critical review of clinical and pathophysiological aspects. Doc Ophthalmol. 1993;84(4):309-33.

🗗 1L2A6. HEREDITARY ECTODERMAL DYSPLASIA SYNDROME (SIEMENS SYNDROME; KERATOSIS FOLLICULARIS SPINULOSA SYNDROME; HYPOHIDROTIC ECTODERMAL DYSPLASIA; CHRIST-SIEMENS-TOURAINE SYNDROME; WEECH SYNDROME; ANHIDROTIC ECTODERMAL DYSPLASIA; ICHTHYOSIS FOLLICULARIS)

General

Autosomal recessive inheritance; strong male preponderance (about 95%); linked to X-chromosome.

Ocular

Complete loss of eyebrows (madarosis); follicular keratosis; blepharitis; entropion or ectropion; reduced tear formation or epiphora; myopia; keratoconjunctivitis; corneal erosions and ulcers (recurrent); corneal dystrophy; cataract; increased periorbital pigmentation; mongoloid lid slant; photophobia; absence of iris; luxation of lens; papillary abnormalities.

Clinical

Mental retardation; dry skin and anhidrosis (reduced number of sweat glands); hypotrichosis; follicular hyperkeratosis (neck, palms, soles); hypohidrosis.

Laboratory

Diagnosis is made by clinical findings.

Treatment

- *Corneal dystrophy*: Mild cases can be observed and soft contact lenses are helpful; penetrating keratoplasty (PK) may be necessary, graft recurrences treated by superficial keratectomy, phototherapeutic keratectomy or repeat PK.
- *Cataract*: Change in glasses can sometimes improve a patient's visual function temporarily; however the most common treatment is cataract surgery.

🗗 BIBLIOGRAPHY

1. Shah KN. (2012). Ectodermal dysplasia. [online] Available from www.emedicine.com/derm/TOPIC114.HTM. [Accessed September, 2013].

🗗 1L2B1. BELL'S PALSY (IDIOPATHIC FACIAL PARALYSIS)

General

Unilateral facial nerve paralysis of sudden onset and gradual recovery involving the nerve as it runs through the fallopian canal; etiology unknown; more common in adults.

Ocular

Corneal ulcer; paralysis of seventh nerve; ectropion; lagophthalmos; ptosis; epiphora; decreased visual acuity; diplopia; ocular irritation; exposure keratitis.

Clinical

Aching in the ear or mastoid; tingling or numbness of cheek or mouth; alteration of taste; hyperacusis; epiphora; facial weakness; most commonly and frequently affected cranial nerve with herpes zoster is the facial nerve.

Laboratory

It is not diagnosed by clinical findings.

Treatment

Most patients recover without treatment. If spontaneous recovery does not occur, the most widely accepted treatment is corticosteroids.

🗗 BIBLIOGRAPHY

1. Taylor DC, Khoromi S, Zachariah SB. (2012). Bell palsy. [online] Available from www.emedicine.com/neuro/TOPIC413.HTM. [Accessed September, 2013].

⊟ 1L2B2. GUILLAIN-BARRÉ SYNDROME (LANDRY PARALYSIS; ACUTE INFECTIOUS NEURITIS; ACUTE POLYRADICULITIS; ACUTE FEBRILE POLYNEURITIS; ACUTE IDIOPATHIC POLYNEURITIS; INFLAMMATORY POLYRADICULONEUROPATHY; LANDRY-GUILLAIN-BARRÉ-STROHL SYNDROME; POSTINFECTIOUS POLYNEURITIS)

General

Etiology unknown; occurs from age 16–50 years.

Ocular

Facial nerve paralysis with paralytic ectropion of the lower eyelid; mild-to-complete external ophthalmoplegia; optic neuritis; papilledema; ptosis; anisocoria; nystagmus; dyschromatopsia; scotoma; bilateral tonic pupils.

Clinical

Polyneuritis involving facial peripheral motor nerves and spinal cord; facial diplegia; bladder incontinence; variable degrees of paralysis, usually beginning in lower extremities; tendon reflexes absent; involvement of respiratory muscles possible; paresthesia (symmetrical).

Laboratory

Cytomegalovirus (CMV), Epstein-Barr virus and human immunodeficiency virus (HIV) have been most closely associated with this condition.

Treatment

Plasma exchange have shown to be beneficial. Corneal exposure is treated with topical therapy or lateral tarsorrhaphies if warranted.

⊟ BIBLIOGRAPHY

1. Andary MT, Oleszek JL, Cha-Kim A. (2012). Guillain-Barre Syndrome. [online] Available from www.emedicine.com/pmr/TOPIC48.HTM. [Accessed September, 2013].

⊟ 1L2B3. LAGOPHTHALMOS

General

Inability to close eyelids caused by projection of the eye in orbit, inadequate vertical dimensions of either lid, contraction of the eyelid retractors or malfunction of the orbicularis oculi.

Clinical

None.

Ocular

Decreased visual acuity, pain, dry eye syndrome, corneal erosion, corneal ulceration, endophthalmitis, inability to close eyelids.

Laboratory

Diagnosis is made by clinical findings.

Treatment

Topical lubricants, punctal plugs or thermal occlusion of punctum may be useful. Tarsorrhaphy with upper eyelid retraction may require upper lid levator recession and graded Müllerectomy; facial nerve palsy—gold weight implant.

⊟ BIBLIOGRAPHY

1. Roy FH, Fraunfelder FW, Fraunfelder FT. Roy and Fraunfelder's Current Ocular Therapy, 6th edition. London, UK: Elsevier; 2008.

1L2B4. ECTROPION

General

Outward turning of eyelid which can be congenital or acquired.

Clinical

Facial abnormalities.

Ocular

Eyelid turning outward, exposure keratopathy, ocular irritation or infection.

Laboratory

Diagnosis is made by clinical findings.

Treatment

- Topical ocular lubricants.
  - Congenital: Full thickness skin graft with canthal tendon tightening.
  - Involutional: Tighten the lid by resecting full-thickness wedge-medial spindle procedure for punctal eversion. Paralytic may require a fascia lata sling procedure if it does not resolve in 3–6 months.

BIBLIOGRAPHY

1. Ing E. (2012). Ectropion. [online] Available from www.emedicine.com/oph/TOPIC211.HTM. [Accessed September, 2013].

1L2C1. AMENDOLA SYNDROME

General

Observed in Sao Paulo, Brazil; all ethnic groups are affected; endemic form of pemphigus foliaceus; possibly caused by environmental agents; autoimmune disease mediated by autoantibodies of the immunoglobulin G (IgG) class, IgG4 subclass.

Ocular

Blisters around eyebrows; entropion; ectropion; trichiasis; iritis.

Clinical

Brazilian pemphigus (fogo selvagem, "wild fire"), which resembles, because of its appearance, pemphigus foliaceus; fever; chills.

Laboratory

Diagnosis is made by clinical findings.

Treatment

- *Entropion*: Topical antibiotics and lubricants, temporary sutures to evert the eyelid, lateral cantholysis with subconjunctival incision just inferior to the tarsus. Inferior retractors are isolated and reattached to anterior inferior portion of tarsus with multiple interrupted sutures.
- *Iritis*: Oral steroids if not responsive to topical steroids, immunosuppressants if bilateral disease that does not respond to oral steroids, periocular steroids for unilateral or posterior uveitis. Vitrectomy can be used for severe vitreous opacification. Cryotherapy and laser photocoagulation may be used for localized pars plana exudates.

BIBLIOGRAPHY

1. Amendola F. Cataracta No Pemfigo Foliaceo (nota previa). Rev Paul Med. 1945;26:286.
2. Korting GW. The skin and the eye: a dermatologic correlation of diseases of the periorbital region. Philadelphia: WB Saunders; 1973. pp. 82.
3. Magalini SI, Scrascia, E. Dictionary of Medical Syndromes, 2nd edition. Philadelphia: JB Lippincott; 1981.
4. Sampaio SA, Rivitti EA, Aoki V, et al. Brazilian pemphigus foliaceus, endemic pemphigus foliaceus or fogo selvagem (wild fire). Dermatol Clin. 1994;12:765-76.

◫ 1L2C2. BLASTOMYCOSIS

General

Chronic fungal disease caused by *Blastomyces dermatitidis*.

Ocular

Hypopyon; mycotic keratitis; corneal ulcer; choroidal granuloma; nodules of iris; cicatrization of eyelid; ectropion; descemetocele; panophthalmitis; recurrent papillomatous lesion upper lid; granulomatous conjunctivitis.

Clinical

Granulomatous lesions of skin, lung, bone, or any part of the body.

Laboratory

Periodic acid-Schiff and Gomori methenamine-silver stains.

Treatment

Therapeutic approaches involve the use of oral azoles, primarily itraconazole. Ocular treatment may include surgical draining of the lid in addition to antifungal therapy.

◫ BIBLIOGRAPHY

1. Steele RW. (2011). Pediatric blastomycosis. [online] Available from www.emedicine.com/ped/TOPIC254.HTM. [Accessed September, 2013].

◫ 1L2C3. HARLEQUIN SYNDROME (BULLOUS ICHTHYOSIFORM ERYTHRODERMA; COLLODION BABY; CONGENITAL ICHTHYOSIS; EPIDERMOLYTIC HYPERKERATOSIS; ICHTHYOSIS; ICHTHYOSIS VULGARIS; LAMELLAR ICHTHYOSIS; NONBULLOUS ICHTHYOSIFORM ERYTHRODERMA; XERODERMA; X-LINKED ICHTHYOSIS)

General

Autosomal inherited disorder; affects both sexes; normal at birth; onset within first 7 days.

Ocular

Keratopathy; corncal scarring; keratitis; conjunctivitis; lagophthalmos; photophobia; ectropion; lid erythema; lacrimation.

Clinical

At birth, the skin surface is moist, red, and tender; within several days, thick verrucous scales form.

Laboratory

Diagnosis is made by clinical findings.

Treatment

Treatment is primarily surgical. Patients with bilateral and visually disabling corneal opacity, PK is recommended.

◫ BIBLIOGRAPHY

1. Chua CN, Ainsworth J. Ocular management of harlequin syndrome: photo essay. Arch Ophthalmol. 2001;119:454-5.
2. Frost P. Disorders of cornification. In: Moschella SL, Hurley HJ (Eds). Dermatology. Philadelphia: WB Saunders; 1975. pp. 1056-84.
3. Magalini SI, Scrascia E. Dictionary of Medical Syndromes, 2nd edition. Philadelphia: JB Lippincott; 1981.
4. Orth DH, Fretzin DF, Abramson V. Collodion baby with transient bilateral lid ectropion. Review of ocular manifestations of ichthyosis. Arch Ophthalmol. 1974;91:206-7.
5. Roy FH, Fraunfelder FW, Fraunfelder FT. Roy and Fraunfelder's Current Ocular Therapy, 6th edition. Philadelphia: WB Saunders; 2008.

⊟ 1L2C10. KABUKI MAKEUP SYNDROME (NIIKAWA-KUROKI SYNDROME)

General

Etiology unknown; originally termed Kabuki makeup syndrome because dysmorphic facies resembled the stylized makeup worn by Kabuki actors; also seen in ethnic groups other than Japanese.

Ocular

Ectropion of lower eyelid; long palpebral fissures; sparse lateral half of eyebrows; highly arched eyebrows.

Clinical

Prominent ears; cleft or highly arched palates; brachydactyly; dermatoglyphics; pad-like swelling of fingertips; short stature; mental retardation; susceptibility to infection; characteristic facies; developmental delay; mental and growth retardation with specific craniofacial malformations including a depressed nasal tip; musculoskeletal abnormalities, evolving phenotype over time suggesting an underlying defect of the connective tissue.

Laboratory

Diagnosis is made by clinical findings.

Treatment

Lubrication and moisture shields are helpful if significant corneal exposure exists from the ectropion. If symptoms warrant, a surgical procedure may be necessary for the ectropion—lateral tarsal strip—horizontal lid laxity is a component of most ectropion cases.

⊟ BIBLIOGRAPHY

1. Kaiser-Kupfer MI, Mulvihill JJ, Klein KL, et al. The Niikawa-Kuroki (Kabuki make-up) syndrome in an American black. Am J Ophthalmol. 1986;102:667-8.
2. Kuroki Y, Suzuki Y, Chyo H, et al. A new malformation syndrome of long palpebral fissure, large ears, depressed nasal tip and skeletal anomalies associated with postnatal dwarfism and mental retardation. J Pediatr. 1981;99:570-3.
3. Niikawa N, Matsuura N, Fukushima Y, et al. Kabuki make-up syndrome: a syndrome of mental retardation, unusual facies, large and protruding ears and postnatal growth deficiency. J Pediatr. 1981;99:565-9.
4. Sheikh TM, Qasi QH, Beller E. Niikawa-Kuroki syndrome (Kabuki make-up syndrome) in a Hispanic child. Pediatr Res. 1986;20:340A.

⊟ 1L2C11. HANSEN DISEASE (LEPROSY)

General

Communicable disease caused by *Mycobacterium leprae*.

Ocular

Keratitis; leukoma; pannus; corneal ulcer; uveitis; iris atrophy; dacryocystitis; anisocoria; multiple pupils; decreased or absent pupillary reaction to light; paralysis of seventh nerve; episcleritis; blepharospasm; lagophthalmos; madarosis; secondary glaucoma; decreased IOP; subconjunctival fibrosis; punctate epithelial keratopathy; posterior subcapsular cataract; corneal hypesthesia; prominent corneal nerves; iridocyclitis; foveal avascular keratitis; scleritis; interstitial keratitis; iris pearls; dry eye.

Clinical

Disease affects primarily the skin, mucous membrane, and peripheral nerves.

Laboratory

Skin biopsy specimens contain vacuolated macrophages, few lymphocytes, and numerous acid-fast bacilli often in clumps or globi.

Treatment

The World Health Organization (WHO) recommends multiple drug therapy (MDT) for all forms of leprosy. MDT 14 consists of rifampin, ofloxacin, and minocycline.

⊟ BIBLIOGRAPHY

1. Kim EC. (2011) Ocular manifestations of leprosy. [online] Available from www.emedicine.com/oph/TOPIC743.HTM. [Accessed September, 2013].

🖥 1L2C12. ORBITAL FRACTURE, APEX

General

It affects the most posterior portion of the pyramidal-shaped orbit, positioned at the craniofacial junction. Usually associated with blunt or penetrating trauma to the face or skull.

Clinical

Intracranial or facial trauma.

Ocular

Visual loss; optic neuropathy; optic nerve sheath hematoma; optic nerve impingement; optic nerve compression; retrobulbar hemorrhage; extraocular muscle nerve palsy; diplopia; afferent pupil defect; periocular ecchymosis; proptosis.

Laboratory

CT scan is most appropriate to make diagnosis.

Treatment

In cases that involve decreased vision and optic nerve injury, medical or surgical nerve decompression should be considered. Corticosteroids should be the initial treatment and if it is not effective, surgical intervention is necessary.

🖥 BIBLIOGRAPHY

1. Patel B, Taylor SF. (2012). Apex orbital fracture. [online] Available from emedicine.medscape.com/article/1218196-overview. [Accessed September, 2013].

🖥 1L2C13. KERATODERMIA PALMARIS ET PLANTARIS (PALMOPLANTAR KERATODERMIA; KERATOSIS PALMOPLANTARIS)

General

Autosomal recessive; hereditary disorder; diffuse or focal thickening of the palms and soles.

Ocular

Hyperkeratosis of lid and cornea; ectropion; leukoma; corneal ulceration; pronounced photophobia; hereditary optic atrophy; epiphora; conjunctivitis.

Clinical

Localized or disseminated hyperkeratotic changes of the palms and soles with a tendency toward fissure and secondary infection.

Laboratory

Clinical.

Treatment

- *Ectropion*: Topical ocular lubricants.
  - Congenital: Full thickness skin graft with canthal tendon tightening.
  - Involutional: Tighten lid by resecting full-thickness wedge-medial spindle procedure for punctal eversion. Paralytics may require a fascia lata sling procedure if does not resolve in 3–6 months.
- *Corneal ulceration*: Corneal cultures may be taken and treatment initiated. Treatment include a broad spectrum of antibiotics and cycloplegic drops.

🖥 BIBLIOGRAPHY

1. Kingsbery MY, Lee RA, James WD. (2013). Keratosis Palmaris et Plantaris. [online] Available from www.emedicine.com/derm/TOPIC589.HTM. [Accessed September, 2013].

🖥 1L2C15. PSORIASIS (PSORIASIS VULGARIS)

General

Chronic skin disease of unknown etiology; both sexes affected; onset at any age; disease peaks at puberty; strong human leukocyte antigen (HLA) association resulting in heritable disease susceptibility.

Ocular

Desquamative psoriatic plaques of lids resulting in madarosis, trichiasis, or ectropion; corneal plaques; xerosis, symblepharon; keratitis; chronic corneal ulceration; phthisis bulbi; iritis.

Clinical

Thick, dry, elevated red patches of skin covered with coarse silvery scales that usually affect areas of skin not exposed to sun, such as scalp, sacrum, elbows, and knees; positive association with Sjögren syndrome and keratitis sicca.

Laboratory

Diagnosis is made by clinical findings.

Treatment

The simplest treatment of psoriasis is daily sun exposure, sea bathing, topical moisturizers, and relaxation. Moisturizers, such as petrolatum jelly, are helpful. Anthralin, coal or wood tar, corticosteroids, salicylic acid, phenolic compounds, and calcipotriene (a vitamin D analog) also may be effective. Ocular lubricants and punctal occlusion, oral and topical corticosteroids are sometimes beneficial.

BIBLIOGRAPHY

1. Meffert J, Arffa R, Gordon R, et al. (2012). Psoriasis. [online] Available from www.emedicine.com/oph/TOPIC483.HTM. [Accessed September, 2013].

1L2C17. MYCOSIS FUNGOIDES SYNDROME (SÉZARY SYNDROME; MALIGNANT CUTANEOUS RETICULOSIS SYNDROME)

General

Lymphoma characterized by abnormal lymphocytes having hyperchromatic, hyperconvoluted nuclei; malignant, cutaneous T-cell lymphoma, which initially presents as a nonspecific erythematous cutaneous eruption that progresses to form plaques and tumors.

Ocular

Thick and swollen eyelids; ectropion; blepharitis; loss of eyelashes; keratoconjunctivitis; uveitis; retinal edema and exudates; papilledema; exophthalmos; retinal hemorrhage; endophthalmitis; pupillary dilatation; scleritis; corneal opacity; optic disk swelling.

Clinical

Pruritus followed by thickening and edema of the skin; dermatitis exfoliativa; eczema; pyoderma; pigmentary changes of body and extremities (mottled appearance); hyperhidrosis.

Laboratory

Blood work, biopsy.

Treatment

- *Ectropion*: Topical ocular lubricants.
  - Congenital: Full thickness skin graft with canthal tendon tightening.
  - Involutional: Tighten lid by resecting full-thickness wedge-medial spindle procedure for punctal eversion. Paralytic may require a fascia lata sling procedure if does not resolve in 3–6 months.

- *Blepharitis*: Oral tetracyclines, Omega-3 fatty acids, flax seed oil or fish oil. Ocular therapy include eyelid scrubs, warm compresses, bacitracin ointment to lid margins, topical cyclosporine A and preservative-free lubricants.
- *Uveitis*: Topical steroids and cycloplegic medication should be the initial treatment choice. Oral steroids if not responsive to topical steroids, immunosuppressants if bilateral disease that does not respond to oral steroids, periocular steroids for unilateral or posterior uveitis. Vitrectomy can be used for severe vitreous opacification. Cryotherapy and laser photocoagulation may be used for localized pars plana exudates.
- *Papilledema*: Underlying cause should be determined and treated. Systemic acetazolamide is the medical therapy of choice.
- *Exophthalmos*: Reversing the problem which is causing the exophthalmos is the treatment of choice and will minimize the ocular complications. Ocular lubricants are beneficial for control of the corneal exposure.

BIBLIOGRAPHY

1. Deutsch AR, Duckworth JK. Mycosis fungoides of upper lid. Am J Ophthalmol. 1968;65:884-8.
2. Forester HC. Mycosis fungoides with intraocular involvement. Trans Am Acad Ophthalmol Otolaryngol. 1960;64:308.
3. Leitch RJ, Rennie IG, Parsons MA. Ocular involvement in mycosis fungoides. Br J Ophthalmol. 1993;77:126-7.
4. Meekins B, Proia AD, Klintworth GK. Cutaneous T-cell lymphoma presenting as a rapidly enlarging ocular adnexal tumor. Ophthalmology. 1985;92:1288-93.
5. Roy FH, Fraunfelder FW, Fraunfelder FT. Roy and Fraunfelder's Current Ocular Therapy, 6th edition. Philadelphia: WB Saunders; 2008.

1L2C22. ZINSSER-ENGMAN-COLE SYNDROME (DYSKERATOSIS CONGENITA WITH PIGMENTATION; COLE-RAUSCHKOLB-TOOMEY SYNDROME) ECTROPION

General

Variant of Fanconi familial aplastic anemia; recessively inherited with male linkage; consanguinity; onset between ages 5 years and 13 years.

Ocular

Ectropion; chronic blepharitis; obstruction of lacrimal puncta; conjunctival keratinization; bullous conjunctivitis; epiphora; nasolacrimal duct obstruction; loss of lashes; cataract; glaucoma; strabismus; abnormal fundi.

Clinical

Congenital dyskeratosis with pigmentation of "marble" configuration or "gun metal" appearance; atrophic areas and telangiectasis; dystrophy of nails; vesicular and bullous lesions of oral cavity followed by ulceration; mucosal atrophy; leukoplakia; aplastic anemia; defect of teeth; physical and mental development may be retarded; tufts of hairs on the limbs; keratinized basal cell; papillomas on the trunk.

Laboratory

Screen for bone marrow, neurologic, pulmonary and mucosal malignancies. CBC, chest radiography, pulmonary function test, and stool test for occult blood. Mutation analysis test.

Treatment

Anabolic steroids for bone marrow failure. Stem cell transplantation is the long-term curative option.

BIBLIOGRAPHY

1. Robles DT, Olson JM, Chan EF, et al. (2013). Dyskeratosis congenital. [online] Available from www.emedicine.com/derm/TOPIC111.HTM. [Accessed September, 2013].

1L2D1. DANBOLT-CLOSS SYNDROME (ACRODERMATITIS ENTEROPATHICA; BRANDT SYNDROME)

General

Etiology unknown; autosomal recessive; occurs in both sexes with onset in early infancy; characterized by intermittent simultaneous occurrence of diarrhea and dermatitis with failure to thrive.

Ocular

Loss of eyebrows; blepharitis; ectropion; loss of eyelashes; photophobia; conjunctivitis; scattered superficial corneal opacities; keratitis; lacrimal punctal stenosis; corneal sup-erficial punctate lesions, nebulous subepithelial opacities and linear epithelial erosions.

Clinical

Symmetrical skin eruptions on hands, feet, elbows, knees, and buttocks usually dry up to an erythematosquamous type; glossitis and stomatitis; alopecia; paronychia with nail dystrophy; gastrointestinal disturbances; diarrhea (intermittent).

Laboratory

Determining hair, urine, and parotid saliva zinc levels as well as serum alkaline phosphatase activity (which lowers later in the disease) may be helpful.

Treatment

Oral zinc supplementation per day for life.

BIBLIOGRAPHY

1. Dela Rosa KM, Satter EK. (2011). Acrodermatitis enteropathica. [online] Available from www.emedicine.com/derm/TOPIC5.HTM. [Accessed September, 2013].

1L2D2. ELSCHNIG SYNDROME I (MEIBOMIAN CONJUNCTIVITIS)

General

Chronic inflammations; characteristic foamy secretion; benign.

Ocular

Conjunctivitis; foamy secretion; ocular irritation; photophobia; minimal visual impairment.

Clinical

Hyperplasia of tarsal glands.

Laboratory

Diagnosis is made by clinical findings.

Treatment

Symptomatic control may include cold compresses, artificial tears; nonsteroidal and occasionally steroidal drops to relieve itching.

BIBLIOGRAPHY

1. Elschnig A. Belt ray Artiologie und Therapie der chronischen Conjunctivitis. Dtsch Med Wochenschr. 1908;34:1133-5.
2. Magalini SI, Scrascia E. Dictionary of Medical Syndromes, 2nd edition. Philadelphia, PA: Lippincott Williams & Wilkins; 1981.

1L2E1. KAPOSI DISEASE (KAPOSI SARCOMA; KAPOSI HEMORRHAGIC SARCOMA; MULTIPLE IDIOPATHIC HEMORRHAGIC SARCOMA; KAPOSI VARICELLIFORM ERUPTION)

General

Vascular tumor of unknown cause; seen most often in males, Jews, and those from eastern Europe, the southern Mediterranean, and Africa; HIV-related Kaposi syndrome is the most common type of cancer seen in acquired immunodeficiency syndrome patients.

Ocular

Ocular adnexa, varicelliform eruption, including lids, conjunctivae, lacrimal glands, and orbit may be involved; hemorrhage; extensive injection and thickening of conjunctival tissues; conjunctival involvement more evident in bulbar conjunctiva.

Clinical

Vascular sarcomas usually occur on the legs, although widespread cutaneous and visceral tumors may develop; secondary malignancies are very common; lymphedema.

Laboratory

Diagnosis is histopathologic.

Treatment

Cutaneous or conjunctival biopsy of the lesion may be necessary for a definitive diagnosis.

BIBLIOGRAPHY

1. Freudenthal J, Yuhan KR, You TT. (2012). Ophthalmologic manifestations of Kaposi sarcoma. [online] Available from www.emedicine.com/oph/TOPIC481.HTM. [Accessed September, 2013].

1L2E2. LEIOMYOMA

General

Rare, benign tumor that arises from smooth muscle; usually well encapsulated.

Ocular

Pigmented tumor of ciliary body; proptosis; distorted pupil; ectropion; iris tumor; glaucoma; cataract; preferential location: ciliary body, peripheral choroid, supraciliary or suprachoroidal space; it has a predilection for younger patients and females.

Clinical

Metastases have not been described.

Laboratory

Diagnosis is made on histologic examination.

Treatment

Excise the leiomyoma from the iris and ciliary body if tumors increase in size.

BIBLIOGRAPHY

1. Roque MR, Roque BL. (2012). Iris leiomyoma. [online] Available from www.emedicine.com/oph/TOPIC589.HTM. [Accessed August, 2013].

1M. EHLERS-DANLOS SYNDROME (FIBRODYSPLASIA ELASTICA GENERALISATA; CUTIS HYPERELASTICA; MEEKEREN-EHLERS-DANLOS SYNDROME; INDIAN RUBBER MAN SYNDROME; CUTIS LAXA)

General

Present at birth; autosomal dominant; two groups: cutaneous and articular; syndrome is one of the three primary disorders of elastic tissue [other two disorders are pseudoxanthoma elasticum (Grönblad-Strandberg syndrome) and senile elastosis]; inherited disorder of collagen biosynthesis.

Ocular

Hyperelasticity of palpebral skin; easy eversion of upper lid; ptosis; epicanthal folds; hypotony of extraocular muscles; strabismus; microcornea; thinning of cornea with keratoconus; thinning of sclera (blue sclera); subluxation of lens; angioid streaks; chorioretinal hemorrhages; retinitis proliferans with secondary detachment; macular degeneration; myopia; ruptured globe after minor trauma; limbus-to-limbus corneal thinning; acute hydrops; cornea plana; keratoglobus.

Clinical

Cutaneous manifestations include thin, atrophic, fragile skin, cutaneous hyperelasticity and pseudomolluscoid tumors; articular manifestations include excessive articular laxity and luxations; hypermobile joints.

Laboratory

Biochemical studies can detect alterations in collagen molecules in cultured skin fibroblasts. Molecular [deoxyribonucleic acid (DNA)]-based testing is available. Diagnosis may by urinary analyte assay and clinical examination is the most common.

Treatment

Ascorbic acid therapy, in the event of skin lacerations seriously consider alternatives to sutures, including adhesive strips and wound glues, monitor for cardiac conditions and scoliosis.

BIBLIOGRAPHY

1. Steiner RD. (2011). Genetics of Ehlers-Danlos syndrome. [online] Available from www.emedicine.com/ped/TOPIC654.HTM. [Accessed September, 2013].

1N. ENTROPION (INVERSION OF LID MARGIN)

1. *Congenital*, including congenital epiblepharon-inferior oblique insufficiency; ectrodactyly, ectodermal dysplasia, cleft lip-palate syndrome, including with and without lower eyelid retractor insertion
   †A. Inferior oblique insuffieciency syndrome
   B. Dental-ocular-cutaneous syndrome
   C. Siemen syndrome (anhidrotic ectodermal dysplasia)
2. *Acquired*
   †A. *Spastic entropion*: Acute, affecting lower lid, precipitated by acute inflammation or prolonged patching
   B. *Mechanical entropion*

1. Anophthalmos
2. Enophthalmos
†3. Microphthalmos
4. Lymphedema
†C. *Senile entropion*: Relative enophthalmos secondary to fat atrophy
D. *Cicatricial entropion*: Physical and chemical burns of conjunctiva and cicatrizing diseases, including trachoma and leprosy
  †1. Chronic cicatricial conjunctivitis
  2. *Leprosy (Hansen disease)
  †3. Radiation
  4. Thermal burns
  †5. Trachoma
  †6. Following cryosurgery of the eyelid

7. Amendola syndrome
8. Variola

Treatment

Ocular ointments are helpful in protection and providing comfort to the eye.

BIBLIOGRAPHY

1. DeBacker C, Dryden RM. (2011). Entropion. [online] Available from www.emedicine.com/oph/TOPIC212.HTM. [Accessed September, 2013].

---

†Indicates a general entry and therefore has not been described in detail in the text

---

1N1B. DENTAL-OCULAR-CUTANEOUS SYNDROME

General

Abnormal tooth roots; distinctive features separate this syndrome from oculodentodigital or faciodentodigital syndromes.

Ocular

Entropion lower eyelids; glaucoma (juvenile type).

Clinical

Unusual upper lip with lack of "cupid's bow" and thickening and widening of the philtrum; syndactyly; cutaneous hyperpigmentation overlying the interphalangeal joints; clinodactyly; single conical roots in all primary teeth and permanent first molars; scant body hair; horizontal ridging of fingernails.

Laboratory

X-rays.

Treatment

- *Entropion*: Topical antibiotics and lubricants, temporary sutures to evert the eyelid, lateral cantholysis with subconjunctival incision just inferior to the tarsus. Inferior retractors are isolated and reattached to anterior' inferior portion of tarsus with multiple interrupted sutures.
- *Glaucoma*: Glaucoma medication should be the first plan of action. If medication is unsuccessful, a filtering surgical procedure with or without antimetabotites may be beneficial.

BIBLIOGRAPHY

1. Ackerman JL, Ackerman AL, Ackerman AB. A new dental ocular and cutaneous syndrome. Int J Dermatol. 1973;12:285-9.

1N1C. HEREDITARY ECTODERMAL DYSPLASIA SYNDROME (SIEMENS SYNDROME; KERATOSIS FOLLICULARIS SPINULOSA SYNDROME; HYPOHIDROTIC ECTODERMAL DYSPLASIA; CHRIST-SIEMENS-TOURAINE SYNDROME; WEECH SYNDROME; ANHIDROTIC ECTODERMAL DYSPLASIA; ICHTHYOSIS FOLLICULARIS)

General

Autosomal recessive inheritance; strong male preponderance (about 95%); linked to X-chromosome.

Ocular

Complete loss of eyebrows (madarosis); follicular keratosis; blepharitis; entropion or ectropion; reduced tear formation or epiphora; myopia; keratoconjunctivitis; corneal erosions and ulcers (recurrent); corneal dystrophy; cataract; increased periorbital pigmentation; mongoloid lid slant; photophobia; absence of iris; luxation of lens; papillary abnormalities.

Clinical

Mental retardation; dry skin and anhidrosis (reduced number of sweat glands); hypotrichosis; follicular hyperkeratosis (neck, palms, soles); hypohidrosis.

Laboratory

Diagnosis is made by clinical findings.

Treatment

- *Corneal dystrophy*: Mild cases can be observed and soft contact lenses are helpful; PK may be necessary; graft recurrences treated by superficial keratectomy; phototherapeutic keratectomy or repeat PK.
- *Cataract*: Change in glasses can sometimes improve a patient's visual function temporarily; however the most common treatment is cataract surgery.

BIBLIOGRAPHY

1. Shah KN. (2012). Ectodermal dysplasia. [online] Available from www.emedicine.com/derm/TOPIC114.HTM. [Accessed September, 2013].

1N2B1. ANOPHTHALMOS

General

Primary optic vesicle fails to develop.

Clinical

None.

Ocular

Small orbit with narrowed palpebral fissure and shrunken fornix.

Laboratory

CT and MRI of orbit and brain; B-scan ultrasound imaging.

Treatment

Orbital expansion with serial implants in the growing orbit, increased horizontal length of palpebral fissure, dermis fat graft, inflatable silicone expander.

BIBLIOGRAPHY

1. Mamalis N, Ollerton AJ. (2012). Anophthalmos. [online] Available from www.emedicine.com/oph/TOPIC572.HTM. [Accessed September, 2013].

1N2B2. GENERAL FIBROSIS SYNDROME (CONGENITAL ENOPHTHALMOS WITH OCULAR MUSCLE FIBROSIS AND PTOSIS; CONGENITAL FIBROSIS OF THE INFERIOR RECTUS WITH PTOSIS; STRABISMUS FIXUS; VERTICAL RETRACTION SYNDROME (CONGENITAL FIBROSIS SYNDROME)

General

Present from birth; familial history; apparent autosomal dominant transmission; sex-linked recessive transmission is also reported.

Ocular

Ptosis; enophthalmos; disk hypoplasia; astigmatism; esotropia; exotropia; hypotropia; nystagmus; visual loss; positive forced duction test; may be associated with Marcus Gunn jaw-winking and synergistic divergence in attempted right gaze.

Clinical

None.

Laboratory

Neuroimaging is the most essential laboratory study.

Treatment

Surgically approximating normal orbital bone positions before addressing soft tissue volume loss.

BIBLIOGRAPHY

1. Soparkar CN. (2012). Enophthalmos. [online] Available from www.emedicine.com/oph/TOPIC617.HTM. [Accessed September, 2013].

1N2B4. LYMPHEDEMA

General

Abnormal accumulation of lymph in the extremities; occurs from multiple causes.

Ocular

Conjunctival chemosis; ectropion; ptosis; strabismus; hyperpigmentation of eyelids; chorioretinal dysplasia; distichiasis; eyelid lymphedema.

Clinical

Abnormal lymphatic drainage; painless swelling; fibrosis of skin and subcutaneous tissues; skin becomes thickened, brown, multiple papillary projections (lymphostatic verrucosis); microcephaly; lymphedema.

Laboratory

Lymphangiography, CT, MRI, Doppler ultrasonography.

Treatment

The goal of conservative therapy is to eliminate protein stagnation and to restore normal lymphatic circulation. Compression garments, intermittent pneumatic pump compression therapy, weight loss, avoiding even minor trauma, and avoiding constrictive clothing are all useful.

BIBLIOGRAPHY

1. Rossy KM, Scheinfeld NS. (2013). Lymphedema. Available from www.emedicine.com/med/TOPIC2722.HTM. [Accessed September, 2013].

1N2D2. HANSEN DISEASE (LEPROSY)

General

Communicable disease caused by *M. leprae.*

Ocular

Keratitis; leukoma; pannus; corneal ulcer; uveitis; iris atrophy; dacryocystitis; anisocoria; multiple pupils; decreased or absent pupillary reaction to light; paralysis of seventh nerve; episcleritis; blepharospasm; lagophthalmos; madarosis; secondary glaucoma; decreased IOP; subconjunctival fibrosis; punctate epithelial keratopathy; posterior subcapsular cataract; corneal hypesthesia; prominent corneal nerves; iridocyclitis; foveal avascular keratitis; scleritis; interstitial keratitis; iris pearls; dry eye.

Clinical

Disease affects primarily the skin, mucous membrane, and peripheral nerves.

Laboratory

Skin biopsy specimens contain vacuolated macrophages, few lymphocytes, and numerous acid-fast bacilli often in clumps or globi.

Treatment

The WHO recommends MDT for all forms of leprosy. MDT 14 consists of rifampin, ofloxacin, and minocycline.

BIBLIOGRAPHY

1. Kim EC. (2011). Ocular manifestations of leprosy. [online] Available from www.emedicine.com/oph/TOPIC743.HTM. [Accessed September, 2013].

🖥 1N2D4. TRACHOMA

General

Most common in rural communities of the Middle East, Africa, Asia, and South and Central America; caused by *Chlamydia trachomatis*; associated with poor sanitation and medical care.

Ocular

Chronic keratoconjunctivitis; papillae follicles; keratitis; opacities of cornea; scars of palpebral conjunctiva; ptosis; tearing; entropion.

Clinical

Rhinitis; otitis media; upper respiratory tract infection.

Laboratory

Most endemic areas, lab tests are unavailable. Commercial polymerase chain reaction (PCR) based assay has high sensitivity and specificity.

Treatment

Tetracycline eye ointment for 6 weeks or a single dose azithromycin systemically.

🖥 BIBLIOGRAPHY

1. Solomon AW. (2011). Trachoma. [online] Available from www.emedicine.com/oph/TOPIC118.HTM. [Accessed September, 2013].

🖥 1N2D7. AMENDOLA SYNDROME

General

Observed in Sao Paulo, Brazil; all ethnic groups are affected; endemic form of pemphigus foliaceus; possibly caused by environmental agents; autoimmune disease mediated by autoantibodies of the IgG class, IgG4 subclass.

Ocular

Blisters around eyebrows; entropion; ectropion; trichiasis; iritis.

Clinical

Brazilian pemphigus (fogo selvagem, "wild fire"), which resembles, because of its appearance, pemphigus foliaceus; fever; chills.

Laboratory

Diagnosis is made by clinical findings.

Treatment

- *Entropion*: Topical antibiotics and lubricants, temporary sutures to evert the eyelid, lateral cantholysis with subconjunctival incision just inferior to the tarsus. Inferior retracters are isolated and reattached to anterior inferior portion of tarsus with multiple interrupted sutures.
- *Iritis*: Oral steroids if not responsive to topical steroids, immunosuppressants if bilateral disease that does not respond to oral steroids, periocular steroids for unilateral or posterior uveitis. Vitrectomy can be used for severe vitreous opacification. Cryotherapy and laser photocoagulation may be used for localized pars plana exudates.

🖥 BIBLIOGRAPHY

1. Amendola F. Cataracta No Pemfigo Foliaceo (nota previa). Rev Paul Med. 1945;26:286.
2. Korting GW. The skin and the eye: a dermatologic correlation of diseases of the periorbital region. Philadelphia: WB Saunders; 1973. pp. 82.
3. Magalini SI, Scrascia, E. Dictionary of Medical Syndromes, 2nd edition. Philadelphia: JB Lippincott; 1981.
4. Sampaio SA, Rivitti EA, Aoki V, et al. Brazilian pemphigus foliaceus, endemic pemphigus foliaceus or fogo selvagem (wild fire). Dermatol Clin. 1994;12:765-76.

⊟ 1N2D8. SMALLPOX (VARIOLA)

General

Highly contagious cutaneous disease caused by viral infection.

Ocular

Conjunctivitis; keratitis; corneal ulcer; hypopyon; endophthalmitis; congenital corneal clouding; albinotic spots on iris; choroiditis; vitreous opacities; papillitis; extraocular muscle palsies; entropion; dacryocystitis; chorioretinitis; optic neuritis; and vesicles of the eyelid; preauricular adenopathy; eyelid ulcerating pustules; several conditions predispose to the spread of vaccinia, including eczema, hypogammaglobulinemia, steroid therapy, and acquired immunodeficiency syndrome (AIDS).

Clinical

Fever, headache, and vomiting prior to appearance of the rash on the face, upper trunk, and down to the extremities.

Laboratory

Brick-shaped virions viewed with electron microscopy examination, virus culture from live cells, or DNA analysis using PCR and smallpox skin specimen should be collected.

Treatment

No known treatment is effective.

⊟ BIBLIOGRAPHY

1. Hussain AN, Hussain F, Alam M, et al. (2011). Smallpox. [online] Available from www.emedicine.com/med/TOPIC3545.HTM. [Accessed September, 2013].

⊟ 1O. EPICANTHUS (FOLD OF SKIN OVER INNER CANTHUS OF EYE)

†1. *Types*
   A. Epicanthus inversus: Fold arises in the lower lid and extends upward to a point slightly above the inner canthus; it is accompanied by long medial canthal tendons, blepharophimosis, and ptosis-autosomal dominant.
   B. Epicanthus palpebralis (common type): Epicanthal fold arises from the upper lid above the tarsal region and extends to the lower margin of the orbit.
   C. Epicanthus supraciliaris (unusual type): Epicanthal fold arises near brow and runs toward tear sac.
   D. Epicanthus tarsalis (Mongolian eye): Epicanthal fold arises from the tarsal (lid) fold and loses itself in the skin close to the inner canthus-autosomal dominant.

2. *Associated conditions*
   A. Aminopterin-induced syndrome
   B. Basal cell nevus syndrome (Gorlin syndrome)
   C. Bassen-Kornzweig syndrome (familial hypolipoproteinemia)
   †D. Bilateral renal agenesis
   E. Blepharophimosis, ptosis, epicanthus inversus syndrome
   F. Bonnevie-Ullrich syndrome (pterygolymphangiectasia)
   G. Carpenter syndrome (acrocephalopolysyndactyly II)
   H. Cat-eye syndrome (partial G-trisomy syndrome)
   †I. Cerebrofacioarticular syndrome of van Maldergen
   J. Cerebrohepatorenal syndrome (Smith-Lemli-Opitz syndrome)
   K. Chondrodystrophia (Conradi syndrome)
   L. Chromosome long-arm deletion syndrome
   M. Chromosome deletion (deletion 18) Craniocarpotarsal syndrome (whistling face syndrome)
   N. Chromosome partial short-arm deletion syndrome (Wolf syndrome)
   †O. Chromosome short-arm deletion syndrome
   P. Chromosome 13q partial deletion syndrome
   Q. Congenital facial paralysis (Möbius syndrome)
   S. Craniosynostosis-radial aplasia (Baller-Gerold syndrome)
   T. Cri-du-chat syndrome (Cry of the cat syndrome)
   U. Dubowitz syndrome
   V. Down syndrome (trisomy 21, mongolism)
   W. Drummond syndrome (idiopathic hypercalcemia, blue diaper syndrome)
   X. Ehlers-Danlos syndrome (fibrodysplasia elastica generalisata)
   Y. 18q syndrome

Z. Familial blepharophimosis
AA. Fetal alcohol syndrome
BB. Freeman-Sheldon syndrome (whistling face syndrome)
CC. 4Q syndrome
DD. Gansslen syndrome (hematologic-metabolic bone disorder)
EE. Greig syndrome (ocular hypertelorism syndrome)
FF. Hurler syndrome (dysostosis multiplex)
†GG. Infantile hypercalcemia
HH. Jacobs syndrome (triple X syndrome)
II. Klinefelter XXY syndrome (gynecomastia-aspermatogenesis syndrome)
JJ. Kohn-Romano syndrome (ptosis, blepharophimosis, epicanthus inversus, and telecanthus)
KK. Komoto syndrome (congenital eyelid tetrad)
LL. Laurence-Moon-Bardet-Biedl syndrome (retinitis pigmentosa-polydactyly-adiposogenital)
MM. LEOPARD syndrome (multiple lentigines syndrome)
NN. Leroy syndrome (mucopolysaccharide excretion)
OO. Little syndrome (nail patella syndrome)
PP. Michel syndrome
QQ. Mohr-Claussen syndrome (similar to orodigitofacial syndrome)
RR. Noonan syndrome (Turner syndrome in males)
SS. Oculocerebrorenal syndrome (Lowe syndrome)
TT. Oculodentodigital dysplasia (microphthalmos syndrome)

UU. Potter syndrome (renofacial syndrome)
VV. Ring chromosome syndrome
†WW. Ring chromosome (microcephaly, hypertelorism, epicanthus)
†XX. Ring chromosome in the D group (13-15)
YY. Robinow-Silverman-Smith syndrome
ZZ. Rubinstein-Taybi syndrome (broad thumbs syndrome)
AAA. Schonenberg syndrome (dwarf-cardiopathy syndrome)
BBB. Smith syndrome (facioskeletogenital dysplasia)
CCC. Thrombocytopenia absent radius (TAR) syndrome
DDD. Thalassemia
EEE. Trisomy syndrome (Edward syndrome)
FFF. Turner syndrome (gonadal dysgenesis)
GGG. Waardenburg syndrome (embryonic fixation syndrome)
HHH. X-linked mental retardation syndrome
III. XXXXX syndrome

🗗 BIBLIOGRAPHY

1. McKusick VA. Mendelian Inheritance in Man, 12th edition. Baltimore: Johns Hopkins University Press; 1998.
2. Roy FH. Ocular Syndromes and Systemic Diseases, 6th edition. New Delhi: Jaypyee Brothers Medical Publishers; 2013.

---

†Indicates a general entry and therefore has not been described in detail in the text

🗗 10.2A. AMINOPTERIN-INDUCED SYNDROME

General

Teratogenic effect of aminopterin and derivatives on fetus; present at birth; usually fetal or postnatal death.

Ocular

Hypertelorism.

Clinical

Small body; microcephaly; hypoplasia of cranial bones; broad nasal bridge; micrognathia; cleft palate; low-set ears; mesomelic; hypodactyly; talipes equinovarus.

Laboratory

Diagnosis is made by clinical findings.

Treatment

None.

🗗 BIBLIOGRAPHY

1. Draper JC, Cox KW, Matthews KJ. (2013). Teratology and drug use during pregnancy. [online] Available from www.emedicine.com/med/TOPIC3242.HTM. [Accessed September, 2013].

⊡ 10.2B. BASAL CELL NEVUS SYNDROME (NEVOID BASAL CELL CARCINOMA SYNDROME; NEVOID BASALIOMA SYNDROME; GORLIN SYNDROME; GORLIN-GOLTZ SYNDROME; MULTIPLE BASAL CELL NEVI SYNDROME)

General

Autosomal dominant; onset of skin lesions in childhood, usually at puberty.

Ocular

Basal cell carcinomas of eyelids; strabismus; hypertelorism; congenital cataracts; choroidal colobomas; glaucoma; medullated nerve fibers; prominence of supraorbital ridges; corneal leukoma; basalioma of the skin; coloboma of the choroid and optic nerve.

Clinical

Basal cell tumors with facial involvement; shallow pits of the skin of the hands and feet; jaw cysts; rib anomalies; kyphoscoliosis and fusion of vertebrae; medulloblastoma; frontal and temporoparietal bossing and broad nasal root.

Laboratory

CT scanning, ultrasonography, or MRI to evaluate neoplasms. Endoscopy to evaluate for the degree of polyposis and survey for malignant transformation is done.

Treatment

Patients may require medical attention for craniofacial, vertebral, dental and ophthalmologic abnormalities, in addition to diagnosis and treatment of potential neoplasia.

⊡ BIBLIOGRAPHY

1. Hsu EK, Mamula P, Ruchelli ED. (2011). Intestinal polyposis syndromes. [online] Available from www.emedicine.com/ped/TOPIC828.HTM. [Accessed August, 2013].

⊡ 10.2C. BASSEN-KORNZWEIG SYNDROME (ABETALIPOPROTEINEMIA; ACANTHOCYTOSIS; FAMILIAL HYPOLIPOPROTEINEMIA)

General

Inability to absorb and transport lipids; predominant in males; autosomal recessive inheritance; acanthocytosis, a peculiar burr cell malformation of the red blood cells; the basic defect is thought to be an inability to synthesize the apolipoprotein B peptide of low-density and very-low-density lipoproteins.

Ocular

Ptosis (may be present); nystagmus; progressive external ophthalmoplegia; retinitis pigmentosa (usually atypical); retinopathy develops with age after 10–14 years; optic atrophy occasionally; epicanthal folds; cataract; optic nerve pallor; hypopigmentation of retina; macular degeneration; dyschromatopsia.

Clinical

Steatorrhea; hypocholesterolemia; neurologic disorder with ataxia (similar to Friedreich ataxia); areflexia; Babinski sign; muscle weakness (facial, lingual; proximal and distal); slurred speech; lordosis; kyphosis.

Laboratory

Most patients will exhibit acanthocytosis on peripheral blood smear.

Treatment

Medical care is symptomatic and supportive.

⊡ BIBLIOGRAPHY

1. Gross KV, Lorenzo N. (2012). Neuroacanthocytosis syndromes. [online] Available from www.emedicine.com/neuro/TOPIC502.HTM. [Accessed September, 2013].

⛶ 10.2E. BLEPHAROPHIMOSIS SYNDROME (SIMOSA SYNDROME)

General

Dominantly inherited tetrad of ptosis, epicanthus inversus, telecanthus and blepharophimosis.

Ocular

Scarred or contracted in the secondary blepharophimosis because of ocular pemphigus or trachoma; ectropion; epicanthus inversus; lacrimal puncta displacement; ptosis; telecanthus; optic nerve coloboma; angle dysgenesis; optic nerve hypoplasia; amblyopia; strabismus.

Clinical

Low-set ears; low nasal bridge.

Laboratory

Diagnosis is made by clinical findings.

Treatment

The ptosis is corrected by frontalis fixation at an early age. Canthoplasties may be performed to improve the blepharophimosis. The considerable epicanthus is usually best left until early adolescence, since the degree of this problem tends to diminish with time and the skin becomes easier to move.

⛶ BIBLIOGRAPHY

1. Bashour M. (2012). Ptosis blepharoplasty. [online] Available from www.emedicine.com/ent/TOPIC97.HTM. [Accessed September, 2013].

⛶ 10.2F. TURNER SYNDROME (TURNER-ALBRIGHT SYNDROME; GONADAL DYSGENESIS; GENITAL DWARFISM SYNDROME; ULLRICH-TURNER SYNDROME; BONNEVIE-ULLRICH SYNDROME; PTERYGOLYMPHANGIECTASIA SYNDROME; ULLRICH-BONNEVIE SYNDROME) CATARACT, POSTERIOR

General

Ovarian or gonadal agenesis; 45 chromosomes with an XO sex-chromosome constitution; females; rare in males; onset in childhood.

Ocular

Exophthalmos; hypertelorism; ptosis; epicanthal folds; blue sclera; corneal nebulae; cataracts; conjunctival lymphedema; keratoconus.

Clinical

Webbed neck (pterygium colli); diminished growth; mandibulofacial disproportion; cubitus valgus; masculine chest and trunk; late appearance of pubic and axillary hair; congenital deafness; mental retardation; coarctation of aorta.

Laboratory

Karyotyping is needed for diagnosis. Y-chromosomal test; Luteinizing hormone (LH) and follicle-stimulating hormone (FSH) levels, thyroid function test, fasting glucose levels, echocardiography and MRI.

Treatment

Growth hormone therapy is used to prevent short stature. Estrogen replacement therapy is usually started by the age of 12–15 years.

⛶ BIBLIOGRAPHY

1. Postellon DC, Daniel MS. (2012). Turner syndrome. [online] Available from emedicine.medscape.com/article/949681-overview. [Accessed September, 2013].

10.2G. CARPENTER SYNDROME (ACROCEPHALOPOLYSYNDACTYLY TYPE II)

General

Hereditary; transmitted as an autosomal recessive trait; severe form of Apert syndrome; normal intelligence has been reported with this syndrome; polysyndactyly is not an absolute requirement for this diagnosis.

Ocular

Lateral displacement of inner canthus; epicanthal folds; microcornea; corneal opacities.

Clinical

Acrocephalopolysyndactyly; brachydactyly; peculiar facies; obesity; mental retardation; hypogonadism; generalized aminoaciduria; cryptorchidism; hypogenitalism.

Laboratory

Skull radiography, cranial CT.

Treatment

Carefully monitoring for signs and symptoms of elevated intracranial pressure is important. Surgery typically is indicated for increased intracranial pressure or for cosmetic reasons.

BIBLIOGRAPHY

1. Sheth RD, Ranalli N, Aldana P, et al. (2012). Pediatric craniosynostosis. [online] Available from www.emedicine.com/neuro/TOPIC80.HTM. [Accessed September, 2013].

10.2H. CAT'S-EYE SYNDROME (SCHACHENMANN SYNDROME; SCHMID-FRACCARO SYNDROME; PARTIAL TRISOMY G SYNDROME)

General

Causative factor is one extra chromosome, a G chromosome, which may be from a 13-15 or 21-22 chromosome; although the ocular findings of the syndrome are similar to the D 13-15 trisomy group, the systemic manifestations usually are less severe; this syndrome is associated with a supernumerary bisatellited marker chromosome derived from duplicated regions of 22pter'22q11.2; partial cat's-eye syndrome is characterized by the absence of coloboma.

Ocular

Hypertelorism; microphthalmos; antimongoloid slant of palpebral fissures; strabismus; inferior vertical iris coloboma (cat eye); cataract; choroidal coloboma; epicanthal folds.

Clinical

Anal atresia; preauricular fistulae (bilateral); umbilical hernia; heart anomalies.

Laboratory

Chromosome analysis.

Treatment

- *Cataract*: Change in glasses can sometimes improve a patient's visual function temporarily; however the most common treatment is cataract surgery.
- *Strabismus*: Equalized vision with correct refractive error; surgery may be helpful in patients with diplopia.

BIBLIOGRAPHY

1. Collins JF. Handbook of Clinical Ophthalmology. New York: Masson; 1982.

⊟ 10.2J. SMITH-LEMLI-OPITZ SYNDROME (CEREBROHEPATORENAL SYNDROME)

General

Autosomal recessive; similarities with trisomy 18 syndrome; prognosis poor, with death in early infancy (*see* Zellweger Syndrome); onset in fetal life; prevalent in males; reduced myelination in the cerebral hemispheres, cranial nerves, and peripheral nerves secondary to a defective cholesterol biosynthesis.

Ocular

Joining of the eyebrows (synophrys); ptosis (bilateral); pronounced epicanthal folds; strabismus; nystagmus; cataract; optic nerve demyelinization.

Clinical

Mental retardation; microcephaly; hypertonia; low-set ears; high-arched palate; failure to thrive; vomiting; hypospadias; cryptorchidism; metatarsus adductus.

Laboratory

Examination via slit lamp may reveal strabismus, cataracts, ptosis, and/or optic nerve abnormalities. Fetal ultrasonography, sterol analysis, MRI or CT scanning may reveal brain malformations. Renal ultrasonography is used to identify renal anomalies. Abdominal ultrasonography and barium swallow may help rule out pyloric stenosis.

Treatment

No treatment has proven effective for patients with Smith-Lemli-Opitz.

⊟ BIBLIOGRAPHY

1. Steiner RD. (2013). Smith-Lemli-Opitz Syndrome. [online] Available from www.emedicine.com/ped/TOPIC2117.HTM. [Accessed September, 2013].

⊟ 10.2K. CONRADI SYNDROME (MULTIPLE EPIPHYSEAL DYSPLASIA CONGENITA; DYSPLASIA EPIPHYSEALIS CONGENITA; CHONDRODYSTROPHIA FOETALIS HYPOPLASTICA; CALCINOSIS UNIVERSALIS; CONGENITAL CALCIFYING CHONDRODYSTROPHY; STIPPLED EPIPHYSES SYNDROME; CONRADI-HÜNERMANN SYNDROME; CHONDRODYSPLASIA PUNCTATA)

General

Autosomal recessive; manifestations within the first 6 months of life; epiphyseal stippling present at birth; perinatal manifestations include disorganization of the spine, premature echogenicity of femoral epiphyses, and frontal bossing with depressed nasal bridge.

Ocular

Hypertelorism; heterochromia iridis (rare); bilateral total congenital cataract appearing at or shortly after birth; primary optic atrophy (rare); bilateral corneal punctate erosions.

Clinical

Short limbs (mainly proximal part) resulting in "short-limbed dwarfism"; deformities of hip, knee, and elbow joints by contraction and immobility, and possible transformation of muscles into fibrous tissue as a result; congenital heart defect with calcium deposits in the cardiac valves; skin anomalies (dyskeratosis); mental retardation.

Laboratory

Clinical.

Treatment

- *Cataract*: Change in glasses can sometimes improve a patient's visual function temporarily; however the most common treatment is cataract surgery.
- *Corneal erosion*: Goal of therapy is regenerating or repairing the epithelial basement membrane to restore the adhesion between the epithelium and the anterior stroma, topical lubrication therapy bandage soft contact lenses, debridement of the epithelium and basement membrane, or anterior stromal micropuncture may be useful.

⊟ BIBLIOGRAPHY

1. Bellson FA. Optic nerve hypoplasia in chondrodysplasia punctata. J Pediatr Ophthalmol. 1977;14:144-7.
2. Conradi E. Vorzeitiges Auftreten von Knochenund Eigenartigen Verkalkungskernen bei Chondrodystrophia Fotalis Hypoplastica. Histologische un Rontgenuntersuchungen. Jahrb Kinderhk. 1914;80:86.
3. Happle R. Cataracts as a marker of genetic heterogeneity in chondrodysplasia punctata. Clin Genet. 1981;19:64-6.
4. Massey JY, Roy FH. Ocular manifestations of Conradi disease. Arch Ophthalmol. 1974;92:524-6.
5. Pryde PG, Bawle E, Brandt F, et al. Prenatal diagnosis of nonrhizomelic chondrodysplasia punctata (Conradi-Hunermann syndrome). Am J Med Genet. 1993;47:426-31.
6. Spierer A, Neumann D. Corneal changes in chondrodysplasia punctata syndrome. Ann Ophthalmol. 1993;25:356-8.

⊟ 10.2L. CHROMOSOME 18 PARTIAL DELETION (LONG-ARM) SYNDROME [MONOSOMY 18 PARTIAL (LONG-ARM) SYNDROME; DE GROUCHY SYNDROME]

General

Deletion of approximately one half of the long arm of chromosome 18.

Ocular

Hypertelorism; epicanthal folds; narrow palpebral fissure; nystagmus (horizontal); strabismus; myopia; astigmatism; glaucoma; oval pupils; microcornea; posterior staphyloma; oblique disk; optic nerve staphyloma; optic nerve atrophy; microphthalmia; corneal opacities; iris hypoplasia; corectopia.

Clinical

Dwarfism; mental retardation; microcephaly; midface dysplasia; prominent antihelix and antitragus; congenital cardiac disease; abnormal, spindle-shaped fingers; genital defects.

Laboratory

Clinical.

Treatment

- *Glaucoma*: Glaucoma medication should be the first plan of action. If medication is unsuccessful, a filtering surgical procedure with or without antimetabotites may be beneficial.
- *Strabismus*: Equalized vision with correct refractive error; surgery may be helpful in patient with diplopia.

⊟ BIBLIOGRAPHY

1. de Grouchy J, Royer P, Salmon C, et al. Deletion Partielle des Bras Longs du Chromosome 18. Pathol Biol (France). 1964;12:579-82.

⊟ 10.2M. FREEMAN-SHELDON SYNDROME (CRANIO-CARPO-TARSAL DYSPLASIA; WHISTLING FACE SYNDROME)

General

Rare; autosomal dominant and recessive inheritance as well as sporadic cases (genetic heterogeneity).

Ocular

Eyes deeply sunken (enophthalmos); hypertelorism; blepharophimosis; ptosis; antimongoloid slanting of lid fissures; esotropia.

Clinical

Small nose with narrow nostrils and long philtrum; alae nasi often bent, simulating colobomas; nasolabial folds present only near the nose; microstomia; high-arched palate and small mandible; flexion contractures of fingers; excessive bulging of central part of cheeks when whistling.

Laboratory

No specific laboratory studies, imaging, or diagnostic procedures are valuable.

Treatment

Various reconstructive procedures may be necessary.

BIBLIOGRAPHY

1. Freeman EA, Sheldon JH. Cranio-carpotarsal dystrophy: an undescribed congenital malformation. Arch Dis Child. 1938;13:277.
2. McKusick VA. Mendelian Inheritance in man: A Catalog of Human Genes and Genetic Disorders, 12th edition. Baltimore: The Johns Hopkins University Press; 1998.
3. O'Keefe M, Crawford JS, Young JD, et al. Ocular abnormalities in the Freeman-Sheldon syndrome. Am J Ophthalmol. 1986;102:346-8.
4. Wang TR, Lin SJ. Further evidence for genetic heterogeneity of whistling face or Freeman-Sheldon syndrome in a Chinese family. Am J Genet. 1987;28:471-5.
5. Weinstein S, Gorlin RJ. Cranio-carpotarsal dystrophy or the whistling face syndrome. Am J Dis Child. 1969;117:427-33.

10.2N. WOLF SYNDROME (MONOSOMY 4 PARTIAL SYNDROME; CHROMOSOME 4 PARTIAL DELETION SYNDROME; HIRSCHHORN-COOPER SYNDROME) PTOSIS

General

Partial deletion of chromosome 4 of the B group; short life expectancy; present from birth (*see* Cri-Du-Chat syndrome).

Ocular

Hypertelorism; antimongoloid slanting of palpebral fissures; ptosis; nystagmus; strabismus; iris coloboma; retinal coloboma.

Clinical

Microcephaly; mental retardation; seizures; ear malformations; hypospadias; beaked nose; broad nasal root; cleft lip and palate; hypotonia.

Laboratory

High-resolution cytogenetic studies, conventional cytogenetic, fluorescence in situ hybridization.

Treatment

No known treatment exist for the underlying disorder.

BIBLIOGRAPHY

1. Chen H. (2013). Wolf-Hirschhorn syndrome. [online] Available from www.emedicine.com/ped/TOPIC2446.HTM. [Accessed September, 2013].

10.2P. CHROMOSOME 13Q PARTIAL DELETION (LONG-ARM SYNDROME; 13Q SYNDROME)

General

No hereditary factor.

Ocular

Microphthalmos; antimongoloid slant of lid fissures; bilateral epicanthus; esotropia; cataract; choroidal coloboma; ptosis; retinoblastoma.

Clinical

Genital malformations; meningocele; short neck; small mouth; mental and physical retardation; small head; short stature; broad nasal bridge; simian crease; microcephaly; high nasal bridge; thumb hypoplasia.

Laboratory

The red blood cells are usually normochromic normocytic. An elevated white blood cell (WBC) count (> 12,000/μL) occurs in approximately 60% of patients.

Treatment

Phlebotomy is the mainstay of therapy for this disease. The object is to remove excess cellular elements, mainly red blood cells, to improve the circulation of blood by lowering the blood viscosity.

BIBLIOGRAPHY

1. Besa EC, Woermann UJ. (2012). Polycythemia vera. [online] Available from www.emedicine.com/med/TOPIC1864.HTM. [Accessed September, 2013].

⊟ 10.2Q. MÖBIUS II SYNDROME (CONGENITAL FACIAL DIPLEGIA; CONGENITAL PARALYSIS OF THE SIXTH AND SEVENTH NERVES; CONGENITAL OCULO FACIAL PARALYSIS; VON GRAEFES SYNDROME)

General

Congenital; possibly failure of development of facial nerve cells or primary defect of muscles deriving from first two brachial arches or both; recovery in a few weeks or non-progressive permanent paralysis of face; asymmetrical; if incomplete, usually spares lower face and platysma.

Ocular

Proptosis; ptosis; weakness of abductor muscles; normal convergence; limitation to internal rotation in lateral movements; esotropia.

Clinical

Facial diplegia; deafness; loss of vestibular responses; webbed fingers or toes; clubfoot.

Laboratory

Diagnosis is made by clinical findings.

Treatment

Ptosis: If visual acuity is affected most cases require surgical correction and there are several procedures that may be used including levator resection, repair or advancement and Fasanella-Servat.

⊟ BIBLIOGRAPHY

1. Abbott RL, Metz HS, Weber AA. Saccadic velocity studies in Möbius syndrome. Ann Ophthalmol. 1978;10:619-23.
2. Fenichel GM. Congenital facial asymmetry (aplasia of facial muscles). In: Fenichel GM (ed). Clinical pediatric neurology, 2nd edition. Philadelphia: WB Saunders; 1993. pp. 341-2.
3. Kawai M, Momoi T, Fujii T, et al. The syndrome of Möbius sequence, peripheral neuropathy, and hypogonadotropic hypogonadism. Am J Med Genet. 1990;37:578-82.
4. Menkes JH, Kenneth T. Möbius syndrome. In: Menkes JH (ed). Textbook of child neurology, 5th edition. Baltimore: Williams & Wilkins; 1995. pp. 309-10.
5. Merz M, Wójtowicz S. The Möbius syndrome. Report of electromyographic examinations in two cases. Am J Ophthalmol. 1967;63(4):837-40.
6. Möbius PJ. über angeborene doppelseitige Abducens-Facial-islahmung. Munch Med Wochenschr. 1888;35:91-108.
7. Pucket CL, Beg SA. Facial reanimation in Möbius syndrome. South Med J. 1978;71:1498-501.

⊟ 10.2S. BALLER-GEROLD SYNDROME (CRANIOSYNOSTOSIS RADIAL APLASIA)

General

Autosomal recessive inheritance.

Ocular

Ocular hypertelorism; epicanthic folds.

Clinical

High nasal bridge; low philtrum; dysplastic ears; radius hypoplastic or absent; ulna short and bowed; carpal bones missing or fused; thumb hypoplastic or missing; craniosynostosis; anal, urogenital, cardiac, CNS, and vertebral defects; agenesis of frontal and parietal bones; midline facial angioma; scrotally positioned anus; microcephaly; erythroblastosis of the liver; pancreatic islet cell hypertrophy.

Laboratory

Diagnosis is made with clinical findings.

Treatment

Surgery before age of 6 months to repair bilateral craniosynostosis.

⊟ BIBLIOGRAPHY

1. Baller F. Radiuasplasie und Inzucht. Z Mensch Vererb Konstitutionsl Lehre. 1950;29:782-90.
2. Dallapiccola B, Zelante L, Mingarelli R, et al. Baller-Gerold syndrome: case report and Clinical and radiological review. Am J Med Genet. 1992;42:365-8.
3. Lin AE, McPherson E, Nwokoro NA, et al. Further delineation of the Baller-Gerold syndrome. Am J Med Genet. 1993;45:519-24.
4. Magalini SI, Scrascia E. Dictionary of Medical Syndromes, 2nd edition. Philadelphia: JB Lippincott; 1981.
5. Van Maldergem L, Verloes A, Lejeune L, et al. The Baller-Gerold syndrome. J Med Genet. 1992;29:266-8.

10.2T. CRI-DU-CHAT SYNDROME [CAT-CRY (5P-) SYNDROME; CRYING CAT SYNDROME; BI DELETION SYNDROME; LEJEUNE SYNDROME]

General

Short arm deletion of a no. 5 chromosome (5p-); increased inheritance risk; 13% have one parent with balanced translocation; female preponderance 2:1 (*see* Wolf Syndrome).

Ocular

Hypertelorism; epicanthal folds; antimongoloid slanting of palpebral fissures; strabismus; increased tortuosity of retinal vessels.

Clinical

High-pitched, plaintive cry by an infant (reminiscent of a crying cat); mental retardation; broad nasal root; micrognathia or retrognathia; low-set ears; simian crease; congenital heart defect; small larynx and epiglottis.

Laboratory

Conventional cytogenetic studies, skeletal radiography, MRI, echocardiography.

Treatment

No treatment exists for the underlying disorder. Correction of congenital heart defects may be indicated.

⊡ BIBLIOGRAPHY

1. Chen H. (2013). Cri-du-chat Syndrome. [online] Available from www.emedicine.com/ped/TOPIC504.HTM. [Accessed September, 2013].

10.2U. DUBOWITZ SYNDROME (DWARFISM-ECZEMA-PECULIAR FACIES)

General

Affects both sexes; congenital; may be autosomal recessive inheritance.

Ocular

Hypertelorism; lateral telecanthus; palpebral ptosis; short palpebral tissues.

Clinical

Eczema; sparse hair; cleft palate; hypospadia; microcephaly; low birth weight; mild mental retardation; characteristic face; short stature; spontaneous keloids; intrauterine growth retardation.

Laboratory

Bone marrow biopsy, quantitative hemoglobin electrophoresis, cytogenetic studies, HLA.

Treatment

Management involves supportive care that includes transfusion, treatment of infections, and a search for an allogeneic stem cell donor.

⊡ BIBLIOGRAPHY

1. Dixon N, Castellino SM, Howard SC. (2011). Pediatric myelodysplasia. [online] Available from www.emedicine.com/ped/TOPIC1526.HTM. [Accessed September, 2013].

10.2V. DOWN SYNDROME (MONGOLISM; TRISOMY G; TRISOMY 21 SYNDROME; MONGOLOID IDIOCY)

General

Trisomy of chromosome 21.

Ocular

Hypertelorism; epicanthus; blepharitis; ectropion; nystagmus; esotropia; high myopia (30%); hyperopia; color blindness; yellow spots on the iris; hypoplasia of the iris; blepharoconjunctivitis; lens opacities (50%); keratoconus (may be acute); corneal hydrops; corneal ectasia; corneal edema; leukoma; lateral displacement of canaliculi and puncta; megaloblepharon; euryblepharon; decreased accommodation; Leber congenital amaurosis.

Clinical

Mental retardation; skeletal abnormalities; overextension of joints; deformed and low-set ears; short fifth finger; transverse palmar crease; fissured tongue; heart anomalies.

Laboratory

Amniocentesis during second trimester to check mothers who have low α-fetoprotein serum values, prenatal echography, craniofacial X-ray to check features and echocardiography.

Treatment

Primary care provider should coordinate the multisystemic evaluation. Awareness of systemic and ocular findings is essential for managing patients.

BIBLIOGRAPHY

1. Izquierdo NJ, Townsend W. (2011). Ophthalmologic manifestations of Down syndrome. [online] Available from www.emedicine.com/oph/TOPIC522.HTM. [Accessed August, 2013].

10.2W. DRUMMOND SYNDROME (IDIOPATHIC HYPERCALCEMIA; BLUE DIAPER SYNDROME)

General

Autosomal recessive; manifests itself in infancy; defective intestinal transport of tryptophan, which oxidizes to indigo blue and stains the diaper blue.

Ocular

Sclerosis of optic foramina (occasionally); prominent epicanthal folds; nystagmus; strabismus; peripheral retinal atrophy; papilledema; optic atrophy; microcornea; hypoplasia of the optic nerve; abnormal eye movements.

Clinical

Dwarfism; osteosclerosis; craniostenosis; depressed bridge of nose; "elfin-like" face; mental retardation; anorexia; vomiting; constipation.

Laboratory

Measurement of serum phosphate, alkaline phosphatase, serum chloride, serum bicarbonate, and urinary calcium.

Treatment

Treatment depends on the severity of symptoms and the underlying cause.

BIBLIOGRAPHY

1. Agraharkar M, Dellinger OD, Gangakhedkar AK. (2012). Hypercalcemia. [online] Available from www.emedicine.com/med/TOPIC1068.HTM. [Accessed September, 2013].

10.2X. EHLERS-DANLOS SYNDROME (FIBRODYSPLASIA ELASTICA GENERALISATA; CUTIS HYPERELASTICA; MEEKEREN-EHLERS-DANLOS SYNDROME; INDIAN RUBBER MAN SYNDROME; CUTIS LAXA)

General

Present at birth; autosomal dominant; two groups: cutaneous and articular; syndrome is one of the three primary disorders of elastic tissue [other two disorders are pseudoxanthoma elasticum (Grönblad-Strandberg syndrome) and senile elastosis]; inherited disorder of collagen biosynthesis.

Ocular

Hyperelasticity of palpebral skin; easy eversion of upper lid; ptosis; epicanthal folds; hypotony of extraocular muscles; strabismus; microcornea; thinning of cornea with keratoconus; thinning of sclera (blue sclera); subluxation of lens; angioid streaks; chorioretinal hemorrhages; retinitis proliferans with secondary detachment; macular degeneration; myopia; ruptured globe after minor trauma; limbus-to-limbus corneal thinning; acute hydrops; cornea plana; keratoglobus.

Clinical

Cutaneous manifestations include thin, atrophic, fragile skin, cutaneous hyperelasticity and pseudomolluscoid tumors; articular manifestations include excessive articular laxity and luxations; hypermobile joints.

Laboratory

Biochemical studies can detect alterations in collagen molecules in cultured skin fibroblasts. Molecular (DNA)-based testing is available. Diagnosis may by urinary analyte assay and clinical examination is the most common.

Treatment

Ascorbic acid therapy, in the event of skin lacerations seriously consider alternatives to sutures, including adhesive strips and wound glues, monitor for cardiac conditions and scoliosis.

BIBLIOGRAPHY

1. Steiner RD. (2011). Genetics of Ehlers-Danlos syndrome. [online] Available from www.emedicine.com/ped/TOPIC654.HTM. [Accessed September, 2013].

10.2Y. 18Q- SYNDROME (18Q DELETION SYNDROME)

General

Chromosome 18q deletion syndrome.

Ocular

Macular "fibrosis"; optic disk abnormalities with tractional retinal detachment, retinal degeneration, and tilting of the optic disk.

Clinical

Microcephaly; short stature; hypotonia; hypothyroidism; diabetes mellitus; short neck; sensorineural hearing loss; sensorimotor axonal neuropathy; mild-to-moderate mental retardation; chronic arthritis; seizures.

Laboratory

Clinical.

Treatment

Retinal detachment: Scleral buckle, pneumatic retinopexy and vitrectomy may be used to close all the breaks.

BIBLIOGRAPHY

1. Gordon MF, Bressman S, Brin MF, et al. Dystonia in a patient with deletion of 18q. Mov Disord. 1995;10:496-9.
2. Hansen US, Herline T. Chronic arthritis in a boy with 18q-syndrome. J Rheumatol. 1994;21:1958-9.
3. Smith A, Caradus V, Henry JG. Translocation 46X6 t(17;18)(q25;q21) in a mentally retarded boy with progressive eye abnormalities. Clin Genet. 1979;16:156-62.

10.2Z. ABERFELD SYNDROME (SCHWARTZ-JAMPEL SYNDROME; CONGENITAL BLEPHAROPHIMOSIS ASSOCIATED WITH GENERALIZED MYOPATHY SYNDROME; OCULAR AND FACIAL ABNORMALITIES SYNDROME)

General

Etiology is not known; autosomal recessive inheritance, although there are reports of dominant inheritance; progressive disorder.

Ocular

Blepharophimosis; exotropia; myopia; congenital cataracts; microcornea.

Clinical

Myopathy; bone deformities; arachnodactyly; dwarfism; hypoplastic facial bones; hypertrichosis; kyphoscoliosis.

Laboratory

Physicians might consider referring suspected cases to genetic clinics that have affiliations with groups actively research so that genetic studies can be performed. Muscle biopsy findings are consistent with a myopathy.

Treatment

The goal is to reduce the abnormal muscle activity that causes stiffness. Botulinum toxin therapy may be considered for the treatment of blepharospasm. However, if ptosis is present this is contraindicated. Some medications that have been found useful in myotonic disorders include the anticonvulsants and the antiarrhythmics.

BIBLIOGRAPHY

1. Ault J, Berman SA, Dinnerstein E. (2012). Schwartz-Jampel syndrome. [online] Available from www.emedicine.com/neuro/TOPIC337.HTM. [Accessed September, 2013].

⊟ 10.2AA. FETAL ALCOHOL SYNDROME

General

Dysgenesis in children born to alcoholic mothers; both sexes affected; onset from birth.

Ocular

Antimongoloid slant of lid fissures; lateral displacement of inner canthi; ptosis; epicanthi; strabismus; myopia; optic nerve hypoplasia; diffuse corneal clouding; iridocorneal abnormalities with central corneal edema; lens opacification; motility disorders.

Clinical

Growth retardation; delayed development (physical and intellectual); maxillary hypoplasia; micrognathia; large, low-set ears; abnormal motor function; irritability; microcephaly; cerebral nervous system dysfunctions; abnormal philtrum; flattened nasal bridge; cardiovascular defects; thin upper lip.

Laboratory

If suspected, consult a subspecialist (e.g. geneticist, developmentalist) to confirm the diagnosis.

Treatment

Treat for associated birth defects and intervention for potential cognitive and behavioral abnormalities. Vitrectomy may be necessary.

⊟ BIBLIOGRAPHY

1. Vaux KK, Chambers C. (2012). Fetal alcohol syndrome. [online] Available from www.emedicine.com/ped/TOP-IC767.HTM. [Accessed September, 2013].

⊟ 10.2BB. FREEMAN-SHELDON SYNDROME (CRANIO-CARPO-TARSAL DYSPLASIA; WHISTLING FACE SYNDROME)

General

Rare; autosomal dominant and recessive inheritance as well as sporadic cases (genetic heterogeneity).

Ocular

Eyes deeply sunken (enophthalmos); hypertelorism; blepharophimosis; ptosis; antimongoloid slanting of lid fissures; esotropia.

Clinical

Small nose with narrow nostrils and long philtrum; alae nasi often bent, simulating colobomas; nasolabial folds present only near the nose; microstomia; high-arched palate and small mandible; flexion contractures of fingers; excessive bulging of central part of cheeks when whistling.

Laboratory

No specific laboratory studies, imaging, or diagnostic procedures are valuable.

Treatment

Various reconstructive procedures may be necessary.

⊟ BIBLIOGRAPHY

1. Freeman EA, Sheldon JH. Cranio-carpotarsal dystrophy: an undescribed congenital malformation. Arch Dis Child. 1938;13:277.
2. McKusick VA. Mendelian Inheritance in Man: A Catalog of Human Genes and Genetic Disorders, 12th edition. Baltimore: The Johns Hopkins University Press; 1998.
3. O'Keefe M, Crawford JS, Young JD, et al. Ocular abnormalities in the Freeman-Sheldon syndrome. Am J Ophthalmol. 1986;102:346-8.
4. Wang TR, Lin SJ. Further evidence for genetic heterogeneity of whistling face or Freeman-Sheldon syndrome in a Chinese family. Am J Genet. 1987;28:471-5.
5. Weinstein S, Gorlin RJ. Cranio-carpotarsal dystrophy or the whistling face syndrome. Am J Dis Child. 1969;117:427-33.

⊟ 10.2CC. 4Q- SYNDROME (4Q DELETION SYNDROME)

General

Chromosome 4q deletion syndrome.

Ocular

Hypertelorism, epicanthal folds.

Clinical

Depressed nasal bridge; short nasal septum with upturned nose, cleft lip and palate; micrognathia; low-set malformed ears; short neck; distally placed nipples; sacral dimple; hypospadias; dysplastic nails; overriding toes; simian creases; hypoplasia of gall bladder; cardiac defects; mental retardation.

Laboratory

Diagnosis is made by clinical findings.

Treatment

See hypertelorism and epicanthal folds.

⊟ BIBLIOGRAPHY

1. Robertson SP, O'Day K, Banker A. The 4q- syndrome: delineating of the minimal critical region to within band 4q31. Clin Genet. 1998;53:70-73.
2. Townes PL, White M, DiMarzo SV. 4q- syndrome. Am J Dis Child. 1979;133:383-5.
3. Yu CW, Chen H, Baucum RW, et al. Terminal deletion of the long arm of chromosome 4. Report of a case of 46,XY,del(4)(q31) and review of 4q- syndrome. Ann Genet. 1981;24:158-61.

⊟ 10.2DD. GANSSLEN SYNDROME (FAMILIAL HEMOLYTIC ICTERUS; HEMATOLOGIC-METABOLIC BONE DISORDER)

General

Autosomal dominant inheritance; occurs mainly in Caucasians.

Ocular

Hypertelorism; microphthalmos; epicanthus; narrowing of palpebral fissure; lid hemorrhages; myopia; dyschromatopsia; hypochromic heterochromia; scleral icterus; conjunctival hemorrhages; retinal pallor and edema in advanced stages; dilated retinal arteries and veins; round retinal hemorrhages in deeper retinal layers; retinal exudates and macular star.

Clinical

Splenomegaly; hemolytic crises; dental deformities; brachydactyly; polydactyly; congenital hip luxation; oxycephaly; deformities of the outer ear and otosclerosis.

Laboratory

Indirect Coomb's test and direct antibody test results are positive in the mother and affected newborn; serial maternal antibody titers are monitored until a critical titer of 1:32, which indicates that a high risk of fetal hydrops.

Treatment

Early exchange transfusion with type-O Rh-negative fresh RBCs with intensive phototherapy is usually required.

⊟ BIBLIOGRAPHY

1. Ganser SJ. Uber Einen Eigenarrigen Hysterischen Dammerzustand. Arch Psychiatr Nervenkrankh. 1898;30:633.
2. Magalini SI, Scrascia E. Dictionary of Medical Syndromes, 2nd edition. Philadelphia: JB Lippincott; 1981.

⊟ 10.2EE. GREIG SYNDROME (OCULAR HYPERTELORISM SYNDROME; HYPERTELORISM; PRIMARY EMBRYONIC HYPERTELORISM; HYPERTELORISM OCULARIS)

General

Condition is rare; sporadic or hereditary; autosomal dominant or sex linked; if not associated with mental deficiency, then adequate mental and physical development is found.

Ocular

Hypertelorism (wide spacing of orbits); enophthalmos; epicanthus; deformities of eyelids and brows; defects of the palpebral fissure; bilateral sixth nerve paralysis;

esotropia; astigmatism; optic atrophy by tension on the optic nerve; strabismus.

Clinical

Skull may show mild malformations, including bitemporal eminences and decreased anteroposterior diameter; harelip; high-arched palate; cleft palate; broad and flat nasal root; mental impairment.

Laboratory

Diagnosis is made by clinical findings.

Treatment

Minor degrees of deformity (referred to as telecanthus) can be corrected by removing a small amount of bone in the midline. A limited frontal craniotomy is performed in the midline osteotomy.

BIBLIOGRAPHY

1. Jackson IT, Malhotra G. (2012). Congenital syndromes. [online] Available from www.emedicine.com/plastic/TOPIC183.HTM. [Accessed September, 2013].

10.2FF. HURLER SYNDROME (PFAUNDLER-HURLER SYNDROME; GARGOYLISM; DYSOSTOSIS MULTIPLEX; MPS IH SYNDROME; SYSTEMIC MUCOPOLYSACCHARIDOSIS TYPE IH; MUCOPOLYSACCHARIDOSIS IH)

General

Autosomal recessive inheritance; in addition to corneal opacities and enlargement of the head at birth, other symptoms become apparent at the end of the 1st year; death occurs usually before 20 years; gross excess of chondroitin sulfate band, heparitin sulfate in the urine (*see* Hunter Syndrome; Sanfilippo-Good Syndrome; Morquio-Brailsford Syndrome; Scheie Syndrome; Maroteaux-Lamy Syndrome). Jensen suggested that the pathogenesis of the various mucopolysaccharidoses is the same but that the variations in the defective enzymes cause the different types; most common mucopolysaccharidosis (MPS), decreased iduronidase.

Ocular

Proptosis; hypertelorism; thick, enlarged lids; esotropia; diffuse haziness of the cornea at birth progressive to milky opacity; retinal pigmentary changes may exist; macular edema and absence of foveal reflex; optic atrophy; megalocornea; bushy eyebrows; coarse eyelashes; mucopolysaccharide deposits of iris, lens, and sclera; enlarged optic foramen; retinal detachment; anisocoria; buphthalmos; nystagmus; secondary open-angle glaucoma; progressive retinopathy with vascular narrowing; hyperpigmentation of the fundus; bone spicule; papilledema.

Clinical

Dorsolumbar kyphosis; head deformities with depressed nose bridge; short cervical spine; short limbs; macroglossia; enlarged liver and spleen; short stature; facial dysmorphism; progressive psychomotor retardation.

Laboratory

Blood smears-abnormal cytoplasmic inclusions in lymphocytes; urine: increased excretion of dermatan sulfate and heparin sulfate.

Treatment

- *Macular edema*: Use of corticosteroids, carbonic anhydrase inhibitors and nonsteroidal anti-inflammatory drugs (NSAIDs) are the mainstay of treatment. If traditional therapy is not effective, intraocular injections of Avastin® may be helpful. In cases that have vitreous strand tugging against the macula, pars plana vitrectomy may be necessary.
- *Retinal detachment*: Scleral buckle, pneumatic retinopexy and vitrectomy may be used to close all the breaks.
- *Glaucoma*: Glaucoma medication should be the first plan of action. If medication is unsuccessful, a filtering surgical procedure with or without antimetabolites may be beneficial.
- *Papilledema*: Underlying cause should be determined and treated. Systemic acetazolamide is the medical therapy of choice.

BIBLIOGRAPHY

1. Banikazemi M. (2012). Genetics of mucopolysaccharidosis type I. [online] Available from www.emedicine.com/ped/TOPIC1031.HTM. [Accessed September, 2013].

⊡ 10.2HH. JACOBS SYNDROME (TRIPLE X SYNDROME; XXX SYNDROME; SUPER FEMALE SYNDROME)

General

It is caused by sex chromosomal anomaly with 44 autosomal and 3X sex chromosomes; due to nondisjunction; often associated with autosomal trisomies; majority of cases are asymptomatic.

Ocular

Hypertelorism; epicanthus; mongoloid slanted lid fissure; strabismus.

Clinical

Microcephaly; oligophrenia, occasionally with secondary amenorrhea; abnormal dentition; high-arched palate; hypogenitalism; occasionally mental retardation; early menopause.

Laboratory

Diagnosis is made by clinical findings.

Treatment

Strabismus can be treated with appropriate surgical procedure.

⊡ BIBLIOGRAPHY

1. Jacobs PA, Baikie AG, Brown WM, et al. Evidence for the existence of the human "superfemale." Lancet. 1959;2: 423-5.
2. Kohn G, Winter JS, Mellman WJ, et al. Trisomy X in three children. J Pediatr. 1968;72:248-52.

⊡ 10.2II. KLINEFELTER SYNDROME (GYNECOMASTIA-ASPERMATOGENESIS SYNDROME; XXY SYNDROME; XXXY SYNDROME; XXYY SYNDROME; REIFENSTEIN-ALBRIGHT SYNDROME)

General

Occurrence in 1% of retarded males; phenotypically males with positive female sex chromatin; karyotype shows 47 chromosomes, 44 autosomes, and 3 sex chromosomes with the complement XXY.

Ocular

Anophthalmos; coloboma; corneal opacities.

Clinical

Testicular hypoplasia; sterility; gynecomastia; eunuchoid physique; mental retardation; association with progressive systemic sclerosis and systemic lupus erythematosus.

Laboratory

May be diagnosed prenatally based on cytogenetic analysis of a fetus. If not diagnosed prenatally, the 47,XXY karyotype may manifest as various subtle age-related clinical signs that may prompt chromosomal evaluation.

Treatment

Treatment should address three major facets of the disease: (1) hypogonadism, (2) gynecomastia, and (3) psychosocial problems.

⊡ BIBLIOGRAPHY

1. Chen H. (2013). Klinefelter syndrome. [online] Available from www.emedicine.com/ped/TOPIC1252.HTM. [Accessed August, 2013].

⊡ 10.2JJ. KOHN-ROMANO SYNDROME (BPES SYNDROME)

General

Autosomal dominant transmittance; tetrad with telecanthus, ptosis, epicanthus inversus, and blepharophimosis; male preponderance; location of the abnormal gene responsible for this syndrome has been postulated to be a 3q2.

Ocular

Telecanthus; ptosis; epicanthus inversus; blepharophimoses; divergent strabismus; nystagmus; esotropia; anomalies of the lacrimal punctum; reduced corneal diameter.

Clinical

Highly arched palate; low-set ears with deformed pinnas.

Laboratory

Diagnosis is made by clinical findings.

Treatment

See ptosis, strabismus, lacrimal punctum obstruction.

⊟ BIBLIOGRAPHY

1. Suh DW. (2012). Congenital Ptosis. [online] Available from www.emedicine.com/oph/TOPIC345.HTM. [Accessed August, 2013].

⊟ 10.2KK. KOMOTO SYNDROME (CONGENITAL EYELID TETRAD; CET)

General

Autosomal dominant; all races affected; most patients are of normal intelligence.

Ocular

Ptosis; epicanthus inversus; blepharophimosis; telecanthus.

Clinical

None.

Laboratory

Diagnosis is made by clinical findings.

Treatment

Ptosis: If visual acuity is affected, most cases require surgical correction and there are several procedures that may be used including levator resection, repair or advancement and Fasanella-Servat.

⊟ REFERENCES

1. Bergin DJ, La Piana FG. Natural history of the congenital eyelid tetrad (Komoto's syndrome). Ann Ophthalmol. 1981;13:1145-8.
2. Komoto J. Veber die Operation be; Hereditaren Phimosis Congenita mit Ptosis. Nippon Ganka Gakkai 1920; 24, and Klin Monatsbl Augenheilkd. 1921;66:952.

⊟ 10.2LL. LAURENCE-MOON-BARDET-BIEDL SYNDROME (BARDET-BIEDL SYNDROME; RETINITIS PIGMENTOSA-POLYDACTYLY-ADIPOSOGENITAL SYNDROME)

General

Recessive, autosomal dominant, and recessive sex-linked gene; male preponderance; onset in childhood; cases of Laurence-Moon belong to the group of heredoataxias.

Ocular

Ptosis; epicanthus; nystagmus; strabismus; night blindness; myopia; hypermetropia; iris coloboma; RP "bone corpuscles"; macular degeneration; attenuation of retinal vessels; choroidal atrophy; optic nerve atrophy; cataract; microphthalmia; keratoconus.

Clinical

Obesity (Fröhlich type); hypogenitalism; reduced intelligence and mental retardation; turricephaly; shortness of stature; atresia ani; genu valgum; congenital heart disease; polydactyly; body hair scant or absent; pseudogynecomastia.

Laboratory

Chromosomal analysis is recommended to confirm chromosomal sex and to evaluate for associated genetic syndromes.

Treatment

Consultation by pediatric endocrinologist and pediatric urologist is usually necessary.

⊟ BIBLIOGRAPHY

1. Telander DG, de Beus A, Small KW. (2012). Retinitis pigmentosa. [online] Available from www.emedicine.com/oph/TOPIC704.HTM. [Accessed September, 2013].

⊟ 10.2MM. MULTIPLE LENTIGINES SYNDROME (LEOPARD SYNDROME)

General

Familial occurrence; classic features include lentigines (small focal hyperpigmentations of skin), electrocardiographic conduction abnormalities, ocular hypertelorism, pulmonary stenosis, abnormal genitalia, retardation of growth, and deafness (LEOPARD).

Ocular

Hypertelorism; exophthalmos; epicanthal folds; strabismus; nystagmus; keratoconus.

Clinical

Lowset ears; receding chin; deafness; lentigines; pulmonary stenosis; genital abnormalities; growth retardation; skeletal malformations (bony fusion involving cervical vertebrae, ossicles, carpal and tarsal bones, scoliosis); hyposmia; heart murmur; mental retardation; hypospadias; congenital heart defect; thoracic deformities; respiratory insufficiency.

Laboratory

CT scanning or MRI, skeletal radiography, echocardiography.

Treatment

Cryosurgery and laser treatment may be helpful; beta-adrenergic receptor or calcium channel blocking agents.

⊟ BIBLIOGRAPHY

1. Jozwiak S, Schwartz RA. (2012). LEOPARD Syndrome. [online] Available from www.emedicine.com/derm/TOPIC627.HTM. [Accessed September, 2013].

⊟ 10.2NN. LEROY SYNDROME

General

Possible mild increase in mucopolysaccharide excretion.

Ocular

Nasal epicanthic folds; corneal opacities.

Clinical

High, narrow forehead; narrow nasal bridge.

Laboratory

Urine spot tests are readily available to screen for mucopolysaccharidoses (MPSs), full skeletal survey.

Treatment

Enzyme replacement therapy (ERT) and bone marrow transplantation (BMT) can be useful.

⊟ BIBLIOGRAPHY

1. Roth KS, Rizzo WB, McGovern MM. (2012). I-Cell Disease (Mucolipidosis Type II). [online] Available from www.emedicine.com/ped/TOPIC1150.HTM. [Accessed September, 2013].

🗗 10.2OO. LITTLE SYNDROME (NAIL-PATELLA SYNDROME; HEREDITARY OSTEO-ONYCHO-DYSPLASIA; HOOD SYNDROME)

General

Inherited as autosomal dominant; affects males and females equally.

Ocular

Hypertelorism; ptosis; epicanthus; microcornea; keratoconus; sclerocornea; cataract; microphakia; light pigmentation of iris root with dark pigmented "clover-leaf" spots, referred to as the Lester line, not seen in all cases.

Clinical

Absent or hypoplastic patella; hypoplastic or dislocated head of radius; exostosis of skull bones; bilateral horns of iliac crests; longitudinal ridging of fingernails; glomerulonephritis; renal involvement; bilateral antecubital pterygia; arthrogryposis; disorder has been mapped to the long arm of chromosome 9; sensorineural hearing loss.

Laboratory

Conduct urinalysis, along with a microscopic analysis, to check for proteinuria and hematuria. Radiography findings reveal iliac horns. MRI to identify abnormal muscle insertions; renal biopsy.

Treatment

Renal dialysis and transplantation are necessary.

🗗 BIBLIOGRAPHY

1. Hoover-Fong J, McIntosh I, Sweeney E. (2012). Genetics of nail-patella syndrome. [online] Available from www.emedicine.com/ped/TOPIC1546.HTM. [Accessed September, 2013].

🗗 10.2PP. MICHEL SYNDROME

General

Autosomal dominant, characterized by agenesis of the inner ear.

Clinical

Profound but not total congential deafness.

Ocular

Telecanthus.

Laboratory

Diagnosis is made by clinical findings.

Treatment

Ocular—none.

🗗 BIBLIOGRAPHY

1. Ghazli K, Merite-Drancy A, Marsot-Dupuch K, et al. A report of two familial cases of Michel syndrome (bilateral agenesis of the inner ear). Ann Otolaryngol Chir Cervicofac. 1998;115:29-34.

🗗 10.2QQ. MOHR-CLAUSSEN SYNDROME (ORAL-FACIAL-DIGITAL SYNDROME TYPE II; OFD SYNDROME; OROFACIODIGITAL SYNDROME II)

General

Rare; autosomal recessive; certain features similar to Papillon-Leage-Psaume, Carpenter, Laurence-Moon-Bardet-Biedl, and Ellis-Van Creveld syndromes.

Ocular

Epicanthus; bridged chorioretinal colobomata.

Clinical

Clefts and fibroma of tongue; polydactylia; broad nasal bridge; narrow-arched palate; short humerus, femur, and tibia; irregular teeth; hypotonia; mental retardation; deafness; thin and fair hair; cerebellar atrophy.

Laboratory

Clinical.

Treatment

None—ocular.

🗗 BIBLIOGRAPHY

1. Annerén G, Gustavson KH, Jòzwiak S, et al. Abnormalities of the cerebellum in oro-facio-digital syndrome II (Mohr syndrome). Clin Genet. 1990;38:69-73.
2. Claussen O. Et Arvelig Syndrome Omfattende Tungemisdannelse og Polydaktyli. Nord Med. 1946;30:1147.
3. Geeraets WJ. Ocular Syndromes, 3rd edition. Philadelphia: Lea & Febiger; 1976.

🗗 10.2RR. NOONAN SYNDROME (MALE TURNER SYNDROME)

General

Similar to Turner syndrome, but with normal chromosomal analysis; X-linked dominant inheritance; X-linked dominant phenotype.

Ocular

Hypertelorism; exophthalmos; ptosis (unilateral or bilateral); antimongoloid-slanting palpebral fissure; myopia; keratoconus; optic disk coloboma.

Clinical

Valvular pulmonary stenosis; short stature; webbed neck; low hairline in the back; cubitus valgus; deformed chest wall; micrognathia; low-set ears; mild mental retardation.

Laboratory

Xl deficiency, bleeding diatheses, karyotyping test, cardiac examination.

Treatment

Growth hormone therapy.

🗗 BIBLIOGRAPHY

1. Ibrahim J, McGovern MM. (2013). Noonan syndrome. [online] Available from www.emedicine.com/ped/TOPIC1616.HTM. [Accessed September, 2013].

🗗 10.2SS. LOWE SYNDROME (OCULO-CEREBRO-RENAL SYNDROME)

General

Essential enzyme or protein abnormality is unknown; sex-linked recessive trait (male incidence only); onset in early infancy.

Ocular

Nystagmus; congenital glaucoma; miotic pupils; no pupillary reaction; ectropion uveae; malformation of the anterior chamber angle and of the iris; Schlemm's canal may be absent with imperfect angle cleavage; blue sclera; cloudy cornea; cataracts; megalocornea; corneal dystrophy; buphthalmos; microphthalmos; microphakia; mydriasis; strabismus; lens punctate cortical opacities.

Clinical

Mental, psychomotor, and growth retardation; aminoaciduria; albuminuria; glycosuria; renal tubular acidosis; rickets; osteomalacia; muscular hypotony; hyporeflexia; hyperactivity with bizarre choreoathetoid movements and screaming.

Laboratory

Urine-aminoaciduria, proteinuria, calciuria, phosphaturia; serum-elevated acid phosphate; imaging studies—brain MRI—mild ventriculomegaly (one-third cases); ocular ultrasound—if dense cataract, rule out mass or retinal detachment posterior.

Treatment

Monitor and treat for glaucoma. If glaucoma develops, IOP lowering agents must be used. Often, these patients require surgical intervention with goniotomy, trabeculotomy, or a drainage filtration device. Congenital cataracts should be removed, ideally in the first 6 weeks of life, to optimize the visual potential.

🗗 BIBLIOGRAPHY

1. Alcorn DM. (2012). Oculocerebrorenal syndrome. [online] Available from www.emedicine.com/oph/TOPIC516.HTM. [Accessed September, 2013].

🗗 1O.2TT. MEYER-SCHWICKERATH-WEYERS SYNDROME (MICROPHTHALMOS SYNDROME; OCULODENTODIGITAL DYSPLASIA)

General

Etiology unknown; two types recognized: (I) dysplasia oculodentodigitalis and (II) dyscraniopygophalangie; type I is characterized by microphthalmia with possible iris pathology and glaucoma, oligodontia and brown pigmentation of teeth, camptodactyly, and possible absence of middle phalanx of second to fifth toes; type II consists of severe microphthalmos to anophthalmos, polydactyly, and developmental anomalies of nose and oral cavity; both sexes affected; present from birth; abnormal cerebral white matter.

Ocular

Microphthalmos; hypotrichosis; glaucoma; iris anomalies (eccentric pupil; changes in normal iris texture; remnants of pupillary membrane along iris margins); microcornea; hypertelorism; myopia; hyperopia; keratoconus.

Clinical

Thin, small nose with anteverted nostrils and hypoplastic alae; syndactyly; camptodactyly (fourth and fifth fingers); anomalies of middle phalanx of fifth finger and toe; hypoplastic teeth; wide mandible; alveolar ridge; sparse hair growth; visceral malformations.

Laboratory

Diagnosis is made by clinical findings.

Treatment

- *Glaucoma*: Glaucoma medication should be the first plan of action. If medication is unsuccessful, a filtering surgical procedure with or without antimetabotites may be beneficial.
- *Keratoconus*: Spectacle correction, hard contacts, avoid eye rubbing. If hydrops occur, discontinue contact lens, use NaCl drops and ointment, patching, and short course of steroids. As disease advances, PK, deep anterior lamellar keratoplasty intacs with laser grooves or collagen stabilization of cornea.

🗗 BIBLIOGRAPHY

1. Geeraets WK. Ocular Syndromes, 3rd edition. Philadelphia: Lea & Febiger; 1976.
2. Gutmann DH, Zackai EH, McDonald-McGinn DM, et al. Oculodentodigital dysplasia syndrome associated with abnormal cerebral white matter. Am J Med Genet. 1991;41: 18-20.
3. McKusick VA. Mendelian Inheritance in Man: A Catalog of Human Genes and Genetic Disorders, 12th edition. Baltimore: The Johns Hopkins University Press; 1998.

🗗 1O.2UU. POTTER SYNDROME (RENAL AGENESIS SYNDROME; RENOFACIAL SYNDROME)

General

Unknown etiology; may be severe form of the trisomy 18 syndrome; results from prolonged oligohydramnios of any cause.

Ocular

Hypertelorism; pronounced epicanthal folds extending down the cheeks; antimongoloid slant of palpebral fissure.

Clinical

Flat bridge of the nose; low-set ears; facial deformities; micrognathia; pulmonary hypoplasia; cystic dysplasia of kidney to agenesis; oligohydramnios; clubbing of hands and feet; spina bifida; prominent infracanthal folds; flattened beaked nose; creased skin; positional deformities of the limbs.

Laboratory

Serum electrolyte tests to evaluate electrolyte problems such as hyponatremia, hypernatremia, hyperkalemia, hypocalcemia, hyperphosphatemia, and/or metabolic acidosis, which may be present in neonates with renal failure, Doppler ultrasonography.

Treatment

The renal function and respiratory status of neonates born with Potter syndrome must be assessed. Associated anomalies of the gastrointestinal, cardiovascular, and musculoskeletal systems should also be evaluated. Once the long-term prognosis of survival is determined, resuscitation and management plans should be addressed.

🗗 BIBLIOGRAPHY

1. Gupta S, Araya CE. (2012). Potter Syndrome. [online] Available from www.emedicine.com/ped/TOPIC1878.HTM. [Accessed September, 2013].

🗗 10.2VV. RING CHROMOSOME 6 (ANIRIDIA, CONGENITAL GLAUCOMA, AND HYDROCEPHALUS)

General

Rare disorder associated with various congenital anomalies; autosomal dominant with recessive sporadically reported.

Ocular

Microphthalmia; aniridia; congenital uveal ectropion; Rieger anomaly; congenital glaucoma; corneal clouding; prominent Schwalbe's line with attached iris strands; hypopigmented fundi; hypoplasia of iris stroma; strabismus; ptosis; nystagmus; megalocornea; iris coloboma; optic atrophy; hypertelorism; antimongoloid slant of palpebral fissures; ectopic pupils; angle anomalies; posterior embryotoxon; microcornea; colobomatous.

Clinical

Hydrocephalus; agenesis of corpus callosum; congenital heart defects; mental retardation; low-set malformed ears; broad nasal bridge; micrognathia; short neck; hand anomalies; high-arched palate; widely spaced nipples; deformity of feet; respiratory distress syndrome; hyperbilirubinemia; hypocalcemia; anemia; seizure; bulging anterior fontanel.

Laboratory

Diagnosis is made by clinical findings.

Treatment

Ptosis: If visual acuity is affected, most cases require surgical correction and there are several procedures that may be used including levator resection, repair or advancement and Fasanella-Servat.

🗗 BIBLIOGRAPHY

1. Bateman JB. Chromosomal anomalies and the eye. In: Wright KW (Ed). Pediatric Ophthalmology and Strabismus. St Louis: Mosby; 1995. p. 595.
2. Chitayat D, Hahm SY, Iqbal MA, et al. Ring chromosome 6: report of a patient and literature review. Am J Med Genet. 1987;26(1):145-51.
3. deLuise UP, Anderson DR. Primary infantile glaucoma (congenital glaucoma). Surv Ophthalmol. 1983;28(1):1-19.
4. Levin H, Ritch R, Barathur R, et al. Aniridia, congenital glaucoma, and hydrocephalus in a male infant with ring chromosome 6. Am J Med Genet. 1986;25(2):281-7.

🗗 10.2YY. ROBINOW-SILVERMAN-SMITH SYNDROME (ACHONDROPLASTIC DWARFISM; MESOMELIC DWARFISM; ROBINOW DWARFISM)

General

Autosomal dominant; both sexes affected; present from birth.

Ocular

Hypertelorism; epicanthal folds.

Clinical

Dwarfism; shortened forearms; bulging forehead; depressed nasal bridge; hypoplastic mandible; small, upturned nose; micrognathia; crowded teeth; penile hypoplasia.

Laboratory

Radiography, CT scan, MRI, and ultrasound.

Treatment

No specific treatment exists.

🗗 BIBLIOGRAPHY

1. Khan AN, Rahim R, MacDonald S. (2013). Achondroplasia imaging. [online] Available from www.emedicine.com/radio/TOPIC809.HTM. [Accessed September, 2013].

⊟ 1O.2ZZ. RUBINSTEIN-TAYBI SYNDROME (OPTIC ATROPHY)

General

Inheritance polygenic or multifactorial; rare.

Ocular

Antimongoloid slant of lid fissure; epicanthus; long eyelashes and highly arched brows; strabismus; myopia; hyperopia; iris coloboma; cataract; optic atrophy; ptosis; retinal detachment.

Clinical

Motor and mental retardation; broad thumbs and toes; highly arched palate; allergies; heart murmurs; anomalies of size, shape, and position of ears; dwarfism; cryptorchidism.

Laboratory

CT scan, MRI, chromosomal karyotype analysis, fluorescence in situ hybridization and CBP gene analysis.

Treatment

Physical therapy, speech and feeding therapy. Cardiothoracic intervention may be needed in patients with congenital heart defect.

⊟ BIBLIOGRAPHY

1. Mijuskovic ZP, Karadaglic D, Stojanov L. (2013). Dermatologic Manifestations of Rubinstein-Taybi Syndrome. [online] Available from www.emedicine.com/derm/TOPIC711.HTM. [Accessed September, 2013].

⊟ 1O.2AAA. SCHONENBERG SYNDROME (DWARF-CARDIOPATHY SYNDROME) BLEPHAROPHYMOSIS

General

Consanguinity and familial occurrence; etiology obscure.

Ocular

Blepharophimosis; epicanthal folds; pseudoptosis.

Clinical

Dwarfism (proportionate); congenital heart disease.

Laboratory

Clinical.

Treatment

None.

⊟ BIBLIOGRAPHY

1. Geeraets WJ. Ocular Syndromes, 3rd edition. Philadelphia: Lea & Febiger; 1976.
2. Schonenberg H. Uber ein Neues Kombinationsbild Multipler Abartungen. (Minderwuchs, Vitium Cordis, Beiderseitige Congenitale Ptose.) Ann Pediatr. 1954;182:229-40.

⊟ 1O.2BBB. SMITH SYNDROME (FACIO-SKELETO-GENITAL DYSPLASIA)

General

Autosomal recessive; more common in males.

Ocular

Ptosis; antimongoloid slant; epicanthus.

Clinical

Microcephaly; high-arched palate; large, low-set ears; mental retardation; broad nose; hypoplastic mandible; pedal syndactyly.

Laboratory

Clinical.

Treatment

Ptosis: If visual acuity is affected, most cases require surgical correction and there are several procedures that may be used including levator resection, repair or advancement and Fasanella-Servat.

🗗 BIBLIOGRAPHY

1. Aita JA. Congenital facial anomalies with neurologic defects. Springfield, IL: Charles C Thomas; 1969. pp. 246.
2. Magalini SI, Scrascia E. Dictionary of Medical Syndromes, 2nd edition. Philadelphia: JB Lippincott; 1981.

🗗 1O.2CCC. TAR SYNDROME (THROMBOCYTOPENIA-ABSENT RADIUS SYNDROME)

General

Bilateral absence of the radius and hypomegakaryocytic thrombocytopenia.

Ocular

May have cataracts, glaucoma, megalocornea, and blue sclera.

Clinical

Patients have foreshortened forearms and radially deviated hands; infrequently associated with mental retardation (7%); also may have lower extremity deformity.

Laboratory

CBC count, genetic testing, ultrasonography and bone marrow biopsy.

Treatment

Platelet transfusion is the most important treatment.

🗗 BIBLIOGRAPHY

1. Wu JK, Wong MP, Williams S. (2012). Thrombocytopenia-absent radius syndrome. [online] Available from www.emedicine.com/ped/TOPIC2237.HTM. [Accessed September, 2013].

🗗 1O.2DDD. COOLEY ANEMIA (THALASSEMIA; THALASSEMIA MAJOR; THALASSEMIA MINOR)

General

Autosomal dominant in synthesis of α or β chain of hemoglobin; most prevalent in Mediterranean and Oriental populations.

Ocular

Retinal hemorrhages; angioid streaks; macular vascular abnormalities; pigmented chorioretinal scars (black sunbursts); occlusion of peripheral retinal arteries; vitreous hemorrhages.

Clinical

Hemolytic anemia; hypochromic anemia.

Laboratory

Blood—hypochromic, microcystic anemia

Treatment

Goals of medical therapy are correction of anemia, suppression of erythropoiesis, and inhibition of increased gastrointestinal iron.

🗗 BIBLIOGRAPHY

1. Takeshita K. (2012). Beta thalassemia. [online] Available from www.emedicine.com/med/TOPIC438.HTM. [Accessed September, 2013].

⊟ 1O.2EEE. TRISOMY 18 SYNDROME (E SYNDROME; EDWARDS SYNDROME) CONGENITAL GLAUCOMA

General

Chromosome 18 present in triplicate; more common in females (3:1); age of mother over 40 years; onset from fetal life.

Ocular

Unilateral ptosis; epicanthal folds; congenital glaucoma; corneal opacities; lens opacities; optic atrophy.

Clinical

Low-set ears; micrognathia; high-arched palate; prominent occiput; cryptorchidism; failure to thrive; ventricular septal defect; hypertonicity with rigidity in flexion of limbs; mental retardation; umbilical and inguinal hernias.

Laboratory

Cytogenetic test, echocardiography, ultrasonography, and skeletal radiography are used to detect any abnormalities.

Treatment

Treat infections as appropriate. For feeding difficulties, nasogastric and gastrostomy supplementation is recommended.

⊟ BIBLIOGRAPHY

1. Chen H. (2013). Trisomy 18. [online] Availble from www.emedicine.com/ped/TOPIC652.HTM. [Accessed August, 2013].

⊟ 1O.2FFF. TURNER SYNDROME (TURNER-ALBRIGHT SYNDROME; GONADAL DYSGENESIS; GENITAL DWARFISM SYNDROME; ULLRICH-TURNER SYNDROME; BONNEVIE-ULLRICH SYNDROME; PTERYGOLYMPHANGIECTASIA SYNDROME; ULLRICH-BONNEVIE SYNDROME) CATARACT, POSTERIOR

General

Ovarian or gonadal agenesis; 45 chromosomes with an XO sex-chromosome constitution; females; rare in males; onset in childhood.

Ocular

Exophthalmos; hypertelorism; ptosis; epicanthal folds; blue sclera; corneal nebulae; cataracts; conjunctival lymphedema; keratoconus.

Clinical

Webbed neck (pterygium colli); diminished growth; mandibulofacial disproportion; cubitus valgus; masculine chest and trunk; late appearance of pubic and axillary hair; congenital deafness; mental retardation; coarctation of aorta.

Laboratory

Karyotyping is needed for diagnosis. Y-chromosomal test; LH and FSH levels, thyroid function test, fasting glucose levels, echocardiography and MRI.

Treatment

Growth hormone therapy is used to prevent short stature. Estrogen replacement therapy is usually started by the age of 12–15 years.

⊟ BIBLIOGRAPHY

1. Postellon DC, Daniel MS. (2012). Turner syndrome. [online] Available from emedicine.medscape.com/article/949681-overview. [Accessed September, 2013].

10.2GGG. WAARDENBURG SYNDROME (VAN DER HOEVE-HALBERSTAM-WAARDENBURG SYNDROME; WAARDENBURG-KLEIN SYNDROME; EMBRYONIC FIXATION SYNDROME; INTEROCULO-IRIDODERMATO-AUDITIVE DYSPLASIA; PIEBALDISM) HYPERTELORISM

General

Irregular dominant inheritance; developmental fault in neural crest with absence of the organ of Corti, aplasia of the spiral ganglion, and pigmentary changes; no sex preference; onset at birth.

Ocular

Hyperplasia of the medial portions of the eyebrows; hypertelorism; blepharophimosis; strabismus; heterochromia iridis; aniridia; microcornea; cornea plana; microphakia; abnormal fundus pigmentation; hypoplasia of optic nerve; synophrys; poliosis; hypopigmentation and hypoplasia of retina and choroid; epicanthus; lateral displacement of inferior puncta; lenticonus; underdevelopment of orbital bones; lateral displacement of inner canthi; hypopigmented iris.

Clinical

Congenital deafness; unilateral deafness or deaf-mutism; broad and high nasal root with absent nasofrontal angle; albinotic hair strain (unilateral); faint patches of skin pigmentation; pituitary tumor; nasal atresia; white forelock.

Laboratory

Molecular testing and audiology.

Treatment

Genetic counseling, audiology and otolaryngology management.

BIBLIOGRAPHY

1. Schwartz RA, Bawle EV, Jozwiak S. (2013). Genetics of Waardenburg syndrome. [online] Available from www.emedicine.com/ped/TOPIC2422.HTM. [Accessed September, 2013].

10.2HHH. X-LINKED MENTAL RETARDATION SYNDROME (XLMR) GLAUCOMA

General

X-linked mental retardation syndrome, of which many types may exist.

Ocular

Glaucoma may be found in some patients; optic atrophy has been noted.

Clinical

Short stature; small hands and feet; seizures; cleft palate; "coarse" facial appearance; brachydactyly.

Laboratory

Clinical.

Treatment

Glaucoma: Glaucoma medication should be the first plan of action. If medication is unsuccessful, a filtering surgical procedure with or without antimetabotites may be beneficial.

BIBLIOGRAPHY

1. Armfield K, Nelson R, Lubs HA, et al. X-linked mental retardation syndrome with short stature, small hands and feet, seizures, cleft palate, and glaucoma is linked to Xq28. Am J Med Genet. 1999;85:236-42.
2. Carpenter NJ, Qu Y, Curtis M, et al. X-linked mental retardation syndrome with characteristic "coarse" facial appearance, brachydactyly, and short stature maps to proximal Xq. Am J Med Genet. 1999;85:230-5.

⊟ 10.2III. XXXXX SYNDROME (PENTA X SYNDROME, TETRA X SYNDROME) HYPERTELORISM

General

Congenital syndrome due to aneuploidy.

Ocular

Epicanthal folds; hypertelorism; antimongoloid (upward slant) of palpebral fissures.

Clinical

Growth retardation, bilateral.

Laboratory

Urine microscopic analysis, blood test for creatinine, urea, and electrolytes, renal ultrasonography.

Treatment

No drug therapy is currently available for this condition.

⊟ BIBLIOGRAPHY

1. Swiatecka-Urban A. (2013). Multicystic renal dysplasia. [online] Available from www.emedicine.com/ped/TOPIC1493.HTM. [Accessed September, 2013].

⊟ 1P. FACIAL PALSY (BELL'S PALSY)

Facial palsy is defined as paralysis of facial muscles supplied by the seventh nerve; orbicularis oculi paralysis may result in epiphora and ectropion.

†1. Congenital
†2. Birth injury with nerve crushed at exit of stylomastoid foramen
3. Myogenic paralysis
  †A. Myotonic atrophia
  †B. Facioscapulohumeral type of muscular dystrophy
  C. Myasthenia gravis (Erb-Goldflam syndrome)
  †D. Hypokalemia, periodic
  †E. Curare poisoning
  F. Botulism
  G. Congenital facial diplegia (Möbius syndrome)
  †H. Infants, from maternal ingestion of thalidomide
  I. Kugelberg-Welander syndrome
4. Neurologic paralysis
  A. *Supranuclear paralysis*: Upper face, including orbicularis relatively unaffected with affected lower face
    1. *Voluntary movement*: Pyramidal fibers involved, such as in Weber syndrome, with contralateral hemiplegia of face and limbs and ipsilateral oculomotor paralysis
    †2. Weakness or abolition of the emotional movements of the face with retention of full voluntary activity, such as with lesion of anterior part of frontal lobe or near optic thalamus
  B. *Peripheral paralysis*: Involvement of upper and lower face

1. Pontine lesion: Associated structures involved include sixth nerve, conjugate ocular deviation to the same side, ipsilateral paralysis of jaw muscles, and pyramidal tract in paralysis of limb of opposite side
  a. Acute nuclear lesions, such as with anterior poliomyelitis, Landry paralysis, or degenerative conditions
  b. Foville syndrome: Ipsilateral sixth nerve with loss of conjugate deviation to same side and hemiplegia of the opposite limbs
  c. Millard-Gubler syndrome: Ipsilateral sixth nerve paralysis and hemiplegia of the opposite limbs
  †d. Parotid gland surgery
  †e. Progressive muscular atrophy
  f. Syringobulbia
  †g. Tumors
  †h. Vascular lesions
2. Posterior fossa-associated with nerve deafness, loss of taste on anterior two thirds of tongue, and occasionally diminution of tears
  †a. Acoustic neuroma
  b. Coloboma, heart disease, atresia choanae, retarded growth and retarded development or CNS anomalies, genital hypoplasia, and ear anomalies or deafness (CHARGE) syndrome association
  c. Facial neuritis due to polyneuritis cranialis, beriberi, encephalitis, diabetes, or intrathecal anesthesia

†d. Fracture of the skull

e. Meningitis, including syphilitic and tuberculous

†f. Preauricular cyst associated with congenital cholesteatoma

†g. Tumors of facial nerve

3. *Petrous temporal bone*: Associated with decreased lacrimation and salivary secretion, loss of taste on anterior two thirds of tongue, and intensified sensation of loud noises

a. Arteriosclerosis

b. Bell palsy: Inflammation of facial nerve of unknown cause

†c. Cephalic tetanus

†d. Diabetes mellitus (Willis disease)

e. Fractures

f. Herpes zoster, spread from geniculate ganglion

g. Hypertension

h. Nerve leprosy (Hansen disease)

†i. Otitis media

j. Secondary syphilis

4. Facial lesions at or beyond the stylomastoid foramen

†a. Fracture of the ramus of the mandible

b. Melkersson-Rosenthal syndrome (Melkersson idiopathic fibroedema)

c. Neoplasia or inflammatory swelling of parotid, such as in uveoparotid fever (Heerfordt disease) and Mikulicz disease

†d. Supporting lymph nodes behind the angle of the jaw

Treatment

- By definition, Bell's palsy is idiopathic. Possible etiologies include infections (herpetic, Lyme disease, Epstein-Barr viral infection, HIV, and mycoplasma), inflammation, and microvascular disease (diabetes mellitus and hypertension).

- The use of corticosteroids for Bell palsy is still controversial. However, a short course of high-dose corticosteroids in the 1st week of onset may be effective in improving the patient's prognosis.

---

†Indicates a general entry and therefore has not been described in detail in the text

- Although the use of oral antiviral agents (e.g. acyclovir, valacyclovir) is also controversial, these drugs are used in the early treatment of Bell palsy.

- In most cases, topical ocular lubrication (with artificial tears during the day and lubricating ophthalmic ointment at night, or occasionally ointment day and night) is sufficient to prevent the complications of corneal exposure.

- Occluding the eyelids by using tape or by applying a patch for 1 or 2 days may help to heal corneal erosions. Care must be taken to prevent worsening the abrasion with the tape or a patch by ensuring that the eyelid is securely closed.

- External eyelid weights are available to improve mechanical blink. The weights are attached to the upper lid with an adhesive and are available in different skin tones.

- Clear plastic wrap, cut to 8 cm × 10 cm and applied with generous amounts of ointment as a night time occlusive bandage, may be required.

- Lower-lid ectropion or droop can temporarily be helped by applying tape below the lid margin in the center of the lower lid; pull the lid laterally and upward to anchor on the orbital rim.

- Punctal plugs may be helpful if dryness of the cornea is a persistent problem.

- Botulinum toxin can be injected transcutaneously or subconjunctivally at the upper border of the tarsus and aimed at the levator muscle to produce complete ptosis and to protect the cornea.

- Botulinum toxin may help in relaxing the facial muscles after they have developed mass contraction, though the results are not as satisfying as in patients with Bell palsy as in patients with idiopathic hemifacial spasm.

- Surgery to decompress the facial nerve is controversial when performed in patients with complete Bell palsy.

BIBLIOGRAPHY

1. Caputo WE, Sinert RH. (2013). Lyme disease in emergency medicine. [online] Available from www.emedicine.com/emerg/TOPIC588.HTM. [Accessed August, 2013].
2. Gulevich S. (2012). Hemifacial spasm. [online] Available from www.emedicine.com/neuro/TOPIC154.HTM. [Accessed September, 2013].
3. Janniger CK, Eastern JS, Hospenthal DR, et al. (2013). Herpes zoster. [online] Available from www.emedicine.com/med/TOPIC1007.HTM. [Accessed September, 2013].
4. Kelsch RD. (2012). Fissured tongue. [online] Available from www.emedicine.com/derm/TOPIC665.HTM. [Accessed September, 2013].

5. Lin HC, Quan D. (2012). Diabetic neuropathy. [online] Available from www.emedicine.com/pmr/TOPIC40.HTM. [Accessed September, 2013].

6. Lipton JM, Alter BP. (2013). Fanconi anemia. [online] Available from www.emedicine.com/ped/TOPIC3022.HTM. [Accessed September, 2013].

7. Miravalle AA. (2012). Ramsay hunt syndrome. [online] Available from www.emedicine.com/neuro/TOPIC420.HTM. [Accessed September, 2013].

8. Nervi SJ. (2011). Catscratch disease. [online] Available from www.emedicine.com/med/TOPIC304.HTM. [Accessed September, 2013].

9. Orkwis HK, Conologue TD, Meffert J. (2012). Lamellar ichthyosis. Available from www.emedicine.com/derm/TOPIC190.HTM. [Accessed September, 2013].

10. Szudek J, Joshi AS, Sadeghi N, et al. Intratemporal tumors of the facial nerve. [online] Available from www.emedicine.com/ent/TOPIC245.HTM. [Accessed September, 2013].

11. Taylor DC, Khoromi S, Zachariah SB. (2012). Bell palsy. [online] Available from emedicine.medscape.com/article/1146903-overview. [Accessed August, 2013].

12. Weinblatt ME. (2013). Pediatric acute myelocytic leukemia. [online] Available from www.emedicine.com/ped/TOPIC1301.HTM. [Accessed September, 2013].

13. White-McCrimmon RY, Maurelus K. (2013). Emergent Management of Guillain-Barre Syndrome. [online] Available from www.emedicine.com/emerg/TOPIC222.HTM. [Accessed September, 2013].

14. Yakobi R. (2013). Acute complications of sarcoidosis. [online] Available from www.emedicine.com/emerg/TOPIC516.HTM. [Accessed September, 2013].

15. Zaidman GW. (2011). Ophthalmic aspects of lyme disease overview of lyme disease. [online] Available from www.emedicine.com/oph/TOPIC262.HTM. [Accessed September, 2013].

🖰 1P.3C. ERB-GOLDFLAM SYNDROME (ERB II SYNDROME; HOPPE-GOLDFLAM DISEASE; PSEUDOPARALYTIC SYNDROME; MYASTHENIA GRAVIS)

General

Occurs at any age; more frequent between ages 20–40 years; more females affected than males; progressive; spontaneous; symptoms improve or resolve with rest in early stages of disease (*see* myasthenia gravis, neonatal or infantile); caused by autoantibodies against the acetylcholine receptor at the neuromuscular junction, leading to abnormal fatigability and weakness of skeletal muscle.

Ocular

Transient diplopia; ptosis of upper eyelids.

Clinical

Excessive fatigability of musculature; symptoms appear and increase as day progresses; expressionless face; sagging jaw; difficulty in chewing and talking; nasal regurgitation.

Laboratory

Ice test—crushed ice in surgical glove over ptotic eyelid for 2 minutes and watch for brief elevation of eyelid; Tensilon test and prostigmin test may result in the elevation of ptotic eyelid or improved strabismus in individuals with myasthenia gravis.

Treatment

Adrenal corticosteroids are frequently used. In some cases, mycophenolate mofetil, cyclosporine and cyclophosphamide may be useful. Patching one eye or using prisms may be helpful.

🖰 BIBLIOGRAPHY

1. Erb W. Zur Casuistick der Bulbaren La hmungen. Arch Psychiatr Vervenkr. 1879;9:325-50.

2. Roy FH, Fraunfelder FT, Fraunfelder FW. Roy and Fraunfelder's Current Ocular Therapy, 6th edition. London, UK: Elsevier; 2008.

3. Goldflam S. Vebereinen Scheinbar Keilbaren Bulbarparalytischem Symptom Complex mit Betheiligung der Extremitaten. Dtsch Z Nerven. 1983;4:312-52.

4. Kim JH, Hwang JM, Hwang YS, et al. Childhood ocular myasthenia gravis. Ophthalmology. 2003;110(7):1458-62.

5. Lepore FE, Sanborn GE, Slevin JT. Pupillary dysfunction in myasthenia gravis. Ann Neurol. 1979;6(1):29-33.

6. Sommer N, Melms A, Weller M, et al. Ocular myasthenia gravis. A critical review of clinical and pathophysiological aspects. Doc Ophthalmol. 1993;84(4):309-33.

1P.3F. BOTULISM

General

It is caused by a toxin-producing strain of *Clostridium botulinum*; it occurs primarily after the ingestion of contaminated food; the organism can produce a neurotoxin, the effect of which can be life threatening.

Ocular

Absent optokinetic nystagmus, absent vertical gaze; marked limitation of horizontal gaze; ptosis; diplopia; decreased tear secretion; mydriasis; paralysis of accommodation; nystagmus; optic atrophy; optic neuritis; extraocular muscle paresis.

Clinical

Dizziness; severe respiratory impairment; gastrointestinal disturbances; dysphagia; dysarthria; postural hypotension.

Laboratory

Toxin assay for early diagnosis, whereas later cases are more likely to yield a positive specimen culture.

Treatment

Antitoxin appears to be the only effective medication. Supportive care such as ventilation and parenteral nutrition are necessary for the duration of the paralytic illness.

BIBLIOGRAPHY

1. Patel B, Taylor SF. (2012). Ophthalmologic manifestations of botulism. [online] Available from www.emedicine.com/oph/TOPIC493.HTM. [Accessed September, 2013].

1P.3G. MÖBIUS II SYNDROME (CONGENITAL FACIAL DIPLEGIA; CONGENITAL PARALYSIS OF THE SIXTH AND SEVENTH NERVES; CONGENITAL OCULOFACIAL PARALYSIS; VON GRAEFES SYNDROME)

General

Congenital; possibly failure of development of facial nerve cells or primary defect of muscles deriving from first two brachial arches or both; recovery in a few weeks or nonprogressive permanent paralysis of face; asymmetrical; if incomplete, usually spares lower face and platysma.

Ocular

Proptosis; ptosis; weakness of abductor muscles; normal convergence; limitation to internal rotation in lateral movements; esotropia.

Clinical

Facial diplegia; deafness; loss of vestibular responses; webbed fingers or toes; clubfoot.

Laboratory

Diagnosis is made by clinical findings.

Treatment

Ptosis: If visual acuity is affected most cases require surgical correction and there are several procedures that may be used including levator resection, repair or advancement and Fasanella-Servat.

BIBLIOGRAPHY

1. Abbott RL, Metz HS, Weber AA. Saccadic velocity studies in Möbius syndrome. Ann Ophthalmol. 1978;10:619-23.
2. Fenichel GM. Congenital facial asymmetry (aplasia of facial muscles). In: Fenichel GM (Ed). Clinical pediatric neurology, 2nd edition. Philadelphia: WB Saunders; 1993. pp. 341-2.
3. Kawai M, Momoi T, Fujii T, et al. The syndrome of Möbius sequence, peripheral neuropathy, and hypogonadotropic hypogonadism. Am J Med Genet. 1990;37:578-82.
4. Menkes JH, Kenneth T. Möbius syndrome. In: Menkes JH (Ed). Textbook of Child Neurology, 5th edition. Baltimore: Williams & Wilkins; 1995. pp. 309-10.
5. Merz M, Wójtowicz S. The Möbius syndrome. Report of electromyographic examinations in two cases. Am J Ophthalmol. 1967;63(4):837-40.
6. Möbius PJ. über angeborene doppelseitige Abducens-Facialislahmung. Munch Med Wochenschr. 1888;35:91-108.
7. Pucket CL, Beg SA. Facial reanimation in Möbius syndrome. South Med J. 1978;71:1498-501.

⯐ 1P.3I. KUGELBERG-WELANDER SYNDROME (JUVENILE MUSCULAR ATROPHY)

General

Autosomal recessive; juvenile spinal muscular atrophy; affects both sexes; onset in late childhood or adolescence.

Ocular

Ptosis; ophthalmoplegia; exotropia; orbicularis oculi paresis.

Clinical

Slowly progressive proximal muscle atrophy; lower extremities usually are affected first, with the upper limbs being affected late; frequently, fasciculation; proximal muscle weakness, especially of the lower extremities; elevated serum creatine kinase levels.

Laboratory

Routine genetic testing only detects patients with the homozygous deletion; ultrasound of the muscles had been used to assess neurogenic atrophy.

Treatment

No cure is known. Treatment is focused on symptomatic control and preventative rehabilitation.

⯐ BIBLIOGRAPHY

1. Oleszek JL, Vallee SE, Dichiaro M, et al. (2011). Kugelberg Welander spinal muscular atrophy. [online] Available from http://www.emedicine.com/pmr/TOPIC62.HTM. [Accessed September, 2013].

⯐ 1P.4A1. WEBER SYNDROME (WEBER-DUBLER SYNDROME; CEREBELLAR PEDUNCLE SYNDROME; ALTERNATING OCULOMOTOR PARALYSIS; VENTRAL MEDIAL MIDBRAIN SYNDROME) PTOSIS

General

Lesion of the peduncle (crus), pons or medulla, which interrupts the third nerve before it emerges from the peduncle and interrupts fibers in the pyramidal tract above the level of the third nuclei; hemorrhage and thrombosis; tumor of the pituitary region, extending posteriorly; also may result in secondary to cerebrovascular disease.

Ocular

Ptosis; homolateral third nerve palsy (usually complete); fixed, dilated pupil.

Clinical

Contralateral hemiplegia; contralateral paralysis of face and tongue (supranuclear type).

Laboratory

Diagnosis is made by clinical findings.

Treatment

Ptosis: If visual acuity is affected, most cases require surgical correction and there are several procedures that may be used including levator resection, repair or advancement and Fasanella-Servat.

⯐ BIBLIOGRAPHY

1. Kistler JP, Ropper AH, Martin JB. Cerebrovascular diseases. In: Isselbacher KJ, Braunwald E, Wilson JD, Martin JB, Fauci A, Kasper DL (Eds). Harrison's Principles of Internal Medicine, 13th edition. New York: McGraw-Hill; 1994.
2. Miller NR (Ed). Walsh and Hoyt's Clinical Neuro-Ophthalmology, 44th edition. Baltimore, USA: Williams & Wilkins; 1995.
3. Newman NJ. Third, fourth and sixth-nerve lesions and the cavernous sinus. In: Albert DM, Jakobiec FA (Eds). Albert & Jakobiec's Principles and Practice of Ophthalmology: Clinical Practice, 5th edition. Philadelphia, PA: WB Saunders; 1994.
4. Weber H. A contribution to the pathology of the crura cerebri. Med Chir Trans. 1863;46:121-40.1.
5. Wolf BS, Newman CM, Khilnani MT. The posterior inferior cerebellar artery on vertebral angiography. Am J Roentgenol Radium Ther Nucl Med. 1962;87:322-37.

🗗 1P.4B1A. GUILLAIN-BARRÉ SYNDROME (LANDRY PARALYSIS; ACUTE INFECTIOUS NEURITIS; ACUTE POLYRADICULITIS; ACUTE FEBRILE POLYNEURITIS; ACUTE IDIOPATHIC POLYNEURITIS; INFLAMMATORY POLYRADICULONEUROPATHY; LANDRY-GUILLAIN-BARRÉ-STROHL SYNDROME; POSTINFECTIOUS POLYNEURITIS)

General

Etiology unknown; occurs from age 16–50 years.

Ocular

Facial nerve paralysis with paralytic ectropion of the lower eyelid; mild-to-complete external ophthalmoplegia; optic neuritis; papilledema; ptosis; anisocoria; nystagmus; dyschromatopsia; scotoma; bilateral tonic pupils.

Clinical

Polyneuritis involving facial peripheral motor nerves and spinal cord; facial diplegia; bladder incontinence; variable degrees of paralysis, usually beginning in lower extremities; tendon reflexes absent; involvement of respiratory muscles possible; paresthesia (symmetrical).

Laboratory

Cytomegalovirus, Epstein-Barr virus and HIV have been most closely associated with this condition.

Treatment

Plasma exchange have shown to be beneficial. Corneal exposure is treated with topical therapy or lateral tarsorrhaphies if warranted.

🗗 BIBLIOGRAPHY

1. Andary MT, Oleszek JL, Cha-Kim A. (2012). Guillain-Barre Syndrome. [online] Available from www.emedicine.com/pmr/TOPIC48.HTM. [Accessed September, 2013].

🗗 1P.4B1B. FOVILLE SYNDROME (FOVILLE PEDUNCULAR SYNDROME)

General

Pontine area tumor, hemorrhage, tuberculoma, multiple sclerosis, or unilateral obstruction of paramedian branches may cause clinical manifestations.

Ocular

Paralysis of cranial nerve VI; paralysis of conjugate movement to the side of the lesion; abduction or horizontal gaze deficit.

Clinical

Peripheral facial palsy; contralateral hemiplegia; headache; ipsilateral: facial weakness, loss of taste, facial analgesia, Homer syndrome and deafness.

Laboratory

CT and MRI.

Treatment

See neurologist.

🗗 BIBLIOGRAPHY

1. Bedi HK, Devpura JC, Bomb BS. Clinical tuberculoma of pons presenting as Foville's syndrome. J Indian Med Assoc. 1973;61(4):184-5.
2. Foville AL. Note sur une Paralysie Peu Connue des Certains Muscles de l'Oeil, et Sa Liaison avec Quelques Points de l'Anatomie et la Physiologic de la Protuberance Annulaire. Bull Soc Anat (Paris). 1858;33:393.
3. Geeraets WJ. Ocular Syndromes, 3rd edition. Philadelphia, USA: Lea & Febiger; 1976.
4. Newman NJ. Third, fourth, and sixth nerve lesions and the cavernous sinus. In: Albert DM, Jakobiec FA, Miller JW, Azar DT, Blodi BA (Eds). Albert & Jakobiec's Principles and Practice of Ophthalmology, 3rd edition. Philadelphia, USA: WB Saunders; 1994. p. 2458.

1P.4B1C. MILLARD-GUBLER SYNDROME (ABDUCENS-FACIAL HEMIPLEGIA ALTERNANS)

General

Vascular, infectious, or tumorous lesion at the base of the pons affecting the nuclei of the sixth and seventh nerves and fibers of the pyramidal tract; demyelinating disease.

Ocular

Diplopia; esotropia; paralysis external rectus muscle (often bilateral); in unilateral cases, there is deviation of eyes to side opposite lesion and inability to move them toward side of lesion; abduction of eye prevented by destruction of sixth nerve nucleus; opposite eye cannot be voluntarily adducted but can converge and move in this position by rotatory and caloric stimulation.

Clinical

Ipsilateral facial paralysis; contralateral hemiplegia of arm and leg from involvement of pyramidal tract.

Laboratory/Diplopia

None.

Treatment/Diplopia

Occluding one eye, Fresnel prism, anticholinergic agent and corticosteroids may be needed in the treatment of myasthenia gravis.

BIBLIOGRAPHY

1. Geeraets WJ. Ocular Syndromes, 3rd edition. Philadelphia, USA: Lea & Febiger; 1976.
2. Gubler A. De l'Hemiplegie Alterne Envisagee Comme Signe de Lesion de la Protuberance Annulaire et Comme Preuve de la Decussation des Nerfs Faciaux. Gaz Hebd Med Chir. 1856;3:749,789,811.
3. Minderhoud JM. Diagnostic significance of symptomatology in brain stem ischaemic infarction. Eur Neurol. 1971;5(6):343-53.
4. Newman NJ. Third, fourth and sixth nerve lesions and the cavernous sinus. In: Albert DM, Jakobiec FA, Miller JW, Azar DT, Blodi BA (Eds). Albert & Jakobiec's Principles and Practice of Ophthalmology, 3rd edition. Philadelphia, USA: WB Saunders; 1994. p. 2458.

1P.4B1F. PASSOW SYNDROME (BREMER STATUS DYSRAPHICUS; STATUS DYSRAPHICUS SYNDROME; SYRINGOMYELIA; SYRINGOBULBIA)

General

Congenital nonclosure of the neural tube; familial occurrence or may be sporadic; insidious onset in 2nd to 3rd decade of life.

Ocular

Enophthalmos; ptosis; rotatory nystagmus; heterochromia iridis; anterior uveitis; corneal anesthesia; neuroparalytic keratitis; paralysis of third, fifth, sixth, and seventh cranial nerves; Horner syndrome; anisocoria; papilledema; optic atrophy; zonular cataract (*see* Horner Syndrome).

Clinical

Anesthesia over area of first division of trigeminal nerve; facial hemiatrophy; facial nerve paralysis; muscular weakness; cervical ribs; kyphoscoliosis; spina bifida; unilateral numbness of fingers; loss of deep reflexes; insensitivity to pain and temperature in affected areas; neurogenic bladder.

Laboratory

MRI, CT.

Treatment

Suboccipital and cervical decompression, laminectomy and syringotomy, shunts, fourth ventriculostomy, terminal ventriculostomy and neuroendoscopic surgery may be considered.

BIBLIOGRAPHY

1. Al-Shatoury HA, Galhom AA, Wagner FC. (2012). Syringomyelia. [online] Available from emedicine.medscape.com/article/1151685-overview. [Accessed September, 2013].

⊟ 1P.4B2B. CHARGE ASSOCIATION (MULTIPLE CONGENITAL ANOMALIES SYNDROME; COLOBOMA, HEART DISEASE, ATRESIA, RETARDED GROWTH, GENITAL HYPOPLASIA, EAR MALFORMATION ASSOCIATION)

General

Syndrome consists of four of six major manifestations of ocular coloboma, heart disease, atresia, retarded growth and development, genital hypoplasia, and ear malformations with or without hearing loss.

Ocular

Blepharoptosis; iris coloboma; optic nerve coloboma; macular hypoplasia; lacrimal canalicular atresia; nasolacrimal duct obstruction.

Clinical

Microcephaly; brachycephaly; malformed ear; bilateral finger contractures; heart disease; genital hypoplasia; heart disease; choanal atresia; retarded growth; hearing loss; facial nerve palsies; mental retardation.

Laboratory

CHD7 mutation analysis is diagnostic in 58–71% of individuals who meet the clinical criteria, head CT and MRI, cranial ultrasound.

Treatment

Secure airway, stabilize the patient, exclude major life-threatening congenital anomalies and transfer the individual with coloboma of the eye, heart defects, atresia of the nasal choanae, retardation of growth and/or development, genital and/or urinary abnormalities, and ear abnormalities and deafness (CHARGE) syndrome to a specialist center with pediatric otolaryngologist and other subspecialty services.

⊟ BIBLIOGRAPHY

1. Tegay DH, Yedowitz JC. (2012). CHARGE syndrome. [online] Available from www.emedicine.com/ped/TOPIC367.HTM. [Accessed September, 2013].

⊟ 1P.4B2C. WERNICKE SYNDROME I (SUPERIOR HEMORRHAGIC POLIOENCEPHALOPATHIC SYNDROME; HEMORRHAGIC POLIOENCEPHALITIS SUPERIOR SYNDROME; ENCEPHALITIS HEMORRHAGICA SUPERIORIS; AVITAMINOSIS B; THIAMINE DEFICIENCY; BERIBERI; GAYET-WERNICKE SYNDROME; WERNICKE-KORSAKOFF SYNDROME) PTOSIS

General

Lack of vitamin B or thiamine; focal vascular lesions in the gray matter around third and fourth ventricles and Sylvian aqueduct; alcoholics (adults); beriberi of all ages.

Ocular

Ptosis; acute bilateral nuclear ophthalmoplegia; complete ophthalmoplegia; retinal hemorrhages; optic atrophy; optic neuritis; conjunctivitis; blepharitis; nutritional amblyopia; central scotoma; papilledema; nystagmus; absolute pupillary paralysis or Argyll Robertson pupils; accommodative palsy.

Clinical

Early prostration; lethargy; irritability; stupor; delirium; mental disturbances to Korsakoff psychosis; ataxia; tremors; peripheral neuritis; anorexia; vomiting; insomnia; perspiration; tachycardia; hallucinations; retrograde amnesia; apathy; anxiety; fear; defective concentration; cardiomyopathy.

Laboratory

Electrolyte studies, serum thiamine levels, CBC. Evaluation of hypoxemia, hypercarbia, acidosis, or alkalosis. Serum/urine toxin drug screen and liver enzymes.

Treatment

Parenteral thiamine is the treatment of choice.

⊟ BIBLIOGRAPHY

1. Xiong GL, Kenedi CA. (2013). Wernicke-Korsakoff syndrome. [online] Available from www.emedicine.com/med/TOPIC2405.HTM. [Accessed September, 2013].

⊟ 1P.4B2E. ACQUIRED LUES (SYPHILIS; ACQUIRED SYPHILIS; LUES VENEREA; MALUM VENEREUM)

General

Causative agent, *Treponema pallidum*, usually transmitted sexually.

Ocular

Conjunctival chancroid; conjunctivitis; keratitis; blepharitis; ptosis; iris atrophy; hippus; dacryocystitis; optic nerve atrophy; optic neuritis; periostitis; episcleritis; scleritis; nystagmus; uveitis; vitreous hemorrhages; paralysis of sixth nerve; papilledema; retinal hemorrhages; retinitis proliferans; oculogyric crisis; neuroretinitis; papilledema (associated with aseptic meningitis); diffuse or multifocal chorioretinitis; vertical supranuclear gaze palsy; Benedikt syndrome.

Clinical

Primary lesion associated with regional lymphadenopathy; secondary bacteremic stage associated with generalized mucocutaneous lesions; tertiary stage characterized by destructive mucocutaneous, musculoskeletal, or parenchymal lesions, aortitis, or CNS disease; syphilis and HIV infection often coexist in the same patient who experiences a higher incidence and greater severity of neurologic and ocular manifestations; a significant percentage of patients infected with HIV-I and *T. pallidum* become seronegative to syphilis testing.

Laboratory

Serologic nontreponemal tests include Venereal Disease Research Laboratory (VDRL) and rapid plasma reagin (RPR).

Treatment

The goals are to reduce morbidity and to prevent complications. Penicillin is the antibiotic of choice for treating syphilis. Ocular syphilis should be treated the same as patients with neurosyphilis.

⊟ BIBLIOGRAPHY

1. Majmudar PA. (2011). Interstitial keratitis overview of interstitial keratitis. [online] Available from www.emedicine.com/oph/TOPIC453.HTM. [Accessed September, 2013].
2. Euerle B, Chandrasekar PH, Diaz MM, et al. (2012). Syphilis. [online] Available from www.emedicine.com/med/TOPIC2224.HTM. [Accessed September, 2013].

⊟ 1P.4B2E. TUBERCULOSIS

General

Communicable disease caused by the acid-fast bacillus *Mycobacterium tuberculosis*.

Ocular

Conjunctivitis; subconjunctival nodules (tuberculomas); keratitis; pannus; corneal ulcer; blepharitis; cellulitis; meibomianitis; uveitis; dacryocystitis; chronic orbital cellulitis; retinitis; scleritis; scleral perforation; hypopyon; vitreous hemorrhages; optic neuritis; optic atrophy; tuberculous panophthalmitis; choroidal tubercles; intraorbital extraocular lesions.

Clinical

Pulmonary infection; pyuria; hematuria; epididymitis; dysuria; flank pain; distorted calyces; productive cough.

Laboratory

Acid-fast bacillus culture of body fluids including vitreous and aqueous. PCR is 89% positive for pulmonary infection.

Treatment

A course of chemotherapy (isoniazid, rifampin, pyrazinamide and ethambutol or streptomycin) for a period of 6 months is the recommended therapy.

BIBLIOGRAPHY

1. Collins JK. Handbook of Clinical Ophthalmology. New York: Masson; 1982.
2. DeVoe AG, Locatcher-Khorazo D. The external manifestations of ocular tuberculosis. Trans Am Ophthalmol Soc. 1964;62:203-12.
3. D'Souza P, Garg R, Dhaliwal RS, et al. Orbital tuberculosis. Int Ophthalmol. 1994;18:149-52.
4. Gupta V, Gupta A, Arora S, et al. Presumed tubercular serpiginous like choroiditis. Ophthalmology. 2003;110:17 44-9.
5. Patkar S, Singhania BK, Agrawal A. Intraorbital extraocular tuberculosis: a report of three cases. Surg Neurol. 1994; 42:320-1.
6. Roy FH, Fraunfelder FW, Fraunfelder FT. Roy and Fraunfelder's Current Ocular Therapy, 6th editon. Philadelphia: WB Saunders; 2008.
7. Tejada P, Mendez MJ, Negreira S. Choroidal tubercles with tuberculous meningitis. Int Ophthalmol. 1994;18:115-8.

1P.4B3A. ARTERIOSCLEROSIS

General

Thickening and induration of the arterial wall; prominent in the elderly.

Ocular

Increased arterial light reflex, copper/silver wire arteries; arteriovenous crossing changes; arterial caliber variation/irregularity; arterial straightening or tortuosity; intimal hyperplasia, medial atrophy, atherosclerotic fibrous plaques and calcifications of the internal elastic lamina observed in aged human orbital arteries.

Clinical

Increased collagen deposition in small- and medium-sized arteries with progressive replacement of the smooth muscle in the vessel walls; arterial wall changes at arteriovenous crossings.

Laboratory

Diagnosis is made by clinical findings.

Treatment

None.

BIBLIOGRAPHY

1. Büchi ER, Schiller P, Felice M, et al. Common histopathological changes in aged human orbital arteries. Int Ophthalmol. 1993;17:37-42.
2. Collins JF. Handbook of Clinical Ophthalmology. New York: Masson; 1982. p. 269.

1P.4B3B. BELL'S PALSY (IDIOPATHIC FACIAL PARALYSIS)

General

Unilateral facial nerve paralysis of sudden onset and gradual recovery involving the nerve as it runs through the fallopian canal; etiology unknown; more common in adults.

Ocular

Corneal ulcer; paralysis of seventh nerve; ectropion; lagophthalmos; ptosis; epiphora; decreased visual acuity; diplopia; ocular irritation; exposure keratitis.

Clinical

Aching in the ear or mastoid; tingling or numbness of cheek or mouth; alteration of taste; hyperacusis; epiphora; facial weakness; most commonly and frequently affected cranial nerve with herpes zoster is the facial nerve.

Laboratory

It is not diagnosed by clinical findings.

Treatment

Most patients recover without treatment. If spontaneous recovery does not occur, the most widely accepted treatment is corticosteroids.

BIBLIOGRAPHY

1. Taylor DC, Khoromi S, Zachariah SB. (2012). Bell palsy. [online] Available from www.emedicine.com/neuro/TOPIC413.HTM. [Accessed September, 2013].

1P.4B3F. HERPES ZOSTER

General

It is caused by varicella zoster virus; about 75% of cases occur in persons over age of 45 years; condition is more frequent with advancing age and in patients who are immunocompromised by drugs or disease; in particular, an increasing number of patients with herpes zoster ophthalmicus are immunosuppressed.

Ocular

Conjunctivitis; keratitis; recurrent corneal ulcer; neuralgia; zoster rash of eyelids; uveitis; iris atrophy; scleritis; cataract; optic neuritis; paralysis of third nerve; proptosis; paralysis of lids; orbital apex syndrome; retinitis; neurotrophic keratitis; acute retinal necrosis; progressive outer retinal necrosis; ocular motor nerve pareses; tonic pupil; encephalitis; vasculitis.

Clinical

Local lesions involving the posterior or root ganglia; nerve damage; tissue scarring.

Laboratory

Diagnosed mostly on the basis of the characteristic pain and appearance of the dermatomal rashes.

Treatment

Antiviral agents, systemic corticosteroids, antidepressants, and adequate pain control. Immunocompetent adults aged 60 years or older, benefit from receipt of the herpes zoster vaccine and have a lower incidence of herpes zoster.

BIBLIOGRAPHY

1. Diaz MM, Foster CS, Walton RC, et al. (2011). Herpes zoster ophthalmicus. [online] Available from www.emedicine.com/oph/TOPIC257.HTM. [Accessed September, 2013].
2. Ghaznawi N, Virdi A, Dayan A, et al. Herpes zoster ophthalmicus: comparison of disease in patients 60 years and older versus younger than 60 years. Ophthalmology. 2011;118(11):2242-50.
3. Ho J, Xirasagar S, Lin H. Increased risk of a cancer diagnosis after herpes zoster ophthalmicus: a nationwide population-based study. Ophthalmology. 2011;118(6):1076-81.
4. Tseng HF, Smith N, Harpaz R, et al. Herpes zoster vaccine in older adults and the risk of subsequent herpes zoster disease. JAMA. 2011;305(2):160-6.

1P.4B3G. HYPERTENSION

General

Elevated blood pressure.

Ocular

Retinal arterial narrowing; arteriosclerosis; hemorrhages; retinal edema; cotton-wool spots; fatty exudates; optic disk edema; exudative retinal detachment; optic neuropathy; swollen optic nerve; central retinal vein occlusion; branch retinal vein occlusion; choroidal ischemia.

Clinical

Systemic hypertension; patchy loss of muscle tone in vessel walls; vascular decompensation.

Laboratory

Diagnosis is made from clinical findings; complete blood count (CBC), serum electrolytes, serum creatinine, serum glucose, uric acid and urinalysis, lipid profile (total cholesterol, low-density lipoprotein and high-density lipoprotein and triglycerides).

Treatment

Lifestyle modifications: Weight loss, stop smoking, exercise, reduce stress, limit alcohol intake, reduce sodium intake, maintain adequate calcium and potassium intake. Refer to internist for drug therapy.

🖶 BIBLIOGRAPHY

1. Madhur MS, Riaz K, Dreisbach AW, et al. (2012). Hypertension. [online] Available from www.emedicine.com/med/TOPIC1106.HTM. [Accessed January, 2013].

🖶 1P.4B3H. HANSEN DISEASE (LEPROSY)

General

Communicable disease caused by *M. leprae*.

Ocular

Keratitis; leukoma; pannus; corneal ulcer; uveitis; iris atrophy; dacryocystitis; anisocoria; multiple pupils; decreased or absent pupillary reaction to light; paralysis of seventh nerve; episcleritis; blepharospasm; lagophthalmos; madarosis; secondary glaucoma; decreased IOP; subconjunctival fibrosis; punctate epithelial keratopathy; posterior subcapsular cataract; corneal hypesthesia; prominent corneal nerves; iridocyclitis; foveal avascular keratitis; scleritis; interstitial keratitis; iris pearls; dry eye.

Clinical

Disease affects primarily the skin, mucous membrane, and peripheral nerves.

Laboratory

Skin biopsy specimens contain vacuolated macrophages, few lymphocytes, and numerous acid-fast bacilli often in clumps or globi.

Treatment

The WHO recommends MDT for all forms of leprosy. MDT 14 consists of rifampin, ofloxacin, and minocycline.

🖶 BIBLIOGRAPHY

1. Kim EC. (2011) Ocular manifestations of leprosy. [online] Available from www.emedicine.com/oph/TOPIC743.HTM. [Accessed September, 2013].

🖶 1P.4B3J. ACQUIRED LUES (SYPHILIS; ACQUIRED SYPHILIS; LUES VENEREA; MALUM VENEREUM)

General

Causative agent, *T. pallidum*, usually transmitted sexually.

Ocular

Conjunctival chancroid; conjunctivitis; keratitis; blepharitis; ptosis; iris atrophy; hippus; dacryocystitis; optic nerve atrophy; optic neuritis; periostitis; episcleritis; scleritis; nystagmus; uveitis; vitreous hemorrhages; paralysis of sixth nerve; papilledema; retinal hemorrhages; retinitis proliferans; oculogyric crisis; neuroretinitis; papilledema (associated with aseptic meningitis); diffuse or multifocal chorioretinitis; vertical supranuclear gaze palsy; Benedikt syndrome.

Clinical

Primary lesion associated with regional lymphadenopathy; secondary bacteremic stage associated with generalized mucocutaneous lesions; tertiary stage characterized by destructive mucocutaneous, musculoskeletal, or parenchymal lesions, aortitis, or CNS disease; syphilis and HIV infection often coexist in the same patient who experiences a higher incidence and greater severity of neurologic and ocular manifestations; a significant percentage of patients infected with HIV-I and *T. pallidum* become seronegative to syphilis testing.

Laboratory

Serologic nontreponemal tests include VDRL and RPR.

Treatment

The goals are to reduce morbidity and to prevent complications. Penicillin is the antibiotic of choice for treating syphilis. Ocular syphilis should be treated the same as patients with neurosyphilis.

⊟ BIBLIOGRAPHY

1. Majmudar PA. (2011). Interstitial keratitis overview of interstitial keratitis. [online] Available from www.emedicine.com/oph/TOPIC453.HTM. [Accessed September, 2013].
2. Euerle B, Chandrasekar PH, Diaz MM, et al. (2012). Syphilis. [online] Available from www.emedicine.com/med/TOPIC2224.HTM. [Accessed September, 2013].

⊟ 1P.4B4B. MELKERSSON-ROSENTHAL SYNDROME (MELKERSSON IDIOPATHIC FIBROEDEMA; MIESCHER CHEILITIS GRANULOMATOSIS)

General

Occurrence in childhood or youth; possible etiologies include viral infection, tuberculosis, sarcoidosis and allergic reactions (all affecting parasympathetic cells in geniculate ganglia); facial palsy resembles Bell palsy; possible localization of this disorder to the gene at 9p11 has been reported.

Ocular

Lagophthalmos; lid edema; lacrimation is secondary to the "crocodile tear" phenomenon from aberrant seventh nerve regeneration; exposure keratitis and corneal ulcers; corneal opacities.

Clinical

Chronic edema of face and lips; peripheral facial palsy (may be bilateral), which may precede edema by weeks to years; furrowed tongue; granulomatous cheilitis and glossitis; lingua plicata.

Laboratory

Lip biopsy or facial tissues.

Treatment

Daily compressions may provide improvement.

⊟ BIBLIOGRAPHY

1. Scully C. (2012). Cheilitis granulomatosa. [online] Available from www.emedicine.com/derm/TOPIC72.HTM. [Accessed September, 2013].

⊟ 1P.4B4C. HEERFORDT SYNDROME (UVEOPAROTID FEVER; UVEOPAROTITIS; UVEOPAROTITIC PARALYSIS)

General

It occurs in young adults, more frequently in females than in males; usual cause is sarcoidosis.

Ocular

Band keratopathy; keratoconjunctivitis sicca; uveitis; optic atrophy; papilledema; episcleritis; snowball opacity of vitreous; retinal vasculitis; proptosis; cataract; paralysis of seventh nerve; sarcoid nodules of eyelid, iris, ciliary body, choroid, and sclera; dacryoadenitis.

Clinical

Parotid gland swelling; facial paralysis; lymphadenopathy; splenomegaly; cutaneous nodules; facial nerve palsy.

Laboratory

Biopsy of liver, skin, lymph nodes or conjunctiva show noncaseating epithelioid cell follicles; X-ray shows lung changes; low tuberculin sensitivity; elevated angiotensin-converting enzyme (ACE) level.

Treatment

Systemic corticosteroids are the treatment of choice.

⏚ BIBLIOGRAPHY

1. Dahl AA. (2011). Ophthalmologic manifestations of sarcoidosis. [online] Available from www.emedicine.com/oph/TOPIC451.HTM. [Accessed September, 2013].

⏚ 1P.4B4C. MIKULICZ-RADECKI SYNDROME (MIKULICZ SYNDROME; DACRYOSIALOADENOPATHY; MIKULICZ-SJÖGREN SYNDROME)

General

Not an individual disease but a manifestation of tuberculosis, syphilis, leukemia, lymphosarcoma, sarcoidosis, Hodgkin disease, mumps, Waldenström macroglobulinemia, or lymphoma; exhibits a chronic course with frequent recurrences; milder form of Sjögren syndrome (*see* Schaumann Syndrome).

Ocular

Bilateral painless enlargement of lacrimal glands with bulging of upper lid; decreased or absent lacrimation; conjunctivitis; uveitis; optic atrophy; optic neuritis; phlyctenules; keratoconjunctivitis; dacryoadenitis; retinal candlewax spots; periphlebitis.

Clinical

Symmetrical, perhaps marked, enlargement of salivary glands; dryness of mouth and pharynx; hoarseness; neurologic complications.

Laboratory

Diagnosis is made by clinical findings.

Treatment

Identify cause.

⏚ BIBLIOGRAPHY

1. Meyer D, Yanoff M, Hanno H, et al. Differential diagnosis in Mikulicz's syndrome, Mikulicz's disease, and similar disease entities. Am J Ophthalmol. 1971;71(2):516-24.
2. Von Mikulicz-Radecki J. Ueber eine Eigenartige Symmetrische Erkrankung der Thranen und Mundspeicheldrusen. Beitr Chirurg Festschr Gewid T Billroth Stuttgart. 1892;610-30.

⏚ 1Q. FLOPPY EYELID SYNDROME

General

Origin unknown; more common in males; overweight; X-chromosome-linked inheritance pattern or possible hormonal influence; it has been postulated that the degenerative changes in the tarsus may result from the combination of local pressure-induced lid ischemia and systemic hypoventilation.

Ocular

Easily everted, floppy upper eyelid and papillary conjunctivitis of the upper palpebral conjunctiva; upper eyelid everts during sleep, resulting in irritation, papillary conjunctivitis and conjunctival keratinization; most distinct feature is rubbery, malleable upper tarsus; keratoconus; punctate keratopathy; blepharoptosis; lash ptosis.

Clinical

Obesity; sleep apnea.

Laboratory

Conjunctival scrapings reveal keratinized epithelial cells. Bacterial cultures are important.

Treatment

Full-thickness upper and lower eyelid resection.

BIBLIOGRAPHY

1. Ezra DG, Beaconsfield M, Sira M, et al. Long-term outcomes of surgical approaches to the treatment of floppy eyelid syndrome. Ophthalmology. 2010;117(4):839-46.
2. Ezra DG, Beaconsfield M, Sira M, et al. The associations of floppy eyelid syndrome: a case control study. Ophthalmology. 2010;117(4):831-8.
3. Chatziralli IP, Sergentanis TN. Risk factors for intraoperative floppy iris syndrome: a meta-analysis. Ophthalmology. 2011;118(4):730-5.
4. Blaydon SM. (2011). Floppy eyelid syndrome. [online] Available from www.emedicine.com/oph/TOPIC605.HTM. [Accessed January, 2013].

1R. GRANULOMA FACIALE

General

Uncommon disease; etiology unknown; characterized by single or multiple cutaneous nodules usually occurring on the face; asymptomatic; most common in males; seen in whites, rarely in Blacks and Japanese.

Ocular

Unusual eyelid nodules.

Clinical

Cutaneous nodules most often on face but may appear anywhere; lesions are soft, elevated, well-circumscribed nodules, from a few millimeters to several centimeters in size; extrafacial lesions are extremely rare but have been reported.

Laboratory

Skin biopsy of a representative lesion.

Treatment

A variety of surgical procedures may be used in the management of granuloma faciale. Scarring may occur with many of these, so the pulsed dye laser is preferred.

BIBLIOGRAPHY

1. Wiederkehr M, Schwartz RA. (2011). Granuloma faciale. [online] Available from www.emedicine.com/derm/TOPIC170.HTM. [Accessed September, 2013].

1S. HORNER SYNDROME

Horner syndrome comprises paralysis of sympathetic nerve supply with lid ptosis, miosis, apparent enophthalmos, frequently dilatation of the vessels with absence of sweating (anhidrosis) on homolateral side; the pupil demonstrates a decreased sensitivity to cocaine and hypersensitivity to adrenalin and may have heterochromia with congenital Horner syndrome.

1. *Region of first neuron*: Lesions of hypothalamus and diencephalic region also suggest diabetes insipidus, disturbed temperature regulation, adiposogenital syndrome, and autonomic epidemic epilepsy of Penfield.
   A. Arnold-Chiari malformation
   B. Basal meningitis, such as in syphilis
   C. Base-of-skull tumors (e.g. melanoma)
   D. Multiple sclerosis
   †E. Pituitary tumor
   †F. Tumor of the third ventricle
   †G. Midbrain, such as in syphilis
   †H. Pons, such as in intrapontine hemorrhage
   I. Medulla, such as in Wallenberg syndrome (lateral medullary syndrome): Thrombosis of posterior inferior cerebellar artery
   J. Cervical region
      1. Syringomyelia
      †2. Tumor
      †3. Injury as traumatic dislocation of cervical vertebrae or dissection of the vertebral artery
      4. Syphilis (acquired lues)
      5. Poliomyelitis
      6. Meningitis
      †7. Amyotrophic lateral sclerosis
      8. Related to scleroderma and facial hemiatrophy
      †9. Vascular malformation such as agenesis of internal carotid artery

2. *Region of second neuron*
   A. Spinal birth injury: Klumpke paralysis with injured lower brachial plexus
   †B. Cervical rib
   C. Thoracic lesions
      1. Pancoast tumor: In apex of lung, such as carcinoma or tuberculosis
      †2. Aneurysm of aorta, subclavian, or carotid artery
      †3. Central venous catheterization
      †4. Mediastinal tumors
      5. Lymphadenopathy of Hodgkin disease, leukemia, lymphosarcoma, or tuberculosis
      †6. Stellate ganglion block
      †7. Tube thoracostomy
   †D. Neck
      *1. Enlarged lymph gland, tumors, aneurysm, and thyroid gland
      2. Carcinoma of esophagus
      3. Retropharyngeal tumors
      4. Neuroma of sympathetic chain
      5. Intraoral trauma with damage to internal carotid plexus
      6. Thin intervertebral foramina of spinal cord, such as in pachymeningitis, hypertrophic spinal arthritis, ruptured intervertebral disk, and meningeal tumors
      7. Traction of sternocleidomastoid muscle, such as from positioning on operating table
      8. Complications of tonsillectomy
      9. Mandibular tooth abscess
      *10. Lesions of middle ear, such as in acute purulent otitis media and petromastoid operation
      *11. Carotid artery dissection
      12. Internal carotid artery occlusion
3. *Region of third neuron*
   †A. Aneurysm of internal carotid and its branches
   B. Paratrigeminal syndrome (Raeder syndrome)
   C. Cavernous sinus syndrome (Foix syndrome)
   †D. Tumors of cysts of orbit
   †E. Drugs can affect any region and include the following:
      - Acetophenazine
      - Alseroxylon
      - Bupivacaine
      - Butaperazine
      - Carphenazine
      - Chloroprocaine
      - Chlorpromazine
      - Deserpidine
      - Diacetylmorphine
      - Diethazine
      - Ethopropazine
      - Etidocaine
      - Fluphenazine
      - Guanethidine
      - Influenza virus vaccine
      - Levodopa
      - Lidocaine
      - Mepivacaine
      - Mesoridazine
      - Methdilazine
      - Methotrimeprazine
      - Oral contraceptives
      - Perazine
      - Pericyazine
      - Perphenazine
      - Piperacetazine
      - Prilocaine
      - Procaine
      - Prochlorperazine
      - Promazine
      - Promethazine
      - Propiomazine
      - Propoxycaine
      - *Rauwolfia serpentina*
      - Rescinnamine
      - Reserpine
      - Syrosingopine
      - Thiethylperazine
      - Thiopropazate
      - Thioproperazine
      - Thioridazine
      - Trifluoperazine
      - Triflupromazine
      - Trimeprazine
   F. Cluster headaches (migrainous neuralgia)
   G. Herpes zoster
   H. Migraine
   I. Fetal varicella syndrome

Treatment

See as needed.

*Indicates most frequent
†Indicates a general entry and therefore has not been described in detail in the text

BIBLIOGRAPHY

1. Aytug S, Shapiro LE. (2012). Hurthle cell carcinoma. [online] Available from www.emedicine.com/med/TOPIC1045. HTM. [Accessed September, 2013].
2. Bardorf CM, Stavern GV, Garcia-Valenzuela E. (2013). Horner syndrome. [online] Available from www.emedicine.com/oph/TOPIC336.HTM. [Accessed September, 2013].
3. Bruce JN, Fusco DJ, Feldstein NA, et al. (2013). Ependymoma. [online] Available from www.emedicine.com/med/TOPIC700.HTM. [Accessed September, 2013].
4. Dave J, Bessette MJ, Setnik G. (2013). Torsade de Pointes. [online] Available from www.emedicine.com/med/TOPIC2286.HTM. [Accessed September, 2013].
5. D'Silva KJ, May SK. (2012). Pancoast syndrome. [online] Available from www.emedicine.com/med/TOPIC3576. HTM. [Accessed September, 2013].
6. Eggenberger ER. (2012). Anisocoria. [online] Available from www.emedicine.com/oph/TOPIC160.HTM. [Accessed September, 2013].
7. Eskandari MK, Pearce WH. (2012). Upper extremity occlusive disease. [online] Available from www.emedicine.com/med/TOPIC2776.HTM. [Accessed September, 2013].
8. Guerrero M, Williams SC. (2013). Pancoast tumor imaging. [online] Available from www.emedicine.com/radio/TOPIC515.HTM. [Accessed September, 2013].
9. Gurme M, Quan D, Oskarsson BE. (2012). Idiopathic orthostatic hypotension and other autonomic failure syndrome. [online] Available from www.emedicine.com/neuro/TOPIC609.HTM. [Accessed September, 2013].
10. Kattah JC, Tsung AT, Hanovnikian JV. (2013). Pituitary tumors. [online] Available from www.emedicine.com/neuro/TOPIC312.HTM. [Accessed September, 2013].
11. Kaye V, Brandstate ME. (2011). Vertebrobasilar stroke overview of vertebrobasilar stroke. [online] Available from www.emedicine.com/pmr/TOPIC143.HTM. [Accessed September, 2013].
12. Kidwell CS, Burgess RE. (2011). Dissection syndrome. [online] Available from www.emedicine.com/neuro/TOPIC99.HTM. [Accessed September, 2013].
13. Lacayo NJ, Davis KA. (2012). Pediatric neuroblastoma. [online] Available from www.emedicine.com/ped/TOPIC1570.HTM. [Accessed August, 2013].
14. Lo SS, Lee N, Karimi S, et al. (2011). Imaging in nasopharyngeal squamous cell carcinoma. [online] Available from www.emedicine.com/radio/TOPIC551.HTM. [Accessed September, 2013].
15. Ramachandran TS, Ramachandran A. (2012). Temporal/giant cell arteritis. [online] Available from www.emedicine.com/neuro/TOPIC592.HTM. [Accessed September, 2013].
16. Schechter SH. (2012). Raeder paratrigeminal syndrome. [online] Available from www.emedicine.com/neuro/TOPIC331.HTM. [Accessed September, 2013].
17. Schwartz RA, Altman R, Kihiczak G. (2013). Hyperhidrosis. [online] Available from www.emedicine.com/derm/TOPIC893.HTM. [Accessed September, 2013].
18. Sharma S, Maycher B. (2011). Imaging in non-small cell lung cancer. [online] Available from www.emedicine.com/radio/TOPIC406.HTM. [Accessed September, 2013].
19. Vandenakker-Albanese C, Zhao H. (2012). Brown-sequard syndrome. [online] Available from www.emedicine.com/pmr/TOPIC17.HTM. [Accessed September, 2013].
20. Vaphiades MS. (2013). Pituitary apoplexy. [online] Available from www.emedicine.com/oph/TOPIC471.HTM. [Accessed September, 2013].

1S.1A. ARNOLD-CHIARI SYNDROME (PLATYBASIA SYNDROME; CEREBELLOMEDULLARY MALFORMATION SYNDROME; BASILAR IMPRESSIONS)

General

Malformation of the hindbrain; developmental deformity of the occipital bone and upper cervical spine; recognized in children or adults; clinical picture may be indistinguishable from that of Dandy-Walker syndrome in infants.

Ocular

Horizontal, vertical and rotary forms of nystagmus; vertical nystagmus in both upgaze and downgaze is most common; papilledema; esotropia; Duane's retraction syndrome (association); oscillopsia.

Clinical

Hydrocephalus; cerebellar ataxia; bilateral pyramidal tract signs.

Laboratory

CT scans are used most commonly for the diagnosis of hydrocephalus and for the evaluation of suspected shunt malfunction.

Treatment

Early recognition and treatment is important because of the potential life-threatening symptoms. Early surgical intervention, especially in infants may prevent irreversible changes and death.

BIBLIOGRAPHY

1. Incesu L, Khosla A, Aiello MR. (2011). Imaging in Chiari II malformation. [online] Available from www.emedicine.com/radio/TOPIC150.HTM. [Accessed September, 2013].

⊟ 1S.1B. ACQUIRED LUES (SYPHILIS; ACQUIRED SYPHILIS; LUES VENEREA; MALUM VENEREUM)

General

Causative agent, *T. pallidum*, usually transmitted sexually.

Ocular

Conjunctival chancroid; conjunctivitis; keratitis; blepharitis; ptosis; iris atrophy; hippus; dacryocystitis; optic nerve atrophy; optic neuritis; periostitis; episcleritis; scleritis; nystagmus; uveitis; vitreous hemorrhages; paralysis of sixth nerve; papilledema; retinal hemorrhages; retinitis proliferans; oculogyric crisis; neuroretinitis; papilledema (associated with aseptic meningitis); diffuse or multifocal chorioretinitis; vertical supranuclear gaze palsy; Benedikt syndrome.

Clinical

Primary lesion associated with regional lymphadenopathy; secondary bacteremic stage associated with generalized mucocutaneous lesions; tertiary stage characterized by destructive mucocutaneous, musculoskeletal, or parenchymal lesions, aortitis, or CNS disease; syphilis and HIV infection often coexist in the same patient who experiences a higher incidence and greater severity of neurologic and ocular manifestations; a significant percentage of patients infected with HIV-I and *T. pallidum* become seronegative to syphilis testing.

Laboratory

Serologic nontreponemal tests include VDRL and RPR.

Treatment

The goals are to reduce morbidity and to prevent complications. Penicillin is the antibiotic of choice for treating syphilis. Ocular syphilis should be treated the same as patients with neurosyphilis.

⊟ BIBLIOGRAPHY

1. Majmudar PA. (2011). Interstitial keratitis overview of interstitial keratitis. [online] Available from www.emedicine.com/oph/TOPIC453.HTM. [Accessed September, 2013].

⊟ 1S.1C. IRIS MELANOMA

General

Malignant neoplasm.

Clinical

None.

Ocular

Iris melanoma, ectropion uvea, sector cataract, sentinel vessels, heterochromia, hyphema, chronic uveitis, glaucoma.

Laboratory

Diagnosis is made by clinical findings.

Treatment

Resection with iridectomy/iridocyclectomy or radiotherapy and enucleation.

⊟ BIBLIOGRAPHY

1. Waheed NK, Foster CS. (2012). Iris melanoma. [online] Available from www.emedicine.com/oph/TOPIC405.HTM. [Accessed September, 2013].

⊟ 1S.1D. DISSEMINATED SCLEROSIS (MULTIPLE SCLEROSIS)

General

Disseminated demyelination affecting white matter of the brain, spinal cord, and optic nerves; etiology unknown.

Ocular

Nystagmus; ptosis; myokymia; optic atrophy; papillitis; optic neuritis; anisocoria; Argyll Robertson pupil; Marcus Gunn pupil; hippus, decreased or absent papillary reaction to light; periphlebitis; visual field defects; gaze palsy; paralysis of third or sixth nerve; uveitis; oscillopsia; Uhthoff symptom (reduction of visual acuity with exercise or ocular hyperthermia); pars planitis; retinal venous sheathing; retinitis; granulomatous uveitis.

Clinical

Incoordination; paresthesia; spasticity; tic douloureux; urinary frequency and infections; progressive disability; paralysis; death.

Laboratory

MRI, cerebrospinal fluid (CSF) positive for oligoclonal band, albumin and IgG index; brainstem auditory evoked response (BAER) and somato-sensory evoked potentials (SEP).

Treatment

Patients with MS may require multiple consultations to rule out other causes for their symptoms. Drugs such as immunodulator, immunosuppressors, anti-Parkinson agent, CNS stimulants are all used in the management of the disease.

⊟ BIBLIOGRAPHY

1. Luzzio C, Dangond F. (2013). Multiple sclerosis. [online] Available from www.emedicine.com/neuro/topic228.htm. [Accessed September, 2013].

⊟ 1S.1I. WALLENBERG SYNDROME (DORSOLATERAL MEDULLARY SYNDROME; LATERAL BULBAR SYNDROME) PTOSIS

General

Occlusion of the posterior inferior cerebellar artery; onset after age 40 years; similar to Babinski-Nageotte syndrome but crossed hemiparesis is absent; nystagmus is produced by involvement of the vestibular nuclei or posterior longitudinal bundle.

Ocular

Enophthalmos; ptosis; spontaneous homolateral or contralateral horizontal or torsional nystagmus; miosis; Horner syndrome; skew deviation; impaired contralateral pursuit; saccadic abnormalities; gaze-holding abnormalities.

Clinical

Nausea; vertigo; difficulty in swallowing and speaking; ipsilateral ataxia; muscular hypotonicity; ipsilateral loss of pain and temperature sense of the face; neurotrophic skin ulcers; contralateral hypalgesia; facial weakness.

Laboratory

CT scan.

Treatment

Seek neurological assistance. Ptosis evaluation.

⊟ BIBLIOGRAPHY

1. Brazis PW. Ocular motor abnormalities in Wallenberg's lateral medullary syndrome. Mayo Clin Proc. 1992;67:365-8.
2. Hornsten G. Wallenberg's syndrome. I. General symptomatology with reference to visual disturbances and imbalance. Acta Neural Scand. 1974;50:434-46.
3. Marcoux C, Malfait Y, Pirard C, et al. Neurotrophic ulcer following Wallenberg's syndrome. Dermatology. 1993;186:301-2.
4. Sacco RL, Freddo L, Bello JA, et al. Wallenberg's lateral medullary syndrome. Clinical-magnetic resonance imaging correlations. Arch Neurol. 1993;50:609-14.
5. Silfverskiold BP. Skew deviation in Wallenberg's syndrome. Acta Neurol Scand. 1966;41:381-6.
6. Wallenberg A. Anatomische Befunde in Einem als "Akute Bulbaraffektion (Embolie der Arteria Cerebellar. Post. Inf. Sinist.)" Beschriebenen Falle. Arch F Psychiatr. 1901;34.

1S.1J1. PASSOW SYNDROME (BREMER STATUS DYSRAPHICUS; STATUS DYSRAPHICUS SYNDROME; SYRINGOMYELIA; SYRINGOBULBIA)

General

Congenital nonclosure of the neural tube; familial occurrence or may be sporadic; insidious onset in 2nd to 3rd decade of life.

Ocular

Enophthalmos; ptosis; rotatory nystagmus; heterochromia iridis; anterior uveitis; corneal anesthesia; neuroparalytic keratitis; paralysis of third, fifth, sixth, and seventh cranial nerves; Horner syndrome; anisocoria; papilledema; optic atrophy; zonular cataract (*see* Horner Syndrome).

Clinical

Anesthesia over area of first division of trigeminal nerve; facial hemiatrophy; facial nerve paralysis; muscular weakness; cervical ribs; kyphoscoliosis; spina bifida; unilateral numbness of fingers; loss of deep reflexes; insensitivity to pain and temperature in affected areas; neurogenic bladder.

Laboratory

MRI, CT.

Treatment

Suboccipital and cervical decompression, laminectomy and syringotomy, shunts, fourth ventriculostomy, terminal ventriculostomy and neuroendoscopic surgery may be considered.

BIBLIOGRAPHY

1. Al-Shatoury HA, Galhom AA, Wagner FC. (2012). Syringomyelia. [online] Available from emedicine.medscape.com/article/1151685-overview. [Accessed September, 2013].

1S.1J4. ACQUIRED LUES (SYPHILIS; ACQUIRED SYPHILIS; LUES VENEREA; MALUM VENEREUM)

General

Causative agent, *T. pallidum*, usually transmitted sexually.

Ocular

Conjunctival chancroid; conjunctivitis; keratitis; blepharitis; ptosis; iris atrophy; hippus; dacryocystitis; optic nerve atrophy; optic neuritis; periostitis; episcleritis; scleritis; nystagmus; uveitis; vitreous hemorrhages; paralysis of sixth nerve; papilledema; retinal hemorrhages; retinitis proliferans; oculogyric crisis; neuroretinitis; papilledema (associated with aseptic meningitis); diffuse or multifocal chorioretinitis; vertical supranuclear gaze palsy; Benedikt syndrome.

Clinical

Primary lesion associated with regional lymphadeno pathy; secondary bacteremic stage associated with generalized mucocutaneous lesions; tertiary stage characterized by destructive mucocutaneous, musculoskeletal, or parenchymal lesions, aortitis, or CNS disease; syphilis and HIV infection often coexist in the same patient who experiences a higher incidence and greater severity of neurologic and ocular manifestations; a significant percentage of patients infected with HIV-I and *T. pallidum* become seronegative to syphilis testing.

Laboratory

Serologic nontreponemal tests include VDRL and RPR.

Treatment

The goals are to reduce morbidity and to prevent complications. Penicillin is the antibiotic of choice for treating syphilis. Ocular syphilis should be treated the same as patients with neurosyphilis.

BIBLIOGRAPHY

1. Majmudar PA. (2011). Interstitial keratitis overview of interstitial keratitis. [online] Available from www.emedicine.com/oph/TOPIC453.HTM. [Accessed September, 2013].

🖩 1S.1J5. POLIOMYELITIS (INFANTILE PARALYSIS)

General

Acute viral infection characterized by varying degrees of neuronal injury, with special localization in the anterior horns and motor nuclei of the brainstem.

Ocular

Diplopia; nystagmus; paralysis of third, fourth, and sixth nerves; paresis of seventh nerve; papilledema; visual agnosia; Homer's syndrome; pupillary paralysis; optic neuritis; ophthalmoparesis; transient visual loss; internuclear ophthalmoplegia; papillary disturbances, spasm of near reflex.

Clinical

Flaccid paralysis of many muscle groups; death from asphyxia and involvement of vital centers in the brainstem.

Laboratory

Obtain specimens from the cerebrospinal fluid (CSF), stool and throat for viral cultures.

Treatment

No antivirals are effective against polioviruses. The treatment of poliomyelitis is mainly supportive and will involve physical therapist and rehabilitation therapist, pulmonologist, neurologist, immunologist and infectious diseases specialist.

🖩 BIBLIOGRAPHY

1. Estrada B. (2012). Pediatric poliomyelitis. [online] Available from www.emedicine.com/ped/TOPIC1843.HTM. [Accessed September, 2013].

🖩 1S.1J6. MENINGOCOCCEMIA (NEISSERIA MENINGITIDES; MENINGITIS)

General

Systemic bacterial infection caused by *Neisseria meningitides*; can be present chronically in patients with immune deficiencies including deficient complement levels.

Ocular

Photophobia; conjunctivitis; chemosis; keratitis; uveitis; panophthalmitis; retinal endophlebitis; macular edema; papillitis; optic neuritis; paresis of sixth or seventh nerve; nystagmus; miosis; hippus; cortical blindness; papilledema (rare); conjunctival petechiae; strabismus.

Clinical

Meningitis; fever; malaise; joint pain; splenic enlargement.

Laboratory

Cultures from blood, spinal fluid, or joint fluid.

Treatment

Treat with antibiotics promptly.

🖩 BIBLIOGRAPHY

1. Javid MH, Ahmed SH. (2012). Meningococcemia. [online] Available from www.emedicine.com/med/TOPIC1445.HTM. [Accessed September, 2013].

🖩 1S.1J8. PROGRESSIVE SYSTEMIC SCLEROSIS (SCLERODERMA; SYSTEMIC SCLERODERMA)

General

Chronic connective tissue disease of unknown etiology; chronic and usually progressive disorder; typical onset is in 3rd–5th decade; ratio of women to men is 4:1; primary sites of pathology are the arterioles and capillaries of affected organs.

Ocular

Marginal corneal ulcers; shortened fornices of the conjunctiva; ptosis; cotton-wool patches of retina; papilledema; retinal hemorrhages; cicatrization of conjunctiva and cornea; blepharitis; blepharospasm; thready, tenacious yellow-white conjunctival discharge; hypertrophy of lacrimal gland; episcleritis; ocular myositis; Sjögren syndrome; uveitis; vitreous haze; keratitis sicca; decreased corneal sensation; iritis; ischemic choroidopathy; iris sectorial atrophy; blepharophimosis; heterochromia; keratoconus; central retinal vein occlusion; branch retinal vein occlusion.

Clinical

Vascular insufficiency; Raynaud's phenomenon; malaise; weight loss; stiffness; fever; polyarticular arthritis; diffuse edema of the hands; calcinosis; esophageal involvement; sclerodactyly; telangiectasis; esophageal stricture; renal failure; diffuse interstitial fibrosis.

Laboratory

No specific test establishes diagnosis. Hypergammaglobulinemia—50% of cases ANA increased in 40–70% cases.

Treatment

Skin thickening can be treated with D-penicillamine and other experimental drugs. Pruritus can be treated with moisturizers and histamine. Raynaud's phenomenon can be treated with calcium channel blockers. Renal crisis episodes are best prevented and treated with the aggressive use of angiotensin-converting enzyme (ACE) inhibitors. Myositis may be treated cautiously with steroids.

⊟ BIBLIOGRAPHY

1. Jimenez SA, Cronin PM, Koenig AS, et al. (2012). Scleroderma. [online] Available from www.emedicine.com/med/TOPIC2076.HTM. [Accessed September, 2013].

⊟ 1S.2A. DEJERINE-KLUMPKE SYNDROME (LOWER RADICULAR SYNDROME; KLUMPKE SYNDROME; KLUMPKE PARALYSIS)

General

Lesion involving the inferior roots of the brachial plexus with nerves derived from the eighth cervical and first thoracic root.

Ocular

Enophthalmos; ptosis; narrowed palpebral fissure; miosis.

Clinical

Paralysis and atrophy of the small muscles of forearm and hand (flexor carpi ulnaris, flexor digitorum, interossei, thenar, hypothenar); decreased sensation or increased sensibility on the inner side of the forearm.

Laboratory

Neurologic evaluation, CT, MRI

Treatment

Primary exploration and repair of brachial plexus. Secondary deformities may require surgical intervention and therapy.

⊟ BIBLIOGRAPHY

1. Bienstock A, Kim JY. (2011). Brachial Plexus Hand Surgery. [online] Available from www.emedicine.com/plastic/TOPIC450.HTM. [Accessed September, 2013].

⊟ 1S.2C1. PANCOAST SYNDROME (HARE SYNDROME; SUPERIOR PULMONARY SULCUS SYNDROME)

General

Mass occupying lesion in pulmonary apex; erosion of first three ribs frequent; primary bronchogenic carcinoma most frequent cause; symptomatology similar to lower radicular (Dejerine-Klumpke) syndrome and scalenus anticus (Naffziger) syndrome; Horner syndrome caused by involvement of sympathetic chain (also can be caused by locally invasive fungus such as *Cryptococcus neoformans* or lymphomatoid granulomatosis.

Ocular

Mild enophthalmos; ptosis; narrowing of the palpebral fissure; miosis.

Clinical

Pulmonary apical tumor; severe shoulder pain; paresthesias, pain, and paresis of the homolateral arm with atrophy of arm and hand muscles.

Laboratory

Imaging and biopsy are the cornerstones of diagnosis.

Treatment

Radiation and chemotherapy; surgical treatment of choice is complete removal of the tumor by en bloc chest wall resection combined with lobectomy and node staging.

BIBLIOGRAPHY

1. D'Silva KJ, May SK. (2012). Pancoast Syndrome. [online] Available from emedicine.medscape.com/article/284011-overview. [Accessed September, 2013].

1S.2C5. HODGKIN DISEASE

General

Hodgkin disease begins in the lymph nodes and usually spreads in a predictable fashion along contiguous chains of nodes; etiology may be viral; prevalent in males.

Ocular

Keratitis; uveitis; cataract; retinal hemorrhages; vasculitis; Horner syndrome; cortical blindness; papilledema; paralysis of oculomotor nerve; episcleritis; visual field defects; infiltration of choroid, conjunctiva, lacrimal gland, and orbit; papillitis; retrobulbar neuritis; opsoclonus-myoclonus; keratitis sicca; infiltrative optic neuropathy; association with Vogt-Koyanagi-Harada syndrome; bilateral serous detachments of the macula.

Clinical

Painless cervical, axillary, or inguinal lymph node swelling; fever; weight loss; anemia; generalized pruritus.

Laboratory

Biopsy of lymph glands is diagnostic.

Treatment

The goal of therapy is to induce a complete remission with radiation therapy, chemotherapy or BMT.

BIBLIOGRAPHY

1. Lash BW, Dessain SK, Argiris A. (2012). Hodgkin lymphoma. [online] Available from www.emedicine.com/med/TOPIC1022.HTM. [Accessed September, 2013].

1S.2C5. LEUKEMIA

General

Acute or chronic blood disorder.

Ocular

Engorgement of conjunctival vessels; papillary hypertrophy; aggregations of tumor cells in conjunctiva, choroid and orbit; secondary glaucoma; retinal venous engorgement and tortuosity with pronounced constrictions; retinal hemorrhages; retinal detachment; cotton-wool spots; macular edema; papilledema; optic atrophy; optic neuritis; paralysis of extraocular muscles; hypopyon; vitreous opacities; retinal sea fans; perilimbal subconjunctival infiltrates; corneal leukemic infiltration (rare); shallow serous retinal detachments; hyphema; iris neovascularization; central retinal vein occlusion; vitreous infiltrates.

Clinical

Frequent involvement of CNS; intracranial hemorrhage; thrombocytopenia; rising white cell count.

Laboratory

CBC and differential, bone marrow aspiration, immunophenotyping, chromosomal analysis.

Treatment

Chemotherapy with or without radiotherapy.

⊟ BIBLIOGRAPHY

1. Wu L, Evans T, Martinez J. (2012). Leukemias. [online] Available from www.emedicine.com/oph/TOPIC489.HTM. [Accessed January, 2013].

⊟ 1S.2C5. TUBERCULOSIS

General

Communicable disease caused by the acid-fast bacillus *M. tuberculosis*.

Ocular

Conjunctivitis; subconjunctival nodules (tuberculomas); keratitis; pannus; corneal ulcer; blepharitis; cellulitis; meibomianitis; uveitis; dacryocystitis; chronic orbital cellulitis; retinitis; scleritis; scleral perforation; hypopyon; vitreous hemorrhages; optic neuritis; optic atrophy; tuberculous panophthalmitis; choroidal tubercles; intraorbital extraocular lesions.

Clinical

Pulmonary infection; pyuria; hematuria; epididymitis; dysuria; flank pain; distorted calyces; productive cough.

Laboratory

Acid-fast bacillus culture of body fluids including vitreous and aqueous. PCR is 89% positive for pulmonary infection.

Treatment

A course of chemotherapy (isoniazid, rifampin, pyrazinamide and ethambutol or streptomycin) for a period of 6 months is the recommended therapy.

⊟ BIBLIOGRAPHY

1. Collins JK. Handbook of Clinical Ophthalmology. New York: Masson; 1982.
2. DeVoe AG, Locatcher-Khorazo D. The external manifestations of ocular tuberculosis. Trans Am Ophthalmol Soc. 1964;62:203-12.
3. D'Souza P, Garg R, Dhaliwal RS, et al. Orbital tuberculosis. Int Ophthalmol. 1994; 18:149-52.
4. Gupta V, Gupta A, Arora S, et al. Presumed tubercular serpiginous like choroiditis. Ophthalmology. 2003;110:1744-9.
5. Patkar S, Singhania BK, Agrawal A. Intraorbital extraocular tuberculosis: a report of three cases. Surg Neurol 1994; 42:320-1.
6. Roy FH, Fraunfelder FW, Fraunfelder FT. Roy and Fraunfelder's Current Ocular Therapy, 6th editon. Philadelphia: WB Saunders; 2008.
7. Tejada P, Mendez MJ, Negreira S. Choroidal tubercles with tuberculous meningitis. Int Ophthalmol. 1994;18:115-8.

⊟ 1S.3B. RAEDER SYNDROME (PARATRIGEMINAL PARALYSIS; HORTON HEADACHE; HISTAMINE CEPHALALGIA; CILIARY NEURALGIA; CLUSTER HEADACHE; PERIODIC MIGRAINOUS NEURALGIA)

General

Interruption of sympathetic fibers about the carotid artery and involvement of the fifth nerve; meningioma and aneurysm of the internal carotid artery are the most frequent causes; prominent in males; possible pathogenetic mechanism of this condition is an ischemic injury of the gasserian ganglion.

Ocular

Mild enophthalmos; mild ptosis (unilateral); epiphora; scotoma possible; hypotonia; unilateral miosis; increased tear secretion; periocular pain; Homer syndrome.

Clinical

Facial pain; occasionally weakness of the jaw muscles; headaches (V-region); hypertension; associated inflammatory processes are not infrequent.

Laboratory

Brain scan to rule out meningioma and basilar artery aneurysm.

Treatment

Oxygen inhalation and sumatriptan subcutaneous is useful in acute attacks.

🖫 BIBLIOGRAPHY

1. Bardorf CM, van Stavern G, Garcia-Valenzuela E. (2012). Horner syndrome. [online] Available from www.emedicine.com/oph/TOPIC336.HTM. [Accessed August, 2013].

🖫 1S.3C. FOIX SYNDROME (CAVERNOUS SINUS SYNDROME; HYPOPHYSEAL-SPHENOIDAL SYNDROME; CAVERNOUS SINUS NEURALGIA SYNDROME; GODTFREDSEN SYNDROME; CAVERNOUS SINUS-NASOPHARYNGEAL TUMOR SYNDROME; CAVERNOUS SINUS THROMBOSIS)

General

Causes include tumor of lateral sinus wall or sphenoid bone, intracranial aneurysm, cavernous and lateral sinus thrombosis, or lesions; multiple myeloma; may result from infarctions or cancer or be idiopathic.

Ocular

Proptosis; severe ocular and periorbital pain; lid edema; paresis or paralysis of cranial nerves III, IV, V, and VI; corneal anesthesia; optic atrophy.

Clinical

Postauricular edema; trigeminal neuralgia; deviation of the tongue toward paralyzed side; patients usually have prominent manifestations of sepsis and paranasal sinus; local skin infections are the most common cause.

Laboratory

CT, MRI

Treatment

Radiotherapy, anticoagulation, high-dose antibiotic therapy.

🖫 BIBLIOGRAPHY

1. Kattah JC, Pula JH. (2012). Cavernous sinus syndromes. [online] Available from www.emedicine.com/neuro/topic572.htm. [Accessed September, 2013].

🖫 1S.3F. RAEDER SYNDROME (PARATRIGEMINAL PARALYSIS; HORTON HEADACHE; HISTAMINE CEPHALALGIA; CILIARY NEURALGIA; CLUSTER HEADACHE; PERIODIC MIGRAINOUS NEURALGIA)

General

Interruption of sympathetic fibers about the carotid artery and involvement of the fifth nerve; meningioma and aneurysm of the internal carotid artery are the most frequent causes; prominent in males; possible pathogenetic mechanism of this condition is an ischemic injury of the gasserian ganglion.

Ocular

Mild enophthalmos; mild ptosis (unilateral); epiphora; scotoma possible; hypotonia; unilateral miosis; increased tear secretion; periocular pain; Homer syndrome.

Clinical

Facial pain; occasionally weakness of the jaw muscles; headaches (V-region); hypertension; associated inflammatory processes are not infrequent.

Laboratory

Brain scan to rule out meningioma and basilar artery aneurysm.

Treatment

Oxygen inhalation and sumatriptan subcutaneous is useful in acute attacks.

🖶 BIBLIOGRAPHY

1. Bardorf CM, van Stavern G, Garcia-Valenzuela E. (2012). Horner syndrome. [online] Available from www.emedicine.com/oph/TOPIC336.HTM. [Accessed August, 2013].

🖶 1S.3G. HERPES ZOSTER

General

It is caused by varicella zoster virus; about 75% of cases occur in persons over age of 45 years; condition is more frequent with advancing age and in patients who are immunocompromised by drugs or disease; in particular, an increasing number of patients with herpes zoster ophthalmicus are immunosuppressed.

Ocular

Conjunctivitis; keratitis; recurrent corneal ulcer; neuralgia; zoster rash of eyelids; uveitis; iris atrophy; scleritis; cataract; optic neuritis; paralysis of third nerve; proptosis; paralysis of lids; orbital apex syndrome; retinitis; neurotrophic keratitis; acute retinal necrosis; progressive outer retinal necrosis; ocular motor nerve pareses; tonic pupil; encephalitis; vasculitis.

Clinical

Local lesions involving the posterior or root ganglia; nerve damage; tissue scarring.

Laboratory

Diagnosed mostly on the basis of the characteristic pain and appearance of the dermatomal rashes.

Treatment

Antiviral agents, systemic corticosteroids, antidepressants, and adequate pain control. Immunocompetent adults aged 60 years or older, benefit from receipt of the herpes zoster vaccine and have a lower incidence of herpes zoster.

🖶 BIBLIOGRAPHY

1. Ghaznawi N, Virdi A, Dayan A, et al. Herpes zoster ophthalmicus: comparison of disease in patients 60 years and older versus younger than 60 years. Ophthalmology. 2011;118(11):2242-50.
2. Tseng HF, Smith N, Harpaz R, et al. Herpes zoster vaccine in older adults and the risk of subsequent herpes zoster disease. JAMA. 2011;305(2):160-6.

🖶 1S.3H. MIGRAINE (VASCULAR HEADACHE)

General

Recurrent attacks of pain in the head; usually unilateral; often familial.

Ocular

Abnormal visual sensations; scotoma generally restricted to one-half of the visual field; complete blindness; unilateral transient visual loss; photopsia; branch retinal artery occlusions; anisocoria.

Clinical

Nausea; vomiting; anorexia; sensory, motor, and mood disturbances; fluid imbalance; headache.

Laboratory

Investigation studies; rule out comorbid disease, exclude other causes of headaches such as structural and/or metabolic; neurological examination; lumbar puncture (LP) followed by CT scan or MRI.

Treatment

Treatment is based on the severity of the case.

BIBLIOGRAPHY

1. Chawla J, Blanda M, Braswell R, et al. (2011). Migraine headache. [online] Available from www.emedicine.com/neuro/TOPIC218.HTM. [Accessed September, 2013].

1S.31. CONGENITAL VARICELLA SYNDROME

General

Varicella passed in utero from mother to fetus.

Ocular

Microphthalmia; microcornea; persistent hyperplastic primary vitreous.

Clinical

Urinary tract infection; neurogenic bladder.

Laboratory

Clinical.

Treatment

See persistent hyperplastic primary vitreous.

BIBLIOGRAPHY

1. Anderson WE. (2011). Varicella-zoster virus. [online] Available from www.emedicine.com/med/TOPIC2361.HTM. [Accessed September, 2013].

1T. HYPOMELANOSIS OF ITO SYNDROME (INCONTINENTIA PIGMENTI ACHROMIANS; SYSTEMATIZED ACHROMIC NEVUS)

General

Probable autosomal dominant transmission; cutaneous abnormality consisting of bizarre, patterned, macular hypopigmentation over variable portions of the body with multiple associated defects in other body systems; abnormal chromosome constitutions.

Ocular

Iridal heterochromia; myopia; esotropia; microphthalmia; hypertelorism; nystagmus; strabismus; corneal opacity; choroidal atrophy; exotropia; small optic nerve; hypopigmentation of the fundus; corneal asymmetry; pannus; atrophic irides with irregular pupillary margins; cataract; retinal detachment.

Clinical

Cutaneous manifestations consist of macular hypopigmented whorls, streaks, and patches in a bilateral or unilateral distribution affecting almost any portion of the body surface; 50% have associated noncutaneous abnormalities, including CNS dysfunction (seizure, delayed development) and musculoskeletal anomalies.

Laboratory

Diagnosis is made by clinical findings.

Treatment

No treatment is necessary for the cutaneous findings except makeup for cosmetic purposes. Other symptoms should be treated by specific specialists.

BIBLIOGRAPHY

1. Ratz JL, Gross N. (2012). Hypomelanosis of Ito. [online] Available from www.emedicine.com/derm/TOPIC186.HTM. [Accessed September, 2013].

🗗 1U. LAGOPHTHALMOS

General

Inability to close eyelids caused by projection of the eye in orbit, inadequate vertical dimensions of either lid, contraction of the eyelid retractors or malfunction of the orbicularis oculi.

Clinical

None.

Ocular

Decreased visual acuity, pain, dry eye syndrome, corneal erosion, corneal ulceration, endophthalmitis, inability to close eyelids.

Laboratory

Diagnosis is made by clinical findings.

Treatment

Topical lubricants, punctal plugs or thermal occlusion of punctum may be useful. Tarsorrhaphy with upper eyelid retraction may require upper lid levator recession and graded Müllerectomy; facial nerve palsy—gold weight implant.

🗗 BIBLIOGRAPHY

1. Roy FH, Fraunfelder FW, Fraunfelder FT. Roy and Fraunfelder's Current Ocular Therapy, 6th edition. London, UK: Elsevier; 2008.

🗗 1V. LID MYOKYMIA

General

Usually unilateral, persist for months, benign, self-limited.

Clinical

Stress, fatigue, excessive caffeine or alcohol intake.

Ocular

Spontaneous fascicular eyelid tremor without muscular atrophy or weakness.

Laboratory

Diagnosis is made by clinical findings.

Treatment

Reassurance and reduction of precipitating factors, botulinum toxin type A, oral quinine or baclofen.

🗗 BIBLIOGRAPHY

1. Lam BL. (2011). Eyelid myokymia. [online] Available from www.emedicine.com/oph/TOPIC607.HTM. [Accessed September, 2013].

🗗 1W. MADAROSIS (LOSS OF LASHES)

General

Loss of eyelashes caused by systemic or topical infections and inflammation, eyelid tumors, the hysteric plucking of hairs, surgery and trauma.

Clinical

May have emotional problems in alopecia artefacta.

Ocular

Loss of lashes is frequent in only one segment of lid.

Laboratory

Diagnosis is made by clinical findings.

Treatment

Lid hygiene; lid scrubs with baby shampoo and topical antibiotics; eyeliner and false eyelashes; transplantation of lashes to area missing lashes.

🗗 BIBLIOGRAPHY

1. Roy FH, Fraunfelder FW, Fraunfelder FT. Roy and Fraunfelder's Current Ocular Therapy, 6th edition. London, UK: Elsevier; 2008.

1X. MARCUS GUNN SYNDROME (JAW-WINKING SYNDROME; CONGENITAL TRIGEMINOOCULOMOTOR SYNKINESIS)

General

Familial occurrence rare, although dominant inheritance has been reported; symptoms are caused by abnormal connections between external pterygoid muscle and levator palpebrae, with supranuclear or supranuclear-nuclear involvement (*See* Marin Amat syndrome).

Ocular

Unilateral congenital ptosis in more than 90% of cases; 10% have spontaneous onset, usually in older persons; lid elevates rapidly when mouth is opened or mandible is moved to one or the other side; left eye seems to be more frequently affected than right eye; high incidences of strabismus (36%) and amblyopia (34%); bilateral jaw-winking; decreased abduction.

Clinical

Stimulation of ipsilateral pterygoid with chewing, opening of mouth, sucking or contralateral jaw thrusts.

Laboratory

Diagnosis is made by clinical findings.

Treatment

Treat amblyopia; if mild ptosis and mild jaw-winking, consider Muller's muscle conjunctival resection; severe jaw-winking, release levator and perform a frontalis sling usually bilaterally; unilateral ptosis mild jaw-winking, consider levator release and advance frontalis muscle to the superior tarsus.

BIBLIOGRAPHY

1. Blaydon SM. (2011). Marcus Gunn jaw-winking syndrome. [online] Available from www.emedicine.com/oph/TOPIC 608.HTM. [Accessed January, 2013].
2. Demirci H, Frueh BR, Nelson CC. Marcus Gunn jaw-winking synkinesis. Ophthalmology. 2010;117(7):1447-52.

1Y. MARIN AMAT SYNDROME (INVERTED MARCUS GUNN PHENOMENON)

General

Intrafacial connection between the orbicularis oculi and external pterygoid muscles; occurs primarily after peripheral facial palsy.

Ocular

When mouth is opened and/or mandible is moved to side opposite to ptosis, closure of the eye occurs; increased tearing during mastication.

Clinical

Signs of old facial palsy are usually recognizable.

Laboratory

Diagnosis is made by clinical findings.

Treatment

If amblyopia is noted, occlusion therapy is needed.

BIBLIOGRAPHY

1. Blaydon SM. (2011). Marcus Gunn jaw-winking syndrome. [online] Available from www.emedicine.com/oph/TOPIC608.HTM. [Accessed September, 2013].

🔲 1Z. MELKERSSON-ROSENTHAL SYNDROME (MELKERSSON IDIOPATHIC FIBROEDEMA; MIESCHER CHEILITIS GRANULOMATOSIS)

General

Occurrence in childhood or youth; possible etiologies include viral infection, tuberculosis, sarcoidosis and allergic reactions (all affecting parasympathetic cells in geniculate ganglia); facial palsy resembles Bell palsy; possible localization of this disorder to the gene at 9p11 has been reported.

Ocular

Lagophthalmos; lid edema; lacrimation is secondary to the "crocodile tear" phenomenon from aberrant seventh nerve regeneration; exposure keratitis and corneal ulcers; corneal opacities.

Clinical

Chronic edema of face and lips; peripheral facial palsy (may be bilateral), which may precede edema by weeks to years; furrowed tongue; granulomatous cheilitis and glossitis; lingua plicata.

Laboratory

Lip biopsy or facial tissues.

Treatment

Daily compressions may provide improvement.

🔲 BIBLIOGRAPHY

1. Scully C. (2012). Cheilitis granulomatosa. [online] Available from www.emedicine.com/derm/TOPIC72.HTM. [Accessed September, 2013].

🔲 1AA. ERB-GOLDFLAM SYNDROME (ERB II SYNDROME; HOPPE-GOLDFLAM DISEASE; PSEUDOPARALYTIC SYNDROME; MYASTHENIA GRAVIS)

General

Occurs at any age; more frequent between ages 20–40 years; more females affected than males; progressive; spontaneous; symptoms improve or resolve with rest in early stages of disease (*see* myasthenia gravis, neonatal or infantile); caused by autoantibodies against the acetylcholine receptor at the neuromuscular junction, leading to abnormal fatigability and weakness of skeletal muscle.

Ocular

Transient diplopia; ptosis of upper eyelids.

Clinical

Excessive fatigability of musculature; symptoms appear and increase as day progresses; expressionless face; sagging jaw; difficulty in chewing and talking; nasal regurgitation.

Laboratory

Ice test—crushed ice in surgical glove over ptotic eyelid for 2 minutes and watch for brief elevation of eyelid; Tensilon test and prostigmin test may result in the elevation of ptotic eyelid or improved strabismus in individuals with myasthenia gravis.

Treatment

Adrenal corticosteroids are frequently used. In some cases, mycophenolate mofetil, cyclosporine and cyclophosphamide may be useful. Patching one eye or using prisms may be helpful.

🔲 BIBLIOGRAPHY

1. Erb W. Zur Casuistick der Bulbaren La hmungen. Arch Psychiatr Vervenkr. 1879;9:325-50.
2. Roy FH, Fraunfelder FT, Fraunfelder FW. Roy and Fraunfelder's Current Ocular Therapy, 6th edition. London, UK: Elsevier; 2008.
3. Goldflam S. Vebereinen Scheinbar Keilbaren Bulbarparalytischem Symptom Complex mit Betheiligung der Extremitaten. Dtsch Z Nerven. 1983;4:312-52.
4. Kim JH, Hwang JM, Hwang YS, et al. Childhood ocular myasthenia gravis. Ophthalmology. 2003;110(7):1458-62.
5. Lepore FE, Sanborn GE, Slevin JT. Pupillary dysfunction in myasthenia gravis. Ann Neurol. 1979;6(1):29-33.
6. Sommer N, Melms A, Weller M, et al. Ocular myasthenia gravis. A critical review of clinical and pathophysiological aspects. Doc Ophthalmol. 1993;84(4):309-33.

1BB. OCULOPHARYNGEAL SYNDROME (PROGRESSIVE MUSCULAR DYSTROPHY WITH PTOSIS AND DYSPHAGIA; OCULOPHARYNGEAL MUSCULAR DYSTROPHY)

General

Etiology unknown; autosomal dominant inheritance; no CNS pathology; muscles of pharynx, hypopharynx, and proximal third of esophagus involved with myopathy; onset late in life; progressive hereditary myopathy in which the levator palpebrae and pharyngeal muscles are selectively involved; progressive usually symmetrical blepharoptosis with or without dysphagia appears in the 5th decade.

Ocular

Ptosis.

Clinical

Dysphagia; occasionally weakness of facial muscles.

Laboratory/Ocular

Diagnosis is made by clinical findings.

Treatment

Ptosis: If visual acuity is affected, most cases require surgical correction and there are several procedures that may be used including levator resection, repair or advancement and Fasanella-Servat.

BIBLIOGRAPHY

1. Codère F. Oculopharyngeal muscular dystrophy. Can J Ophthalmol. 1993;28(1):1-2.
2. Duranceau A, Forand MD, Fauteux JP. Surgery in oculopharyngeal muscular dystrophy. Am J Surg. 1980;139(1):33-9.
3. Jordan DR, Addison DJ. Surgical results and pathological findings in the oculopharyngeal dystrophy syndrome. Can J Ophthalmol. 1993;28(1):15-8.
4. Molgat YM, Rodrigue D. Correction of blepharoptosis in oculopharyngeal muscular dystrophy: review of 91 cases. Can J Ophthalmol. 1993;28(1):11-4.
5. Murphy SF, Drachman DB. The oculopharyngeal syndrome. JAMA. 1968;203(12):1003-8.
6. Taylor EW. Progressive vagus-glossopharyngeal paralysis with ptosis: contribution to a group of family diseases. J Nerv Ment Dis. 1915;42(3):129-39.

1CC. PALPEBRAL COLOBOMA-LIPOMA SYNDROME (NASOPALPEBRAL LIPOMA-COLOBOMA)

General

Autosomal dominant; described in a Venezuelan family.

Ocular

Coloboma of upper and lower lids at junction between their middle and inner thirds; fat deposits of both upper lids; malposition of lacrimal puncta; hypertelorism; telecanthus.

Clinical

Broad nasal bridge; fatty accumulations on nasal bridge and nasolabial area; maxillary hypoplasia.

Laboratory

Diagnosis is made by clinical findings.

Treatment

Corneal protection is the primary goal in the medical treatment of eyelid colobomas. The eyelid coloboma is large; immediate surgical closure is usually needed to prevent corneal compromise.

BIBLIOGRAPHY

1. Bashour M. (2012). Eyelid coloboma. [online] Available from www.emedicine.com/oph/TOPIC673.HTM. [Accessed September, 2013].

⊟ 1DD. PIERRE-ROBIN SYNDROME (ROBIN SYNDROME; MICROGNATHIA-GLOSSOPTOSIS SYNDROME)

General

Etiology unknown; manifestations at birth; pathogenesis based on arrested fetal development; history of intrauterine disturbance in early pregnancy (25% of cases); also increased incidence in offspring of mother's age 35 years or older; pathogenesis is thought to be incomplete development of the first brachial arch, which forms the maxilla and mandible.

Ocular

Microphthalmos; proptosis; ptosis; high myopia; glaucoma; cataract (rare); retinal disinsertion; megalocornea; iris atrophy; blue sclera; esotropia; conjunctivitis; distichiasis; vitreoretinal degeneration; retinal detachments.

Clinical

Micrognathia; cleft palate; glossoptosis; cyanosis; facial expression bird-like with flat base of nose and high-arched deformed palate with or without cleft; difficulty in breathing.

Laboratory

Diagnosis is made by clinical findings.

Treatment

Multidisciplinary approach is required to manage the complex features involved in the care of these children and their families.

⊟ BIBLIOGRAPHY

1. Tewfik TL, Trinh N, Teebi AS. (2012). Pierre Robin syndrome. [online] Available from www.emedicine.com/ent/TOPIC150.HTM. [Accessed January, 2013].

⊟ 1EE. COMPREHENSIVE PTOSIS CLASSIFICATION

Ptosis is drooping of the upper eyelid. Two muscles are required for normal elevation of the eyelid. The first and stronger muscle is the levator palpebrae superioris, innervated by the superior division of the oculomotor nerve (cranial nerve III). The second muscle, Müller's muscle, is responsible for 1–2 mm of lid elevation and is supplied by the sympathetic fibers originating in the superior cervical ganglion.

Traditionally ptosis has been categorized as congenital or acquired. A mechanistic classification has been used to distinguish types of ptosis. Ptosis may be divided into myogenic, neurogenic, aponeurotic, mechanical, protective and pseudoptosis causes.

Congenital ptosis is usually myogenic and thought to result from abnormal development of the levator muscle (fibrofatty replacement of the normal striated muscle fibers). Myogenic causes include any disorder with reduced or absent levator palpebral muscle function.

Neurogenic causes of ptosis rarely occur with congenital ptosis. Neurogenic include cranial nerve III dysfunction with partial or complete ptosis depend on the site and degree of nerve involvement.

No congenital causes of aponeurotic ptosis are found. Mechanical causes of congenital ptosis are unusual.

The comprehensive ptosis classification will consist of congenital and acquired types. The congenital types will have all myogenic, neurogenic and mechanical types in an alphabetic listing.

Congenital: Present at birth—amblyopia may occur.

A. Myogenic ptosis: Abnormal development of levator palpebral superious muscle, secondary to maldevelopment. It can be unilateral or bilateral and is generally characterized by reduced levator muscle function, lid lag on down gaze, poor or absent lid crease and lagophthalmos (incomplete closure).
   1. Aarskog syndrome (faciogenital dysplasia)
   2. Acrorenocular syndrome
   3. Alacrima congenital with distichiasis
   4. Albers-Schonberg syndrome (marble bone disease)
   5. Amyloidosis (Lubarsch-Pick syndrome)
   6. Apert syndrome (acrocephalosyndactylia syndrome)

†7. Autosomal recessive external ophthalmoplegia

8. Autosomal recessive retinitis pigmentosa

9. Axenfeld-Schurenberg syndrome (cyclic oculomotor paralysis)—during spasm, lid is raised.

10. Baraitser-Winter syndrome

11. Bassen-Kornzweig syndrome (abetalipoproteinemia)

12. Blepharophimosis syndrome

13. Bonnet-Dechaume-Blanc syndrome (neuroretinoangiomatosis, Turner syndrome)

14. Bonnevie-Ullrich syndrome (pterygolymphangiectasia)

15. Brown syndrome (superior oblique tendon sheath syndrome)

16. Carpenter syndrome (acrocephalopolysyndactyly II)

17. Cerebral palsy

18. Chromosome 11 long-arm deletion syndrome

19. Chromosome 18 (long arm) syndrome

20. Chromosome 18 (short arm) syndrome

21. Congenital fibrosis of the inferior rectus with ptosis

22. Congenital progressive external ophthalmoplegia

†23. Congenital ptosis
   a. Ptosis with blepharochimosis—dominant
   b. Ptosis due to ophthalmoplegia—autosomal dominant

24. Craniocarpotarsal dysplasia (Cranio-Carpo-Tarsal dysplasia; whistling face syndrome, Freeman-Sheldon syndrome)

25. Cretinism (juvenile hypothyroidism)

26. Cri-du-chat syndrome (cry of the cat syndrome)

27. Crouzon syndrome (craniofacial dysostosis)

28. Dandy-Walker syndrome (atresia of foramen of Magendie)

29. de Lange syndrome (congenital muscular hypertrophy-cerebral syndrome)

30. Dubowitz syndrome (dwarfism-eczema-peculiar facies)

†31. Duck-bill lips, low-set ears

32. Ehlers-Danlos syndrome (fibrodysplasia elastic generalisata)

33. Engelmann syndrome (osteopathia hyperostotica scleroticans multiplex infantalis)

34. Enophthalmos
   a. Arthrogryposis (amyoplasia congenital)
   b. Cockayne syndrome (dwarfism with retinal atrophy and deafness)
   c. Cryptophthalmia syndrome
   d. Duane retraction syndrome
   e. Freeman-Sheldon syndrome (craniocarpotarsal dysplasia)
   f. General fibrosis syndrome (congenital fibrosis syndrome)
   g. Greig syndrome (ocular hypertelorism syndrome)
   h. Hemifacial microsomia syndrome (Francois-Haustrate syndrome)
   i. Klippel-Trenaunay-Weber syndrome (angio-osteohypertrophy syndrome)
   j. Krause syndrome (congenital encephalo-ophthalmic dysplasia; encephalo-ophthalmic syndrome)
   k. Maple syrup urine disease (branched-chain ketoaciduria)
   l. Morquio syndrome (MPS IV)
   m. Neurofibromatosis
   n. Parry-Romberg syndrome (progressive facial hemiatrophy)
   o. Passow syndrome (Bremer status dysraphicus)

35. Epidermal nevus syndrome (ichthyosis hystrix)

36. Fabry syndrome

37. Gillum-Anderson syndrome (dominant blepharoptosis, high myopia)

38. Hemangiomas—strabismus, amblyopia

39. Hereditary cerebellar ataxia of Pierre-Marie syndrome; (von Bekhterev disease)

40. Hunter syndrome [mucopolysaccharidosis (MPS) II]

41. Hurler disease (MPSI)

42. Hyperammonemia

43. Kiloh-Nevin syndrome (muscular dystrophy of external ocular muscles)

44. Kohn-Romano syndrome (blepharoptosis, blepharophimosis, epicanthus inversus, telecanthus)

45. Komoto syndrome (congenital eyelid tetrad)

46. Kugelberg-Welander syndrome (progressive proximal muscle atrophy)

47. Laurence-Moon-Bardet-Biedl syndrome (retinitis pigmentosa-poydactyly-adiposogenital syndrome)

48. Leigh disease

49. Little syndrome (nail-patella syndrome)

50. MERRF syndrome

51. Microphthalmia
   a. Microphthalmia associated with the following:
      †1. Cataract—dominant inheritance
      2. Coloboma—dominant and sex-linked inheritance

3. Congenital spastic diplegia—X-linked

†4. Ectopic pupils—dominant inheritance

†5. Glaucoma—recessive inheritance

†6. Harelip and cleft palate—autosomal recessive

†7. High hypermetropia—recessive inheritance

†8. Malformation of hands and feet—autosomal recessive

†9. Polydactyly—autosomal recessive

10. Retinitis pigmentosa and glaucoma—dominant inheritance

b. Colobomatous microphthalmia

1. X-linked

a. Aicardi syndrome

b. Bloch-Sulzberger syndrome (incontinentia pigmenti)

c. Goltz syndrome (focal dermal hypoplasia)

d. Lenz microphthalmia syndrome

2. Autosomal recessive

†a. Cohen syndrome

b. Ellis-van Creveld syndrome

c. Hepatic fibrosis, polycystic kidneys, colobomas, and encephalopathy; Joubert syndrome

†d. Humeroradial synostosis

e. Kartagener syndrome

f. Laurence–Moon–Bardet–Biedl syndrome

g. Marinesco-Sjögren syndrome

h. Meckel syndrome

i. Micro syndrome

j. Sjögren-Larsson syndrome

k. Warburg syndrome

3. Autosomal dominant

a. Congenital contractural arachnodactyly

b. Crouzon syndrome

c. Stickler syndrome

d. Treacher Collins syndrome

e. Tuberous sclerosis

f. Zellweger syndrome

4. Chromosomal abnormalities

a. Deletions 4p and 4r

b. Deletions 11q

c. Deletions 13q

d. Deletions 18q; deletion syndrome; chromosome 18q syndrome

†e. Deletions XO

†f. Duplications 9q, 13q

†g. Ring D syndrome

h. Triploidy

i. Trisomy 8

j. Trisomy 9q

k. Trisomy 13

l. Trisomy 18

m. Trisomy XXX, XYY

5. Unknown cause

a. Amniogenic band syndrome (Streeter dysplasia)

b. Cat's-eye syndrome, Schmid-Fraccaro syndrome, Trisomy 21, Schachenmann syndrome, partial Trisomy G syndrome

c. Coloboma, heart disease, atresia choanae, retarded growth and retarded growth development or central nervous system anomalies, genital hypoplasia, and ear anomalies, or deafness (CHARGE) syndrome

d. Dyscraniopygophalangea (Ullrich syndrome)

e. Frontonasal dysplasia (median cleft face syndrome)

f. Goldenhar syndrome (oculoauriculovertebral syndrome)

g. Hemifacial microsomia syndrome

h. Linear sebaceous nevus syndrome

i. Rubinstein-Taybi syndrome

†j. Noncolobomatous microphthalmia

6. X-linked

a. Anderson-Warburg syndrome

b. Forsius-Eriksson syndrome (Aland disease)

c. Lowe syndrome (oculocerebrorenal syndrome)

7. Autosomal recessive

a. Cerebrooculofacioskeletal syndrome (COFS syndrome)

b. Conradi syndrome

c. Cross syndrome

d. Diamond-Blackfan syndrome

e. Fanconi syndrome

f. Obesity-cerebral-ocular-skeletal anomalies syndrome

8. Autosomal dominant

a. Blatt syndrome

b. Gansslen syndrome

c. Hypomelanosis of Ito syndrome

d. Leri syndrome

e. Myotonic dystrophy

f. Rieger syndrome

9. Chromosomal abnormalities

a. Duplication 10q

b. Trisomy 21q syndrome

c. Chromosome deletion X

10. Unknown cause

a. Arachnoidal cyst; Beals syndrome; congenital controchural arachnodactyly

b. Gorlin-Chaudhry-Moss syndrome

c. Hallerman-Streiff syndrome

d. Hutchinson-Gilford syndrome (progeria)

e. Krause syndrome (encephaloophthalmic)

f. Meyer-Schwickerath and Weyers syndrome

g. Pierre Robin syndrome

h. Retinal disinsertion syndrome

i. Sabin-Feldman syndrome

j. Weyers syndrome

11. Infectious etiology

a. Congenital rubella (Gregg syndrome)

b. Congenital spherocytic anemia

c. Congenital toxoplasmosis

d. Cytomegalovirus

e. Epstein-Barr syndrome

f. Varicella

12. Intoxicants syndrome

a. Fetal alcohol effects

b. Maternal phenylketonuria fetal effects

Nanophthalmos

52. Mobius II syndrome (congenital paralysis of the sixth and seventh nerves)

53. Morquio syndrome (keratosulfaturia)

†54. Myopathy, centronuclear with external ophthalmoplegia

55. Myotonic dystrophy syndrome (Curschmann-Steinert syndrome)

†56. Myotubular myopathy

57. Neurofibromatosis (Von Recklinghausen syndrome)

58. Nonne-Milroy-Meige disease (congenital trophedema)

59. Noonan syndrome (male Turner syndrome)

60. Oculopharyngeal muscular dystrophy

61. Orodigital-facial syndrome (Papillon-Léage-Psaume syndrome)

62. Pachydermoperiostosis (Touraine-Solente-Gole syndrome)

63. Parry Romberg syndrome (progressive facial hemiatrophy)

64. Shy-Gonatas syndrome (similar to Hunter and Refsum syndrome)

65. Smith-Lemli-Opitz syndrome (cerebrohepatorenal syndrome)

66. Smith syndrome (facioskeletogenital dysplasia)

67. Strabismus and ectopic pupils (ectopic lentis with ectopia of pupil)

68. Syringomyelia (Passow syndrome)

†69. 3p syndrome

70. Treft syndrome

71. Tunbridge-Paley disease

72. Van Bogaert-Hozay syndrome, posterior lumbosacral with ptosis—autosomal dominant

73. Waardenburg syndrome (embryonic fixation syndrome)

A. Neurogenic ptosis: Involvement of the nerve to the levator palpebral superioris

1. Arteriovenous fistula

†2. Congenital cranial nerve III dysfunction—palsy III nerve muscle

3. Horner syndrome (cervical sympathetic paralysis)

4. Marcus Gunn syndrome (jaw-winking syndrome)

5. Marin Amat syndrome (inverted Marcus Gunn syndrome)

6. Misdirected third nerve syndrome

7. Riley-Day syndrome (congenital familial dysautonomia)

8. Von Herrenschwand syndrome (sympathetic heterochromia)

B. Mechanical ptosis may have "s" shaped ptosis, structural change to narrow lid fissure

1. Periorbital tumor

2. Neuroma, neurofibroma

3. Cicatricial skin changes

Acquired ptosis is divided into myogenic, neurogenic, aponeurotic, mechanical, protective and pseudoptosis causes.

†C. Myogenic causes include any disorder with reduced or absent levator palpebral muscle function secondary to dystrophy, degeneration or injury to the levator muscle.

1. Neurogenic causes of ptosis include cranial nerve III dysfunction (with partial or complete ptosis) depending on the site and degree of nerve involvement.

2. Aponeurotic acquired ptosis is the most common cause of acquired ptosis. Stretching of the levator aponeurosis or dehiscence of insertion onto the tarsal place is acquired ptosis.

3. Characterized by normal levator function, a high lid crease, deep symmetrical tarsal sulcus and increased ptosis on down gaze.

4. Mechanical acquired ptosis includes cicatricial changes, lid masses, blepharochalasis, brow ptosis, and microphthalmos or enophthalmos.

5. Protective ptosis is droopy lid from eye pain or photophobia.

6. Pseudoptosis occurs with lid retraction of contralateral eyelid.

7. Acquired

D. Myogenic ptosis: Any disorder with reduced or absent levator palpebrae muscle function secondary to dystrophy, degeneration, or injury to the levator muscle.

1. Amyloid degeneration
2. Botulinum toxin—extraocular muscle palsy
3. Brown syndrome (superior oblique tendon sheath syndrome)
†4. Corticosteroid ptosis—prolonged use of topical corticosteroid therapy
†5. Drugs, including the following:
   - Adenine arabinoside
   - Adrenal cortex injection
   - Alcohol
   - Aldosterone
   - Allobarbital
   - Amobarbital
   - Amodiaquine
   - Aprobarbital
   - Aurothioglucose
   - Aurothioglycanide
   - Barbital
   - Betamethasone
   - Butabarbital
   - Butalbital
   - Butallylonal
   - Butethal
   - Carbon dioxide
   - Cabromal
   - Chloral hydrate
   - Chloroquine
   - Cocaine
   - Cortisone
   - Cyclobarbital
   - Cyclopentyl allylbarbituric acid
   - Cyclopentobarbital
   - Desoxycorticosterone
   - Dexamethasone
   - Dextrothyroxine
   - Digitalis
   - Dimethyl tubocurarine
   - Diphtheria and tetanus toxoids and pertussis (DPT)
   - Disulfiram
   - Flurocortisone
   - Fluorometholone
   - Flu-prednisolone
   - F3T
   - Gold Au-198
   - Gold sodium thiomalate
   - Heptabarbital
   - Hexethal
   - Hexobarbital
   - Hydrocortisone
   - Hydroxy3-methyl-glutaryl-CoA
   - Hydroxychloroquine
   - Idoxuridine
   - Isocarboxazid
   - Isosorbide dinitrate
   - Loxapine
   - Measles virus vaccine (live)
   - Medrysone
   - Mephenesin
   - Mephobarbital
   - Metharbital
   - Methitural
   - Methohexital
   - Methyl alcohol
   - Methylpentynol
   - Methylprednisolone
   - Nalidixic acid
   - Opium
   - Oral contraceptives
   - Paramethasone
   - Pentobarbital
   - Phencyclidine
   - Phenelzine
   - Phenobarbital
   - Phenoxybenzamine
   - Prednisolone
   - Prednisone
   - Primidone
   - Probarbital
   - Secobarbital
   - Succinylcholine
   - Sulthiame
   - Talbutal
   - Tetraethylammonium
   - Thiamylal
   - Thiopental
   - Tolazoline
   - Tranylcypromine
   - Triamcinolone

- Trichloroethylene
- Trifluorthymidine
- Tubocurarine
- Vidarabine
- Vinbarbital
- Vinblastine
- Vincristine

6. Enophthalmos
   †a. Apparent enophthalmos with horizontal conjugate gaze
   b. Associated syndromes
      1. Cestan-Chenais syndrome (lesion in the lateral portion of medulla oblongata)
      2. Craniocervical syndrome (whiplash injury)
      3. Cretinism (hypothyroidism)
      4. Dejean syndrome (orbital floor syndrome)
      5. Dejerine-Klumpke syndrome (thalamic hyperesthetic anesthesia)
      6. Horner syndrome (cervical sympathetic paralysis syndrome)
      7. Krause syndrome (encephaloophthalmic syndrome)
      8. Naffziger syndrome (scalenus anticus syndrome)
      9. Pancoast syndrome (superior pulmonary sulcus syndrome)
      10. Raeder syndrome (paratrigeminal paralysis)
      11. Retroparotid space syndrome
      12. Silent sinus syndrome
      13. Vernet syndrome (jugular foramen syndrome)
      14. Wallenberg syndrome (dorsolateral medullary syndrome)
      a. Iatrogenic
         1. Orbital decompression
         2. Sinus surgery
         †a. Liver or gall bladder disease: (chronic or severe), usually in right eye owing to increased tone of orbicularis muscle and extraocular muscles.
         †b. Metastatic adenocarcinoma of orbit
         †c. Neurofibromatosis: Pulsating enophthalmos
         †d. Orbital varices: Transient exophthalmos with fat atrophy
         †e. Senility (common)
         f. Superior sulcus deformity
            †1. Atrophy of the orbital tissues
            †2. Herniated orbital fat secondary to an orbital fracture

†3. Levator detachment with ptosis
†4. Migration of muscle cone implant
†5. Traumatic bony loss
6. Typhoid fever (abdominal typhus)
†7. Wasting disease: Loss of orbital fat
8. Hyperthyroidism
†9. Late spontaneous unilateral ptosis
†10. Mascara ptosis: Due to subconjunctival deposit of mascara
11. Myasthenia gravis
†12. Myopathic ptosis
†13. Muscular atrophy
14. Pregnancy: Myopia; visual field defects; corneal edema
†15. Senility: Loss of general muscle tone and atrophy of orbital fat
†16. Trauma to levator muscle without affecting its aponeurosis or innovation

E. Neurogenic acquired ptosis: Includes cranial nerve III dysfunction (with partial or complete ptosis depending on the site and degree of nerve involvement.
   1. Guillain-Barre syndrome including Miller-Fisher
   2. Horner syndrome
      a. *Region of first neuron*: Lesions of hypothalamus and diencephalic region also suggest diabetes insipidus, disturbed temperature regulation, adiposogenital syndrome, and autonomic epidemic epilepsy of Penfield.
         1. Arnold-Chiari malformation
         2. Basal meningitis, such as in syphilis
         †3. Base-of-skull tumors (e.g. melanoma)
         †4. Multiple sclerosis
         †5. Pituitary tumor
         †6. Tumor of the third ventricle
         †7. Midbrain, such as in syphilis
         †8. Pons, such as in intrapontine hemorrhage
         9. Medulla, such as in Wallenberg syndrome (lateral medullary syndrome)
         10. Cervical region
            a. Syringomyelia
            †b. Tumor
            †c. Injury as traumatic dislocation of cervical vertebrae or dissection of the vertebral artery
         d. Syphilis (acquired lues)
         e. Poliomyelitis
         f. Meningitis: Photophobia; conjunctivitis; chemosis; keratitis; uveitis

†g. Amyotrophic lateral sclerosis

h. Related to scleroderma and facial hemiatrophy

†i. Vascular malformation such as agenesis of internal carotid artery

j. Region of second neuron

  1. Spinal birth injury: Klumpke paralysis with injured lower brachial plexus

  †2. Cervical rib

  3. Thoracic lesions

  a. *Pancoast tumor*: In apex of lung, such as carcinoma or tuberculosis

  †b. Aneurysm of aorta, subclavian, or carotid artery

  †c. Central venous catheterization

  †d. Mediastinal tumors

  e. Lymphadenopathy of Hodgkin disease, leukemia lymphosarcoma, or tuberculosis

  †f. Stellate ganglion block

  †g. Tube thoracostomy

†5. Neck

a. Enlarged lymph gland, tumors, aneurysm, and thyroid gland

b. Carcinoma of esophagus

c. Retropharyngeal tumors

d. Neuroma of sympathetic chain

e. Intraoral trauma with damage to internal carotid plexus

f. Thin intervertebral foramina of spinal cord, such as in pachymeningitis, hypertrophic spinal arthritis, ruptured intervertebral disk, and meningeal tumors

g. Traction of sternocleidomastoid muscle, such as from positioning on operating table

h. Complications of tonsillectomy

i. Mandibular tooth abscess

j. Lesions of middle ear, such as in acute purulent otitis media and petromastoid operation

k. Carotid artery dissection

l. Internal carotid artery occlusion

C. Region of third neuron

†1. Aneurysm of internal carotid and its branches

2. Paratrigeminal syndrome (Raeder syndrome)

3. Cavernous sinus syndrome (Foix syndrome)

†4. Tumors or cysts of orbit

†5. Drugs can affect any region and include the following:

- Acetophenazine
- Alseroxylon
- Bupivacaine
- Butaperazine
- Carphenazine
- Chloroprocaine
- Chlorpromazine
- Deserpidine
- Diacetylmorphine
- Diethazine
- Ethorpropazine
- Etidocaine
- Fluphenazine
- Guanethidine
- Influenza virus vaccine
- Levodopa
- Ledocaine
- Mepivacaine
- Mesoridazine
- Methdilazine
- Methotrimeprazine
- Oral contraceptives
- Perazine
- Pericyazine
- Perphenazine
- Piperacetazine
- Prilocaine
- Procaine
- Prochlorperazine
- Promazine
- Promethazine
- Propiomazine
- Propoxycaine
- *Rauwolfia serpentina*
- Rescinnamine
- Reserpine
- Syrosingopine
- Thiethylperazine
- Thiopropazate
- Thioproperazine
- Thioridazine
- Trifluoperazine
- Triflupromazine
- Trimeprazine

6. Cluster headaches (migrainous neuralgia)

7. Herpes zoster

8. Migraine—abnormal visual sensations; scotoma generally restricted to one half of the visual field

9. Varicella

  3. Paralysis of third Nerve (oculomotor nerve)

  A. Intracerebral

1. Lesion of red nucleus (Benedikt syndrome)
2. Myasthenia gravis and mesencephalic cavernous angioma
3. Nuclear types: Pareses of a single or a few extraocular muscles supplied by the oculomotor nerve in one or both eyes; there may or may not be papillary disturbances
   †a. Mydriasis; sluggish papillary reaction
   †b. Pinealomas
   c. Parinaud syndrome; Sylvian aqueduct syndrome; pineal syndrome
   d. Axenfeld-Schurenberg syndrome; cyclic oculomotor paralysis
   e. Bruns syndrome; postural change syndrome
   f. Claude syndrome; inferior nucleus rubber syndrome
   g. Congenital vertical retracton syndrome
   h. Nothnagel syndrome; ophthalmoplegia-cerebellar ataxia syndrome
†4. Occlusion of basilar artery
5. Recurrent third nerve palsy secondary to vascular spasm of migraine
6. Syndrome of cerebral peduncle (Weber syndrome)
7. Tumors
a. Intracranial
   1. Amebic dysentery
   2. Aneurysm rupture at base of brain—third nerve paralysis, pain around the face (fifth verve), and headache
   3. Botulism
   4. Chickenpox
   5. Craniopharyngioma—paresis of third or sixth nerve; optic nerve atrophy; optic neuritis; papilledema
   6. Dengue fever
   7. Devic syndrome (optical myelitis)
   8. Diphtheria
   9. Encephalitis, acute
   10. Hepatitis
   11. Influenza
   12. Lockjaw (tetanus)
   13. Lymphoma
   14. Malaria
   15. Measles immunization
   16. Meningococcal meningitis
   17. Multiple sclerosis (disseminated sclerosis)
   18. Ophthalmic migraine
   19. Periarteritis nodosa
   20. Poliomyelitis
   21. Polyneuritis because of toxins such as alcohol, lead, arsenic, and carbon monoxide; dinitrophenol or carbon disulfide poisoning; or diabetes mellitus,

†B. Herpes zoster or mumps
   22. Rabies
   23. Relapsing polychondritis
   24. Smallpox vaccination
   25. Subdural hematoma
   26. Syphilis (acquired lues)
   27. Temporal arteritis syndrome (Hutchinson-Horton-Magath-Brown syndrome)
   28. Tuberculosis

†C. Lesions affecting exit from cranial cavity

D. Cavernous sinus syndrome
   a. Aneurysm (arteriovenous fistula syndrome)
   b. Carotid-cavernous fistula
   †c. Cavernous sinus thrombosis
   †d. Extension from lateral sinus thrombosis
   †e. Extension of nasopharyngeal tumor
   †f. Pituitary adenoma—lateral extension
   g. Tolosa-Hunt syndrome (painful ophthalmoplegia)

E. Superior orbital fissure syndrome
   h. Aneurysm of internal carotid artery syndrome (foramen lacerum syndrome)
   †i. Occlusion of superior ophthalmic vein
   †j. Skull fractures or hemorrhage
   k. Sphenoid sinus suppuration (sphenocavernous syndrome)
   l. Temporal syndrome (Gradenigo syndrome)
   m. Tumors, such as sphenoid ridge meningioma (Rochon-Duvigneaud syndrome), nasopharyngeal tumor, metastatic carcinoma, rhabdomyosarcoma, chordoma, and sarcoma
   n. Albers-Schönberg syndrome (marble bone disease, osteopetrosis)
   †o. Associated with aspirin poisoning
   p. Hodgkin disease
   q. Lupus erythematosus (Kaposi-Libman-Sacks syndrome)
   r. Myasthenia gravis (masquerade)
   s. Passow syndrome (status dysraphicus syndrome)
   t. Porphyria cutanea tarda
   u. Sarcoid (Schaumann syndrome)

F. Aponeurogenic acquired ptosis: Caused by stretching of the levator aponeurotic or dehiscence of its insertion onto the tarsal plate.

†1. Aging
2. Trauma
   - Air-blast injury
   - Botulinum toxin treatment of strabismus and blepharospasm
   - Eyelid laceration
   - Foreign bodies lying in the roof of the orbit
   - Fracture of orbital roof, also following contusion with resulting hematoma but without fracture
   - Infratemporal fossa foreign body
   - Postsurgical ptosis
     1. Anterior transposition
     2. Cataract operation
     3. Enucleation
     4. Orbital operation
     5. Radial keratotomy
     6. Prolonged hard contact lens wear
G. Mechanical acquired ptosis—a structural change that narrows the lid aperture
   1. Blepharochalasis
   †2. Brow ptosis
   †3. Contact lens migration
   4. Conjunctivitis
   a. Acute mucopurulent—epidemic pink eye; marked hyperemia; mucopurulent discharge
   1. Gram-positive group
   a. *Pneumococcus*—hypopyon; conjunctivitis; keratitis; corneal ulcer; endophthalmitis
   b. *Staphylococcus*—eyelid lesions and punctuate staining of the lower cornea may occur
   2. Gram-negative group

Haemophilus aegyptius (Koch-Weeks bacillus)—conjunctivitis; corneal opacity; corneal ulcer

H. Influenzae—Subconjunctival hemorrhage; keratitis; tendonitis

   3. Associated with exanthems and viral infections
      a. German measles (Gregg syndrome)
      b. Measles (rubeola)
      c. Mumps
      d. Reiter syndrome (conjunctivourethrosynovial syndrome)
      †e. Scarlet fever—blepharitis; scarlatinal rash of lid; gangrene of lid
   4. Fungus
      a. *Candida albicans*
      †b. *Leptothrix*
   5. Lyell disease
   6. Relapsing polychondritis
   7. Sjögren syndrome (secretoinhibitor syndrome)
   †8. Etiology: Obscure in many cases

Chronic mucopurulent conjunctivitis
1. Infective element: Lids or lacrimal apparatus
   †a. Monilia species
   b. Morax-Axenfeld diplobacillus (angular conjunctivitis)—hypopyon; keratitis; corneal marginal ulcer
   c. Pubic lice
   d. *Staphylococcus*—uveitis; hypopyon; cellulitis of lids
   e. *Streptothrix foersteri*
2. Allergic: Cosmetic
3. Irritative
   a. Associated infections or irritation of lids, lacrimal apparatus, nose, or skin
   b. Deficiency of lacrimal secretions
   c. Direct irritants: Foreign body, mascara, dust, wind, smog, insecticides, chlorinated water, and many others
   d. Exposure: Ectropion, facial paralysis, exophthalmos, and others
   e. Eyestrain
   f. Metabolic conditions: Gout, alcoholism, or prolonged digestive disturbances
   g. Overtreatment by drugs: Antibiotics, miotics, mydriatics

Membranous Conjunctivitis
2. Chemical irritants
   a. Acids, such as acetic or lactic
   b. Alkalis, such as ammonia or lime
   c. Metallic salts, such as silver nitrate or copper sulfate
†3. *Corynebacterium diphtheriae*
†4. Ligneous conjunctivitis—chronic, cause unknown
†5. *Pneumococcus*
†6. *Streptococcus*—conjunctivitis; corneal ulcer; blepharitis
7. Uncommon
   a. Actinomyces
   b. Epidemic keratoconjunctivitis (type adenovirus)
   c. Glander syndrome
   e. *Neisseria catarrhalis*
   f. *Pseudomonas aeruginosa*
   g. Herpes simplex
   h. Variola

Acute Follicular Conjunctivitis
8. Adenovirus conjunctivitis; pharyngoconjunctival fever—EKC has been reported worldwide from virus serotypes (the most common are 8, 11, and 19); pharyngoconjunctival fever (PCF) is usually caused by serotypes 3, 4, and 7.
   a. Epidemic keratoconjunctivitis—because of adenovirus type (rarely occurs in children)—chemosis; subconjunctival hemorrhages.

9. Inclusion conjunctivitis; chlamydia—adult inclusion conjunctivitis (AIC) (begins 2 days after exposure to organisms may be bilateral, no systemic symptoms, and a unilateral or bilateral preauricular node is often present.

10. Primary herpetic keratoconjunctivitis—conjunctival reaction may be follicular or pseudomembranous.

11. Newcastle disease (fowl-pox) conjunctivitis—usually seen in poultry handlers, veterinarians (caused by a paramyxovirus: single-stranded RNA virus that causes respiratory infections); lid edema; decrease accommodation and visual acuity.

12. Influenza virus A—Tenonitis; cellulites of orbit and lid; dacryocystitis

13. Herpes zoster

14. Cat-scratch fever (Parinaud oculoglandular syndrome)

†15. Echovirus keratoconjunctivitis

16. Trachoma (sometimes)

17. Bacterial
    a. *Moraxella*
    b. *Streptococcus*
    c. *Treponema* organisms

†18. Mesantoin use

19. Chlamydia epizootic (feline pneumonitis)

†20. Ophthalmomyiasis

†21. Acute hemorrhagic conjunctivitis—chemosis; seromucous discharge; keratitis

22. Neonatal inclusion conjunctivitis

†23. Unknown types—a case that resists etiologic classification is encountered occasionally; it is probable that other viruses occasionally produce acute follicular conjunctivitis

24. Associated with regional adenitis
    a. Angelucci syndrome (critical allergic conjunctivitis syndrome)
    b. Anoxic overwear syndrome
    c. Benjamin-Allen syndrome (brachial arch syndrome)
    d. Floppy eyelid syndrome
    e. Giant papillary conjunctivitis syndrome
    †f. Inclusion conjunctivitis in adults—acute mucopurulent follicular inflammation, persisting as long as several months, sometimes with scarring
    g. Syndrome of Beal
    †h. Chronic follicular conjunctivitis—(lymphoid follicles cobblestoning) of conjunctiva with long-term course

25. Chronic follicular conjunctivitis: Axenfeld's type (orphan's)—frequently found in institutionalized children; almost asymptomatic; long duration (to months or longer); no keratitis; cause unknown

†26. Chronic follicular conjunctivitis, toxic type
    a. Bacterial origin, such as that due to a diplobacillus or other microorganism
    b. Drugs, including the following:
       • Acyclovir
       • Adenine arabinoside
       • Amphotericin B
       • Apraclonidine
       • Atropine
       • Carbachol
       • Clonidine
       • Demecarium
       • Diatrizoate meglumine and sodium
       • Diisopropyl fluorophosphates
       • Dipivefrin
       • DPE
       • Echothiophate
       • Eserine
       • F3T
       • Framycetin
       • Gentamicin
       • Homatropine
       • Hyaluronidase
       • Idoxuridine
       • Isoflurophate
       • Ketorolac tromethamine
       • Methscopolamine
       • Neomycin
       • Neostigmine
       • Physostigmine
       • Pilocarpine
       • Scopolamine
       • Sulfacetamide
       • Sulfamethizole
       • Sulfisoxazole
       • Trifluorothymidine
       • Trifluridine
       • Vidarabine

†27. Chronic follicular conjunctivitis with epithelial keratitis—differentiated from Axenfeld type by shorter duration (to months) and by epithelial keratitis involving upper third of cornea; epidemic in schools; can be transmitted by mascara pencil; cause unknown

28. Ectodermal syndrome (Rothmund syndrome)

†29. Folliculosis—associated general lymphoid hypertrophy

30. Molluscum contagiosum
31. Neurocutaneous syndrome (ectodermal dysgenesis)
32. Parinaud syndrome
†33. Postoperative PK or cataract surgery sutures
†34. Sebaceous carcinoma with papillary conjunctivitis—blepharitis; madarosis; meibomianitis
35. Trachoma
36. Use of hard and soft contact lens
†37. Use of ocular prostheses
38. With generalized lymphadenopathy
    Cicatricial conjunctivitis (scarring of conjunctiva)
39. General—a postinfectious type of membranous conjunctivitis such as *C. diphtheriae*, streptococcal conjunctivitis, autoimmune or presumably autoimmune sarcoidosis, scleroderma, pemphigoid, lichen planus, atopic blepharoconjunctivitis, miscellaneous causes and linear IgA dermatosis.
40. Upper lid
    a. Trachoma
41. Lower lid
    a. Acne rosacea
    b. Chemical (especially alkali)
    c. *Chlamydia* organisms (psittacosis-lymphogranuloma group)
    d. Chronic cicatricial conjunctivitis—occurs in the elderly; has a chronic course; may have concurrent skin and mucous membrane lesions—entropion, trichiasis, corneal opacity
    e. Congenital syphilis
    f. Dermatitis herpetiformis
    g. Epidemic keratoconjunctivitis—chemosis, blepharospasm, corneal ulcer
    h. Epidermolysis acuta toxica (Lyell syndrome)
    i. Epidermolysis bullosa
    j. Erythema multiforme (Stevens-Johnson disease)—hypopyon, iritis, corneal ulcers
    k. Erythroderma ichthyosiforme
    l. Exfoliative dermatitis
    m. Fuchs-Lyell syndrome
    n. Hydroa vacciniforme
    o. Impetigo
    p. Lamellar ichthyosis
    q. Ocular pemphigoid
    r. Paraneoplastic lichen planus—conjunctivitis, keratin plaque on bulbar conjunctiva
    †s. Radium burn
    t. Reiter syndrome (conjunctivourethrosynovial syndrome)—epiphoria, iritis
    u. Sjögren syndrome
    v. Staphylococcal granuloma—uveitis, hypopyon
    w. Syphilis
    x. Systemic scleroderma
    y. Vaccinia
42. Drugs, including the following:
    • Demecarium bromide
    • Echothiophate iodide
    • Idoxuridine
    • Penicillamine
    • Pilocarpine
    • Practolol
    • Thiabendazole
    • Timolol
    • Topical ocular epinephrine
    †a. Purulent—swelling of lids; copious secretion of pus; marked tendency to corneal involvement and even possible loss of the eye.
    †b. Gram-positive group
    c. *Listeria monocytogenes:* Conjunctivitis, keratitis, corneal abscess and ulcer, blepharitis, uveitis
    d. *Pneumococcus:* Hypopyon, conjunctivitis, keratitis, corneal ulcer, orbital cellulitis
    e. *Staphylococcus:* Hypopyon; keratitis; cellulites of lid
    f. *Streptococcus*: Conjunctivitis; corneal ulcer; blepharitis; gangrene of lid
6. Gram-negative group
    †a. Aerobacter aerogenes
    †b. Enterobacteriaceae
    c. *Escherichia coli:* Uveitis; hyphema; cornea edema
    d. *Haemophilus influenzae biotype III*—corneal opacity; corneal ulcer; cellulites of lid
    e. *Klebsiella pneumoniae*—conjunctivitis, chronic dacryocystitis, lid inflammation
    f. *Moraxella lacunata*—catarrhal angular conjunctivitis; corneal ulcer
    g. *Neisseria gonorrhoeae*
    h. *Neisseria meningitis*—photophobia; chemosis; uveitis; macular edema
    i. *Proteus* species
    j. *Pseudomonas* species
    †k. *Serratia marcescens*
7. *Vaccinia virus*—pustules of lids; edema of lids; orbital cellulitis
8. Fungus
    a. *Actinomyces*
    b. *Candida*
    c. *Nocardia*
9. *Wiskott-Aldrich syndrome*—X-linked, corneal ulcer, papilledema, peripapillary hemorrhages
10. Floppy eyelid syndrome

†11. *Orbital malignancy*—infiltrating the upper orbital tissue

†12. Orbital neurofibromatosis

13. Tumor
   a. Molluscum contagiosum—small, greasy-appearing elevation that is usually umbilicated or any other granuloma
   †b. Neoplasm
      1. *Basal cell epithelioma*—common; may be a red, circumscribed, growth involving the lid margin or may have an umbilicated center (rodent ulcer)
      2. *Squamous cell or Zeis cell epithelioma*—hard pearly appearing lesion, usually without increased vascularity
      †3. *Meibomian gland carcinoma*—resembles a chalazion, foamy secretion, ocular irritation, photophobia
      †4. *Metastatic tumors of the lid*—respiratory tract, breast, skin (melanoma), gastrointestinal tract, or kidney
      †5. *Keratoacanthoma*—benign, hemispherical, eleva-ted tumor with a central keratin-filled crater; develops within several months
      6. *Hemangioma*—rubor of vascular tumor, usually having a smooth surface with tufts of vessels near the surface; hemangiomas of lids or orbits; ptosis
      †7. Benign mixed tumor of the lacrimal (palpebral) gland
      †8. *Trichilemmoma*—conjunctivitis, retinal hemorrhage, dyschromatopsia
      9. *Lymphangioma*: Conjunctival hemorrhage; cellulites of lids
      10. Juvenile xanthogranuloma
      11. Malignant melanoma
      12. Rhabdomyosarcoma
         Metaplasia or hyperplasia
         †1. Trichoepithelioma
         2. *Syringomyelia*: Enophthalmos; rotatory nystagmus; heterochromia iridis
         †3. Sebaceous adenoma
         4. *Papilloma*—smooth, rounded, or pedunculated elevation—papillary conjunctivitis; psuedopterygium
         5. *Nevus*—usually pigmented, raised and smooth surfaced; however, may be papillomatous or contain hair

      †6. Benign calcifying epithelioma
      †7. Inverted follicular keratosis
      †8. *Blue nevus*—Blue-black and velvet-like in appearance; subconjunctival hemangioma with overlying fibrosis
      †9. Freckles
      10. Lentigo simplex
      †11. Solar lentigo
      †12. Melasma
      13. Sinus extension such as mucocele of frontal sinus
      Cyst
         1. Sebaceous
         †2. Soporiferous
         †3. Traumatic
         †4. Congenital inclusion
         5. Lipoid proteinosis
         †6. Pseudotumor of lid-encysted contact lens—proptosis; lesions of orbit; lacrimal gland
         7. Amyloidosis (Lubarsch-Pick syndrome)
         8. *Protective ptosis*—occurs when the patient has pain or photophobia. Protective ptosis in caused by a corneal abrasion, foreign body or other disease of the corneal surface.
         †9. *Pseudoptosis*—may be associated with lid retraction of the contralateral eyelid. Because both eyelids receive equal amounts of neural stimulation, retraction of one lid causes a reduced need for activity of that levator muscle. This reduced stimulation is also supplied to the contralateral eye resulting in pseudoptosis. The lack of support of the upper lid by a small eye or prosthetic eye may also allow the upper lid to assume a lower than normal position even though the levator and Müller muscles are functioning normally.

⊟ BIBLIOGRAPHY

1. Fraunfelder FW, Richards AB. Diplopia, Blepharoptosis and Ophthalmoplegia and 3-Hydroxy-3 Methyl-Glutaryl-CoA Reductase Inhibitor Use. Ophthalmology. 2008;115:2282-5.
2. Roy FH. Comprehensive ptosis classification. Ann Ophthalmol. 2005;37:5-22.

---

†Indicates a general entry and therefore has not been described in detail in the text

🗗 1EE.A1. AARSKOG-SCOTT SYNDROME (FACIOGENITAL DYSPLASIA)

General

Sex-linked; characterized by ocular hypertelorism, anteve–rted nostrils, broad upper lip, and saddlebag scrotum.

Ocular

Ptosis, hypertelorism.

Clinical

Hyperextensibility of fingers; genu recurvatum; flat feet; hypermobility in cervical spine with neurologic deficit; cleft lip and palate; anteverted nostrils; broad upper lip; abnormal penoscrotal relations; "saddlebag scrotum".

Treatment

Primary goal is to prevent the development of a severe deformity rather.

Laboratory

Full and detailed physical examination; a radiologic evaluation is essential. Standard posteroanterior and lateral views are used for the initial evaluation.

🗗 BIBLIOGRAPHY

1. Bawle E, Tyrkus M, Lipman S, et al. Aarskog-Scott syndrome: full male and female expression with an X autosome translocation. Am J Med Genet. 1984;17:595-602.
2. Mckusick VA. Mendelian Inheritance in Man, 12th edition. Baltimore: The Johns Hopkins University Press; 1998.
3. Scott EI. Unusual facies, joint hypermobility, genital anomaly and shory stature: a new dysmorphic syndrome. Birth defects. 1971;6:240-6.

🗗 1EE.A2. ACRORENOOCULAR SYNDROME

General

Autosomal dominant; Duane syndrome with radial defects.

Ocular

Complete coloboma; coloboma of optic nerve; ptosis and Duane anomaly.

Clinical

Renal anomalies; hypoplasia of distal part of thumb with lack of motion at phalangeal joint; renal ectopia without fusion; bladder diverticula; malrotation of both kidneys; absence of kidney; clubhand or absence of thumb.

Laboratory

Diagnosis is made by clinical findings.

Treatment

If visual acuity is affected most cases require surgical correction and there are several procedures that may be used including levator resection, repair or advancement and Fasanella-Servat.

🗗 BIBLIOGRAPHY

1. Halal F, Homsy M, Perreault G. Acro-renal-ocular syndrome: autosomal dominant thumb hypoplasia; renal ectopia and eye defect. Am J Med Genet. 1984;17:753-62.
2. McKusick VA. Mendelian Inheritance in Man: A Catalog of Human Genes and Genetic Disorders, 12th edition. Baltimore: The Johns Hopkins University Press;1998.
3. Online Mendelian Inheritance in Man, OMIM. McKusick-Nathans Institute for Genetic Medicine, Johns Hopkins University and National Center for Biotechnology Information, National Library of Medicine, February 12, 2007. Available from www.ncbi.nlm.nih.gov/omim. [Accessed September, 2013].

⊟ IEE.A3. ALACRIMA

General

Autosomal recessive; wide spectrum of lacrimal secretory disorders that are mostly congenital in origin. Symptoms of these disorders can range from a complete absence of tears to hyposecretion of tears; symptoms of rarer disorders include a selective absence of tearing in response to emotional stimulation but a normal secretory response to mechanical stimulation. It may be associated with syndromes such as Riley-Day, anhidrotic ectodermal dysplasia, Sjögren and Allgrove.

Clinical

Decreased salivation and sweating; osteoporosis; short stature; adrenocortical insufficiency.

Ocular

Foreign body sensation; photophobia, decreased visual acuity; absence of tears; chronic blepharoconjunctivitis; hyperemia; thick mucoid discharge; keratinization; pannus; corneal ulcers or perforation; tonic pupils; optic atrophy.

Laboratory

CT scan of orbits to determine aplastic lacrimal glands; Schirmer testing; conjunctival and lacrimal gland biopsy.

Treatment

Artificial tears, gels and ointments are used as the primary treatment. Permanent or temporary punctal occlusion can be effective. Tarsorrhaphy may be necessary if the corneal health has been compromised.

⊟ BIBLIOGRAPHY

1. DeAngelis DD, Hurwitz J. (2012). Alacrima. [online] Available from emedicine.medscape.com/article/1210539-overview. [Accessed September, 2013].

⊟ 1EE.A4. ALBERS-SCHONBERG DISEASE (MARBLE BONE DISEASE; OSTEOSCLEROSIS FRAGILIS GENERALISATA; OSTEOPETROSIS; OSTEOPOIKILOSIS; OSTEOSCLEROSIS CONGENITA DIFFUSA)

General

Simple recessive inheritance, also dominant transmission; benign form is asymptomatic in about 50% of cases and known under the synonym Henck-Assmann syndrome; prognosis is poor for malignant form, with death usually in infancy.

Ocular

Oculomotor paralysis; cranial nerve VII palsy; optic atrophy; ptosis; exophthalmos; papilledema; nystagmus; anisocoria; congenital cataracts; hypertelorism; visual loss in infancy; nasolacrimal duct obstruction; keratoconus.

Clinical

Cartilage and bone thickening; multiple fractures; hyperchromic anemia; osteomyelitis; severe forms: jaundice, hepatosplenomegaly, skeleton sclerosis, lymphadenopathy, and hydrocephalus in infants; mild forms: nerve compression, fractures, and milder form of anemia; pancytopenia from marrow obliteration; low serum calcium; elevated phosphorus.

Laboratory

Radiologic features are usually diagnostic. Patients usually have generalized osteosclerosis. Bones may be uniformly sclerotic, but alternating sclerotic and lucent bands may be noted in iliac wings and near ends of long bones. The bones might be club-like or appear like a bone within bone.

Treatment

- *Infantile therapy*: Vitamin D appears to help by stimulating dormant osteoclasts and thus stimulate bone resorption. Large doses of calcitriol, along with restricted calcium intake, sometimes improve osteopetrosis dramatically.
- *Adult therapy*: No specific medical treatment exists for the adult type.

⊟ BIBLIOGRAPHY

1. Blank R, Bhargava A. (2012). Osteopetrosis. [online] Available from www.emedicine.com/med/TOPIC1692.HTM. [Accessed September, 2013].

IEE.A5. LUBARSCH-PICK SYNDROME (PRIMARY AMYLOIDOSIS; IDIOPATHIC AMYLOIDOSIS; AMYLOIDOSIS)

General

Rare condition of unknown etiology; inherited as a dominant trait, with male preponderance; characterized by amyloid accumulation in muscles and in gastrointestinal and genitourinary tracts.

Ocular

Internal and external ophthalmoplegia; diminished lacrimation; amyloid deposits in conjunctival, episcleral, and ciliary vessels; vitreous opacities; amyloid deposits in the corneal stroma; retinal hemorrhages and perivascular exudates; paralysis of extraocular muscles; pseudopodia lentis; strabismus fixus convergens; keratoconus.

Clinical

Peripheral neuropathy (extremities); heart failure; defective hepatic and renal functions with hepatosplenomegaly; waxy skin lesions; muscular weakness (progressive); multiple myeloma; hoarseness; chronic gastrointestinal symptoms.

Laboratory

Biopsy-stain with Congo red demonstrates apple-green birefringence under polarized light; distinctive fibrillar ultrastructure.

Treatment

Deoxydoxorubicin had demonstrated some clinical benefit.

BIBLIOGRAPHY

1. Biswas J, Badrinath SS, Rao NA. Primary nonfamilial amyloidosis of the vitreous. A light microscopic and ultrastructural study. Retina. 1992;12(3):251-3.
2. Goebel HH, Friedman AH. Extraocular muscle involvement in idiopathic primary amyloidosis. Am J Ophthalmol. 1971;71(5):1121-7.

1EE.A6. APERT SYNDROME (ACROCEPHALOSYNDACTYLISM SYNDROME; ACROCRANIO-DYSPHALANGIA; ACRODYSPLASIA; SPHENOACROCRANIO-SYNDACTYLY; ABSENT-DIGITS-CRANIAL-DEFECTS SYNDROME)

General

Inherited; most often recessive, sometimes dominant; an extreme form of Apert syndrome has been described as Carpenter syndrome, with the latter being familial and transmitted as an autosomal recessive.

Ocular

Shallow orbit; exophthalmos; hypertelorism; ptosis; strabismus; nystagmus; ophthalmoplegia; hyperopia; exposure keratitis; cataracts; ectopia lentis; medullated nerve fibers; retinal detachment; papilledema with subsequent optic atrophy; keratoconus.

Clinical

Oxycephaly (tower skull); syndactyly (symmetrically); synostoses and synarthroses of shoulder and elbows frequent; agenesis of spinal bones and limbs; headaches; hypertelorism; hypoplastic maxilla; acrocephaly; abnormality of sutures.

Laboratory

CT is the most useful radiological examination in identifying skull shape and presence or absence of involved sutures. MRI reveals the anatomy of the soft-tissue structures and associated brain abnormalities.

Treatment

Medical treatment involves fitting patient with hearing aids, providing airway management and psychological counseling. Surgical care involves early release of the coronal suture and fronto-orbital advancement and reshaping to reduce dysmorphic and unwanted skull growth changes.

BIBLIOGRAPHY

1. Chen H. (2013). Apert syndrome. [online] Available from www.emedicine.com/ped/TOPIC122.HTM. [Accessed September, 2013].

🖶 1EE.A8. RETINITIS PIGMENTOSA

General

Inherited progressive retinal disorder may have changes in ear or kidney.

Clinical

Hearing and kidney defects can be associated with the disease.

Ocular

Waxy-pole optic nerve, bonespickle pigmentation, posterior subcapsular cataract, visual field defect.

Laboratory

Diagnosis is made by clinical findings. A diagnostic genetic test is available and differentiates between simplex retinitis pigmentosa (RP) and autosomal recessive RP.

Treatment

Vitamin A 15,000 IU/day is thought to slow the decline of retinal function, dark sunglasses for outdoor use, surgery for cataract, genetic counseling.

🖶 BIBLIOGRAPHY

1. Clark GR, Crowe P, Muszynska D, et al. Development of a diagnostic genetic test for simplex and autosomal recessive retinitis pigmentosa. Ophthalmology. 2010;117:2169-77.e3.
2. Telander DG, de Beus A, Small KW. (2013). Retinitis pigmentosa. [online] Available from www.emedicine.com/oph/TOPIC704.HTM. [Accessed September, 2013].

🖶 1EE.A9. AXENFELD-SCHURENBERG SYNDROME (CYCLIC OCULOMOTOR PARALYSIS)

General

Congenital manifestation; frequently unilateral.

Ocular

Cyclic oculomotor paralysis (paralysis alternating with spasm); during periods of paralysis, lid exhibits ptosis and affected eye is abducted; during spasm, lid is raised, deviation of affected eye is either inward or outward, and pupil is fixed and contracted.

Laboratory

Diagnosis is made by clinical findings.

Treatment

Prism therapy; surgical: Muscle surgery on the affected muscle, and occlusion at the involved eye to relief diplopia.

🖶 BIBLIOGRAPHY

1. Axenfeld T, Schurenberg L. Beitrage zur Kenntnis der Angeborenen Beweglichkeitsdefekte des Auges. Klin Monastbl Augenheilkd. 1901;39:64.
2. Hamed LM. Oculomotor palsy with cyclic spasm. In: Margo CE, Mames R, Hamed LM (Eds). Diagnostic Problems in Clinical Ophthalmology, illustrated edition. Philadelphia, PA: WB Saunders; 1994. p. 712.
3. Levy MR. Cyclic oculomotor paralysis with optic atrophy. Am J Ophthalmol. 1968;65(5):766-9.

⊟ 1EE.A10. BARAITSER-WINTER SYNDROME

General

X-linked mental retardation, macrosomia, macrocephaly, and obesity syndrome.

Ocular

Ptosis; hypertelorism; down-slanting palpebral fissures.

Clinical

May be confused with Noonan syndrome; phenotypic features appear to be variable.

Laboratory

Clinical.

Treatment

If visual acuity is affected, most cases require surgical correction and there are several procedures that may be used including levator resection, repair or advancement and Fasanella-Servat.

⊟ BIBLIOGRAPHY

1. Megarbana A, Le Merrer M, Kallab K. Ptosis, down-slanting palpebral fissures, hypertelorism, seizures, and mental retardation: a possible new MCA/MR syndrome. Clin Dysmorphol. 1997;6;239-44.
2. Verloes A. Iris coloboma, ptosis, hypertelorism, and mental retardation: Baraitser-Winter syndrome or Noonan syndrome? J Med Genet. 1993;30:425-6.

⊟ 1EE.A11. BASSEN-KORNZWEIG SYNDROME (ABETALIPOPROTEINEMIA; ACANTHOCYTOSIS; FAMILIAL HYPOLIPOPROTEINEMIA)

General

Inability to absorb and transport lipids; predominant in males; autosomal recessive inheritance; acanthocytosis, a peculiar burr cell malformation of the red blood cells; the basic defect is thought to be an inability to synthesize the apolipoprotein β peptide of low-density and very-low-density lipoproteins.

Ocular

Ptosis (may be present); nystagmus; progressive external ophthalmoplegia; retinitis pigmentosa (usually atypical); retinopathy develops with age after 10–14 years; optic atrophy occasionally; epicanthal folds; cataract; optic nerve pallor; hypopigmentation of retina; macular degeneration; dyschromatopsia.

Clinical

Steatorrhea; hypocholesterolemia; neurologic disorder with ataxia (similar to Friedreich ataxia); areflexia; Babinski sign; muscle weakness (facial, lingual; proximal and distal); slurred speech; lordosis; kyphosis.

Laboratory

Most patients will exhibit acanthocytosis on peripheral blood smear.

Treatment

Medical care is symptomatic and supportive.

⊟ BIBLIOGRAPHY

1. Gross KV, Lorenzo N. (2012). Neuroacanthocytosis syndromes. [online] Available from www.emedicine.com/neuro/TOPIC502.HTM. [Accessed September, 2013].

1EE.A12. BLEPHAROPHIMOSIS SYNDROME (SIMOSA SYNDROME)

General

Dominantly inherited tetrad of ptosis, epicanthus inversus, telecanthus, and blepharophimosis.

Ocular

Scarred or contracted in secondary blepharophimosis because of ocular pemphigus or trachoma; ectropion; epicanthus inversus; lacrimal puncta displacement; ptosis; telecanthus; optic nerve coloboma; angle dysgenesis; optic nerve hypoplasia; amblyopia; strabismus.

Clinical

Low-set ears; low nasal bridge.

Laboratory

Diagnosis is made by clinical findings.

Treatment

The ptosis is corrected by frontalis fixation at an early age. Canthoplasties may be performed to improve the blepharophimosis. The considerable epicanthus is usually best left until early adolescence, since the degree of this problem tends to diminish with time, and the skin becomes more easy to move.

BIBLIOGRAPHY

1. Bashour M. (2012). Ptosis Blepharoplasty. [online] Available from www.emedicine.com/ent/TOPIC97.HTM. [Accessed September, 2013].

1EE.A13. BONNET-DECHAUME-BLANC SYNDROME (CEREBRORETINAL ARTERIOVENOUS ANEURYSM SYNDROME; NEURORETINOANGIOMATOSIS SYNDROME; WYBURN-MASON SYNDROME)

General

Dominant inheritance; unilateral or bilateral arteriovenous aneurysm of the midbrain with ipsilateral retinal angioma and skin nevi; severity and extent of symptoms depend on location of cerebral aneurysm and structures it may involve; not regarded as hereditary; incidence is equal in men and women; usually becomes symptomatic at the age of 30 years.

Ocular

Exophthalmos; ptosis; strabismus; nystagmus; hemianopsia due to lesion in optic tract or pulvinar; sluggish pupils; anisocoria; retinal arteriovenous aneurysm; varicosity of retinal veins; arteriovenous angiomas; papilledema; optic atrophy of fellow eye; vitreous hemorrhage; rubeosis iridis; optic neuropathy secondary to compression by vascular malformation; proptosis; partial ophthalmoplegia.

Clinical

Arteriovenous angiomas of the thalamus and mesencephalon; facial vascular and pigmented nevi, usually in the trigeminal distribution; psychic disturbances; slow and scanning speech; hydrocephalus; headache; dizziness; hemiplegia; congenital defects of bone, muscle, kidneys and gastrointestinal tract.

Laboratory

MRI, magnetic resonance angiography (MRA), fluorescein angiography.

Treatment

Referral for neurologic evaluation is indicated since intracranial vascular malformations are associated more commonly with larger retinal vascular lesions. Stability of the retinal lesions limits the need for ocular treatment.

BIBLIOGRAPHY

1. Bidwell AE. (2012). Wyburn-Mason syndrome. [online] Available from www.emedicine.com/oph/TOPIC357.HTM. [Accessed September, 2013].

🗗 1EE.A14. TURNER SYNDROME (TURNER-ALBRIGHT SYNDROME; GONADAL DYSGENESIS; GENITAL DWARFISM SYNDROME; ULLRICH-TURNER SYNDROME; BONNEVIE-ULLRICH SYNDROME; PTERYGOLYMPHANGIECTASIA SYNDROME; ULLRICH-BONNEVIE SYNDROME) CATARACT, POSTERIOR

General

Ovarian or gonadal agenesis; 45 chromosomes with an XO sex-chromosome constitution; females; rare in males; onset in childhood.

Ocular

Exophthalmos; hypertelorism; ptosis; epicanthal folds; blue sclera; corneal nebulae; cataracts; conjunctival lymphedema; keratoconus.

Clinical

Webbed neck (pterygium colli); diminished growth; mandibulofacial disproportion; cubitus valgus; masculine chest and trunk; late appearance of pubic and axillary hair; congenital deafness; mental retardation; coarctation of aorta.

Laboratory

Karyotyping is needed for diagnosis. Y-chromosomal test; LH and FSH levels, thyroid function test, fasting glucose levels, echocardiography and MRI.

Treatment

Growth hormone therapy is used to prevent short stature. Estrogen replacement therapy is usually started by the age of 12–15 years.

🗗 BIBLIOGRAPHY

1. Postellon DC, Daniel MS. (2012). Turner syndrome. [online] Available from emedicine.medscape.com/article/949681-overview. [Accessed September, 2013].

🗗 1EE.A15. BROWN SYNDROME (SUPERIOR OBLIQUE TENDON SHEATH SYNDROME)

General

Etiology unknown; affects both sexes; present from birth; may be congenital or acquired (secondary to trauma, orbital surgery, or injections, or following delivery).

Ocular

Bilateral ptosis with associated backward head tilt; widening of palpebral fissure with attempted upward gaze; ocular movements show failure in the direction of superior oblique action; may be associated with underaction of the inferior oblique; adduction or abduction restricted or completely abolished; choroidal coloboma.

Laboratory

Diagnosis is made by clinical findings.

Treatment

Once systemic disease is excluded, patients' inflammation can be treated with anti-inflammatory medication. Oral ibuprofen is a good first-line choice. Local steroid injections in the area of the trochlea and oral corticosteroids can be used for inflammation. Once the inflammatory disease process is controlled, patients with inflammatory Brown syndrome may show spontaneous resolution. Congenital Brown syndrome is unlikely to improve spontaneously; therefore, surgery is important to consider as an option.

🗗 BIBLIOGRAPHY

1. Wright KW, Salvador MG. (2012). Brown syndrome. [online] Available from www.emedicine.com/oph/TOPIC552.HTM. [Accessed September, 2013].
2. Suh DW, Oystreck DT, Hunter DG. Long-term results of an intraoperative adjustable superior oblique tendon suture spacer using nonabsorbable suture for Brown Syndrome. Ophthalmology. 2008;115(10):1800-4.

⊟ 1EE.A16. CARPENTER SYNDROME (ACROCEPHALOPOLYSYNDACTYLY TYPE II)

General

Hereditary; transmitted as an autosomal recessive trait; severe form of Apert syndrome; normal intelligence has been reported with this syndrome; polysyndactyly is not an absolute requirement for this diagnosis.

Ocular

Lateral displacement of inner canthus; epicanthal folds; microcornea; corneal opacities.

Clinical

Acrocephalopolysyndactyly; brachydactyly; peculiar facies; obesity; mental retardation; hypogonadism; generalized aminoaciduria; cryptorchidism; hypogenitalism.

Laboratory

Skull radiography, cranial CT.

Treatment

Careful monitoring for signs and symptoms of elevated intracranial pressure is important. Surgery typically is indicated for increased intracranial pressure or for cosmetic reasons.

⊟ BIBLIOGRAPHY

1. Sheth RD, Ranalli N, Aldana P, et al. (2012). Pediatric craniosynostosis. [online] Available from www.emedicine.com/neuro/TOPIC80.HTM. [Accessed September, 2013].

⊟ 1EE.A17. CEREBRAL PALSY

General

Group of diverse nonprogressive syndromes resulting from injury to the motor centers of the brain; lesions may occur prenatally, in infancy or in childhood up to age of 5 years or more; constitutes the most common cause of permanent physical handicap in children.

Ocular

Strabismus; ptosis; congenital cataract; optic nerve atrophy; papilledema; iris coloboma; nystagmus; uveitis; paresis of extraocular muscles; blepharospasm; leukoma.

Clinical

Systemic abnormalities such as mental retardation, seizures, microcephalus, hydrocephalus, speech delays, and behavioral or emotional disturbances; motor defect; central visual impairment due to cerebral cortex and white matter malformation.

Laboratory

No diagnosis is made by clinical findings.

Treatment

Multiple medical complications require orthopedics, neurologists and rehabilitation medicine specialists.

⊟ BIBLIOGRAPHY

1. Abdel-Hamid HZ, Zeldin AS, Bazzano AT, et al. (2011). Cerebral palsy. [online] Available from www.emedicine.com/neuro/TOPIC533.HTM. [Accessed September, 2013].

🗗 1EE.A18. CHROMOSOME 11 LONG-ARM DELETION SYNDROME

General

Patients with deletion of the long arm of chromosome 11 exhibit a distinctive countenance; female preponderance.

Ocular

Colobomas of the choroid, retina, and iris; retinal reduplication; retinal dysplasia; epicanthus; blepharoptosis; abnormal slanting of the interpalpebral fissures; bilateral uveal colobomas; hypertelorism; avascular retina (bilateral); abnormal pattern of retinal vessels.

Clinical

Keeled forehead; small carp-shaped mouth; low-set ears; highly arched palate; long upper lip with absent philtrum; short neck; widely spaced nipples; flexion contractures of the knees and elbows; hypoplastic nails; broad thumbs with low insertion; deeply pigmented skin on buttocks, lower back, and abdomen and in inguinal regions, axillas, and clavicular areas; congenital heart disease.

Laboratory

Clinical.

Treatment

Ocular: None.

🗗 BIBLIOGRAPHY

1. Ferry AP, Marchevsky A, Strauss L. Ocular abnormalities in deletion of the long arm of chromosome 11. Ann Ophthalmol. 1981;13:1373-7.
2. Uto H, Shigeto M, Tanaka H, et al. A case of 11q- syndrome associated with abnormalities of the retinal vessels. Ophthalmologica. 1994;208:233-6.

🗗 1EE.A19. CHROMOSOME 18 PARTIAL DELETION (LONG-ARM) SYNDROME [MONOSOMY 18 PARTIAL (LONG-ARM) SYNDROME; DE GROUCHY SYNDROME]

General

Deletion of approximately one half of the long arm of chromosome 18.

Ocular

Hypertelorism; epicanthal folds; narrow palpebral fissure; nystagmus (horizontal); strabismus; myopia; astigmatism; glaucoma; oval pupils; microcornea; posterior staphyloma; oblique disk; optic nerve staphyloma; optic nerve atrophy; microphthalmia; corneal opacities; iris hypoplasia; corectopia.

Clinical

Dwarfism; mental retardation; microcephaly; midface dysplasia; prominent antihelix and antitragus; congenital cardiac disease; abnormal, spindle-shaped fingers; genital defects.

Laboratory

Clinical.

Treatment

- *Glaucoma*: Glaucoma medication should be the first plan of action. If medication is unsuccessful, a filtering surgical procedure with or without antimetabotites may be beneficial.
- *Strabismus*: Equalized vision with correct refractive error; surgery may be helpful in patient with diplopia

🗗 BIBLIOGRAPHY

1. de Grouchy J, Royer P, Salmon C, et al. Deletion Partielle des Bras Longs du Chromosome 18. Pathol Biol (France). 1964;12:579-82.

⊟ IEE.A20. CHROMOSOME 18 PARTIAL DELETION (SHORT-ARM) SYNDROME [MONOSOMY 18 PARTIAL (SHORT-ARM) SYNDROME]

General

Deletion of the short arm of chromosome 18 (note similarity of clinical features to those of the Cri-du-Chat syndrome or B1 deletion syndrome) (*see* Cri-du-Chat syndrome).

Ocular

Hypertelorism; epicanthal folds; ptosis; mongolian or antimongolian slant; strabismus; eccentric pupil; cataract; corneal opacities; concentric visual field defects.

Clinical

Short stature; mental retardation; low-set ears; dysphagia; moon face; oliguria; arhinencephaly; microcephaly; congenital alopecia; flat bridge of nose; pyramidal tract signs; weakness and focal dystonia of the lower extremities.

Laboratory

Clinical.

Treatment

- *Ptosis*: If visual acuity is affected, most cases require surgical correction and there are several procedures that may be used including levator resection, repair or advancement and Fasanella-Servat.
- *Strabismus*: Equalized vision with correct refractive error; surgery may be helpful in patient with diplopia.

⊟ BIBLIOGRAPHY

1. Bühler E, Bühler U, Stalder G. Partial monosomy 18 and anomaly of thyroxine synthesis. Lancet. 1964;1:170-1.
2. Levenson JE, Crandall BF, Sparkes RS. Partial deletion syndromes of chromosome 18. Ann Ophthalmol. 1971;3:756-60.
2. Yanoff M, Rorke LB, Niederer BS. Ocular and cerebral abnormalities in chromosome 18 deletion defect. Am J Ophthalmol. 1970;10:391-402.

⊟ 1EE.A21. GENERAL FIBROSIS SYNDROME [CONGENITAL ENOPHTHALMOS WITH OCULAR MUSCLE FIBROSIS AND PTOSIS; CONGENITAL FIBROSIS OF THE INFERIOR RECTUS WITH PTOSIS; STRABISMUS FIXUS; VERTICAL RETRACTION SYNDROME (CONGENITAL FIBROSIS SYNDROME)]

General

Present from birth; familial history; apparent autosomal dominant transmission; sex-linked recessive transmission is also reported.

Ocular

Ptosis; enophthalmos; disk hypoplasia; astigmatism; esotropia; exotropia; hypotropia; nystagmus; visual loss; positive forced duction test; it may be associated with Marcus Gunn jaw-winking and synergistic divergence in attempted right gaze.

Clinical

None.

Laboratory

Neuroimaging is the most essential laboratory study.

Treatment

Surgically approximating normal orbital bone positions, before addressing soft tissue volume loss.

⊟ BIBLIOGRAPHY

1. Soparkar CN. (2012). Enophthalmos. [online] Available from www.emedicine.com/oph/TOPIC617.HTM. [Accessed September, 2013].

🗗 1EE.A22. OPHTHALMOPLEGIA, PROGRESSIVE EXTERNAL

General

Autosomal recessive; progressive limitation of ocular motility with clinical sparing of pupillary function; underlying pathogenesis is secondary to a mitochondrial cytopathy; appearance of ragged-red fibers in the abnormal muscles is primarily caused by mitochondrial accumulations beneath the plasma membrane and between the myofibrils.

Ocular

Oculopharyngeal muscular dystrophy; retinitis pigmentosa; progressive external ophthalmoplegia; some patients show only ptosis and ophthalmoplegia; most patients have multisystem involvement.

Clinical

Heart block; ataxia.

Laboratory

Thyroid studies, acetylcholine receptor antibody. MRI, CT and ultrasound may show enlarged extraocular muscles.

Treatment

If ptosis is present, lid crutches may be helpful or ptosis surgery. Strabismus surgery may be helpful in patients with diplopia.

🗗 BIBLIOGRAPHY

1. Roy H. (2011). Chronic progressive external ophthalmoplegia. [online] Available from www.emedicine.com/oph/ TOPIC510.HTM. [Accessed September, 2013].

🗗 1EE.A24. FREEMAN-SHELDON SYNDROME (CRANIO-CARPO-TARSAL DYSPLASIA; WHISTLING FACE SYNDROME)

General

Rare; autosomal dominant and recessive inheritance as well as sporadic cases (genetic heterogeneity).

Ocular

Eyes deeply sunken (enophthalmos); hypertelorism; ble–pharophimosis; ptosis; antimongoloid slanting of lid fissures; esotropia.

Clinical

Small nose with narrow nostrils and long philtrum; alae nasi often bent, simulating colobomas; nasolabial folds present only near the nose; microstomia; high-arched palate and small mandible; flexion contractures of fingers; excessive bulging of central part of cheeks when whistling.

Laboratory

No specific laboratory studies, imaging, or diagnostic procedures are valuable.

Treatment

Various reconstructive procedures may be necessary.

🗗 BIBLIOGRAPHY

1. Freeman EA, Sheldon JH. Cranio-carpotarsal dystrophy: an undescribed congenital malformation. Arch Dis Child. 1938;13:277.
2. McKusick VA. Mendelian Inheritance in Man: A Catalog of Human Genes and Genetic Disorders, 12th edition. Baltimore: The Johns Hopkins University Press; 1998.
3. O'Keefe M, Crawford JS, Young JD, et al. Ocular abnormalities in the Freeman-Sheldon syndrome. Am J Ophthalmol. 1986;102:346-8.
4. Wang TR, Lin SJ. Further evidence for genetic heterogeneity of whistling face or Freeman-Sheldon syndrome in a Chinese family. Am J Genet. 1987;28:471-5.
5. Weinstein S, Gorlin RJ. Cranio-carpotarsal dystrophy or the whistling face syndrome. Am J Dis Child. 1969;117:427-33.

🖹 1EE.A25. CRETINISM (HYPOTHYROID GOITER; HYPOTHYROIDISM; JUVENILE HYPOTHYROIDISM; MYXEDEMA)

General

Deficient thyroid function.

Ocular

Blepharitis; ptosis; enophthalmos; temporal madarosis; decreased tear secretion; glaucoma; proptosis; optic atrophy; optic neuritis; blue dot cataract; conjunctivitis; scleritis; optic disk hemorrhage and arcuate scotoma associated with glaucoma.

Clinical

Myxedema; larynx and tongue swollen; hoarse speech; dry, yellowish skin; slow pulse; mental retardation; infertility; pericardial effusion; cardiac enlargement; physical development retarded.

Laboratory

Clinical.

Treatment

- *Blepharitis*: Oral tetracyclines, omega-3 fatty acids, flax seed oil or fish oil. Ocular therapy include eyelid scrubs, warm compresses, bacitracin ointment to lid margins, topical cyclosporine A and preservative free lubricants.
- *Ptosis*: If visual acuity is affected, most cases require surgical correction and there are several procedures that may be used including levator resection, repair or advancement and Fasanella-Servat
- *Glaucoma*: Glaucoma medication should be the first plan of action. If medication is unsuccessful, a filtering surgical procedure with or without antimetabotites may be beneficial.
- *Cataract*: Change in glasses can sometimes improve a patient's visual function temporarily; however the most common treatment is cataract surgery.

🖹 BIBLIOGRAPHY

1. Daniel MS, Postellon DC. (2013). Congenital hypothyroidism. [online] Available from www.emedicine.com/ped/TOPIC501.HTM. [Accessed September, 2013].

🖹 1EE.A26. CRI-DU-CHAT SYNDROME [CAT-CRY (5P-) SYNDROME; CRYING CAT SYNDROME; BI DELETION SYNDROME; LEJEUNE SYNDROME]

General

Short arm deletion of a no. 5 chromosome (5p-); increased inheritance risk; 13% have one parent with balanced translocation; female preponderance 2:1 (*see* Wolf Syndrome).

Ocular

Hypertelorism; epicanthal folds; antimongoloid slanting of palpebral fissures; strabismus; increased tortuosity of retinal vessels.

Clinical

High-pitched, plaintive cry by an infant (reminiscent of a crying cat); mental retardation; broad nasal root; micrognathia or retrognathia; low-set ears; simian crease; congenital heart defect; small larynx and epiglottis.

Laboratory

Conventional cytogenetic studies, skeletal radiography, MRI, echocardiography.

Treatment

No treatment exists for the underlying disorder. Correction of congenital heart defects may be indicated.

🖹 BIBLIOGRAPHY

1. Chen H. (2013). Cri-du-chat Syndrome. [online] Available from www.emedicine.com/ped/TOPIC504.HTM. [Accessed September, 2013].

1EE.A27. CROUZON SYNDROME (DYSOSTOSIS CRANIOFACIALIS; OXYCEPHALY; CRANIOFACIAL DYSOSTOSIS; PARROT-HEAD SYNDROME; MÖBIUS-CROUZON SYNDROME; HEREDITARY CRANIOFACIAL DYSOSTOSIS)

General

Autosomal dominant; manifestations present at birth.

Ocular

Bilateral exophthalmos; hypertelorism (wide interpupillary distance); obliquity of palpebral fissures with outer canthus slanting downward; nystagmus; exotropia; upper field defects due to pressure upon the optic nerve on its lower part; bluish sclera; exposure keratitis in extreme exophthalmos; cataract; papilledema; secondary optic atrophy; corneal dystrophy; ptosis; strabismus; keratoconus.

Clinical

Prognathism; maxillary hypoplasia with short upper lip; synostosis of coronal and lambda sutures; parrot-beaked nose (psittachosrhina); widening temporal fossae; headaches.

Laboratory

Skull, spine, and hand radiography is usually necessary to confirm the diagnosis.

Treatment

Neurosurgical procedure is recommended in cases of intracranial hypertension leading to further optic atrophy.

BIBLIOGRAPHY

1. Chen H. (2013). Genetics of Crouzon syndrome. [online] Available from www.emedicine.com/ped/TOPIC511.HTM. [Accessed September, 2013].

1EE.A28. DANDY-WALKER SYNDROME (ATRESIA OF THE FORAMEN OF MAGENDIE)

General

Manifested in infants; malformation and stenosis of the foramina of Luschka and Magendie; dilation of fourth ventricle.

Ocular

Ptosis; sixth nerve paralysis; papilledema.

Clinical

Hydrocephalus (varies in severity) with enlargement of the skull and thinning of the bone predominantly in occipital region; loss of tendon reflexes; basilar impression; scoliosis; hydromelia.

Laboratory

CT, MRI, ultrasound, angiography.

Treatment

Shunt to treat associated hydrocephalus.

BIBLIOGRAPHY

1. Incesu L, Khosla A. (2013). Imaging in Dandy-Walker malformation. [online] Available from www.emedicine.com/radio/TOPIC206.HTM. [Accessed September, 2013].

🗗 1EE.A29. DE LANGE SYNDROME (I) (CONGENITAL MUSCULAR HYPERTROPHY CEREBRAL SYNDROME; BRACHMANN-DE LANGE SYNDROME)

General

Etiology not known; autosomal recessive inheritance.

Ocular

Antimongoloid slant of palpebral fissures; mild exophthalmos; hypertrichosis of eyebrows; long eyelashes; telecanthus; ptosis; blepharophimosis; nystagmus on lateral gaze; constant coarse nystagmus; strabismus; alternating exotropia; high myopia; anisocoria; chronic conjunctivitis; blue sclera; pallor of optic disk.

Clinical

Mental retardation; growth retardation; extrapyramidal motor disturbances; multiple skeletal abnormalities with congenital muscular hypertrophy; long philtrum; thin lips; crescent-shaped mouth.

Laboratory

Molecular diagnosis with screening of the nipped-B-like (NIPBL) gene, X-ray, ultrasonography, echocardiography

Treatment

Early intervention for feeding problems, hearing and visual impairment, congenital heart disease, and urinary system abnormalities and psychomotor delay.

🗗 BIBLIOGRAPHY

1. Tekin M, Bodurtha J. (2011). Cornelia De Lange syndrome. [online] Available from www.emedicine.com/ped/TOPIC482.HTM. [Accessed September, 2013].

🗗 1EE.A30. DUBOWITZ SYNDROME (DWARFISM-ECZEMA-PECULIAR FACIES)

General

Affects both sexes; congenital; may be autosomal recessive inheritance.

Ocular

Hypertelorism; lateral telecanthus; palpebral ptosis; short palpebral tissues.

Clinical

Eczema; sparse hair; cleft palate; hypospadia; microcephaly; low birth weight; mild mental retardation; characteristic face; short stature; spontaneous keloids; intrauterine growth retardation.

Laboratory

Bone marrow biopsy, quantitative hemoglobin electrophoresis, cytogenetic studies, HLA.

Treatment

Management involves supportive care that includes transfusion, treatment of infections, and a search for an allogeneic stem cell donor.

🗗 BIBLIOGRAPHY

1. Dixon N, Castellino SM, Howard SC. (2011). Pediatric Myelodysplasia. [online] Available from www.emedicine.com/ped/TOPIC1526.HTM. [Accessed September, 2013].

🗗 1EE.A31. DUCK-BILL LIPS AND PTOSIS

General

Autosomal dominant.

Ocular

Ptosis; strabismus; hypertelorism.

Clinical

Short philtrum; duck-bill lips; low-set ears; broad forehead; slightly anteverted nose and flat nasal bridge; slightly wide-spaced teeth and high-arched palate; slightly receding chin; slightly wide-set nipples; two phalanges in both fifth fingers; impaired speech.

Laboratory

Diagnosis is made by clinical findings.

Treatment

Observation in mild cases with no abnormal head position or amblyopia. More severe cases may require levator muscle resection, frontalis suspension procedure, Fasanella-Servat procedure, Müller muscle-conjunctival resection.

BIBLIOGRAPHY

1. Suh DW. (2012). Congenital ptosis. [online] Available from www.emedicine.com/oph/TOPIC345.HTM. [Accessed September, 2013].

1EE.A32. EHLERS-DANLOS SYNDROME (FIBRODYSPLASIA ELASTICA GENERALISATA; CUTIS HYPERELASTICA; MEEKEREN-EHLERS-DANLOS SYNDROME; INDIAN RUBBER MAN SYNDROME; CUTIS LAXA)

General

Present at birth; autosomal dominant; two groups: cutaneous and articular; syndrome is one of the three primary disorders of elastic tissue [other two disorders are pseudoxanthoma elasticum (Grönblad-Strandberg syndrome) and senile elastosis]; inherited disorder of collagen biosynthesis.

Ocular

Hyperelasticity of palpebral skin; easy eversion of upper lid; ptosis; epicanthal folds; hypotony of extraocular muscles; strabismus; microcornea; thinning of cornea with keratoconus; thinning of sclera (blue sclera); subluxation of lens; angioid streaks; chorioretinal hemorrhages; retinitis proliferans with secondary detachment; macular degeneration; myopia; ruptured globe after minor trauma; limbus-to-limbus corneal thinning; acute hydrops; cornea plana; keratoglobus.

Clinical

Cutaneous manifestations include thin, atrophic, fragile skin, cutaneous hyperelasticity and pseudomolluscoid tumors; articular manifestations include excessive articular laxity and luxations; hypermobile joints.

Laboratory

Biochemical studies can detect alterations in collagen molecules in cultured skin fibroblasts. Molecular (DNA) based testing is available. Diagnosis may by urinary analyte assay and clinical examination is the most common.

Treatment

Ascorbic acid therapy, in the event of skin lacerations seriously consider alternatives to sutures, including adhesive strips and wound glues, monitor for cardiac conditions and scoliosis.

BIBLIOGRAPHY

1. Steiner RD. (2011). Genetics of Ehlers-Danlos syndrome. [online] Available from www.emedicine.com/ped/TOPIC654.HTM. [Accessed September, 2013].

1EE.A33. ENGELMANN SYNDROME [OSTEOPATHIA HYPEROSTOTICA (SCLEROTICANS) MULTIPLEX INFANTILIS; DIAPHYSEAL DYSPLASIA; CAMURATI-ENGELMANN DISEASE; HEREDITARY MULTIPLE DIAPHYSEAL SCLEROSIS; JUVENILE PAGET DISEASE]

General

Etiology unknown; progressive resorption and deposits of bone with thickening of periosteum and changes of cortex as evident by diagnostic X-ray studies in the intermediate portion of the long bones.

Ocular

Exophthalmos; hypertelorism (secondary); ptosis; lagophthalmos; lateral rectus palsy; convergence insufficiency; epiphora; cataract; tortuous retinal vessels; papilledema; optic atrophy.

Clinical

Pain in extremities; poorly developed musculature; waddling gait; delayed ambulation; scaly skin; delayed dentition; deafness; hypogonadism; pain in both legs; aching in the forearms; episodic temporofrontal and occipital headache.

Laboratory

Clinical.

Treatment

- *Exophthalmos*: Reversing the problem which is causing the exophthalmos is the treatment of choice and will minimize the ocular complications. Ocular lubricants are beneficial for control of the corneal exposure.
- *Ptosis*: If visual acuity is affected, most cases require surgical correction and there are several procedures that may be used including levator resection, repair or advancement and Fasanella-Servat.

- *Cataract*: Change in glasses can sometimes improve a patient's visual function temporarily; however the most common treatment is cataract surgery.
- *Papilledema*: Underlying cause should be determined and treated. Systemic acetazolamide is the medical therapy of choice.

BIBLIOGRAPHY

1. Brodrick JD. Luxation of the globe in Engelmann's disease. Am J Ophthalmol. 1977;83:870-3.
2. De Vits A, Keymeulen B, Bossuyt A, et al. Progressive diaphyseal dysplasia (Camurati-Engelmann's disease). Improvement of clinical signs and of bone scintigraphy during pregnancy. Clin Nucl Med. 1994;19:104-7.
3. Engelmann G. Ein Fall von Osteopathia Hyperostotica (Scleroticans) Infantilis. Fortschr Geb Roentgen Strahl. 1929;39:1101.
4. Morse PH, Walsh FB, McCormick JR. Ocular findings in hereditary diaphyseal dysplasia (Engelmann's disease). Am J Ophthalmol. 1969;68:100.
5. Roy FH, Fraunfelder FW, Fraunfelder FT. Roy and Fraunfelder's Current Ocular Therapy, 6th edition. Philadelphia: WB Saunders; 2008.

1EE.A34A. ARTHROGRYPOSIS MULTIPLEX CONGENITA

General

Heterogeneous group of disorders of multiple proposed etiologies; often one manifestation of a complex of congenital anomalies; probable autosomal recessive transmission; found in Eskimos; affects more males than females; characterized by decreased fetal joint mobility secondary to neuropathic disease, myopathic disease, or some other cause.

Ocular

Congenital bilateral cataract; associated with ophthalmoplegia, retinopathy, goniodysgenesis, and infantile glaucoma, as well as Duane retraction syndrome.

Clinical

Multiple articular rigidities; hypoplasia of adjacent muscle groups; soft tissue shortening; duck-like waddle; muscle atrophy.

Laboratory

In general, laboratory tests are not extremely useful.

Treatment

Goals include lower-limb alignment and establishment of stability for ambulation and upper-limb function for self-care. Early vigorous physical therapy to stretch contractures is very important to promote active range of motion.

BIBLIOGRAPHY

1. Chen H. (2013). Arthrogryposis. [online] Available from www.emedicine.com/ped/TOPIC142.HTM. [Accessed September, 2013].

⊟ 1EE.A34B. COCKAYNE SYNDROME (DWARFISM WITH RETINAL ATROPHY AND DEAFNESS; MICKEY MOUSE SYNDROME)

General

Autosomal recessive; onset in 2nd year of life; wide spectrum of symptoms and severity of the disease suggest that biochemical and genetic heterogeneity exist.

Ocular

Enophthalmos; cataracts; pigmentary degeneration of retina; optic atrophy; band keratopathy; exotropia; nystagmus; absence of foveal reflex; corneal dystrophy; corneal perforation; anhidrosis; exposure keratitis; decreased blinking.

Clinical

Dwarfism (nanism) with disproportionately long limbs, large hands, and large feet; kyphosis; deformed limbs; thickened skull; intracranial calcifications; mental retardation; prognathism; deafness (often partial); precociously senile appearance; sensitivity to sunlight, with skin pigmentation and scarring; dental caries.

Laboratory

Brain CT scan may reveal calcifications and cortical atrophy.

Treatment

Photoprotection with sunscreens and clothing are useful. Cochlear implantation can help to minimize the effects of auditory impairment.

⊟ BIBLIOGRAPHY

1. Imaeda S. (2012). Cockayne syndrome. [online] Available from www.emedicine.com/derm/TOPIC717.HTM. [Accessed September, 2013]

⊟ 1EE.A34C. CRYPTOPHTHALMIA SYNDROME (CRYPTOPHTHALMOS SYNDACTYLY SYNDROME; FRASER SYNDROME)

General

Autosomal recessive.

Ocular

Microphthalmia; epibulbar dermoid; cryptophthalmos; enophthalmia; eyebrows partially or completely missing; skin from forehead completely covers one or both eyes, but the globes can be palpated beneath the skin; in unilateral cases, the fellow eye may present lid coloboma; buphthalmos; conjunctival sac partially or totally obliterated; absence of trabeculae, Schlemm canal, and ciliary muscles; cornea is differentiated from the sclera; lens anomalies from complete absence to hypoplasia, dislocation, and calcification.

Clinical

Syndactyly (finger, toes; about 40%); coloboma of alae nasi and nostrils; urogenital abnormalities, including pseudohermaphroditism and renal hypoplasia; abnormal, bizarre hairline; narrow external auditory meatus and malformation of ossicles; cleft lip and palate may occur; atresia or hypoplasia of larynx in some cases; hoarse voice; dysplastic pinna; meatal stenosis; glottic web and subglottic stenosis.

Laboratory

CT and MRI.

Treatment

Ocular—none.

⊟ BIBLIOGRAPHY

1. Mamalis N, Ollerton AJ. (2012). Anophthalmos. [online] Available from www.emedicine.com/oph/TOPIC572.HTM. [Accessed September, 2013].

⏚ 1EE.A34D. DUANE SYNDROME (RETRACTION SYNDROME; STILLING SYNDROME; TURK-STILLING SYNDROME)

General

Autosomal dominant; more frequent in females; manifestations in infancy; was thought to be secondary to fibrosis of the LR muscle or abnormal check ligaments; now established to be due to congenital aberrant innervation affecting third and seventh cranial nerves.

Ocular

Narrowing of palpebral fissure on adduction, widening on abduction; primary global retraction; deficiency of medial and lateral recti motility; limitation of abduction in affected eye usually is complete; retraction of the globe with attempted adduction varies from 1 mm to 10 mm; convergence insufficiency; heterochromia irides; left eye is more frequently involved.

Clinical

Associated Klippel-Feil syndrome; malformation of face, ears and teeth.

Laboratory

Diagnosis is made by clinical findings.

Treatment

Indications for surgery include anomalous head position, strabismus in primary gaze, significant upshoot or downshoot in adduction and cosmetically significant palpebral fissure. Duane retraction syndrome type 1 (DRS-1) (absent abduction, esotropia in primary position and head turn toward the affected side to fuse) medial rectus recession of the affected eye; DRS with exotropia—recess LR of involved side. Retraction of the globe—recess medial and lateral rectus of involved eye. Upshoots and downshoots—recess the LR.

⏚ BIBLIOGRAPHY

1. Verma A. (2011). Duane syndrome. [online] Available from www.emedicine.com/oph/TOPIC326.HTM. [Accessed September, 2013].

⏚ 1EE.A34E. FREEMAN-SHELDON SYNDROME (CRANIO-CARPO-TARSAL DYSPLASIA; WHISTLING FACE SYNDROME)

General

Rare; autosomal dominant and recessive inheritance as well as sporadic cases (genetic heterogeneity).

Ocular

Eyes deeply sunken (enophthalmos); hypertelorism; blepharophimosis; ptosis; antimongoloid slanting of lid fissures; esotropia.

Clinical

Small nose with narrow nostrils and long philtrum; alae nasi often bent, simulating colobomas; nasolabial folds present only near the nose; microstomia; high-arched palate and small mandible; flexion contractures of fingers; excessive bulging of central part of cheeks when whistling.

Laboratory

No specific laboratory studies, imaging, or diagnostic procedures are valuable.

Treatment

Various reconstructive procedures may be necessary.

⏚ BIBLIOGRAPHY

1. Freeman EA, Sheldon JH. Cranio-carpotarsal dystrophy: an undescribed congenital malformation. Arch Dis Child. 1938;13:277.
2. McKusick VA. Mendelian Inheritance in Man: A Catalog of Human Genes and Genetic Disorders, 12th edition. Baltimore: The Johns Hopkins University Press; 1998.
3. O'Keefe M, Crawford JS, Young JD, et al. Ocular abnormalities in the Freeman-Sheldon syndrome. Am J Ophthalmol. 1986;102:346-8.
4. Wang TR, Lin SJ. Further evidence for genetic heterogeneity of whistling face or Freeman-Sheldon syndrome in a Chinese family. Am J Genet. 1987;28:471-5.
5. Weinstein S, Gorlin RJ. Cranio-carpotarsal dystrophy or the whistling face syndrome. Am J Dis Child. 1969;117: 427-33.

1EE.A34F. GENERAL FIBROSIS SYNDROME (CONGENITAL ENOPHTHALMOS WITH OCULAR MUSCLE FIBROSIS AND PTOSIS; CONGENITAL FIBROSIS OF THE INFERIOR RECTUS WITH PTOSIS; STRABISMUS FIXUS; VERTICAL RETRACTION SYNDROME (CONGENITAL FIBROSIS SYNDROME)

General

Present from birth; familial history; apparent autosomal dominant transmission; sex-linked recessive transmission is also reported.

Ocular

Ptosis; enophthalmos; disk hypoplasia; astigmatism; esotropia; exotropia; hypotropia; nystagmus; visual loss; positive forced duction test; it may be associated with Marcus Gunn jaw-winking and synergistic divergence in attempted right gaze.

Clinical

None.

Laboratory

Neuroimaging is the most essential laboratory study.

Treatment

Surgically approximating normal orbital bone positions, before addressing soft tissue volume loss.

BIBLIOGRAPHY

1. Soparkar CN. (2012). Enophthalmos. [online] Available from www.emedicine.com/oph/TOPIC617.HTM. [Accessed September, 2013].

1EE.A34G. GREIG SYNDROME (OCULAR HYPERTELORISM SYNDROME; HYPERTELORISM; PRIMARY EMBRYONIC HYPERTELORISM; HYPERTELORISM OCULARIS)

General

Condition is rare; sporadic or hereditary; autosomal dominant or sex linked; if not associated with mental deficiency, then adequate mental and physical development is found.

Ocular

Hypertelorism (wide spacing of orbits); enophthalmos; epicanthus; deformities of eyelids and brows; defects of the palpebral fissure; bilateral sixth nerve paralysis; esotropia; astigmatism; optic atrophy by tension on the optic nerve; strabismus.

Clinical

Skull may show mild malformations, including bitemporal eminences and decreased anteroposterior diameter; harelip; high-arched palate; cleft palate; broad and flat nasal root; mental impairment.

Laboratory

Diagnosis is made by clinical findings.

Treatment

Minor degrees of deformity (referred to as telecanthus) can be corrected by removing a small amount of bone in the midline. A limited frontal craniotomy is performed in the midline osteotomy.

BIBLIOGRAPHY

1. Jackson IT, Malhotra G. (2012). Congenital syndromes. [online] Available from www.emedicine.com/plastic/TOPIC183.HTM. [Accessed September, 2013].

⊟ 1EE.A34H. HEMIFACIAL MICROSOMIA SYNDROME (UNILATERAL FACIAL AGENESIS; OTOMANDIBULAR DYSOSTOSIS; FRANCOIS-HAUSTRATE SYNDROME)

General

No inheritance pattern; left side of face seems to be more frequently involved; facial asymmetry usually most obvious finding; both sexes affected; alteration of intrauterine environment is possible cause.

Ocular

Microphthalmos; congenital cystic ophthalmia; enophthalmos; strabismus; cataract; colobomata of iris, choroid, and retina.

Clinical

Microtia; macrostomia; failure of development of mandibular ramus and condyle; external auditory meatus may be absent; single or numerous ear tags; hypoplasia of facial muscles unilaterally; pulmonary agenesis (ipsilateral side); associated with Goldenhar syndrome.

Laboratory

X-ray, CT and MRI.

Treatment

Silastic implants remain one of the most common materials used for malar and submalar augmentation.

⊟ BIBLIOGRAPHY

1. Francois J, Haustrate L. Anomalies Colobomateuses du Globe Oculaire et Syndrome du Premier arc. Ann Ocul. 1954;187:340.
2. Geeraets WJ. Ocular Syndromes, 3rd edition. Philadelphia: Lea & Febiger; 1976.
3. Kobrynski L, Chitayat D, Zahed L, et al. Trisomy 22 and facioauriculovertebral (Goldenhar) sequence. Am J Med Genet. 1993;46:68-71.
4. Magalini SI, Scrascia E. Dictionary of Medical Syndromes, 2nd edition. Philadelphia: JB Lippincott; 1981.

⊟ 1EE.A34I. KLIPPEL-TRENAUNAY-WEBER SYNDROME (PARKES-WEBER SYNDROME; ANGIO-OSTEO-HYPERTROPHY SYNDROME)

General

Most frequently inherited as irregular dominant; however, reported to be recessive with parent consanguinity; association of Klippel-Trenaunay-Weber syndrome and Sturge-Weber syndrome has been reported.

Ocular

Enophthalmos; unilateral hydrophthalmos; conjunctival telangiectasia; atypical iris coloboma; cataract; irregular and dilated retinal vessels; choroidal angiomas; exudative outer retinal vascular masses.

Clinical

Vascular nevi; varicose vessels; capillary angiomas; lymphangioma; arteriovenous aneurysm; hypertrophy of soft tissues and bones (local); phlebitis; thrombosis; syndactyly; polydactyly; early eruption of teeth; hemifacial hypertrophy.

Laboratory

Ultrasound, MRI, angiography and X-ray.

Treatment

Compression stockings or pneumatic pumps are usually successful. Surgical intervention (resection or ligation of abnormal blood vessels) is sometimes necessary.

⊟ BIBLIOGRAPHY

1. Buehler B. (2012). Genetics of Klippel-Trenaunay-Weber Syndrome. [online] Available from www.emedicine.com/ped/TOPIC1253.HTM. [Accessed September, 2013].

🗗 1EE.A34J. KRAUSE SYNDROME (CONGENITAL ENCEPHALO-OPHTHALMIC DYSPLASIA; ENCEPHALO-OPHTHALMIC SYNDROME)

General

No hereditary factors involved; no predilection for either sex; more frequent in premature infants; death frequently from intercurrent infections.

Ocular

Microphthalmos; enophthalmos; ptosis; strabismus; secondary glaucoma; iris atrophy; anterior and posterior synechiae; scleral atrophy; persistent remnants of hyaloid's artery; intraocular hemorrhages and exudates; cyclitic membranes; cataracts; retinal hypoplasia and hyperplasia; choroidal and retinal malformation; retinal glial membranes; retinal detachment; choroidal atrophy; optic nerve malformation; optic atrophy.

Clinical

Congenital cerebral dysplasia; hydrocephalus or microcephaly; mental retardation; heterotopia.

Laboratory

Clinical.

Treatment

- *Ptosis*: If visual acuity is affected most cases require surgical correction and there are several procedures that may be used including levator resection, repair or advancement and Fasanella-Servat.
- *Strabismus*: Equalized vision with correct refractive error; surgery may be helpful in patient with diplopia.
- *Glaucoma*: Glaucoma medication should be the first plan of action. If medication is unsuccessful, a filtering surgical procedure with or without antimetabolites may be beneficial.
- *Cataract*: Change in glasses can sometimes improve a patient's visual function temporarily; however the most common treatment is cataract surgery.
- *Vitreous hemorrhage*: If possible, the source of the bleeding needs to be isolated and treated with laser. Vitrectomy may be necessary.
- *Retinal detachment*: Scleral buckle, pneumatic retinopexy and vitrectomy may be used to close all the breaks.

🗗 BIBLIOGRAPHY

1. Krause AC. Congenital encephalo-ophthalmic dysplasia. Arch Ophthalmol. 1946;36:387-94.
2. Miller M, Robbins J, Fishman R, et al. A chromosomal anomaly with multiple ocular defects. Am J Ophthalmol. 1963;55:901.

🗗 1EE.A34K. BRANCHED-CHAIN KETOACIDURIA (MAPLE SYRUP URINE DISEASE)

General

Deficiency in the oxidative decarboxylation of the corresponding α-ketoacids; possibly autosomal recessive inheritance; both sexes affected; onset in 1st week of life.

Ocular

Ptosis; epicanthal folds; hypertelorism; prominence of supraorbital ridges; cataract; strabismus; decreased or absent pupillary reaction to light; horizontal nystagmus; optic atrophy; ophthalmoplegia.

Clinical

Maple syrup odor of urine; neurologic symptoms; death may follow promptly or the patient may live for a decade during which severe mental retardation is apparent; vomiting; failure to thrive; absence of grasping reflex; generalized rigidity; hypoglycemic crisis; cortical blindness.

Laboratory

Plasma amino acids (elevation of branched-chain amino acids, detection of alloisoleucine). The detection of alloisoleucine is diagnostic.

Treatment

The mainstay in the treatment is dietary restriction of branched-chain amino acids.

🗗 BIBLIOGRAPHY

1. Bodamer OA, Lee B. (2012). Maple Syrup Urine Disease. [online] Available from www.emedicine.com/ped/TOPIC1368.HTM. [Accessed September, 2013].

⊟ 1EE.A34L. MORQUIO SYNDROME (MORQUIO-BRAILSFORD SYNDROME; BRAILSFORD-MORQUIO DYSTROPHY; FAMILIAL OSSEOUS DYSTROPHY; KERATOSULFATURIA; MPS IV; MUCOPOLYSACCHARIDOSIS IV; SPONDYLOEPI-PHYSEAL DYSPLASIA; OSTEOCHONDRODYSTROPHIA DEFORMANS; INFANTILE HEREDITARY CHONDRODYSPLASIA; HEREDITARY POLY TOPIC ENCHONDRAL DYSOSTOSIS; HEREDITARY OSTEOCHONDRODYSTROPHY; ECCENTRO-OSTEOCHONDRODYSPLASIA; DYSOSTOSIS ENCHONDRALIS META-EPIPHYSARIA; MORQUIO-ULLRICH SYNDROME; ATYPICAL CHONDRODYSTROPHY; CHONDRODYSTROPHIA TARDA; CHONDRO-OSTEODYSTROPHY)

General

Autosomal recessive dystrophy of cartilage and bone; slight predilection for males; apparent between ages 4 and 10 years; excess production of keratosulfate (*see* Hurler Syndrome; Hunter Syndrome; Sanfilippo-Good Syndrome; Scheie Syndrome; Maroteaux-Lamy Syndrome); autosomal recessive; abnormal N-acetylgalactosamine-G-sulfate sulfatase.

Ocular

Enophthalmos; ptosis; excessive tear secretion; ocular hypotony; miosis; occasionally hazy cornea; bushy eyebrows; optic nerve atrophy; moderate-to-late corneal clouding.

Clinical

Dwarfism; skeletal deformities (progressive); delayed ossification of epiphyses; decreased muscle tone; deafness; weak extremities; waddling gait; coarse broad mouth; spaced teeth; aortic regurgitation; normal intelligence.

Laboratory

Blood-Reilly's granules in leukocytes; X-ray—flat vertebrae and odontoid hypoplasia.

Treatment

Treatment is limited to supportive care.

⊟ BIBLIOGRAPHY

1. Bittar T, Washington ER. (2012). Mucopolysaccharidosis. [online] Available from www.emedicine.com/orthoped/TOPIC203.HTM. [Accessed September, 2013].

⊟ 1EE.A34M. VON RECKLINGHAUSEN SYNDROME (NEUROFIBROMATOSIS TYPE I; NEURINOMATOSIS)

General

Dominant inheritance activated at puberty, during pregnancy and at menopause; strong evidence supports the existence of neurofibromatosis type I (NF-I) as a tumor suppressor gene.

Ocular

Proptosis; displacement of the globe; pulsation of the globe; ptosis; elephantiasis of the lids; pigment spots on lids; hydrophthalmos; nodular swelling of corneal nerves; cataracts; optic atrophy; choroidal melanoma; neurofibroma of the choroid, iris, eyelid and ciliary body; enlarged optic foramen; underdevelopment of orbital bones; café-au-lait spots on fundus; hamartoma of retina; congenital glaucoma; focal iris nodules; choroidal nevi; optic nerve gliomas; orbital neurofibroma; keratoconus.

Clinical

Café-au-lait skin pigmentations; fibroma molluscum; lipomas and sebaceous adenomas; schwannomas; growth abnormalities; spontaneous fractures; facial hemihypertrophy.

Laboratory

T2-weighted MRI images demonstrate multiple bright lesions in the basal ganglia, cerebellum, and brain in 80% optic nerve gliomas often develop perineural arachnoidal hyperplasia, which appears as an expanded CSF space around the nerve.

Treatment

Oral ketotifen may reduce the pain, tenderness and itchiness associated with neurofibromas.

⊟ BIBLIOGRAPHY

1. Dahl AA. (2011). Ophthalmologic manifestations of neurofibromatosis type. [online] Available from www.emedicine.com/oph/TOPIC338.HTM. [Accessed September, 2013].

⊟ 1EE.A34N. ROMBERG SYNDROME (PARRY-ROMBERG SYNDROME; PROGRESSIVE HEMIFACIAL ATROPHY; PROGRESSIVE FACIAL HEMIATROPHY; FACIAL HEMIATROPHY) ENOPHTHALMUS

General

Autosomal dominant; irritation in the peripheral trophic sympathetic system; onset in the 2nd decade; both sexes affected.

Ocular

Enophthalmos; outer canthus lowered; absence of nasal portion of eyebrow; ptosis; paresis of ocular muscles; miosis; iritis; iridocyclitis; heterochromia iridis; keratitis; neuroparalytic keratitis; cataracts; choroiditis; Fuchs' heterochromic cyclitis; retinal vascular abnormalities; association with Coats syndrome and exudative stellate neuroretinopathy; scleral melting.

Clinical

Atrophy of soft tissue on one side of the face, including tongue; trigeminal neuralgia and/or paresthesia; alopecia and poliosis not uncommon.

Laboratory/Ocular

Neuroimaging, CT scan of the orbits, MRI and bone scans.

Treatment/Ocular

Chemotherapy, ionizing radiation or immunosuppressive treatments.

⊟ BIBLIOGRAPHY

1. Aracena T, Roca FP, Barragan M. Progressive hemifacial atrophy (Parry-Romberg syndrome): report of two cases. Ann Ophthalmol. 1979;11:953-8.
2. Gass JD, Harbin TS, Del Piero EJ. Exudative stellate neuroretinopathy and Coats' syndrome in patients with progressive hemifacial atrophy. Eur J Ophthalmol. 1991; 1:2-10.
3. Hoang-Xuan T, Foster CS, Jakobiec FA, et al. Romberg's progressive hemifacial atrophy: an association with scleral melting. Cornea. 1991;10:361-6.
4. La Hey E, Baarsma GS. Fuchs' heterochromic cyclitis and retinal vascular abnormalities in progressive hemifacial atrophy. Eye. 1993;7:426-8.
5. Parry CH. Collections from Unpublished Papers, Volume I. London: Underwood; 1825.
6. Romberg MH. Trophoneurosen. Klin Ergebn. Berlin: A. Forster; 1846.

⊟ 1EE.A34O. PASSOW SYNDROME (BREMER STATUS DYSRAPHICUS; STATUS DYSRAPHICUS SYNDROME; SYRINGOMYELIA; SYRINGOBULBIA)

General

Congenital nonclosure of the neural tube; familial occurrence or may be sporadic; insidious onset in 2nd to 3rd decade of life.

Ocular

Enophthalmos; ptosis; rotatory nystagmus; heterochromia iridis; anterior uveitis; corneal anesthesia; neuroparalytic keratitis; paralysis of third, fifth, sixth, and seventh cranial nerves; Horner syndrome; anisocoria; papilledema; optic atrophy; zonular cataract (*see* Horner Syndrome).

Clinical

Anesthesia over area of first division of trigeminal nerve; facial hemiatrophy; facial nerve paralysis; muscular weakness; cervical ribs; kyphoscoliosis; spina bifida; unilateral numbness of fingers; loss of deep reflexes; insensitivity to pain and temperature in affected areas; neurogenic bladder.

Laboratory

MRI, CT.

Treatment

Suboccipital and cervical decompression, laminectomy and syringotomy, shunts, fourth ventriculostomy, terminal ventriculostomy and neuroendoscopic surgery may be considered.

🖵 BIBLIOGRAPHY

1. Al-Shatoury HA, Galhom AA, Wagner FC. (2012). Syringomyelia. [online] Available from emedicine.medscape.com/article/1151685-overview. [Accessed September, 2013].

🖵 1EE.A35. EPIDERMAL NEVUS SYNDROME (ICHTHYOSIS HYSTRIX)

General

One or a combination of the following epidermal nevi described as nevus unius lateris, ichthyosis hystrix, linear nevus sebaceous, or congenital acanthosis nigricans; autosomal dominant.

Ocular

Blepharoptosis and fibroma on bulbar conjunctiva; antimongoloid eyelid fissures; eyelid colobomata; horizontal and rotary nystagmus; esotropia; conjunctival tumors; corneal opacities; corectopia and colobomata of the iris.

Clinical

Somatic anomalies involving the skeletal and central nervous system; anomalies of bone formation; atrophy; ankylosis; vitamin D-resistant rickets; bone cysts; mental retardation; cortical atrophy; hydrocephalus; focal and grand mal epilepsy; cerebrovascular tumors; cortical blindness.

Laboratory

Histologic examination, EEG, MRI.

Treatment

Vitamin D analogs may work by inhibiting epidermal proliferation, promoting keratinocyte differentiation, and/or exerting immunosuppressive effects on lymphoid cells.

🖵 BIBLIOGRAPHY

1. Schwartz RA, Jozwiak S. (2013). Epidermal nevus syndrome. [online] Available from www.emedicine.com/derm/TOPIC732.HTM. [Accessed September, 2013].

🖵 1EE.A36. FABRY DISEASE (ANGIOKERATOMA CORPORIS DIFFUSUM SYNDROME; DIFFUSE ANGIOKERATOSIS; FABRY-ANDERSON SYNDROME; GLYCOSPHINGOLIPID LIPIDOSIS; GLYCOSPHINGOLIPIDOSIS)

General

Lipoid storage disorder; X-linked recessive inheritance; lack of α-galactosidase A enzyme.

Ocular

Swelling of eyelids; varicosities of palpebral and bulbar conjunctiva; corneal dystrophy; corneal opacities; increased tortuosity of retinal vessels and aneurysmal dilatations; cornea verticillata; cataract; central retinal artery occlusion; internuclear paralysis of extraocular muscles; papilledema; tortuosity and caliber irregularity of conjunctival vessels; characteristic cream-colored whorl-like opacity in deep part of corneal epithelium; posterior cataract; occasional edema of optic disk and retina.

Clinical

Angiokeratoma of the skin with small, grouped papular lesions mainly over the scrotum, thighs, buttocks, sacral area, umbilical area, and lips; elevated blood pressure; disturbance in sweat secretion; pain in arms and legs; enlarged heart; albuminuria.

Laboratory

Reduced α-galactosidase A level in plasma; elevated trihexosyl ceramide levels in urine and plasma.

Treatment

Primarily surgical and is usually a corneal transplant. After surgery, treatment of amblyopia and optical therapy can be helpful.

BIBLIOGRAPHY

1. Banikazemi M, Desnick RJ, Astrin KH. (2012). Genetics of Fabry disease. [online] Available from www.emedicine.com/ped/TOPIC2888.HTM. [Accessed September, 2013].

1EE.A37. GILLUM-ANDERSON SYNDROME

General

Genetic defect responsible for weakness in the orbital connective tissue; proposed connective tissue defect of sclera, zonules, and levator aponeurosis.

Ocular

Dislocated lenses; high myopia; bilateral ptosis typical for levator disinsertions; ectopia lentis.

Laboratory

Diagnosis is made by clinical findings.

Treatment

Treatment of a lens dislodged into the anterior chamber is initially pharmacological with mydriasis/cycloplegia (to permit posterior migration of the lens behind the iris) in conjunction with ocular massage through a closed lid to promote this posterior migration. Surgical treatment will then be needed to prevent further complications.

BIBLIOGRAPHY

1. Eifrig CW. (2013). Ectopia Lentis. [online] Available from www.emedicine.com/oph/TOPIC55.HTM. [Accessed September, 2013].

1EE.A38. HEMANGIOMA

General

It can occur throughout the body, but particularly in the head; primary intraosseous orbital hemangiomas is rare; capillary hemangioma of the orbit and eyelids generally is unilateral.

Ocular

Hemangiomas of lids or orbit; ptosis; strabismus; amblyopia; proptosis; optic atrophy; hypermetropia; cavernous hemangiomas are the most common benign orbital tumors of adults.

Clinical

Ipsilateral hemangiomas of the brain and meninges.

Laboratory

Neuroimaging can be of great assistance in making the diagnosis.

Treatment

Most of these lesions regress on their own; there is no need for intervention. If spontaneous regression does not occur, corticosteroids, in various formulations, may be considered. Topical application of timolol has been useful in some cases.

BIBLIOGRAPHY

1. Karmel M. Topical timolol for capillary hemangioma. Eyenet. 2010.
2. Seiff S, Zwick OM, DeAngelis DD, et al. (2011). Capillary hemangioma. [online] Available from www.emedicine.com/oph/TOPIC691.HTM. [Accessed September, 2013].

🔲 1EE.A39. VON BEKHTEREV-STRUMPELL SYNDROME (MARIE-STRUMPELL SPONDYLITIS; ANKYLOSING SPONDYLITIS; PIERRE-MARIE SYNDROME; BEKHTEREV DISEASE; RHEUMATOID SPONDYLITIS) OPTIC ATROPHY

General

Variant of RA; etiology unknown; autosomal dominant; male preponderance; onset at age 20–40 years; although genetic background determines susceptibility to uveitis, the disease pattern suggests the possibility of random environmental triggers unrelated to the course of the underlying rheumatologic disorder.

Ocular

Nongranulomatous anterior uveitis; optic nerve atrophy (occasionally); hypopyon; band keratopathy; spontaneous hyphema.

Clinical

Spondylitis of vertebra and sacroiliac joints; ankylosis; general arthralgia; kyphosis; scoliosis; displaced head and total rigidity of spine.

Laboratory

Histocompatibility antigen human leukocyte antigen (HLA-B27) and a negative rheumatoid factor and ANA; X-ray evidence of narrowing of sacroiliac joint space and sclerosis.

Treatment

Oral NSAIDs, urethritis in Reiter's disease should be treated with tetracycline, topical steroids and cycloplegic agents.

🔲 BIBLIOGRAPHY

1. Vives MJ, Garfin SR. (2011). Rheumatoid arthritis of the cervical spine overview of rheumatoid spondylitis. [online] Available from www.emedicine.com/orthoped/TOPIC551. HTM. [Accessed September, 2013].

🔲 1EE.A40. HUNTER SYNDROME (MPS II SYNDROME; MUCOPOLYSACCHARIDOSIS II; SYSTEMIC MUCOPOLYSACCHARIDOSIS TYPE II)

General

Sex-linked recessive inheritance; clinically less severe than Hurler syndrome (MPS I) with a longer life span (into adulthood); similar to MPS I (Hurler syndrome), with chondroitin sulfate B and heparitin sulfate excreted in excess in the urine (*see* Sanfilippo-Good Syndrome; Morquio-Brailsford Syndrome; Scheie Syndrome; Maroteaux-Lamy Syndrome); X-linked recessive inheritance; decreased iduronate sulfatase.

Ocular

Visual fields may be constricted; splitting or absence of Bowman membrane in the periphery; stromal haze may be present; pigmentary degeneration of the retina; night blindness; narrowed retinal vessels and central choroidal sclerosis; bushy eyebrows; coarse eyelashes; ptosis; optic atrophy; papilledema; proptosis; angle-closure glaucoma; corneal clouding; scleral thickening; uveal effusion.

Clinical

Dwarfism; stiff joints; hepatosplenomegaly; gargoyle-like facies.

Laboratory

Urine-dermatan and heparin sulfate; serum-assay of iduronate 2-sulfatase (IDS) activity; assay for activity of sulfoiduronate sulfatase in fibroblasts.

Treatment

The relevant enzyme (IDS in the case of MPS type II) can be given in the form of ERT or by BMT; surgical intervention for chronic hydrocephalus, nerve entrapment (carpal tunnel syndrome), abdominal wall hernias, tracheostomy, and joint contractures.

BIBLIOGRAPHY

1. Braverman NE, Fenton CL, Conover-Walker MK. (2011). Genetics of Mucopolysaccharidosis Type II. Available from www.emedicine.com/ped/TOPIC1029.HTM. [Accessed September, 2013].

1EE.A41. HURLER SYNDROME (PFAUNDLER-HURLER SYNDROME; GARGOYLISM; DYSOSTOSIS MULTIPLEX; MPS IH SYNDROME; SYSTEMIC MUCOPOLYSACCHARIDOSIS TYPE IH; MUCOPOLYSACCHARIDOSIS IH)

General

Autosomal recessive inheritance; in addition to corneal opacities and enlargement of the head at birth, other symptoms become apparent at the end of the 1st year; death occurs usually before 20 years; gross excess of chondroitin sulfate band, heparitin sulfate in the urine (*see* Hunter Syndrome; Sanfilippo-Good Syndrome; Morquio-Brailsford Syndrome; Scheie Syndrome; Maroteaux-Lamy Syndrome). Jensen suggested that the pathogenesis of the various mucopolysaccharidoses is the same but that the variations in the defective enzymes cause the different types; most common MPS, decreased iduronidase.

Ocular

Proptosis; hypertelorism; thick, enlarged lids; esotropia; diffuse haziness of the cornea at birth progressive to milky opacity; retinal pigmentary changes may exist; macular edema and absence of foveal reflex; optic atrophy; megalocornea; bushy eyebrows; coarse eyelashes; mucopolysaccharide deposits of iris, lens, and sclera; enlarged optic foramen; retinal detachment; anisocoria; buphthalmos; nystagmus; secondary open-angle glaucoma; progressive retinopathy with vascular narrowing; hyperpigmentation of the fundus; bone spicule; papilledema.

Clinical

Dorsolumbar kyphosis; head deformities with depressed nose bridge; short cervical spine; short limbs; macroglossia; enlarged liver and spleen; short stature; facial dysmorphism; progressive psychomotor retardation.

Laboratory

Blood smears-abnormal cytoplasmic inclusions in lymphocytes; urine: increased excretion of dermatan sulfate and heparin sulfate.

Treatment

- *Macular edema*: Use of corticosteroids, carbonic anhydrase inhibitors and NSAIDs are the mainstay of treatment. If traditional therapy is not effective, intraocular injections of Avastin® may be helpful. In cases that have vitreous strand tugging against the macula, pars plana vitrectomy may be necessary.
- *Retinal detachment*: Scleral buckle, pneumatic retinopexy and vitrectomy may be used to close all the breaks.
- *Glaucoma*: Glaucoma medication should be the first plan of action. If medication is unsuccessful, a filtering surgical procedure with or without antimetabolites may be beneficial.
- *Papilledema*: Underlying cause should be determined and treated. Systemic acetazolamide is the medical therapy of choice.

BIBLIOGRAPHY

1. Banikazemi M. (2012). Genetics of mucopolysaccharidosis type I. [online] Available from www.emedicine.com/ped/TOPIC1031.HTM. [Accessed September, 2013].

🗗 1EE.A42. HYPERAMMONEMIA I (CARBAMYL PHOSPHATE SYNTHETASE DEFICIENCY; HYPERAMMONEMIA II; ORNITHINE TRANSCARBAMYLASE DEFICIENCY; HYPERAMMONEMIA-HYPERORNITHINEMIA-HOMOCITRULLINURIA SYNDROME)

General

Hyperammonemias I and II are due to errors at or near the "start" of the urea cycle; in hyperammonemia I, a decrease in the activity of the enzyme carbamyl phosphate synthetase, responsible for the first step of the cycle, results in the accumulation of excess ammonia; in hyperammonemia II, the defect is in ornithine transcarbamylase; type II occurs only in infants.

Ocular

Ptosis and visual loss; retinal depigmentation and chorioretinal thinning.

Clinical

Vomiting; screaming; confusion; lethargy; ataxia; mental retardation; atrophy of cerebral cortex; decreased vibration sense; bucco-faciolingual dyspraxia; learning difficulties; widespread manifestations in the central and peripheral nervous systems.

Laboratory

Plasma ornithine is increased at the time of presentation, which differentiates hyperornithinemia-hyperammonemia-homocitrullinemia (HHH) syndrome from other urea-cycle disorders.

Treatment

Ornithine supplementation, arginine supplementation, sodium benzoate and sodium phenylacetate may reduce ammonia levels; crisis might be managed with short-term protein restriction and intravenous fluids that contain large amounts of glucose.

🗗 BIBLIOGRAPHY

1. Frye RE, Benke PJ. (2013). Genetics of Hyperammonemia-Hyperornithinemia-Homocitrullinemia Syndrome. [online] Available from www.emedicine.com/ped/TOPIC1058.HTM. [Accessed September, 2012].

🗗 1EE.A43. KILOH-NEVIN SYNDROME (MUSCULAR DYSTROPHY OF EXTERNAL OCULAR MUSCLES; OCULAR MYOPATHY)

General

Etiology unknown; autosomal dominant.

Ocular

Ptosis; orbicularis muscle weakness; ocular myopathy; diplopia progressing to bilateral myopathic ophthalmoplegia; may be associated with pigmentary retinopathy and heart block (*see* Kearns-Sayre syndrome).

Clinical

Progressive muscular dystrophy in which facial muscles may be involved; occasionally, hereditary ataxia; pain; myokymia.

Laboratory

Diagnosis is made by clinical findings.

Treatment

Topical keratolytics, systemic and topical retinoids, potent topical steroids.

🗗 BIBLIOGRAPHY

1. Duszowa J, Koraszewska-Matuszewska B, Niebrój TK. The Kiloh-Nevin syndrome. Klin Oczna. 1974;44:805-7.
2. Kiloh LG, Nevin S. Progressive dystrophy of the external ocular muscles. Brain. 1951;74:115.

🗗 1EE.A44. KOHN-ROMANO SYNDROME (BPES SYNDROME)

General

Autosomal dominant transmittance; tetrad with telecanthus, ptosis, epicanthus inversus, and blepharophimosis; male preponderance; location of the abnormal gene responsible for this syndrome has been postulated to be a 3q2.

Ocular

Telecanthus; ptosis; epicanthus inversus; blepharophimoses; divergent strabismus; nystagmus; esotropia; anomalies of the lacrimal punctum; reduced corneal diameter.

Clinical

Highly arched palate; low-set ears with deformed pinnas.

Laboratory

Diagnosis is made by clinical findings.

Treatment

See ptosis, strabismus, lacrimal punctum obstruction.

🗗 BIBLIOGRAPHY

1. Suh DW. (2012). Congenital Ptosis. [online] Available from www.emedicine.com/oph/TOPIC345.HTM. [Accessed September, 2013].

🗗 1EE.A45. KOMOTO SYNDROME (CONGENITAL EYELID TETRAD; CET)

General

Autosomal dominant; all races affected; most patients are of normal intelligence.

Ocular

Ptosis; epicanthus inversus; blepharophimosis; telecanthus.

Clinical

None.

Laboratory

Diagnosis is made by clinical findings.

Treatment

Ptosis: If visual acuity is affected, most cases require surgical correction and there are several procedures that may be used including levator resection, repair or advancement and Fasanella-Servat.

🗗 BIBLIOGRAPHY

1. Bergin DJ, La Piana FG. Natural history of the congenital eyelid tetrad (Komoto's syndrome). Ann Ophthalmol. 1981;13:1145-8.
2. Komoto J. Veber die Operation be; Hereditaren Phimosis Congenita mit Ptosis. Nippon Ganka Gakkai 1920; 24, and Klin Monatsbl Augenheilkd. 1921;66:952.

🗗 1EE.A46. KUGELBERG-WELANDER SYNDROME (JUVENILE MUSCULAR ATROPHY)

General

Autosomal recessive; juvenile spinal muscular atrophy; affects both sexes; onset in late childhood or adolescence.

Ocular

Ptosis; ophthalmoplegia; exotropia; orbicularis oculi paresis.

Clinical

Slowly progressive proximal muscle atrophy; lower extremities usually are affected first, with the upper limbs being affected late; frequently, fasciculation; proximal muscle weakness, especially of the lower extremities; elevated serum creatine kinase levels.

Laboratory

Routine genetic testing only detects patients with the homozygous deletion; ultrasound of the muscles had been used to assess for neurogenic atrophy.

Treatment

No cure is known. Treatment is focused on symptomatic control and preventative rehabilitation.

🗗 BIBLIOGRAPHY

1. Oleszek JL, Vallee SE, Dichiaro M, et al. (2011). Kugelberg Welander Spinal Muscular Atrophy. [online] Available from www.emedicine.com/pmr/TOPIC62.HTM. [Accessed September, 2013].

🗗 1EE.A47. LAURENCE-MOON-BARDET-BIEDL SYNDROME (BARDET-BIEDL SYNDROME; RETINITIS PIGMENTOSA-POLYDACTYLY-ADIPOSOGENITAL SYNDROME)

General

Recessive, autosomal dominant, and recessive sex-linked gene; male preponderance; onset in childhood; cases of Laurence-Moon-Bardet-Biedl belong to the group of heredoataxias.

Ocular

Ptosis; epicanthus; nystagmus; strabismus; night blindness; myopia; hypermetropia; iris coloboma; RP "bone corpuscles"; macular degeneration; attenuation of retinal vessels; choroidal atrophy; optic nerve atrophy; cataract; microphthalmia; keratoconus.

Clinical

Obesity (Fröhlich type); hypogenitalism; reduced intelligence and mental retardation; turricephaly; shortness of stature; atresia ani; genu valgum; congenital heart disease; polydactyly; body hair scant or absent; pseudogynecomastia.

Laboratory

Chromosomal analysis is recommended to confirm chromosomal sex and to evaluate for associated genetic syndromes.

Treatment

Consultation by pediatric endocrinologist and pediatric urologist is usually necessary.

🗗 BIBLIOGRAPHY

1. Telander DG, de Beus A, Small KW. (2012). Retinitis pigmentosa. [online] Available from www.emedicine.com/oph/TOPIC704.HTM. [Accessed September, 2013].

🗗 1EE.A48. LEIGH SYNDROME (SUBACUTE NECROTIZING ENCEPHALOMYELOPATHY; INFANTILE SUBACUTE NECROTIZING ENCEPHALOMYELOPATHY; HYPERPYRUVICEMIA WITH HYPER-ALPHA-ALANINEMIA; GANGLIOSIDOSIS G_{M2} TYPE 3)

General

Autosomal recessive; metabolic disease occurring in infancy and childhood with increased levels of serum lactate, serum pyruvates, blood α-ketoglutarate, and aminoaciduria; course is remittent with early neuro-ophthalmologic manifestations and psychomotor retardation; the later the onset of clinical manifestations, the longer the survival time; acute form in young infants, subacute form in older infants, and chronic course in juveniles; mutation at nt8993 of mitochondrial DNA has been reported as a common cause of Leigh syndrome; biochemical analysis revealed cytochrome c oxidase deficiency with this condition.

Ocular

Nystagmoid movements or nystagmus; disconjugate ocular movements due to tegmental involvement of brainstem; degrees of visual impairment, depending on pathologic changes involving optic nerves and tracts; optic nerve atrophy; oculomotor palsy; supranuclear gaze palsy; blindness.

Clinical

Spasticity of extremities; ataxia; muscular weakness; hemiparesis; progressive mental deterioration; hearing defects; dysphagia; dyspnea; mild hypotonia; slow development; intermittent abnormal respiratory rhythm; cranial nerve palsies.

Laboratory

Diagnosis is made by clinical findings.

Treatment

None—ocular.

⊟ BIBLIOGRAPHY

1. Revilla FJ, Raghavan R. (2013). Ataxia with Identified Genetic and Biochemical Defects. [online] Available from www.emedicine.com/neuro/TOPIC556.HTM. [Accessed September, 2013].

⊟ 1EE.A49. LITTLE SYNDROME (NAIL-PATELLA SYNDROME; HEREDITARY OSTEO-ONYCHO-DYSPLASIA; HOOD SYNDROME)

General

Inherited as autosomal dominant; affects males and females equally.

Ocular

Hypertelorism; ptosis; epicanthus; microcornea; keratoconus; sclerocornea; cataract; microphakia; light pigmentation of iris root with dark pigmented "clover-leaf" spots, referred to as the Lester line, not seen in all cases.

Clinical

Absent or hypoplastic patella; hypoplastic or dislocated head of radius; exostosis of skull bones; bilateral horns of iliac crests; longitudinal ridging of fingernails; glomerulonephritis; renal involvement; bilateral antecubital pterygia; arthrogryposis; disorder has been mapped to the long arm of chromosome 9; sensorineural hearing loss.

Laboratory

Conduct urinalysis, along with a microscopic analysis, to check for proteinuria and hematuria. Radiography findings reveal iliac horns. MRI to identify abnormal muscle insertions; renal biopsy.

Treatment

Renal dialysis and transplantation are necessary.

⊟ BIBLIOGRAPHY

1. Hoover-Fong J, McIntosh I, Sweeney E. (2012). Genetics of nail-patella syndrome. [online] Available from www.emedicine.com/ped/TOPIC1546.HTM. [Accessed September, 2013].

⊟ 1EE.A50. MERRF SYNDROME

General

Associated with mitochondrial tRNA [Leu(UUR)] A3243G mutation.

Ocular

Optic neuropathy; pigmentary retinopathy, ophthalmoparesis, and ptosis.

Clinical

Mitochondrial encephalomyopathy; lactic acidosis; stroke-like episodes.

Laboratory/Ocular

Erythrocyte sedimentation rate, C-reactive protein.

Treatment/Ocular

Prednisone.

⊟ BIBLIOGRAPHY

1. Hwang JM, Park HW, Kim SJ. Optic neuropathy associated with mitochondrial tRNA[Leu(UUR)] A3243G mutation. Ophthalmic Genet. 1997;18:101-5.

⊟ 1EE.A51A2. COLOBOMATOUS, MICROPHTHALMIA AND MICROCORNEA SYNDROME

General

Autosomal dominant pattern of inheritance with complete penetrance.

Ocular

Bilateral inferonasal coloboma; axial enlargement; myopia; iridocorneal angle abnormalities; elevated IOP.

Clinical

None.

Laboratory

Diagnosis is made by clinical findings.

Treatment

See glaucoma.

⊟ BIBLIOGRAPHY

1. Toker E, Elcioglu N, Ozcan E, et al. Colobomatous macrophthalmia with microcornea syndrome: report of a new pedigree. Am J Med Genet. 2003;121A(1):25-30.

⊟ 1EE.A51A3. SJÖGREN-LARSSON SYNDROME (OLIGOPHRENIA ICHTHYOSIS SPASTIC DIPLEGIA SYNDROME)

General

Rare; autosomal recessive; consanguinity; loss of neurons and gliosis throughout gray matter; autosomal recessively inherited disorder characterized by the triad of congenital ichthyosis, spastic diplegia or tetraplegia, and mental retardation.

Ocular

Hypertelorism; ichthyosis of lid; chorioretinitis with macular and perimacular pigment degeneration or bright, glistening intraretinal dots; atypical retinitis pigmentosa; blepharitis; conjunctivitis; keratitis; tan/white areas of retinal pigment epithelium loss; maculopathy.

Clinical

Oligophrenia idiocy; ichthyosis (congenital); spastic disorders; epilepsy; speech defect.

Laboratory

Measurement of fatty aldehyde dehydrogenase (FALDH) or fatty alcohol: NAD+ oxidoreductase on cultured skin fibroblast.

Treatment

Moisturizing creams and keratolytic agent such as alpha-hydroxyacid, salicylic acid, and urea. Standard anticonvulsant are used to treat recurrent seizures. Surgery procedures such as tendon lengthening, adduction release, dorsal root rhizotomy may help some patients with SLS.

⊟ BIBLIOGRAPHY

1. Rizzo WB. (2012). Genetics of Sjogren-Larsson syndrome. [online] Available from www.emedicine.com/ped/TOPIC2111.HTM. [Accessed September, 2013].
2. Rob L, Veen VD, Fuijkschot J, et.al. Patients with Sjögren-Larsson syndrome lack macular pigment. Ophthalmology. 2010;117:966-71.

⊟ 1EE.A51A10. RETINITIS PIGMENTOSA

General

Inherited progressive retinal disorder may have changes in ear or kidney.

Clinical

Hearing defect and kidney defect can be associated with the disease.

Ocular

Waxy-pole optic nerve, bonespickle pigmentation, posterior subcapsular cataract, visual field defect.

Laboratory

Diagnosis is made by clinical findings. A diagnostic genetic test is available and differentiates between simplex retinitis pigmentosa (RP) and autosomal recessive RP.

Treatment

Vitamin A 15,000 IU/day is thought to slow the decline of retinal function, dark sunglasses for outdoor use, surgery for cataract, genetic counseling.

⊟ BIBLIOGRAPHY

1. Clark GR, Crowe P, Muszynska D, et al. Development of a diagnostic genetic test for simplex and autosomal recessive retinitis pigmentosa. Ophthalmology. 2010;117:2169-77.e3.
2. Telander DG, de Beus A, Small KW. (2013). Retinitis pigmentosa. [online] Available from www.emedicine.com/oph/TOPIC704.HTM. [Accessed September, 2013].

⊟ 1EE.A51B1A. AICARDI SYNDROME

General

All symptoms present at birth; cause unknown; all findings progress with age; shows X-linked dominant inheritance.

Ocular

Microphthalmia; lid twitching; absent pupillary reflexes; round retinal lacunae up to disk size look likc holes with retinal vessels crossing over them; funnel-shaped disk; chorioretinitis.

Clinical

Infantile spasms (tonic seizures in flexion); epileptic seizures; cyanosis; mental anomaly; vertebral anomalies; telangiectasia; hypotonia; head deformities with biparietal bossing, occipital flattening, and plagiocephaly; defects of corpus callosum; cortical heterotopia; characteristic electroencephalogram; dilated intracranial ventricle with leukomalacia.

Laboratory

Generally diagnosis is made by clinical findings. Neuroimaging can delineate the degree of CNS dysgenesis and help to evaluate other potential etiologies of intractable epilepsy and developmental delay.

Treatment

Consultation with a child neurologist is recommended. Use of traditional epilepsy therapies for seizure manifestations is recommended.

⊟ BIBLIOGRAPHY

1. Davis RG, DiFazio MP. (2012). Aicardi syndrome. [online] Available from www.emedicine.com/ped/TOPIC58.HTM. [Accessed September, 2013].

⊟ 1EE.A51B1B. BLOCH-SULZBERGER SYNDROME (INCONTINENTIA PIGMENTI; SIEMENS-BLOCH-SULZBERGER SYNDROME)

General

Familial disorder affecting ectoderm; manifestations at birth; female predominance; X-linked dominant phenotype; disturbance of skin pigmentation.

Ocular

Orbital mass; retrolental fibroplasia; pseudoglioma; strabismus; blue sclera; cataract; optic nerve atrophy; papillitis; nystagmus; chorioretinitis; anomalies of chamber angle; neo–vascularization of retina; retinal hemorrhages and edema; microphthalmia; tractional retinal detachment.

Clinical

Dental and skeletal anomalies common; neurologic abno–rmalities; recurrent inflammatory lesions; skin melanin pigmentation on the trunk: (marble cake); occipital lobe infarct; neonatal infarction of the macula.

Laboratory

CT scan or MRI of the brain should be performed.

Treatment

No specific treatment. Lesions should be left intact and kept clean and meticulous dental care is very important.

⊟ BIBLIOGRAPHY

1. Chang CH. (2012). Neurologic manifestations of incontinentia pigmenti. [online] Available from www.emedicine.com/neuro/TOPIC169.HTM. [Accessed September, 2013].

⊟ 1EE.A51B1C. GOLTZ SYNDROME (FOCAL DERMAL HYPOPLASIA SYNDROME)

General

X-linked dominant inheritance; lethal in males; skin manifestations present at birth.

Ocular

Microphthalmia; strabismus; coloboma of iris and/or choroid; epiphora; blue sclera; nystagmus; anophthalmos; keratoconus.

Clinical

Skin atrophy and linear pigmentation; telangiectasias of trunk and extremities; superficial, localized fatty skin deposits; multiple papillomas of mucous membranes and periorificial skin (oral, genital, anal); anomalies of extremities with syndactyly, oligodactyly, adactyly; hypohidrosis; paper-thin nails may be present; spina bifida; hypoplasia of right clavicle; umbilical or inguinal hernia.

Laboratory

Radiography may reveal osteopathia striata.

Treatment

Flashlamp-pumped pulse dye laser may ameliorate the pruritic symptoms that sometimes are noted in affected skin and improve the clinical appearance of the telangiectatic and erythematous skin lesions. Papillomas frequently require repeated surgical intervention.

⊟ BIBLIOGRAPHY

1. Goltz RW, Castelo-Soccio L. (2012). Focal dermal hypoplasia syndrome. [online] Available from emedicine.medscape.com/article/1110936-overview. [Accessed September, 2013].

🗗 1EE.A51B1D. LENZ MICROPHTHALMIA SYNDROME

General

X-linked recessive; female carriers.

Ocular

Microphthalmia; microcornea; ocular coloboma; colobomatous microphthalmia.

Clinical

Skeletal abnormalities of vertebral column, clavicles, and limbs; severe renal dysgenesis and hydroureters; dental anomalies; hypospadias and bilateral cryptorchidism; severe speech impairment; shortness of stature; long, cylindrical, and thin thorax; sloping shoulders; flat feet.

Laboratory

Diagnosis is made by clinical findings.

Treatment

None—ocular.

🗗 BIBLIOGRAPHY

1. Antoniades K, Tzouvelekis G, Doudou A, et al. A sporadic case of Lenz microphthalmia syndrome. Ann Ophthalmol. 1993;25:342-5.
2. Herrmann J, Optiz JM. The Lenz microphthalmia syndrome. Birth Defects. 1969;5:138-48.

🗗 1EE.A51B2B. ELLIS-VAN CREVELD SYNDROME (CHONDROECTODERMAL DYSPLASIA)

General

Autosomal recessive inheritance; occurs in the Amish; associated with *de novo* chromosomal abnormality: deletion of 12 (p11.21p12.2).

Ocular

Esotropia; iris coloboma; congenital cataract.

Clinical

Bilateral polydactyly; short and plump limbs; genu valgum; talipes (equinovarus, calcaneovalgus); thoracic constriction; fusion of middle part of upper lip to maxillary gingival margin; dental anomalies: number, shape, spacing; congenital heart defect in about 50% of patients; dystrophic fingernails; genital anomalies; mild mental retardation; short stature; hypoplastic hair and skin; oligodontia; small thoracic cage; hypoplastic pelvis; cone-shaped epiphyses of hands.

Laboratory

Clinical.

Treatment

- *Esotropia*: Equalized vision with correct refractive error; surgery may be helpful in patient with diplopia.
- *Retinal detachment*: Scleral buckle, pneumatic retinopexy and vitrectomy may be used to close all the breaks.

🗗 BIBLIOGRAPHY

1. Chen H. (2013). Ellis-van Creveld Syndrome. [online] Available from www.emedicine.com/ped/TOPIC660.HTM. [Accessed September, 2013].

1EE.A51B2C. JOUBERT SYNDROME (FAMILIAL CEREBELLAR VERMIS AGENESIS)

General

Autosomal recessive; both sexes affected; onset in early infancy.

Ocular

Choroidal coloboma; nystagmus; ocular fibrosis, telecanthus.

Clinical

Episodic hyperpnea; apnea; ataxia; psychomotor retardation; rhythmic protrusion of tongue; mental retardation; micrognathia; complex cardiac malformation; cutaneous dimples over wrists and elbows.

Laboratory

Urine culture, renal ultrasonography, dimercaptosuccinic acid (DMSA) renal scanning.

Treatment

Lifetime follow-up is required whether or not involution has occurred or a nephrectomy.

BIBLIOGRAPHY

1. Swiatecka-Urban A. (2011). Multicystic renal dysplasia. [online] Available from www.emedicine.com/ped/TOPIC1493.HTM. [Accessed September, 2013].

1EE.A51B2E. KARTAGENER SYNDROME (SINUSITIS-BRONCHIECTASIS-SITUS INVERSUS SYNDROME; BRONCHIECTASIS-DEXTROCARDIA-SINUSITIS; KARTAGENER TRIAD)

General

Autosomal recessive; onset in early infancy; occasionally dominant; finding of various structural defects in patients with this condition suggests that there are several genetic determinants.

Ocular

Myopia; glaucoma; conjunctival melanosis; iris coloboma; tortuous and dilated retinal vessels; retinal pigmentary degeneration; pseudopapillitis.

Clinical

Immotile cilia; situs inversus; bronchiectasis; sinusitis; various cardiovascular and renal abnormalities; dyspnea; productive cough; recurrent respiratory infections; palpitation; otitis media; nasal speech; conductive hearing loss; nasal polyps; situs inversus viscerum with hepatic dullness on left side.

Laboratory

High-resolution CT scan of the chest is the most sensitive modality for documenting early and subtle abnormalities within airways and pulmonary parenchyma when compared to routine chest radiographs.

Treatment

Antibiotics, intravenous or oral and continuous or intermittent, are used to treat upper and lower airway infections. Obstructive lung disease, if present, should be treated with inhaled bronchodilators and aggressive pulmonary toilet. Tympanostomy tubes are required to reduce conductive hearing loss and recurrent infections.

BIBLIOGRAPHY

1. Bent JP, Willis EB. (2013). Kartagener syndrome. [online] Available from www.emedicine.com/med/TOPIC1220.HTM. [Accessed September, 2013].

🗗 1EE.A51B2F. LAURENCE-MOON-BARDET-BIEDL SYNDROME (BARDET-BIEDL SYNDROME; RETINITIS PIGMENTOSA-POLYDACTYLY-ADIPOSOGENITAL SYNDROME)

General

Recessive, autosomal dominant, and recessive sex-linked gene; male preponderance; onset in childhood; cases of Laurence-Moon-Bardet-Biedl belong to the group of heredoataxias.

Ocular

Ptosis; epicanthus; nystagmus; strabismus; night blindness; myopia; hypermetropia; iris coloboma; RP "bone corpuscles"; macular degeneration; attenuation of retinal vessels; choroidal atrophy; optic nerve atrophy; cataract; microphthalmia; keratoconus.

Clinical

Obesity (Fröhlich type); hypogenitalism; reduced intelligence and mental retardation; turricephaly; shortness of stature; atresia ani; genu valgum; congenital heart disease; polydactyly; body hair scant or absent; pseudogynecomastia.

Laboratory

Chromosomal analysis is recommended to confirm chromosomal sex and to evaluate for associated genetic syndromes.

Treatment

Consultation by pediatric endocrinologist and pediatric urologist is usually necessary.

🗗 BIBLIOGRAPHY

1. Telander DG, de Beus A, Small KW. (2012). Retinitis pigmentosa. [online] Available from www.emedicine.com/oph/TOPIC704.HTM. [Accessed September, 2013].

🗗 1EE.A51B2G. MARINESCO-SJÖGREN SYNDROME (CONGENITAL SPINOCEREBELLAR ATAXIA-CONGENITAL CATARACT-OLIGOPHRENIA SYNDROME)

General

Autosomal recessive trait; onset when child learns to walk; mitochondrial disease.

Ocular

Cataracts; aniridia; rotary and horizontal nystagmus; nystagmus; strabismus; optic atrophy.

Clinical

Cerebellar ataxia; oligophrenia; small stature; scoliosis; genu valgum; restricted extensibility of the knee; defects of fingers and toes; mental retardation; hair sparse; hypersalivation; sensorineural hearing loss.

Laboratory

Diagnosis is made by clinical findings.

Treatment

Cataracts: Change in glasses can sometimes improve a patient's visual function temporarily; however, the most common treatment is cataract surgery.

🗗 BIBLIOGRAPHY

1. Dotti MT, Bardelli AM, De Stefano N, et al. Optic atrophy in Marinesco-Sjögren syndrome: an additional ocular feature: Report of three cases in two families. Ophthalmic Genet. 1993;14(1):5-7.
2. Gillespie FD. Aniridia, cerebellar ataxia, and oligophrenia in siblings. Arch Ophthalmol. 1965;73(3):338-41.

⊟ 1EE.A51B2H. MECKEL SYNDROME (DYSENCEPHALIA SPLANCHNOCYSTIC SYNDROME; GRUBER SYNDROME)

General

Autosomal recessive; ocular manifestations are similar to those of trisomy 13–15 syndrome.

Ocular

Cryptophthalmos; clinical anophthalmos; microphthalmos; mongoloid slant of lid fissures; sclerocornea; microcornea; partial aniridia; cataract; retinal dysplasia; posterior staphyloma; optic nerve hypoplasia.

Clinical

Sloping forehead; posterior encephalocele; short neck; polydactyly and syndactyly (hands and feet); polycystic kidneys; cryptorchidism; cleft lip and palate; CNS abnormalities, including the Dandy-Walker malformation.

Laboratory

Chromosome analysis, MRI.

Treatment

Cardiac surgery may be warranted.

⊟ BIBLIOGRAPHY

1. Jayakar PB, Spiliopoulos M, Jayakar A. (2011). Meckel-Gruber syndrome. [online] Available from www.emedicine.com/ped/TOPIC1390.HTM. [Accessed September, 2013].

⊟ 1EE.A51B2I. MICRO SYNDROME

General

Autosomal recessive microcephaly and microcornea; Muslim Pakistani inheritance; present at birth; consanguinity; autosomal recessive.

Ocular

Microcornea; congenital cataract; retinal dystrophy; optic nerve atrophy; ptosis; microphakia; microphthalmos; nuclear cataract; atonic pupils.

Clinical

Severe mental retardation; hypothalamic hypogenitalism; hypoplasia of the corpus callosum; short stature; cortical visual impairment; microcephaly; developmental delay.

Laboratory/Congenital Cataracts

Dilated examination, TORCH titers and VDRL test.

Treatment/Congenital Cataracts

Cataract surgery is the treatment of choice.

⊟ BIBLIOGRAPHY

1. Ainsworth JR, Morton JE, Good P, et al. Micro syndrome in Muslim Pakistan children. Ophthalmology. 2001;108: 491-7.
2. Mégarbané A, Choueiri R, Bleik J, et al. Microcephaly, microphthalmia, congenital cataract, optic atrophy, short stature, hypotonia. Severe psychomotor retardation, and cerebral malformations: a second family with micro syndrome or a new syndrome? J Med Genet. 1999;36:637-40.
3. Rodriguez C, Rufo M, Gomez de Terreros I. A second family with micro syndrome. Clin Dysmorphol. 1999;8:241-5.
4. Warburg M, Sjö O, Fledelius HC, et al. Autosomal recessive microcephaly, microcornea, congenital cataract, mental retardation, optic atrophy, and hypogenitalism: micro syndrome. Am J Dis Child. 1993;147:1309-12.

1EE.A51B2J. SJÖGREN-LARSSON SYNDROME (OLIGOPHRENIA ICHTHYOSIS SPASTIC DIPLEGIA SYNDROME)

General

Rare; autosomal recessive; consanguinity; loss of neurons and gliosis throughout gray matter; autosomal recessively inherited disorder characterized by the triad of congenital ichthyosis, spastic diplegia or tetraplegia, and mental retardation.

Ocular

Hypertelorism; ichthyosis of lid; chorioretinitis with macular and perimacular pigment degeneration or bright, glistening intraretinal dots; atypical retinitis pigmentosa; blepharitis; conjunctivitis; keratitis; tan/white areas of retinal pigment epithelium loss; maculopathy.

Clinical

Oligophrenia idiocy; ichthyosis (congenital); spastic disorders; epilepsy; speech defect.

Laboratory

Measurement of fatty aldehyde dehydrogenase (FALDH) or fatty alcohol: NAD+ oxidoreductase on cultured skin fibroblast.

Treatment

Moisturizing creams and keratolytic agent such as alpha-hydroxyacid, salicylic acid, and urea. Standard anticonvulsant are use to treat recurrent seizures. Surgery procedures such as tendon lengthening, adduction release, dorsal root rhizotomy may help some patients with SLS.

BIBLIOGRAPHY

1. Rizzo WB. (2012). Genetics of Sjogren-Larsson syndrome. [online] Available from www.emedicine.com/ped/TOPIC2111.HTM. [Accessed September, 2013].
2. Rob L, Veen VD, Fuijkschot J, et.al. Patients with Sjögren-Larsson syndrome lack macular pigment. Ophthalmology. 2010;117:966-71.

1EE.A51B2K. WALKER-WARBURG SYNDROME (CEREBROOCULAR DYSPLASIA-MUSCULAR DYSTROPHY; WARBURG SYNDROME; COD-MD SYNDROME; FUKUYAMA CONGENITAL MUSCULAR DYSTROPHY; HARD + OR - E SYNDROME) CATARACT

General

Rare; encompassing a triad of brain, eye, and muscle abnormalities; probably autosomal recessive.

Ocular

Microphthalmia; cataract; immature anterior chamber angle; retinal dysplasia; retinal detachment; persistent hyperplastic primary vitreous; optic nerve hypoplasia; iris coloboma; opaque cornea; myopia; orbicularis weakness; irregular gray subretinal mottling; optic atrophy.

Clinical

Cerebral and cerebellar agyria-micropolygyria; cortical disorganization; glial mesodermal proliferation; neuronal heterotopias; hypoplasia of nerve tracts; hydrocephalus; encephalocele; muscular dystrophy; seizures; mental retardation; hypotonia; abnormal facies.

Laboratory

MRI, creatine kinases levels, electromyography and nerve conduction study.

Treatment

No specific treatment is available.

BIBLIOGRAPHY

1. Lopate G. (2013). Congenital Muscular Dystrophy. [online] Available from www.emedicine.com/neuro/TOPIC549.HTM. [Accessed September, 2013].

1EE.A51B3A. MARFAN SYNDROME (DOLICHOSTENOMELIA; ARACHNODACTYLY; HYPERCHONDROPLASIA; DYSTROPHIA MESODERMALIS CONGENITA)

General

Hypoplastic form of dystrophia mesodermalis congenita; autosomal dominant; affects both sexes. It has been demonstrated that an abnormality of the gene coding for the connective tissue protein fibrillin is responsible for chronic Marfan syndrome.

Ocular

Exotropia; nystagmus; paralysis of accommodation; myopia (axial or lenticular); iridodonesis; miosis; persistent pupillary membrane; blue sclera; spherophakia; lens dislocation; cataract; megalocornea; retinal detachment (less frequently); pigmentary retinopathy; colobomata of macula, iris, optic nerve, and uveal tract (less frequently); keratoconus; central retinal artery occlusion; rhegmatogenous retinal detachment; syringoma.

Clinical

Arachnodactyly; skeletal anomalies; asymmetric thorax; dolichocephaly and high-arched palate; dissecting aneurysm; mitral valve prolapse; prominent ears; kyphoscoliosis; pectus excavatum; flat feet; hammer toes; pulmonary and kidney defects.

Laboratory

Genetic testing, molecular studies.

Treatment

- *Keratoconus*: Spectacle correction, hard contacts, avoid eye rubbing. If hydrops occur, discontinue contact lens, use sodium chloride (NaCl) drops and ointment, patching, and short course of steroids. As disease advances, PK, deep anterior lamellar keratoplasty intacs with laser grooves or collagen stabilization of cornea.
- *Cataract*: Change in glasses can sometimes improve a patient's visual function temporarily; however the most common treatment is cataract surgery.
- *Glaucoma*: Glaucoma medication should be the first plan of action. If medication is unsuccessful, a filtering surgical procedure with or without antimetabolites may be beneficial.
- *Strabismus*: Equalized vision with correct refractive error; surgery may be helpful in patient with diplopia.

BIBLIOGRAPHY

1. Chen H. (2011). Genetics of Marfan syndrome. [online] Available from www.emedicine.com/ped/TOPIC1372.HTM. [Accessed September, 2013].

1EE.A51B3B. CROUZON SYNDROME (DYSOSTOSIS CRANIOFACIALIS; OXYCEPHALY; CRANIOFACIAL DYSOSTOSIS; PARROT-HEAD SYNDROME; MÖBIUS-CROUZON SYNDROME; HEREDITARY CRANIOFACIAL DYSOSTOSIS)

General

Autosomal dominant; manifestations present at birth.

Ocular

Bilateral exophthalmos; hypertelorism (wide interpupillary distance); obliquity of palpebral fissures with outer canthus slanting downward; nystagmus; exotropia; upper field defects due to pressure upon the optic nerve on its lower part; bluish sclera; exposure keratitis in extreme exophthalmos; cataract; papilledema; secondary optic atrophy; corneal dystrophy; ptosis; strabismus; keratoconus.

Clinical

Prognathism; maxillary hypoplasia with short upper lip; synostosis of coronal and lambda sutures; parrot-beaked nose (psittachosrhina); widening temporal fossae; headaches.

Laboratory

Skull, spine, and hand radiography is usually necessary to confirm the diagnosis.

Treatment

Neurosurgical procedure is recommended in cases of intracranial hypertension leading to further optic atrophy.

BIBLIOGRAPHY

1. Chen H. (2013). Genetics of Crouzon syndrome. [online] Available from www.emedicine.com/ped/TOPIC511.HTM. [Accessed September, 2013].

⊡ 1EE.A51B3C. STICKLER SYNDROME (HEREDITARY PROGRESSIVE ARTHRO-OPHTHALMOPATHY)

General

Autosomal dominant; onset in childhood; severe and debilitating connective tissue disorder inherited as an autosomal dominant syndrome with a variable phenotype; linkage analysis has provided statistical evidence for linkage of collagen type II (COL2A1) gene with this syndrome in some but not all families.

Ocular

Phthisis bulbi; glaucoma; chronic uveitis; keratopathy; complicated cataracts; chorioretinal degeneration; total retinal detachment during 1st decade of life; myopia; giant retinal tears.

Clinical

Bony enlargement of joints with abnormal development of the articular surfaces and premature degenerative changes; hypermobility of joints with abnormality in connective tissues supporting the joints; possible skeletal deformities.

Laboratory

Bone radiographs and a full genetic evaluation is appropriate.

Treatment

The primary concern is airway obstruction. Tracheotomy tube is effective in bypassing the obstruction. If feeding difficulties, special cleft nursing bottles are available. If this is not enough, gavage or feeding tubes can provide temporary nutrition.

⊡ BIBLIOGRAPHY

1. Tolarova MM. (2012). Pierre Robin Malformation. [online] Available from www.emedicine.com/ped/TOPIC2680. HTM. [Accessed September, 2013].

⊡ 1EE.A51B3D. FRANCESCHETTI SYNDROME (FRANCESCHETTI-ZWAHLEN-KLEIN SYNDROME; TREACHER COLLINS SYNDROME; MANDIBULOFACIAL DYSOSTOSIS; MANDIBULOFACIAL SYNDROME; EYELID-MALAR-MANDIBLE SYNDROME; OCULOVERTEBRAL SYNDROME; BERRY SYNDROME; FRANCESCHETTI-ZWAHLEN SYNDROME; ZWAHLEN SYNDROME; BILATERAL FACIAL AGENESIS; BERRY-FRANCESCHETTI-KLEIN SYNDROME; FRANCESCHETTI-KLEIN SYNDROME; FRANCESCHETTI SYNDROME (II); TREACHER COLLINS-FRANCESCHETTI SYNDROME; WEYERS-THIER SYNDROME)

General

Irregular dominant inheritance; Weyers-Thier syndrome has similar features, except it is a unilateral variant; prevalent in Caucasians.

Ocular

Microphthalmia; oblique position of eyes with lateral downward slope of palpebral fissures; temporal lower lid coloboma; lack of cilia on middle third of lower lid; iris coloboma; underdeveloped orbicularis oculi muscle; cataract; optic disk hypoplasia.

Clinical

Fish-like face with sunken cheek bones, receding chin, and large, wide mouth; absent or malformed external ears with auricular appendages; high palate and possible harelip; hypoplastic zygomatic arch with absence of normal malar eminences; prolonged hairline on the cheek; deafness; micrognathia; glossoptosis; cleft palate.

Laboratory

Full craniofacial CT scan (axial and coronal slices from the top of the skull through the cervical spine), brain MRI.

Treatment

Operative repair is based upon the anatomic deformity and timing of correction is done according to physiologic need and development.

🗗 BIBLIOGRAPHY

1. Tolarova MM, Wong GB, Varma S. (2012). Mandibulofacial Dysostosis (Treacher Collins Syndrome). [online] Available from www.emedicine.com/ped/TOPIC1364.HTM. [Accessed September, 2013].

🗗 1EE.A51B3E. BOURNEVILLE SYNDROME (BOURNEVILLE-PRINGLE SYNDROME; TUBEROUS SCLEROSIS; EPILOIA)

General

Irregular dominant inheritance; more frequent in females; most patients die before age 24 years.

Ocular

Vitreous often cloudy; lens opacities; retinal mushroom-like tumor of grayish-white color; yellowish-white plaques with small hemorrhages and cystic changes in retina; papilledema; disk drusen; cerebral astrocytoma; 40–50% of patients have normal intelligence.

Clinical

Grand mal, petit mal, or Jacksonian seizures (manifest in first 2 years of life); mental changes from feeble minded-ness to imbecility and idiocy; skin changes arranged usually about nose and cheeks (adenoma sebaceum); congenital tumors of kidney (hypernephroma or tubular adenoma) and heart (rhabdomyoma); cerebral astrocytoma.

Laboratory

Brain MRI is recommended for the detection and follow-up imaging of cortical tubers.

Treatment

A neurologist should be consulted to assist with seizure management and anticonvulsant medication.

🗗 BIBLIOGRAPHY

1. Schwartz RA, Jozwiak S, Pedersen R. (2013). Genetics of tuberous sclerosis. [online] Available from www.emedicine.com/ped/TOPIC2796.HTM. [Accessed September, 2013].

🗗 1EE.A51B3F. ZELLWEGER SYNDROME (CEREBROHEPATORENAL SYNDROME OF ZELLWEGER)

General

Rare; congenital; lethal disease; prevalent in females; demyelination of cerebral white matter, spinal cord, and peripheral spinal cord and peripheral nerves; enzymatic defects cause myelin deficiency (*see* Smith-Lemli-Opitz Syndrome); severe multisevere multisystem disorder resul-ting from defective biogenesis of the peroxisome causes death within the 1st year.

Ocular

Hypertelorism; microphthalmia; nystagmus; glaucoma; hemimydriasis; corneal opacities; cataract; narrowing of retinal vessels; pigment irregularities and areas of depig-mentation; retinal holes without detachment; tapetoreti-nal detachment; tapetoretinal degeneration; irregular border-lined optic disks; gray-colored disks; hypoplastic supraorbital ridges; optic atrophy.

Clinical

Hypotony; hepatomegaly; albuminuria; mental retarda-tion; failure to thrive; vomiting; seizures; low birth weight; jaundice; short stature; broad nose; hypospadias; cryptor-chidism; septal defect; craniofacial dysmorphic features; high forehead; renal cyst; psychomotor retardation; hepat-osplenomegaly; severe hearing impairment.

Laboratory

Diagnosis is made by clinical findings.

Treatment

Multisystem disorder will involve separate specialities to treat the specific disorders.

BIBLIOGRAPHY

1. Fenichel F, Fenichel GM. Cerebrohepatorenal syndrome (Zellweger syndrone). In: Fenichel GM (Ed). Clinical Pediatric Neurology, 2nd edition. Philadelphia: WB Saunders; 1993. p. 151.
2. Bowen P, Lee CS, Zellweger H, et al. A familial syndrome of multiple congenital defects. Bull Johns Hopkins Hosp. 1964;114:402-14.

1EE.A51B4A. 4Q SYNDROME

General

Chromosome 4q deletion syndrome.

Ocular

Hypertelorism, epicanthal folds.

Clinical

Depressed nasal bridge; short nasal septum with up-turned nose, cleft lip and palate; micrognathia; low-set malformed ears; short neck; distally placed nipples; sacral dimple; hypospadias; dysplastic nails; overriding toes; simian creases; hypoplasia of gall bladder; cardiac defects; mental retardation.

Laboratory

Diagnosis is made by clinical findings.

Treatment

See hypertelorism and epicanthal fold.

BIBLIOGRAPHY

1. Robertson SP, O'Day K, Banker A. The 4q- syndrome: delineating of the minimal critical region to within band 4q31. Clin Genet. 1998;53:70-73.
2. Townes PL, White M, DiMarzo SV. 4q- syndrome. Am J Dis Child. 1979;133:383-5.
3. Yu CW, Chen H, Baucum RW, et al. Terminal deletion of the long arm of chromosome 4. Report of a case of 46,XY,del(4)(q31) and review of 4q- syndrome. Ann Genet. 1981;24:158-61.

1EE.A51B4B. 11Q- SYNDROME

General

Chromosome II deletion syndrome.

Ocular

Telecanthus/hypertelorism; rarely, congenital glaucoma, cyclopia.

Clinical

Psychomotor retardation, trigonocephaly, broad depressed nasal bridge, micrognathia, low-set abnormal ears, cardiac anomalies, hand and foot anomalies, renal agenesis, anal atresia, supratentorial white matter abnormality on CT or MRI; microphallus; holoprosencephaly; female preponderance.

Laboratory

Clinical.

Treatment

See congenital glaucoma.

BIBLIOGRAPHY

1. Helmuth RA, Weaver DD, Wills ER. Holoprosencephaly, ear abnormalities, congenital heart defect, and microphallus in a patient with 11q- mosaicism. Am J Med Genet. 1989;32:178-81.
2. Ishida Y, Watanabe N, Ishihara Y, et al. The 11q- syndrome with mosaic partial deletion of 11q. Acta Paediatr Jpn. 1992;34:592-6.
3. Leegte B, Kerstjens-Frederikse WS, Deelstra K, et al. 11q-syndrome: three cases and a review of the literature. Genet Couns. 1999;10:305-13.

🖵 1EE.A51B4C. 13Q-SYNDROME (13Q DELETION SYNDROME)

General

Chromosome 13q deletion syndrome.

Ocular

Retinoblastoma; telecanthus; hypertelorism; optic nerve hypoplasia; retinal dysplasia.

Clinical

Holoprosencephaly; abnormal lower extremity configuration; atrial septal defect; microcephaly; ambiguous genitalia; hypotonia; low-set ears; growth retardation; mild mental retardation; intestinal atresia.

Laboratory/Ocular

Diagnosis is made by clinical findings.

Treatment

Retinoblastoma: External beam radiation therapy is recommended on patients with significant vitreous seeding. Radioactive isotope plaques and chemotherapy are also an option. Removal of the tumor is the standard management for retinoblastoma.

🖵 BIBLIOGRAPHY

1. Nishikawa A, Mitomori T, Matsuura A, et al. A 13q-syndrome with extensive intestinal atresia. Acta Paediatr Scand. 1985;74:305-8.
2. Santolaya J, McCorquodale MM, Torres W, et al. Ultrasonographic prenatal diagnosis of the 13q- syndrome. Fetal Diagn Ther. 1993;8:261-7.
3. Stoll C, Alembik Y. A patient with 13q-syndrome with mild mental retardation and with growth retardation. Ann Genet. 1998; 41:209-12.
4. Weichselbaum RR, Zakov ZN, Albert DM, et al. New findings in the chromosome 13 long-arm deletion syndrome and retinoblastoma. Ophthalmology. 1979;86:1191-201.

🖵 1EE.A51B4D. 18Q- SYNDROME (18Q DELETION SYNDROME)

General

Chromosome 18q deletion syndrome.

Ocular

Macular "fibrosis"; optic disk abnormalities with tractional retinal detachment, retinal degeneration, and tilting of the optic disk.

Clinical

Microcephaly; short stature; hypotonia; hypothyroidism; diabetes mellitus; short neck; sensorineural hearing loss; sensorimotor axonal neuropathy; mild-to-moderate mental retardation; chronic arthritis; seizures.

Laboratory

Clinical.

Treatment

Retinal detachment: Scleral buckle, pneumatic retinopexy and vitrectomy may be used to close all the breaks.

🖵 BIBLIOGRAPHY

1. Gordon MF, Bressman S, Brin MF, et al. Dystonia in a patient with deletion of 18q. Mov Disord. 1995;10:496-9.
2. Hansen US, Herline T. Chronic arthritis in a boy with 18q-syndrome. J Rheumatol. 1994;21:1958-9.
3. Smith A, Caradus V, Henry JG. Translocation 46X6 t(17;18) (q25;q21) in a mentally retarded boy with progressive eye abnormalities. Clin Genet. 1979;16:156162.

⬚ 1EE.A51B4H. TRIPLOIDY SYNDROME (IRIS COLOBOMA)

General

Extra set of chromosomes due to diandry or digyny; still-birth or early neonatal death.

Ocular

Iris coloboma; microphthalmia; hypertelorism.

Clinical

Large placenta; prenatal growth deficits; large fontanels; syndactyly; heart defects; cleft lip; genital, brain, ear, and kidney malformations; meningomyelocele; micrognathia.

Laboratory/Ocular

Diagnosis is made by clinical findings.

Treatment

None.

⬚ BIBLIOGRAPHY

1. Arvidsson CG, Hamberg H, Johnsson H, et al. A boy with complete triploidy and unusually long survival. Acta Paediatr Scand. 1986;75:507-10.
2. Crane JP, Beaver HA, Cheung SW. Antenatal ultrasound findings in fetal triploidy syndrome. J Ultrasound Med. 1985;4:519-24.
3. Kaufman MH. New insights into triploidy and tetraploidy, from an analysis of model systems for these conditions. Hum Reprod. 1991;6:8-16.
4. Magalim SI, Scrascia E. Dictionary of Medical Syndromes, 2nd edition. Philadelphia: JB Lippincott; 1981.
5. O'Brien WF, Knuppel RA, Kousseff B, et al. Elevated maternal serum alpha-fetoprotein in triploidy. Obstet Gynecol. 1988;71:994-5.
6. Rubenstein JB, Swayne LC, Dise CA, et al. Placental changes in fetal triploidy syndrome. J Ultrasound Med. 1986;5:545-50.
7. Strobel SL, Brandt JT. Abnormal hematologic features in a live-born female with triploidy. Arch Pathol Lab Med. 1985;109:775-7.
8. Walker S, Andrews J, Gregson NM, et al. Three further cases of triploidy in man surviving to birth. J Med Genet. 1973;10:135-41.

⬚ 1EE.A51B4I. TRISOMY 8 MOSAICISM SYNDROME (EXOTROPIA)

General

Chromosomally abnormal cell line with each cell containing an extra chromosome 8; other cell lines normal; both sexes affected; present from birth.

Ocular

Strabismus; hypertelorism; deep-set eyes.

Clinical

Mild-to-moderate mental retardation; low-set or malformed ears; broad, bulbous nose; palatal deformity; congenital cardiovascular disorders; hydronephrosis; cryptorchidism; poor coordination; prominent forehead; enlarged nares; full lips; cupped ears; camptodactyly of fingers and toes; reported as a nonrandom secondary change in myxoid liposarcoma.

Laboratory/Ocular

Diagnosis is made by clinical findings.

Treatment

Strabismus: Equalized vision with correct refractive error; surgery may be helpful in patients with diplopia.

⬚ BIBLIOGRAPHY

1. Fineman RM, Ablow RC, Howard RO, et al. Trisomy 8 mosaicism syndrome. Pediatrics. 1975;56:762-7.
2. Geeraets WJ. Ocular Syndromes, 3rd edition. Philadelphia: Lea & Febiger; 1976.

⊟ 1EE.A51B4J. TRISOMY 9Q SYNDROME (HYPERTELORISM)

General

Congenital mental retardation syndrome due to 9p trisomy.

Ocular

Hypertelorism; deep-set eyes; antimongoloid (up-slanting) eyes.

Clinical

Mental retardation; short stature; down-turned corners of the mouth; slightly or moderately bulbous nose; moderately large ears; nail dysplasia and hypoplasias; clinodactyly; abnormal dermatoglyphs.

Laboratory

Clinical.

Treatment

None.

⊟ BIBLIOGRAPHY

1. Centerwall WR, Miller KS, Reeves LM. Familial "partial 9q" trisomy: six cases and four carriers in three generations. J Med Genet. 1976;13:57-61.
2. Wahlstrom J, Gustavasson KH. Trisomy 9p syndrome in siblings. Clin Genet. 1978;13:511.
3. Young RS, Reed T, Hodes ME, et al. The dermatoglyphic and clinical features of the 9p trisomy and partial 9p monosomy syndromes. Hum Genet. 1985;62:31-9.

⊟ 1EE.A51B4K. TRISOMY 13 SYNDROME (TRISOMY DL SYNDROME, PATAU SYNDROME, REESE SYNDROME) IRIS COLOBOMA

General

Extra chromosome in the D group; fatal in the first few months of life; trisomy 13–15 resembles trisomy D1.

Ocular

Anophthalmia; microphthalmia; iris coloboma; cataracts; retinal dysplasia; optic nerve coloboma; optic atrophy; iris dyplasia; calcified lens; retinal detachment; optic nerve hypoplasia; orbital cysts.

Clinical

Apneic spells; developmental deficiency of the nervous system; seizures (minor motor); deafness; cleft lip and palate; hemangiomata; horizontal palmar creases; hyperconvex fingernails; interventricular septal defects; renal abnormalities; cardiovascular changes; respiratory involvement; gastrointestinal disease; urogenital involvement; cerebral hypoplasia with hydrocephalus; mental retardation.

Laboratory

Immediate conventional cytogenetic test. Ultrasonography for any anomalies. Trisomy 13 is best identified through cytogenetic study of amniotic fluid.

Treatment

Surgical care is usually withheld for the first few months of life.

⊟ BIBLIOGRAPHY

1. Best RG, Gregg AR. (2012). Patau syndrome. [online] Available from www.emedicine.com/ped/TOPIC1745.HTM. [Accessed September, 2013].

🗗 1EE.A51B4L. TRISOMY 18 SYNDROME (E SYNDROME; EDWARDS SYNDROME) CONGENITAL GLAUCOMA

General

Chromosome 18 present in triplicate; more common in females (3:1); age of mother over 40 years; onset from fetal life.

Ocular

Unilateral ptosis; epicanthal folds; congenital glaucoma; corneal opacities; lens opacities; optic atrophy.

Clinical

Low-set ears; micrognathia; high-arched palate; prominent occiput; cryptorchidism; failure to thrive; ventricular septal defect; hypertonicity with rigidity in flexion of limbs; mental retardation; umbilical and inguinal hernias.

Laboratory

Cytogenetic test, echocardiography, ultrasonography, and skeletal radiography are used to detect any abnormalities.

Treatment

Treat infections as appropriate. For feeding difficulties nasogastric and gastrostomy supplementation is recommended.

🗗 BIBLIOGRAPHY

1. Chen H. (2013). Trisomy 18. [online] Availble from www.emedicine.com/ped/TOPIC652.HTM. [Accessed September, 2013].

🗗 1EE.A51B4M. XXXXY SYNDROME (HYPERTELORISM)

General

49 chromosome anomaly; characterized by mental retardation; hypoplastic male genitalia; proximal radioulnar synostosis.

Ocular

Upward slanting of palpebral fissures; strabismus; hypertelorism.

Clinical

Microcephaly; mongoloid facies; high-arched palate; cubitus valgus; in-curving fifth fingers and toes; depressed nasal bridge; nasal speech; prominent lower lip; broad chin; round face configuration; small chest; depressed sternum; wide-spaced nipples; genu valgum; flat feet; no facial or pubic hair; small testes; poor scrotal development; girdle obesity; tremor; excessive dribbling; withdrawal; irritability; proximal radioulnar synostosis; vertebral anomalies; Parkinsonism.

Laboratory

Chromosome studies.

Treatment

Strabismus: Equalized vision with correct refractive error; surgery may be helpful in patient with diplopia.

🗗 BIBLIOGRAPHY

1. Hecht F. Observation on the natural history of 49,XXXXY individuals. Am J Med Genet. 1982;13:335-6.

⊟ 1EE.A51B5A. AMNIOGENIC BAND SYNDROME (RING CONSTRICTION; STREETER DYSPLASIA)

General

It is caused by fetus swallowing one or more of the free-floating strands that result from amniotic rupture; the tension of these strands intraorally and extraorally produces secondary tears and deformations; no hereditary factor known.

Ocular

Upward slant of palpebral fissures; bilateral upper and lower lid colobomas; telecanthus; bilateral corneal opacities; microphthalmos; strabismus; hypertelorism; epibulbar choristoma; unilateral chorioretinal defects or lacuna (rare).

Clinical

Craniofacial and limb abnormalities.

Laboratory

Diagnosis is made by clinical findings.

Treatment

Equalized vision with correct refractive error; surgery may be helpful in patient with strabismus.

⊟ BIBLIOGRAPHY

1. Braude LS, Miller M, Cuttone J. Ocular abnormalities in the anmiogenic band syndrome. Br J Ophthalmol. 1981;65: 299-303.
2. Hashemi K, Traboulsi EI, Chavis R, et al. Chorioretinal lacuna in the anmiotic band syndrome. J Pediatr Ophthalmol Strabismus. 1991;28:238-9.
3. Miller MT, Deutsch TA, Cronin C, et al. Amniotic bands as a cause of ocular anomalies. Am J Ophthalmol. 1987;104: 270-9.
4. Murata T, Hashimoto S, Ishibashi T, et al. A case of anmiotic band syndrome with bilateral epibulbar choristoma. Br J Ophthalmol. 1992;76:685-7.
5. Streeter GL. Focal deficiencies in fetal tissues and their relation to intrauterine amputation. Contrib Embryol Carney Inst. 1930;22:1-44.

⊟ 1EE.A51B5B. CAT'S-EYE SYNDROME (SCHACHENMANN SYNDROME; SCHMID-FRACCARO SYNDROME; PARTIAL TRISOMY G SYNDROME)

General

Causative factor is one extra chromosome, a G chromosome, which may be from a 13-15 or 21-22 chromosome; although the ocular findings of the syndrome are similar to the D 13-15 trisomy group, the systemic manifestations usually are less severe; this syndrome is associated with a supernumerary bisatellited marker chromosome derived from duplicated regions of 22pter'22q11.2; partial cat's-eye syndrome is characterized by the absence of coloboma.

Ocular

Hypertelorism; microphthalmos; antimongoloid slant of palpebral fissures; strabismus; inferior vertical iris coloboma (cat eye); cataract; choroidal coloboma; epicanthal folds.

Clinical

Anal atresia; preauricular fistulae (bilateral); umbilical hernia; heart anomalies.

Laboratory

Chromosome analysis.

Treatment

- *Cataract*: Change in glasses can sometimes improve a patient's visual function temporarily; however the most common treatment is cataract surgery.
- *Strabismus*: Equalized vision with correct refractive error; surgery may be helpful in patients with diplopia.

⊟ BIBLIOGRAPHY

1. Collins JF. Handbook of Clinical Ophthalmology. New York: Masson; 1982.
2. Cory CC, Jamison DL. The cat eye syndrome. Arch Ophthalmol. 1974;92:259.
3. Liehr T, Pfeiffer RA, Trautmann U. Typical and partial cat eye syndrome: identification of the marker chromosome by FISH. Clin Genet. 1992;42:91-6.
4. Mears AJ, Duncan AM, Budarf ML, et al. Molecular characterization of the marker chromosome associated with cat eye syndrome. Am J Hum Genet. 1994;55:134-43.
5. Peterson RA. Schmid-Fraccaro syndrome ("cat's eye" syndrome): partial trisomy of G chromosome. Arch Ophthalmol. 1973;90:287.
6. Schachenmann G, Schmid W, Fraccaro M, et al. Chromosomes in coloboma and anal atresia. Lancet. 1965;2:290.
7. Walknowska J, Peakman D, Weleber RG. Cytogenetic investigation of cat-eye syndrome. Am J Ophthalmol. 1977;84:477-86.

🗗 1EE.A51B5C. CHARGE ASSOCIATION (MULTIPLE CONGENITAL ANOMALIES SYNDROME; COLOBOMA, HEART DISEASE, ATRESIA, RETARDED GROWTH, GENITAL HYPOPLASIA, EAR MALFORMATION ASSOCIATION)

General

Syndrome consists of four of six major manifestations of ocular coloboma, heart disease, atresia, retarded growth and development, genital hypoplasia, and ear malformations with or without hearing loss.

Ocular

Blepharoptosis; iris coloboma; optic nerve coloboma; macular hypoplasia; lacrimal canalicular atresia; nasolacrimal duct obstruction.

Clinical

Microcephaly; brachycephaly; malformed ear; bilateral finger contractures; heart disease; genital hypoplasia; heart disease; choanal atresia; retarded growth; hearing loss; facial nerve palsies; mental retardation.

Laboratory

CHD7 mutation analysis is diagnostic in 58–71% of individuals who meet the clinical criteria, head CT and MRI, cranial ultrasound.

Treatment

Secure airway, stabilize the patient, exclude major life-threatening congenital anomalies and transfer the individual with coloboma of the eye, heart defects, atresia of the nasal choanae, retardation of growth and/or development, genital and/or urinary abnormalities, and ear abnormalities and deafness (CHARGE) syndrome to a specialist center with pediatric otolaryngologist and other subspecialty services.

🗗 BIBLIOGRAPHY

1. Tegay DH, Yedowitz JC. (2012). CHARGE syndrome. [online] Available from www.emedicine.com/ped/TOPIC367.HTM. [Accessed September, 2013].

🗗 1EE.A51B5D. ULLRICH SYNDROME (ULLRICH-FEICHTIGER SYNDROME; DYSCRANIOPYLOPHALANGY) CORNEAL ULCER

General

Belongs to trisomy 13–15; unknown etiology; sporadic occurrence.

Ocular

Microphthalmia to anophthalmia; hypertelorism; narrow lid fissures; strabismus; glaucoma; aniridia; cloudy cornea; corneal ulcers; chorioretinal coloboma.

Clinical

Hypoplastic mandible; broad nose; polydactyly; spina bifida; bicornuate uterus or septa vagina; congenital heart disease.

Laboratory/Ocular

ANA test, serum muscle enzyme levels.

Treatment/Ocular/Corneal Ulcer

Topical cycloplegic agents, topical cyclosporin and topical antibiotics.

🗗 BIBLIOGRAPHY

1. Geeraets WJ. Ocular Syndromes, 3rd edition. Philadelphia: Lea & Febiger; 1976.

⊟ 1EE.51B5E. FRONTONASAL DYSPLASIA SYNDROME (MEDIAN CLEFT FACE SYNDROME)

General

Congenital disorder without genetic background; condition may present a variety of facial malformations, depending on the stage of embryonic development at which interference occurs.

Ocular

Hypertelorism; anophthalmia or microphthalmia; significant refractive errors; strabismus; nystagmus; eyelid ptosis; optic nerve hypoplasia; optic nerve colobomas; cataract; corneal dermoid; inflammatory retinopathy.

Clinical

Broad nasal root may be associated with median nasal groove and cleft of nose and/or upper lip; cleft of ala nasi (unilateral or bilateral); V-shaped hair prolongation into forehead.

Laboratory

CT, MRI and physical examination.

Treatment

Reconstruction surgery may be warranted.

⊟ BIBLIOGRAPHY

1. Kinsey JA, Streeten BW. Ocular abnormalities in the medial cleft face syndrome. Am J Ophthalmol. 1977;83:261.
2. Roarty JD, Pron GE, Siegel-Bartelt J, et al. Ocular manifestations of frontonasal dysplasia. Plast Reconstr Surg. 1994;93:25-30.
3. Sedano HO, Cohen MM, Jirasek J, et al. Frontonasal dysplasia. J Pediatr. 1970;76:906-13.
4. Weaver D, Bellinger D. Bifid nose associated with midline cleft of the upper lip: case report. Arch Otolaryngol. 1946;44:480.

⊟ 1EE.51B5F. GOLDENHAR SYNDROME (OCULO-AURICULO-VERTEBRAL DYSPLASIA; GOLDENHAR-GORLIN SYNDROME)

General

Most cases have been sporadic, but cases of autosomal dominant and recessive inheritance have been reported; male preponderance (60%); present at birth.

Ocular

Anophthalmia; colobomata of choroid, iris, and eyelid; antimongolian slant of lid fissure; epibulbar dermoid or lipodermoids of conjunctiva, cornea, and orbit; tilted optic disk; nerve hypoplasia; microphthalmia; macular heterotopia; tortuous retinal vessels.

Clinical

Frontal bulging of the skull; receding chin; malar hypoplasia; micrognathia and macrostomia; auricular appendices (single or multiple); multiple vertebral anomalies; preauricular fistulas; mental retardation.

Laboratory

Clinical.

Treatment

Dermoids: Surgery for function or cosmesis.

⊟ BIBLIOGRAPHY

1. Tewfik TL, Al-Noury KI. (2013). Manifestations of craniofacial syndromes. [online] Available from www.emedicine.com/ent/TOPIC319.HTM. [Accessed September, 2013].

1EE.51B5G. HEMIFACIAL MICROSOMIA SYNDROME (UNILATERAL FACIAL AGENESIS; OTOMANDIBULAR DYSOSTOSIS; FRANCOIS-HAUSTRATE SYNDROME)

General

No inheritance pattern; left side of face seems to be more frequently involved; facial asymmetry usually most obvious finding; both sexes affected; alteration of intrauterine environment is possible cause.

Ocular

Microphthalmos; congenital cystic ophthalmia; enophthalmos; strabismus; cataract; colobomata of iris, choroid, and retina.

Clinical

Microtia; macrostomia; failure of development of mandibular ramus and condyle; external auditory meatus may be absent; single or numerous ear tags; hypoplasia of facial muscles unilaterally; pulmonary agenesis (ipsilateral side); associated with Goldenhar syndrome.

Laboratory

X-ray, CT and MRI.

Treatment

Silastic implants remain one of the most common materials used for malar and submalar augmentation.

BIBLIOGRAPHY

1. Francois J, Haustrate L. Anomalies Colobomateuses du Globe Oculaire et Syndrome du Premier arc. Ann Ocul. 1954;187:340.
2. Geeraets WJ. Ocular Syndromes, 3rd edition. Philadelphia: Lea & Febiger; 1976.
3. Kobrynski L, Chitayat D, Zahed L, et al. Trisomy 22 and facioauriculovertebral (Goldenhar) sequence. Am J Med Genet. 1993;46:68-71.
4. Magalini SI, Scrascia E. Dictionary of Medical Syndromes, 2nd edition. Philadelphia: JB Lippincott; 1981.

1EE.51B5H. LINEAR NEVUS SEBACEUS OF JADASSOHN (NEVUS SEBACEUS OF JADASSOHN; JADASSOHN-TYPE ANETODERMA; ORGANOID NEVUS SYNDROME; SEBACEUS NEVUS SYNDROME)

General

Skin nevus caused by failure of separation of skin appendages from adjacent epithelium during the 3rd month of gestation.

Ocular

Proptosis; epibulbar lipodermoids; colobomata of eyelids, iris, and choroid; antimongoloid fissures; ocular motor palsies; nystagmus; teratomas of orbit and aberrant lacrimal glands; corneal vascularization; vision defects; conjunctival dermolipomas; choristomas of conjunctiva, sclera; corneal vascularization/opacification; colobomas of uvea, retina, optic disk, and lids; optic nerve hypoplasia; microphthalmia; anophthalmia; hemangioma of the sclera/conjunctiva.

Clinical

Circumscribed lesions of the face and scalp with excessively large sebaceous glands; papillomatous epidermal hyperplasia; seizures; skeletal abnormalities, particularly in skull; failure to thrive; convulsion; mental retardation.

Laboratory

Epidermis shows papillomatous hyperplasia. In the dermis, the numbers of mature sebaceous glands are increased. Ectopic apocrine glands are often found in the deep dermis beneath sebaceous glands.

Treatment

Photodynamic therapy with topical aminolevulinic acid. Full-thickness skin excision is usually required, and topical destruction.

BIBLIOGRAPHY

1. Al Hammadi A, Lebwohl MG. (2012). Nevus Sebaceus. [online] Available from www.emedicine.com/derm/TOPIC296.HTM. [Accessed September, 2013].

⊟ 1EE.51B5I. RUBINSTEIN-TAYBI SYNDROME (OPTIC ATROPHY)

General

Inheritance polygenic or multifactorial; rare.

Ocular

Antimongoloid slant of lid fissure; epicanthus; long eyelashes and highly arched brows; strabismus; myopia; hyperopia; iris coloboma; cataract; optic atrophy; ptosis; retinal detachment.

Clinical

Motor and mental retardation; broad thumbs and toes; highly arched palate; allergies; heart murmurs; anomalies of size, shape, and position of ears; dwarfism; cryptorchidism.

Laboratory

CT scan, MRI, chromosomal karyotype analysis, fluorescence in situ hybridization and CBP gene analysis.

Treatment

Physical therapy, speech and feeding therapy. Cardiothoracic intervention may be needed in patients with congenital heart defect.

⊟ BIBLIOGRAPHY

1. Mijuskovic ZP, Karadaglic D, Stojanov L. (2013). Dermatologic Manifestations of Rubinstein-Taybi Syndrome. [online] Available from www.emedicine.com/derm/TOPIC711.HTM. [Accessed September, 2013].

⊟ 1EE.51B6A. ANDERSEN-WARBURG SYNDROME (WHITNALL-NORMAN SYNDROME; OLIGOPHRENIA MICROPHTHALMOS SYNDROME; NORRIE DISEASE; ATROPHIA OCULI CONGENITAL FETAL IRITIS SYNDROME; CONGENITAL PROGRESSIVE OCULO-ACOUSTICO-CEREBRAL DYSPLASIA)

General

Sex-linked inheritance; gross deformation of both eyes; only males affected; onset at birth; putative gene for Norrie disease has been isolated and mapped to Xp11.3.

Ocular

Bilateral microphthalmos with extensive destruction of all ocular structures often resembling a pseudotumor; blindness at birth; iris atrophy; iritis; corneal opacification and lenticular destruction with a mass visible behind the lens as long as the lens is still clear; malformed retina and choroid with retinal pseudotumors; retinal detachment; retrolental vascular mass.

Clinical

Mental retardation ranging from imbecility to idiocy (may begin at any age) in about two-thirds of the cases; deafness of differing severity with onset between ages 9 years and 45 years.

Laboratory

Diagnosis is made by clinical findings.

Treatment

Topical treatment for iritis; retinal detachment surgery and vitrectomy may be necessary. Immediate laser treatment is recommended following birth.

⊟ BIBLIOGRAPHY

1. Andersen SR, Warburg M. Norrie's disease: congenital bilateral pseudotumor of the retina with recessive X-chromosomal inheritance; Preliminary Report. Arch Ophthalmol. 1961;66(5):614-8.

⊞ 1EE.51B6B. FORSIUS-ERIKSSON SYNDROME (ALAND DISEASE)

General

Associated with the natives of the Aland Islands; sex-linked inheritance; consanguinity versus mutant gene; affects males only; it has been considered a variety of incomplete congenital stationary night blindness.

Ocular

Microphthalmos; irregular latent nystagmus; myopia; astigmatism; dyschromatopsia; tapetoretinal degeneration; primary foveal hypoplasia or dysplasia; nystagmus.

Clinical

Prematurity; impaired hearing; mental retardation; epilepsy.

Laboratory

Diagnosis is made by clinical findings.

Treatment

Genetic counseling.

⊞ BIBLIOGRAPHY

1. Forsius H, Eriksson AW. Ein Neues Augensyndrom mit X-chromosomaler Transmission. Eine Sippe mit Fundusalbinismus, Foveahypoplasie, Nystagmus, Myopic, Astigmatismus und Dyschromatopsie. Klin Monatsbl Augenheilkd. 1964;144:447.
2. McKusick VA. Mendelian Inheritance in Man: A Catalog of Human Genes and Genetic Disorders. 12th edition. Baltimore: The Johns Hopkins University Press; 1998.

⊞ 1EE.51B6C. LOWE SYNDROME (OCULO-CEREBRO-RENAL SYNDROME)

General

Essential enzyme or protein abnormality is unknown; sex-linked recessive trait (male incidence only); onset in early infancy.

Ocular

Nystagmus; congenital glaucoma; miotic pupils; no pupillary reaction; ectropion uveae; malformation of the anterior chamber angle and of the iris; Schlemm canal may be absent with imperfect angle cleavage; blue sclera; cloudy cornea; cataracts; megalocornea; corneal dystrophy; buphthalmos; microphthalmos; microphakia; mydriasis; strabismus; lens punctate cortical opacities.

Clinical

Mental, psychomotor, and growth retardation; aminoaciduria; albuminuria; glycosuria; renal tubular acidosis; rickets; osteomalacia; muscular hypotony; hyporeflexia; hyperactivity with bizarre choreoathetoid movements and screaming.

Laboratory

Urine–aminoaciduria, proteinuria, calciuria, phosphaturia; serum–elevated acid phosphate; imaging studies–brain MRI–mild ventriculomegaly (one third cases); ocular ultrasound–if dense cataract, rule out mass or retinal detachment posterior.

Treatment

Monitor and treat for glaucoma. If glaucoma develops, IOP-lowering agents must be used. Often, these patients require surgical intervention with goniotomy, trabeculotomy, or a drainage filtration device. Congenital cataracts should be removed, ideally in the first 6 weeks of life, to optimize the visual potential.

⊞ BIBLIOGRAPHY

1. Alkorn DM. (2012). Oculocerebrorenal syndrome. [online] Available from www.emedicine.com/oph/TOPIC516.HTM. [Accessed October, 2013].

⊟ 1EE.51B7A. CEREBRO-OCULO-FACIO-SKELETAL SYNDROME (COFS SYNDROME)

General

Inherited as autosomal recessive disorder; death within the first 3 years of life; feeding difficulties secondary to incoordination of the swallowing mechanism.

Ocular

Microphthalmia; blepharophimosis; cataracts.

Clinical

Microcephaly; hypotonia; prominent nasal root; large ear pinnae; flexion contractures at elbows and knees; camptodactylia; osteoporosis; kyphosis; scoliosis; congenital muscular dystrophy.

Laboratory

Clinical.

Treatment

Change in glasses can sometimes improve a patient's visual function temporarily; however the most common treatment is cataract surgery.

⊟ BIBLIOGRAPHY

1. Geeraets WJ. Ocular Syndromes, 3rd edition. Philadelphia: Lea & Febiger; 1976.
2. Gershoni-Baruch R, Ludatscher RM, Lichtig C, et al. Cerebrooculo-facio-skeletal syndrome: further delineation. Am J Med Genet. 1991;41:74-7.
3. Lowry RB, MacLean R, McLean DM, et al. Cataracts, microcephaly, kyphosis and limited joint movement in two siblings. A new syndrome. J Pediatr. 1971;79:282.
4. McKusick VA. Mendelian Inheritance in Man: A Catalog of Human Genes and Genetic Disorders, 12th edition. Baltimore: The Johns Hopkins University Press; 1998.
5. Online Mendelian Inheritance in Man, OMIM. McKusick-Nathans Institute for Genetic Medicine, Johns Hopkins University and National Center for Biotechnology Information, National Library of Medicine, February 12, 2007. Available from www.ncbi.nlm.nih.gov/omim. [Accessed September, 2013].
6. Pena SD, Shokeir MK. Autosomal recessive cerebro-oculo-facio-skeletal (COFS) syndrome. Clin Genet. 1974;5:285.

⊟ 1EE.51B7B. CONRADI SYNDROME (MULTIPLE EPIPHYSEAL DYSPLASIA CONGENITA; DYSPLASIA EPIPHYSEALIS CONGENITA; CHONDRODYSTROPHIA FOETALIS HYPOPLASTICA; CALCINOSIS UNIVERSALIS; CONGENITAL CALCIFYING CHONDRODYSTROPHY; STIPPLED EPIPHYSES SYNDROME; CONRADI-HÜNERMANN SYNDROME; CHONDRODYSPLASIA PUNCTATA)

General

Autosomal recessive; manifestations within the first 6 months of life; epiphyseal stippling present at birth; perinatal manifestations include disorganization of the spine, premature echogenicity of femoral epiphyses, and frontal bossing with depressed nasal bridge.

Ocular

Hypertelorism; heterochromia iridis (rare); bilateral total congenital cataract appearing at or shortly after birth; primary optic atrophy (rare); bilateral corneal punctate erosions.

Clinical

Short limbs (mainly proximal part) resulting in "short-limbed dwarfism"; deformities of hip, knee, and elbow joints by contraction and immobility, and possible transformation of muscles into fibrous tissue as a result; congenital heart defect with calcium deposits in the cardiac valves; skin anomalies (dyskeratosis); mental retardation.

Laboratory

Clinical.

Treatment

- *Cataract*: Change in glasses can sometimes improve a patient's visual function temporarily; however the most common treatment is cataract surgery.
- *Corneal erosion*: Goal of therapy is regenerating or repairing the epithelial basement membrane to restore the adhesion between the epithelium and the anterior stroma, topical lubrication therapy, bandage soft contact lenses, debridement of the epithelium and basement membrane, or anterior stromal micropuncture may be useful.

BIBLIOGRAPHY

1. Bellson FA. Optic nerve hypoplasia in chondrodysplasia punctata. J Pediatr Ophthalmol. 1977;14:144-7.
2. Conradi E. Vorzeitiges Auftreten von Knochenund Eigenartigen Verkalkungskernen bei Chondrodystrophia Fotalis Hypoplastica. Histologische un Rontgenuntersuchungen. Jahrb Kinderhk. 1914;80:86.
3. Happle R. Cataracts as a marker of genetic heterogeneity in chondrodysplasia punctata. Clin Genet. 1981;19:64-6.
4. Massey JY, Roy FH. Ocular manifestations of Conradi disease. Arch Ophthalmol. 1974;92:524-6.
5. Pryde PG, Bawle E, Brandt F, et al. Prenatal diagnosis of non-rhizomelic chondrodysplasia punctata (Conradi-Hunermann syndrome). Am J Med Genet. 1993;47:426-31.
6. Spierer A, Neumann D. Corneal changes in chondrodysplasia punctata syndrome. Ann Ophthalmol. 1993;25:356-8.

1EE.51B7C. OCULOCEREBRAL SYNDROME WITH HYPOPIGMENTATION (AMISH OCULOCEREBRAL SYNDROME; CROSS SYNDROME)

General

Autosomal recessive.

Ocular

Spastic ectropion; microphthalmos; enophthalmos; microcornea; corneal opacification; corneal vascularization; palpebral conjunctival injection; narrow lid fissures; aniridia; nystagmus; bilateral optic atrophy.

Clinical

Spastic diplegia; cutaneous hypopigmentation; mental retardation; hypogonadism; growth retardation; developmental defects of the CNS such as cystic malformation of the posterior fossa of the Dandy-Walker type.

Laboratory

Diagnosis is made by clinical findings.

Treatment

See enophthalmos.

BIBLIOGRAPHY

1. Cross HE, McKusick VA, Breen W, et al. A new oculocerebral syndrome with hypopigmentation. J Pediatr. 1967;70(3):398-406.
2. De Jong G, Fryns JP. Oculocerebral syndrome with hypopigmentation (Cross syndrome): the mixed pattern of hair pigmentation as an important diagnostic sign. Genet Couns. 1991;2(3):151-5.
3. Lerone M, Possagno A, Taccone A, et al. Oculocerebral syndrome with hypopigmentation (Cross syndrome): report of a new case. Clin Genet. 1992;41(2):87-9.
4. Pinsky L, DiGeorge AM, Harley RD, et al. Microphthalmos, corneal opacity, mental retardation, and spastic cerebral palsy: An oculocerebral syndrome. J Pediatr. 1965;67(3):387-98.

1EE.51B7D. DIAMOND BLACKFAN SYNDROME

General

Rare, congenital hematologic disorder characterized by isolated erythroid hypoplasia (hypoplastic anemia).

Ocular

Strabismus, hypertelorism, microphthalmos, and infantile glaucoma.

Clinical

May have musculoskeletal abnormalities.

Laboratory

Hemoglobin studies, imaging studies may be helpful in revealing occult malformations.

Treatment

Packed red cell transfusions may be necessary.

BIBLIOGRAPHY

1. Huang LH, Portwine C, Miller R. (2012). Transient Erythroblastopenia of Childhood. [online] Available from www.emedicine.com/ped/TOPIC2279.HTM. [Accessed September, 2013].

☐ 1EE.51B7E. FANCONI SYNDROME (TONI-FANCONI SYNDROME; AMINO DIABETES; HYPOCHLOREMIC-GLYCOSURIC OSTEONEPHROPATHY SYNDROME; DE TONI-FANCONI SYNDROME)

General

Autosomal recessive inheritance; hematologic manifestations mainly in young patients; in adults the syndrome resembles Milkman's syndrome with disorder of calcium and phosphorus metabolism; chronic organic acidosis in Fanconi syndrome due to an inborn error of protein metabolism.

Ocular

Massive retinal hemorrhage may be present secondary to blood dyscrasia; bilateral anterior uveitis.

Clinical

Ecchymoses and mucous membrane hemorrhages; skin hyperpigmentation; osteomalacia; pseudo fractures; deformities of radius and absence of thumbs; hypophosphatemia.

Laboratory

Diagnosis is made by clinical findings.

Treatment

Treat the underlying cause as quickly as possible, vitrectomy.

☐ BIBLIOGRAPHY

1. Fanconi G, Turler U. Kogenitale Kleinhirnatrophie mit Supranuklearen Storungen der Motilitat der Augenmuskein. Helv Paediatr Acta. 1951;6:475-83.
2. Geeraets WJ. Ocular Syndromes, 3rd edition. Philadelphia: Lea & Febiger; 1976.
3. Tsilou ET, Giri N, Weinstein S, et al. Ocular and orbital manifestations of the inherited bone marrow failure syndromes: Fanconi anemia and dyskeratosis congenita. Ophthalmology. 2010;117:615-22.

☐ 1EE.51B7F. OBESITY-CEREBRAL-OCULAR-SKELETAL ANOMALIES SYNDROME

General

Rare, autosomal recessive disease; similar to Prader-Willi and Laurence-Moon-Bardet-Biedl syndromes.

Ocular

Microphthalmia; antimongoloid slant of lid fissure; asymmetrical size of fissure; strabismus; myopia; iris and chorioretinal colobomata; mottled retina; prominent choroidal vessels.

Clinical

Obesity (mid-childhood onset); hypotonia; mental retardation; craniofacial anomalies with microcephaly; tapering extremities; hyperextensibility at elbows and proximal interphalangeal joints; cubitus valgus; genu valgum; Simian creases; syndactyly.

Laboratory

Diagnosis is made by clinical findings.

Treatment

Strabismus: Equalized vision with correct refractive error; surgery may be helpful in patient with diplopia.

☐ BIBLIOGRAPHY

1. Cohen MM, Hall BD, Smith DW, et al. A new syndrome with hypotonia, obesity, mental deficiency, and facial, oral, ocular, and limb anomalies. J Pediatr. 1973;83(2):280-4.
2. Hall BD, Smith DW. Prader-Willi syndrome: A resumé of 32 cases including an instance of affected first cousins, one of whom is of normal stature and intelligence. J Pediatr. 1972;81(2):286-93.

⊟ 1EE.51B8A. BLATT SYNDROME (CRANIO-ORBITO-OCULAR DYSRAPHIA)

General

Autosomal dominant; characterized by distichiasis and anisometropia; both sexes are affected; present from birth.

Ocular

Hypertelorism; microphthalmos; distichiasis with the Meibomian glands usually absent; anisometropia.

Clinical

Meningocele or meningoencephalocele; cranial deformities; malformations of facial bones.

Laboratory

Diagnosis is made by clinical findings.

Treatment

Distichiasis: Symptomatic–therapeutic contact lenses as well as lubricating drops and ointments. Epilation with electrolysis cryosurgery; double freeze-thaw down to –20°C; lid splitting procedure.

⊟ BIBLIOGRAPHY

1. Blatt N. [Cranio-orbito-ocular dysraphia and meningocele]. Rev Otoneuroophtalmol. 1961;33:185-232.
2. Duke-Elder S (Ed). System of Ophthalmology. St Louis: CV Mosby; 1976.
3. Magalini SI, Scrascia E. Dictionary of Medical Syndromes, 2nd edition. Philadelphia, PA: Lippincott Williams and Wilkins; 1981.

⊟ 1EE.51B8B. GANSSLEN SYNDROME (FAMILIAL HEMOLYTIC ICTERUS; HEMATOLOGIC-METABOLIC BONE DISORDER)

General

Autosomal dominant inheritance; occurs mainly in Caucasians.

Ocular

Hypertelorism; microphthalmos; epicanthus; narrowing of palpebral fissure; lid hemorrhages; myopia; dyschromatopsia; hypochromic heterochromia; scleral icterus; conjunctival hemorrhages; retinal pallor and edema in advanced stages; dilated retinal arteries and veins; round retinal hemorrhages in deeper retinal layers; retinal exudates and macular star.

Clinical

Splenomegaly; hemolytic crises; dental deformities; brachydactyly; polydactyly; congenital hip luxation; oxycephaly; deformities of the outer ear and otosclerosis.

Laboratory

Indirect Coomb's test and direct antibody test results are positive in the mother and affected newborn; serial maternal antibody titers are monitored until a critical titer of 1:32, which indicates high risk of fetal hydrops.

Treatment

Early exchange transfusion with type-O Rh-negative fresh RBCs with intensive phototherapy is usually required.

⊟ BIBLIOGRAPHY

1. Ganser SJ. Uber Einen Eigenarrigen Hysterischen Dammerzustand. Arch Psychiatr Nervenkrankh. 1898;30:633.
2. Magalini SI, Scrascia E. Dictionary of Medical Syndromes, 2nd edition. Philadelphia: JB Lippincott; 1981.

⊡ 1EE.51B8C. HYPOMELANOSIS OF ITO SYNDROME (INCONTINENTIA PIGMENTI ACHROMIANS; SYSTEMATIZED ACHROMIC NEVUS)

General

Probable autosomal dominant transmission; cutaneous abnormality consisting of bizarre, patterned, macular hypopigmentation over variable portions of the body with multiple associated defects in other body systems; abnormal chromosome constitutions.

Ocular

Iridal heterochromia; myopia; esotropia; microphthalmia; hypertelorism; nystagmus; strabismus; corneal opacity; choroidal atrophy; exotropia; small optic nerve; hypopigmentation of the fundus; corneal asymmetry; pannus; atrophic irides with irregular pupillary margins; cataract; retinal detachment.

Clinical

Cutaneous manifestations consist of macular hypopigmented whorls, streaks, and patches in a bilateral or unilateral distribution affecting almost any portion of the body surface; 50% have associated noncutaneous abnormalities, including CNS dysfunction (seizure, delayed development) and musculoskeletal anomalies.

Laboratory

Diagnosis is made by clinical findings.

Treatment

No treatment is necessary for the cutaneous findings except makeup for cosmetic purposes. Other symptoms should be treated by specific specialists.

⊡ BIBLIOGRAPHY

1. Ratz JL, Gross N. (2012). Hypomelanosis of Ito. [online] Available from www.emedicine.com/derm/TOPIC186. HTM. [Accessed September, 2013].

⊡ 1EE.51B8D. LERI SYNDROME (PLEONOSTEOSIS SYNDROME; CARPAL TUNNEL SYNDROME)

General

Autosomal dominant type of congenital osseous dystrophy; early epiphyseal bone formation of extremities; Morton metatarsalgia syndrome may result; onset in early infancy.

Ocular

Microphthalmia; anophthalmia; oculomotor paralysis; corneal clouding; cataract.

Clinical

Dwarfism (disproportionate); articular deformities; cutaneous deformities; carpal tunnel syndrome (median nerve compression); deformities of thumbs and great toes; laryngeal stenosis.

Laboratory

Clinical.

Treatment

- *Cataract*: Change in glasses can sometimes improve a patient's visual function temporarily; however the most common treatment is cataract surgery.
- *Corneal clouding*: Check for elevated IOP. Medical treatment includes the use of hyperosmotic drops, non-steroidal and steroid eye drops. Corneal transplant may be necessary.

⊡ BIBLIOGRAPHY

1. Fuller DA. (2012). Orthopedic Surgery for Carpal Tunnel Syndrome. [online] Available from www.emedicine.com/orthoped/TOPIC455.HTM. [Accessed September, 2013].

1EE.51B8E. MYOTONIC DYSTROPHY SYNDROME (MYOTONIA ATROPHICA SYNDROME; DYSTROPHIA MYOTONICA; CURSCHMANN-STEINERT SYNDROME)

General

Rare autosomal dominant disease; onset at the age of 20 years; condition is worsened by administration of neostigmine (Prostigmin); associated with an unstable DNA sequence composed of varying numbers of CTG triplet repeats (which allows a specific molecular test for this disorder).

Ocular

Mild ptosis (occasionally); myotonic cataract with small, dot-like subcapsular cortical opacities during early stage, with polychromatic properties on biomicroscopic examination; corneal epithelial dystrophy; loss of corneal sensitivity; tapetoretinal degeneration; macular red spot; macular degeneration; chorioretinitis; pilomatrixomas; ocular hypotony; pattern pigmentary changes; abnormal saccades.

Clinical

Progressive muscular atrophy with selection of certain muscles (mainly sternocleidomastoid, temporalis, dorsiflexor muscles of the ankle, anterior oblique); myotonia; bland facial expression; speech disturbance due to involvement of vocal cords and palatal muscles; dysphagia; endocrine disturbances.

Laboratory

Diagnosis is made by clinical findings.

Treatment

- *Ptosis*: If visual acuity is affected, most cases require surgical correction and there are several procedures that may be used including levator resection, repair or advancement and Fasanella-Servat.
- *Cataract*: Change in glasses can sometimes improve a patient's visual function temporarily; however, the most common treatment is cataract surgery.
- *Corneal dystrophy*: Mild cases—can be observed and soft contact lenses are helpful; PK may be necessary; graft recurrences are treated by superficial keratectomy, PTK or repeat PK.
- *Macular degeneration*: No treatment is available for non-neovascular age-related macular degeneration (AMD). Preventative therapy includes no smoking, control of hypertension, cholesterol, and blood sugar, exercise and vitamins. Neovascular AMD treatment consists of laser, avastin and lucentis.

BIBLIOGRAPHY

1. Brooke NM, Cwik VE. Myotonic dystrophy. In: Bradley WG (Ed). Neurology in Clinical Practice: Principles of Diagnosis and Management, 2nd edition. Boston, USA: Butterworth-Heinemann; 1995. pp. 2020-2.
2. Gjertsen IK, Sandvig KU, Eide N, et al. Recurrence of secondary opacification and development of a dense posterior vitreous membrane in patients with myotonic dystrophy. J Cataract Refract Surg. 2003;29(1):213-6.
3. Kimizuka Y, Kiyosawa M, Tamai M, et al. Retinal changes in myotonic dystrophy. Clinical and follow-up evaluation. Retina. 1993;13(2):129-35.
4. Koca MR, Horn F, Korth M. Alterations of saccadic eye movements in myotonic dystrophy. Graefes Arch Clin Exp Ophthalmol. 1992;230(5):437-41.
5. Kuwabara T, Lessell S. Electron microscopic study of extraocular muscles in myotonic dystrophy. Am J Ophthalmol. 1976;82(2):303-9.
6. Mausolf FA, Burns CA, Burian IIM. Morphologic and functional retinal changes in myotonic dystrophy unrelated to quinine therapy. Am J Ophthalmol. 1972;74(6):1141-3.
7. Meyer E, Navon D, Auslender L, et al. Myotonic dystrophy: pathological study of the eyes. Ophthalmologica. 1980;181(3-4):215-20.
8. Reardon W, MacMillan JC, Myring J, et al. Cataract and myotonic dystrophy: the role of molecular diagnosis. Br J Ophthalmol. 1993;77(9):579-83.
9. Rosa N, Lanza M, Borrelli M, et al. Low intraocular pressure resulting from ciliary body detachment in patients with myotonic dystrophy. Ophthalmology. 2011;118(2):260-4.

⊟ 1EE.51B8F. RIEGER SYNDROME (AXENFELD-RIEGER SYNDROME; DYSGENESIS MESODERMALIS CORNEAE ET IRIDES; DYSGENESIS MESOSTROMALIS; AXENFELD POSTERIOR EMBRYOTOXON-JUVENILE GLAUCOMA)

General

Autosomal dominant; neural crest abnormality; 50% of patients develop glaucoma.

Ocular

Microphthalmia; congenital glaucoma; iris hypoplasia; deformed and acentric pupil; anterior synechiae; aniridia; microcornea; corneal opacities in Descemet's membrane parallel to the limbus; dislocated lens; optic atrophy; cataract; strabismus; ptosis; hypertelorism; keratoconus; posterior embryotoxon; broad iris processes to embryotoxon; iris stromal hypoplasia; corectopia; polycoria; secondary glaucoma.

Clinical

Face wide; hypodontia; underdeveloped maxilla; teeth deformities; myotonic dystrophy; facial anomalies: maxillary hypoplasia, protrusion of the lower lip, broad, flat nose; dental anomalies include absent teeth, pig-like incisors and decreased crown size; hypospadias.

Laboratory

Diagnosis is made by clinical findings.

Treatment/Ocular

Congenital glaucoma can be treated with beta-blockers, prostaglandin analogs and carbonic anhydrase inhibitors. Surgery such as goniotomy or trabeculectomy can be used if IOP is not controlled.

⊟ BIBLIOGRAPHY

1. Eagle RC. Congenital, developmental and degenerative disorders of the iris and ciliary body. In: Albert DM, Jakobiec FA (Eds). Albert & Jakobiec's Principles and Practice of Ophthalmology: Clinical Practice, 3rd edition. Philadelphia, PA: WB Saunders; 1994. pp. 367-87.
2. Montes JG, Montes JC. Syndrome de Rieger, anomalie de axenfeld con glaucoma Juvenil familiar. Arch Soc Ophth Hisp Am. 1967;27:93.
3. Rieger H. Beitrage zur Kenntnis seltener Missbildungen der Iris. Graefes Arch Clin Esp Ophthalmol. 1935;133:602.
4. Wesley RK, Baker JD, Golnick AL. Rieger's syndrome: (oligodontia and primary mesodermal dysgenesis of the iris) clinical features and report of an isolated case. J Pediatr Ophthalmol Strabismus. 1978;15(2):67-70.

⊟ 1EE.51B9A. TRISOMY 10Q SYNDROME (10Q+ SYNDROME) OPTIC DISK

General

Chromosome 10q trisomy (duplication) syndrome.

Ocular

Microphthalmia; deep-set eyes; epicanthus; bilateral, enlarged, gray optic disks; distended retinal vessels; bilateral punctate yellow deposits near the macula and optic disk.

Clinical

Mental retardation; microcephaly; prominent forehead; upturned nose; bow shaped mouth; micrognathia; thick and flat helices of the ears; long slender limbs.

Laboratory

Clinical.

Treatment

None—ocular.

⊟ BIBLIOGRAPHY

1. Neely K, Mets MB, Wong P, et al. Ocular findings in partial trisomy 10q syndrome. Am J Ophthalmol. l988;106:82-7.

⊟ 1EE.51B9B. TRISOMY 21Q- SYNDROME (21Q DELETION SYNDROME)

General

Chromosome 21q deletion syndrome.

Ocular

Blepharochalasis; microphthalmia with persistent hypoplastic primary vitreous.

Clinical

Mental and physical retardation; generalized hypertonia; high nasal bridge; micrognathia; malformed ears with preauricular pits, and overlying fingers.

Laboratory

Amniocentesis, fetal chromosome analysis, and prenatal echography.

Treatment

Knowing the systemic and ocular findings is important in the treatment of patients with trisomy 21.

⊟ BIBLIOGRAPHY

1. Izquierdo NJ, Townsend W. (2011). Ophthalmologic Manifestations of Down Syndrome. [online] Available from www.emedicine.com/oph/TOPIC522.HTM. [Accessed September, 2013].

⊟ 1EE.51B9C. X CHROMOSOMAL DELETION (OPTIC ATROPHY)

General

Deletion of proximal part of long arm of the X chromosome; deletion covers part of region Xq21.1-Xq21.31, the locus for choroideremia; congenital deafness; probable mental retardation.

Ocular

Choroideremia, translucent pigment epithelium; peripheral hyperpigmentation; diffuse choriocapillary layer and retinal pigment epithelium; decreased night vision; optic atrophy; excessive myopia; nystagmus.

Clinical

Congenital deafness; mental retardation; corpus callosum agenesia; cleft lip and palate; anhidrotic ectodermal dysplasia; agammaglobulinemia.

Laboratory

Chromosome studies.

Treatment

None.

⊟ BIBLIOGRAPHY

1. Bleeker-Wagemakers LM, Friedrich U, Gal A, et al. Close linkage between Norrie disease: a cloned DNA sequence from the proximal short arm and the centromere of the X-chromosome. Hum Genet. 1987;71:211-4.
2. Rosenberg T, Niebuhr E, Yang HM, et al. Choroideremia, congenital deafness and mental retardation in a family with an X chromosomal deletion. Ophthalmic Paediatr Genet. 1987;8:139-43.

⊟ 1EE.51B10A. BEAL SYNDROME

General

Transient unilateral disease; becoming bilateral later, then resolving within 2 weeks.

Ocular

Acute follicular conjunctivitis (lymphoid follicles; cobblestoning of conjunctiva with rapid onset).

Clinical

No purulent discharge; associated with regional adenitis.

Laboratory

Clinical.

Treatment

Symptomatic control may include cold compresses, artificial tears; nonsteroidal and occasionally steroidal drops to relieve itching.

⊟ BIBLIOGRAPHY

1. Ostler HB, Schachter J, Dawson CR. Acute follicular conjunctivitis of epizootic origin. Arch Ophthalmol. 1969;82:587-91.
2. Thygeson P. Follicular conjunctivitis: infectious diseases of the conjunctiva and cornea. In: Symposium of the New Orleans Academy of Ophthalmology. St. Louis: CV Mosby; 1965. p.103.

⊟ 1EE.51B10B. GORLIN-CHAUDHRY-MOSS SYNDROME

General

Etiology unknown.

Ocular

Microphthalmia; hypertelorism; depressed supraorbital ridges; inability to open or close lids fully because of incomplete lid development; antimongoloid, oblique palpebral fissures; sparse eyelash development; lid defect (notching); horizontal nystagmus at extreme lateral gaze; limited upper gaze; astigmatism; marked hyperopia; corneal scars (possibly due to exposure keratitis); keratoconus.

Clinical

Craniofacial dysostosis; saddled appearance of upper face; high-arched, narrow palate; dental anomalies (size, number, position); hypertrichosis; hypoplasia of labia majora; patent ductus arteriosus; normal mental development; fatigue; frontal headache.

Laboratory

Diagnosis is made by clinical findings.

Treatment

In patients with bilateral and visually disabling corneal opacity, PK is recommended.

⊟ BIBLIOGRAPHY

1. Scheinfeld NS, Freilich BD, Freilich J. (2013). Congenital Clouding of the Cornea. [online] Available from www.emedicine.com/oph/TOPIC771.HTM. [Accessed September, 2013].

1EE.51B10C. HALLERMANN-STREIFF SYNDROME (DYSCEPHALIC-MANDIBULO-OCULO-FACIAL SYNDROME; OCULO-MANDIBULO-DYSCEPHALY; ULLRICH-FREMERY-DOHNA SYNDROME; FRANCOIS DYSCEPHALIC SYNDROME; MANDIBU-LO-OCULO-FACIAL DYSCEPHALY SYNDROME; FRANCOIS-HALLERMANN-STREIFF SYNDROME; HALLERMANN-STREIFF-FRANCOIS SYNDROME; AUDRY I SYNDROME; DOHNA SYNDROME; FRANCOIS SYNDROME (1); DYSCEPHALY-TEETH ABNORMA-LITY-DWARFISM; DYSCEPHALIA OCULOMANDIBULARIS-HYPOTRICHOSIS; MANDIBULO-OCULAR DYSCEPHALIA HYPOTRICHOSIS; FREMERY-DOHNA SYNDROME; OCULO-MANDIBULO-FACIAL DYSCEPHALY)

General

Rare; familial occurrence and consanguinity; males and females are equally affected.

Ocular

Microphthalmos (bilateral); proptosis; nystagmus; strabismus; cataracts; bilateral optic atrophy; coloboma of optic disk, choroid, and iris; keratoglobus; microcornea; antimongoloid slant; iris atrophy; uveitis; blue sclera; persistent pupillary membrane; secondary glaucoma.

Clinical

Malformations of skull (brachycephaly), facial skeleton and jaws; erupted teeth at birth; diminished hair growth; hyperextensibility of joints; short stature; skin atrophy; mental deficiency; predisposition to upper airway compromise; obstructive sleep apnea.

Laboratory

Diagnosis is made by clinical findings.

Treatment

- *Cataract*: Change in glasses can sometimes improve a patient's visual function temporarily; however the most common treatment is cataract surgery.
- *Strabismus*: Equalized vision with correct refractive error; surgery may be helpful in patients with diplopia.
- *Uveitis*: Topical steroids and cycloplegic medication should be the initial treatment of choice. Oral steroids should be given if not responsive to topical steroids, immunosuppressants if bilateral disease that does not respond to oral steroids, periocular steroids for unilateral or posterior uveitis. Vitrectomy can be used for severe vitreous opacification. Cryotherapy and laser photocoagulation may be used for localized pars plana exudates.
- *Glaucoma*: Glaucoma medication should be the first plan of action. If medication is unsuccessful, a filtering surgical procedure with or without antimetabolites may be beneficial.

BIBLIOGRAPHY

1. François J, Victoria-Troncoso V. François' dyscephalic syndrome and skin manifestations. Ophthalmologica. 1981;183(2):63-7.
2. Roy FH, Fraunfelder FW, Fraunfelder FT. Roy and Fraunfelder's Current Ocular Therapy, 6th edition. Philadelphia, PA: WB Saunders; 2008.
3. Hallermann W. Vogelgesicht und Cataracta Congenita. Klin Monatsbl Augenheilkd. 1948;113:315-8.
4. Ronen S, Rozenmann Y, Isaacson M, et al. The early management of baby with Hallermann-Streiff-Francois syndrome. J Pediatr Ophthalmol Strabismus. 1979;16(2):119-21.
5. Spaepen A, Schrander-Stumpel C, Fryns JP, et al. Hallermann-Streiff syndrome: clinical and psychological findings in children. Nosologic overlap with oculodentodigital dysplasia? Am J Med Genet. 1991;41(4):517-20.
6. Streiff EB. Dysmorphic Mandibulo-faciale (Tete d'Oiseau) et al. Alterations Oculaires. Ophthalmologica. 1950;120 (1-2):79-83.

🗗 1EE.51B10D. HUTCHINSON-GILFORD SYNDROME (PROGERIA)

General

Inheritance unknown; belongs to group of ectodermal dysplasias (*see* Werner Syndrome-Progeria of Adults); elevated hyaluronic acid of unknown etiology, likely sporadic dominant mutation.

Ocular

Microphthalmia; hypotrichosis; microcornea; cataract.

Clinical

Appearance of "old age" in children; short stature to dwarfism; dyscephaly; atrophy of skin and subcutaneous adipose tissue; aplasia of maxilla; oligodontia; arteriosclerosis (premature); progeria.

Laboratory

Radiography findings usually manifest within the 1st or 2nd year of life and most commonly involve the skull, thorax, long bones, and phalanges.

Treatment

No effective therapy is available. Careful monitoring and referral to the proper specialists is important.

🗗 BIBLIOGRAPHY

1. Shah KN. (2013). Hutchinson-Gilford Progeria. [online] Available from www.emedicine.com/derm/TOPIC731. HTM. [Accessed September, 2013].

🗗 1EE.51B10E. KRAUSE SYNDROME (CONGENITAL ENCEPHALO-OPHTHALMIC DYSPLASIA; ENCEPHALO-OPHTHALMIC SYNDROME)

General

No hereditary factors involved; no predilection for either sex; more frequent in premature infants; death frequently from intercurrent infections.

Ocular

Microphthalmos; enophthalmos; ptosis; strabismus; secondary glaucoma; iris atrophy; anterior and posterior synechiae; scleral atrophy; persistent remnants of hyaloid's artery; intraocular hemorrhages and exudates; cyclitic membranes; cataracts; retinal hypoplasia and hyperplasia; choroidal and retinal malformation; retinal glial membranes; retinal detachment; choroidal atrophy; optic nerve malformation; optic atrophy.

Clinical

Congenital cerebral dysplasia; hydrocephalus or microcephaly; mental retardation; heterotopia.

Laboratory

Clinical.

Treatment

- *Ptosis*: If visual acuity is affected most cases require surgical correction and there are several procedures that may be used including levator resection, repair or advancement and Fasanella-Servat.
- *Strabismus*: Equalized vision with correct refractive error, surgery may be helpful in patient with diplopia.
- *Glaucoma*: Glaucoma medication should be the first plan of action. If medication is unsuccessful, a filtering surgical procedure with or without antimetabolites may be beneficial.
- *Cataract*: Change in glasses can sometimes improve a patient's visual function temporarily; however the most common treatment is cataract surgery.
- *Vitreous hemorrhage*: If possible the source of the bleeding needs to be isolated and treated with laser. Vitrectomy may be necessary.
- *Retinal detachment*: Scleral buckle, pneumatic retinopexy and vitrectomy may be used to close all the breaks.

🗗 BIBLIOGRAPHY

1. Krause AC. Congenital encephalo-ophthalmic dysplasia. Arch Ophthalmol. 1946;36:387-94.
2. Miller M, Robbins J, Fishman R, et al. A chromosomal anomaly with multiple ocular defects. Am J Ophthalmol. 1963;55:901.

🗗 1EE.51B10F. MEYER-SCHWICKERATH-WEYERS SYNDROME (MICROPHTHALMOS SYNDROME; OCULODENTODIGITAL DYSPLASIA)

General

Etiology unknown; two types recognized: (I) dysplasia oculodentodigitalis and (II) dyscraniopygophalangie; type I is characterized by microphthalmia with possible iris pathology and glaucoma, oligodontia and brown pigmentation of teeth, camptodactyly, and possible absence of middle phalanx of second to fifth toes; type II consists of severe microphthalmos to anophthalmos, polydactyly, and developmental anomalies of nose and oral cavity; both sexes affected; present from birth; abnormal cerebral white matter.

Ocular

Microphthalmos; hypotrichosis; glaucoma; iris anomalies (eccentric pupil; changes in normal iris texture; remnants of pupillary membrane along iris margins); microcornea; hypertelorism; myopia; hyperopia; keratoconus.

Clinical

Thin, small nose with anteverted nostrils and hypoplastic alae; syndactyly; camptodactyly (fourth and fifth fingers); anomalies of middle phalanx of fifth finger and toe; hypoplastic teeth; wide mandible; alveolar ridge; sparse hair growth; visceral malformations.

Laboratory

Diagnosis is made by clinical findings.

Treatment

- *Glaucoma*: Glaucoma medication should be the first plan of action. If medication is unsuccessful, a filtering surgical procedure with or without antimetabolites may be beneficial.
- *Keratoconus*: Spectacle correction, hard contacts, avoid eye rubbing. If hydrops occur, discontinue contact lens, use NaCl drops and ointment, patching, and short course of steroids. As disease advances, PK, deep anterior lamellar keratoplasty intacs with laser grooves or collagen stabilization of cornea.

🗗 BIBLIOGRAPHY

1. Geeraets WK. Ocular Syndromes, 3rd edition. Philadelphia: Lea & Febiger; 1976.
2. , Gutmann DH, Zackai EH, McDonald-McGinn DM, et al. Oculodentodigital dysplasia syndrome associated with abnormal cerebral white matter. Am J Med Genet. 1991; 41:18-20.
3. McKusick VA. Mendelian Inheritance in Man: A Catalog of Human Genes and Genetic Disorders, 12th edition. Baltimore: The Johns Hopkins University Press; 1998.

🗗 1EE.51B10G. PIERRE-ROBIN SYNDROME (ROBIN SYNDROME; MICROGNATHIA-GLOSSOPTOSIS SYNDROME)

General

Etiology unknown; manifestations at birth; pathogenesis based on arrested fetal development; history of intrauterine disturbance in early pregnancy (25% of cases); also increased incidence in offspring of mother's age 35 years or older; pathogenesis is thought to be incomplete development of the first brachial arch, which forms the maxilla and mandible.

Ocular

Microphthalmos; proptosis; ptosis; high myopia; glaucoma; cataract (rare); retinal disinsertion; megalocornea; iris atrophy; blue sclera; esotropia; conjunctivitis; distichiasis; vitreoretinal degeneration; retinal detachments.

Clinical

Micrognathia; cleft palate; glossoptosis; cyanosis; facial expression bird-like with flat base of nose and high-arched deformed palate with or without cleft; difficulty in breathing.

Laboratory

Diagnosis is made by clinical findings.

Treatment

Multidisciplinary approach is required to manage the complex features involved in the care of these children and their families.

⊟ BIBLIOGRAPHY

1. Tewfik TL, Trinh N, Teebi AS. (2012). Pierre Robin syndrome. [online] Available from www.emedicine.com/ent/TOPIC150.HTM. [Accessed September, 2013].

⊟ 1EE.51B10H. RETINAL DISINSERTION SYNDROME (KERATOCONUS)

General

None.

Ocular

Subluxation of the lens; microphthalmos; bilateral keratoconus; retinal detachment.

Clinical

None.

Laboratory

Diagnosis is made by clinical findings.

Treatment

Spectacle correction, hard contacts, avoid eye rubbing. If hydrops occur, discontinue contact lens, use NaCl drops and ointment, patching, and short course of steroids. As disease advances, PK, deep anterior lamellar keratoplasty intacs with laser grooves or collagen stabilization of cornea. Subluxation of the lens—careful phacoemulsification, topical steroids to control ocular inflammation.

⊟ BIBLIOGRAPHY

1. Ryan SJ (Ed). Retina (Volume III), 2nd edition. St. Louis: Mosby; 1994.
2. Hovland KR, Schepens CL, Freeman HM. Developmental giant retinal tears associated with lens coloboma. Arch Ophthalmol. 1968;80:325-31.

⊟ 1EE.51B10I. SABIN-FELDMAN SYNDROME (CHORIORETINITIS)

General

Etiology unknown; similar to toxoplasmosis; results of toxoplasma dye and complement fixation tests are negative; onset in early infancy.

Ocular

Microphthalmia; strabismus; fixed pupils; posterior lenticonus; microcornea; chorioretinitis or atrophic degenerative chorioretinal changes; optic atrophy.

Clinical

Cerebral calcifications (infrequent); convulsions (frequent); microcephaly; hydrocephalus.

Laboratory

Clinical.

Treatment

Lens extraction with irrigation-aspiration.

⊟ BIBLIOGRAPHY

1. Geeraets WJ. Ocular Syndromes, 3rd edition. Philadelphia: Lea & Febiger; 1976.
2. Sabin AB, Feldman HA. Chorioretinopathy associated with other evidence of cerebral damage in childhood: a syndrome of unknown etiology separable from congenital toxoplasmosis. J Pediatr. 1949;35:296.

🖻 1EE.51B10J. WEYERS SYNDROME (2) (WEYERS IV SYNDROME; LRIDODENTAL DYSPLASIA; DENTOIRIDEAL DYSPLASIA; DYSGENESIS IRIDODENTALIS; DYSGENESIS MESODERMALIS CORNEAE ET IRIDES WITH DIGODONTIA) CORNEAL OPACITY

General

Present from birth; hereditary; etiology unknown.

Ocular

Dysplasia; small perforation of iris; pupillary synechiae; microphthalmia; corneal opacity.

Clinical

Dwarfism; myotonic dystrophy; microdontia; oligodontia; hypoplasia of dental enamel.

Laboratory

Clinical.

Treatment

None.

🖻 BIBLIOGRAPHY

1. Magalini SI, Scrascia E. Dictionary of Medical Syndromes, 2nd edition. Philadelphia: JB Lippincott; 1981. p. 864.
2. Weyers H. Dysgenesis Irido-dentalis. Ein Neues Syndrome mit obweichdendem Chromosomalen Geschlecht bei Weiblichen Merkmalträgern. Presented at the Meeting of Deutsche Gessellschaft fuer Kinderheilkunde, Kassel, Germany: 1960.

🖻 1EE.51B11A. RUBELLA SYNDROME (CONGENITAL RUBELLA SYNDROME; GERMAN MEASLES; GREGG SYNDROME)

General

Rubella infection of the mother during first trimester of pregnancy; ocular disease is the most commonly found abnormality in patients with congenital rubella syndrome (75%), multiorgan disease is common (greater than 75%); no significant association has been found between gestational age and time of maternal infection and incidence of individual ocular conditions.

Ocular

Nystagmus; glaucoma; corneal haziness; cataracts; retinal pigmentary changes; appearance and central distribution of lesions are quite distinguishable from retinitis pigmentosa; retinopathy is not progressive and has little, if any, effect on vision; waxy atrophy of optic disk; conjunctivitis; megalocornea or microcornea; buphthalmos; microphthalmos; uveitis; iris atrophy; spherophakia; strabismus.

Clinical

Low-birth weight; diarrhea; pneumonia; urinary infection; hearing loss; heart disease; hepatosplenomegaly; mental retardation; inguinal hernias; ataxia; cardiac abnormalities.

Laboratory

Diagnosis is made by clinical findings. If in doubt, a rising titer of IgM will indicate a recent infection.

Treatment

Treatment for rubella of the eye centers on glaucoma and cataract.

🖻 BIBLIOGRAPHY

1. Lombardo PC. (2011). Dermatologic manifestations of rubella. [online] Available from www.emedicine.com/derm/TOPIC380.HTM. [Accessed September, 2013].

1EE.51B11B. CONGENITAL SPHEROCYTIC ANEMIA (CONGENITAL HEMOLYTIC JAUNDICE; HEREDITARY SPHEROCYTOSIS)

General

Hereditary deficiency of erythrocyte glucose-6-phosphate after exposure to certain drugs, chemicals, and foods such as fava beans.

Ocular

Congenital cataract; ring-shaped pigmentary deposits of cornea; tortuosity of retinal vessels; mongoloid palpebral aperture; microphthalmos.

Clinical

Leukemia; anemia.

Laboratory

The most sensitive test is the incubated osmotic fragility test performed after incubating RBCs for 18–24 hours under sterile conditions.

Treatment

The treatment involves presplenectomy care, splenectomy, and postsplenectomy complications.

BIBLIOGRAPHY

1. Gonzalez G, Eichner ER. (2012). Hereditary spherocytosis. [online] Available from www.emedicine.com/med/TOPIC2147.HTM. [Accessed September, 2013].

1EE.51B11C. OCULAR TOXOPLASMOSIS (TOXOPLASMIC RETINOCHOROIDITIS; TOXOPLASMOSIS)

General

Parasite infestation caused by *Toxoplasma gondii*; cell-mediated immunity is believed to be the major defence mechanism against *Toxoplasma* infection; ocular toxoplasmosis occurs in approximately 1% of patients with AIDS; AIDS-related toxoplasma retinochoroiditis may have several atypical clinical manifestations.

Ocular

Keratitis; uveitis; optic atrophy; papillitis; anisocoria; persistent pupillary membrane; focal retinochoroiditis; scleritis; cataract; microphthalmos; myopia; nystagmus; esotropia.

Clinical

Cysts are seen in many organs, including brain and muscle; hydrocephalus; intracerebral calcification; various CNS complaints.

Laboratory

Serologic tests for anti-*T. gondii*. Antibodies are common.

Treatment

Triple drug therapy: pyrimethamine, sulfadiazine and prednisone. Pyrimethamine should be combined with folinic acid. Surgical care includes photocoagulation, cryotherapy or vitrectomy.

BIBLIOGRAPHY

1. Wuh L. (2011). Ophthalmologic Manifestations of Toxoplasmosis. [online] Available from www.emedicine.com/oph/TOPIC707.HTM. [Accessed September, 2013].
2. Lasave AF, Llopis MD, Muccioli C, et al. Intravitreal clindamycin and dexamethasone for zone 1 toxoplasmic retinochoroiditis at twenty-four months. Ophthalmology. 2010;1831-8.

🗗 1EE.51B11D. CYTOMEGALOVIRUS RETINITIS

General

Cytomegalovirus is a ubiquitous DNA virus that infects the majority of adults and generally, only an issue in immuno-compromised individuals such as those with AIDS, transplant and those on immunosuppressive medication.

Clinical

AIDS, transplantation patients; myalgia, cervical lymphadenopathy; hepatitis.

Ocular

Decreased visual acuity; blindness; retinitis; retinal detachment; retinal breaks; necrotic retina.

Laboratory

Laboratory testing is performed to determine the cause; ultrasound is done to evaluate for retinal detachment; dilated fundus examination.

Treatment

Intravitreal ganciclovir implant or injection may be used; retinal detachment surgery may be necessary.

🗗 BIBLIOGRAPHY

1. Altaweel M, Youssef PN, Reed MD. (2012). CMV retinitis. [online] Available from emedicine.medscape.com/article/1227228-overview. [Accessed September, 2013].

🗗 1EE.51B11E. INFECTIOUS MONONUCLEOSIS (MONONUCLEOSIS; EPSTEIN-BARR VIRUS, ACUTE; ACUTE EPSTEIN-BARR VIRUS, GLANDULAR FEVER)

General

Asymptomatic in childhood; manifested in late adolescence of early adulthood; associated with Burkitt lymphoma and nasopharyngeal carcinoma.

Ocular

Conjunctivitis; ptosis; hippus; dacryocystitis; episcleritis; hemianopsia; nystagmus; retinal and subconjunctival hemorrhages; optic neuritis; orbital edema; scotoma; paralysis of extraocular muscles; uveitis; peripheral choroiditis; keratitis; papilledema; scleritis; retrobulbar neuritis, Sjögren syndrome; retinitis, choroiditis.

Clinical

Fever; widespread lymphadenopathy; pharyngitis; hepatic involvement; presence of atypical lymphocytes and heterophile antibodies in the blood; fatigue.

Treatment

A self-limited illness that does not usually require specific therapy. Splenic rupture is an acute abdominal emergency that usually requires surgical intervention.

🗗 BIBLIOGRAPHY

1. Cunha BA. (2011). Infectious Mononucleosis. [online] Available from www.emedicine.com/med/TOPIC1499.HTM. [Accessed September, 2013].

🗗 1EE.51B11F. CHICKENPOX (VARICELLA)

General

Acute exanthematous disease; highly contagious; children between ages between 2 and 8 years.

Ocular

Conjunctival ulcer; corneal ulcer; descemetocele; corneal opacity; keratitis; paresis of third, fourth and sixth nerves; optic neuritis; papilledema; retinitis; hemorrhagic retinopathy; uveitis; cataract; paralytic mydriasis; phthisis bulbi; unifocal choroiditis; dendritic keratitis; acute retinal necrosis (in a patient with AIDS); disciform keratitis.

Clinical

Fever; malaise; rash; pruritus.

Laboratory

Diagnosis is made by clinical findings.

Treatment

Isolation oral antihistamines, such as diphenhydramine and hydroxyzine, are used for severe pruritus and acetaminophen is recommended for the reduction of fever.

⊟ BIBLIOGRAPHY

1. Bechtel KA, Chatterjee A, Lichenstein R, et al. (2013). Pediatric chickenpox. [online] Available from www.emedicine. com/emerg/TOPIC367.HTM. [Accessed September, 2013].

⊟ 1EE.51B12A. FETAL ALCOHOL SYNDROME

General

Dysgenesis in children born to alcoholic mothers; both sexes affected; onset from birth.

Ocular

Antimongoloid slant of lid fissures; lateral displacement of inner canthi; ptosis; epicanthi; strabismus; myopia; optic nerve hypoplasia; diffuse corneal clouding; iridocorneal abnormalities with central corneal edema; lens opacification; motility disorders.

Clinical

Growth retardation; delayed development (physical and intellectual); maxillary hypoplasia; micrognathia; large, low-set ears; abnormal motor function; irritability; microcephaly; cerebral nervous system dysfunctions; abnormal philtrum; flattened nasal bridge; cardiovascular defects; thin upper lip.

Laboratory

If suspected, consult a subspecialist (e.g. geneticist, developmentalist) to confirm the diagnosis.

Treatment

Treat for associated birth defects and intervention for potential cognitive and behavioral abnormalities. Vitrectomy may be necessary.

⊟ BIBLIOGRAPHY

1. Vaux KK, Chambers C. (2012). Fetal alcohol syndrome. [online] Available from www.emedicine.com/ped/TOPIC767.HTM. [Accessed September, 2013].

⊟ 1EE.51B12B. FOLLING SYNDROME (PHENYLKETONURIA; PHENYLPYRUVIC OLIGOPHRENIA; IKIOTIA PHENYLKETONURIA SYNDROME)

General

Rare; autosomal recessive; phenylalanine cannot be converted to tyrosine; poor prognosis without early diet therapy; both sexes affected.

Ocular

Blue sclera; severe photophobia; corneal opacities; cataracts (controversial); partial ocular albinism; macular atrophy.

Clinical

Phenylketonuria; oligophrenia; partial albinism; muscle hypertonicity; hyper-reflexia of tendons; epilepsy; microcephaly; mousy odor of habitus; fair skin.

Laboratory

Newborn screening, low-grade elevations of phenylalanine may require repeat screening. More significant elevations may require definitive testing and/or referral to a metabolic treatment facility experienced with phenylketonuria (PKU).

Treatment

Most patients are treated in a specialty metabolic clinic, usually under the auspices of a genetics or pediatric endocrinology clinic. Treatment consists of dietary restriction of phenylalanine with tyrosine supplementation.

⊟ BIBLIOGRAPHY

1. Arnold GL, Steiner RD. (2013). Phenylketonuria. [online] Available from www.emedicine.com/ped/TOPIC1787.HTM. [Accessed September, 2013].

1EE.52. MÖBIUS II SYNDROME (CONGENITAL FACIAL DIPLEGIA; CONGENITAL PARALYSIS OF THE SIXTH AND SEVENTH NERVES; CONGENITAL OCULOFACIAL PARALYSIS; VON GRAEFES SYNDROME)

General

Congenital; possibly failure of development of facial nerve cells or primary defect of muscles deriving from first two brachial arches or both; recovery in a few weeks or non-progressive permanent paralysis of face; asymmetrical; if incomplete, usually spares lower face and platysma.

Ocular

Proptosis; ptosis; weakness of abductor muscles; normal convergence; limitation to internal rotation in lateral movements; esotropia.

Clinical

Facial diplegia; deafness; loss of vestibular responses; webbed fingers or toes; clubfoot.

Laboratory

Diagnosis is made by clinical findings.

Treatment

Ptosis: If visual acuity is affected most cases require surgical correction and there are several procedures that may be used including levator resection, repair or advancement and Fasanella-Servat.

BIBLIOGRAPHY

1. Abbott RL, Metz HS, Weber AA. Saccadic velocity studies in Möbius syndrome. Ann Ophthalmol. 1978;10:619-23.
2. Fenichel GM. Congenital facial asymmetry (aplasia of facial muscles). In: Fenichel GM (ed). Clinical pediatric neurology, 2nd edition. Philadelphia: WB Saunders; 1993. pp. 341-2.
3. Kawai M, Momoi T, Fujii T, et al. The syndrome of Möbius sequence, peripheral neuropathy, and hypogonadotropic hypogonadism. Am J Med Genet. 1990;37:578-82.
4. Menkes JH, Kenneth T. Möbius syndrome. In: Menkes JH (ed). Textbook of child neurology, 5th edition. Baltimore: Williams & Wilkins; 1995. pp. 309-10.
5. Merz M, Wójtowicz S. The Möbius syndrome. Report of electromyographic examinations in two cases. Am J Ophthalmol. 1967;63(4):837-40.
6. Möbius PJ. über angeborene doppelseitige Abducens-Facial-islahmung. Munch Med Wochenschr. 1888;35:91-108.
7. Pucket CL, Beg SA. Facial reanimation in Möbius syndrome. South Med J. 1978;71(12):1498-501.

1EE.53. MORQUIO SYNDROME (MORQUIO-BRAILSFORD SYNDROME; BRAILSFORD-MORQUIO DYSTROPHY; FAMILIAL OSSEOUS DYSTROPHY; KERATOSULFATURIA; MPS IV; MUCOPOLYSACCHARIDOSIS IV; SPONDYLOEPI-PHYSEAL DYSPLASIA; OSTEOCHONDRODYSTROPHIA DEFORMANS; INFANTILE HEREDITARY CHONDRODYSPLASIA; HEREDITARY POLY TOPIC ENCHONDRAL DYSOSTOSIS; HEREDITARY OSTEOCHONDRODYSTROPHY; ECCENTRO-OSTEOCHONDRODYSPLASIA; DYSOSTOSIS ENCHONDRALIS META-EPIPHYSARIA; MORQUIO-ULLRICH SYNDROME; ATYPICAL CHONDRODYSTROPHY; CHONDRODYSTROPHIA TARDA; CHONDRO-OSTEODYSTROPHY)

General

Autosomal recessive dystrophy of cartilage and bone; slight predilection for males; apparent between ages 4 and 10 years; excess production of keratosulfate (*see* Hurler Syndrome; Hunter Syndrome; Sanfilippo-Good Syndrome; Scheie Syndrome; Maroteaux-Lamy Syndrome); autosomal recessive; abnormal N-acetylgalactosamine-G-sulfate sulfatase.

Ocular

Enophthalmos; ptosis; excessive tear secretion; ocular hypotony; miosis; occasionally hazy cornea; bushy eyebrows; optic nerve atrophy; moderate-to-late corneal clouding.

Clinical

Dwarfism; skeletal deformities (progressive); delayed ossification of epiphyses; decreased muscle tone; deafness; weak extremities; waddling gait; coarse broad mouth; spaced teeth; aortic regurgitation; normal intelligence.

Laboratory

Blood-Reilly's granules in leukocytes; X-ray—flat vertebrae and odontoid hypoplasia.

Treatment

Treatment is limited to supportive care.

🖫 BIBLIOGRAPHY

1. Bittar T, Washington ER. (2012). Mucopolysaccharidosis. [online] Available from www.emedicine.com/orthoped/TOPIC203.HTM. [Accessed September, 2013].

🖫 1EE.55. MYOTONIC DYSTROPHY SYNDROME (MYOTONIA ATROPHICA SYNDROME; DYSTROPHIA MYOTONICA; CURSCHMANN-STEINERT SYNDROME)

General

Rare autosomal dominant disease; onset at the age of 20 years; condition is worsened by administration of neostigmine (Prostigmin); associated with an unstable DNA sequence composed of varying numbers of CTG triplet repeats (which allows a specific molecular test for this disorder).

Ocular

Mild ptosis (occasionally); myotonic cataract with small, dot-like subcapsular cortical opacities during early stage, with polychromatic properties on biomicroscopic examination; corneal epithelial dystrophy; loss of corneal sensitivity; tapetoretinal degeneration; macular red spot; macular degeneration; chorioretinitis; pilomatrixomas; ocular hypotony; pattern pigmentary changes; abnormal saccades.

Clinical

Progressive muscular atrophy with selection of certain muscles (mainly sternocleidomastoid, temporalis, dorsiflexor muscles of the ankle, anterior oblique); myotonia; bland facial expression; speech disturbance due to involvement of vocal cords and palatal muscles; dysphagia; endocrine disturbances.

Laboratory

Diagnosis is made by clinical findings.

Treatment

- *Ptosis*: If visual acuity is affected, most cases require surgical correction and there are several procedures that may be used including levator resection, repair or advancement and Fasanella-Servat.
- *Cataract*: Change in glasses can sometimes improve a patient's visual function temporarily; however, the most common treatment is cataract surgery.

- *Corneal dystrophy*: Mild cases—can be observed and soft contact lenses are helpful; PK may be necessary; graft recurrences are treated by superficial keratectomy, PTK or repeat PK.
- *Macular degeneration*: No treatment is available for non-neovascular AMD. Preventative therapy includes no smoking, control of hypertension, cholesterol, and blood sugar, exercise and vitamins. Neovascular AMD treatment consists of laser, avastin and lucentis.

🖫 BIBLIOGRAPHY

1. Brooke NM, Cwik VE. Myotonic dystrophy. In: Bradley WG (Ed). Neurology in Clinical Practice: Principles of Diagnosis and Management, 2nd edition. Boston, USA: Butterworth-Heinemann; 1995. pp. 2020-2.
2. Gjertsen IK, Sandvig KU, Eide N, et al. Recurrence of secondary opacification and development of a dense posterior vitreous membrane in patients with myotonic dystrophy. J Cataract Refract Surg. 2003;29(1):213-6.
3. Kimizuka Y, Kiyosawa M, Tamai M, et al. Retinal changes in myotonic dystrophy. Clinical and follow-up evaluation. Retina. 1993;13(2):129-35.
4. Koca MR, Horn F, Korth M. Alterations of saccadic eye movements in myotonic dystrophy. Graefes Arch Clin Exp Ophthalmol. 1992;230(5):437-41.
5. Kuwabara T, Lessell S. Electron microscopic study of extraocular muscles in myotonic dystrophy. Am J Ophthalmol. 1976;82(2):303-9.
6. Mausolf FA, Burns CA, Burian HM. Morphologic and functional retinal changes in myotonic dystrophy unrelated to quinine therapy. Am J Ophthalmol. 1972;74(6):1141-3.
7. Meyer E, Navon D, Auslender L, et al. Myotonic dystrophy: pathological study of the eyes. Ophthalmologica. 1980;181(3-4):215-20.
8. Reardon W, MacMillan JC, Myring J, et al. Cataract and myotonic dystrophy: the role of molecular diagnosis. Br J Ophthalmol. 1993;77(9):579-83.
9. Rosa N, Lanza M, Borrelli M, et al. Low intraocular pressure resulting from ciliary body detachment in patients with myotonic dystrophy. Ophthalmology. 2011;118(2):260-4.

⊟ 1EE.57. VON RECKLINGHAUSEN SYNDROME (NEUROFIBROMATOSIS TYPE I; NEURINOMATOSIS)

General

Dominant inheritance activated at puberty, during pregnancy and at menopause; strong evidence supports the existence of neurofibromatosis type I (NF-I) as a tumor suppressor gene.

Ocular

Proptosis; displacement of the globe; pulsation of the globe; ptosis; elephantiasis of the lids; pigment spots on lids; hydrophthalmos; nodular swelling of corneal nerves; cataracts; optic atrophy; choroidal melanoma; neurofibroma of the choroid, iris, eyelid and ciliary body; enlarged optic foramen; underdevelopment of orbital bones; café-au-lait spots on fundus; hamartoma of retina; congenital glaucoma; focal iris nodules; choroidal nevi; optic nerve gliomas; orbital neurofibroma; keratoconus.

Clinical

Café-au-lait skin pigmentations; fibroma molluscum; lipomas and sebaceous adenomas; schwannomas; growth abnormalities; spontaneous fractures; facial hemihypertrophy.

Laboratory

T2-weighted MRI images demonstrate multiple bright lesions in the basal ganglia, cerebellum, and brain in 80% optic nerve gliomas often develop perineural arachnoidal hyperplasia, which appears as an expanded CSF space around the nerve.

Treatment

Oral ketotifen may reduce the pain, tenderness and itchiness associated with neurofibromas.

⊟ BIBLIOGRAPHY

1. Dahl AA. (2011). Ophthalmologic manifestations of neurofibromatosis type. [online] Available from www.emedicine.com/oph/TOPIC338.HTM. [Accessed September, 2013].

⊟ 1EE.58. NONNE-MILROY-MEIGE DISEASE (CHRONIC HEREDITARY LYMPHEDEMA; MILROY DISEASE; MEIGE DISEASE; MEIGE-MILROY SYNDROME; NONNE-MILROY SYNDROME; CHRONIC HEREDITARY EDEMA; CHRONIC HEREDITARY TROPHEDEMA; CHRONIC TROPHEDEMA; ELEPHANTIASIS CONGENITA HEREDITARIA; FAMILIAL HEREDITARY EDEMA; HEREDITARY EDEMA; IDIOPATHIC HEREDITARY LYMPHEDEMA; PSEUDOEDEMATOUS HYPODERMAL HYPERTROPHY; PSEUDOELEPHANTIASIS NEUROARTHRITICA; OROMANDIBULAR DYSTONIA; BLEPHAROSPASM-OROMANDIBULAR DYSTONIA; CONGENITAL TROPHEDEMA; TROPHOLYMPHEDEMA; TROPHONEUROSIS; ELEPHANTIASIS ARABUM CONGENITA)

General

Autosomal dominant; prevalent in females; two types: praecox at birth to 35 years and tarda after age 35 years.

Ocular

Lid and conjunctival edema; blepharoptosis; distichiasis; strabismus; buphthalmos; ectropion.

Clinical

Lymphedema; mandibulofacial dysostosis; unilateral or bilateral edema of ankle ascending to the knee and eventually above; rough, pigmented skin over swollen parts.

Laboratory

Clincal findings.

Treatment

Prevention of infection and control local complications.

BIBLIOGRAPHY

1. Rossy KM, Scheinfeld NS. (2013). Lymphedema. [online] Available from www.emedicine.com/med/TOPIC1482. HTM. [Accessed September, 2013].

1EE.59. NOONAN SYNDROME (MALE TURNER SYNDROME)

General

Similar to Turner syndrome, but with normal chromosomal analysis; X-linked dominant inheritance; X-linked dominant phenotype.

Ocular

Hypertelorism; exophthalmos; ptosis (unilateral or bilateral); antimongoloid-slanting palpebral fissure; myopia; keratoconus; optic disk coloboma.

Clinical

Valvular pulmonary stenosis; short stature; webbed neck; low hairline in the back; cubitus valgus; deformed chest wall; micrognathia; low-set ears; mild mental retardation.

Laboratory

Xl deficiency, bleeding diatheses, karyotyping test, cardiac examination.

Treatment

Growth hormone therapy.

BIBLIOGRAPHY

1. Ibrahim J, McGovern MM. (2013). Noonan syndrome. [online] Available from www.emedicine.com/ped/TOPIC1616.HTM. [Accessed September, 2013].

1EE.60. OCULOPHARYNGEAL SYNDROME (PROGRESSIVE MUSCULAR DYSTROPHY WITH PTOSIS AND DYSPHAGIA; OCULOPHARYNGEAL MUSCULAR DYSTROPHY)

General

Etiology unknown; autosomal dominant inheritance; no CNS pathology; muscles of pharynx, hypopharynx, and proximal third of esophagus involved with myopathy; onset late in life; progressive hereditary myopathy in which the levator palpebrae and pharyngeal muscles are selectively involved; progressive usually symmetrical blepharoptosis with or without dysphagia appears in the 5th decade.

Ocular

Ptosis.

Clinical

Dysphagia; occasionally weakness of facial muscles.

Laboratory/Ocular

Diagnosis is made by clinical findings.

Treatment

Ptosis: If visual acuity is affected, most cases require surgical correction and there are several procedures that may be used including levator resection, repair or advancement and Fasanella-Servat.

BIBLIOGRAPHY

1. Codère F. Oculopharyngeal muscular dystrophy. Can J Ophthalmol. 1993;28(1):1-2.
2. Duranceau A, Forand MD, Fauteux JP. Surgery in oculopharyngeal muscular dystrophy. Am J Surg. 1980;139(1):33-9.
3. Jordan DR, Addison DJ. Surgical results and pathological findings in the oculopharyngeal dystrophy syndrome. Can J Ophthalmol. 1993;28(1):15-8.
4. Molgat YM, Rodrigue D. Correction of blepharoptosis in oculopharyngeal muscular dystrophy: review of 91 cases. Can J Ophthalmol. 1993;28(1):11-4.
5. Murphy SF, Drachman DB. The oculopharyngeal syndrome. JAMA. 1968;203(12):1003-8.
6. Taylor EW. Progressive vagus-glossopharyngeal paralysis with ptosis: contribution to a group of family diseases. J Nerv Ment Dis. 1915;42(3):129-39.

1EE.61. PAPILLON-LEAGE-PSAUME SYNDROME (ORO-DIGITAL-FACIAL SYNDROME; LINGUOFACIAL DYSPLASIA OF GROB; GORLIN SYNDROME; DYSPLASIA LINGUOFACIALIS; OFD SYNDROME; ORO-DIGITAL-FACIAL DYSOSTOSIS; GROB LINGUOFACIAL DYSPLASIA)

General

Familial with strong female preponderance; transmitted as a dominant; partial trisomy has been suggested for the 6-12 (C) chromosome.

Ocular

Hypertelorism; displaced medial and lateral canthi; anti-mongoloid slanting of palpebral fissures; exotropia; see-saw winking.

Clinical

Clefts of jaws and tongue due to abnormalities in development of frenulum; syndactyly; polydactyly; alopecia; white, hamartomatous patches of midline of tongue; mental retardation; bradydactyly; hypoplastic nasal cartilages; seborrheic changes; dystopia canthus; pseudocleft of upper lip; alopecia; missing mandibular lateral incisors.

Laboratory

Patients with suspected Gorlin syndrome undergo biopsy with samples obtained from several suspicious skin lesions.

Treatment

Wide range of congenital anomalies. May need to be treated by a wide range of specialists, including dermatologists, dentists, cardiologists, oncologists, and orthopedic surgeons. Patients most commonly present to a dermatologist because of skin nodules.

BIBLIOGRAPHY

1. Berg D, Olson JM. (2013). Nevoid Basal Cell Carcinoma Syndrome. [online] Available from www.emedicine.com/ped/TOPIC890.HTM. [Accessed September, 2013].

1EE.62. TOURAINE-SOLENTE-GOLE SYNDROME (PACHYDERMOPERIOSTOSIS; ACROPACHYDERMA; AUDRY II SYNDROME; BRUGSCH SYNDROME; FRIEDRICH-ERB-ARNOLD SYNDROME; HEHLINGER SYNDROME)

General

Rare; hereditary; predominant in males; onset in puberty to 3rd decade.

Ocular

Elephantiasis of the lids caused by Meibomian gland cysts and connective tissue hypertrophy; ptosis.

Clinical

Thick and furrowed skin of forehead, face, scalp, hands, and feet; hyperhidrosis of hands and feet; increased subcutaneous secretion; enormous hands and feet; watch crystal-like nails; cylindrical arms and legs; effusions of ankles, knees, and other joints; finger clubbing; facial enlargement; periostitis; cutaneous mucinosis.

Laboratory

Levels of thyrotropin and growth hormone should be tested. Radionucleotide bone imaging.

Treatment

Nonsteroidal anti-inflammatory drugs or corticosteroids may provide comfort from the polyarthritis. Vagotomy may alleviate the swelling and articular pain.

BIBLIOGRAPHY

1. Schwartz RA, Goyal S, Richards GM, et al. (2013). Pachydermoperiostosis. [online] Available from www.emedicine.com/derm/TOPIC815.HTM. [Accessed September, 2013].

🖥 1EE.63. ROMBERG SYNDROME (PARRY-ROMBERG SYNDROME; PROGRESSIVE HEMIFACIAL ATROPHY; PROGRESSIVE FACIAL HEMIATROPHY; FACIAL HEMIATROPHY) ENOPHTHALMUS

General

Autosomal dominant; irritation in the peripheral trophic sympathetic system; onset in the 2nd decade; both sexes affected.

Ocular

Enophthalmos; outer canthus lowered; absence of nasal portion of eyebrow; ptosis; paresis of ocular muscles; miosis; iritis; iridocyclitis; heterochromia iridis; keratitis; neuroparalytic keratitis; cataracts; choroiditis; Fuchs' heterochromic cyclitis; retinal vascular abnormalities; association with Coats syndrome and exudative stellate neuroretinopathy; scleral melting.

Clinical

Atrophy of soft tissue on one side of the face, including tongue; trigeminal neuralgia and/or paresthesia; alopecia and poliosis not uncommon.

Laboratory/Ocular

Neuroimaging, CT scan of the orbits, MRI and bone scans.

Treatment/Ocular

Chemotherapy, ionizing radiation or immunosuppressive treatments.

🖥 BIBLIOGRAPHY

1. Aracena T, Roca FP, Barragan M. Progressive hemifacial atrophy (Parry-Romberg syndrome): report of two cases. Ann Ophthalmol. 1979;11:953-8.
2. Gass JD, Harbin TS, Del Piero EJ. Exudative stellate neuroretinopathy and Coats' syndrome in patients with progressive hemifacial atrophy. Eur J Ophthalmol. 1991;1:2-10.
3. Hoang-Xuan T, Foster CS, Jakobiec FA, et al. Romberg's progressive hemifacial atrophy: an association with scleral melting. Cornea. 1991;10:361-6.
4. La Hey E, Baarsma GS. Fuchs' heterochromic cyclitis and retinal vascular abnormalities in progressive hemifacial atrophy. Eye. 1993;7:426-8.
5. Parry CH. Collections from Unpublished Papers, Volume I. London: Underwood; 1825.
6. Romberg MH. Trophoneurosen. Klin Ergebn. Berlin: A. Forster; 1846.

🖥 1EE.64. SHY-GONATAS SYNDROME

General

Unknown etiology; similar to Hunter and Refsum syndromes; accumulation of lipids in muscles simulates gargoylism; present from birth.

Ocular

Mild proptosis; hypertelorism; ptosis; external ophthalmoplegia (progressive); concentric visual field constriction; keratopathy with possible corneal ulcer; lattice-like white opacities in the area of Bowman membrane; retinal pigmentary degeneration (atypical retinitis pigmentosa) with difficulties with night vision.

Clinical

Weakness of extremities (proximal); myopathy and neuropathy; cerebellar ataxia.

Laboratory

Clinical.

Treatment

- *Ptosis*: If visual acuity is affected most cases require surgical correction and there are several procedures that may be used including levator resection, repair or advancement and Fasanella-Servat.
- *Corneal ulcer*: Corneal cultures may be taken and treatment initiated. Treatment includes a broad spectrum of antibiotics and cycloplegic drops.

🖥 BIBLIOGRAPHY

1. Geeraets WJ. Ocular Syndromes, 3rd edition. Philadelphia: Lea & Febiger; 1976.

2. Gonatas NK. A generalized disorder of nervous system, skeletal muscle and heart resembling Refsum's disease and Hurler's syndrome. II. Ultrastructure. Am J Med. 1967;42:169-78.

3. Shy GM, Silberberg DH, Appel SH, et al. A generalized disorder of nervous system, skeletal muscle and heart resembling Refsum's disease and Hurler's syndrome. I. Clinical, pathologic and biochemical characteristics. Am J Med. 1967;42:163-8.

1EE.65. SMITH-LEMLI-OPITZ SYNDROME (CEREBROHEPATORENAL SYNDROME)

General

Autosomal recessive; similarities with trisomy 18 syndrome; prognosis poor, with death in early infancy (*see* Zellweger Syndrome); onset in fetal life; prevalent in males; reduced myelination in the cerebral hemispheres, cranial nerves, and peripheral nerves secondary to a defective cholesterol biosynthesis.

Ocular

Joining of the eyebrows (synophrys); ptosis (bilateral); pronounced epicanthal folds; strabismus; nystagmus; cataract; optic nerve demyelinization.

Clinical

Mental retardation; microcephaly; hypertonia; low-set ears; high-arched palate; failure to thrive; vomiting; hypospadias; cryptorchidism; metatarsus adductus.

Laboratory

Examination via slit lamp may reveal strabismus, cataracts, ptosis, and/or optic nerve abnormalities. Fetal ultrasonography, sterol analysis, MRI or CT scanning may reveal brain malformations. Renal ultrasonography is used to identify renal anomalies. Abdominal ultrasonography and barium swallow may help to rule out pyloric stenosis.

Treatment

No treatment has proven effective for patients with Smith-Lemli-Opitz.

BIBLIOGRAPHY

1. Steiner RD. (2013). Smith-Lemli-Opitz Syndrome. [online] Available from www.emedicine.com/ped/TOPIC2117.HTM. [Accessed September, 2013].

1EE.66. SMITH SYNDROME (FACIO-SKELETO-GENITAL DYSPLASIA)

General

Autosomal recessive; more common in males.

Ocular

Ptosis; antimongoloid slant; epicanthus.

Clinical

Microcephaly; high-arched palate; large, low-set ears; mental retardation; broad nose; hypoplastic mandible; pedal syndactyly.

Laboratory

Clinical.

Treatment

Ptosis: If visual acuity is affected most cases require surgical correction and there are several procedures that may be used including levator resection, repair or advancement and Fasanella-Servat.

BIBLIOGRAPHY

1. Aita JA. Congenital facial anomalies with neurologic defects. Springfield, IL: Charles C Thomas; 1969. pp. 246.
2. Magalini SI, Scrascia E. Dictionary of Medical Syndromes, 2nd edition. Philadelphia: JB Lippincott; 1981.

1EE.67. ECTOPIA LENTIS WITH ECTOPIA OF PUPIL (ECTOPIA LENTIS ET PUPILLAE)

General

Autosomal recessive.

Ocular

Lens and pupil displaced in opposite directions; bilateral cataracts; acute intermittent IOP crises; persistent pupillary membrane; poor pupillary dilation.

Clinical

None.

Laboratory

Perform appropriate diagnostic and laboratory evaluation-cardiac evaluation for Marfan syndrome; check serum and urine levels of homocysteine or methionine for homocystinuria.

Treatment

Repair of an impending dissecting aortic aneurysm, treatment of glaucoma, lensectomy.

BIBLIOGRAPHY

1. Eifrig CW. (2013). Ectopia Lentis. [online] Available from www.emedicine.com/oph/TOPIC55.HTM. [Accessed September, 2013].

1EE.68. PASSOW SYNDROME (BREMER STATUS DYSRAPHICUS; STATUS DYSRAPHICUS SYNDROME; SYRINGOMYELIA; SYRINGOBULBIA)

General

Congenital nonclosure of the neural tube; familial occurrence or may be sporadic; insidious onset in 2nd to 3rd decade of life.

Ocular

Enophthalmos; ptosis; rotatory nystagmus; heterochromia iridis; anterior uveitis; corneal anesthesia; neuroparalytic keratitis; paralysis of third, fifth, sixth, and seventh cranial nerves; Horner syndrome; anisocoria; papilledema; optic atrophy; zonular cataract (*see* Horner Syndrome).

Clinical

Anesthesia over area of first division of trigeminal nerve; facial hemiatrophy; facial nerve paralysis; muscular weakness; cervical ribs; kyphoscoliosis; spina bifida; unilateral numbness of fingers; loss of deep reflexes; insensitivity to pain and temperature in affected areas; neurogenic bladder.

Laboratory

MRI, CT.

Treatment

Suboccipital and cervical decompression, laminectomy and syringotomy, shunts, fourth ventriculostomy, terminal ventriculostomy and neuroendoscopic surgery may be considered.

BIBLIOGRAPHY

1. Al-Shatoury HA, Galhom AA, Wagner FC. (2012). Syringomyelia. [online] Available from emedicine.medscape.com/article/1151685-overview. [Accessed September, 2013].

⊟ 1EE.70. TREFT SYNDROME (OPTIC ATROPHY)

General

Autosomal dominant; usually appears by age 11 years.

Ocular

Optic atrophy; visual loss; ptosis; ophthalmoplegia.

Clinical

Hearing loss by age 14 years; myopathic changes; balance difficulty.

Laboratory

Diagnosis is made by clinical findings.

Treatment

Optic atrophy: Intravenous steroids may be used with optic neuritis or ischemic neuropathy. Stem cell treatment may be the future treatment of choice.

⊟ BIBLIOGRAPHY

1. McKusick VA. Mendelian Inheritance in Man: A Catalog of Human Genes and Genetic Disorders, 12th edition. Baltimore: The Johns Hopkins University Press; 1998.
2. McKusick-Nathans Institute for Genetic Medicine, Johns Hopkins University and National Center for Biotechnology Information, National Library of Medicine. (2007). Online Mendelian Inheritance in Man, OMIM. [online] Available from www.ncbi.nlm.nih.gov/omim. [Accessed September, 2013].
3. Treft RL, Sanborn GE, Carey J, et al. Dominant optic atrophy, deafness, ptosis, ophthalmoplegia, dystaxia, and myopathy: a new syndrome. Ophthalmology. 1984;91:908-15.

⊟ 1EE.71. TUNBRIDGE-PALEY DISEASE (OPTIC ATROPHY)

General

Onset in childhood; familial; optic atrophy and deafness seen in conjunction with juvenile diabetes mellitus.

Ocular

Optic atrophy; ptosis; retinal pigmentation.

Clinical

Hearing loss; perceptive deafness; juvenile diabetes mellitus; neurogenic bladder; Friedreich ataxia; Refsum syndrome; amentia; epilepsy; Laurence-Moon-Biedl-Bardet syndrome.

Laboratory

Clinical.

Treatment

Ptosis: If visual acuity is affected most cases require surgical correction and there are several procedures that may be used including levator resection, repair or advancement and Fasanella-Servat.

⊟ BIBLIOGRAPHY

1. Ikkos DG, Fraser GR, Matsouki-Gavra E, et al. Association of juvenile diabetes mellitus, primary optic atrophy, and perceptive hearing loss in three sibs, with additional idiopathic diabetes insipidus in one case. Acta Endocrinol. 1970;65:95-102.
2. Konigsmark BW, Knox DL, Hussels IE, et al. Dominant congenital deafness and progressive optic nerve atrophy. Arch Ophthalmol. 1974;91:99-103.
3. Tunbridge RE, Paley RG. Primary optic atrophy in diabetes mellitus. Diabetes. 1956;5:295-6.

🗗 1EE.72. VAN BOGAERT-HOZAY SYNDROME (ESOTROPIA)

General

Manifest after age 3 years; similar to Rubinstein-Taybi syndrome; etiology unknown; affects both sexes.

Ocular

Hypertelorism; hypoplastic cilia and eyebrows; ptosis; esotropia; astigmatism; myopia.

Clinical

Facial dysplasia; broad nasal bridge and zygomatic arch; flat, wide nose; arched palate; skeletal anomalies with short, thick phalangeal joints; finger and toes appear infantile; flat nasal bridge; thickened cheeks; deformed ears; micrognathia.

Laboratory/Ocular

Diagnosis is made by clinical findings.

Treatment

Hypertelorism: The primary correction involves orbital reconstruction and the nasal deformity correction that is universally associated with this deformity.

🗗 BIBLIOGRAPHY

1. Hozay J. Sur une Dystrophic Familiale Particuliere. Inhibition Precoce de la Croissance et Osteolyse Non Mutilante Acrales avec Dysmorphie Faciale. Rev Neural. 1953;89:245.
2. McKusick VA. Mendelian Inheritance in Man: A Catalog of Human Genes and Genetic Disorders, 12th edition. Baltimore: The Johns Hopkins University Press; 1998.
3. McKusick-Nathans Institute for Genetic Medicine, Johns Hopkins University and National Center for Biotechnology Information, National Library of Medicine. (2007). Online Mendelian Inheritance in Man, OMIM. [online] Available from www.ncbi.nlm.nih.gov/omim. [Accessed September, 2013].
4. Roy FH, Summitt RL, Hiatt RL, et al. Ocular manifestations of the Rubinstein-Taybi syndrome. Arch Ophthalmol. 1968; 79:272-8.
5. van Bogaert L. Essai de Classement et d'lnterpretation de Quelques Acro-osteolyses Mutilantes et Non Mutilantes Actuellement Connues. Acta Neural Psychiatr Belg. 1953; 53:90.

🗗 1EE.73. WAARDENBURG SYNDROME (VAN DER HOEVE-HALBERSTAM-WAARDENBURG SYNDROME; WAARDENBURG-KLEIN SYNDROME; EMBRYONIC FIXATION SYNDROME; INTEROCULO-IRIDODERMATO-AUDITIVE DYSPLASIA; PIEBALDISM) HYPERTELORISM

General

Irregular dominant inheritance; developmental fault in neural crest with absence of the organ of Corti, aplasia of the spiral ganglion, and pigmentary changes; no sex preference; onset at birth.

Ocular

Hyperplasia of the medial portions of the eyebrows; hypertelorism; blepharophimosis; strabismus; heterochromia iridis; aniridia; microcornea; cornea plana; microphakia; abnormal fundus pigmentation; hypoplasia of optic nerve; synophrys; poliosis; hypopigmentation and hypoplasia of retina and choroid; epicanthus; lateral displacement of inferior puncta; lenticonus; underdevelopment of orbital bones; lateral displacement of inner canthi; hypopigmented iris.

Clinical

Congenital deafness; unilateral deafness or deaf-mutism; broad and high nasal root with absent nasofrontal angle; albinotic hair strain (unilateral); faint patches of skin pigmentation; pituitary tumor; nasal atresia; white forelock.

Laboratory

Molecular testing and audiology.

Treatment

Genetic counseling, audiology and otolaryngology management.

🗗 BIBLIOGRAPHY

1. Schwartz RA, Bawle EV, Jozwiak S. (2013). Genetics of Waardenburg syndrome. [online] Available from www.emedicine.com/ped/TOPIC2422.HTM. [Accessed September, 2013].

⎘ 1EE.73A1. ARTERIOVENOUS FISTULA (ARTERIOVENOUS ANEURYSM; ARTERIOVENOUS ANGIOMA; ARTERIOVENOUS MALFORMATION; CIRSOID ANEURYSM; RACEMOSE HEMANGIOMA; VARICOSE ANEURYSM)

General

Abnormal communications between arteries and veins that allow arterial blood to enter the vein directly without traversing a capillary network; may be congenital or secondary to penetrating trauma or blunt trauma.

Ocular

Uveitis; chemosis and neovascularization of conjunctiva; bullous keratopathy; eyelid edema; ptosis; exophthalmos; iris atrophy; papilledema; retinal hemorrhages; cataract; paresis of third or sixth nerves; glaucoma; upper lid tumor; total choroidal detachment; leaking retinal macroaneurysms; central retinal vein occlusion; iris neovascularization.

Clinical

Cerebral hemorrhage; death; substernal pain; dyspnea; varicose veins.

Laboratory

Orbital ultrasonography, CT and six-vessel cranial digital subtraction angiography.

Treatment

Obtain emergent neurosurgical consultation for definitive treatment.

⎘ BIBLIOGRAPHY

1. Zebian RC, Kazzi AA. (2013). Emergent management of subarachnoid hemorrhage. [online] Available from www.emedicine.com/emerg/topic559.htm. [Accessed September, 2013].

⎘ 1EE.73A3. HORNER SYNDROME (BERNARD-HORNER SYNDROME; CERVICAL SYMPATHETIC PARALYSIS SYNDROME; CLAUDE-BERNARD-HORNER SYNDROME; HORNER OCULOPUPILLARY SYNDROME)

General

Paralysis of cervical sympathetic; hypothalamic lesion with first neuron involved or lesion in the pons or cervical portion of cord; syndrome present in Babinski-Nageotte, Cestan-Chenais, Dejerine-Klumpke, Pancoast, Raeder, and Wallenberg syndromes (*see* Babinski-Nageotte syndrome; Cestan-Chenais syndrome; Dejerine-Klumpke syndrome; Pancoast syndrome; Raeder syndrome; Wallenberg syndrome).

Ocular

Enophthalmos; ptosis or narrowing of palpebral fissure; ocular hypotony; miosis (degree of miosis depends on the site of lesion; most pronounced when roots of cranial nerves VII and VIII, and first thoracic nerve are involved); hypochromic heterochromia (children more than adults); pupil does not dilate with cocaine.

Clinical

Anhidrosis on ipsilateral side of face and neck; transitory rise in facial temperature; hemifacial atrophy; it may result from a variety of conditions, including cluster headache, parasellar neoplasms or aneurysms, internal carotid dissection or occlusion, and Tolosa-Hunt syndrome.

Laboratory

Pharmacologic testing is very helpful in the diagnosis of Horner syndrome; cocaine or apraclonidine (instilled in an eye with intact sympathetic innervation) causes the pupil to dilate. A sympathetically denervated pupil dilates poorly to cocaine, regardless of the level of the sympathetic interruption because of the absence of endogenous norepinephrine in the synapse.

Treatment

Surgical and medical care is dependent upon the particular etiology. Potential surgical care includes neurosurgical care for aneurysm-related Horner syndrome and vascular surgical care for etiologies such as carotid artery dissection/aneurysm.

BIBLIOGRAPHY

1. Bardorf CM, Stavern GV, Garcia-Valenzuela E. (2012). Horner syndrome. [online] Available from www.emedicine.com/oph/TOPIC336.HTM. [Accessed September, 2013].

⊞ 1EE.73A4. MARCUS GUNN SYNDROME (JAW-WINKING SYNDROME; CONGENITAL TRIGEMINOOCULOMOTOR SYNKINESIS)

General

Familial occurrence rare, although dominant inheritance has been reported; symptoms are caused by abnormal connections between external pterygoid muscle and levator palpebrae, with supranuclear or supranuclear-nuclear involvement (*See* Marin Amat syndrome).

Ocular

Unilateral congenital ptosis in more than 90% of cases; 10% have spontaneous onset, usually in older persons; lid elevates rapidly when mouth is opened or mandible is moved to one or the other side; left eye seems to be more frequently affected than right eye; high incidences of strabismus (36%); amblyopia (34%); bilateral jaw-winking; decreased abduction.

Clinical

Stimulation of ipsilateral pterygoid with chewing, opening of mouth, sucking or contralateral jaw thrusts.

Laboratory

Diagnosis is made by clinical findings.

Treatment

Treat amblyopia; if mild ptosis and mild jaw-winking, consider Muller's muscle conjunctival resection; severe jaw-winking, release levator and perform a frontalis sling usually bilaterally; unilateral ptosis mild jaw-winking, consider levator release and advance frontalis muscle to the superior tarsus.

BIBLIOGRAPHY

1. Blaydon SM. (2011). Marcus Gunn jaw-winking syndrome. [online] Available from www.emedicine.com/oph/TOPIC608.HTM. [Accessed September, 2013].
2. Demirci H, Frueh BR, Nelson CC. Marcus Gunn jaw-winking synkinesis. Ophthalmology. 2010;117(7):1447-52.

⊞ 1EE.73A5. MARIN AMAT SYNDROME (INVERTED MARCUS GUNN PHENOMENON)

General

Intrafacial connection between the orbicularis oculi and external pterygoid muscles; occurs primarily after peripheral facial palsy.

Ocular

When mouth is opened and/or mandible is moved to side opposite to ptosis, closure of the eye occurs; increased tearing during mastication.

Clinical

Signs of old facial palsy are usually recognizable.

Laboratory

Diagnosis is made by clinical findings.

Treatment

If amblyopia is noted, occlusion therapy is needed.

BIBLIOGRAPHY

1. Blaydon SM. (2011). Marcus Gunn jaw-winking syndrome. [online] Available from www.emedicine.com/oph/TOPIC608.HTM. [Accessed September, 2013].

🗗 1EE.73A6. MISDIRECTED THIRD NERVE SYNDROME

General

May occur with a variety of inflammatory infections and parainfections, vascular lesions, tumors, and degenerative and demyelinating diseases that may involve the nerve anywhere; may occur as primary aberrant regeneration without prior history of acute oculomotor nerve palsy.

Ocular

Bizarre eyelid movements that may accompany various eye movements; lid may rise as the medial rectus, the inferior rectus, or the superior rectus muscle contracts; iridoplegia; ptosis.

Clinical

None.

Laboratory

Diagnosis is made by clinical findings.

Treatment

Ptosis: If visual acuity is affected most cases require surgical correction and there are several procedures that may be used including levator resection, repair or advancement and Fasanella-Servat.

🗗 BIBLIOGRAPHY

1. Beard C. Misdirected third nerve syndrome. In: Mosby CV (Ed). Ptosis, 3rd edition. St. Louis: CV Mosby; 1981. p. 115.
2. Harley RD (Ed). Pediatric Ophthalmology, 4th edition. Philadelphia: WB Saunders; 1998.
3. Lepore FE, Glaser JS. Misdirection revisited: a critical appraisal of acquired oculomotor nerve synkinesis. Arch Ophthalmol. 1980;98:2206-9.
4. Miller NR (Ed). Walsh and Hoyt's Clinical Neuro-Ophthalmology, vol. III. 4th editon. Baltimore: Williams & Wilkins, 1988.
5. Roy FH. Ocular Differential Diagnosis, 9th edition. New Delhi: Jaypee Brothers Medical Publishers; 2012.
6. Schatz NJ, Savino PJ, Corbett JJ. Primary aberrant oculomotor regeneration: a sign of intracavernous meningioma. Arch Neurol. 1977;34:29-32.

🗗 1EE.73A7. RILEY-DAY SYNDROME (CONGENITAL FAMILIAL DYSAUTONOMIA)

General

Autosomal recessive; it occurs in Ashkenazi Jewish population; impaired catechol metabolism; manifested in first few days of life; it is characterized by developmental loss of neurons from the sensory and autonomic nervous systems.

Ocular

Congenital failure of tear production; corneal anesthesia; neuroparalytic keratitis; keratitis sicca; corneal ulcers; optic atrophy.

Clinical

Excessive salivation; failure to thrive; recurrent respiratory infections; diarrhea; insensitivity to pain; spontaneous fractures; pandysautonomia; orthostatic hypotension; gastrointestinal paresis; decreased fungiform papillae on the tongue.

Laboratory

DNA test is used to confirm the diagnosis.

Treatment

Artificial drops and/or gels are useful in any dry eye condition. Tarsorrhaphy is an effective treatment of the decompensated neurotrophic cornea.

🗗 BIBLIOGRAPHY

1. D'Amico RA, Axelrod FB. (2011). Familial dysautonomia. [online] Available from www.emedicine.com/oph/TOPIC678.HTM. [Accessed September, 2013].

⊟ 1EE.73A8. VON HERRENSCHWAND SYNDROME (SYMPATHETIC HETEROCHROMIA) PTOSIS

General

Congenital anomaly; heterochromia with Horner syndrome; sympathetic palsy from cervical ribs, tumor of the thyroid gland, enlarged cervical lymph nodes, scars following tuberculosis, or syringomyelia in apex of the pleura.

Ocular

Enophthalmos; ptosis; heterochromia (ipsilateral iris); miosis; iris on the side of the sympathetic denervation usually shows subtle hypochromia.

Clinical

Decreased sweating on ipsilateral side of face as part of the sympathetic paralysis.

Laboratory

CT scan of neck.

Treatment

Seek specialist assistance.

⊟ BIBLIOGRAPHY

1. Durham DG. Congenital heredity in Homer's syndrome. Arch Ophthalmol. 1958;60:939.
2. Eagle RC. Congenital, developmental and degenerative disorders of the iris and ciliary body. In: Albert DM, Jakobiec FA (Eds). Principles and Practice of Ophthalmology. Philadelphia: WB Saunders; 1994. p. 367.
3. Margo CE, Hamed LM. Horner's syndrome. In: Margo CE, Mames R, Hamed LM (Eds). Diagnostic problems in Clinical Ophthalmology. Philadelphia: WB Saunders; 1994. p. 729.
4. Volpe JJ (Ed). Brachial plexus injury. Neurology of the Newborn, 3rd edition. Philadelphia: WB Saunders; 1995. p. 781-4.
5. von Herrenschwand F. Zur Sympathikusheterochromie. Klin Wochenschr. 1923;2:1059.

⊟ 1EE.73B4. BLEPHAROCHALASIS

General

Rare, with recurrent episodic painless periorbital edema.

Clinical

None.

Ocular

Skin of the lids is thin and baggy.

Laboratory

Diagnosis is made by clinical findings.

Treatment

Cold compress may be of some use. Surgical—excise the redundant skin, reposition the ectopic lacrimal gland and reconstruct lateral canthal tendon.

⊟ BIBLIOGRAPHY

1. Roy FH, Fraunfelder FW, Fraunfelder FT. Roy and Fraunfelder's Current Ocular Therapy, 6th edition. London, UK: Elsevier; 2008.

⊟ 1EE.73D1. LUBARSCH-PICK SYNDROME (PRIMARY AMYLOIDOSIS; IDIOPATHIC AMYLOIDOSIS; AMYLOIDOSIS)

General

Rare condition of unknown etiology; inherited as a dominant trait, with male preponderance; characterized by amyloid accumulation in muscles and in gastrointestinal and genitourinary tracts.

Ocular

Internal and external ophthalmoplegia; diminished lacrimation; amyloid deposits in conjunctival, episcleral, and ciliary vessels; vitreous opacities; amyloid deposits in the corneal stroma; retinal hemorrhages and perivascular exudates; paralysis of extraocular muscles; pseudopodia lentis; strabismus fixus convergens; keratoconus.

Clinical

Peripheral neuropathy (extremities); heart failure; defective hepatic and renal functions with hepatosplenomegaly; waxy skin lesions; muscular weakness (progressive); multiple myeloma; hoarseness; chronic gastrointestinal symptoms.

Laboratory

Biopsy-stain with Congo red demonstrates apple-green birefringence under polarized light; distinctive fibrillar ultrastructure.

Treatment

Deoxydoxorubicin had demonstrated some clinical benefit.

BIBLIOGRAPHY

1. Biswas J, Badrinath SS, Rao NA. Primary nonfamilial amyloidosis of the vitreous. A light microscopic and ultrastructural study. Retina. 1992;12(3):251-3.
2. Goebel HH, Friedman AH. Extraocular muscle involvement in idiopathic primary amyloidosis. Am J Ophthalmol. 1971;71(5):1121-7.
3. Lubarsch O. Zur Kenntnis Ungewohnlicher Amyloidablagerungen. Virchows Arch Pathol Anat. 1929; 271:867.
4. Magalini SI, Scrascia E. Dictionary of Medical Syndromes, 2nd edition. Philadelphia: JB Lippincott; 1981.
5. Sharma P, Gupta NK, Arora R, et al. Strabismus fixus convergens secondary to amyloidosis. J Pediatr Ophthalmol Strabismus. 1991;28:236-7.
6. Wong VG, McFarlin DE. A case of primary familial amyloidosis. Arch Ophthalmol. 1967;78:208-13.

1EE.73D2. BOTULISM

General

It is caused by a toxin-producing strain of *C. botulinum;* it occurs primarily after the ingestion of contaminated food; the organism can produce a neurotoxin, the effect of which can be life threatening.

Ocular

Absent optokinetic nystagmus, absent vertical gaze; marked limitation of horizontal gaze; ptosis; diplopia; decreased tear secretion; mydriasis; paralysis of accommodation; nystagmus; optic atrophy; optic neuritis; extraocular muscle paresis.

Clinical

Dizziness; severe respiratory impairment; gastrointestinal disturbances; dysphagia; dysarthria; postural hypotension.

Laboratory

Toxin assay for early diagnosis, whereas later cases are more likely to yield a positive specimen culture.

Treatment

Antitoxin appears to be the only effective medication. Supportive care such as ventilation and parenteral nutrition are necessary for the duration of the paralytic illness.

BIBLIOGRAPHY

1. Patel B, Taylor SF. (2012). Ophthalmologic manifestations of botulism. [online] Available from www.emedicine.com/oph/TOPIC493.HTM. [Accessed September, 2013].

1EE.73D3. BROWN SYNDROME (SUPERIOR OBLIQUE TENDON SHEATH SYNDROME)

General

Etiology unknown; affects both sexes; present from birth; may be congenital or acquired (secondary to trauma, orbital surgery, or injections, or following delivery).

Ocular

Bilateral ptosis with associated backward head tilt; widening of palpebral fissure with attempted upward gaze; ocular movements show failure in the direction of superior oblique action; may be associated with underaction of the inferior oblique; adduction or abduction restricted or completely abolished; choroidal coloboma.

Laboratory

Diagnosis is made by clinical findings.

Treatment

Once systemic disease is excluded, patients' inflammation can be treated with anti-inflammatory medication. Oral ibuprofen is a good first-line choice. Local steroid injections in the area of the trochlea and oral corticosteroids can be used for inflammation. Once the inflammatory disease process is controlled, patients with inflammatory Brown syndrome may show spontaneous resolution. Congenital Brown syndrome is unlikely to improve spontaneously; therefore, surgery is important to consider as an option.

BIBLIOGRAPHY

1. Wright KW, Salvador MG. (2012). Brown syndrome. [online] Available from www.emedicine.com/oph/TOPIC552.HTM. [Accessed September, 2013].
2. Suh DW, Oystreck DT, Hunter DG. Long-term results of an intraoperative adjustable superior oblique tendon suture spacer using nonabsorbable suture for Brown Syndrome. Ophthalmology. 2008;115(10):1800-4.

1EE.73D6B1. CESTAN-CHENAIS SYNDROME [CESTAN (1) SYNDROME]

General

Combination of Babinski-Nageotte and Avellis syndromes; lesion in the lateral portion of medulla oblongata.

Ocular

Enophthalmos; ptosis; nystagmus; miosis.

Clinical

Pharyngolaryngeal or glossopharyngeal paralysis; cerebellar hemiataxia; disturbance of sensibility; contralateral side of lesion.

Laboratory

CT, MRI, transcranial Doppler, ECG.

Treatment

Rehabilitation services have been shown to play a critical role in recovery. Physical, occupational, and speech therapy consultations are necessary.

BIBLIOGRAPHY

1. Kaye V, Brandstater ME. (2011). Vertebrobasilar Stroke Overview of Vertebrobasilar Stroke. [online] Available from www.emedicine.com/pmr/TOPIC143.HTM. [Accessed September, 2013].

1EE.73D6B2. CRANIOCERVICAL SYNDROME (WHIPLASH INJURY)

General

Disturbed accommodation is due to a central lesion rather than a peripheral lesion of the ciliary muscle; Horner syndrome observed where a palsy of the cervical sympathetics occurs (*see* Horner Syndrome).

Ocular

General ocular pain; enophthalmos; mild ptosis; reduced ability to accommodate; disturbance in ocular movements; primarily those extraocular muscles innervated by the oculomotor nerve are involved; convergence insufficiency; nystagmus (gaze direction and vestibular, central, peripheral, and mixed type); vestibular impairment in more than 50% of cases; asthenopia; fogging; double vision; miosis; mydriasis; retinal arteriolar pressure may show changes in systolic and diastolic pressure and be more pronounced than changes in the brachial blood pressure; decreased stereoacuity; vitreous detachment.

Clinical

Headache; vertigo; dizziness; neck and back pain.

Laboratory

Radiographs in the neutral, flexed, and extended positions, should be obtained and the degree of movement measured.

Treatment

Physical therapy; cervical fusion should be considered with great caution and only after aggressive nonsurgical care has failed; intra-articular facet joint injections and medial branch blocks.

BIBLIOGRAPHY

1. Windsor RE, Hankley D, Cone-Sullivan LA, et al. (2012). Cervical Facet Syndrome. [online] Available from www.emedicine.com/sports/TOPIC20.HTM. [Accessed September, 2013].

1EE.73D6B3. CRETINISM (HYPOTHYROID GOITER; HYPOTHYROIDISM; JUVENILE HYPOTHYROIDISM; MYXEDEMA)

General

Deficient thyroid function.

Ocular

Blepharitis; ptosis; enophthalmos; temporal madarosis; decreased tear secretion; glaucoma; proptosis; optic atrophy; optic neuritis; blue dot cataract; conjunctivitis; scleritis; optic disk hemorrhage and arcuate scotoma associated with glaucoma.

Clinical

Myxedema; larynx and tongue swollen; hoarse speech; dry, yellowish skin; slow pulse; mental retardation; infertility; pericardial effusion; cardiac enlargement; physical development retarded.

Laboratory

Clinical.

Treatment

- *Blepharitis*: Oral tetracyclines, omega-3 fatty acids, flax seed oil or fish oil. Ocular therapy include eyelid scrubs, warm compresses, bacitracin ointment to lid margins, topical cyclosporine A and preservative free lubricants.
- *Ptosis*: If visual acuity is affected, most cases require surgical correction and there are several procedures that may be used including levator resection, repair or advancement and Fasanella-Servat.
- *Glaucoma*: Glaucoma medication should be the first plan of action. If medication is unsuccessful, a filtering surgical procedure with or without antimetabotites may be beneficial.
- *Cataract*: Change in glasses can sometimes improve a patient's visual function temporarily; however the most common treatment is cataract surgery.

BIBLIOGRAPHY

1. Daniel MS, Postellon DC. (2013). Congenital hypothyroidism. [online] Available from www.emedicine.com/ped/TOPIC501.HTM. [Accessed September, 2013].

1EE.73D6B4. DEJEAN SYNDROME (ORBITAL FLOOR SYNDROME)

General

Usually secondary to a traumatic lesion involving the floor of the orbit.

Ocular

Enophthalmos; exophthalmos; lid hematoma; diplopia due to displacement of the globe or restricted function of the inferior rectus and/or inferior oblique muscles; orbital emphysema.

Clinical

Severe pain in superior maxillary region; numbness in area of first and second branches of trigeminal nerve; nausea and vomiting.

Laboratory

CT and MRI of orbit.

Treatment

Repair orbital floor fracture.

⊟ BIBLIOGRAPHY

1. Roy FH. Ocular Syndromes and Systemic Diseases, 4th edition. Philadelphia: Lippincott Williams & Wilkins; 2007.

⊟ 1EE.73D6B5. DEJERINE-KLUMPKE SYNDROME (LOWER RADICULAR SYNDROME; KLUMPKE SYNDROME; KLUMPKE PARALYSIS)

General

Lesion involving the inferior roots of the brachial plexus with nerves derived from the eighth cervical and first thoracic root.

Ocular

Enophthalmos; ptosis; narrowed palpebral fissure; miosis.

Clinical

Paralysis and atrophy of the small muscles of forearm and hand (flexor carpi ulnaris, flexor digitorum, interossei, thenar, hypothenar); decreased sensation or increased sensibility on the inner side of the forearm.

Laboratory

Neurologic evaluation, CT, MRI

Treatment

Primary exploration and repair of brachial plexus. Secondary deformities may require surgical intervention and therapy.

⊟ BIBLIOGRAPHY

1. Bienstock A, Kim JY. (2011). Brachial Plexus Hand Surgery. [online] Available from www.emedicine.com/plastic/TOPIC450.HTM. [Accessed September, 2013].

⊟ 1EE.73D6B6. HORNER SYNDROME (BERNARD-HORNER SYNDROME; CERVICAL SYMPATHETIC PARALYSIS SYNDROME; CLAUDE-BERNARD-HORNER SYNDROME; HORNER OCULOPUPILLARY SYNDROME)

General

Paralysis of cervical sympathetic; hypothalamic lesion with first neuron involved or lesion in the pons or cervical portion of cord; syndrome present in Babinski-Nageotte, Cestan-Chenais, Dejerine-Klumpke, Pancoast, Raeder, and Wallenberg syndromes (*see* Babinski-Nageotte syndrome; Cestan-Chenais syndrome; Dejerine-Klumpke syndrome; Pancoast syndrome; Raeder syndrome; Wallenberg syndrome).

Ocular

Enophthalmos; ptosis or narrowing of palpebral fissure; ocular hypotony; miosis (degree of miosis depends on the site of lesion; most pronounced when roots of cranial nerves VII and VIII, and first thoracic nerve are involved); hypochromic heterochromia (children more than adults); pupil does not dilate with cocaine.

Clinical

Anhidrosis on ipsilateral side of face and neck; transitory rise in facial temperature; hemifacial atrophy; it may result from a variety of conditions, including cluster headache, parasellar neoplasms or aneurysms, internal carotid dissection or occlusion, and Tolosa-Hunt syndrome.

Laboratory

Pharmacologic testing is very helpful in the diagnosis of Horner syndrome; cocaine or apraclonidine (instilled in an eye with intact sympathetic innervation) causes the pupil to dilate. A sympathetically denervated pupil dilates poorly to cocaine, regardless of the level of the sympathetic interruption because of the absence of endogenous norepinephrine in the synapse.

Treatment

Surgical and medical care is dependent upon the particular etiology. Potential surgical care includes neurosurgical care for aneurysm-related Horner syndrome and vascular surgical care for etiologies such as carotid artery dissection/aneurysm.

🗗 BIBLIOGRAPHY

1. Bardorf CM, Stavern GV, Garcia-Valenzuela E. (2012). Horner syndrome. [online] Available from www.emedicine.com/oph/TOPIC336.HTM. [Accessed September, 2013].

🗗 1EE.73D6B7. KRAUSE SYNDROME (CONGENITAL ENCEPHALO-OPHTHALMIC DYSPLASIA; ENCEPHALO-OPHTHALMIC SYNDROME)

General

No hereditary factors involved; no predilection for either sex; more frequent in premature infants; death frequently from intercurrent infections.

Ocular

Microphthalmos; enophthalmos; ptosis; strabismus; secondary glaucoma; iris atrophy; anterior and posterior synechiae; scleral atrophy; persistent remnants of hyaloid's artery; intraocular hemorrhages and exudates; cyclitic membranes; cataracts; retinal hypoplasia and hyperplasia; choroidal and retinal malformation; retinal glial membranes; retinal detachment; choroidal atrophy; optic nerve malformation; optic atrophy.

Clinical

Congenital cerebral dysplasia; hydrocephalus or microcephaly; mental retardation; heterotopia.

Laboratory

Clinical.

Treatment

- *Ptosis*: If visual acuity is affected most cases require surgical correction and there are several procedures that may be used including levator resection, repair or advancement and Fasanella-Servat.
- *Strabismus*: Equalized vision with correct refractive error; surgery may be helpful in patient with diplopia.
- *Glaucoma*: Glaucoma medication should be the first plan of action. If medication is unsuccessful, a filtering surgical procedure with or without antimetabotites may be beneficial
- *Cataract*: Change in glasses can sometimes improve a patient's visual function temporarily; however the most common treatment is cataract surgery.
- *Vitreous hemorrhage*: If possible the source of the bleeding needs to be isolated and treated with laser. Vitrectomy may be necessary
- *Retinal detachment*: Scleral buckle, pneumatic retinopexy and vitrectomy may be used to close all the breaks.

🗗 BIBLIOGRAPHY

1. Krause AC. Congenital encephalo-ophthalmic dysplasia. Arch Ophthalmol. 1946;36:387-94.
2. Miller M, Robbins J, Fishman R, et al. A chromosomal anomaly with multiple ocular defects. Am J Ophthalmol. 1963;55:901.

🗗 1EE.73D6B8. NAFFZIGER SYNDROME (SCALENUS ANTICUS SYNDROME)

General

Compression of brachial plexus and subclavian artery by scalenus anticus muscle; symptoms vary from mild, with remissions and exacerbations, to severe.

Ocular

Enophthalmos; ptosis (unilateral); small pupil.

Clinical

Weakness of ipsilateral hand grip; reduced ipsilateral biceps reflex; diminution of pulse volume on affected side; numbness and coldness in hand and fingers.

Laboratory

Diagnosis is made by clinical findings.

Treatment

Ptosis: If visual acuity is affected most cases require surgical correction and there are several procedures that may be used including levator resection, repair or advancement and Fasanella-Servat.

BIBLIOGRAPHY

1. Aligne C, Barral X. Rehabilitation of patients with thoracic outlet syndrome. Ann Vasc Surg. 1992;6:381-9.
2. Atasoy E. Thoracic outlet compression syndrome. Orthop Clin North Am. 1996;27:265-303.
3. Davies AH, Walton J, Stuart E, et al. Surgical management of the thoracic outlet syndrome. Br J Surg. 1991;78:1193-5.
4. Geeraets WJ. Ocular Syndromes, 3rd edition. Philadelphia: Lea & Febiger; 1976.
5. Karas SE. Thoracic outlet syndrome. Clin Sports Med. 1990;9:297-310.
6. Naffziger HD. Scalenus anticus (Naffziger) syndrome. Am J Surg. 1935;28:669.
7. Pfaltz CR, Richter HR. Syndrome of vertebrobasilar insufficiency: etiology and pathogenesis of the cochleovestibular symptoms m cerebral circulation disorders. 1969;193: 190-200.

1EE.73D6B9. PANCOAST SYNDROME (HARE SYNDROME; SUPERIOR PULMONARY SULCUS SYNDROME)

General

Mass occupying lesion in pulmonary apex; erosion of first three ribs frequent; primary bronchogenic carcinoma most frequent cause; symptomatology similar to lower radicular (Dejerine-Klumpke) syndrome and scalenus anticus (Naffziger) syndrome; Horner syndrome caused by involvement of sympathetic chain (also can be caused by locally invasive fungus such as *C. neoformans* or lymphomatoid granulomatosis.

Ocular

Mild enophthalmos; ptosis; narrowing of the palpebral fissure; miosis.

Clinical

Pulmonary apical tumor; severe shoulder pain; paresthesias, pain, and paresis of the homolateral arm with atrophy of arm and hand muscles.

Laboratory

Imaging and biopsy are the cornerstones of diagnosis

Treatment

Radiation and chemotherapy; surgical treatment of choice is complete removal of the tumor by en bloc chest wall resection combined with lobectomy and node staging.

BIBLIOGRAPHY

1. D'Silva KJ, May SK. (2012). Pancoast Syndrome. [online] Available from emedicine.medscape.com/article/284011-overview. [Accessed September, 2013].

1EE.73D6B1O. RAEDER SYNDROME (PARATRIGEMINAL PARALYSIS; HORTON HEADACHE; HISTAMINE CEPHALALGIA; CILIARY NEURALGIA; CLUSTER HEADACHE; PERIODIC MIGRAINOUS NEURALGIA)

General

Interruption of sympathetic fibers about the carotid artery and involvement of the fifth nerve; meningioma and aneurysm of the internal carotid artery are the most frequent causes; prominent in males; possible pathogenetic mechanism of this condition is an ischemic injury of the gasserian ganglion.

Ocular

Mild enophthalmos; mild ptosis (unilateral); epiphora; scotoma possible; hypotonia; unilateral miosis; increased tear secretion; periocular pain; Homer syndrome.

Clinical

Facial pain; occasionally weakness of the jaw muscles; headaches (V-region); hypertension; associated inflammatory processes are not infrequent.

Laboratory

Brain scan to rule out meningioma and basilar artery aneurysm.

Treatment

Oxygen inhalation and sumatriptan subcutaneous is useful in acute attacks.

⊟ BIBLIOGRAPHY

1. Bardorf CM, van Stavern G, Garcia-Valenzuela E. (2012). Horner syndrome. [online] Available from www.emedicine.com/oph/TOPIC336.HTM. [Accessed September, 2013].

⊟ 1EE.73D6B11. RETROPAROTID SPACE SYNDROME (VILLARET SYNDROME; POSTERIOR RETROPAROTID SPACE SYNDROME) ENOPHTHALMOS

General

Lesions (traumatic, inflammatory, tumors) involving cranial nerves IX to XII and the cervical sympathetic [*see* Jugular Foramen Syndrome (Vernet Syndrome)].

Ocular

Enophthalmos; ptosis; lagophthalmos; epiphora; miosis; may produce sympathetic overactivity resulting in increased sympathetic outflow (i.e. pupillary dilation, widened palpebral fissure, and facial sweating).

Clinical

Homolateral paralysis of cranial nerves IX to XII, with dysphagia and loss of taste in posterior third of the tongue; dysphonia; paralysis of sternocleidomastoid and trapezium muscles; paralysis cranial nerve VII occasionally.

Laboratory

Clinical.

Treatment

Ptosis: If visual acuity is affected most cases require surgical correction and there are several procedures that may be used including levator resection, repair or advancement and Fasanella-Servat.

⊟ BIBLIOGRAPHY

1. Garrett D, Ansell LV, Story JL. Villaret's syndrome: a report of two cases. Surg Neurol. 1993;39:282-5.
2. Geeraets WJ. Ocular Syndromes, 3rd edition. Philadelphia: Lea & Febiger; 1976.
3. Magalini SI, Scrascia E. Dictionary of Medical Syndromes, 2nd edition. Philadelphia: JB Lippincott; 1981.
4. Villaret M. Le Syndrome Nerveux de l'Espace Retro-parotidien Posterieur. Rev Neurol. 1916;23:188.

⊟ 1EE.73D6B12. SILENT SINUS SYNDROME

General

Spontaneous enophthalmos and hypoglobus associated with a small, ipsilateral maxillary sinus.

Ocular

Enophthalmos; hypoglobus.

Clinical

Patients usually undergo painless progressive sinking of the eye.

Laboratory

Imaging of maxillary sinus.

Treatment

Sinus surgery.

⊟ BIBLIOGRAPHY

1. Davidson JK, Soparkar CN, Williams JB, et al. Negative sinus pressure and normal predisease imaging in silent sinus syndrome. Arch Ophthalmol. 1999;117:1653-4.

2. Eto RT, House JM. Enophthalmos: a sequela of maxillary sinusitis. AJNR Am J Neuroradiol. 1995;16:939-41.

3. Kass ES, Salman S, Montgomery WW. Manometric study of complete ostial occlusion in chronic maxillary atelectasis. Laryngoscope. 1996;106:1255-8.

4. Rose, GE, Sandy C, Hallberg L, et al. Clinical and radiologic characteristics of the imploding antrum or silent sinus syndrome. Ophthalmology. 2003;110:811-8.

5. Scharf KE, Lawson W, Shapiro JM, et al. Pressure measurements in the normal and occluded rabbit maxillary sinus. Laryngoscope. 1995;105:570-4.

6. Soparkar CN, Patrinely JR, Cuaycong MJ, et al. The silent sinus syndrome. Ophthalmology. 1994;101:772-8.

1EE.73D6B13. JUGULAR FORAMEN SYNDROME (VERNET SYNDROME)

General

Injuries, aneurysms, and tumors (more commonly due to metastatic lesion than primary neoplasms) affecting the foramen jugulare are the primary causes for the syndrome to develop; if sympathetic fibers surrounding the carotid artery are involved, this will produce Horner triad; note similarity of clinical findings of Villaret syndrome or "retroparotid space syndrome", which may include epiphora and lagophthalmos and in which cranial nerves IX to XII and the cervical sympathetics are involved.

Ocular

Enophthalmos; ptosis; miosis.

Clinical

Paralysis of the ninth, tenth, and eleventh cranial nerves with resulting impairment of related function, that is, dysphagia, loss of taste on the posterior third of the tongue, and nasal regurgitation; anhidrosis; paralysis of the sternocleidomastoid muscle and part of the trapezium (upper portion); hoarseness; tachycardia; dysarthria; weight loss.

Laboratory

CT, MRI, carotid arteriography.

Treatment

Anticoagulation or thrombolytic therapy is useful. Severe neurological deterioration may require open thrombectomy and local thrombolytic therapy.

BIBLIOGRAPHY

1. McElveen WA, Keegan aP. (2012). Cerebral Venous Thrombosis. [online] Available from www.emedicine.com/neuro/TOPIC642.HTM. [Accessed September, 2013].

1EE.73D6B14. WALLENBERG SYNDROME (DORSOLATERAL MEDULLARY SYNDROME; LATERAL BULBAR SYNDROME) PTOSIS

General

Occlusion of the posterior inferior cerebellar artery; onset after age 40 years; similar to Babinski-Nageotte syndrome but crossed hemiparesis is absent; nystagmus is produced by involvement of the vestibular nuclei or posterior longitudinal bundle.

Ocular

Enophthalmos; ptosis; spontaneous homolateral or contralateral horizontal or torsional nystagmus; miosis; Horner syndrome; skew deviation; impaired contralateral pursuit; saccadic abnormalities; gaze-holding abnormalities.

Clinical

Nausea; vertigo; difficulty in swallowing and speaking; ipsilateral ataxia; muscular hypotonicity; ipsilateral loss of pain and temperature sense of the face; neurotrophic skin ulcers; contralateral hypalgesia; facial weakness.

Laboratory

CT scan.

Treatment

Seek neurological assistance. Ptosis evaluation.

BIBLIOGRAPHY

1. Brazis PW. Ocular motor abnormalities in Wallenberg's lateral medullary syndrome. Mayo Clin Proc. 1992;67:365-8.
2. Hornsten G. Wallenberg's syndrome. I. General symptomatology with reference to visual disturbances and imbalance. Acta Neural Scand. 1974;50:434-46.
3. Marcoux C, Malfait Y, Pirard C, et al. Neurotrophic ulcer following Wallenberg's syndrome. Dermatology. 1993;186:301-2.
4. Sacco RL, Freddo L, Bello JA, et al. Wallenberg's lateral medullary syndrome. Clinical-magnetic resonance imaging correlations. Arch Neurol. 1993;50:609-14.
5. Silfverskiold BP. Skew deviation in Wallenberg's syndrome. Acta Neurol Scand. 1966;41:381-6.
6. Wallenberg A. Anatomische Befunde in Einem als "Akute Bulbaraffektion (Embolie der Arteria Cerebellar. Post. Inf. Sinist.)" Beschriebenen Falle. Arch F Psychiatr. 1901;34.

1EE.73D6B14A2F6. ABDOMINAL TYPHUS (ENTERIC FEVER; TYPHOID FEVER)

General

Causative agent, *Salmonella typhi.*

Ocular

Conjunctivitis; chemosis; corneal ulcer; tenonitis; paralysis of extraocular muscles; endophthalmitis; panophthalmitis; optic neuritis; retinal detachment; central scotoma; central retinal artery emboli; iritis with or without hypopyon; choroiditis; retinal hemorrhages; bilateral optic neuritis; abnormal ocular motility (likely secondary to thrombotic infarcts affecting the ocular motor nerve nuclei, fascicles, brainstem, or cerebral hemispheres).

Clinical

Fever; headache; bradycardia; splenomegaly; maculopapular rash; leukopenia; encephalitis. Salmonella may produce an illness characterized by fever and bacteremia without any other manifestations of enterocolitis or enteric fever, which is particularly common in patients with AIDS.

Laboratory

Gram-negative bacillus isolation from blood culture (50–70% of cases). Positive stool culture is less frequent.

Treatment

Early detection, antibiotic therapy and adequate fluids, electrolytes, and nutrition reduce the rate of complications and reduce the case-fatality rate.

BIBLIOGRAPHY

1. Brusch JL. (2011). Typhoid fever. [online] Available from www.emedicine.com/med/TOPIC2331.HTM. [Accessed September, 2013].

1EE.73D6B14A2F8. BASEDOW SYNDROME (GRAVES DISEASE; HYPERTHYROIDISM; THYROTOXICOSIS; EXOPHTHALMIC GOITER; PARRY DISEASE)

General

Diffuse toxic goiter; inherited as a simple autosomal recessive; penetrance greater in females; however, dominant mode of inheritance and variable penetrance are possible; uncommon in either sex before the age of 15 years.

Ocular

Exophthalmos; swelling of eyelids and discoloration of upper eyelids; lid lag (von Graefe's sign); globe lag (Koeber's sign); lid trembling on gentle closure (Rosenbach's sign); reduced blinking (Stellwag's sign); retraction of upper lid; difficulty in everting upper lid (Gifford's sign); convergence weakness (Möbius's sign); impaired fixation on extreme lateral gaze (Suker's sign); possible external ophthalmoplegia (Ballet's sign); Dalrymple's sign (staring appearance); tearing; photophobia; epiphora; prolapse of lacrimal gland; neuroretinal edema; tortuous vessels; papilledema and papillitis; anisocoria; keratitis; increased IOP on upgaze; decreased visual acuity; enlargement of the extraocular muscles; increased volume of the extraorbital fat; superior rectus muscle enlargement; decreased venous outflow.

Clinical

Tachycardia; anxiety; insomnia; loss of weight; hyperhidrosis; restlessness; myocarditis (toxic); atrial fibrillation.

Laboratory

Visual field testing, forced duction testing for restrictive myopathy, CT, MRI, T4 and thyroid-stimulating hormone, thyroid-stimulating immunoglobulins.

Treatment

There is no immediate treatment; the disease is self-limited but prolonged course over 1 or more years. Five percent of patients may require surgical intervention which could be orbital decompression, strabismus surgery, lid-lengthening surgery or blepharoplasty.

BIBLIOGRAPHY

1. Ing E. (2012). Thyroid-associated orbitopathy. [online] Available from www.emedicine.com/oph/TOPIC237.HTM. [Accessed September, 2013].
2. Regensburg NI, Wiersinga WM, Berendschot TT, et al. Do subtypes of Graves' orbitopathy exist? Ophthalmology. 2011;118:191-6.

1EE.73D6B14A2F11. ERB-GOLDFLAM SYNDROME (ERB II SYNDROME; HOPPE-GOLDFLAM DISEASE; PSEUDOPARALYTIC SYNDROME; MYASTHENIA GRAVIS)

General

Occurs at any age; more frequent between ages 20 and 40 years; more females affected than males; progressive; spontaneous; symptoms improve or resolve with rest in early stages of disease (*see* myasthenia gravis, neonatal or infantile); caused by autoantibodies against the acetylcholine receptor at the neuromuscular junction, leading to abnormal fatigability and weakness of skeletal muscle.

Ocular

Transient diplopia; ptosis of upper eyelids.

Clinical

Excessive fatigability of musculature; symptoms appear and increase as day progresses; expressionless face; sagging jaw; difficulty in chewing and talking; nasal regurgitation.

Laboratory

Ice test—crushed ice in surgical glove over ptotic eyelid for 2 minutes and watch for brief elevation of eyelid; Tensilon test and prostigmin test may result in the elevation of ptotic eyelid or improved strabismus in individuals with myasthenia gravis.

Treatment

Adrenal corticosteroids are frequently used. In some cases, mycophenolate mofetil, cyclosporine and cyclophosphamide may be useful. Patching one eye or using prisms may be helpful.

BIBLIOGRAPHY

1. Erb W. Zur Casuistick der Bulbaren La hmungen. Arch Psychiatr Vervenkr. 1879;9:325-50.
2. Roy FH, Fraunfelder FT, Fraunfelder FW. Roy and Fraunfelder's Current Ocular Therapy, 6th edition. London, UK: Elsevier; 2008.
3. Goldflam S. Vebereinen Scheinbar Keilbaren Bulbarparalytischem Symptom Complex mit Betheiligung der Extremitaten. Dtsch Z Nerven. 1983;4:312-52.
4. Kim JH, Hwang JM, Hwang YS, et al. Childhood ocular myasthenia gravis. Ophthalmology. 2003;110(7):1458-62.
5. Lepore FE, Sanborn GE, Slevin JT. Pupillary dysfunction in myasthenia gravis. Ann Neurol. 1979;6(1):29-33.
6. Sommer N, Melms A, Weller M, et al. Ocular myasthenia gravis. A critical review of clinical and pathophysiological aspects. Doc Ophthalmol. 1993;84(4):309-33.

⊟ 1EE.73D6B14A2F14. PREGNANCY

General

Pregnancy results in hormonal changes that produce ocular effects; symptoms resolve at end of pregnancy term.

Ocular

Myopia; visual field defects; corneal edema; acute ischemic optic neuropathy; central serous retinopathy; glaucoma; ptosis; diabetic retinopathy; Krukenberg spindles; transient blindness; serous retinal detachment; retinal artery occlusion; retinal vein occlusion; disseminated intravascular coagulopathy; uveal melanoma.

Clinical

Nausea; headaches; hypertension; benign intracranial hypertension; preeclampsia; toxemia; fluid retention.

Laboratory

Home pregnancy test that utilize the modern immunometric assay. Transvaginal ultrasound and transabdominal ultrasound are also useful.

Treatment

Most ocular symptoms resolve at the end of pregnancy. Obstetrician should be consulted before topical medications are prescribed.

⊟ BIBLIOGRAPHY

1. Somani S, Bhatti A, Ahmed II. (2011). Pregnancy Special Considerations. [online] Available from www.emedicine.com/oph/TOPIC747.HTM. [Accessed September, 2013].

⊟ 1EE.73E1. GUILLAIN-BARRÉ SYNDROME (LANDRY PARALYSIS; ACUTE INFECTIOUS NEURITIS; ACUTE POLYRADICULITIS; ACUTE FEBRILE POLYNEURITIS; ACUTE IDIOPATHIC POLYNEURITIS; INFLAMMATORY POLYRADICULONEUROPATHY; LANDRY-GUILLAIN-BARRÉ-STROHL SYNDROME; POSTINFECTIOUS POLYNEURITIS)

General

Etiology unknown; occurs from age 16–50 years.

Ocular

Facial nerve paralysis with paralytic ectropion of the lower eyelid; mild-to-complete external ophthalmoplegia; optic neuritis; papilledema; ptosis; anisocoria; nystagmus; dyschromatopsia; scotoma; bilateral tonic pupils.

Clinical

Polyneuritis involving facial peripheral motor nerves and spinal cord; facial diplegia; bladder incontinence; variable degrees of paralysis, usually beginning in lower extremities; tendon reflexes absent; involvement of respiratory muscles possible; paresthesia (symmetrical).

Laboratory

Cytomegalovirus, Epstein-Barr virus and HIV have been most closely associated with this condition.

Treatment

Plasma exchange have shown to be beneficial. Corneal exposure is treated with topical therapy or lateral tarsorrhaphies if warranted.

⊟ BIBLIOGRAPHY

1. Andary MT, Oleszek JL, Cha-Kim A. (2012). Guillain-Barre Syndrome. [online] Available from www.emedicine.com/pmr/TOPIC48.HTM. [Accessed September, 2013].

⊟ 1EE.73E2. HORNER SYNDROME (BERNARD-HORNER SYNDROME; CERVICAL SYMPATHETIC PARALYSIS SYNDROME; CLAUDE-BERNARD-HORNER SYNDROME; HORNER OCULOPUPILLARY SYNDROME)

General

Paralysis of cervical sympathetic; hypothalamic lesion with first neuron involved or lesion in the pons or cervical portion of cord; syndrome present in Babinski-Nageotte, Cestan-Chenais, Dejerine-Klumpke, Pancoast, Raeder, and Wallenberg syndromes (*see* Babinski-Nageotte syndrome; Cestan-Chenais syndrome; Dejerine-Klumpke syndrome; Pancoast syndrome; Raeder syndrome; Wallenberg syndrome).

Ocular

Enophthalmos; ptosis or narrowing of palpebral fissure; ocular hypotony; miosis (degree of miosis depends on the site of lesion; most pronounced when roots of cranial nerves VII and VIII, and first thoracic nerve are involved); hypochromic heterochromia (children more than adults); pupil does not dilate with cocaine.

Clinical

Anhidrosis on ipsilateral side of face and neck; transitory rise in facial temperature; hemifacial atrophy; it may result from a variety of conditions, including cluster headache, parasellar neoplasms or aneurysms, internal carotid dissection or occlusion, and Tolosa-Hunt syndrome.

Laboratory

Pharmacologic testing is very helpful in the diagnosis of Horner syndrome; cocaine or apraclonidine (instilled in an eye with intact sympathetic innervation) causes the pupil to dilate. A sympathetically denervated pupil dilates poorly to cocaine, regardless of the level of the sympathetic interruption because of the absence of endogenous norepinephrine in the synapse.

Treatment

Surgical and medical care is dependent upon the particular etiology. Potential surgical care includes neurosurgical care for aneurysm-related Horner syndrome and vascular surgical care for etiologies such as carotid artery dissection/aneurysm.

⊟ BIBLIOGRAPHY

1. Bardorf CM, Stavern GV, Garcia-Valenzuela E. (2012). Horner syndrome. [online] Available from www.emedicine.com/oph/TOPIC336.HTM. [Accessed September, 2013].

⊟ 1EE.73E2A. LAURENCE-MOON-BARDET-BIEDL SYNDROME (BARDET-BIEDL SYNDROME; RETINITIS PIGMENTOSA-POLYDACTYLY-ADIPOSOGENITAL SYNDROME)

General

Recessive, autosomal dominant, and recessive sex-linked gene; male preponderance; onset in childhood; cases of Laurence-Moon-Bardet-Biedl belong to the group of heredoataxias.

Ocular

Ptosis; epicanthus; nystagmus; strabismus; night blindness; myopia; hypermetropia; iris coloboma; RP "bone corpuscles"; macular degeneration; attenuation of retinal vessels; choroidal atrophy; optic nerve atrophy; cataract; microphthalmia; keratoconus.

Clinical

Obesity (Fröhlich type); hypogenitalism; reduced intelligence and mental retardation; turricephaly; shortness of stature; atresia ani; genu valgum; congenital heart disease; polydactyly; body hair scant or absent; pseudogynecomastia.

Laboratory

Chromosomal analysis is recommended to confirm chromosomal sex and to evaluate for associated genetic syndromes.

Treatment

Consultation by pediatric endocrinologist and pediatric urologist is usually necessary.

⊟ BIBLIOGRAPHY

1. Telander DG, de Beus A, Small KW. (2012). Retinitis pigmentosa. [online] Available from www.emedicine.com/oph/TOPIC704.HTM. [Accessed September, 2013].

⊟ 1EE.73E2A. DIENCEPHALIC SYNDROME (DIENCEPHALIC EPILEPSY SYNDROME; AUTONOMIC EPILEPSY SYNDROME; PENFIELD SYNDROME; ANTERIOR DIENCEPHALIC AUTONOMIC EPILEPSY SYNDROME)

General

Occurs in males at ages 6–7 years; caused by hypothalamic dysfunction and a localized epileptic stimulus originating in the dorsal nucleus of the thalamus.

Ocular

Proptosis (occasionally); excessive lacrimation; pupillary abnormalities.

Clinical

Abdominal pain; headache; irritability; rapid pulse; elevated blood pressure; salivation; hiccup; chills; dyspnea (Cheyne-Stokes); seizures (possible); sudden onset of vasodilation of the skin (cervical sympathetic).

Laboratory

Brain MRI, head CT, EEG.

Treatment

Anticonvulsant medication.

⊟ BIBLIOGRAPHY

1. Nouri S. (2013). Epilepsy and the Autonomic Nervous System. [online] Available from www.emedicine.com/neuro/TOPIC658.HTM. [Accessed September, 2013].

⊟ 1EE.73E2.A1. ARNOLD-CHIARI SYNDROME (PLATYBASIA SYNDROME; CEREBELLOMEDULLARY MALFORMATION SYNDROME; BASILAR IMPRESSIONS)

General

Malformation of the hindbrain; developmental deformity of the occipital bone and upper cervical spine; recognized in children or adults; clinical picture may be indistinguishable from that of Dandy-Walker syndrome in infants.

Ocular

Horizontal, vertical and rotary forms of nystagmus; vertical nystagmus in both upgaze and downgaze is most common; papilledema; esotropia; Duane's retraction syndrome (association); oscillopsia.

Clinical

Hydrocephalus; cerebellar ataxia; bilateral pyramidal tract signs.

Laboratory

CT scans are used most commonly for the diagnosis of hydrocephalus and for the evaluation of suspected shunt malfunction.

Treatment

Early recognition and treatment is important because of the potential life-threatening symptoms. Early surgical intervention, especially in infants may prevent irreversible changes and death.

⊟ BIBLIOGRAPHY

1. Incesu L, Khosla A, Aiello MR. (2011). Imaging in Chiari II malformation. [online] Available from www.emedicine.com/radio/TOPIC150.HTM. [Accessed September, 2013].

⊟ 1EE.73E2.A2. ACQUIRED LUES (SYPHILIS; ACQUIRED SYPHILIS; LUES VENEREA; MALUM VENEREUM)

General

Causative agent, *T. pallidum*, usually transmitted sexually.

Ocular

Conjunctival chancroid; conjunctivitis; keratitis; blepharitis; ptosis; iris atrophy; hippus; dacryocystitis; optic nerve atrophy; optic neuritis; periostitis; episcleritis; scleritis; nystagmus; uveitis; vitreous hemorrhages; paralysis of sixth nerve; papilledema; retinal hemorrhages; retinitis proliferans; oculogyric crisis; neuroretinitis; papilledema (associated with aseptic meningitis); diffuse or multifocal chorioretinitis; vertical supranuclear gaze palsy; Benedikt syndrome.

Clinical

Primary lesion associated with regional lymphadenopathy; secondary bacteremic stage associated with generalized mucocutaneous lesions; tertiary stage characterized by destructive mucocutaneous, musculoskeletal, or parenchymal lesions, aortitis, or CNS disease; syphilis and HIV infection often coexist in the same patient who experiences a higher incidence and greater severity of neurologic and ocular manifestations; a significant percentage of patients infected with HIV-I and *T. pallidum* become seronegative to syphilis testing.

Laboratory

Serologic nontreponemal tests include VDRL and RPR.

Treatment

The goals are to reduce morbidity and to prevent complications. Penicillin is the antibiotic of choice for treating syphilis. Ocular syphilis should be treated the same as patients with neurosyphilis.

⊟ BIBLIOGRAPHY

1. Majmudar PA. (2011). Interstitial Keratitis Overview of Interstitial Keratitis. [online] Available from www.emedicine.com/oph/TOPIC453.HTM. [Accessed September, 2013].
2. Euerle B, Chandrasekar PH, Diaz MM, et al. (2012). Syphilis. [online] Available from www.emedicine.com/med/TOPIC2224.HTM. [Accessed September, 2013].

⊟ 1EE.73E2.A9. WALLENBERG SYNDROME (DORSOLATERAL MEDULLARY SYNDROME; LATERAL BULBAR SYNDROME) PTOSIS

General

Occlusion of the posterior inferior cerebellar artery; onset after age 40 years; similar to Babinski-Nageotte syndrome but crossed hemiparesis is absent; nystagmus is produced by involvement of the vestibular nuclei or posterior longitudinal bundle.

Ocular

Enophthalmos; ptosis; spontaneous homolateral or contralateral horizontal or torsional nystagmus; miosis; Horner syndrome; skew deviation; impaired contralateral pursuit; saccadic abnormalities; gaze-holding abnormalities.

Clinical

Nausea; vertigo; difficulty in swallowing and speaking; ipsilateral ataxia; muscular hypotonicity; ipsilateral loss of pain and temperature sense of the face; neurotrophic skin ulcers; contralateral hypalgesia; facial weakness.

Laboratory

CT scan.

Treatment

Seek neurological assistance. Ptosis evaluation.

⊟ BIBLIOGRAPHY

1. Brazis PW. Ocular motor abnormalities in Wallenberg's lateral medullary syndrome. Mayo Clin Proc. 1992;67:365-8.
2. Hornsten G. Wallenberg's syndrome. I. General symptomatology with reference to visual disturbances and imbalance. Acta Neural Scand. 1974;50:434-46.
3. Marcoux C, Malfait Y, Pirard C, et al. Neurotrophic ulcer following Wallenberg's syndrome. Dermatology. 1993;186:301-2.
4. Sacco RL, Freddo L, Bello JA, et al. Wallenberg's lateral medullary syndrome. Clinical-magnetic resonance imaging correlations. Arch Neurol. 1993;50:609-14.
5. Silfverskiold BP. Skew deviation in Wallenberg's syndrome. Acta Neurol Scand. 1966;41:381-6.
6. Wallenberg A. Anatomische Befunde in Einem als "Akute Bulbaraffektion (Embolie der Arteria Cerebellar. Post. Inf. Sinist.)" Beschriebenen Falle. Arch F Psychiatr. 1901;34.

⊟ 1EE.73E2.A10A. PASSOW SYNDROME (BREMER STATUS DYSRAPHICUS; STATUS DYSRAPHICUS SYNDROME; SYRINGOMYELIA; SYRINGOBULBIA)

General

Congenital nonclosure of the neural tube; familial occurrence or may be sporadic; insidious onset in 2nd to 3rd decade of life.

Ocular

Enophthalmos; ptosis; rotatory nystagmus; heterochromia iridis; anterior uveitis; corneal anesthesia; neuroparalytic keratitis; paralysis of third, fifth, sixth, and seventh cranial nerves; Horner syndrome; anisocoria; papilledema; optic atrophy; zonular cataract (*see* Horner Syndrome).

Clinical

Anesthesia over area of first division of trigeminal nerve; facial hemiatrophy; facial nerve paralysis; muscular weakness; cervical ribs; kyphoscoliosis; spina bifida; unilateral numbness of fingers; loss of deep reflexes; insensitivity to pain and temperature in affected areas; neurogenic bladder.

Laboratory

MRI, CT.

Treatment

Suboccipital and cervical decompression, laminectomy and syringotomy, shunts, fourth ventriculostomy, terminal ventriculostomy and neuroendoscopic surgery may be considered.

⊟ BIBLIOGRAPHY

1. Al-Shatoury HA, Galhom AA, Wagner FC. (2012). Syringomyelia. [online] Available from emedicine.medscape.com/article/1151685-overview. [Accessed September, 2013].

⊟ 1EE.73E2.A10D. ACQUIRED LUES (SYPHILIS; ACQUIRED SYPHILIS; LUES VENEREA; MALUM VENEREUM)

General

Causative agent, *T. pallidum*, usually transmitted sexually.

Ocular

Conjunctival chancroid; conjunctivitis; keratitis; blepharitis; ptosis; iris atrophy; hippus; dacryocystitis; optic nerve atrophy; optic neuritis; periostitis; episcleritis; scleritis; nystagmus; uveitis; vitreous hemorrhages; paralysis of sixth nerve; papilledema; retinal hemorrhages; retinitis proliferans; oculogyric crisis; neuroretinitis; papilledema (associated with aseptic meningitis); diffuse or multifocal chorioretinitis; vertical supranuclear gaze palsy; Benedikt syndrome.

Clinical

Primary lesion associated with regional lymphadenopathy; secondary bacteremic stage associated with generalized mucocutaneous lesions; tertiary stage characterized by destructive mucocutaneous, musculoskeletal, or parenchymal lesions, aortitis, or CNS disease; syphilis and HIV infection often coexist in the same patient who experiences a higher incidence and greater severity of neurologic and ocular manifestations; a significant percentage of patients infected with HIV-I and *T. pallidum* become seronegative to syphilis testing.

Laboratory

Serologic nontreponemal tests include VDRL and RPR.

Treatment

The goals are to reduce morbidity and to prevent complications. Penicillin is the antibiotic of choice for treating syphilis. Ocular syphilis should be treated the same as patients with neurosyphilis.

BIBLIOGRAPHY

1. Majmudar PA. (2011). Interstitial Keratitis Overview of Interstitial Keratitis. [online] Available from www.emedicine.com/oph/TOPIC453.HTM. [Accessed September, 2013].
2. Euerle B, Chandrasekar PH, Diaz MM, et al. (2012). Syphilis. [online] Available from www.emedicine.com/med/TOPIC2224.HTM. [Accessed September, 2013].

1EE.73E2.A10E. POLIOMYELITIS (INFANTILE PARALYSIS)

General

Acute viral infection characterized by varying degrees of neuronal injury, with special localization in the anterior horns and motor nuclei of the brainstem.

Ocular

Diplopia; nystagmus; paralysis of third, fourth, and sixth nerves; paresis of seventh nerve; papilledema; visual agnosia; Homer's syndrome; pupillary paralysis; optic neuritis; ophthalmoparesis; transient visual loss; internuclear ophthalmoplegia; papillary disturbances, spasm of near reflex.

Clinical

Flaccid paralysis of many muscle groups; death from asphyxia and involvement of vital centers in the brainstem.

Laboratory

Obtain specimens from the CSF, stool and throat for viral cultures.

Treatment

No antivirals are effective against polioviruses. The treatment of poliomyelitis is mainly supportive and will involve physical therapist and rehabilitation therapist, pulmonologist, neurologist, immunologist and infectious diseases specialist.

BIBLIOGRAPHY

1. Estrada B. (2012). Pediatric poliomyelitis. [online] Available from www.emedicine.com/ped/TOPIC1843.HTM. [Accessed September, 2013].

1EE.73E2.A10F. MENINGOCOCCEMIA (NEISSERIA MENINGITIDES; MENINGITIS)

General

Systemic bacterial infection caused by *N. meningitides*; can be present chronically in patients with immune deficiencies including deficient complement levels.

Ocular

Photophobia; conjunctivitis; chemosis; keratitis; uveitis; panophthalmitis; retinal endophlebitis; macular edema; papillitis; optic neuritis; paresis of sixth or seventh nerve; nystagmus; miosis; hippus; cortical blindness; papilledema (rare); conjunctival petechiae; strabismus.

Clinical

Meningitis; fever; malaise; joint pain; splenic enlargement.

Laboratory

Cultures from blood, spinal fluid, or joint fluid.

Treatment

Treat with antibiotics promptly.

BIBLIOGRAPHY

1. Javid MH, Ahmed SH. (2012). Meningococcemia. [online] Available from www.emedicine.com/med/TOPIC1445.HTM. [Accessed September, 2013].

1EE.73E2.A10H. PROGRESSIVE SYSTEMIC SCLEROSIS (SCLERODERMA; SYSTEMIC SCLERODERMA)

General

Chronic connective tissue disease of unknown etiology; chronic and usually progressive disorder; typical onset is in 3rd to 5th decade; ratio of women to men is 4:l; primary sites of pathology are the arterioles and capillaries of affected organs.

Ocular

Marginal corneal ulcers; shortened fornices of the conjunctiva; ptosis; cotton-wool patches of retina; papilledema; retinal hemorrhages; cicatrization of conjunctiva and cornea; blepharitis; blepharospasm; thready, tenacious yellow-white conjunctival discharge; hypertrophy of lacrimal gland; episcleritis; ocular myositis; Sjögren syndrome; uveitis; vitreous haze; keratitis sicca; decreased corneal sensation; iritis; ischemic choroidopathy; iris sectorial atrophy; blepharophimosis; heterochromia; keratoconus; central retinal vein occlusion; branch retinal vein occlusion.

Clinical

Vascular insufficiency; Raynaud's phenomenon; malaise; weight loss; stiffness; fever; polyarticular arthritis; diffuse edema of the hands; calcinosis; esophageal involvement; sclerodactyly; telangiectasis; esophageal stricture; renal failure; diffuse interstitial fibrosis.

Laboratory

No specific test establishes diagnosis. Hypergammaglobulinemia—50% of cases ANA increased in 40–70% cases.

Treatment

Skin thickening can be treated with D-penicillamine and other experimental drugs. Pruritus can be treated with moisturizers and histamine. Raynaud's phenomenon can be treated with calcium channel blockers. Renal crisis episodes are best prevented and treated with the aggressive use of ACE inhibitors. Myositis may be treated cautiously with steroids.

BIBLIOGRAPHY

1. Jimenez SA, Cronin PM, Koenig AS, et al. (2012). Scleroderma. [online] Available from www.emedicine.com/med/TOPIC2076.HTM. [Accessed September, 2013].

1EE.73E2.A10J1. DEJERINE-KLUMPKE SYNDROME (LOWER RADICULAR SYNDROME; KLUMPKE SYNDROME; KLUMPKE PARALYSIS)

General

Lesion involving the inferior roots of the brachial plexus with nerves derived from the eighth cervical and first thoracic root.

Ocular

Enophthalmos; ptosis; narrowed palpebral fissure; miosis.

Clinical

Paralysis and atrophy of the small muscles of forearm and hand (flexor carpi ulnaris, flexor digitorum, interossei, thenar, hypothenar); decreased sensation or increased sensibility on the inner side of the forearm.

Laboratory

Neurologic evaluation, CT, MRI

Treatment

Primary exploration and repair of brachial plexus. Secondary deformities may require surgical intervention and therapy.

BIBLIOGRAPHY

1. Bienstock A, Kim JY. (2011). Brachial Plexus Hand Surgery. [online] Available from www.emedicine.com/plastic/TOPIC450.HTM. [Accessed September, 2013].

⊡ 1EE.73E2.A10J3A. PANCOAST SYNDROME (HARE SYNDROME; SUPERIOR PULMONARY SULCUS SYNDROME)

General

Mass occupying lesion in pulmonary apex; erosion of first three ribs frequent; primary bronchogenic carcinoma most frequent cause; symptomatology similar to lower radicular (Dejerine-Klumpke) syndrome and scalenus anticus (Naffziger) syndrome; Horner syndrome caused by involvement of sympathetic chain (also can be caused by locally invasive fungus such as *C. neoformans* or lymphomatoid granulomatosis.

Ocular

Mild enophthalmos; ptosis; narrowing of the palpebral fissure; miosis.

Clinical

Pulmonary apical tumor; severe shoulder pain; paresthesias, pain, and paresis of the homolateral arm with atrophy of arm and hand muscles.

Laboratory

Imaging and biopsy are the cornerstones of diagnosis.

Treatment

Radiation and chemotherapy; surgical treatment of choice is complete removal of the tumor by en bloc chest wall resection combined with lobectomy and node staging.

⊡ BIBLIOGRAPHY

1. D'Silva KJ, May SK. (2012). Pancoast Syndrome. [online] Available from emedicine.medscape.com/article/284011-overview. [Accessed September, 2013].

⊡ 1EE.73E2.A10J3E. HODGKIN DISEASE

General

Hodgkin disease begins in the lymph nodes and usually spreads in a predictable fashion along contiguous chains of nodes; etiology may be viral; prevalent in males.

Ocular

Keratitis; uveitis; cataract; retinal hemorrhages; vasculitis; Horner syndrome; cortical blindness; papilledema; paralysis of oculomotor nerve; episcleritis; visual field defects; infiltration of choroid, conjunctiva, lacrimal gland, and orbit; papillitis; retrobulbar neuritis; opsoclonus myoclonus; keratitis sicca; infiltrative optic neuropathy; association with Vogt-Koyanagi-Harada syndrome; bilateral serous detachments of the macula.

Clinical

Painless cervical, axillary, or inguinal lymph node swelling; fever; weight loss; anemia; generalized pruritus.

Laboratory

Biopsy of lymph glands is diagnostic.

Treatment

The goal of therapy is to induce a complete remission with radiation therapy, chemotherapy or BMT.

⊡ BIBLIOGRAPHY

1. Lash BW, Dessain SK, Argiris A. (2012). Hodgkin Lymphoma. [online] Available from www.emedicine.com/med/TOPIC1022.HTM. [Accessed September, 2013].

⊡ 1EE.73E2.A10J3E. LEUKEMIA

General

Acute or chronic blood disorder.

Ocular

Engorgement of conjunctival vessels; papillary hypertrophy; aggregations of tumor cells in conjunctiva, choroid and orbit; secondary glaucoma; retinal venous engorgement and tortuosity with pronounced constrictions; retinal hemorrhages; retinal detachment; cotton-wool spots; macular edema; papilledema; optic atrophy; optic neuritis; paralysis of extraocular muscles; hypopyon; vitreous opacities; retinal sea fans; perilimbal subconjunctival infiltrates; corneal leukemic infiltration (rare); shallow serous retinal detachments; hyphema; iris neovascularization; central retinal vein occlusion; vitreous infiltrates.

Clinical

Frequent involvement of CNS; intracranial hemorrhage; thrombocytopenia; rising white cell count.

Laboratory

CBC and differential, bone marrow aspiration, immunophenotyping, chromosomal analysis.

Treatment

Chemotherapy with or without radiotherapy.

⊡ BIBLIOGRAPHY

1. Wu L, Evans T, Martinez J. (2012). Leukemias. [online] Available from www.emedicine.com/oph/TOPIC489.HTM. [Accessed January, 2013].

⊡ 1EE.73C3. FOIX SYNDROME (CAVERNOUS SINUS SYNDROME; HYPOPHYSEAL-SPHENOIDAL SYNDROME; CAVERNOUS SINUS NEURALGIA SYNDROME; GODTFREDSEN SYNDROME; CAVERNOUS SINUS-NASOPHARYNGEAL TUMOR SYNDROME; CAVERNOUS SINUS THROMBOSIS)

General

Causes include tumor of lateral sinus wall or sphenoid bone, intracranial aneurysm, cavernous and lateral sinus thrombosis, or lesions; multiple myeloma; may result from infarctions or cancer or be idiopathic.

Ocular

Proptosis; severe ocular and periorbital pain; lid edema; paresis or paralysis of cranial nerves III, IV, V, and VI; corneal anesthesia; optic atrophy.

Clinical

Postauricular edema; trigeminal neuralgia; deviation of the tongue toward paralyzed side; patients usually have prominent manifestations of sepsis and paranasal sinus; local skin infections are the most common cause.

Laboratory

CT, MRI.

Treatment

Radiotherapy, anticoagulation, high-dose antibiotic therapy.

⊡ BIBLIOGRAPHY

1. Kattah JC, Pula JH. (2012). Cavernous sinus syndromes. [online] Available from www.emedicine.com/neuro/topic572.htm. [Accessed September, 2013].

1EE.73C6. RAEDER SYNDROME (PARATRIGEMINAL PARALYSIS; HORTON HEADACHE; HISTAMINE CEPHALALGIA; CILIARY NEURALGIA; CLUSTER HEADACHE; PERIODIC MIGRAINOUS NEURALGIA)

General

Interruption of sympathetic fibers about the carotid artery and involvement of the fifth nerve; meningioma and aneurysm of the internal carotid artery are the most frequent causes; prominent in males; possible pathogenetic mechanism of this condition is an ischemic injury of the gasserian ganglion.

Ocular

Mild enophthalmos; mild ptosis (unilateral); epiphora; scotoma possible; hypotonia; unilateral miosis; increased tear secretion; periocular pain; Homer syndrome.

Clinical

Facial pain; occasionally weakness of the jaw muscles; headaches (V-region); hypertension; associated inflammatory processes are not infrequent.

Laboratory

Brain scan to rule out meningioma and basilar artery aneurysm.

Treatment

Oxygen inhalation and sumatriptan subcutaneous is useful in acute attacks.

BIBLIOGRAPHY

1. Bardorf CM, van Stavern G, Garcia-Valenzuela E. (2012). Horner syndrome. [online] Available from www.emedicine.com/oph/TOPIC336.HTM. [Accessed September, 2013].

1EE.73C7. HERPES ZOSTER

General

Caused by varicella zoster virus; about 75% of cases occur in persons over age of 45 years; condition is more frequent with advancing age and in patients who are immunocompromised by drugs or disease; in particular, an increasing number of patients with herpes zoster ophthalmicus are immunosuppressed.

Ocular

Conjunctivitis; keratitis; recurrent corneal ulcer; neuralgia; zoster rash of eyelids; uveitis; iris atrophy; scleritis; cataract; optic neuritis; paralysis of third nerve; proptosis; paralysis of lids; orbital apex syndrome; retinitis; neurotrophic keratitis; acute retinal necrosis; progressive outer retinal necrosis; ocular motor nerve pareses; tonic pupil; encephalitis; vasculitis.

Clinical

Local lesions involving the posterior or root ganglia; nerve damage; tissue scarring.

Laboratory

Diagnosed mostly on the basis of the characteristic pain and appearance of the dermatomal rashes.

Treatment

Antiviral agents, systemic corticosteroids, antidepressants, and adequate pain control. Immunocompetent adults aged 60 years or older, benefit from receipt of the herpes zoster vaccine and have a lower incidence of herpes zoster.

BIBLIOGRAPHY

1. Diaz MM, Foster CS, Walton RC, et al. (2011). Herpes zoster ophthalmicus. [online] Available from www.emedicine.com/oph/TOPIC257.HTM. [Accessed September, 2013].
2. Ghaznawi N, Virdi A, Dayan A, et al. Herpes zoster ophthalmicus: comparison of disease in patients 60 years and older versus younger than 60 years. Ophthalmology. 2011;118(11):2242-50.
3. Ho J, Xirasagar S, Lin H. Increased risk of a cancer diagnosis after herpes zoster ophthalmicus: a nationwide population-based study. Ophthalmology. 2011;118(6):1076-81.
4. Tseng HF, Smith N, Harpaz R, et al. Herpes zoster vaccine in older adults and the risk of subsequent herpes zoster disease. JAMA. 2011;305(2):160-6.

1EE.73C8. MIGRAINE (VASCULAR HEADACHE)

General

Recurrent attacks of pain in the head; usually unilateral; often familial.

Ocular

Abnormal visual sensations; scotoma generally restricted to one-half of the visual field; complete blindness; unilateral transient visual loss; photopsia; branch retinal artery occlusions; anisocoria.

Clinical

Nausea; vomiting; anorexia; sensory, motor, and mood disturbances; fluid imbalance; headache.

Laboratory

Investigation studies; rule out comorbid disease, exclude other causes of headaches such as structural and/or metabolic; neurological examination; LP followed by CT or MRI.

Treatment

Treatment is based on the severity of the case.

BIBLIOGRAPHY

1. Chawla J, Blanda M, Braswell R, et al. (2011). Migraine headache. [online] Available from www.emedicine.com/neuro/TOPIC218.HTM. [Accessed September, 2013].

1EE.73C9. CHICKENPOX (VARICELLA)

General

Acute exanthematous disease; highly contagious; children between ages of 2 and 8 years.

Ocular

Conjunctival ulcer; corneal ulcer; descemetocele; corneal opacity; keratitis; paresis of third, fourth and sixth nerves; optic neuritis; papilledema; retinitis; hemorrhagic retinopathy; uveitis; cataract; paralytic mydriasis; phthisis bulbi; unifocal choroiditis; dendritic keratitis; acute retinal necrosis (in a patient with AIDS); disciform keratitis.

Clinical

Fever; malaise; rash; pruritus.

Laboratory

Diagnosis is made by clinical findings.

Treatment

Isolation oral antihistamines, such as diphenhydramine and hydroxyzine, are used for severe pruritus and acetaminophen is recommended for use for the reduction of fever.

BIBLIOGRAPHY

1. Bechtel KA, Chatterjee A, Lichenstein R, et al. (2013). Pediatric chickenpox. [online] Available from www.emedicine.com/emerg/TOPIC367.HTM. [Accessed September, 2013].

1EE.73C9.3. OCULOMOTOR PARALYSIS (III NERVE PALSY)

General

Congenital or acquired; may occur in association with trochlear nerve palsy.

Clinical

Diabetes, neurological.

Ocular

Exotropia, hypotropia, diplopia, paralysis of the ciliary muscles and iris sphincter, dilated pupil, blepharoptosis, pseudoptosis.

Laboratory

Diagnosis is made by clinical findings.

Treatment

Prism therapy; surgical—muscle surgery on the affected muscle, and occlusion at the involved eye to relief diplopia.

BIBLIOGRAPHY

1. Goodwin J. (2012). Oculomotor nerve palsy. [online] Available from www.emedicine.com/oph/TOPIC183.HTM. [Accessed September, 2013].

1EE.73C9.3A1. BENEDIKT SYNDROME (TEGMENTAL SYNDROME)

General

Lesion of the inferior nucleus tuber with obstruction of the third nerve; arteriosclerotic occlusion of branches of the basilar artery, trauma and hemorrhages in the midbrain, and neoplasm most common causes.

Ocular

Homolateral paralysis of cranial nerve III (oculomotor); involves associated movements of convergence, elevation, and depression of the eyes; loss of reflex to light and accommodation, diplopia.

Clinical

Unilateral hyperkinesis; contralateral hemiparesis, coarse tremor of upper extremity (greatly increased during movement), hemihypesthesia, and absent deep sensibility; ipsilateral ataxia. There is at least one reported case of an HIV-positive patient with Benedikt syndrome who had elevated toxoplasma IgG titers.

Laboratory

CT, MRI, transcranial Doppler.

Treatment

Ocular: Patients who do not recover from third cranial nerve palsy after 6–12 months may become candidates for eye muscle resection or recession to treat persistent and stable-angle diplopia.

BIBLIOGRAPHY

1. Kaye V, Brandstate ME. (2011). Vertebrobasilar Stroke Overview of Vertebrobasilar Stroke. [online] Available from www.emedicine.com/pmr/TOPIC143.HTM. [Accessed September, 2013].
2. Goodwin J. (2012). Oculomotor Nerve Palsy. [online] Available from www.emedicine.com/oph/TOPIC183.HTM. [Accessed September, 2013].

1EE.73C9.3A2. ERB-GOLDFLAM SYNDROME (ERB II SYNDROME; HOPPE-GOLDFLAM DISEASE; PSEUDOPARALYTIC SYNDROME; MYASTHENIA GRAVIS)

General

Occurs at any age; more frequent between ages 20 and 40 years; more females affected than males; progressive; spontaneous; symptoms improve or resolve with rest in early stages of disease (*see* myasthenia gravis, neonatal or infantile); caused by autoantibodies against the acetylcholine receptor at the neuromuscular junction, leading to abnormal fatigability and weakness of skeletal muscle.

Ocular

Transient diplopia; ptosis of upper eyelids.

Clinical

Excessive fatigability of musculature; symptoms appear and increase as day progresses; expressionless face; sagging jaw; difficulty in chewing and talking; nasal regurgitation.

Laboratory

Ice test—crushed ice in surgical glove over ptotic eyelid for 2 minutes and watch for brief elevation of eyelid; Tensilon test and prostigmin test may result in the elevation of ptotic eyelid or improved strabismus in individuals with myasthenia gravis.

Treatment

Adrenal corticosteroids are frequently used. In some cases, mycophenolate mofetil, cyclosporine and cyclophosphamide may be useful. Patching one eye or using prisms may be helpful.

BIBLIOGRAPHY

1. Erb W. Zur Casuistick der Bulbaren La hmungen. Arch Psychiatr Vervenkr. 1879;9:325-50.
2. Roy FH, Fraunfelder FT, Fraunfelder FW. Roy and Fraunfelder's Current Ocular Therapy, 6th edition. London, UK: Elsevier; 2008.
3. Goldflam S. Vebereinen Scheinbar Keilbaren Bulbarparalytischem Symptom Complex mit Betheiligung der Extremitaten. Dtsch Z Nerven. 1983;4:312-52.
4. Kim JH, Hwang JM, Hwang YS, et al. Childhood ocular myasthenia gravis. Ophthalmology. 2003;110(7):1458-62.
5. Lepore FE, Sanborn GE, Slevin JT. Pupillary dysfunction in myasthenia gravis. Ann Neurol. 1979;6(1):29-33.
6. Sommer N, Melms A, Weller M, et al. Ocular myasthenia gravis. A critical review of clinical and pathophysiological aspects. Doc Ophthalmol. 1993;84(4):309-33.

1EE.73C9.3A3C. PARINAUD SYNDROME (DIVERGENCE PARALYSIS; SUBTHALAMIC SYNDROME; PARALYSIS OF VERTICAL MOVEMENTS; PRETECTAL SYNDROME)

General

Various causes, including pineal tumor, supranuclear lesions, vascular lesions, inflammation, hemorrhages, midbrain lesions, lesion of posterior white commissure of pons, red nucleus, or superior cerebellar peduncle; combination of Parinaud and von Monakow syndromes is known as Gruner-Bertolotti syndrome, which consists of paralysis in upward gaze, tremors, hemiplegia, and sensory disturbances.

Ocular

Retraction of lids with lesion in mesencephalic gray matter and ptosis with lesions more anteriorly; paralysis of conjugate upward movement of the eye without paralysis of convergence; occasionally paralysis of upward and downward movement; spasm with convergence insufficiency; contralateral hemianopsia occurs when the lateral geniculate body becomes involved in case of infiltrating tumor; wide pupils that fail to react to light but sometimes react during accommodation (Holmes); papilledema (usually severe).

Clinical

Vertigo; contralateral cerebellar ataxia and choreoathetoid movement if lesion involves superior cerebellar peduncle after decussation.

Laboratory

Diagnosis is made by clinical findings; CT and MRI.

Treatment

Papilledema: Underlying cause should be determined and treated. Systemic acetazolamide is the medical therapy of choice.

BIBLIOGRAPHY

1. Zee C, Yao Z, Go JL, et al. (2011). Imaging in Pineal Germinoma. [online] Available from www.emedicine.com/radio/TOPIC554.HTM. [Accessed September, 2013].

⊟ 1EE.73C9.3A3D. AXENFELD-SCHURENBERG SYNDROME (CYCLIC OCULOMOTOR PARALYSIS)

General

Congenital manifestation; frequently unilateral.

Ocular

Cyclic oculomotor paralysis (paralysis alternating with spasm); during periods of paralysis, lid exhibits ptosis and affected eye is abducted; during spasm, lid is raised, deviation of affected eye is either inward or outward, and pupil is fixed and contracted.

Laboratory

Diagnosis is made by clinical findings.

Treatment

Prism therapy; surgical—muscle surgery on the affected muscle, and occlusion at the involved eye to relief diplopia.

⊟ BIBLIOGRAPHY

1. Axenfeld T, Schurenberg L. Beitrage zur Kenntnis der Angeborenen Beweglichkeitsdefekte des Auges. Klin Monastbl Augenheilkd. 1901;39:64.
2. Hamed LM. Oculomotor palsy with cyclic spasm. In: Margo CE, Mames R, Hamed LM (Eds). Diagnostic Problems in Clinical Ophthalmology, illustrated edition. Philadelphia, PA: WB Saunders; 1994. p. 712.
3. Levy MR. Cyclic oculomotor paralysis with optic atrophy. Am J Ophthalmol. 1968;65(5):766-9.
4. Purvin V. Oculomotor palsy in children. In: Margo CE, Mames R, Hamed LM (Eds). Diagnostic Problems in Clinical Ophthalmology. Philadelphia: WB Saunders; 1994. pp. 682-3.

⊟ 1EE.73C9.3A3E. BRUNS SYNDROME (POSTURAL CHANGE SYNDROME)

General

Caused by tumors of the third, fourth, or lateral ventricle or by lesions of the midline in the brain.

Ocular

Partial ophthalmoplegia (third nerve paralysis) and gaze paralysis; oculomotor paresis associated with postural change of head or body; amaurosis or transient blindness; flashes of light.

Clinical

Severe paroxysmal headache; nausea and vomiting; vertigo; irregular respiration; apnea; syncope; tachycardia; free-floating cysts within the fourth ventricle may produce intermittent foramen obstruction and Bruns syndrome; Kramer reported a patient with a free-floating cysticercus cyst with this condition.

Laboratory

Computed tomography scan of head.

Treatment

Consultation with a neurologist.

⊟ BIBLIOGRAPHY

1. Geeraets WJ. Ocular syndromes, 3rd edition. Philadelphia, USA: Lea & Febiger;1969.
2. Bruns O. Neuropathologische Demonstrationen. Neurol Centralbl. 1902;21:561.

1EE.73C9.3A3F. CLAUDE SYNDROME (INFERIOR NUCLEUS RUBER SYNDROME; RUBROSPINAL-CEREBELLAR-PEDUNCLE SYNDROME)

General

Paramedian mesencephalic lesion starting in midbrain; often occlusion of terminal branches of the paramedian arteries supplying the inferior portion of the nucleus ruber.

Ocular

Paralysis of ipsilateral oculomotor and trochlear nerves (III, IV).

Clinical

It may be associated with motor hemiplegia.

Laboratory

Diagnosis is made by clinical findings.

Treatment

Prisms may be useful for small deviations. Botulinum toxin may also be useful. For deviation greater than 15 prism diopters, strabismus surgery may be required.

BIBLIOGRAPHY

1. Claude H. Inferior nucleus ruber syndrome. Rev Neurol. 1912;1:311.
2. Cremieux G, Serratrice G. A case of retraction nystagmus associated with Claude's syndrome. Mars Med (Fre). 1972;109:635.
3. Gaymard B, Saudeau D, de Toffol B, et al. Two mesencephalic lacunar infarcts presenting as Claude's syndrome and pure motor hemiparesis. Eur Neurol. 1991;31:152-5.
4. Geeraets WJ. Ocular Syndromes, 3rd edition. Philadelphia, USA: Lea & Febiger; 1969.

1EE.73C9.3A3G. CONGENITAL VERTICAL RETRACTION SYNDROME

General

Congenital.

Ocular

Aberrant regeneration of the oculomotor nerve; concurrent protective eyelid closure; congenital alterations in the extraocular muscle, its insertion and peripheral innervation; nystagmus retractorius; surgical or traumatic rearrangement of orbital structures may account for retraction.

Clinical

None.

Laboratory

Diagnosis is made by clinical findings.

Treatment

None.

BIBLIOGRAPHY

1. Khodadoust AA, von Noorden GK. Bilateral vertical retraction syndrome. A family study. Arch Ophthalmol. 1967;78(5):606-12.
2. Osher RH, Schatz NJ, Duane TD. Acquired orbital retraction syndrome. Arch Ophthalmol. 1980;98(10):1798-802.
3. Pesando P, Nuzzi G, Maraini G. Vertical retraction syndrome. Ophthalmologica. 1978;177(5):254-9.

1EE.73C9.3A3H. NOTHNAGEL SYNDROME (OPHTHALMOPLEGIA-CEREBELLAR ATAXIA SYNDROME)

General

Lesion of superior cerebellar peduncle, red nucleus and emerging oculomotor fibers such as pineal tumor, or tumor or vascular disturbance in corpora quadrigemina or vermis cerebelli (*see* Bruns syndrome).

Ocular

Oculomotor paresis; gaze paralysis most frequently upward, combined with some degree of internal or external ophthalmoplegia.

Clinical

Cerebellar ataxia; poor upper extremity movements; neoplasia; infarction; midbrain lesion.

Laboratory

Computed tomography and MRI of brain.

Treatment

See neurologist.

BIBLIOGRAPHY

1. Magalini SI, Scrascia E. Dictionary of Medical Syndromes, 2nd edition. Philadelphia, PA: Lippincott Williams and Wilkins; 1981.
2. Nothnagel H. Topische Diagnostik Der Gehirnkrankheiten. Berlin, Germany: Nabu Press; 2010. p. 220.

1EE.73C9.5. MIGRAINE (VASCULAR HEADACHE)

General

Recurrent attacks of pain in the head; usually unilateral; often familial.

Ocular

Abnormal visual sensations; scotoma generally restricted to one-half of the visual field; complete blindness; unilateral transient visual loss; photopsia; branch retinal artery occlusions; anisocoria.

Clinical

Nausea; vomiting; anorexia; sensory, motor and mood disturbances; fluid imbalance; headache.

Laboratory

Investigation studies; rule out comorbid disease, exclude other causes of headaches such as structural and/or metabolic; neurological examination; LP followed by CT or MRI.

Treatment

Treatment is based on the severity of the case.

BIBLIOGRAPHY

1. Chawla J, Blanda M, Braswell R, et al. (2011). Migraine headache. [online] Available from www.emedicine.com/neuro/TOPIC218.HTM. [Accessed September, 2013].

1EE.73C9.6. WEBER SYNDROME (WEBER-DUBLER SYNDROME; CEREBELLAR PEDUNCLE SYNDROME; ALTERNATING OCULOMOTOR PARALYSIS; VENTRAL MEDIAL MIDBRAIN SYNDROME) PTOSIS

General

Lesion of the peduncle (crus), pons or medulla, which interrupts the third nerve before it emerges from the peduncle and interrupts fibers in the pyramidal tract above the level of the third nuclei; hemorrhage and thrombosis; tumor of the pituitary region, extending posteriorly; also may result in secondary to cerebrovascular disease.

Ocular

Ptosis; homolateral third nerve palsy (usually complete); fixed, dilated pupil.

Clinical

Contralateral hemiplegia; contralateral paralysis of face and tongue (supranuclear type).

Laboratory

Diagnosis is made by clinical findings.

Treatment

Ptosis: If visual acuity is affected, most cases require surgical correction and there are several procedures that may be used including levator resection, repair or advancement and Fasanella-Servat.

🗗 BIBLIOGRAPHY

1. Kistler JP, Ropper AH, Martin JB. Cerebrovascular diseases. In: Isselbacher KJ, Braunwald E, Wilson JD, Martin JB, Fauci A, Kasper DL (Eds). Harrison's Principles of Internal Medicine, 13th edition. New York: McGraw-Hill; 1994. pp. 2242-3.
2. Miller NR (Ed). Walsh and Hoyt's Clinical Neuro-Ophthalmology, 44th edition. Baltimore, USA: Williams & Wilkins; 1995. pp. 238-44.
3. Newman NJ. Third, fourth and sixth-nerve lesions and the cavernous sinus. In: Albert DM, Jakobiec FA (Eds). Albert & Jakobiec's Principles and Practice of Ophthalmology: Clinical Practice, 5th edition. Philadelphia, PA: WB Saunders; 1994. pp. 245-51.
4. Weber H. A contribution to the pathology of the crura cerebri. Med Chir Trans. 1863;46:121-40.1.
5. Wolf BS, Newman CM, Khilnani MT. The posterior inferior cerebellar artery on vertebral angiography. Am J Roentgenol Radium Ther Nucl Med. 1962;87:322-37.

🗗 1EE.73C9.7A1. AMEBIASIS (AMEBIC DYSENTERY, ENTAMOEBA HISTOLYTICA)

General

Caused by *Entamoeba histolytica*; *E. histolytica* cysts in stools are diagnostic.

Ocular

Conjunctivitis; iridocyclitis; hypopyon; central choroiditis; retinal hemorrhages; retinal perivasculitis; macular edema; corneal ulceration; granulomatous and nongranulomatous uveitis; vitreous hemorrhage.

Clinical

Chronic dysentery; abscesses of liver and brain; toxic megacolon.

Laboratory

Enzyme immunoassay (EIA) is the best test for making the specific diagnosis of *E. histolytica*.

Treatment

Metronidazole is considered as the drug of choice for symptomatic, invasive disease. Asymptomatic intestinal infection may be treated with iodoquinol, paromomycin, or diloxanide furoate.

🗗 BIBLIOGRAPHY

1. Lacasse A, Cleveland KO, Cantey JR, et al. Amebiasis. [online] Availble from www.emedicine.com/ped/TOPIC80.HTM. [Accessed September, 2013].

🗗 1EE.73C9.7A2. OCULOMOTOR PARALYSIS (III NERVE PALSY)

General

Congenital or acquired; may occur in association with trochlear nerve palsy.

Clinical

Diabetes, neurological.

Ocular

Exotropia, hypotropia, diplopia, paralysis of the ciliary muscles and iris sphincter, dilated pupil, blepharoptosis, pseudoptosis.

Laboratory

Diagnosis is made by clinical findings.

Treatment

Prism therapy; surgical—muscle surgery on the affected muscle, and occlusion at the involved eye to relief diplopia.

🗗 BIBLIOGRAPHY

1. Goodwin J. (2012). Oculomotor nerve palsy. [online] Available from www.emedicine.com/oph/TOPIC183.HTM. [Accessed September, 2013].

⊟ 1EE.73C9.7A3. BOTULISM

General

It is caused by a toxin-producing strain of *C. botulinum*; it occurs primarily after the ingestion of contaminated food; the organism can produce a neurotoxin, the effect of which can be life threatening.

Ocular

Absent optokinetic nystagmus, absent vertical gaze; marked limitation of horizontal gaze; ptosis; diplopia; decreased tear secretion; mydriasis; paralysis of accommodation; nystagmus; optic atrophy; optic neuritis; extraocular muscle paresis.

Clinical

Dizziness; severe respiratory impairment; gastrointestinal disturbances; dysphagia; dysarthria; postural hypotension.

Laboratory

Toxin assay for early diagnosis, whereas later cases are more likely to yield a positive specimen culture.

Treatment

Antitoxin appears to be the only effective medication. Supportive care such as ventilation and parenteral nutrition are necessary for the duration of the paralytic illness.

⊟ BIBLIOGRAPHY

1. Patel B, Taylor SF. (2012). Ophthalmologic manifestations of botulism. [online] Available from www.emedicine.com/oph/TOPIC493.HTM. [Accessed September, 2013].

⊟ 1EE.73C9.7A4. CHICKENPOX (VARICELLA)

General

Acute exanthematous disease; highly contagious; children between ages of 2 years and 8 years.

Ocular

Conjunctival ulcer; corneal ulcer; descemetocele; corneal opacity; keratitis; paresis of third, fourth and sixth nerves; optic neuritis; papilledema; retinitis; hemorrhagic retinopathy; uveitis; cataract; paralytic mydriasis; phthisis bulbi; unifocal choroiditis; dendritic keratitis; acute retinal necrosis (in a patient with AIDS); disciform keratitis.

Clinical

Fever; malaise; rash; pruritus.

Laboratory

Diagnosis is made by clinical findings.

Treatment

Isolation oral antihistamines, such as diphenhydramine and hydroxyzine, are used for severe pruritus and acetaminophen is recommended for use for the reduction of fever.

⊟ BIBLIOGRAPHY

1. Bechtel KA, Chatterjee A, Lichenstein R, et al. (2013). Pediatric chickenpox. [online] Available from www.emedicine.com/emerg/TOPIC367.HTM. [Accessed September, 2013].

🗗 1EE.73C9.7A5. CRANIOPHARYNGIOMA

General

Benign congenital tumors arising from epithelial remnants of Rathke's pouch; most common non-glial intracranial tumors in childhood; second most common sellar-para-sellar tumor primarily in children or young adults; 35% of cases occur in patients over age of 40 years.

Ocular

Paresis of third or sixth nerve; optic nerve atrophy; optic neuritis; papilledema; dilation of pupil; diplopia; hemianopia; nystagmus; scotoma; visual field defects; visual loss.

Clinical

Hydrocephalus; infantilism; diabetes insipidus; abnormal sexual development; headaches; acute aseptic meningitis.

Laboratory

Cranial CT and MRI are the current imaging standards.

Treatment

Although controversial, aggressive surgical treatment to attempt gross total resection is sometimes considered. Second option is planned limited surgery followed by radiotherapy.

🗗 BIBLIOGRAPHY

1. Bobustuc GC, Groves MD, Fuller GN, et al. (2012). Craniopharyngioma. [online] Available from www.emedicine.com/neuro/TOPIC584.HTM. [Accessed September, 2013].

🗗 1EE.73C9.7A6. DENGUE FEVER

General

Endemic over the tropics and subtropics; caused by four distinct serogroups of dengue viruses, types 1–4, Group B arboviruses; transmitted solely by mosquitoes of the genus *Aedes*.

Ocular

Lid edema; conjunctivitis; ocular and retrobulbar pain accentuated by ocular movement; dacryoadenitis; keratitis; corneal ulcer; iritis; retinal or vitreous hemorrhages; ocular motor paresis; optic atrophy.

Clinical

Hemorrhagic fever, severe headache; backache; joint pain; rigors; insomnia; anorexia; loss of taste; epistaxis; rashes; maculopapular rash; myalgia; human infection with four serotypes of dengue virus causing two diseases: classic dengue fever and dengue hemorrhagic fever (50% mortality).

Laboratory

Basic metabolic panel, liver function test, coagulation studies, chest X-ray, serial ultrasonography.

Treatment

A self-limited illness, and only supportive care is required. Acetaminophen may be used to treat patients with symptomatic fever. Dengue hemorrhagic fever warrant closer observation. Rehydration with intravenous fluids, plasma expander, transfusion and shock therapy may be necessary.

🗗 BIBLIOGRAPHY

1. Shepherd SM, Hinfey PB, Shoff WH. (2012). Dengue. [online] Available from www.emedicine.com/med/TOPIC528.HTM. [Accessed September, 2013].

🗗 1EE.73C9.7A7. DEVIC SYNDROME (OPHTHALMOENCEPHALOMYELOPATHY; OPTIC MYELITIS; NEUROMYELITIS OPTICA)

General

Etiology unknown; frequent between the ages of 20 and 50 years; mortality rate up to 50%; associated with chickenpox.

Ocular

Ptosis is rare; ocular muscle palsy (rare); abducens and oculomotor palsy; paralysis of conjugate gaze; blindness; onset usually very sudden in one eye, followed soon by blindness in the other eye; miosis; bilateral optic neuritis (unilateral involvement is rare); optic atrophy; pupillary dysfunction.

Clinical

Prodromal signs: headache; sore throat; fever and malaise; ascending myelitis with resulting pain, which may be severe; numbness; weakness; paralysis.

Laboratory

Diagnosis is made by clinical findings.

Treatment

Steroids orally or intravenously may be useful.

🗗 BIBLIOGRAPHY

1. Schatz MP, Carter JE. (2011). Childhood Optic Neuritis. [online] Available from www.emedicine.com/oph/TOPIC343.HTM. [Accessed September, 2013].

🗗 1EE.73C9.7A8. DIPHTHERIA

General

Acute infectious disease caused by *C. diphtheriae*; severity is dependent upon the amount of exotoxin absorbed prior to initiation of specific therapy.

Ocular

Conjunctivitis; xerophthalmia; keratitis; corneal ulcer; blepharitis; cellulitis of lid; meibomianitis; ptosis; dacryocystitis; cataract; central retinal artery occlusion; optic neuritis; accommodative spasm or paralysis; convergence paralysis; divergence paralysis; paralysis of third, fourth, or sixth nerve; paralysis of accommodation (in children); ocular motor nerve paresis; choroiditis; cranial neuropathies involving the trigeminal, vagus and hypoglossal cranial nerves; myocarditis.

Clinical

Local inflammatory lesion, with effect on heart, kidneys and nervous system.

Laboratory

Gram-positive rods commonly affect children younger than 10 years.

Treatment

Systemic treatment involves use of diphtheria antitoxin and antibiotics. Ocular treatment includes diphtheria antitoxin and high titer y-globulin preparation. Topical penicillin-G ointment helps to eradicate the bacilli.

🗗 BIBLIOGRAPHY

1. Demirci CS. (2011). Pediatric diphtheria. [online] Available from www.emedicine.com/ped/TOPIC596.HTM. [Accessed September, 2013].

🗗 1EE.73C9.7A9. ENCEPHALITIS, ACUTE

General

In approximately 0.1–0.2% of patients having rubeola (measles), an acute encephalitis is seen within 1 week after the onset of the rash; a case of immunosuppressive encephalitis can present with focal seizures leading to progressive obtundation.

Ocular

Papillitis; optic atrophy; ocular motor palsies; nystagmus; optic neuritis or neuroretinitis.

Clinical

Rise in temperature; drowsiness; irritability; meningismus; vomiting and headache; stupor; convulsions; coma.

Laboratory

Perform head CT, with and without contrast agent, before LP to search for evidence of elevated intracerebral pressure. MRI is useful. Viral serology.

Treatment

Evaluate and treat for shock or hypotension, treat systemic complications, acyclovir.

🗗 BIBLIOGRAPHY

1. Howes DS, Lazoff M. (2013). Encephalitis. [online] Available from www.emedicine.com/emerg/TOPIC163.HTM. [Accessed September, 2013].

🗗 1EE.73C9.7A10. HEPATIC FAILURE

General

Liver failure from infections or toxic or inflammatory causes.

Ocular

Visual field defects; scleral icterus; night blindness; abnormal color vision; eyelid retraction; lid lag; Kayser-Fleischer ring; yellow discoloration of the conjunctiva.

Clinical

Bilirubin accumulation; reduced vitamin A levels.

Laboratory

Diagnosis is made by clinical findings.

Treatment

See internist.

🗗 BIBLIOGRAPHY

1. Nazer H, Nazer D. (2012). Pediatric Fulminant Hepatic Failure. [online] Available from www.emedicine.com/ped/TOPIC808.HTM. [Accessed September, 2013].

🗗 1EE.73C9.7A11. INFLUENZA

General

Acute respiratory infection of specific viral etiology which includes H1N1.

Ocular

Conjunctivitis; subconjunctival hemorrhages; keratitis; tenonitis; ptosis; cellulitis of orbit and lid; dacryocystitis; retinal hemorrhage; cataract; episcleritis; hypopyon; optic neuritis; uveitis; panophthalmitis; vitreal hemorrhage; paralysis of third or fourth nerve; uveitis following vaccination for influenza.

Clinical

Headache; fever; malaise; muscular aching; substernal soreness; nasal stuffiness; nausea.

Laboratory

The standard criterion for diagnosing influenza A and B is a viral culture of nasal-pharyngeal samples, throat samples, or both.

Treatment

Prevention is the most effective therapy. Two new drugs have been marketed recently for treatment of influenza A and B. These are the neuraminidase inhibitors, oseltamivir and zanamivir.

BIBLIOGRAPHY

1. Derlet RW. (2012). Influenza. [online] Available from www.emedicine.com/med/TOPIC1170.HTM. [Accessed September, 2013].

1EE.73C9.7A12. LOCKJAW (TETANUS)

General

Acute infectious disease affecting nervous system; causative agent is *Clostridium tetani*; bacteria enters body through a puncture wound, abrasion, cut, or burn.

Ocular

Chemosis; keratitis; nystagmus; uveitis; corneal ulcer; cellulitis of orbit; hypopyon; panophthalmitis; pupil paralysis; pseudoptosis; blepharospasm; paralysis of third or seventh nerve; may occur following perforating ocular injuries.

Clinical

Severe muscle spasms; dysphagia; trismus; facial palsy; muscle stiffness; irritability.

Laboratory

Gram-positive spore-forming bacteria, laboratory studies are of little value.

Treatment

Passive immunization with human tetanus immune globulin shortens the course of tetanus and may lessen its severity. Benzodiazepines have emerged as the mainstay of symptomatic therapy for tetanus.

BIBLIOGRAPHY

1. Hinfey PB. (2012). Tetanus. [online] Available from www.emedicine.com/med/TOPIC2254.HTM. [Accessed September, 2013].

1EE.73C9.7A13. RETICULUM CELL SARCOMA (NON-HODGKIN LYMPHOMA)

General

Autosomal recessive; large-cell lymphoma with chronic inflammation with a predominance of cells in vitreous cavity; average age at time of diagnosis is 60 years; female to male ratio is approximately 2:1; 80% bilateral (frequently asymmetrical).

Ocular

Chronic uveitis; chorioretinal lesions; mycosis fungoides; necrosis of orbital tissues; phthisis bulbi; endophthalmos; exophthalmos; exudative retinal detachment; iris neovascularization; glaucoma; branch retinal vein occlusion; macular edema; optic neuropathy; vitreous hemorrhage; partial cranial nerve III palsy; multiple retinal pigment epithelium masses.

Clinical

Lymphocytic hyperplasia; fever; anemia; thrombocytopenia; liver and spleen enlargement; associated with immune dysfunction states, such AIDS, or following transplantation.

Laboratory

Computed tomography/MRI scan, HIV evaluation, CBC, LP.

Treatment

Radiation, chemotherapy.

BIBLIOGRAPHY

1. Vinjamaram S, Estrada-Garcia DA, Hernandez-Ilizaliturri FJ, et al. (2012). Non-Hodgkin lymphoma. [online] Available from emedicine.medscape.com/article/203399-overview. [Accessed September, 2013].

🖧 1EE.73C9.7A14. MALARIA

General

Caused by *Plasmodium*, which is transmitted by mosquito bite, blood transfusion, or contaminated needles and syringes.

Ocular

Proliferative retinitis; vascular embolism; keratitis; ocular herpes simplex; blepharitis; optic atrophy; papilledema; papillitis; optic neuritis; anisocoria; Argyll Robertson pupil; vitreal hemorrhages and opacity; cataract; myopia; strabismus; uveitis; scleral icterus; scotoma; lagophthalmos; ptosis; subconjunctival hemorrhages; paralysis of third, fourth, or sixth nerve; epibulbar hemorrhage involving the conjunctiva, episclera, tendinous insertion of the medial rectus.

Clinical

Fever; anemia; splenomegaly; death.

Laboratory

Blood smear.

Treatment

Consult infectious disease specialist.

🖧 BIBLIOGRAPHY

1. Perez-Jorge EV, Herchline TE. (2013). Malaria. [online] Available from www.emedicine.com/med/TOPIC1385.HTM. [Accessed September, 2013].

🖧 1EE.73C9.7A15. MEASLES (MORBILLI; RUBEOLA)

General

Acute, extremely communicable disease that affects young school-aged children; caused by paramyxovirus.

Ocular

Hypopyon; uveitis; conjunctivitis; Koplik (Hirschberg) spots of conjunctiva; keratitis; corneal ulcer; cellulitis of lid; dacryocystitis; congenital cataract; optic atrophy; optic neuritis; strabismus; pigmentary retinopathy; iris prolapse; hemianopsia; secondary glaucoma; central retinal artery occlusion; orbital cellulitis; accommodative spasm; paralysis of sixth nerve; keratoconus.

Clinical

Maculopapular rash; fever.

Laboratory

Diagnosis is made by clinical findings.

Treatment

Good hydration.

🖧 BIBLIOGRAPHY

1. Chen SS. (2011). Measles. [online] Available from www.emedicine.com/derm/TOPIC259.HTM. [Accessed September, 2013].

🖧 1EE.73C9.7A16. MENINGOCOCCEMIA (NEISSERIA MENINGITIDES; MENINGITIS)

General

Systemic bacterial infection caused by *N. meningitides*; can be present chronically in patients with immune deficiencies including deficient complement levels.

Ocular

Photophobia; conjunctivitis; chemosis; keratitis; uveitis; panophthalmitis; retinal endophlebitis; macular edema; papillitis; optic neuritis; paresis of sixth or seventh nerve; nystagmus; miosis; hippus; cortical blindness; papilledema (rare); conjunctival petechiae; strabismus.

Clinical

Meningitis; fever; malaise; joint pain; splenic enlargement.

Laboratory

Cultures from blood, spinal fluid, or joint fluid.

Treatment

Treat with antibiotics promptly.

BIBLIOGRAPHY

1. Javid MH, Ahmed SH. (2012). Meningococcemia. [online] Available from www.emedicine.com/med/TOPIC1445. HTM. [Accessed September, 2013].

1EE.73C9.7A17. DISSEMINATED SCLEROSIS (MULTIPLE SCLEROSIS)

General

Disseminated demyelination affecting white matter of the brain, spinal cord and optic nerves; etiology is unknown.

Ocular

Nystagmus; ptosis; myokymia; optic atrophy; papillitis; optic neuritis; anisocoria; Argyll Robertson pupil; Marcus Gunn pupil; hippus, decreased or absent papillary reaction to light; periphlebitis; visual field defects; gaze palsy; paralysis of third or sixth nerve; uveitis; oscillopsia; Uhthoff symptom (reduction of visual acuity with exercise or ocular hyperthermia); pars planitis; retinal venous sheathing; retinitis; granulomatous uveitis.

Clinical

Incoordination; paresthesia; spasticity; tic douloureux; urinary frequency and infections; progressive disability; paralysis; death.

Laboratory

Magnetic resonance imaging, CSF positive for oligoclonal band, albumin and IgG index; BAER and SEP.

Treatment

Patients with MS may require multiple consultations to rule out other causes for their symptoms. Drugs such as immunomodulators, immunosuppressors, antiparkinson agents, CNS stimulants are all used in the management of the disease.

BIBLIOGRAPHY

1. Luzzio C, Dangond F. (2012). Multiple sclerosis. [online] Available from www.emedicine.com/neuro/topic228.htm. [Accessed September, 2013].

1EE.73C9.7A18. OPHTHALMOPLEGIC MIGRAINE SYNDROME

General

Symptoms produced by ipsilateral herniation of hippocampal gyrus of temporal lobe through incisura tentorii; dependent upon unilateral cerebral edema due to vascular or vasomotor phenomena, intracranial aneurysm, or tumor; incidence may be greater in women with the initial attack in the first decade of life; pathogenesis is unclear, but it is likely secondary to ischemia of the ocular motor nerve.

Ocular

Severe unilateral supraorbital pain; ptosis; transitory partial or complete homolateral oculomotor paralysis; fourth or sixth nerve occasionally involved; retinal hemorrhages; papilledema (may be bilateral); moderate to severe headache with partial to complete cranial nerve III paresis including the pupil; more than one ocular nerve may be affected.

Clinical

Migraine headache, not present in all instances; dizziness; diminution in sense of smell; hypalgesia contralateral side of face; nausea/vomiting may be present; recurrent sinus arrest.

Laboratory

Diagnosis is made by clinical findings.

Treatment

Ptosis: If visual acuity is affected, most cases require surgical correction and there are several procedures that may be used including levator resection, repair or advancement and Fasanella-Servat.

🗗 BIBLIOGRAPHY

1. Bazak I, Margulis T, Shnaider H, et al. Ophthalmoplegic migraine and recurrent sinus arrest. J Neurol Neurosurg Psychiatry. 1991;54:935.
2. Ehlers H. On pathogenesis of ophthalmoplegic migraine. Acta Psychiatr Neurol (Scand). 1928;3:219.
3. Geeraets WJ. Ocular Syndromes, 3rd edition. Philadelphia: Lea & Febiger; 1976.
4. Gulkilik G, Cagatay H, Oba E, et al. Ophthalmoplegic migraine associated with recurrent isolated ptosis. Ann Ophthal. 2010;41:206-12.
5. Raskin NH. Migraine and other headaches. In: Rowland LP (Ed). Merritt's Textbook of Neurology, 9th edition. Baltimore: Williams & Wilkins; 1995. pp. 837-45.
6. Stommel EW, Ward TN, Harris RD. Ophthalmoplegic migraine or Tolosa-Hunt syndrome? Headache. 1994;34:177.
7. Van Pelt W, Andermann F. On the early onset of ophthalmologic migraine. Am J Dis Child. 1964;107:628.
8. Vijayan N. Ophthalmoplegic migraine: ischemic or compressive neuropathy? Headache. 1980;20:300-4.

🗗 1EE.73C9.7A19. KUSSMAUL DISEASE (KUSSMAUL-MAIER DISEASE; NECROTIZING ANGIITIS; PAN; POLYARTERITIS NODOSA)

General

Progressive process of vascular inflammation and necrosis, manifested by numerous nodules along the course of small and medium-sized arteries; lesions are segmental in distribution, have a predilection for bifurcation and involve all but the pulmonary arteries; arteries in gastrointestinal tract, kidneys, and muscles are particularly affected; affects primarily males between ages 20 years and 50 years.

Ocular

Retinal detachment; cotton-wool patches; polyarteritis nodosa (PAN) lesion of arteries; pseudoretinitis pigmentosa; conjunctivitis; corneal ulcer; tenonitis; ptosis; exophthalmos; uveitis; optic atrophy; cataract; scleritis; paralysis of extraocular muscles; neuroretinitis; macular star; peripheral ulcerative keratitis; retinal vasculitis; pseudotumor of the orbit; central retinal artery occlusion.

Clinical

Fever; myalgia; hypertension; gastrointestinal disorders; neuropathy; respiratory infection; weight loss; anginal pain; hemiplegia; convulsion; acute brain syndrome; skin lesions; diffuse erythema; purpura; urticaria; gangrene; tachycardia; pericarditis; aortitis; painful facial swelling; diplopia.

Laboratory

Diagnosis is made by clinical findings.

Treatment

* *Retinal detachment*: Scleral buckle, pneumatic retinopexy and vitrectomy may be used to close all the breaks.
* *Corneal ulcer*: Corneal cultures may be taken and treatment is initiated. Treatment includes a broad spectrum of antibiotics and cycloplegic drops.
* *Uveitis*: Topical steroids and cycloplegic medication should be the initial treatment of choice. Oral steroids if not responsive to topical steroids, immunosuppressants if bilateral disease that does not respond to oral steroids, periocular steroids for unilateral or posterior uveitis. Vitrectomy can be used for severe vitreous opacification. Cryotherapy and laser photocoagulation may be used for localized pars plana exudates.

🗗 BIBLIOGRAPHY

1. Akova YA, Jabbur NS, Foster CS. Ocular presentation of polyarteritis nodosa. Clinical course and management with steroid and cytotoxic therapy. Ophthalmology. 1993;100(12):1775-81.
2. Kussmaul A, Maier R. Ueber Eine Bisher Nicht Beschriebene Eigenthumliche Artenener Krankung (Periarteritis Nodosa), die Mit Morbus Brightii und Rapid Fortschreitender Allgemeiner Muskellahumung Einhergeht. Dtsch Arch Klin Med. 1866;1:484-518.
3. Matsuda A, Chin S, Ohashi T. A case of neuroretinitis associated with long-standing polyarteritis nodosa. Ophthalmologica. 1994;208(3):168-71.
4. Roy FH, Fraunfelder FW, Fraunfelder FT. Roy and Fraunfelder's Current Ocular Therapy, 6th edition. Philadelphia: WB Saunders; 2008.
5. Solomon SM, Solomon JH. Bilateral central retinal artery occlusions in polyarteritis nodosa. Ann Ophthalmol. 1978;10(5):567-9.

🗗 1EE.73C9.7A20. POLIOMYELITIS (INFANTILE PARALYSIS)

General

Acute viral infection characterized by varying degrees of neuronal injury, with special localization in the anterior horns and motor nuclei of the brainstem.

Ocular

Diplopia; nystagmus; paralysis of third, fourth and sixth nerves; paresis of seventh nerve; papilledema; visual agnosia; Homer syndrome; pupillary paralysis; optic neuritis; ophthalmoparesis; transient visual loss; internuclear ophthalmoplegia; papillary disturbances, spasm of near reflex.

Clinical

Flaccid paralysis of many muscle groups; death from asphyxia and involvement of vital centers in the brainstem.

Laboratory

Obtain specimens from the CSF, stool and throat for viral cultures.

Treatment

No antivirals are effective against polioviruses. The treatment of poliomyelitis is mainly supportive and will involve physical therapist and rehabilitation therapist, pulmonologist, neurologist, immunologist and infectious diseases specialist.

🗗 BIBLIOGRAPHY

1. Estrada B. (2012). Pediatric poliomyelitis. [online] Available from www.emedicine.com/ped/TOPIC1843.HTM. [Accessed September, 2013].

🗗 1EE.737A21. HERPES ZOSTER

General

It is caused by varicella zoster virus; about 75% of cases occur in persons over age of 45 years; condition is more frequent with advancing age and in patients who are immunocompromised by drugs or disease; in particular, an increasing number of patients with herpes zoster ophthalmicus are immunosuppressed.

Ocular

Conjunctivitis; keratitis; recurrent corneal ulcer; neuralgia; zoster rash of eyelids; uveitis; iris atrophy; scleritis; cataract; optic neuritis; paralysis of third nerve; proptosis; paralysis of lids; orbital apex syndrome; retinitis; neurotrophic keratitis; acute retinal necrosis; progressive outer retinal necrosis; ocular motor nerve pareses; tonic pupil; encephalitis; vasculitis.

Clinical

Local lesions involving the posterior or root ganglia; nerve damage; tissue scarring.

Laboratory

Diagnosed mostly on the basis of the characteristic pain and appearance of the dermatomal rashes.

Treatment

Antiviral agents, systemic corticosteroids, antidepressants and adequate pain control. Immunocompetent adults aged 60 years or older, benefit from receipt of the herpes zoster vaccine and have a lower incidence of herpes zoster.

🗗 BIBLIOGRAPHY

1. Diaz MM, Foster CS, Walton RC, et al. (2011). Herpes zoster ophthalmicus. [online] Available from www.emedicine.com/oph/TOPIC257.HTM. [Accessed September, 2013].
2. Ghaznawi N, Virdi A, Dayan A, et al. Herpes zoster ophthalmicus: comparison of disease in patients 60 years and older versus younger than 60 years. Ophthalmology. 2011;118(11):2242-50.
3. Ho J, Xirasagar S, Lin H. Increased risk of a cancer diagnosis after herpes zoster ophthalmicus: a nationwide population-based study. Ophthalmology. 2011;118(6):1076-81.
4. Tseng HF, Smith N, Harpaz R, et al. Herpes zoster vaccine in older adults and the risk of subsequent herpes zoster disease. JAMA. 2011;305(2):160-6.

🖵 1EE.73C9.7A21. MUMPS

General

Viral infection.

Ocular

Conjunctivitis; keratitis; corneal ulcer; tenonitis; exophthalmos; microphthalmos; optic atrophy; optic neuritis; papillitis; scleritis; uveitis; cortical blindness; congenital punctal occlusion; paralysis of extraocular muscles; dacryoadenitis; iritis; paralysis of accommodation; internal and external ophthalmoparesis.

Clinical

Affects the parotid glands, but infection of other glandular tissue occurs, including the lacrimal gland and testicles; encephalitis; meningitis.

Laboratory

Mumps virus by acute serologic studies.

Treatment

Generous hydration and alimentation, analgesics for headaches. No antiviral agent is available.

🖵 BIBLIOGRAPHY

1. Defendi GL. (2012). Mumps. [online] Available from www.emedicine.com/ped/TOPIC1503.HTM. [Accessed September, 2013].

🖵 1EE.73C9.7A22. HYDROPHOBIA (LYSSA; RABIES)

General

Acute viral zoonosis of the CNS.

Ocular

Lid retraction; widening of palpebral fissure; retinal hemorrhages; mydriasis; paralysis of third, fourth, fifth, or seventh nerve; bilateral optic neuritis; branch retinal artery occlusion; vaccine-induced autoimmune demyelinative optic neuritis.

Clinical

Fever; headache; nausea; numbness; tingling; acute sensitiveness to sound and light; laryngeal and pharyngeal spasms; increased muscle tonus; convulsions; delirium; coma; death.

Laboratory

Saliva can be tested by virus isolation or reverse transcription followed by PCR. Suspected infectious animal should be quarantined for 10 days.

Treatment

Before the onset of symptoms, both passive and active immunizations are effective for preventing progression to full-blown rabies. In exposures to high-risk species, initiate treatment immediately pending laboratory examination of the animal, if it is caught.

🖵 BIBLIOGRAPHY

1. Gompf SG. (2011). Rabies. [online] Available from www.emedicine.com/med/TOPIC1374.HTM. [Accessed September, 2013].

⊟ 1EE.73C9.7A23. RELAPSING POLYCHONDRITIS (JAKSCH WARTENHOST SYNDROME; MEYENBURG-ALTHERZ-VEHLINGER SYNDROME; VON MEYENBERG II SYNDROME)

General

Episodic, yet generally progressive; onset usually in middle life; possibly caused by lysosomal labilizing factor of endogenous or exogenous toxic nature or immunologic reactions; possible association with Reiter's syndrome.

Ocular

Conjunctivitis; corneal ulcer; exophthalmos; panophthalmitis; phthisis bulbi; proptosis; optic neuritis; papilledema; retinal detachment; blue sclera; episcleritis; scleromalacia; vitreous opacity; cataracts; nystagmus; retinal artery thrombosis; keratoconjunctivitis sicca; secondary glaucoma; scotoma; uveitis; paresis of third or sixth nerve; conjunctival mass (salmon patch); chorioretinitis.

Clinical

Destruction of cartilage and eventual replacement with connective tissue; polyarthritis; chondritis; tracheal collapse; bronchial collapse; anemia; liver dysfunction; death; malaise; fever; dyspnea; changes in pitch of voice; hearing impairment; vertigo; deformed ears; aortic valve insufficiency.

Laboratory

No specific serologic markers.

Treatment

No therapy.

⊟ BIBLIOGRAPHY

1. Compton N, Buckner JH, Harp KI, et al. (2012). Polychondritis. [online] Available from emedicine.medscape.com/article/331475-overview. [Accessed September, 2013].

⊟ 1EE.73C9.7A24. SMALLPOX (VARIOLA)

General

Highly contagious cutaneous disease caused by viral infection.

Ocular

Conjunctivitis; keratitis; corneal ulcer; hypopyon; endophthalmitis; congenital corneal clouding; albinotic spots on iris; choroiditis; vitreous opacities; papillitis; extraocular muscle palsies; entropion; dacryocystitis; chorioretinitis; optic neuritis; and vesicles of the eyelid; preauricular adenopathy; eyelid ulcerating pustules; several conditions predispose to the spread of vaccinia, including eczema, hypogammaglobulinemia, steroid therapy and AIDS.

Clinical

Fever, headache, and vomiting prior to appearance of the rash on the face, upper trunk and down to the extremities.

Laboratory

Brick-shaped virions viewed with electron microscopy examination, virus culture from live cells, or DNA analysis using PCR and smallpox skin specimen should be collected.

Treatment

No known treatment is effective.

⊟ BIBLIOGRAPHY

1. Hussain AN, Hussain F, Alam M, et al. (2011). Smallpox. [online] Available from www.emedicine.com/med/TOPIC3545.HTM. [Accessed September, 2013].

🔲 1EE.73C9.7A26. ACQUIRED LUES (SYPHILIS; ACQUIRED SYPHILIS; LUES VENEREA; MALUM VENEREUM)

General

Causative agent, *T. pallidum*, usually transmitted sexually.

Ocular

Conjunctival chancroid; conjunctivitis; keratitis; blepharitis; ptosis; iris atrophy; hippus; dacryocystitis; optic nerve atrophy; optic neuritis; periostitis; episcleritis; scleritis; nystagmus; uveitis; vitreous hemorrhages; paralysis of sixth nerve; papilledema; retinal hemorrhages; retinitis proliferans; oculogyric crisis; neuroretinitis; papilledema (associated with aseptic meningitis); diffuse or multifocal chorioretinitis; vertical supranuclear gaze palsy; Benedikt syndrome.

Clinical

Primary lesion associated with regional lymphadenopathy; secondary bacteremic stage associated with generalized mucocutaneous lesions; tertiary stage characterized by destructive mucocutaneous, musculoskeletal, or parenchymal lesions, aortitis, or CNS disease; syphilis and HIV infection often coexist in the same patient who experiences a higher incidence and greater severity of neurologic and ocular manifestations; a significant percentage of patients infected with HIV-I and *T. pallidum* become seronegative to syphilis testing.

Laboratory

Serologic nontreponemal tests include VDRL and RPR.

Treatment

The goals are to reduce morbidity and to prevent complications. Penicillin is the antibiotic of choice for treating syphilis. Ocular syphilis should be treated the same as patients with neurosyphilis.

🔲 BIBLIOGRAPHY

1. Euerle B, Chandrasekar PH, Diaz MM, et al. (2012). Syphilis. [online] Available from www.emedicine.com/med/TOPIC2224.HTM. [Accessed September, 2013].
2. Majmudar PA. (2011). Interstitial keratitis overview of interstitial keratitis. [online] Available from www.emedicine.com/oph/TOPIC453.HTM. [Accessed September, 2013].

🔲 1EE.73C9.7A27. TEMPORAL ARTERITIS SYNDROME (CRANIAL ARTERITIS SYNDROME; GIANT CELL ARTERITIS; HUTCHINSON-HORTON-MAGATH-BROWN SYNDROME)

General

Etiology unknown; mainly females; mainly whites; ages 55–80 years; temporal artery shows inflammatory thickening; arteritis of the vessels supplying the optic nerve.

Ocular

Transient ptosis; partial or complete loss of vision on the affected side; retinal detachment; exudates and hemorrhages; narrowing of retinal vessels; obstruction of the central retinal artery; optic atrophy; ischemic optic neuropathy; acute decreased IOP; corneal hypesthesia; palsies of extraocular muscles; hemorrhagic glaucoma; diplopia; hemorrhages on or around the disk.

Clinical

Throbbing headache; hyperalgesia of the scalp; malaise; anorexia; weakness; weight loss; fever; nodular pulmonary nodules; cough; otitis with deafness.

Laboratory

Elevated ESR greater than 50 mm/hour, positive temporal artery biopsy.

Treatment

Systemic corticosteroids are the therapy of choice.

🔲 BIBLIOGRAPHY

1. Allen AW, Biega T, Varma MK. (2012). Temporal arteritis imaging. [online] Available from www.emedicine.com/radio/TOPIC675.HTM. [Accessed September, 2013].
2. Walvick MD, Walvick MP. Giant cell arteritis: laboratory predictors of a positive temporal artery biopsy. Ophthalmology. 2011;118(6):1201-4.

⊟ 1EE.73C9.7A28. TUBERCULOSIS

General

Communicable disease caused by the acid-fast bacillus *M. tuberculosis.*

Ocular

Conjunctivitis; subconjunctival nodules (tuberculomas); keratitis; pannus; corneal ulcer; blepharitis; cellulitis; meibomianitis; uveitis; dacryocystitis; chronic orbital cellulitis; retinitis; scleritis; scleral perforation; hypopyon; vitreous hemorrhages; optic neuritis; optic atrophy; tuberculous panophthalmitis; choroidal tubercles; intraorbital extraocular lesions.

Clinical

Pulmonary infection; pyuria; hematuria; epididymitis; dysuria; flank pain; distorted calyces; productive cough.

Laboratory

Acid-fast bacillus culture of body fluids including vitreous and aqueous. PCR is 89% positive for pulmonary infection.

Treatment

A course of chemotherapy (isoniazid, rifampin, pyrazinamide and ethambutol or streptomycin) for a period of 6 months is the recommended therapy.

⊟ BIBLIOGRAPHY

1. Collins JK. Handbook of Clinical Ophthalmology. New York: Masson; 1982.
2. DeVoe AG, Locatcher-Khorazo D. The external manifestations of ocular tuberculosis. Trans Am Ophthalmol Soc. 1964;62:203-12.
3. D'Souza P, Garg R, Dhaliwal RS, et al. Orbital tuberculosis. Int Ophthalmol. 1994; 18:149-52.
4. Gupta V, Gupta A, Arora S, et al. Presumed tubercular serpiginous like choroiditis. Ophthalmology. 2003;110:1744-9.
5. Patkar S, Singhania BK, Agrawal A. Intraorbital extraocular tuberculosis: a report of three cases. Surg Neurol. 1994; 42:320-1.
6. Roy FH, Fraunfelder FW, Fraunfelder FT. Roy and Fraunfelder's Current Ocular Therapy, 6th editon. Philadelphia: WB Saunders; 2008.
7. Tejada P, Mendez MJ, Negreira S. Choroidal tubercles with tuberculous meningitis. Int Ophthalmol. 1994;18:115-8.

⊟ 1EE.73C9.7D. FOIX SYNDROME (CAVERNOUS SINUS SYNDROME; HYPOPHYSEAL-SPHENOIDAL SYNDROME; CAVERNOUS SINUS NEURALGIA SYNDROME; GODTFREDSEN SYNDROME; CAVERNOUS SINUS-NASOPHARYNGEAL TUMOR SYNDROME; CAVERNOUS SINUS THROMBOSIS)

General

Causes include tumor of lateral sinus wall or sphenoid bone, intracranial aneurysm, cavernous and lateral sinus thrombosis, or lesions; multiple myeloma; may result from infarctions or cancer or be idiopathic.

Ocular

Proptosis; severe ocular and periorbital pain; lid edema; paresis or paralysis of cranial nerves III, IV, V, and VI; corneal anesthesia; optic atrophy.

Clinical

Postauricular edema; trigeminal neuralgia; deviation of the tongue toward paralyzed side; patients usually have prominent manifestations of sepsis and paranasal sinus; local skin infections are the most common cause.

Laboratory

Computed tomography and MRI.

Treatment

Radiotherapy, anticoagulation, high-dose antibiotic therapy.

⊟ BIBLIOGRAPHY

1. Kattah JC, Pula JH. (2012). Cavernous sinus syndromes. [online] Available from www.emedicine.com/neuro/topic572.htm. [Accessed September, 2013].

◫ 1EE.73C9.7DA. ARTERIOVENOUS FISTULA (ARTERIOVENOUS ANEURYSM; ARTERIOVENOUS ANGIOMA; ARTERIOVENOUS MALFORMATION; CIRSOID ANEURYSM; RACEMOSE HEMANGIOMA; VARICOSE ANEURYSM)

General

Abnormal communications between arteries and veins that allow arterial blood to enter the vein directly without traversing a capillary network; may be congenital or secondary to penetrating trauma or blunt trauma.

Ocular

Uveitis; chemosis and neovascularization of conjunctiva; bullous keratopathy; eyelid edema; ptosis; exophthalmos; iris atrophy; papilledema; retinal hemorrhages; cataract; paresis of third or sixth nerves; glaucoma; upper lid tumor; total choroidal detachment; leaking retinal macroaneurysms; central retinal vein occlusion; iris neovascularization.

Clinical

Cerebral hemorrhage; death; substernal pain; dyspnea; varicose veins.

Laboratory

Orbital ultrasonography, CT and six-vessel cranial digital subtraction angiography.

Treatment

Obtain emergent neurosurgical consultation for definitive treatment.

◫ BIBLIOGRAPHY

1. Zebian RC, Kazzi AA. (2013). Emergent management of subarachnoid hemorrhage. [online] Available from www.emedicine.com/emerg/topic559.htm. [Accessed September, 2013].

◫ 1EE.73C9.7DB. CAROTID ARTERY SYNDROME (CAVERNOUS SINUS FISTULA SYNDROME; RED-EYED SHUNT SYNDROME)

General

Seventy-five percent of cases caused by trauma; others occur spontaneously or are congenital; fistula from carotid artery to cavernous sinus.

Ocular

Progressive, pulsating exophthalmos; distended pulsating superior orbital vein; venous congestion of lids; variable ophthalmoplegia, depending on involvement of cranial nerves III to VI; secondary glaucoma; congestion of conjunctiva with chemosis; corneal ulcerations; eversion of the lower lid; loss of corneal sensation; retinal edema; engorgement of retinal veins; papilledema; optic atrophy; ocular bruit that may be subjective and/or objective; diplopia; visual decrease; choroidal folds; dilated superior ophthalmic vein.

Clinical

Severe unilateral headache; buzzing noise.

Laboratory

Orbital ultrasonography, CT, six-vessel cranial digital subtraction angiography—characterization of the arterial supply and venous drainage of fistula.

Treatment

Use of intraocular lowering agent and topical lubrication is the ocular treatment of choice.

◫ BIBLIOGRAPHY

1. Dailey EJ, Holloway JA, Murto RE, et al. Evaluation of ocular signs and symptoms in cerebral aneurysms. Arch Ophthalmol. 1964;71:463-74.
2. Duane TD. Clinical Ophthalmology. Philadelphia: JB Lippincott; 1987.
3. Flaharty PM, Lieb WE, Sergott RC, et al. Color Doppler imaging. A new noninvasive technique to diagnose and monitor carotid cavernous sinus fistulas. Arch Ophthalmol. 1991;109:522-6.

4. Gonshor LG, Kline LB. Choroidal folds and dural cavernous sinus fistula. Arch Ophthalmol. 1991;109:1065-6.
5. Phelps CD, Thompson HS, Ossoinig KC. The diagnosis and prognosis of atypical carotid cavernous fistula. Am J Ophthalmol. 1982;93:423-36.
6. Roy FH, Fraunfelder FW, Fraunfelder FT. Roy and Fraunfelder's Current Ocular Therapy, 6th edition. Philadelphia: WB Saunders; 2008.
7. Travers B. A case of aneurysm by anastomosis in the orbit, cured by ligation of common carotid artery. Med Chir Trans. 1917;2:1-420.

⊟ 1EE.73C9.7DG. TOLOSA-HUNT SYNDROME (PAINFUL OPHTHALMOPLEGIA)

General

Symptoms last from days to weeks; attacks recur at intervals of months or years; inflammatory lesion of cavernous sinus; onset most frequent in fifth decade of life; recurrent Tolosa-Hunt syndrome has been observed in some patients.

Ocular

Steadily "growing" retro-orbital pain; ptosis; involvement of cranial nerves III, IV, VI and first division of V; scintillating scotoma; sluggish pupil reaction to light; corneal sensitivity diminished; optic neuritis.

Clinical

Inflammatory lesions of cavernous sinus.

Laboratory

Magnetic resonance imaging with axial and coronal views of brain, typically showing thickening and enhancement of involved cavernous sinus. Cerebral angiography is done to rule out aneurysm. Blood count, ESR, antinuclear antibody (ANA), antineutrophil cytoplasmic antibody (ANCA) and ACE levels may be abnormal.

Treatment

Corticosteroids are often used to treat the chronic granulomatous inflammation of the cavernous sinus.

⊟ BIBLIOGRAPHY

1. Taylor DC. (2012). Tolosa-Hunt syndrome. [online] Available from www.emedicine.com/neuro/TOPIC373.HTM. [Accessed September, 2013].

⊟ 1EE.73C9.7DH. FORAMEN LACERUM SYNDROME (ANEURYSM OF INTERNAL CAROTID ARTERY SYNDROME)

General

Most commonly caused by congenital aneurysm involving the intradural portion of the carotid artery.

Ocular

Periorbital pain; ptosis; oculomotor paralysis with ptosis, diplopia and internal ophthalmoplegia; cranial nerves IV and VI may be involved; homonymous hemianopia (occasionally); loss of pupillary reflexes for light and accommodation; papilledema; optic atrophy.

Clinical

Meningism; mental disturbances; unilateral frontal or orbital headache; migraine attacks.

Laboratory

Computed tomography, MRI, angiography, MRA.

Treatment

Endovascular balloon occlusion.

⊟ BIBLIOGRAPHY

1. Dailey EJ, Holloway JA, Murto RE, et al. Evaluation of ocular signs and symptoms in cerebral aneurysms. Arch Ophthalmol. 1964;71:463-74.
2. Geeraets WJ. Ocular syndromes, 3rd edition. Philadelphia: Lea & Febiger; 1976.
3. Misra M, Mohanty AB, Rath S. Giant aneurysm of internal carotid artery presenting features of retrobulbar neuritis. Indian J Ophthalmol. 1991;39:28-9.

⬚ 1EE.73C9.7DK. FOIX SYNDROME (CAVERNOUS SINUS SYNDROME; HYPOPHYSEAL-SPHENOIDAL SYNDROME; CAVERNOUS SINUS NEURALGIA SYNDROME; GODTFREDSEN SYNDROME; CAVERNOUS SINUS-NASOPHARYNGEAL TUMOR SYNDROME; CAVERNOUS SINUS THROMBOSIS)

General

Causes include tumor of lateral sinus wall or sphenoid bone, intracranial aneurysm, cavernous and lateral sinus thrombosis, or lesions; multiple myeloma; may result from infarctions or cancer or be idiopathic.

Ocular

Proptosis; severe ocular and periorbital pain; lid edema; paresis or paralysis of cranial nerves III, IV, V, and VI; corneal anesthesia; optic atrophy.

Clinical

Postauricular edema; trigeminal neuralgia; deviation of the tongue toward paralyzed side; patients usually have prominent manifestations of sepsis and paranasal sinus; local skin infections are the most common cause.

Laboratory

Computed tomography and MRI.

Treatment

Radiotherapy, anticoagulation, high-dose antibiotic therapy.

⬚ BIBLIOGRAPHY

1. Kattah JC, Pula JH. (2012). Cavernous sinus syndromes. [online] Available from www.emedicine.com/neuro/topic572.htm. [Accessed September, 2013].

⬚ 1EE.73C9.7DL. GRADENIGO SYNDROME (TEMPORAL SYNDROME; LANNOIS-GRADENIGO SYNDROME)

General

It is caused by extradural abscess of the petrous portion of the temporal bone; good prognosis.

Ocular

Ipsilateral paralysis (cranial nerve VI); transient involvement of cranial nerves III and IV occasionally present; severe pain in area of ophthalmic branch (cranial nerve V); photophobia; lacrimation; reduced corneal sensitivity; optic nerve involvement occasionally present.

Clinical

Inner ear infection with deafness; mastoiditis; facial paresis possible; temperature may be elevated; meningeal signs possible; can occur rarely as a complication of otitis media.

Laboratory

Computed tomography and MRI.

Treatment

See otolaryngologist.

⬚ BIBLIOGRAPHY

1. De Graaf J, Cats H, de Jager AE, et al. Gradenigo's syndrome: a rare complication of otitis media. Clin Neurol Neurosurg. 1988;90(3):237-9.
2. Gradenigro G. A special syndrome of endocranial otitic complications. Ann Otol Rhinol Laryngol. 1904;13:637.
3. Joffe WS. Clinical nerve disease. Int Ophthalmol Clin. 1967;7(4):823-38.

⊞ 1EE.73C9.7DM. ROCHON-DUVIGNEAUD SYNDROME (SUPERIOR ORBITAL FISSURE SYNDROME) OPTIC ATROPHY

General

Inflammatory, traumatic, tumor, or vascular lesions such as meningioma of the sphenoid, carotid aneurysm and arachnoiditis; infections originating in the maxillary sinus.

Ocular

Mild exophthalmos; lid edema; partial or complete ophthalmoplegia (III, IV and VI); decreased corneal sensitivity; papilledema; optic atrophy.

Clinical

Decreased sensitivity in area of nasociliary, lacrimal, frontal, and ophthalmic nerve distribution; may result from a metastatic tumor.

Laboratory

Complete blood count, ESR, thyroid function test, fluorescent treponemal antibody (FTA), ANA, lupus erythematosus (LE) preparation, ANCA, serum protein electrophoresis, Lyme titre, ACE level and HIV titer are helpful. CSF, anti-GQ1b antibodies, and MRI of the brain and the orbits.

Treatment

Corticosteroids are the treatment of choice.

⊞ BIBLIOGRAPHY

1. Falcone F, Lazow SK, Berger JR, et al. Superior orbital fissure syndrome. Secondary to infected dentigerous cyst of the maxillary sinus. NY State Dental J. 1994;60:62-4.
2. Hedstrom J, Parsons J, Maloney PL, et al. Superior orbital fissure syndrome: report of a case. J Oral Surg. 1974; 32:198-201.
3. Phanthumchinda K, Hemachuda T. Superior orbital fissure syndrome as a presenting symptom in hepatocellular carcinoma. J Med Assoc Thailand. 1992;75:62-5.
4. Rochon-Duvigneaud A. Quelques Cas de Paralysie de Tous les Nerfs Orbitaires (Ophtalmoplegie Totale avec Amaurose et Anesthesie dans le Domaine de l'Ophtalmique d'Origine Syphilitique). Arch Ophthalmol. 1896;16:746.

⊞ 1EE.73C9.7DN. ALBERS-SCHONBERG DISEASE (MARBLE BONE DISEASE; OSTEOSCLEROSIS FRAGILIS GENERALISATA; OSTEOPETROSIS; OSTEOPOIKILOSIS; OSTEOSCLEROSIS CONGENITA DIFFUSA)

General

Simple recessive inheritance, also dominant transmission; benign form is asymptomatic in about 50% of cases and known under the synonym Henck-Assmann syndrome; prognosis is poor for malignant form, with death usually in infancy.

Ocular

Oculomotor paralysis; cranial nerve VII palsy; optic atrophy; ptosis; exophthalmos; papilledema; nystagmus; anisocoria; congenital cataracts; hypertelorism; visual loss in infancy; nasolacrimal duct obstruction; keratoconus.

Clinical

Cartilage and bone thickening; multiple fractures; hyperchromic anemia; osteomyelitis; severe forms: jaundice, hepatosplenomegaly, skeleton sclerosis, lymphadenopathy and hydrocephalus in infants; mild forms: nerve compression, fractures and milder form of anemia; pancytopenia from marrow obliteration; low serum calcium; elevated phosphorus.

Laboratory

Radiologic features are usually diagnostic. Patients usually have generalized osteosclerosis. Bones may be uniformly sclerotic, but alternating sclerotic and lucent bands may be noted in iliac wings and near ends of long bones. The bones might be club-like or appear like a bone within bone.

Treatment

- *Infantile therapy*: Vitamin D appears to help by stimulating dormant osteoclasts and thus stimulate bone resorption.

Large doses of calcitriol, along with restricted calcium intake, sometimes improve osteopetrosis dramatically.

- *Adult therapy*: No specific medical treatment exists for the adult type.

BIBLIOGRAPHY

1. Blank R, Bhargava A. (2012). Osteopetrosis. [online] Available from www.emedicine.com/med/TOPIC1692.HTM. [Accessed September, 2013].

1EE.73C9.7DP. HODGKIN DISEASE

General

Hodgkin disease begins in the lymph nodes and usually spreads in a predictable fashion along contiguous chains of nodes; etiology may be viral; prevalent in males.

Ocular

Keratitis; uveitis; cataract; retinal hemorrhages; vasculitis; Horner syndrome; cortical blindness; papilledema; paralysis of oculomotor nerve; episcleritis; visual field defects; infiltration of choroid, conjunctiva, lacrimal gland and orbit; papillitis; retrobulbar neuritis; opsoclonus-myoclonus; keratitis sicca; infiltrative optic neuropathy; association with Vogt-Koyanagi-Harada syndrome; bilateral serous detachments of the macula.

Clinical

Painless cervical, axillary, or inguinal lymph node swelling; fever; weight loss; anemia; generalized pruritus.

Laboratory

Biopsy of lymph glands is diagnostic.

Treatment

The goal of therapy is to induce a complete remission with radiation therapy, chemotherapy or BMT.

BIBLIOGRAPHY

1. Lash BW, Dessain SK, Argiris A. (2012). Hodgkin lymphoma. [online] Available from www.emedicine.com/med/TOPIC1022.HTM. [Accessed September, 2013].

1EE.73C9.7DQ. DISSEMINATED LUPUS ERYTHEMATOSUS (SYSTEMIC LUPUS ERYTHEMATOSUS; LUPUS ERYTHEMATOSUS; KAPOSI-LIBMAN-SACK SYNDROME, SLE)

General

Possible etiology includes viral infections and genetic predisposition; immunologic abnormalities.

Ocular

Keratitis; keratoconjunctivitis sicca; corneal ulcer; optic nerve atrophy; optic neuritis; papilledema; arteritis; central retinal vein occlusion; retinal detachment; microaneurysm; scleritis; uveitis; ptosis; conjunctivitis; paralysis of third nerve; homonymous hemianopsia; multifocal microinfarcts; mydriasis; nystagmus; proptosis; orbital myositis; pseudoretinitis pigmentosa; photophobia.

Clinical

Polyarthritis; morning stiffness; fever; malaise; fatigue; polyserositis; renal disease; CNS disease; anemia; leukopenia; maculopapular rash in a "butterfly" distribution over malar region; alopecia.

Laboratory

Antibodies to double-stranded DNA or the Smith (Sm) antigen or a false-positive serology test for syphilis; positive ANA test that is caused by a medication.

Treatment

Fever, rash, musculoskeletal and serositis manifestations respond to hydroxychloroquine and NSAIDs. Low-to-moderate dose steroids are necessary for acute flares. CNS involvement and renal disease constitute more serious disease and often require high-dose steroids and other immunosuppression agents. Diffuse proliferative lupus nephritis has been treated with cyclophosphamide induction therapy.

⊟ BIBLIOGRAPHY

1. Bartles CM, Muller D. (2012). Systemic erythematosus lupus. [online] Available from www.emedicine.com/med/TOPIC2228.HTM. [Accessed September, 2013].

⊟ 1EE.73C9.7DR. ERB-GOLDFLAM SYNDROME (ERB II SYNDROME; HOPPE-GOLDFLAM DISEASE; PSEUDOPARALYTIC SYNDROME; MYASTHENIA GRAVIS)

General

Occurs at any age; more frequent between ages 20 and 40 years; more females affected than males; progressive; spontaneous; symptoms improve or resolve with rest in early stages of disease (*see* myasthenia gravis, neonatal or infantile); caused by autoantibodies against the acetylcholine receptor at the neuromuscular junction, leading to abnormal fatigability and weakness of skeletal muscle.

Ocular

Transient diplopia; ptosis of upper eyelids.

Clinical

Excessive fatigability of musculature; symptoms appear and increase as day progresses; expressionless face; sagging jaw; difficulty in chewing and talking; nasal regurgitation.

Laboratory

Ice test—crushed ice in surgical glove over ptotic eyelid for 2 minutes and watch for brief elevation of eyelid; Tensilon test and prostigmin test may result in the elevation of ptotic eyelid or improved strabismus in individuals with myasthenia gravis.

Treatment

Adrenal corticosteroids are frequently used. In some cases, mycophenolate mofetil, cyclosporine and cyclophosphamide may be useful. Patching one eye or using prisms may be helpful.

⊟ BIBLIOGRAPHY

1. Erb W. Zur Casuistick der Bulbaren La hmungen. Arch Psychiatr Vervenkr. 1879;9:325-50.
2. Roy FH, Fraunfelder FT, Fraunfelder FW. Roy and Fraunfelder's Current Ocular Therapy, 6th edition. London, UK: Elsevier; 2008.
3. Goldflam S. Vebereinen Scheinbar Keilbaren Bulbarparalytischem Symptom Complex mit Betheiligung der Extremitaten. Dtsch Z Nerven. 1983;4:312-52.
4. Kim JH, Hwang JM, Hwang YS, et al. Childhood ocular myasthenia gravis. Ophthalmology. 2003;110(7):1458-62.
5. Lepore FE, Sanborn GE, Slevin JT. Pupillary dysfunction in myasthenia gravis. Ann Neurol. 1979;6(1):29-33.
6. Sommer N, Melms A, Weller M, et al. Ocular myasthenia gravis. A critical review of clinical and pathophysiological aspects. Doc Ophthalmol. 1993;84(4):309-33.

1EE.73C9.7DS. PASSOW SYNDROME (BREMER STATUS DYSRAPHICUS; STATUS DYSRAPHICUS SYNDROME; SYRINGOMYELIA; SYRINGOBULBIA)

General

Congenital nonclosure of the neural tube; familial occurrence or may be sporadic; insidious onset in second to third decade of life.

Ocular

Enophthalmos; ptosis; rotatory nystagmus; heterochromia iridis; anterior uveitis; corneal anesthesia; neuroparalytic keratitis; paralysis of third, fifth, sixth, and seventh cranial nerves; Horner syndrome; anisocoria; papilledema; optic atrophy; zonular cataract (*see* Horner Syndrome).

Clinical

Anesthesia over area of first division of trigeminal nerve; facial hemiatrophy; facial nerve paralysis; muscular weakness; cervical ribs; kyphoscoliosis; spina bifida; unilateral numbness of fingers; loss of deep reflexes; insensitivity to pain and temperature in affected areas; neurogenic bladder.

Laboratory

Magnetic resonance imaging and CT.

Treatment

Suboccipital and cervical decompression, laminectomy and syringotomy, shunts, fourth ventriculostomy, terminal ventriculostomy and neuroendoscopic surgery may be considered.

BIBLIOGRAPHY

1. Al-Shatoury HA, Galhom AA, Wagner FC. (2012). Syringomyelia. [online] Available from emedicine.medscape.com/article/1151685-overview. [Accessed September, 2013].

1EE.73C9.7DT. PORPHYRIA CUTANEA TARDA

General

Disorder of porphyria metabolism; highest incidence in Bantu population; both sexes affected; onset between ages 40 and 60 years; insidious onset; autosomal dominant; light-sensitive dermatitis in later adult life; associated with excretion of large amounts of uroporphyrin in urine.

Ocular

Synophrys; keratitis; palsies of third and seventh cranial nerves; scleromalacia perforans; optic atrophy; retinal hemorrhages and cotton-wool spots; macular edema; pinguecula; pterygium; brownish pigmentation in conjunctiva and lid margin.

Clinical

Cutaneous manifestations are solar hypersensitivity, vesiculobullous lesions, ulcerations, severe scarring, and hypertrichosis; erythrodontia.

Laboratory

Urinary porphyrin levels are abnormally high, with several hundred to several thousand micrograms excreted in a 24-hour period. Direct immunofluorescence examination can help to differentiate porphyria cutanea tarda (PCT) from immunobullous diseases with dermoepidermal junction cleavage (epidermolysis bullosa acquisita, lupus erythematosus) in which the perivascular Ig deposition found in PCT is not observed.

Treatment

Sunlight avoidance, therapeutic phlebotomy to reduce iron stores, chelation with desferrioxamine; iron-rich foods should be consumed in moderation.

BIBLIOGRAPHY

1. Poh-Fitzpatrick MB. (2012). Porphyria cutanea tarda. [online] Available from www.emedicine.com/derm/TOPIC344.HTM. [Accessed September, 2013].

⊟ 1EE.73C9.7DU. SCHAUMANN SYNDROME (BESNIER-BOECK-SCHAUMANN SYNDROME; BOECK SARCOID; SARCOIDOSIS)

General

Etiology unknown; theories include tuberculosis, hypersensitivity to pine pollen, virus infection; affects blacks most often; chronic course with spontaneous remissions (*see* Heerfordt's syndrome); hilar or paratracheal nodes with erythema nodosum; onset most often in middle and old age; ocular involvement in 20–25% of all cases.

Ocular

Orbital granulomatous mass; bony defects; cutaneous and subcutaneous nodules; myogenic palsy; lacrimal gland adenopathy; decreased tear formation; secondary glaucoma; granulomatous uveitis with iris nodules, cells and flare; mutton fat keratic precipitates; keratitis sicca; vitreous floaters; band-shaped keratitis; complicated cataract; inflammatory retinal exudates; "candle wax drippings"; optic nerve atrophy; neuritis; eyelid nodules; ocular nerve enlargement (granuloma).

Clinical

Lymphadenopathy; hilar nodes; fatigue; cystic, punched-out or reticulated changes in small bones (mainly, hands and feet); muscle wasting; contractures; weakness in legs and arms.

Laboratory

Chest X-ray, CT scan, and MRI of the brain.

Treatment

Glucocorticoids are the treatment of choice.

⊟ BIBLIOGRAPHY

1. Sharma GD. (2011). Pediatric sarcoidosis. [online] Available from www.emedicine.com/ped/TOPIC2043.HTM. [Accessed September, 2013].

⊟ 1EE.73C9.7F2. BOTULISM

General

It is caused by a toxin-producing strain of *C. botulinum*; it occurs primarily after the ingestion of contaminated food; the organism can produce a neurotoxin, the effect of which can be life threatening.

Ocular

Absent optokinetic nystagmus, absent vertical gaze; marked limitation of horizontal gaze; ptosis; diplopia; decreased tear secretion; mydriasis; paralysis of accommodation; nystagmus; optic atrophy; optic neuritis; extraocular muscle paresis.

Clinical

Dizziness; severe respiratory impairment; gastrointestinal disturbances; dysphagia; dysarthria; postural hypotension.

Laboratory

Toxin assay for early diagnosis, whereas later cases are more likely to yield a positive specimen culture.

Treatment

Antitoxin appears to be the only effective medication. Supportive care such as ventilation and parenteral nutrition are necessary for the duration of the paralytic illness.

⊟ BIBLIOGRAPHY

1. Patel B, Taylor SF. (2012). Ophthalmologic manifestations of botulism. [online] Available from www.emedicine.com/oph/TOPIC493.HTM. [Accessed September, 2013].

1EE.73C9.7G1. BLEPHAROCHALASIS

General

Rare, with recurrent episodic painless periorbital edema.

Clinical

None.

Ocular

Skin of the lids is thin and baggy.

Laboratory

Diagnosis is made by clinical findings.

Treatment

Cold compress may be of some use. Surgical—excise the redundant skin, reposition the ectopic lacrimal gland and reconstruct lateral canthal tendon.

BIBLIOGRAPHY

1. Roy FH, Fraunfelder FW, Fraunfelder FT. Roy and Fraunfelder's Current Ocular Therapy, 6th edition. London, UK: Elsevier; 2008.

1EE.73C9.7G4A1A. PNEUMOCOCCAL INFECTIONS (STREPTOCOCCUS PNEUMONIAE INFECTIONS)

General

Gram-positive diplococcus *Streptococcus pneumoniae*; some strains are encapsulated while others are not; ocular infections usually are caused by the encapsulated strains; conjunctivitis and corneal scarring produced in an animal model have been attributed to a hemolytic cytolytic exopeptidase.

Ocular

Hypopyon; conjunctivitis; keratitis; corneal ulcer; endophthalmitis; dacryocystitis; uveitis; orbital cellulitis; secondary glaucoma; ophthalmia neonatorum.

Clinical

Upper respiratory infection; chills; sharp pain in hemithorax; cough with sputum production; fever; headache; gastrointestinal symptoms.

Laboratory

Gram stain demonstrates Gram-positive cocci in pairs. The unattached end of each cocci is slightly pointed outward.

Treatment

Impetigo, oral antibiotics and topical antibiotic ointment; preseptal cellulitis, oral antibiotics; orbital celluliti, need team of infectious diseases, otolaryngology and ophthalmology to develop plan of therapy; dacryocystitis, oral and topical antibiotics, dacryocystorhinostomy may be necessary; conjunctivitis, topical antibiotic; keratitis, topical antibiotics; poststreptococcal reactive arthritis can occur with uveitis, topical steroids and cycloplegics; endophthalmitis, prompt and aggressive therapy with topical, intravitreal and sometimes systemic antibiotics and pars plana vitrectomy; post-refractive surgery keratitis, flap raised, cultured and treated. Occasionally the flap should be amputated.

BIBLIOGRAPHY

1. Muench DF. (2012). Pneumococcal infections. [online] Available from www.emedicine.com/med/TOPIC1848.HTM. [Accessed September, 2013].

⊟ 1EE.73C9.7G41B. STAPHYLOCOCCUS

General

Gram-positive coccus *Staphylococcus aureus*; most common cause of suppurative infection in humans; more common in patients with a previous disorders, such as diabetes, thyroid disease, renal failure, or malnutrition; although most *S. aureus* isolates from other sources are encapsulated, capsules have not been noted in ocular isolates.

Ocular

Uveitis; hypopyon; conjunctivitis; keratitis; cellulitis of lid; meibomianitis; ptosis; blepharitis; endophthalmitis; dacryocystitis; increased IOP; orbital periosteitis.

Clinical

Tissues hypertonic, edematous and painful; lesion liquefies, forming creamy yellow pus; fever; nausea; vomiting; cough; dyspnea; abdominal pain; diarrhea; bloody stools; dehydration; shock.

Laboratory

Aerobic Gram-positive cocci bacteria grow in grape-like clusters. Coagulase positive indicates pathogenicity.

Treatment

Specific antimicrobial therapy is chosen based on the site and severity of the infection and the antimicrobial sensitivities of the organism involved.

⊟ BIBLIOGRAPHY

1. Tolan RW. (2012). Staphylococcus aureus infection. [online] Available from www.emedicine.com/ped/TOPIC2704.HTM. [Accessed September, 2013].

⊟ 1EE.73C9.7G42. HAEMOPHILUS AEGYPTIUS (KOCH-WEEKS BACILLUS)

General

It is caused by Gram-negative Koch-Weeks bacillus in warm climate regions; characterized by a 24 to 48-hour incubation period; now classified as *H. influenzae* biotype III; *H. influenzae* is divided into biotypes based on biochemical reactions (indole production, urease activity, ornithine decarboxylase activity) and into serotypes based on their capsular polysaccharides; common cause of purulent conjunctivitis and preseptal cellulitis in children.

Ocular

Conjunctivitis; corneal opacity; corneal ulcer; phlyctenular keratoconjunctivitis; keratitis; cellulitis of lid; pseudoptosis; uveitis; petechial subconjunctival hemorrhages.

Clinical

Coryza; systemic symptoms are rare.

Laboratory

Poorly staining Gram-negative bacilli or coccobacilli. Culture on chocolate agar.

Treatment

Antibiotics are the mainstay of treatment. Invasive and serious infections are best treated with an intravenous third-generation cephalosporin until antibiotic sensitivities are available.

⊟ BIBLIOGRAPHY

1. Devarajan VR. (2012) Haemophilus influenzae infections. [online] Available from. www.emedicine.com/med/TOPIC936.HTM. [Accessed September, 2013].

1EE.73C9.7G4.2. INFLUENZA

General

Acute respiratory infection of specific viral etiology which includes H1N1.

Ocular

Conjunctivitis; subconjunctival hemorrhages; keratitis; tenonitis; ptosis; cellulitis of orbit and lid; dacryocystitis; retinal hemorrhage; cataract; episcleritis; hypopyon; optic neuritis; uveitis; panophthalmitis; vitreal hemorrhage; paralysis of third or fourth nerve; uveitis following vaccination for influenza.

Clinical

Headache; fever; malaise; muscular aching; substernal soreness; nasal stuffiness; nausea.

Laboratory

The standard criteria for diagnosing influenza A and B is a viral culture of nasal-pharyngeal samples, throat samples, or both.

Treatment

Prevention is the most effective therapy. Two new drugs have been marketed recently for treatment of influenza A and B. These are the neuraminidase inhibitors, oseltamivir and zanamivir.

BIBLIOGRAPHY

1. Derlet RW. (2012). Influenza. [online] Available from www.emedicine.com/med/TOPIC1170.HTM. [Accessed September, 2013].

1EE.73C9.7G4.3A. RUBELLA SYNDROME (CONGENITAL RUBELLA SYNDROME; GERMAN MEASLES; GREGG SYNDROME)

General

Rubella infection of the mother during first trimester of pregnancy; ocular disease is the most commonly found abnormality in patients with congenital rubella syndrome (75%), multiorgan disease is common (> 75%); no significant association has been found between gestational age and time of maternal infection and incidence of individual ocular conditions.

Ocular

Nystagmus; glaucoma; corneal haziness; cataracts; retinal pigmentary changes; appearance and central distribution of lesions are quite distinguishable from retinitis pigmentosa; retinopathy is not progressive and has little, if any, effect on vision; waxy atrophy of optic disk; conjunctivitis; megalocornea or microcornea; buphthalmos; microphthalmos; uveitis; iris atrophy; spherophakia; strabismus.

Clinical

Low-birth weight; diarrhea; pneumonia; urinary infection; hearing loss; heart disease; hepatosplenomegaly; mental retardation; inguinal hernias; ataxia; cardiac abnormalities.

Laboratory

Diagnosis is made by clinical findings. If in doubt, a rising titer of IgM will indicate a recent infection.

Treatment

Treatment for rubella of the eye centers on glaucoma and cataract.

BIBLIOGRAPHY

1. Lombardo PC. (2011). Dermatologic manifestations of rubella. [online] Available from www.emedicine.com/derm/TOPIC380.HTM. [Accessed September, 2013].

1EE.73C9.7G4.3B. MEASLES (MORBILLI; RUBEOLA)

General

Acute, extremely communicable disease that affects young school-aged children; caused by paramyxovirus.

Ocular

Hypopyon; uveitis; conjunctivitis; Koplik (Hirschberg) spots of conjunctiva; keratitis; corneal ulcer; cellulitis of lid; dacryocystitis; congenital cataract; optic atrophy; optic neuritis; strabismus; pigmentary retinopathy; iris prolapse; hemianopsia; secondary glaucoma; central retinal artery occlusion; orbital cellulitis; accommodative spasm; paralysis of sixth nerve; keratoconus.

Clinical

Maculopapular rash; fever.

Laboratory

Diagnosis is made by clinical findings.

Treatment

Good hydration.

BIBLIOGRAPHY

1. Chen SS. (2011). Measles. [online] Available from www.emedicine.com/derm/TOPIC259.HTM. [Accessed September, 2013].

1EE.73C9.7G4.3C. MUMPS

General

Viral infection.

Ocular

Conjunctivitis; keratitis; corneal ulcer; tenonitis; exophthalmos; microphthalmos; optic atrophy; optic neuritis; papillitis; scleritis; uveitis; cortical blindness; congenital punctal occlusion; paralysis of extraocular muscles; dacryoadenitis; iritis; paralysis of accommodation; internal and external ophthalmoparesis.

Clinical

Affects the parotid glands, but infection of other glandular tissue occurs, including the lacrimal gland and testicles; encephalitis; meningitis.

Laboratory

Mumps virus by acute serologic studies.

Treatment

Generous hydration and alimentation, analgesics for headaches. No antiviral agent is available.

BIBLIOGRAPHY

1. Defendi GL. (2012). Mumps. [online] Available from www.emedicine.com/ped/TOPIC1503.HTM. [Accessed September, 2013].

1EE.73C9.7G4.3D. REITER SYNDROME (FIESSINGER-LEROY SYNDROME; CONJUNCTIVO-URETHRO-SYNOVIAL SYNDROME; IDIOPATHIC BLENNORRHEAL ARTHRITIS SYNDROME; POLYARTHRITIS ENTERICA)

General

Etiology unknown; males; onset ages 16–42 years; probably a combined infectious/autoimmune pathogenetic mechanism; reactive arthritis probably associated with infection with many different species of microorganisms; HLA-B27 confers disease susceptibility to infection.

Ocular

Sterile mucopurulent conjunctivitis, usually bilateral; photophobia; epiphora; iritis; keratitis; uveitis; paralysis of extraocular muscles; optic neuritis; secondary glaucoma; hypopyon; hyphema.

Clinical

Skin erythema; genital ulcerations; urethritis with discharge; cystitis with dysuria, abacterial pyuria, and hematuria; arthritis with pain, swelling, heat and effusion; fever; weight loss; fatigue; malaise; fever; diarrhea; oral mucosal lesions; arthralgia.

Laboratory

Giemsa stain may reveal Gram-negative intracellular diplococci associated with gonorrhea. Stool cultures may also be helpful for enteric pathogens. HLA-B27 antigen testing will not provide a diagnosis but may be useful.

Treatment

Systemic antibiotics are useful. Topical corticosteroids and mydriatics should be administered early to minimize tissue damage. NSAIDs may help to reduce ocular inflammation.

⊟ BIBLIOGRAPHY

1. Bashour M. (2012). Ophthalmologic manifestations of reactive arthritis. [online] Available from www.emedicine.com/oph/TOPIC524.HTM. [Accessed September, 2013].

⊟ 1EE.73C9.7G4.4A. CANDIDIASIS

General

Yeast-like opportunistic fungal infection caused by *C. albicans*.

Ocular

Uveitis; hypopyon; conjunctivitis; keratitis; corneal ulcer; blepharitis; endophthalmitis; dacryocystitis; papillitis; retinal atrophy; Roth spot; vitreous abscess; retrobulbar abscess; retinal detachment; panophthalmitis; chorioretinitis; infectious crystalline keratopathy.

Clinical

C. albicans normally is present as an intestinal saprophyte in 35–75% of the human population; in situations of internal environmental change; however, *Candida* can become pathogenic (obesity, diabetes mellitus, malignancy, and other debilitating conditions).

Laboratory

Common yeast from up to 50% of healthy individuals isolate directly from the eye should be attempted to confirm the presence of organism. Blood agar and Sabouraud's dextrose agar may be used; PCR for species identification.

Treatment

Mucocutaneous infection typically responds to topical therapy. Antifungal therapy should be started immediately after necessary cultures have been obtained from all suspected sites of infection. Infectious disease specialists are typically involved in cases of invasive candidiasis.

⊟ BIBLIOGRAPHY

1. Hedayati T. (2012). Candidiasis in emergency medicine. [online] Available from www.emedicine.com/emerg/TOPIC76.HTM. [Accessed September, 2013].

⊟ 1EE.73C9.7G5. SCALDED SKIN SYNDROME (TOXIC EPIDERMAL NECROLYSIS; RITTER DISEASE; TOXIC EPIDERMAL NECROLYSIS OF LYELL; STAPHYLOCOCCAL SCALDED SKIN SYNDROME; LYELL SYNDROME; EPIDERMOLYSIS ACUTA TOXICA; TOXIC EPIDERMAL NECROLYSIS) SYMBLEPHARON

General

Generalized exfoliative dermatitis frequently affecting neonates and resulting from an initial focal staphylococcal infection (i.e. Staphylococcal ophthalmia neonatorum); toxic epidermal necrolysis usually refers to manifestation in the adult secondary to a drug reaction but affects all ages; immunopathogenetic mechanisms probably initiated with drug-skin binding with aberrant immune responses, including complement and IgG deposition with the epidermis and mucosa; recent reports suggest that patients with the AIDS are at higher risk for developing mucocutaneous reactions, such as toxic epidermal necrolysis; mortality rate approximately 30%.

Ocular

Necrotic areas of lids, conjunctiva and cornea; symblepharon; loss of corneal epithelium; corneal ulcer; leukoma; perforation of globe; abolition of lacrimal secretion; conjunctival chemosis; blepharitis; entropion; periorbital swelling; trichiasis; distichiasis; fornix shortening.

Clinical

Widespread reddening and tenderness of the skin followed by the exfoliation of large areas of skin; in children, erythema starts usually around the mouth and spreads over the entire body within hours, followed by blisters and large exudative lesions; fever; shock.

Laboratory

Culture and biopsy of the lesion.

Treatment

Intravenous penicillinase-resistant and antistaphylococcal antibiotics. Cloxacillin is the treatment of choice.

⊟ BIBLIOGRAPHY

1. Lopez-Garcia JS, Jara LR, Garcia-Lozano CI, et al. Ocular features and histopathologic changes during follow-up of toxic epidermal necrolysis. Ophthalmology. 2011; 118:265-71.
2. Kim JH, Benson P. (2012). Dermatologic manifestations of staphylococcal scalded skin syndrome. [online] Available from www.emedicine.com/derm/TOPIC402.HTM. [Accessed September, 2013].

⊟ 1EE.73C9.7G6. RELAPSING POLYCHONDRITIS (JAKSCH WARTENHOST SYNDROME; MEYENBURG-ALTHERZ-VEHLINGER SYNDROME; VON MEYENBERG II SYNDROME)

General

Episodic, yet generally progressive; onset usually in middle life; possibly caused by lysosomal labilizing factor of endogenous or exogenous toxic nature or immunologic reactions; possible association with Reiter's syndrome.

Ocular

Conjunctivitis; corneal ulcer; exophthalmos; panophthalmitis; phthisis bulbi; proptosis; optic neuritis; papilledema; retinal detachment; blue sclera; episcleritis; scleromalacia; vitreous opacity; cataracts; nystagmus; retinal artery thrombosis; keratoconjunctivitis sicca; secondary glaucoma; scotoma; uveitis; paresis of third or sixth nerve; conjunctival mass (salmon patch); chorioretinitis.

Clinical

Destruction of cartilage and eventual replacement with connective tissue; polyarthritis; chondritis; tracheal collapse; bronchial collapse; anemia; liver dysfunction; death; malaise; fever; dyspnea; changes in pitch of voice; hearing impairment; vertigo; deformed ears; aortic valve insufficiency.

Laboratory

No specific serologic markers.

Treatment

No therapy.

⊟ BIBLIOGRAPHY

1. Compton N, Buckner JH, Harp KI, et al. (2012). Polychondritis. [online] Available from emedicine.medscape.com/article/331475-overview. [Accessed September, 2013].

🗗 1EE.73C9.7G7. SJÖGREN SYNDROME (GOUGEROT-SJÖGREN SYNDROME; SECRETOINHIBITOR SYNDROME; SICCA SYNDROME)

General

Etiology unknown; autosomal recessive; occurs in women over 40 years of age; failure of the lacrimal and conjunctival glands to maintain adequate secretion; similarities exist with Mikulicz syndrome; insidious onset; associated with collagen disorders; Epstein-Barr virus infection.

Ocular

Blepharoconjunctivitis; tears show no lysozyme; keratoconjunctivitis sicca; superficial corneal ulcers; thready, tenacious, yellow-white discharge of the conjunctiva; hypertrophy of lacrimal gland; decreased tear secretion with cellular and mucous debris in tear film; cicatrization of cornea and conjunctiva.

Clinical

Dryness of mouth and other mucous membranes; enlarged salivary glands; dysphagia; painless swelling of joints; polyarthritis; dental cavities; vaginitis; laryngitis; rhinitis sicca; hepatomegaly; focal myositis; alopecia; splenomegaly.

Laboratory

Tear osmolarity, fluorecein clearance test and tear function index. Parotid flow rate may determine xerostomia.

Treatment

Artificial tears and lubricating ointments are the treatment of choice. Topical autologous serum eye drops also provide therapeutic benefit.

🗗 BIBLIOGRAPHY

1. Aquavella JV, Williams ZR, Boghani S, et al. (2011). Ophthalmologic manifestations of Sjogren syndrome. [online] Available from www.emedicine.com/oph/TOPIC477.HTM. [Accessed September, 2013].

🗗 1EE.73C9.7G1B. ANGULAR CONJUNCTIVITIS (MORAX-AXENFELD BACILLUS)

General

It is caused by *M. lacunata*, which frequently inhabits the nose.

Ocular

Conjunctivitis; hypopyon; keratitis; uveitis; corneal marginal ulcer.

Laboratory

Diagnosis is made by clinical findings.

Treatment

- *Conjunctivitis*: Antibiotic medication should be used to treat the infection.
- *Corneal ulcer*: Corneal cultures may be taken and treatment is initiated. Treatment includes a broad spectrum of antibiotics and cycloplegic drops.
- *Uveitis*: Topical steroids and cycloplegic medication should be the choice of initial treatment. Oral steroids should be given if not responsive to topical steroids, immunosuppressants if bilateral disease that does not respond to oral steroids, and periocular steroids for unilateral or posterior uveitis. Vitrectomy can be used for severe vitreous opacification. Cryotherapy and laser photocoagulation may be used for localized pars plana exudates.

🗗 BIBLIOGRAPHY

1. Jones DB. Early diagnosis and therapy of bacterial corneal ulcers. Int Ophthalmol Clin. 1973;13(4):1-29.
2. Marioneaux SJ, Cohen EJ, Arentsen JJ, et al. Moraxella keratitis. Cornea. 1991;10(1):21-4.
3. van Bijsterveld OP. Bacterial proteases in Moraxella angular conjunctivitis. Am J Ophthalmol. 1971;72(1):181-4.

⊟ 1EE.73C9.7G1C. PEDICULOSIS AND PHTHIRIASIS

General

Infestation of lice on head, body, or pubic area.

Ocular

Conjunctivitis; keratitis; infestation of lice or nits glued to shafts of eyelashes and eyebrow.

Clinical

Pruritus; skin excoriation; impetigo; pyoderma with lymphadenitis and febrile episodes.

Laboratory

Removal from hair shaft and examination under microscope.

Treatment

Treatments involve spreading an ointment at the base of the eyelashes at night to trap mites as they emerge from their burrow and/or move from one follicle to another.

⊟ BIBLIOGRAPHY

1. Guenther L. (2013). Pediculosis (lice). [online] Available from www.emedicine.com/med/TOPIC1769.HTM. [Accessed September, 2013].

⊟ 1EE.73C9.7G1D. STAPHYLOCOCCUS

General

Gram-positive coccus *S. aureus*; most common cause of suppurative infection in humans; more common in patients with a previous disorders, such as diabetes, thyroid disease, renal failure, or malnutrition; although most *S. aureus* isolates from other sources are encapsulated, capsules have not been noted in ocular isolates.

Ocular

Uveitis; hypopyon; conjunctivitis; keratitis; cellulitis of lid; meibomianitis; ptosis; blepharitis; endophthalmitis; dacryocystitis; increased IOP; orbital periosteitis.

Clinical

Tissues hypertonic, edematous, and painful; lesion liquefies, forming creamy yellow pus; fever; nausea; vomiting; cough; dyspnea; abdominal pain; diarrhea; bloody stools; dehydration; shock.

Laboratory

Aerobic Gram-positive cocci bacteria grow in grape-like clusters. Coagulase positive indicates pathogenicity.

Treatment

Specific antimicrobial therapy is chosen based on the site and severity of the infection and the antimicrobial sensitivities of the organism involved.

⊟ BIBLIOGRAPHY

1. Tolan RW. (2012). Staphylococcus aureus infection. [online] Available from www.emedicine.com/ped/TOPIC2704.HTM. [Accessed September, 2013].

⊟ 1EE.73C9.7G7A. ACTINOMYCOSIS

General

Gram-positive *Actinomyces israelii.*

Ocular

Hypopyon; conjunctivitis; keratitis; corneal ulcer; proptosis; uveitis; dacryocystitis; yellow nodules on conjunctiva and eyelids; occlusion of nasolacrimal canaliculi; canaliculitis; orbital abscess; endophthalmitis (rare).

Clinical

Chronic inflammatory induration and sinus formation.

Laboratory

Canalicular discharge may be sent for Gram stain/Giemsa stain, cultures and sensitivities (i.e. blood agar, Sabouraud, anaerobic) and special stains (i.e. calcofluor white stain).

Treatment

Penicillins and cephalosporins are useful. Subconjunctival penicillin coadministered with systemic iodides and topical sulfacetamide or penicillin can be used.

⊟ BIBLIOGRAPHY

1. Roque MR, Roque BL, Foster CS. (2012). Actinomycosis in ophthalmology. [online] Available from www.emedicine.com/oph/TOPIC491.HTM. [Accessed September, 2013].

⊟ 1EE.73C9.7G7B. EPIDEMIC KERATOCONJUNCTIVITIS

General

Highly communicable; adenovirus types 8 and 19; usually bilateral; epidemic keratoconjunctivitis has been reported worldwide associated with 11 virus serotypes, with serotypes 8, 11, and 19 being the most common responsible ones.

Ocular

Follicular or membranous conjunctivitis; chemosis; subconjunctival hemorrhages; corneal opacity; punctate epithelial keratitis; corneal ulcer; blepharospasm; lid edema; serous discharge; uveitis; epiphora.

Clinical

Submaxillary and cervical lymphadenopathy.

Laboratory

Viral isolation on cell culture from conjunctival scrapings

Treatment

No effective topical or systemic treatment available. Topical steroids may be used if epithelial keratitis occurs.

⊟ BIBLIOGRAPHY

1. Bawazeer A. (2011). Epidemic keratoconjunctivitis. [online] Available from www.emedicine.com/oph/TOPIC677.HTM. [Accessed September, 2013].

⊡ 1EE.73C9.7G7C. GLANDER SYNDROME

General

Serious infection caused by *Malleomyces mallei*; no naturally acquired infections in United States since 1938; transmission from equine animals to man; caused by traumatic inoculations or inhalations; either acute, gangrenous, or chronic ulcerative; fatal usually in 7–10 days.

Ocular

Conjunctivitis; dacryocystitis; ulcerating granulomatous orbital lesions; photophobia; lacrimation.

Clinical

Systemic erythematous pustules; inhalation infection; fever; rigors; generalized myalgia lymphangitis; fatigue, headaches; pleuritic chest pain; diarrhea; lymphadenopathy; splenomegaly; mild leukocytosis; multiple subcutaneous and intramuscular abscesses (often arms and legs); visceral involvement, including pulmonary, pleural, skeletal, hepatic, splenic, meningeal, and intracranial.

Laboratory

White blood cell may be minimally elevated. Elevated liver enzyme levels in Glanders may signify hepatic abscess formation.

Treatment

Initiate rapid administration of supportive care and intravenous antibiotic therapy for severe disease.

⊡ BIBLIOGRAPHY

1. Rega PP. (2013). CBRNE - Glanders and Melioidosis. [online] Available from www.emedicine.com/emerg/TOPIC884.HTM. [Accessed September, 2013].

⊡ 1EE.73C9.7G7E. MENINGOCOCCEMIA (NEISSERIA MENINGITIDES; MENINGITIS)

General

Systemic bacterial infection caused by *Neisseria meningitides*; can be present chronically in patients with immune deficiencies including deficient complement levels.

Ocular

Photophobia; conjunctivitis; chemosis; keratitis; uveitis; panophthalmitis; retinal endophlebitis; macular edema; papillitis; optic neuritis; paresis of sixth or seventh nerve; nystagmus; miosis; hippus; cortical blindness; papilledema (rare); conjunctival petechiae; strabismus.

Clinical

Meningitis; fever; malaise; joint pain; splenic enlargement.

Laboratory

Cultures from blood, spinal fluid, or joint fluid.

Treatment

Treat with antibiotics promptly.

⊡ BIBLIOGRAPHY

1. Javid MH, Ahmed SH. (2012). Meningococcemia. [online] Available from www.emedicine.com/med/TOPIC1445.HTM. [Accessed September, 2013].

⊟ 1EE.73C9.7G7F. PSEUDOMONAS AERUGINOSA INFECTIONS

General

Gram-negative rod with secondary contaminant of superficial wounds; *Pseudomonas* organisms produce a variety of enzymes that cause pathologic changes, including hemolysins and exotoxins as well as a glycocalyx that increases adherence.

Ocular

Hypopyon; conjunctivitis; keratitis; ulcerative abscess of cornea; endophthalmitis; panophthalmitis.

Clinical

Local tissue damage and diminished host resistance, which may occur in ear, lung, skin, and urinary tract.

Laboratory

Complete blood count may reveal leukocytosis with a left shift and bandemia. Positive results on blood culture in the absence of extracardiac sites of infection may indicate pseudomonal endocarditis.

Treatment

Antimicrobials are the mainstay of therapy. Two-drug combination therapy such as an antipseudomonal beta-lactam antibiotic with an aminoglycoside.

⊟ BIBLIOGRAPHY

1. Klaus-Dieter L. (2012). Pseudomonas aeruginosa infections. [online] Available from www.emedicine.com/med/TOPIC1943.HTM. [Accessed September, 2013].

⊟ 1EE.73C9.7G7G. HERPES SIMPLEX

General

Large, complex DNA virus.

Ocular

Conjunctivitis; keratitis; iridocyclitis; corneal ulcer; uveitis; hyphema; hypopyon; iris atrophy; cataract; scleritis; dacryoadenitis; blepharitis; acute retinal necrosis.

Clinical

Recurrent skin vesicles on lids, perioral area, nose and genitalia; meningitis, encephalitis.

Laboratory

Viral cultures.

Treatment

Antiviral therapy, topical or oral, is an effective treatment of epithelial herpes infection.

⊟ BIBLIOGRAPHY

1. Wang JC, Ritterband DC. (2012). Ophthalmologic manifestations of herpes simplex keratitis. [online] Available from www.emedicine.com/oph/TOPIC100.HTM. [Accessed September, 2013].

⊟ 1EE.73C9.7G7H. SMALLPOX (VARIOLA)

General

Highly contagious cutaneous disease caused by viral infection.

Ocular

Conjunctivitis; keratitis; corneal ulcer; hypopyon; endophthalmitis; congenital corneal clouding; albinotic spots on iris; choroiditis; vitreous opacities; papillitis; extraocular muscle palsies; entropion; dacryocystitis; chorioretinitis; optic neuritis; and vesicles of the eyelid; preauricular adenopathy; eyelid ulcerating pustules; several conditions predispose to the spread of vaccinia, including eczema, hypogammaglobulinemia, steroid therapy, and AIDS.

Clinical

Fever, headache, and vomiting prior to appearance of the rash on the face, upper trunk, and down to the extremities.

Laboratory

Brick-shaped virions viewed with electron microscopy examination, virus culture from live cells, or DNA analysis using PCR and smallpox skin specimen should be collected.

Treatment

No known treatment is effective.

⊟ BIBLIOGRAPHY

1. Hussain AN, Hussain F, Alam M, et al. (2011). Smallpox. [online] Available from www.emedicine.com/med/TOPIC3545.HTM. [Accessed September, 2013].

⊟ 1EE.73C9.7G8. ACUTE FOLLICULAR CONJUNCTIVITIS (ADENOVIRAL CONJUNCTIVITIS; PHARYNGOCONJUNCTIVAL FEVER; SYNDROME OF BEAL)

General

It is an infectious disease produced by adenovirus; serotypes 3, 4, 7, 8, 19, 37 and several others may cause acute conjunctivitis with or without upper respiratory tract involvement; epidemic keratoconjunctivitis has been reported worldwide associated with 11 virus serotypes, with serotypes 8, 11 and 19 being the most commonly responsible.

Ocular

Conjunctivitis; chemosis; keratitis; blepharitis; blepharospasm.

Clinical

Fever; pharyngitis; lymph node enlargement; malaise; myalgia; headache; diarrhea.

Laboratory

Laboratory test is generally not useful. Cell cultures from infected areas and adenoviral antibody titer allow for precise identification of serotype.

Treatment

Symptomatic control may include cold compresses, artificial tears; nonsteroidal and occasionally steroidal drops to relieve itching.

⊟ BIBLIOGRAPHY

1. Scott IU. (2012). Pharyngoconjunctival fever. [online] Available from www.emedicine.com/oph/TOPIC501.HTM. [Accessed September, 2013].

⊟ 1EE.73C9.7G8A. EPIDEMIC KERATOCONJUNCTIVITIS

General

Highly communicable; adenovirus types 8 and 19; usually bilateral; epidemic keratoconjunctivitis has been reported worldwide associated with 11 virus serotypes, with serotypes 8, 11, and 19 being the most common responsible ones.

Ocular

Follicular or membranous conjunctivitis; chemosis; subconjunctival hemorrhages; corneal opacity; punctate epithelial keratitis; corneal ulcer; blepharospasm; lid edema; serous discharge; uveitis; epiphora.

Clinical

Submaxillary and cervical lymphadenopathy.

Laboratory

Viral isolation on cell culture from conjunctival scrapings.

Treatment

No effective topical or systemic treatment available. Topical steroids may be used if epithelial keratitis occurs.

⊟ BIBLIOGRAPHY

1. Bawazeer A. (2011). Epidemic keratoconjunctivitis. [online] Available from www.emedicine.com/oph/TOPIC677.HTM. [Accessed September, 2013].

🗗 1EE.73C9.7G9. CHLAMYDIA (INCLUSION CONJUNCTIVITIS; PARATRACHOMA)

General

Organism that infects the epithelium of mucoid surfaces; sexually transmitted; major cause of non-gonococcal urethritis in men and cervicitis in women; major cause of neonatal ophthalmia; *C. trachomatis* is an intracellular bacterium lacking respiratory enzymes that has an affinity for mucosal epithelium; serotypes A through C have been epidemiologically associated with trachoma; serotypes E through K have been associated with genital infection and keratoconjunctivitis in sexually active adults and neonates; other serotypes have been associated with lymphogranuloma venereum and Reiter syndrome.

Ocular

Follicular conjunctivitis; corneal opacities; keratitis; corneal ulcer; lid edema; uveitis.

Clinical

Pneumonia; gastrointestinal disturbances; genital discharge.

Laboratory

Giemsa stain, cell culture—time intensive, direct fluorescent monoclonal antibiotics to stain smears.

Treatment

Three to six weeks of oral tetracycline (500 mg QID), oral doxycycline (100 mg BID), or oral erythromycin stearate (500 mg QID). Simultaneous treatment of all sexual partners is important to prevent reinfection.

🗗 BIBLIOGRAPHY

1. Bashour M. (2012) Ophthalmologic manifestations of Chlamydia. [online] Available from www.emedicine.com/oph/TOPIC494.HTM. [Accessed September, 2013].

🗗 1EE.73C9.7G10. HERPES ZOSTER

General

It is caused by varicella zoster virus; about 75% of cases occur in persons over age of 45 years; condition is more frequent with advancing age and in patients who are immunocompromised by drugs or disease; in particular, an increasing number of patients with herpes zoster ophthalmicus are immunosuppressed.

Ocular

Conjunctivitis; keratitis; recurrent corneal ulcer; neuralgia; zoster rash of eyelids; uveitis; iris atrophy; scleritis; cataract; optic neuritis; paralysis of third nerve; proptosis; paralysis of lids; orbital apex syndrome; retinitis; neurotrophic keratitis; acute retinal necrosis; progressive outer retinal necrosis; ocular motor nerve pareses; tonic pupil; encephalitis; vasculitis.

Clinical

Local lesions involving the posterior or root ganglia; nerve damage; tissue scarring.

Laboratory

Diagnosed mostly on the basis of the characteristic pain and appearance of the dermatomal rashes.

Treatment

Antiviral agents, systemic corticosteroids, antidepressants, and adequate pain control. Immunocompetent adults aged 60 years or older, benefit from receipt of the herpes zoster vaccine and have a lower incidence of herpes zoster.

🗗 BIBLIOGRAPHY

1. Diaz MM, Foster CS, Walton RC, et al. (2011). Herpes zoster ophthalmicus. [online] Available from www.emedicine.com/oph/TOPIC257.HTM. [Accessed September, 2013].
2. Ghaznawi N, Virdi A, Dayan A, et al. Herpes zoster ophthalmicus: comparison of disease in patients 60 years and older versus younger than 60 years. Ophthalmology. 2011;118(11):2242-50.
3. Ho J, Xirasagar S, Lin H. Increased risk of a cancer diagnosis after herpes zoster ophthalmicus: a nationwide population-based study. Ophthalmology. 2011;118(6):1076-81.
4. Tseng HF, Smith N, Harpaz R, et al. Herpes zoster vaccine in older adults and the risk of subsequent herpes zoster disease. JAMA. 2011;305(2):160-6.

⊟ 1EE.73C9.7G11. NEWCASTLE DISEASE (FOWLPOX)

General

Acquired directly by people handling chickens (*see* Parinaud oculoglandular syndrome); self-limiting conjunctivitis caused by a paramyxovirus.

Ocular

Acute follicular conjunctivitis, unilateral; keratitic precipitates; lid edema; decreased accommodation and visual acuity.

Clinical

Fatigue; fever; headache; pulmonary complications; preauricular lymphadenopathy.

Laboratory/Conjunctivitis

Diagnosis is made by clinical findings.

Treatment

Topical antibiotics, cold compresses, artificial tears.

⊟ BIBLIOGRAPHY

1. Gordon S. Viral keratitis and conjunctivitis. Adenovirus and other nonherpetic viral diseases. In: Smolin G, Thoft RA (Eds). The Cornea. Boston: Little, Brown and Company; 1994.
2. Pau H. Differential diagnosis of eye diseases. New York: Thieme; 1987.
3. Roy FH, Fraunfelder FW, Fraunfelder FT. Roy and Fraunfelder's Current Ocular Therapy, 6th edition. Philadelphia: WB Saunders; 2008.

⊟ 1EE.73C9.7G12. INFLUENZA

General

Acute respiratory infection of specific viral etiology which includes H1N1

Ocular

Conjunctivitis; subconjunctival hemorrhages; keratitis; tenonitis; ptosis; cellulitis of orbit and lid; dacryocystitis; retinal hemorrhage; cataract; episcleritis; hypopyon; optic neuritis; uveitis; panophthalmitis; vitreal hemorrhage; paralysis of third or fourth nerve; uveitis following vaccination for influenza.

Clinical

Headache; fever; malaise; muscular aching; substernal soreness; nasal stuffiness; nausea.

Laboratory

The criterion standard for diagnosing influenza A and B is a viral culture of nasal-pharyngeal samples, throat samples, or both.

Treatment

Prevention is the most effective therapy. Two new drugs have been marketed recently for treatment of influenza A and B. These are the neuraminidase inhibitors, oseltamivir and zanamivir.

⊟ BIBLIOGRAPHY

1. Derlet RW. (2012). Influenza. [online] Available from www.emedicine.com/med/TOPIC1170.HTM. [Accessed September, 2013].

⊡ 1EE.73C9.7G13. HERPES ZOSTER

General

It is caused by varicella zoster virus; about 75% of cases occur in persons over age of 45 years; condition is more frequent with advancing age and in patients who are immunocompromised by drugs or disease; in particular, an increasing number of patients with herpes zoster ophthalmicus are immunosuppressed.

Ocular

Conjunctivitis; keratitis; recurrent corneal ulcer; neuralgia; zoster rash of eyelids; uveitis; iris atrophy; scleritis; cataract; optic neuritis; paralysis of third nerve; proptosis; paralysis of lids; orbital apex syndrome; retinitis; neurotrophic keratitis; acute retinal necrosis; progressive outer retinal necrosis; ocular motor nerve pareses; tonic pupil; encephalitis; vasculitis.

Clinical

Local lesions involving the posterior or root ganglia; nerve damage; tissue scarring.

Laboratory

Diagnosed mostly on the basis of the characteristic pain and appearance of the dermatomal rashes.

Treatment

Antiviral agents, systemic corticosteroids, antidepressants, and adequate pain control. Immunocompetent adults aged 60 years or older, benefit from receipt of the herpes zoster vaccine and have a lower incidence of herpes zoster.

⊡ BIBLIOGRAPHY

1. Diaz MM, Foster CS, Walton RC, et al. (2011). Herpes zoster ophthalmicus. [online] Available from www.emedicine.com/oph/TOPIC257.HTM. [Accessed September, 2013].
2. Ghaznawi N, Virdi A, Dayan A, et al. Herpes zoster ophthalmicus: comparison of disease in patients 60 years and older versus younger than 60 years. Ophthalmology. 2011;118(11):2242-50.
3. Ho J, Xirasagar S, Lin H. Increased risk of a cancer diagnosis after herpes zoster ophthalmicus: a nationwide population-based study. Ophthalmology. 2011;118(6):1076-81.
4. Tseng HF, Smith N, Harpaz R, et al. Herpes zoster vaccine in older adults and the risk of subsequent herpes zoster disease. JAMA. 2011;305(2):160-6.

⊡ 1EE.73C9.7G14. PARINAUD OCULOGLANDULAR SYNDROME (PARINAUD CONJUNCTIVA-ADENITIS SYNDROME; CATSCRATCH OCULOGLANDULAR SYNDROME; CATSCRATCH DISEASE; BARTONELLA HENSELAE)

General

Most frequently seen in children; incubation time 7–10 days; caused by small pleomorphic Gram-negative bacillus; good prognosis; affects both sexes; about 90% of patients with this condition have serologic evidence of infection by *Rochalimaea henselae*.

Ocular

Conjunctivitis; retrotarsal conjunctival granulations; formation of granulomata in anterior segment about 3 mm high and 2-6 mm in diameter; inferior fornix usually affected; ulceration common; neuroretinitis; optic neuritis.

Clinical

Tender, red papule at the site of a cat scratch; regional preauricular and cervical lymphadenitis (often only one gland involved); irregular fever for 4–5 days and malaise; fever; parotid gland swelling.

Laboratory

Histopathology of biopsied lymph node of Warthin-Starry silver stain.

Treatment

Symptomatic treatment includes warm compresses, analgesics and antipyretics. Aspiration of lymph node if distention causes pain. Antibiotics may be necessary in severe cases.

⊡ BIBLIOGRAPHY

1. Chi SL, Stinnett S, Eggenberger E, et al. Clinical characteristics in 53 patients with cat scratch optic neuropathy. Ophthalmology. 2012;119:183-7.
2. Nervi SJ. (2011). Catscratch disease. [online] Available from www.emedicine.com/med/TOPIC304.HTM. [Accessed September, 2013].

⊟ 1EE.73C9.7G16. TRACHOMA

General

Most common in rural communities of the Middle East, Africa, Asia, and South and Central America; caused by *C. trachomatis*; associated with poor sanitation and medical care.

Ocular

Chronic keratoconjunctivitis; papillae follicles; keratitis; opacities of cornea; scars of palpebral conjunctiva; ptosis; tearing; entropion.

Clinical

Rhinitis; otitis media; upper respiratory tract infection.

Laboratory

Most endemic areas, laboratory tests are unavailable. Commercial PCR based assay has high sensitivity and specificity.

Treatment

Tetracycline eye ointment for 6 weeks or a single-dose azithromycin systemically.

⊟ BIBLIOGRAPHY

1. Solomon AW. (2011). Trachoma. [online] Available from www.emedicine.com/oph/TOPIC118.HTM. [Accessed September, 2013].
2. Biebesheimer JB, House J, Hong KC, et al. Complete local elimination of infectious trachoma from severely affected communitieis after six biannual mass azithromycin distributions. Ophthalmology. 209;116:2047-50.

⊟ 1EE.73C9.7G17A. MORAXELLA LACUNATA

General

Gram-negative rod; causes chronic angular blepharoconjunctivitis; without treatment, may persist for months or years; normally found in flora of respiratory tract; seen more frequently in alcoholics and those with poor sanitary habits; *Moraxella* organisms produce proteases, although those are not related directly to their pathogenetic mechanism.

Ocular

Catarrhal angular conjunctivitis; corneal ulcer; hypopyon; chronic blepharitis; eczema; lateral canthal skin erythema; iridocyclitis.

Clinical

Alcoholism; impaired nutrition; dermatitis.

Laboratory

Aerobic, oxidase positive, Gram-negative diplococcus or coccobacilli morphologically indistinguishable from *Neisseria*.

Treatment

Artificial tears, cold compresses, antibiotics.

⊟ BIBLIOGRAPHY

1. Baum J, Fedukowicz HB, Jordan A. A survey of Moraxella corneal ulcers in a derelict population. Am J Ophthalmol. 1980;90:476-80.
2. Burd EM. Bacterial keratitis and conjunctivitis. In: Smolin G, Thoft RA (Eds). The Cornea. Boston: Little, Brown and Company; 1994. pp. 20-1.
3. Roy FH, Fraunfelder FW, Fraunfelder FT. Roy and Fraunfelder's Current Ocular Therapy, 6th edition. Philadelphia: WB Saunders; 2008.
4. van Bijsterveld OP. The incidence of Moraxella on mucous membranes and the skin. Am J Ophthalmol. 1972;74:72-6.

🖥 1EE.73C9.7G17B. STREPTOCOCCUS

General

Gram-positive bacteria that can invade any tissue.

Ocular

Conjunctivitis; corneal ulcer; blepharitis; scarlatinal rash of lid; erysipelas dermatitis of lid; gangrene of lid; endophthalmitis; proptosis; dacryocystitis; optic neuritis; orbital cellulitis; uveitis; hypopyon; secondary glaucoma; paralysis of extraocular muscles; infectious crystalline keratopathy; scleritis.

Clinical

Pharyngitis; impetigo; scarlet fever; pneumonia; bacteremia; rheumatic fever; glomerulonephritis.

Laboratory

Gram-positive cocci growing in pairs or chains. Throat culture and sensitivity are useful.

Treatment

Penicillin is the drug of choice.

🖥 BIBLIOGRAPHY

1. Zabawski EJ. (2011). Scarlet fever. [online] Available from www.emedicine.com/emerg/TOPIC518.HTM. [Accessed September, 2013].

🖥 1EE.73C9.7G17C. PINTA (NONVENEREAL TREPONEMATOSIS)

General

It is caused by spirochete *Treponema carateum*; infectious; contagious; found in Mexico, Central America, West Indies, and the northern countries of South America; caused by an organism that is morphologically and antigenically identical to the causative agent of venereal syphilis.

Ocular

Hypopigmentation of eyelid.

Clinical

Cutaneous lesions with marked pigmentary changes; chronic relapsing course.

Laboratory

The nontreponemal and treponemal serologic tests used in diagnosing venereal syphilis are used for serodiagnosis of pinta.

Treatment

After penicillin therapy, lesions become noninfectious in 24 hours.

🖥 BIBLIOGRAPHY

1. Klein NC. (2013). Pinta. [online] Available from www.emedicine.com/med/TOPIC1836.HTM. [Accessed September, 2013].

🖥 1EE.73C9.7G19. CHLAMYDIA (INCLUSION CONJUNCTIVITIS; PARATRACHOMA)

General

Organism that infects the epithelium of mucoid surfaces; sexually transmitted; major cause of non-gonococcal urethritis in men and cervicitis in women; major cause of neonatal ophthalmia; *C. trachomatis* is an intracellular bacterium lacking respiratory enzymes that has an affinity for mucosal epithelium; serotypes A through C have been epidemiologically associated with trachoma; serotypes E through K have been associated with genital infection and keratoconjunctivitis in sexually active adults and neonates; other serotypes have been associated with lymphogranuloma venereum and Reiter syndrome.

Ocular

Follicular conjunctivitis; corneal opacities; keratitis; corneal ulcer; lid edema; uveitis.

Clinical

Pneumonia; gastrointestinal disturbances; genital discharge.

Laboratory

Giemsa stain, cell culture—time intensive, direct fluorescent monoclonal antibiotics to stain smears.

Treatment

Three to six weeks of oral tetracycline (500 mg QID), oral doxycycline (100 mg BID), or oral erythromycin stearate (500 mg QID). Simultaneous treatment of all sexual partners is important to prevent reinfection.

🔲 BIBLIOGRAPHY

1. Bashour M. (2012) Ophthalmologic manifestations of Chlamydia. [online] Available from www.emedicine.com/oph/TOPIC494.HTM. [Accessed September, 2013].

🔲 1EE.73C9.7G22. OPHTHALMIA NEONATORUM (NEONATAL CONJUNCTIVITIS)

General

Conjunctivitis of newborns which may be viral or bacterial in nature. Maternal infection may be a factor.

Clinical

None.

Ocular

Purulent discharge in the first few days of life; can be sight threatening if untreated.

Laboratory

Gram stain—intracellular, Gram-negative—gonococcus, Gram-negative coccobacilli—*H. influenzae*, Gram-positive-*Staphylococcus or Streptococcus*. Giemsa stain or PCR—Chlamydia intracytoplasmic inclusion bodies.

Treatment

Prevention: 2% silver nitrate or topical erythromycin or povidone-iodine drops. Oral and topical antibiotics may be necessary.

🔲 BIBLIOGRAPHY

1. Enzenauer RW, McCourt EA, Jatla KK, et al. (2011). Neonatal conjunctivitis. [online] Available from www.emedicine.com/oph/TOPIC325.HTM. [Accessed September, 2013].

🔲 1EE.73C9.7G24A. ANGELUCCI SYNDROME (CRITICAL ALLERGIC CONJUNCTIVITIS SYNDROME)

General

Etiology unknown; pruriginous cutaneous and mucous reactions that appear and cease rather suddenly.

Ocular

Chemosis; conjunctivitis (papillary type); severe itching and burning; photophobia.

Clinical

Tachycardia; vasomotor lability; excitability; allergies (asthma, urticaria, edema); dystrophic conditions and endocrine disorders are frequently associated findings.

Laboratory

Diagnosis is made by clinical findings.

Treatment

Symptomatic control may include cold compresses, artificial tears; nonsteroidal and occasionally steroidal drops to relieve itching.

🔲 BIBLIOGRAPHY

1. Angelucci A. Di una Sindrome Sconoscita Negli Infermi di Cattarro Primaverile. Arch Ottal Palermo. 1898;4:270-6.
2. Geeraets WJ. Ocular Syndromes, 3rd edition. Philadelphia, PA: Lea & Febiger; 1976.
3. Magalini SI, Scrascia E. Dictionary of Medical Syndromes, 2nd edition. Philadelphia, PA: Lippincott Williams and Wilkins; 1981.

⊟ 1EE.73C9.7G24B. ANOXIC OVERWEAR SYNDROME

General

It is caused by a reduction in oxygen supply due to continuously worn hydrogel lenses; allergic or toxic reactions to preservatives used in the cleaning process.

Ocular

Refractive error changes; endothelial cell changes; physical trauma to the anterior surface of the cornea; corneal neovascularization; giant papillary conjunctivitis; contact lens deposits; acute red eye syndrome.

Laboratory

Diagnosis is made by clinical findings.

Treatment

Observation, topical steroid drops, reduce time individual uses contact lens, corneal laser photocoagulation.

⊟ BIBLIOGRAPHY

1. Binder PS. The physiologic effects of extended wear soft contact lenses. Ophthalmology. 1980;87:745-9.
2. Sarver MD, Baggett DA, Harris MG, et al. Corneal edema with hydrogel lenses and eye closure: effect of oxygen transmissibility. Am J Optom Physiol Opt. 1981;58:386-92.

⊟ 1EE.73C9.7G24C. BENJAMIN-ALLEN SYNDROME

General

Branchial arch syndrome; not hereditary.

Ocular

Bilateral dermoids of conjunctiva; marked follicular hyperplasia of conjunctiva.

Clinical

Lymphadenopathy; cutaneous nevoid lesions; incomplete alopecia; mental retardation; growth retardation.

Laboratory

Diagnosis is made by clinical findings.

Treatment

Symptomatic control may include cold compresses, artificial tears; nonsteroidal and occasionally steroidal drops to relieve itching.

⊟ BIBLIOGRAPHY

1. Benjamin SN, Allen HF Classification of limbal dermoid choristomas and branchial arch anomalies: presentation of an unusual case. Arch Ophthalmol. 1972;87:305-l4.
2. Mattos J, Contreras F, O'Donnell FE. Ring dermoid syndrome. Arch Ophthalmol. 1980;98:1059-61.

⊟ 1EE.73C9.7G24D. FLOPPY EYELID SYNDROME

General

Origin unknown; more common in males; overweight; X-chromosome-linked inheritance pattern or possible hormonal influence; it has been postulated that the degenerative changes in the tarsus may result from the combination of local pressure-induced lid ischemia and systemic hypoventilation.

Ocular

Easily everted, floppy upper eyelid and papillary conjunctivitis of the upper palpebral conjunctiva; upper eyelid everts during sleep, resulting in irritation, papillary conjunctivitis and conjunctival keratinization; most distinct feature is rubbery, malleable upper tarsus; keratoconus; punctate keratopathy; blepharoptosis; lash ptosis.

Clinical

Obesity; sleep apnea.

Laboratory

Conjunctival scrapings reveal keratinized epithelial cells. Bacterial cultures are important.

Treatment

Full-thickness upper and lower eyelid resection.

BIBLIOGRAPHY

1. Ezra DG, Beaconsfield M, Sira M, et al. Long-term outcomes of surgical approaches to the treatment of floppy eyelid syndrome. Ophthalmology. 2010;117(4):839-46.
2. Ezra DG, Beaconsfield M, Sira M, et al. The associations of floppy eyelid syndrome: a case control study. Ophthalmology. 2010;117(4):831-8.
3. Chatziralli IP, Sergentanis TN. Risk factors for intraoperative floppy iris syndrome: a meta-analysis. Ophthalmology. 2011;118(4):730-5.
4. Blaydon SM. (2011). Floppy eyelid syndrome. [online] Available from www.emedicine.com/oph/TOPIC605.HTM. [Accessed September, 2013].

1EE.73C9.7G24E. GIANT PAPILLARY CONJUNCTIVITIS SYNDROME

General

Commonly associated with contact lenses (hard and soft), foreign bodies and ocular prosthesis; immunologic in origin.

Ocular

Ocular irritation; itching of the eye; decreased visual acuity; increased mucous production; papillary changes of the upper tarsal conjunctiva; contact lens coatings; may appear after a lens change from one style to another or by replacement of the previous design; aging of a lens, particularly of a soft contact lens, may be associated; usually bilateral, although it can be markedly asymmetrical.

Clinical

None.

Laboratory

Diagnosis is made by clinical findings.

Treatment

Stop wearing contact lens for 4 weeks, replace contact lens every 6–12 months, topical lubricants and nonsteroidal anti-inflammatory drops.

BIBLIOGRAPHY

1. Weissman BA, Yeung KK. (2011). Giant papillary conjunctivitis. [online] Available from www.emedicine.com/oph/TOPIC87.HTM. [Accessed September, 2013].

1EE.73C9.7G24G. BEAL SYNDROME

General

Transient unilateral disease; becoming bilateral later, then resolving within 2 weeks.

Ocular

Acute follicular conjunctivitis (lymphoid follicles; cobblestoning of conjunctiva with rapid onset).

Clinical

No purulent discharge; associated with regional adenitis.

Laboratory

Diagnosis is made by clinical findings.

Treatment

Symptomatic control may include cold compresses, artificial tears; nonsteroidal and occasionally steroidal drops to relieve itching.

BIBLIOGRAPHY

1. Ostler HB, Schachter J, Dawson CR. Acute follicular conjunctivitis of epizootic origin. Arch Ophthalmol. 1969; 82:587-91.
2. Thygeson P. Follicular conjunctivitis: infectious diseases of the conjunctiva and cornea. In: Symposium of the New Orleans Academy of Ophthalmology. St. Louis: CV Mosby; 1965. p.103.

1EE.73C9.7G25. ANGULAR CONJUNCTIVITIS (MORAX-AXENFELD BACILLUS)

General

It is caused by *M. lacunata*, which frequently inhabits the nose.

Ocular

Conjunctivitis; hypopyon; keratitis; uveitis; corneal marginal ulcer.

Laboratory

Diagnosis is made by clinical findings.

Treatment

- *Conjunctivitis*: Antibiotic medication should be used to treat the infection.
- *Corneal ulcer*: Corneal cultures may be taken and treatment is initiated. Treatment includes a broad spectrum of antibiotics and cycloplegic drops.
- *Uveitis*: Topical steroids and cycloplegic medication should be the choice of initial treatment. Oral steroids should be given if not responsive to topical steroids, immunosuppressants if bilateral disease that does not respond to oral steroids, and periocular steroids for unilateral or posterior uveitis. Vitrectomy can be used for severe vitreous opacification. Cryotherapy and laser photocoagulation may be used for localized pars plana exudates.

BIBLIOGRAPHY

1. Jones DB. Early diagnosis and therapy of bacterial corneal ulcers. Int Ophthalmol Clin. 1973;13(4):1-29.
2. Marioneaux SJ, Cohen EJ, Arentsen JJ, et al. Moraxella keratitis. Cornea. 1991;10(1):21-4.
3. van Bijsterveld OP. Bacterial proteases in Moraxella angular conjunctivitis. Am J Ophthalmol. 1971;72(1):181-4.

1EE.73C9.7G28. ROTHMUND SYNDROME (ROTHMUND-THOMSON SYNDROME; TELANGIECTASIA-PIGMENTATION-CATARACT SYNDROME; ECTODERMAL SYNDROME; CONGENITAL POIKILODERMA WITH JUVENILE CATARACT) KERATOCONUS

General

Autosomal recessive; more common in females (2:1); Werner syndrome in adults has certain similarities to this syndrome; inflammatory phase progresses to atrophy and telangiectasia; onset at age from 3 months to 6 months.

Ocular

Eyebrows may be sparse or absent; hypertelorism; cilia sometimes are diminished or absent; trichiasis; epiphora; cataracts (anterior subcapsular, posterior stellate, or perinuclear type); corneal lesions; retinal hyperpigmentation; keratoconus; strabismus; epibulbar dermoids.

Clinical

Poikiloderma; hypogonadism; hypomenorrhea; head deformity (enlarged with depressed nasal bridge as well as microcephaly); small stature, with short or malformed distal phalanges; aplasia cutis congenita (congenital absence of skin in one or more areas); alopecia.

Laboratory

Skeletal radiograph by age of 5 years.

Treatment

Sun blocker with UVA and UVB should be used often. Keratolytics and retinoids are used to treat hyperkeratotic lesions.

BIBLIOGRAPHY

1. Hsu S, George SJ. (2012). Rothmund-Thomson syndrome. [online] Available from www.emedicine.com/derm/TOPIC379.HTM. [Accessed September, 2013].

⊟ 1EE.73C9.7G30. MOLLUSCUM CONTAGIOSUM

General

Etiologic agent of this disease is a poxvirus that can cause proliferative skin lesions anywhere on the body; commonly found in patients who are immunosuppressed.

Ocular

Lesions of lid, lid margin, conjunctiva, and cornea; conjunctivitis; keratitis; corneal ulcer.

Clinical

Well-defined, pearly appearing papules with umbilicated centers of varying size (3–10 mm); eczematization of the surrounding skin.

Laboratory

Craters have epithelial cells with large eosinophilic intracytoplasmic inclusion bodies (molluscum or Henderson Patterson bodies) when virus particles migrate to the granular layer of the epidermis, the inclusion bodies become basophilic.

Treatment

Topical agents cantharidin, tretinoin, podophllin, trichloroacetic acid, tincture of iodine, silver nitrate or phenol, potassium hydroxide. Systemic agents include griseofulvin, methisazone and cimetidine.

⊟ BIBLIOGRAPHY

1. Bhatia AC. (2012). Molluscum contagiosum. [online] Available from www.emedicine.com/oph/TOPIC500.HTM. [Accessed September, 2013].

⊟ 1EE.73C9.7G31. NEUROCUTANEOUS SYNDROME

General

Triad of linear nevus sebaceous; seizures; mental retardation.

Ocular

Colobomas of irides and choroid; nystagmus; keratoconus; corneal vascularization; optic glioma; epibulbar choristomas; connective tissue nevi of the eyelids.

Clinical

Multiple nevi; seizures; mental retardation; failure to thrive; hydrocephalus; deformities of skull; lipoma of the cranium; alopecia of the scalp.

Laboratory

Diagnosis is made by clinical findings.

Treatment

Spectacle correction, hard contacts, avoid eye rubbing. If hydrops occur, discontinue contact lens, use NaCl drops and ointment, patching, and short course of steroids. As disease advances PK, deep anterior lamellar keratoplasty intacs with laser grooves or collagen stabilization of cornea.

⊟ BIBLIOGRAPHY

1. Kodsi SR, Bloom KE, Egbert JE, et al. Ocular and systemic manifestations of encephalocraniocutaneous lipomatosis. Am J Ophthalmol. 1994;118:77-82.

⊟ 1EE.73C9.7G32. PARINAUD SYNDROME (DIVERGENCE PARALYSIS; SUBTHALAMIC SYNDROME; PARALYSIS OF VERTICAL MOVEMENTS; PRETECTAL SYNDROME)

General

Various causes, including pineal tumor, supranuclear lesions, vascular lesions, inflammation, hemorrhages, midbrain lesions, lesion of posterior white commissure of pons, red nucleus, or superior cerebellar peduncle; combination of Parinaud and von Monakow syndromes is known as Gruner-Bertolotti syndrome, which consists of paralysis in upward gaze, tremors, hemiplegia, and sensory disturbances.

Ocular

Retraction of lids with lesion in mesencephalic gray matter and ptosis with lesions more anteriorly; paralysis of conjugate upward movement of the eye without paralysis of convergence; occasionally paralysis of upward and downward movement; spasm with convergence insufficiency; contralateral hemianopsia occurs when the lateral geniculate body becomes involved in case of infiltrating tumor; wide pupils that fail to react to light but sometimes react during accommodation (Holmes); papilledema (usually severe).

Clinical

Vertigo; contralateral cerebellar ataxia and choreoathetoid movement if lesion involves superior cerebellar peduncle after decussation.

Laboratory

Diagnosis is made by clinical findings, CT and MRI.

Treatment

Papilledema: Underlying cause should be determined and treated. Systemic acetazolamide is the medical therapy of choice.

BIBLIOGRAPHY

1. Zee C, Yao Z, Go JL, et al. (2011). Imaging in pineal germinoma. [online] Available from www.emedicine.com/radio/TOPIC554.HTM. [Accessed September, 2013].

1EE.73C9.7G35. TRACHOMA

General

Most common in rural communities of the Middle East, Africa, Asia, and South and Central America; caused by *C. trachomatis*; associated with poor sanitation and medical care.

Ocular

Chronic keratoconjunctivitis; papillae follicles; keratitis; opacities of cornea; scars of palpebral conjunctiva; ptosis; tearing; entropion.

Clinical

Rhinitis; otitis media; upper respiratory tract infection.

Laboratory

Most endemic areas, laboratory tests are unavailable. Commercial PCR based assay has high sensitivity and specificity.

Treatment

Tetracycline eye ointment for 6 weeks or a single-dose azithromycin systemically.

BIBLIOGRAPHY

1. Biebesheimer JB, House J, Hong KC, et al. Complete local elimination of infectious trachoma from severely affected communitieis after six biannual mass azithromycin distributions. Ophthalmology. 209;116:2047-50.
2. Solomon AW. (2011). Trachoma. [online] Available from www.emedicine.com/oph/TOPIC118.HTM. [Accessed September, 2013].

1EE.73C9.7G36. NEOVASCULARIZATION, CORNEAL CONTACT LENS RELATED

General

Pathologic state in which new blood vessels extending in the corneal stroma from trauma, inflammation, infection, toxic insults secondary to contact lens usage.

Clinical

None.

Ocular

Vessel ingrowth into the cornea, ocular irritation.

Laboratory

Diagnosis is made by clinical findings.

Treatment

Observation, eliminate cause, topical steroid drops, reduced time for an individual using contact lens, corneal laser photocoagulation.

BIBLIOGRAPHY

1. Weissman BA, Yeung KK. (2011). Neovascularization, corneal, CL-related. [online] Available from emedicine.medscape.com/article/1195886-overview. [Accessed September, 2013].

1EE.73C9.7G38. BENIGN MUCOSAL PEMPHIGOID (CHRONIC CICATRICIAL CONJUNCTIVITIS; CICATRICIAL PEMPHIGOID; ESSENTIAL SHRINKAGE OF THE CONJUNCTIVA; MEMBRANE PEMPHIGUS; OCULARPEMPHIGOID)

General

Etiology unknown; involving older age group, especially over 70 years; chronic autoimmune disorder characterized by fibrosis beneath the conjunctival epithelium; associated with the major histocompatibility complex class I alleles, which confer susceptibility to the disease; likely due to a multigene effect and associated with environmental factors; incidence in women is twice as frequent as men, no geographic or racial predilection.

Ocular

Conjunctivitis; absence of goblet cells of conjunctiva; conjunctival ulcer; pannus and keratitis; corneal opacity; entropion; trichiasis; cicatrization of lacrimal ducts; corneal perforation; symblepharon; dry eyes; bilateral involvement (may be asymmetrical); ocular shrinkage; xerosis; conjunctival and corneal bullae.

Clinical

Subepidermal and subepithelial blistering of mucous membranes; blisters may occur in pharyngeal, laryngeal, nasal, anal and genital mucosa.

Laboratory

Diagnosis is made by clinical findings.

Treatment

Subconjunctival injections of steroid or mitomycin may be helpful. Systemic immunomodulators are the major therapeutic plan.

BIBLIOGRAPHY

1. Foster CS, Hamam R, Letko E. (2011). Ophthalmologic manifestations of cicatricial pemphigoid. [online] Available from www.emedicine.com/oph/TOPIC83.HTM. [Accessed September, 2013].

1EE.73C9.7G39. DIPHTHERIA

General

Acute infectious disease caused by *C. diphtheriae*; severity is dependent upon the amount of exotoxin absorbed prior to initiation of specific therapy.

Ocular

Conjunctivitis; xerophthalmia; keratitis; corneal ulcer; blepharitis; cellulitis of lid; meibomianitis; ptosis; dacryocystitis; cataract; central retinal artery occlusion; optic neuritis; accommodative spasm or paralysis; convergence paralysis; divergence paralysis; paralysis of third, fourth, or sixth nerve; paralysis of accommodation (in children); ocular motor nerve paresis; choroiditis; cranial neuropathies involving the trigeminal, vagus, and hypoglossal cranial nerves; myocarditis.

Clinical

Local inflammatory lesion, with effect on heart, kidneys, and nervous system.

Laboratory

Gram-positive rods commonly affect children younger than 10 years

Treatment

Systemic treatment involves use of diphtheria antitoxin and antibiotics. Ocular treatment includes diphtheria antitoxin and high titer y-globulin preparation. Topical penicillin-G ointment helps to eradicate the bacilli.

BIBLIOGRAPHY

1. Demirci CS. (2011). Pediatric diphtheria. [online] Available from www.emedicine.com/ped/TOPIC596.HTM. [Accessed September, 2013].

1EE.73C9.7G39. STREPTOCOCCUS (SCARLET FEVER)

General

Gram-positive bacteria that can invade any tissue.

Ocular

Conjunctivitis; corneal ulcer; blepharitis; scarlatinal rash of lid; erysipelas dermatitis of lid; gangrene of lid; endophthalmitis; proptosis; dacryocystitis; optic neuritis; orbital cellulitis; uveitis; hypopyon; secondary glaucoma; paralysis of extraocular muscles; infectious crystalline keratopathy; scleritis.

Clinical

Pharyngitis; impetigo; scarlet fever; pneumonia; bacteremia; rheumatic fever; glomerulonephritis.

Laboratory

Gram-positive cocci growing in pairs or chains. Throat culture and sensitivity are useful.

Treatment

Penicillin is the drug of choice.

BIBLIOGRAPHY

1. Zabawski EJ. (2011). Scarlet Fever. [online] Available from www.emedicine.com/emerg/TOPIC518.HTM. [Accessed September, 2013].

1EE.73C9.7G39. SCHAUMANN SYNDROME (BESNIER-BOECK-SCHAUMANN SYNDROME; BOECK SARCOID; SARCOIDOSIS)

General

Etiology unknown; theories include tuberculosis, hypersensitivity to pine pollen, virus infection; affects blacks most often; chronic course with spontaneous remissions (*see* Heerfordt's syndrome); hilar or paratracheal nodes with erythema nodosum; onset most often in middle and old age; ocular involvement in 20–25% of all cases.

Ocular

Orbital granulomatous mass; bony defects; cutaneous and subcutaneous nodules; myogenic palsy; lacrimal gland adenopathy; decreased tear formation; secondary glaucoma; granulomatous uveitis with iris nodules, cells and flare; mutton fat keratic precipitates; keratitis sicca; vitreous floaters; band-shaped keratitis; complicated cataract; inflammatory retinal exudates; "candle wax drippings"; optic nerve atrophy; neuritis; eyelid nodules; ocular nerve enlargement (granuloma).

Clinical

Lymphadenopathy; hilar nodes; fatigue; cystic, punched-out or reticulated changes in small bones (mainly, hands and feet); muscle wasting; contractures; weakness in legs and arms.

Laboratory

Chest X-ray, CT scan and MRI of the brain.

Treatment

Glucocorticoids are the treatment of choice.

BIBLIOGRAPHY

1. Sharma GD. (2011). Pediatric sarcoidosis. [online] Available from www.emedicine.com/ped/TOPIC2043.HTM. [Accessed September, 2013].

1EE.73C9.7G39. PROGRESSIVE SYSTEMIC SCLEROSIS (SCLERODERMA; SYSTEMIC SCLERODERMA)

General

Chronic connective tissue disease of unknown etiology; chronic and usually progressive disorder; typical onset is in 3rd to 5th decade; ratio of women to men is 4:1; primary sites of pathology are the arterioles and capillaries of affected organs.

Ocular

Marginal corneal ulcers; shortened fornices of the conjunctiva; ptosis; cotton-wool patches of retina; papilledema; retinal hemorrhages; cicatrization of conjunctiva and cornea; blepharitis; blepharospasm; thready, tenacious yellow-white conjunctival discharge; hypertrophy of lacrimal gland; episcleritis; ocular myositis; Sjögren syndrome; uveitis; vitreous haze; keratitis sicca; decreased corneal sensation; iritis; ischemic choroidopathy; iris sectorial atrophy; blepharophimosis; heterochromia; keratoconus; central retinal vein occlusion; branch retinal vein occlusion.

Clinical

Vascular insufficiency; Raynaud's phenomenon; malaise; weight loss; stiffness; fever; polyarticular arthritis; diffuse edema of the hands; calcinosis; esophageal involvement; sclerodactyly; telangiectasis; esophageal stricture; renal failure; diffuse interstitial fibrosis.

Laboratory

No specific test establishes diagnosis. Hypergammaglobulinemia—50% of cases ANA increased in 40–70% cases.

Treatment

Skin thickening can be treated with D-penicillamine and other experimental drugs. Pruritus can be treated with moisturizers and histamine. Raynaud's phenomenon can be treated with calcium channel blockers. Renal crisis episodes are best prevented and treated with the aggressive use of ACE inhibitors. Myositis may be treated cautiously with steroids.

BIBLIOGRAPHY

1. Jimenez SA, Cronin PM, Koenig AS, et al. (2012). Scleroderma. [online] Available from www.emedicine.com/med/TOPIC2076.HTM. [Accessed September, 2013].

1EE.73C9.7G39. LICHEN PLANUS

General

Conjunctival disorder associated with dermatologic disorder; disappears spontaneously.

Ocular

Conjunctivitis; cicatrizing conjunctivitis; keratin plaque on bulbar conjunctiva.

Clinical

Grayish-white papules; oral lesions may precede skin lesions.

Laboratory

Diagnosis is made by clinical findings.

Treatment

Topical and systemic corticosteroids, systemic immunomodulators.

BIBLIOGRAPHY

1. Foster CS, Hamam R, Letko E. (2011). Ophthalmologic manifestations of cicatricial pemphigoid. [online] Available from www.emedicine.com/oph/TOPIC83.HTM. [Accessed September, 2013].

🗗 1EE.73C9.7G39. BLEPHAROCONJUNCTIVITIS

General

Chronic blepharitis caused by *Staphylococcus*, seborrheic, meibomian seborrhea or seborrheic with secondary meibomianitis.

Clinical

Seborrheic dermatitis.

Ocular

Blepharitis, keratoconjunctivitis.

Laboratory

Eyelid and conjunctival cultures.

Treatment

Ocular: Warm compresses to lids, eyelid scrubs, bacitracin ointment, ocular lubricants and rarely topical steroids. Systemic antibiotics are sometimes necessary in severe cases.

🗗 BIBLIOGRAPHY

1. Roy FH, Fraunfelder FW, Fraunfelder FT. Roy and Fraunfelder's Current Ocular Therapy, 6th edition. London, UK: Elsevier; 2008.

🗗 1EE.73C9.7G39. LINEAR IGA DISEASE

General

Bullous dermatosis with pruritic urticarial lesions with overlying vesicles or bullae; skin lesions heal without scarring; homogeneous deposition of IgA at the dermal-epidermal junction and rarely, deposition of other Ig present; heterogeneous disease with regard to its clinical features, target antigens, and immunogenetics; association with HLA-B8, DR3, Cw7, and the linked rare tumor necrosis factor-a allele; may be induced by amiodarone.

Ocular

Chronic conjunctivitis; subconjunctival fibrosis; symblepharon; chronic progressive conjunctival cicatrization.

Clinical

Recurrent blistering skin disorder consisting of urticarial macules and plaques with vesicular eruptions on trunk and extremities; subepidermal vesiculation.

Laboratory

Diagnosis is made by clinical findings.

Treatment

Conjunctivitis: Symptomatic control may include cold compresses, artificial tears; NSAIDs and occasionally steroidal drops to relieve itching.

🗗 BIBLIOGRAPHY

1. Foster CS, Hamam R, Letko E. (2011). Ophthalmologic manifestations of cicatricial pemphigoid. [online] Available from www.emedicine.com/oph/TOPIC83.HTM. [Accessed September, 2013].

🗗 1EE.73C9.7G40A. TRACHOMA

General

Most common in rural communities of the Middle East, Africa, Asia, and South and Central America; caused by *C. trachomatis*; associated with poor sanitation and medical care.

Ocular

Chronic keratoconjunctivitis; papillae follicles; keratitis; opacities of cornea; scars of palpebral conjunctiva; ptosis; tearing; entropion.

Clinical

Rhinitis; otitis media; upper respiratory tract infection.

Laboratory

Most endemic areas, laboratory tests are unavailable. Commercial PCR based assay has high sensitivity and specificity.

Treatment

Tetracycline eye ointment for 6 weeks or a single-dose azithromycin systemically.

🖶 BIBLIOGRAPHY

1. Biebesheimer JB, House J, Hong KC, et al. Complete local elimination of infectious trachoma from severely affected communitieis after six biannual mass azithromycin distributions. Ophthalmology. 209;116:2047-50.
2. Solomon AW. (2011). Trachoma. [online] Available from www.emedicine.com/oph/TOPIC118.HTM. [Accessed September, 2013].

🖶 1EE.73C9.7G41A. ACNE ROSACEA (ACNE ERYTHEMATOSA; OCULAR ROSACEA)

General

Etiology unknown; usually occurs in women 30–50 years of age; pathogenetic mechanism remains unclear.

Ocular

Conjunctivitis; corneal neovascularization (wedge-shaped); keratitis; meibomianitis; blepharitis; recurrent chalazion; conjunctival hyperemia; superficial punctate keratopathy; corneal vascularization, thinning, perforation, and scarring; episcleritis; scleritis; iritis; nodular conjunctivitis.

Clinical

Symmetrical erythema; papules; pustules; telangiectasia; sebaceous gland hypertrophy of the forehead, malar eminences, and nose.

Laboratory

Diagnosis is made from clinical findings.

Treatment

Systemic antibiotics are useful in most cases.

🖶 BIBLIOGRAPHY

1. Banasikowaska AK, Singh S. (2012). Rosacea. [online] Available from www.emedicine.com/derm/TOPIC377.HTM. [Accessed September, 2013].

🖶 1EE.73C9.7G41B. ALKALINE INJURY OF THE EYE

General

A splash of alkaline solution causes the pH to rise and results in immediate damage to the external ocular tissues. These injuries are frequently seen from household chemicals or farming injuries from liquid ammonia used as fertilizer.

Ocular

Pain; lacrimation; blepharospasm; rise in intraocular pressure; rapid penetration of the cornea and sclera; chemical injury to iris, lens or ciliary body; symblepharon; phthisis bulbi; ankyloblepharon.

Laboratory

Diagnosis is made by clinical findings and history.

Treatment

Immediate copious irrigation, sticky paste of lime should be removed with a cotton-tipped applicator, mydriasis and topical antibiotics, pain medications, treatment of glaucoma with carbonic anhydrase inhibitors, patching and soft contact lenses may facilitate re-epithelialization, insertion of a methyl methacrylate ring may prevent fibrinous adhesions, lysis of adhesions with or without mucous membrane grafts, corneal stem cell transplantation, corneal transplantation, keratoprosthesis and conjunctival autografts.

🖶 BIBLIOGRAPHY

1. Roy FH, Fraunfelder FW, Fraunfelder FT. Roy and Fraunfelder's Current Ocular Therapy, 6th edition. London, UK: Elsevier; 2008.

🔲 1EE.73C9.7G41C. CHLAMYDIA (INCLUSION CONJUNCTIVITIS; PARATRACHOMA)

General

Organism that infects the epithelium of mucoid surfaces; sexually transmitted; major cause of non-gonococcal urethritis in men and cervicitis in women; major cause of neonatal ophthalmia; *C. trachomatis* is an intracellular bacterium lacking respiratory enzymes that has an affinity for mucosal epithelium; serotypes A through C have been epidemiologically associated with trachoma; serotypes E through K have been associated with genital infection and keratoconjunctivitis in sexually active adults and neonates; other serotypes have been associated with lymphogranuloma venereum and Reiter syndrome.

Ocular

Follicular conjunctivitis; corneal opacities; keratitis; corneal ulcer; lid edema; uveitis.

Clinical

Pneumonia; gastrointestinal disturbances; genital discharge.

Laboratory

Giemsa stain, cell culture—time intensive, direct fluorescent monoclonal antibiotics to stain smears.

Treatment

Three to six weeks of oral tetracycline (500 mg QID), oral doxycycline (100 mg BID), or oral erythromycin stearate (500 mg QID). Simultaneous treatment of all sexual partners is important to prevent reinfection.

🔲 BIBLIOGRAPHY

1. Bashour M. (2012). Ophthalmologic manifestations of Chlamydia. [online] Available from www.emedicine.com/oph/TOPIC494.HTM. [Accessed September, 2013].

🔲 1EE.73C9.7G41D. BENIGN MUCOSAL PEMPHIGOID (CHRONIC CICATRICIAL CONJUNCTIVITIS; CICATRICIAL PEMPHIGOID; ESSENTIAL SHRINKAGE OF THE CONJUNCTIVA; MEMBRANE PEMPHIGUS; OCULARPEMPHIGOID)

General

Etiology unknown; involving older age group, especially over 70 years; chronic autoimmune disorder characterized by fibrosis beneath the conjunctival epithelium; associated with the major histocompatibility complex class I alleles, which confer susceptibility to the disease; likely due to a multigene effect and associated with environmental factors; incidence in women is twice as frequent as men, no geographic or racial predilection.

Ocular

Conjunctivitis; absence of goblet cells of conjunctiva; conjunctival ulcer; pannus and keratitis; corneal opacity; entropion; trichiasis; cicatrization of lacrimal ducts; corneal perforation; symblepharon; dry eyes; bilateral involvement (may be asymmetrical); ocular shrinkage; xerosis; conjunctival and corneal bullae.

Clinical

Subepidermal and subepithelial blistering of mucous membranes; blisters may occur in pharyngeal, laryngeal, nasal, anal and genital mucosa.

Laboratory

Diagnosis is made by clinical findings.

Treatment

Subconjunctival injections of steroid or mitomycin may be helpful. Systemic immunomodulators are the major therapeutic plan.

🔲 BIBLIOGRAPHY

1. Foster CS, Hamam R, Letko E. (2011). Ophthalmologic manifestations of cicatricial pemphigoid. [online] Available from www.emedicine.com/oph/TOPIC83.HTM. [Accessed September, 2013].

1EE.73C9.7G41E. CONGENITAL LUES (CONGENITAL SYPHILIS)

General

It is caused by intrauterine transplacental infection of fetus by *T. pallidum* (*see* syphilis).

Ocular

Conjunctivitis; keratitis; dacryocystitis; optic nerve atrophy; periostitis; anisocoria; Argyll Robertson pupil; retinal degeneration; nystagmus; gumma of conjunctiva, eyelids, and orbit; paresis of extraocular muscles; secondary glaucoma; uveitis; iridoschisis.

Clinical

Cutaneous and mucous membrane lesions; periostitis; anemia; hepatosplenomegaly; ectodermal defects; CNS involvement; gummatous lesions.

Laboratory

Fluorescent treponemal antibody-absorption (FTA-ABS) and microhemagglutination assay (MHA-TP) are the standard test. All patients with syphilis should also be tested for HIV.

Treatment

Parenteral penicillin is the preferred treatment for all stages of syphilis. The treatment varies from primary and secondary syphilis, late latent syphilis, tertiary syphilis and neurosyphilis. Ocular treatment includes topical steroids and cycloplegics and it can relieve the symptoms of anterior uveitis and interstitial keratitis. Subconjunctival steroids have been used to relieve recurrent anterior segment inflammation. Severe corneal opacification may require keratoplasty; however, with recurrent inflammation and graft rejection.

BIBLIOGRAPHY

1. Waseem M. (2011). Pediatric syphilis. [online] Available from www.emedicine.com/ped/TOPIC2193.HTM. [Accessed September, 2013].

1EE.73C9.7G41F. DERMATITIS HERPETIFORMIS (DUHRING-BROCQ DISEASE)

General

Malignant; atypical; does not respond well to sulfone or sulfapyridine therapy; uncommon; autoimmune blistering dermatosis; pruritic eruption involving the scalp, buttocks, lower back, and extensor surface of arms; autoantibody is generally of IgA class causing deposition at the dermal-epidermal junction.

Ocular

Bullae of conjunctiva, skin, and mucous membranes; blisters are intraepithelial (acantholysis) and usually do not leave scars; epithelium desquamates in patches; corneal and conjunctival vascularization; symblepharon; cataract.

Clinical

Vesicles; erythema; pruritus; burning; eruption classically involves extensor surface of the knees, elbows, buttocks, sacrum, scapula, and scalp.

Laboratory

Diagnosis is made by clinical findings and skin biopsy.

Treatment

Dapsone and sulfapyridine are the primary medications used for therapy. Avoidance of gluten is also helpful.

BIBLIOGRAPHY

1. Miller JL, Zaman SA. (2013). Dermatitis herpetiformis. [online] Available from www.emedicine.com/derm/TOPIC95.HTM. [Accessed September, 2013].

☐ 1EE.73C9.7G41G. EPIDEMIC KERATOCONJUNCTIVITIS

General

Highly communicable; adenovirus types 8 and 19; usually bilateral; epidemic keratoconjunctivitis has been reported worldwide associated with 11 virus serotypes, with serotypes 8, 11, and 19 being the most common responsible ones.

Ocular

Follicular or membranous conjunctivitis; chemosis; subconjunctival hemorrhages; corneal opacity; punctate epithelial keratitis; corneal ulcer; blepharospasm; lid edema; serous discharge; uveitis; epiphora.

Clinical

Submaxillary and cervical lymphadenopathy.

Laboratory

Viral isolation on cell culture from conjunctival scrapings.

Treatment

No effective topical or systemic treatment available. Topical steroids may be used if epithelial keratitis occurs.

☐ BIBLIOGRAPHY

1. Bawazeer A. (2011). Epidemic keratoconjunctivitis. [online] Available from www.emedicine.com/oph/TOPIC677.HTM. [Accessed September, 2013].

☐ 1EE.73C9.7G41H. SCALDED SKIN SYNDROME (TOXIC EPIDERMAL NECROLYSIS; RITTER DISEASE; TOXIC EPIDERMAL NECROLYSIS OF LYELL; STAPHYLOCOCCAL SCALDED SKIN SYNDROME; LYELL SYNDROME; EPIDERMOLYSIS ACUTA TOXICA; TOXIC EPIDERMAL NECROLYSIS) SYMBLEPHARON

General

Generalized exfoliative dermatitis frequently affecting neonates and resulting from an initial focal staphylococcal infection (i.e. Staphylococcal ophthalmia neonatorum); toxic epidermal necrolysis usually refers to manifestation in the adult secondary to a drug reaction but affects all ages; immunopathogenetic mechanisms probably initiated with drug-skin binding with aberrant immune responses, including complement and IgG deposition with the epidermis and mucosa; recent reports suggest that patients with the AIDS are at higher risk for developing mucocutaneous reactions, such as toxic epidermal necrolysis; mortality rate approximately 30%.

Ocular

Necrotic areas of lids, conjunctiva, and cornea; symblepharon; loss of corneal epithelium; corneal ulcer; leukoma; perforation of globe; abolition of lacrimal secretion; conjunctival chemosis; blepharitis; entropion; periorbital swelling; trichiasis; distichiasis; fornix shortening.

Clinical

Widespread reddening and tenderness of the skin followed by the exfoliation of large areas of skin; in children, erythema starts usually around the mouth and spreads over the entire body within hours, followed by blisters and large exudative lesions; fever; shock.

Laboratory

Culture and biopsy of the lesion.

Treatment

Intravenous penicillinase-resistant and antistaphylococcal antibiotics. Cloxacillin is the treatment of choice.

☐ BIBLIOGRAPHY

1. Lopez-Garcia JS, Jara LR, Garcia-Lozano CI, et al. Ocular features and histopathologic changes during follow-up of toxic epidermal necrolysis. Ophthalmology. 2011;118:265-71.
2. Kim JH, Benson P. (2012). Dermatologic manifestations of staphylococcal scalded skin syndrome. [online] Available from www.emedicine.com/derm/TOPIC402.HTM. [Accessed September, 2013].

⊡ 1EE.73C9.7G41I. GOLDSCHEIDER SYNDROME (WEBER-COCKAYNE SYNDROME; EPIDERMOLYSIS BULLOSA; DOMINANT EPIDERMOLYSIS BULLOSA DYSTROPHIEA ALBOPAPULOIDEA)

General

Rare; Weber-Cockayne syndrome, inherited as an autosomal dominant trait, is actually a milder form without scar formation, whereas Goldscheider syndrome, inherited either autosomal dominant or recessive, shows dystrophic changes with scarring; consanguinity frequent.

Ocular

Blepharitis; shrinkage of conjunctiva; pseudomembrane formation with symblepharon; conjunctivitis; bullous keratitis and subepithelial blisters lead to erosions with subsequent ulcerations and corneal opacities or even perforation; sclera may be similarly involved; lagophthalmos, cicatricial lacrimal stenosis; retinal detachment; cataract; pannus.

Clinical

Vesicular and bullous skin lesions and similar lesions of mucous membranes occur spontaneously or after mild trauma; keloid scars and contraction after healing are common in the dystrophic forms, whereas in the mild form the lesions heal without scarring but may leave some skin pigmentation; growth and mental retardation may be present in the group with recessive inheritance; stenosis of the larynx due to scarring may occur.

Laboratory

Obtain a skin biopsy following a thorough history and physical examination.

Treatment

Wound healing and prevention of infection is the preferred strategy. Esophageal lesions can be managed with phenytoin and oral steroid elixirs to reduce the symptoms of dysphagia. In addition, if oral candidiasis is present, an anticandidal medication is helpful. Patients can experience recurrent blepharitis in one or both eyes along with bullous lesions of the conjunctiva, corneal ulcerations, corneal scarring, obliteration of tear ducts, eyelid lesions and cicatricial conjunctivitis. Corneal erosions are treated with antibiotic ointment and use of cycloplegic agents to reduce ciliary spasm and provide comfort. Avoid using tape to patch the eye because of frequent blistering of the skin under the adhesive. Chronic blepharitis can result in cicatricial ectropion and exposure keratitis. Moisture chambers and ocular lubricants are used commonly for management. This disorder also has been treated with full-thickness skin grafting to the upper eyelid.

⊡ BIBLIOGRAPHY

1. Marinkovich MP. (2012). Epidermolysis bullosa. [online] Available from www.emedicine.com/derm/TOPIC124.HTM. [Accessed September, 2013].

⊡ 1EE.73C9.7G41J. STEVENS-JOHNSON SYNDROME [DERMATOSTOMATITIS; ERYTHEMA MULTIFORME EXUDATIVUM; SYNDROMA MUCOCUTANEO-OCULARE; BAADER DERMATOSTOMATITIS SYNDROME; MUCOSAL-RESPIRATORY SYNDROME; FUCHS (2) SYNDROME; MUCOCUTANEOUS OCULAR SYNDROME]

General

Etiology unknown; affects all ages; most frequently seen in first and third decades of life; prevalent in males; drugs are the most commonly identified etiologic factor in this condition.

Ocular

Hypopyon; iritis; keratitis; corneal ulcers; keratoconjunctivitis sicca; chemosis; conjunctivitis; widespread fibrinoid necrosis of conjunctival vessels; blepharitis; endophthalmitis; phthisis bulbi; uveitis; cataracts; pannus; optic neuritis; keratoconus;

adenoviral conjunctivitis has been reported to have precipitated Stevens-Johnson syndrome; orbital cyst may be a complication.

Clinical

General malaise, headaches, chills, and fever; severe skin and mucous membrane eruptions (erythema multiforme); dorsa of hands and feet are most frequently affected; rhinitis; balanitis; vulvovaginitis; urethritis (nonspecific); cystitis; patients with AIDS are at higher risk of developing Stevens-Johnson syndrome.

Laboratory

No laboratory tests are specific to Stevens-Johnson syndrome. Diagnosis is made by clinical findings.

Treatment

Systemic treatment with steroids is controversial. Antibiotics are used based on clinical course. Eyelid hygiene performed as needed.

BIBLIOGRAPHY

1. Plaza JA, Dronen SC, Foster J, et al. (2011). Erythema multiforme. [online] Available from www.emedicine.com/med/TOPIC727.HTM. [Accessed September, 2013].

1EE.73C9.7G41K. BULLOUS ICHTHYOSIFORM ERYTHRODERMA (COLLODION BABY; CONGENITAL ICHTHYOSIS; EPIDERMOLYTIC HYPERKERATOSIS; ICHTHYOSIS; ICHTHYOSIS VULGARIS; LAMELLAR ICHTHYOSIS; NONBULLOUS ICHTHYOSIFORM ERYTHRODERMA; XERODERMA; X-LINKED ICHTHYOSIS)

General

Autosomal inherited disorder; affects both sexes; normal at birth; onset within first 7 days; X-linked; pathogenesis may be secondary to physicochemical changes of corneal tissues including accumulation of cholesterol sulfate.

Ocular

Keratopathy; corneal scarring; keratitis; conjunctivitis; lagophthalmos; photophobia; ectropion; lid erythema; lacrimation; keratoconus; deep corneal punctate/filiform lesions.

Clinical

At birth, the skin surface is moist, red, and tender; within several days, thick scales form.

Laboratory

Diagnosis is made by clinical findings.

Treatment

Genetic counseling and prenatal diagnosis also can be offered. Newborns with denuded skin are at increased risk for infection, secondary sepsis and electrolyte imbalance and should be transferred to the neonatal intensive care unit (NICU) to be monitored and treated as needed.

BIBLIOGRAPHY

1. Chen TS, Metz BJ. (2012). Epidermolytic hyperkeratosis (bullous congenital ichthyosiform erythroderma). [online] Available from www.emedicine.com/derm/TOPIC590.HTM. [Accessed September, 2013].

⊟ 1EE.73C9.7G41L. CONTACT DERMATITIS (DERMATITIS VENENATA)

General

Reaction of skin due to contact with foreign material; inflammatory disorder of the skin that may result from immunologic hypersensitivity (allergic contact dermatitis) or cutaneous injury not involving immunologic mechanisms (irritant contact dermatitis) from offending topical agents.

Ocular

Keratoconjunctivitis; chemosis; leukoma; corneal ulcer; pruritus of lids.

Clinical

Dermatitis; itching, erythema; vesiculation; edema with weeping and crusting.

Laboratory

Diagnosis is made by clinical findings.

Treatment

Adequate hygiene and avoidance of the contactant may be helpful. Many cases of localized mild contact dermatitis respond well to cool compresses and adequate wound care. Antibiotic therapy may be necessary for secondary infection. Low-strength topical steroids, such as hydrocortisone; may be effective in decreasing inflammation and symptoms associated with very mild contact dermatitis. Systemic steroids are the mainstay of therapy in acute episodes of severe extensive allergic contact dermatitis.

⊟ BIBLIOGRAPHY

1. Crowe MA. (2011). Pediatric contact dermatitis. [online] Available from www.emedicine.com/ped/TOPIC2569. HTM. [Accessed September, 2013].

⊟ 1EE.73C9.7G41M. FUCHS-LYELL SYNDROME (DEBRÉ-LAMY-LYELL SYNDROME; TOXIC EPIDERMAL NECROLYSIS)

General

Allergic reaction with severe manifestations; similar to Fuchs-Salzmann-Terrien syndrome (*see* Fuchs-Salzmann-Terrien syndrome); may result as a reaction to *Staphylococcus aureus* toxin in children or associated with certain medications, including penicillin, sulfa drugs, nonsteroidal anti-inflammatory agents, and allopurinol.

Ocular

Obstruction of nasolacrimal duct; cicatricial changes in conjunctiva and cornea; conjunctivitis; symblepharon; corneal ulceration and possible perforation.

Clinical

Inflammation of mucous membrane with ulcerations; general epidermolysis; cicatricial changes, especially of orifices.

Laboratory

Hematology studies, chemistry to assess fluid and electrolyte losses, liver enzyme tests, coagulation studies.

Treatment

Management requires prompt detection and withdrawal of all potential causative agents, evaluation, and largely supportive care.

⊟ BIBLIOGRAPHY

1. Cohen V, Jellinek SP, Schwartz RA. (2013). Toxic epidermal necrolysis. [online] Available from www.emedicine.com/med/TOPIC2291.HTM. [Accessed September, 2013].

🖰 1EE.73C9.7G41N. HYDROA VACCINIFORME

General

Sensitivity to sunlight.

Ocular

Conjunctivitis; corneal vesiculae; keratitis; cicatricial ectropion.

Clinical

Vesicular skin eruptions in areas exposed to sunlight.

Laboratory

Repetitive, broad-spectrum, UV-A phototesting

Treatment

Consult a dermatologist for evaluation and management of hydroa vacciniforme (HV).

🖰 BIBLIOGRAPHY

1. Sebastian QL, Del Rosario R. (2011). Hydroa vacciniforme. [online] Available from www.emedicine.com/derm/TOPIC181.HTM. [Accessed September, 2013].

🖰 1EE.73C9.7G41O. IMPETIGO

General

Superficial primary pyoderma caused by streptococci and *Staphylococcus aureus*.

Ocular

Pustular, crusting lesions of lids and brows; conjunctivitis; corneal ulcer; cicatricial ankyloblepharon.

Clinical

Thin-roofed vesicles that develop a thin amber crust occur on face and exposed areas of the extremities; extremely common skin infections caused by *S. aureus* in patients infected with HIV.

Laboratory

Diagnosis is made by clinical findings.

Treatment

Antibiotics are the mainstay of therapy and the chosen agent must provide coverage against both *S. aureus* and *S. pyogenes*. Topical antibiotics are used in patients with small or few lesions.

🖰 BIBLIOGRAPHY

1. Lewis LS, Friedman AD. (2013). Impetigo. [online] Available from www.emedicine.com/derm/TOPIC195.HTM. [Accessed September, 2013].

🖰 1EE.73C9.7G41P. BULLOUS ICHTHYOSIFORM ERYTHRODERMA (COLLODION BABY; CONGENITAL ICHTHYOSIS; EPIDERMOLYTIC HYPERKERATOSIS; ICHTHYOSIS; ICHTHYOSIS VULGARIS; LAMELLAR ICHTHYOSIS; NONBULLOUS ICHTHYOSIFORM ERYTHRODERMA; XERODERMA; X-LINKED ICHTHYOSIS)

General

Autosomal inherited disorder; affects both sexes; normal at birth; onset within first 7 days; X-linked; pathogenesis may be secondary to physicochemical changes of corneal tissues including accumulation of cholesterol sulfate.

Ocular

Keratopathy; corneal scarring; keratitis; conjunctivitis; lagophthalmos; photophobia; ectropion; lid erythema; lacrimation; keratoconus; deep corneal punctate/filiform lesions.

Clinical

At birth, the skin surface is moist, red and tender; within several days, thick scales form.

Laboratory

Diagnosis is made by clinical findings.

Treatment

Genetic counseling and prenatal diagnosis also can be offered. Newborns with denuded skin are at increased risk for infection, secondary sepsis, and electrolyte imbalance and should be transferred to the neonatal intensive care unit (NICU) to be monitored and treated as needed.

⊟ BIBLIOGRAPHY

1. Chen TS, Metz BJ. (2012). Epidermolytic hyperkeratosis (bullous congenital ichthyosiform erythroderma). [online] Available from www.emedicine.com/derm/TOPIC590.HTM. [Accessed September, 2013].

⊟ 1EE.73C9.7G41Q. BENIGN MUCOSAL PEMPHIGOID (CHRONIC CICATRICIAL CONJUNCTIVITIS; CICATRICIAL PEMPHIGOID; ESSENTIAL SHRINKAGE OF THE CONJUNCTIVA; MEMBRANE PEMPHIGUS; OCULARPEMPHIGOID)

General

Etiology unknown; involving older age group, especially over 70 years; chronic autoimmune disorder characterized by fibrosis beneath the conjunctival epithelium; associated with the major histocompatibility complex class I alleles, which confer susceptibility to the disease; likely due to a multigene effect and associated with environmental factors; incidence in women is twice as frequent as men, no geographic or racial predilection.

Ocular

Conjunctivitis; absence of goblet cells of conjunctiva; conjunctival ulcer; pannus and keratitis; corneal opacity; entropion; trichiasis; cicatrization of lacrimal ducts; corneal perforation; symblepharon; dry eyes; bilateral involvement (may be asymmetrical); ocular shrinkage; xerosis; conjunctival and corneal bullae.

Clinical

Subepidermal and subepithelial blistering of mucous membranes; blisters may occur in pharyngeal, laryngeal, nasal, anal and genital mucosa.

Laboratory

Diagnosis is made by clinical findings.

Treatment

Subconjunctival injections of steroid or mitomycin may be helpful. Systemic immunomodulators are the major therapeutic plan.

⊟ BIBLIOGRAPHY

1. Foster CS, Hamam R, Letko E. (2011). Ophthalmologic manifestations of cicatricial pemphigoid. [online] Available from www.emedicine.com/oph/TOPIC83.HTM. [Accessed September, 2013].

⊟ 1EE.73C9.7G41R. LICHEN PLANUS

General

Conjunctival disorder associated with dermatologic disorder; disappears spontaneously.

Ocular

Conjunctivitis; cicatrizing conjunctivitis; keratin plaque on bulbar conjunctiva.

Clinical

Grayish-white papules; oral lesions may precede skin lesions.

Laboratory

Diagnosis is made by clinical findings.

Treatment

Topical and systemic corticosteroids, systemic immunomodulators.

🗗 BIBLIOGRAPHY

1. Foster CS, Hamam R, Letko E. (2011). Ophthalmologic manifestations of cicatricial pemphigoid. [online] Available from www.emedicine.com/oph/TOPIC83.HTM. [Accessed September, 2013].

🗗 1EE.73C9.7G41T. REITER SYNDROME (FIESSINGER-LEROY SYNDROME; CONJUNCTIVO-URETHRO-SYNOVIAL SYNDROME; IDIOPATHIC BLENNORRHEAL ARTHRITIS SYNDROME; POLYARTHRITIS ENTERICA)

General

Etiology unknown; males; onset ages 16–42 years; probably a combined infectious/autoimmune pathogenetic mechanism; reactive arthritis probably associated with infection with many different species of microorganisms; HLA-B27 confers disease susceptibility to infection.

Ocular

Sterile mucopurulent conjunctivitis, usually bilateral; photophobia; epiphora; iritis; keratitis; uveitis; paralysis of extraocular muscles; optic neuritis; secondary glaucoma; hypopyon; hyphema.

Clinical

Skin erythema; genital ulcerations; urethritis with discharge; cystitis with dysuria, abacterial pyuria and hematuria; arthritis with pain, swelling, heat and effusion; fever; weight loss; fatigue; malaise; fever; diarrhea; oral mucosal lesions; arthralgia.

Laboratory

Giemsa stain may reveal Gram-negative intracellular diplococci associated with gonorrhea. Stool cultures may also be helpful for enteric pathogens. HLA-B27 antigen testing will not provide a diagnosis but may be useful.

Treatment

Systemic antibiotics are useful. Topical corticosteroids and mydriatics should be administered early to minimize tissue damage. NSAIDs may help to reduce ocular inflammation.

🗗 BIBLIOGRAPHY

1. Bashour M. (2012). Ophthalmologic manifestations of reactive arthritis. [online] Available from www.emedicine.com/oph/TOPIC524.HTM. [Accessed September, 2013].

🗗 1EE.73C9.7G41U. KERATOCONJUNCTIVITIS SICCA AND SJÖGREN'S SYNDROME

General

Autoimmune disease, seen more frequently in females.

Clinical

Xerostomia (dry mouth), dry nasal and genital mucosa.

Ocular

Severe dry eyes, corneal ulceration, corneal perforation, corneal scarring and vascularization.

Laboratory

Biopsy of lip and lachrymal gland positive, anti-nuclear antibody rheumatoid factor (RF) and anti-ro (Sjögren's specific A) and anti-La (Sjögren specific B). Elevated IgG level positive—predication for positive biopsy.

Treatment

Severe cases—immunosuppressive agents as cyclosporin A and corticosteroids. Frequent application of tear substitutes, steroids, punctal plugs, bandage contacts and partial tarsorrhaphy.

🗗 BIBLIOGRAPHY

1. Foster CS, Yuksel E, Anzaar F, et al. (2013). Dry eye syndrome. [online] Available from www.emedicine.com/oph/TOPIC597.HTM. [Accessed September, 2013].

🗗 1EE.73C9.7G41V. STAPHYLOCOCCUS

General

Gram-positive coccus *Staphylococcus aureus*; most common cause of suppurative infection in humans; more common in patients with a previous disorders, such as diabetes, thyroid disease, renal failure, or malnutrition; although most *S. aureus* isolates from other sources are encapsulated, capsules have not been noted in ocular isolates.

Ocular

Uveitis; hypopyon; conjunctivitis; keratitis; cellulitis of lid; meibomianitis; ptosis; blepharitis; endophthalmitis; dacryocystitis; increased IOP; orbital periosteitis.

Clinical

Tissues hypertonic, edematous, and painful; lesion liquefies, forming creamy yellow pus; fever; nausea; vomiting; cough; dyspnea; abdominal pain; diarrhea; bloody stools; dehydration; shock.

Laboratory

Aerobic Gram-positive cocci bacteria grow in grape-like clusters. Coagulase positive indicates pathogenicity.

Treatment

Specific antimicrobial therapy is chosen based on the site and severity of the infection and the antimicrobial sensitivities of the organism involved.

🗗 BIBLIOGRAPHY

1. Tolan RW. (2012). Staphylococcus aureus infection. [online] Available from www.emedicine.com/ped/TOPIC2704.HTM. [Accessed September, 2013].

🗗 1EE.73C9.7G41W. ACQUIRED LUES (SYPHILIS; ACQUIRED SYPHILIS; LUES VENEREA; MALUM VENEREUM)

General

Causative agent, *T. pallidum*, usually transmitted sexually.

Ocular

Conjunctival chancroid; conjunctivitis; keratitis; blepharitis; ptosis; iris atrophy; hippus; dacryocystitis; optic nerve atrophy; optic neuritis; periostitis; episcleritis; scleritis; nystagmus; uveitis; vitreous hemorrhages; paralysis of sixth nerve; papilledema; retinal hemorrhages; retinitis proliferans; oculogyric crisis; neuroretinitis; papilledema (associated with aseptic meningitis); diffuse or multifocal chorioretinitis; vertical supranuclear gaze palsy; Benedikt syndrome.

Clinical

Primary lesion associated with regional lymphadenopathy; secondary bacteremic stage associated with generalized mucocutaneous lesions; tertiary stage characterized by destructive mucocutaneous, musculoskeletal, or parenchymal lesions, aortitis, or CNS disease; syphilis and HIV infection often coexist in the same patient who experiences a higher incidence and greater severity of neurologic and ocular manifestations; a significant percentage of patients infected with HIV-I and *T. pallidum* become seronegative to syphilis testing.

Laboratory

Serologic nontreponemal tests include VDRL and RPR.

Treatment

The goals are to reduce morbidity and to prevent complications. Penicillin is the antibiotic of choice for treating syphilis. Ocular syphilis should be treated the same as patients with neurosyphilis.

🗗 BIBLIOGRAPHY

1. Euerle B, Chandrasekar PH, Diaz MM, et al. (2012). Syphilis. [online] Available from www.emedicine.com/med/TOPIC2224.HTM. [Accessed September, 2013].
2. Majmudar PA. (2011). Interstitial keratitis overview of interstitial keratitis. [online] Available from www.emedicine.com/oph/TOPIC453.HTM. [Accessed September, 2013].

⊟ 1EE.73C9.7G41X. PROGRESSIVE SYSTEMIC SCLEROSIS (SCLERODERMA; SYSTEMIC SCLERODERMA)

General

Chronic connective tissue disease of unknown etiology; chronic and usually progressive disorder; typical onset is in third to fifth decade; ratio of women to men is 4:1; primary sites of pathology are the arterioles and capillaries of affected organs.

Ocular

Marginal corneal ulcers; shortened fornices of the conjunctiva; ptosis; cotton-wool patches of retina; papilledema; retinal hemorrhages; cicatrization of conjunctiva and cornea; blepharitis; blepharospasm; thready, tenacious yellow-white conjunctival discharge; hypertrophy of lacrimal gland; episcleritis; ocular myositis; Sjögren syndrome; uveitis; vitreous haze; keratitis sicca; decreased corneal sensation; iritis; ischemic choroidopathy; iris sectorial atrophy; blepharophimosis; heterochromia; keratoconus; central retinal vein occlusion; branch retinal vein occlusion.

Clinical

Vascular insufficiency; Raynaud's phenomenon; malaise; weight loss; stiffness; fever; polyarticular arthritis; diffuse edema of the hands; calcinosis; esophageal involvement; sclerodactyly; telangiectasis; esophageal stricture; renal failure; diffuse interstitial fibrosis.

Laboratory

No specific test establishes diagnosis. Hypergammaglobulinemia—50% of cases ANA increased in 40–70% cases.

Treatment

Skin thickening can be treated with D-penicillamine and other experimental drugs. Pruritus can be treated with moisturizers and histamine. Raynaud's phenomenon can be treated with calcium channel blockers. Renal crisis episodes are best prevented and treated with the aggressive use of ACE inhibitors. Myositis may be treated cautiously with steroids.

⊟ BIBLIOGRAPHY

1. Jimenez SA, Cronin PM, Koenig AS, et al. (2012). Scleroderma. [online] Available from www.emedicine.com/med/TOPIC2076.HTM. [Accessed September, 2013].

⊟ 1EE.73C9.7G41Y. VACCINIA (KERATITIS)

General

Laboratory virus used for vaccination against smallpox.

Ocular

Pustules of lids; edema of lids; conjunctivitis; orbital cellulitis; keratitis; pannus; corneal perforation; iridocyclitis; central serous retinopathy; perivasculitis; pseudoretinitis pigmentosa; ocular palsies papillitis; optic atrophy.

Clinical

Vesicles; pustules; erythema; fever; malaise; axillary lymphadenopathy; necrosis of skin; vaccinia gangrenosa; encephalomyelitis; drowsiness; vomiting; coma; death.

Laboratory

Immune deficiency workup should be considered as well as imaging studies.

Treatment

Vaccinia immunoglobulin (VIG) can be helpful in selected patients.

⊟ BIBLIOGRAPHY

1. Lee JJ, Diven D, Poonawalla TA, et al. (2012). Vaccinia. [online] Available from www.emedicine.com/med/TOPIC2356.HTM. [Accessed September, 2013].

1EE.73C9.7G42C. LISTERELLOSIS (LISTERIOSIS)

General

It is caused by Gram-positive bacillus *Listeria monocytogenes*. High mortality among pregnant women, their fetuses, and immunocompromised persons with symptoms of abortion, neonatal death, septicemia, meningitis, brain abscesses, endocarditis.

Ocular

Conjunctivitis; keratitis; corneal abscess and ulcer; blepharitis; uveitis; endophthalmitis; cataract; secondary glaucoma.

Clinical

Vomiting; cardiorespiratory distress; diarrhea; hepatosplenomegaly; maculopapular skin lesions.

Laboratory

Histopathology and culture of rash, CT scanning or MRI may be useful in detecting abscesses in the brain or liver.

Treatment

Antibiotics as well as careful monitoring of the patient's temperature, respiratory system, fluid and electrolyte balance, nutrition and cardiovascular support.

BIBLIOGRAPHY

1. Zach T, Anderson-Berry AL. (2013). Listeria infection. [online] Available from www.emedicine.com/ped/TOPIC1319.HTM. [Accessed September, 2013].

1EE.73C9.7G42D. PNEUMOCOCCAL INFECTIONS (STREPTOCOCCUS PNEUMONIAE INFECTIONS)

General

Gram-positive diplococcus *S. pneumoniae*; some strains are encapsulated while others are not; ocular infections usually are caused by the encapsulated strains; conjunctivitis and corneal scarring produced in an animal model have been attributed to a hemolytic cytolytic exopeptidase.

Ocular

Hypopyon; conjunctivitis; keratitis; corneal ulcer; endophthalmitis; dacryocystitis; uveitis; orbital cellulitis; secondary glaucoma; ophthalmia neonatorum.

Clinical

Upper respiratory infection; chills; sharp pain in hemithorax; cough with sputum production; fever; headache; gastrointestinal symptoms.

Laboratory

Gram stain demonstrates Gram-positive cocci in pairs. The unattached end of each cocci is slightly pointed outward.

Treatment

Impetigo, oral antibiotics and topical antibiotic ointment; preseptal cellulitis, oral antibiotics; orbital cellulitis, need team of infectious diseases, otolaryngology and ophthalmology to develop plan of therapy; dacryocystitis, oral and topical antibiotics, dacryocystorhinostomy may be necessary; conjunctivitis, topical antibiotic; keratitis, topical antibiotics; poststreptococcal reactive arthritis can occur with uveitis, topical steroids and cycloplegics; endophthalmitis, prompt and aggressive therapy with topical, intravitreal and sometimes systemic antibiotics and pars plana vitrectomy; postrefractive surgery keratitis, flap raised, cultured and treated. Occasionally the flap should be amputated.

BIBLIOGRAPHY

1. Muench DF. (2012). Pneumococcal infections. [online] Available from www.emedicine.com/med/TOPIC1848.HTM. [Accessed September, 2013].

⊟ 1EE.73C9.7G42E. STAPHYLOCOCCUS

General

Gram-positive coccus *S. aureus*; most common cause of suppurative infection in humans; more common in patients with a previous disorders, such as diabetes, thyroid disease, renal failure, or malnutrition; although most *S. aureus* isolates from other sources are encapsulated, capsules have not been noted in ocular isolates.

Ocular

Uveitis; hypopyon; conjunctivitis; keratitis; cellulitis of lid; meibomianitis; ptosis; blepharitis; endophthalmitis; dacryocystitis; increased IOP; orbital periosteitis.

Clinical

Tissues hypertonic, edematous, and painful; lesion liquefies, forming creamy yellow pus; fever; nausea; vomiting; cough; dyspnea; abdominal pain; diarrhea; bloody stools; dehydration; shock.

Laboratory

Aerobic Gram-positive cocci bacteria grow in grape-like clusters. Coagulase positive indicates pathogenicity.

Treatment

Specific antimicrobial therapy is chosen based on the site and severity of the infection and the antimicrobial sensitivities of the organism involved.

⊟ BIBLIOGRAPHY

1. Tolan RW. (2012). Staphylococcus aureus infection. [online] Available from www.emedicine.com/ped/TOPIC2704.HTM. [Accessed September, 2013].

⊟ 1EE.73C9.7G6C. ESCHERICHIA COLI

General

Gram-negative rod found in the gastrointestinal tract; urinary tract is the usual portal of entry.

Ocular

Uveitis; hyphema; hypopyon; gas bubbles in anterior chamber; purulent conjunctivitis; keratitis; corneal edema; panophthalmitis; endophthalmitis; glaucoma.

Clinical

Diarrhea; gastroenteritis; dehydration.

Laboratory

Anaerobic Gram-negative rod.

Treatment

Antibiotic therapy should start with ampicillin until sensitivity reports return.

⊟ BIBLIOGRAPHY

1. Suh DW. (2011). Ophthalmologic manifestations of Escherichia Coli. [online] Available from www.emedicine.com/oph/TOPIC496.HTM. [Accessed September, 2013].

⊟ 1EE.73C9.7G6D. HAEMOPHILUS INFLUENZAE

General

Gram-negative rod.

Ocular

Conjunctivitis; cellulitis; tenonitis; uveitis; vitreous opacity; pannus; corneal opacity.

Clinical

Pharyngitis; epiglottitis; laryngotracheitis; pneumonia; bronchitis; otitis media; meningitis; cellulitis; septic arthritis; sinusitis.

Laboratory

Gram-negative coccobacillus with eight biotypes and six serotypes. Gram stain and culture.

Treatment

Antibiotics are the mainstay of treatment. Invasive and serious infections are best treated with an intravenous third-generation cephalosporin until antibiotic sensitivities are available.

BIBLIOGRAPHY

1. Devarajan VR. (2012). Haemophilus influenzae infections. [online] Available from www.emedicine.com/med/TOPIC936.HTM. [Accessed September, 2013].

1EE.73C9.7G6E. RHINOSCLEROMA (KLEBSIELLA RHINOSCLEROMATIS)

General

Chronic granulomatous disease; Gram-negative bacillus; cicatricial deformities; chronic progressive granulomatous infection of the upper airways caused by the bacterium *K. rhinoscleromatis*.

Ocular

Conjunctivitis; chronic dacryocystitis; lid inflammation.

Clinical

Granulomas affecting nose and upper respiratory tract causing sclerosis and deformities; airway obstruction; leprosy; paracoccidioidomycosis; sarcoidosis; basal cell carcinoma; Wegener granulomatosis; also may occur in immunocompromised HIV patients.

Laboratory

Culturing in MacConkey agar are positive in only 50–60% of patients. CT scan and MRI are useful.

Treatment

Bronchoscopy can be use as the initial treatment. Long-term antimicrobial and in cases where obstruction is suspected, surgical intervention may be necessary.

BIBLIOGRAPHY

1. Schwartz RA, Goriniene E. (2013). Rhinoscleroma. [online] Available from www.emedicine.com/derm/TOPIC831.HTM. [Accessed September, 2013].

1EE.73C9.7G6F. MORAXELLA LACUNATA

General

Gram-negative rod; causes chronic angular blepharoconjunctivitis; without treatment, may persist for months or years; normally found in flora of respiratory tract; seen more frequently in alcoholics and those with poor sanitary habits; *Moraxella* organisms produce proteases, although those are not related directly to their pathogenetic mechanism.

Ocular

Catarrhal angular conjunctivitis; corneal ulcer; hypopyon, chronic blepharitis; eczema; lateral canthal skin erythema; iridocyclitis.

Clinical

Alcoholism; impaired nutrition; dermatitis.

Laboratory

Aerobic, oxidase positive, Gram-negative diplococcus or coccobacilli morphologically indistinguishable from *Neisseria*.

Treatment

Artificial tears, cold compresses, antibiotics.

BIBLIOGRAPHY

1. Baum J, Fedukowicz HB, Jordan A. A survey of Moraxella corneal ulcers in a derelict population. Am J Ophthalmol. 1980;90:476-80.
2. Burd EM. Bacterial keratitis and conjunctivitis. In: Smolin G, Thoft RA (Eds). The Cornea. Boston: Little, Brown and Company; 1994. pp. 20-1.
3. Roy FH, Fraunfelder FW, Fraunfelder FT. Roy and Fraunfelder's Current Ocular Therapy, 6th edition. Philadelphia: WB Saunders; 2008.
4. van Bijsterveld OP. The incidence of Moraxella on mucous membranes and the skin. Am J Ophthalmol. 1972;74:72-6.

⊟ 1EE.73C9.7G6G. GONORRHEA

General

It is caused by *N. gonorrhoeae*, which is transmitted sexually.

Ocular

Conjunctivitis; eyelid edema; keratitis; uveitis.

Clinical

Pelvic inflammatory disease; arthritis; dermatitis; carditis; meningitis.

Laboratory

Gram-stain smear demonstrates Gram-negative diplo-cocci with polymorphonuclear leukocytes in conjunctival exudates.

Treatment

Therapy consists of systemic antibiotics; topical antibiot-ics are relatively ineffective in the treatment of eye disease. It is important to treat all sexual partners simultaneously to prevent reinfection.

⊟ BIBLIOGRAPHY

1. Wong B. (2012). Gonorrhea. [online] Available from www.emedicine.com/oph/TOPIC497.HTM. [Accessed September, 2013].

⊟ 1EE.73C9.7G6H. MENINGOCOCCEMIA (NEISSERIA MENINGITIDIS; MENINGITIS)

General

Systemic bacterial infection caused by *N. meningitidis*; can be present chronically in patients with immune deficiencies including deficient complement levels.

Ocular

Photophobia; conjunctivitis; chemosis; keratitis; uveitis; panophthalmitis; retinal endophlebitis; macular edema; papillitis; optic neuritis; paresis of sixth or seventh nerve; nystagmus; miosis; hippus; cortical blindness; papilledema (rare); conjunctival petechiae; strabismus.

Clinical

Meningitis; fever; malaise; joint pain; splenic enlargement.

Laboratory

Cultures from blood, spinal fluid, or joint fluid.

Treatment

Treat with antibiotics promptly.

⊟ BIBLIOGRAPHY

1. Javid MH, Ahmed SH. (2013). Meningococcemia. [online] Available from www.emedicine.com/med/TOPIC1445.HTM. [Accessed September, 2013].

⊟ 1EE.73C9.7G6I. PROTEUS SYNDROME

General

A harmarteo neoplastic disorder with variable clinical manifestations.

Ocular

Myopia; band keratopathy; cataract; vitreous hemorrhage; chorioretinal mass; serous retinal detachment.

Clinical

Thickening of the bones of the external auditory meatus and cranial fossa; enlargement of the left internal auditory meatus; deformities of the feet and toes.

Laboratory

Proteus organisms are easily recovered through routine laboratory cultures. An ultrasound of the kidneys or a CT scan should be considered as part of a workup.

Treatment

Traditional treatment includes oral quinolone for 3 days or trimethoprim/sulfamethoxazole.

BIBLIOGRAPHY

1. Struble K. (2011). Proteus infections. [online] Available from www.emedicine.com/med/TOPIC1929.HTM. [Accessed September, 2013].

1EE.73C9.7G6J. PSEUDOMONAS AERUGINOSA

General

Gram-negative rod that is ubiquitous in water, soil and plants. Commonly found in hospital environment.

Clinical

None.

Ocular

Foreign body sensation, conjunctival injection, photophobia and corneal ulceration.

Laboratory

Gram-negative rod on Gram stain and Giemsa stain from corneal ulcer. Culturing contact lens and lens solutions may help to grow organisms.

Treatment

Fortified tobramycin and fortified cefazolin are drugs of choice.

BIBLIOGRAPHY

1. Roy FH, Fraunfelder FW, Fraunfelder FT. Roy and Fraunfelder's Current Ocular Therapy, 6th edition. London: Elsevier; 2008.

1EE.73C9.7G7. VACCINIA (KERATITIS)

General

Laboratory virus used for vaccination against smallpox.

Ocular

Pustules of lids; edema of lids; conjunctivitis; orbital cellulitis; keratitis; pannus; corneal perforation; iridocyclitis; central serous retinopathy; perivasculitis; pseudoretinitis pigmentosa; ocular palsies papillitis; optic atrophy.

Clinical

Vesicles; pustules; erythema; fever; malaise; axillary lymphadenopathy; necrosis of skin; vaccinia gangrenosa; encephalomyelitis; drowsiness; vomiting; coma; death.

Laboratory

Immune deficiency workup should be considered as well as imaging studies.

Treatment

Vaccinia Ig can be helpful in selected patients.

BIBLIOGRAPHY

1. Lee JJ, Diven D, Poonawalla TA, et al. (2012). Vaccinia. [online] Available from www.emedicine.com/med/TOPIC2356.HTM. [Accessed September, 2013].

⊟ 1EE.73C9.7G8A. ACTINOMYCOSIS

General

Gram-positive *Actinomyces israelii.*

Ocular

Hypopyon; conjunctivitis; keratitis; corneal ulcer; proptosis; uveitis; dacryocystitis; yellow nodules on conjunctiva and eyelids; occlusion of nasolacrimal canaliculi; canaliculitis; orbital abscess; endophthalmitis (rare).

Clinical

Chronic inflammatory induration and sinus formation.

Laboratory

Canalicular discharge may be sent for Gram stain/Giemsa stain, cultures and sensitivities (i.e. blood agar, Sabouraud, anaerobic) and special stains (i.e. calcofluor white stain).

Treatment

Penicillins and cephalosporins are useful. Subconjunctival penicillin coadministered with systemic iodides and topical sulfacetamide or penicillin can be used.

⊟ BIBLIOGRAPHY

1. Roque MR, Roque BL, Foster CS. (2012). Actinomycosis in ophthalmology. [online] Available from www.emedicine.com/oph/TOPIC491.HTM. [Accessed September, 2013].

⊟ 1EE.73C9.7G8B. CANDIDIASIS

General

Yeast-like opportunistic fungal infection caused by *C. albicans.*

Ocular

Uveitis; hypopyon; conjunctivitis; keratitis; corneal ulcer; blepharitis; endophthalmitis; dacryocystitis; papillitis; retinal atrophy; Roth spot; vitreous abscess; retrobulbar abscess; retinal detachment; panophthalmitis; chorioretinitis; infectious crystalline keratopathy.

Clinical

C. albicans normally is present as an intestinal saprophyte in 35–75% of the human population; in situations of internal environmental change, however, *Candida* can become pathogenic (obesity, diabetes mellitus, malignancy, and other debilitating conditions).

Laboratory

Common yeast up to 50% of healthy individuals isolate directly from the eye should be attempted to confirm the presence of organism. Blood agar and Sabouraud's dextrose agar may be used; PCR for species identification.

Treatment

Mucocutaneous infection typically responds to topical therapy. Antifungal therapy should be started immediately after necessary cultures have been obtained from all suspected sites of infection. Infectious disease specialists are typically involved in cases of invasive candidiasis.

⊟ BIBLIOGRAPHY

1. Hedayati T. (2012). Candidiasis in emergency medicine. [online] Available from www.emedicine.com/emerg/TOPIC76.HTM. [Accessed September, 2013].

🗗 1EE.73C9.7G8C. NOCARDIOSIS

General

Aerobic actinomycetaceae that may cause a chronic suppurative process; aerobic Gram-positive filamentous bacteria with branching pattern which resemble fungi.

Ocular

Conjunctivitis; keratitis; corneal ulcer; uveitis; lid involvement; orbital cellulitis; endophthalmitis; glaucoma; external ophthalmoplegia; scleritis; canaliculitis; preseptal cellulitis.

Clinical

Granuloma; draining sinuses; brain abscess; meningitis.

Laboratory

Gram-positive filamentous structures with an intermittent or a beaded staining pattern, weakly acid-fast. Organism culture from the infection (i.e. respiratory secretion, skin biopsies, or aspirates from abscesses).

Treatment

Antimicrobial therapy is the treatment of choice.

🗗 BIBLIOGRAPHY

1. DeCroos FC, Garg P, Reddy AK, et al. Optimizing diagnosis and management of nocardia keratitis, scleritis, and endophthalmitis: 11 year microbial and clinical overview. Ophthalmology. 2011;118:1193-200.
2. Greenfield RA. (2011). Nocardiosis. [online] Available from www.emedicine.com/med/TOPIC1644.HTM. [Accessed September, 2013].

🗗 1EE.73C9.7G9. WISKOTT-ALDRICH SYNDROME (CORNEAL ULCER)

General

Sex-linked recessive; early infancy with death in the first decade of life; abnormal immune responses; expression of clusters of differentiation (CD)-43 is defective in this X-chromosome-linked immunodeficiency disorder, suggesting that CD-43 might have a role in T-cell activation.

Ocular

Periorbital hemorrhages; vesicular skin eruptions; blepharitis; lid nodules; episcleritis; scleral icterus; conjunctival hemorrhages and purulent discharge; corneal ulcers; retinal hemorrhages; papilledema; peripapillary hemorrhages.

Clinical

Eczema; epistaxis; purpura; hematemesis; bloody diarrhea; otitis media.

Laboratory

Complete blood count, delayed-type hypersensitivity (DTH) skin test and chest radiographs.

Treatment

Stem cell reconstitution is the main stream of therapy.

🗗 BIBLIOGRAPHY

1. Schwartz RA, Siperstein R. (2013). Pediatric Wiskott-Aldrich syndrome. [online] Available from www.emedicine.com/ped/TOPIC2443.HTM. [Accessed September, 2013].

🗗 1EE.73C9.7G10. FLOPPY EYELID SYNDROME

General

Origin unknown; more common in males; overweight; X-chromosome-linked inheritance pattern or possible hormonal influence; it has been postulated that the degenerative changes in the tarsus may result from the combination of local pressure-induced lid ischemia and systemic hypoventilation.

Ocular

Easily everted, floppy upper eyelid and papillary conjunctivitis of the upper palpebral conjunctiva; upper eyelid everts during sleep, resulting in irritation, papillary conjunctivitis and conjunctival keratinization; most distinct feature is rubbery, malleable upper tarsus; keratoconus; punctate keratopathy; blepharoptosis; lash ptosis.

Clinical

Obesity; sleep apnea.

Laboratory

Conjunctival scrapings reveal keratinized epithelial cells. Bacterial cultures are important.

Treatment

Full-thickness upper and lower eyelid resection.

🗗 BIBLIOGRAPHY

1. Ezra DG, Beaconsfield M, Sira M, et al. Long-term outcomes of surgical approaches to the treatment of floppy eyelid syndrome. Ophthalmology. 2010;117(4):839-46.
2. Ezra DG, Beaconsfield M, Sira M, et al. The associations of floppy eyelid syndrome: a case control study. Ophthalmology. 2010;117(4):831-8.
3. Chatziralli IP, Sergentanis TN. Risk factors for intraoperative floppy iris syndrome: a meta-analysis. Ophthalmology. 2011;118(4):730-5.
4. Blaydon SM. (2011). Floppy eyelid syndrome. [online] Available from www.emedicine.com/oph/TOPIC605.HTM. [Accessed September, 2013].

🗗 1EE.73C9.7G13A. MOLLUSCUM CONTAGIOSUM

General

Etiologic agent of this disease is a poxvirus that can cause proliferative skin lesions anywhere on the body; commonly found in patients who are immunosuppressed.

Ocular

Lesions of lid, lid margin, conjunctiva, and cornea; conjunctivitis; keratitis; corneal ulcer.

Clinical

Well-defined, pearly appearing papules with umbilicated centers of varying size (3–10 mm); eczematization of the surrounding skin.

Laboratory

Craters have epithelial cells with large eosinophilic intracytoplasmic inclusion bodies (molluscum or Henderson Patterson bodies) when virus particles migrate to the granular layer of the epidermis, the inclusion bodies become basophilic.

Treatment

Topical agents cantharidin, tretinoin, podophyllin, trichloroacetic acid, tincture of iodine, silver nitrate or phenol, potassium hydroxide. Systemic agents include griseofulvin, methisazone and cimetidine.

🗗 BIBLIOGRAPHY

1. Bhatia AC. (2012). Molluscum contagiosum. [online] Available from www.emedicine.com/oph/TOPIC500.HTM. [Accessed September, 2013].

🗗 1EE.73C9.7G13.1. BASAL CELL CARCINOMA

General

Most common malignant neoplasm of lids; it can occasionally occur as a primary basal cell cancer of the conjunctiva and in the lacrimal canaliculus.

Ocular

Neoplasm most common on lower lid and medial canthus; lacrimation.

Clinical

Tumors of skin and other regions, including sinuses.

Laboratory

Typical histology findings. Imaging studies only for invading or deep tumor in the medial canthus.

Treatment

Surgery involves local excision; advanced and recurrent tumors are best managed by a multidisciplinary approach involving head and neck surgical oncologists. Photodynamic therapy and cryosurgery are also effective.

🗗 BIBLIOGRAPHY

1. Bader RS, Santacroce L, Diomede L, et al. (2012). Basal cell carcinoma. [online] Available from www.emedicine.com/ent/TOPIC722.HTM. [Accessed September, 2013].

🗗 1EE.73C9.7G13.2. SQUAMOUS CELL CARCINOMA OF EYELID

General

Relatively rare periocular malignancy which usually occurs in the lower eyelid.

Clinical

None.

Ocular

Tumor of the eyelid.

Laboratory

Careful biopsy and histologic examination.

Treatment

Systemic or intralesional chemotherapy, or both has been effective when used in conjunction with surgery or radiation.

🗗 BIBLIOGRAPHY

1. Monroe M. (2012). Head and neck cutaneous squamous cell carcinoma. [online] Available from emedicine.medscape.com/article/1212601-overview. [Accessed September, 2013].

🗗 1EE.73C9.7G13.6. HEMANGIOMA

General

It can occur throughout the body, particularly in the head; primary intraosseous orbital hemangiomas is rare; capillary hemangioma of the orbit and eyelids generally is unilateral.

Ocular

Hemangiomas of lids or orbit; ptosis; strabismus; amblyopia; proptosis; optic atrophy; hypermetropia; cavernous hemangiomas are the most common benign orbital tumors of adults.

Clinical

Ipsilateral hemangiomas of the brain and meninges.

Laboratory

Neuroimaging can be of great assistance in making the diagnosis.

Treatment

Most of these lesions regress on their own; there is no need to intervention. If spontaneous regression does not occur corticosteroids, in various formulations, may be considered. Topical application of timolol has been useful in some cases.

⧉ BIBLIOGRAPHY

1. Karmel M. (2010). Pediatrics update: Topical timolol for capillary hemangioma. [online] Available from www.aao.org/publications/eyenet/201006/news.cfm. [Accessed January, 2014].

⧉ 1EE.73C9.7G13.9. LYMPHANGIOMA

General

Poorly circumscribed infiltrating lesions consisting of lymphatic/dysplastic blood vessels; occurs predominantly in children and young adults.

Ocular

Conjunctival hemorrhages; cellulitis of lid; ptosis; exophthalmos; amblyopia; astigmatism; extraocular muscle imbalance; optic disk edema; retinal striae.

Clinical

Benign tumors of the lymph system.

Laboratory

Ultrasonography lacks specificity and soft-tissue detail; CT images bone deformity and MRI provides superior soft-tissue details.

Treatment

- *Ptosis*: Most cases require surgical correction if visual acuity is affected and there are several procedures that may be used including levator resection, repair or advancement and Fasanella-Servat procedure.
- *Exophthalmos*: Reversing the problem which is causing the exophthalmos is the treatment of choice and will minimize the ocular complications. Ocular lubricants are beneficial for control of the corneal exposure.

⧉ BIBLIOGRAPHY

1. Schwartz RA, Fernandez G. (2012). Lymphangioma. [online] Available from www.emedicine.com/derm/TOPIC866.HTM. [Accessed September, 2013].

⧉ 1EE.73C9.7G13.10. JUVENILE XANTHOGRANULOMA (JXG; NEVOXANTHOENDOTHELIOMA)

General

Childhood disease; unknown etiology.

Ocular

Uveal tract tumor presenting as spontaneous hyphema; secondary glaucoma; uveitis; corneal, lid and epibulbar tumors; proptosis; retinal and choroidal lesions (rare).

Clinical

Multiple benign tumors, primarily of the skin; usually appear in the first 3 years of life; lesions appear as yellow-to-brown papules or nodules.

Laboratory

Diagnostic techniques include biomicroscopy, highfrequency ultrasound and cytologic examination of anterior chamber paracentesis material.

Treatment

Topical, subconjunctival, intralesional and systemic corticosteroids are useful. Low-dose radiation may be the treatment of choice for diffuse uveal lesions. Glaucoma medications should be used in the setting of hyphema and increased IOP.

⧉ BIBLIOGRAPHY

1. Curtis T, Wheeler DT. (2012). Juvenile xanthogranuloma. [online] Available from www.emedicine.com/oph/TOPIC588.HTM. [Accessed September, 2013].

1EE.73C9.7G13.11. MALIGNANT MELANOMA OF THE POSTERIOR UVEA (CHOROIDAL MELANOMA, CILIARY BODY MELANOMA, UVEAL MELANOMA, INTRAOCULAR MELANOMA)

General

Most common primary intraocular tumor in adults.

Clinical

Metastatic melanoma can appear in other parts of the body such as skin or liver.

Ocular

Intraocular tumors of the choroid, iris and ciliary body.

Laboratory

Ultrasonography, fluorescein angiography, indocyanine green angiography.

Treatment

Ocular therapy's goal is to eradicate the tumor before metastasis occurs. Diode laser, brachytherapy, stereotactic, local resection, enucleation and exenteration are all used to achieve this. Systemically intravenous therapy; intrahepatic chemoembolization has been used for isolated liver metastases. Proton beam is used to kill the tumor.

BIBLIOGRAPHY

1. Garcia-Valenzuela E, Pons ME, Puklin JE, et al. (2011). Choroidal melanoma. [online] Available from www.emedicine.com/oph/TOPIC403.HTM [Accessed September, 2013].

1EE.73C9.7G13.12. RHABDOMYOSARCOMA (CORNEAL EDEMA)

General

Most common malignant orbital neoplasm of childhood; usually occurs before age 10 years; more commonly seen in males; rarely may develop in adults; shows evidence of striated muscle differentiation; has been divided into three histopathologic types: (1) embryonal, (2) alveolar and (3) pleomorphic.

Ocular

Choroidal folds; corneal edema; exposure keratitis; rhabdomyosarcoma (RMS) of orbit or extraocular muscles; decreased motility; proptosis; papilledema; orbital edema; enlarged optic foramen; erosion of bony walls of orbit; pupil irregularity; epiphora; glaucoma; visual loss; nasolacrimal duct obstruction; conjunctival mass.

Clinical

Metastasis to the lymph system, bone marrow and lungs; headaches.

Laboratory

Liver, renal and cytogenetic testing; CT and bone scanning; MRI, ultrasonography and echocardiography.

Treatment

Chemotherapy radiation and surgically removing the tumor are used to treat patients with RMS.

BIBLIOGRAPHY

1. Cripe TP. (2011). Pediatric rhabdomyosarcoma. [online] Available from www.emedicine.com/ped/TOPIC2005.HTM. [Accessed September, 2013].

1EE.73C9.7G12.2. PASSOW SYNDROME (BREMER STATUS DYSRAPHICUS; STATUS DYSRAPHICUS SYNDROME; SYRINGOMYELIA; SYRINGOBULBIA)

General

Congenital nonclosure of the neural tube; familial occurrence or may be sporadic; insidious onset in second to third decade of life.

Ocular

Enophthalmos; ptosis; rotatory nystagmus; heterochromia iridis; anterior uveitis; corneal anesthesia; neuroparalytic keratitis; paralysis of third, fifth, sixth, and seventh cranial nerves; Horner syndrome; anisocoria; papilledema; optic atrophy; zonular cataract (*see* Horner Syndrome).

Clinical

Anesthesia over area of first division of trigeminal nerve; facial hemiatrophy; facial nerve paralysis; muscular weakness; cervical ribs; kyphoscoliosis; spina bifida; unilateral numbness of fingers; loss of deep reflexes; insensitivity to pain and temperature in affected areas; neurogenic bladder.

Laboratory

Magnetic resonance imaging and CT.

Treatment

Suboccipital and cervical decompression, laminectomy and syringotomy, shunts, fourth ventriculostomy, terminal ventriculostomy and neuroendoscopic surgery may be considered.

BIBLIOGRAPHY

1. Al-Shatoury HA, Galhom AA, Wagner FC. (2012). Syringomyelia. [online] Available from emedicine.medscape.com/article/1151685-overview. [Accessed September, 2013].

1EE.73C9.7G12.4. PAPILLOMA (WART; VERRUCA)

General

Cutaneous or mucosal tumor of proliferating epithelial and fibrovascular tissues; viral etiology or noninfectious.

Ocular

Papillary conjunctivitis; pseudopterygium; corneal opacity; epithelial keratitis; corneal vascularization; lid ulcers; lacrimal system obstruction; hemorrhages of conjunctiva, lids and lacrimal system.

Clinical

Mulberry or cauliflower-like tumors that may occur on any cutaneous or mucosal surface.

Laboratory

Histologic evaluation is diagnostic.

Treatment

Salicylic acid is a first-line therapy used to treat warts, intralesional immunotherapy using injections, cryosurgery, carbon dioxide lasers, electrodesiccation and curettage or surgical excision.

BIBLIOGRAPHY

1. Shenefelt PD. (2012). Nongenital warts. [online] Available from www.emedicine.com/derm/TOPIC457.HTM. [Accessed September, 2013].

⊡ 1EE.73C9.7G12.5. BASAL CELL NEVUS SYNDROME (NEVOID BASAL CELL CARCINOMA SYNDROME; NEVOID BASALIOMA SYNDROME; GORLIN SYNDROME; GORLIN-GOLTZ SYNDROME; MULTIPLE BASAL CELL NEVI SYNDROME)

General

Autosomal dominant; onset of skin lesions in childhood, usually at puberty.

Ocular

Basal cell carcinomas of eyelids; strabismus; hypertelorism; congenital cataracts; choroidal colobomas; glaucoma; medullated nerve fibers; prominence of supraorbital ridges; corneal leukoma; basalioma of the skin; coloboma of the choroid and optic nerve.

Clinical

Basal cell tumors with facial involvement; shallow pits of the skin of the hands and feet; jaw cysts; rib anomalies; kyphoscoliosis and fusion of vertebrae; medulloblastoma; frontal and temporoparietal bossing and broad nasal root.

Laboratory

Computed tomography scanning, ultrasonography, or MRI to evaluate neoplasms. Endoscopy to evaluate for the degree of polyposis and survey for malignant transformation is done.

Treatment

Patients may require medical attention for craniofacial, vertebral, dental and ophthalmologic abnormalities, in addition to diagnosis and treatment of potential neoplasia.

⊡ BIBLIOGRAPHY

1. Hsu EK, Mamula P, Ruchelli ED. (2011). Intestinal polyposis syndromes. [online] Available from www.emedicine.com/ped/TOPIC828.HTM. [Accessed September, 2013].

⊡ 1EE.73C9.7G12.10. MELANOCYTIC LESIONS OF THE EYELIDS (EPHELIS, LENTIGO, NEOVASCULAR NEVUS, DERMAL MELANOCYTOSIS, MALIGNANT MELANOMA)

General

Congenital or acquired eyelid lesions.

Clinical

Benign lesions—frequently from birth to puberty. Sun exposure increases lesion. Large (1 cm or more) from birth may become melanomas and should be removed.

Ocular

Benign lesions and malignant lesions of the eyelid.

Laboratory

Examination with measurement and serial photography to determine if benign or malignant. Histology or biopsy or excisional biopsy.

Treatment

No treatment necessary for benign lesions. Malignant lesions should be dissected.

⊡ BIBLIOGRAPHY

1. Bashour M, Bassin R, Benchimol M. (2013). Melanocytic lesions of the eyelid. [online] Available from www.emedicine.com/oph/TOPIC715.HTM. [Accessed September, 2013].

⊟ 1EE.73C9.7G12.13. MUCOCELE (PYOCELE)

General

Accumulation and retention of mucoid material within the sinus as a result of continuous or periodic obstruction of the sinus ostium.

Ocular

Paralysis of extraocular muscles; exophthalmos; lacrimation; erosion of bony walls of orbit; decreased visual acuity; diplopia; elevation of lower lid; ptosis; compression optic neuropathy; globe distortion; enophthalmos; epiphora; scleral indentation; choroidal folds; discharging lesion of the upper lid; pseudotelecanthus; spontaneous non-traumatic enophthalmos; local anesthesia.

Clinical

Headaches; epidural abscess; subdural empyema; meningitis; brain abscess; occlusion of nasal passage; loosening of teeth.

Laboratory

Computed tomography scanning helps to outline bony changes; MRI helps to differentiate mucoceles from neoplasms in the paranasal sinuses.

Treatment

Gamma-linolenic acid.

⊟ BIBLIOGRAPHY

1. Flaitz CM, Hicks MJ. (2012). Mucocele and Ranula. [online] Available from www.emedicine.com/derm/TOPIC648. HTM. [Accessed September, 2013].

⊟ 1EE.73C9.7G12.13.1. SEBACEOUS GLAND CARCINOMA

General

Ocular adnexa contains various sebaceous glands from which carcinomas may arise; predilection for the upper lids but may involve both lids; usually in older age groups; slight female preponderance.

Ocular

Blepharitis; madarosis; meibomianitis; sebaceous carcinoma of lids or orbit; orbital edema; proptosis; conjunctivitis; superficial keratitis; lacrimal gland tumor.

Clinical

Metastasis to preauricular or cervical lymph nodes, or submandibular area.

Laboratory

Biopsy diagnostic in chronic non-healing chalazia or suspicious unresolved chronic blepharitis.

Treatment

Mohs' technique appears to have the highest success rate.

⊟ BIBLIOGRAPHY

1. Glassman ML, Bashour M. (2012). Sebaceous gland carcinoma. [online] Available from www.emedicine.com/oph/TOPIC716.HTM. [Accessed September, 2013].

🗗 1EE.73C9.7G12.13.5. URBACH-WIETHE SYNDROME (ROSSLE-URBACH-WIETHE SYNDROME; LIPOPROTEINOSIS; HYALINOSIS CUTIS ET MUCOSAE; LIPOID PROTEINOSIS; PROTEINOSIS-LIPOIDOSIS) DRY EYES

General

Rare autosomal recessive disorder in which hyaline material is deposited in the skin, mucous membranes, and brain; both sexes affected; onset in infancy; relatively benign progressive course; association with diabetes mellitus.

Ocular

Margin of eyelids may show bead-like excrescences with loss of cilia; itching of eyes; dry eyes.

Clinical

Skin about face covered with small, yellowish-white, waxy nodules; alopecia; hoarseness of voice at birth or within first few years of life; tongue large, thick; hyperkeratotic lesions on knees, elbows, and fingers; inability to cry; dry mouth.

Laboratory

Erythrocyte sedimentation rate, polymerase chain amplification and direct neuclotide sequence of the ECM1 gene.

Treatment

No cure is known.

🗗 BIBLIOGRAPHY

1. Cordoro KM, Osleber MF, De Leo VA. (2013). Lipoid proteinosis. [online] Available from www.emedicine.com/derm/TOPIC241.HTM. [Accessed September, 2013].

🗗 1EE.73C9.7G12.13.7. LUBARSCH-PICK SYNDROME (PRIMARY AMYLOIDOSIS; IDIOPATHIC AMYLOIDOSIS; AMYLOIDOSIS)

General

Rare condition of unknown etiology; inherited as a dominant trait, with male preponderance; characterized by amyloid accumulation in muscles and in gastrointestinal and genitourinary tracts.

Ocular

Internal and external ophthalmoplegia; diminished lacrimation; amyloid deposits in conjunctival, episcleral, and ciliary vessels; vitreous opacities; amyloid deposits in the corneal stroma; retinal hemorrhages and perivascular exudates; paralysis of extraocular muscles; pseudopodia lentis; strabismus fixus convergens; keratoconus.

Clinical

Peripheral neuropathy (extremities); heart failure; defective hepatic and renal functions with hepatosplenomegaly; waxy skin lesions; muscular weakness (progressive); multiple myeloma; hoarseness; chronic gastrointestinal symptoms.

Laboratory

Biopsy-stain with Congo red demonstrates apple-green birefringence under polarized light; distinctive fibrillar ultrastructure.

Treatment

Deoxydoxorubicin had demonstrated some clinical benefit.

🗗 BIBLIOGRAPHY

1. Biswas J, Badrinath SS, Rao NA. Primary nonfamilial amyloidosis of the vitreous. A light microscopic and ultrastructural study. Retina. 1992;12(3):251-3.
2. Goebel HH, Friedman AH. Extraocular muscle involvement in idiopathic primary amyloidosis. Am J Ophthalmol. 1971;71(5):1121-7.

⊟ 1EE.737G12.13.8. CORNEAL ABRASIONS, CONTUSIONS, LACERATIONS AND PERFORATIONS

General

Loss of corneal epithelium from direct or indirect injury.

Clinical

None.

Ocular

Photophobia, tearing, eye pain, foreign body sensation, corneal abrasion, laceration or perforation.

Laboratory

Diagnosis is made by clinical findings.

Treatment

Topical antibiotic and cycloplegic agents, pain medication, pressure patching and bandage contact lens.

⊟ BIBLIOGRAPHY

1. Giri G. (2012). Corneoscleral laceration. [online] Available from www.emedicine.com/oph/TOPIC108.HTM. [Accessed September, 2013].
2. Verma A, Khan FH. (2011). Corneal abrasion. [online] Available from www.emedicine.com/oph/TOPIC247.HTM. [Accessed September, 2013].

⊟ 1FF. LOWER LID PTOSIS

General

Generally occurs with age and the excess skin, muscle and fat can begin to sag and bulge below the eye. The orbital septum becomes lax and allows orbital fat through the weak spectum.

Ocular

Saggy, bulging lower eyelids.

Laboratory

Diagnosis is made by clinical findings.

Treatment

Transcutaneous blepharoplasty is used to resect the excessive fat and redundant muscle and skin.

⊟ BIBLIOGRAPHY

1. Kirman CN, Bharti G, Molnar JA. (2013). Lower lid transconjunctival blepharoplasty. [online] Available from emedicine.medscape.com/article/1281800-overview. [Accessed September, 2013].

⊟ 1GG. LID RETRACTION

Lid retraction is defined normally as more than 85% of vertical palpebral fissures and 10 mm or less with the eyelids just concealing the corneoscleral limbus at the 12 O' clock and 6 O' clock meridians.

†1. *Lid retraction with upward movement of eye:*
   A. Congestive dysthyroid disease
   B. Deficiency in upward gaze—following rectus operation or weakness of superior rectus
   C. Excessive stimulation of levator muscles in Bell phenomenon with seventh nerve palsy
   D. Levator muscles receive excessive stimuli from nerve fiber of superior rectus
   E. Pretectal or periaqueductal lesion in midbrain
2. *Lid retraction with downward movement of eye:*
   A. Aberrant regeneration of third nerve of inferior rectus to levator (pseudo-Graefe phenomenon)—elevation of lid in downward gaze
   B. Brown syndrome (superior oblique tendon sheath syndrome)
   C. Extrapyramidal syndrome of postencephalic Parkinsonism and progressive supranuclear palsy
   †D. Failure of levator to relax on downward movement of eye:
      1. Secondary neuromuscular

†2. Mechanical, such as from a scar

†E. Noncongestive type of dysthyroid exophthalmos—lid lag in downward gaze

3. *Lid retraction with horizontal gaze:*
   A. Duane syndrome (retraction syndrome)
   †B. Underaction of lateral rectus muscle and spillover to levator causing widening

4. *Lid retraction because of supranuclear lesions:* Usually bilateral when due to lesion in or about posterior commissure (tucked lids, posterior fossa stare):
   A. Bulbar poliomyelitis
   B. Chorea (Huntington hereditary chorea)
   †C. Closed head injury associated with defective adduction of eyes, coarse nystagmus, nuclear palsy, pyramidal signs
   †D. Coma due to disease of ventral midbrain and pons
   E. Craniostenosis
   F. Epidemic encephalitis
   †G. Hydrocephalic infants
   H. Hydrophobia
   I. Hysteria
   †J. Malingering
   K. Meningitis
   L. Multiple sclerosis (disseminated sclerosis)
   M. Parinaud syndrome (divergence paralysis)
   N. Parkinson disease (paralysis agitans)
   O. Russell syndrome
   P. Sylvian aqueduct syndrome (Koerber-Solus-Elschnig syndrome)
   Q. Syphilis (tabes)
   †R. Tumors of the midbrain; meningiomas of sphenoid wing; sellar, parasellar, and suprasellar tumors; and frontal or temporal lobe tumors
   S. von Economo syndrome (encephalitis lethargica)

5. *Lid retraction because of neuromuscular disease:* Commonly asymmetric or unilateral.
   †A. Drugs:
      1. Phenylephrine and other sympathomimetics
      2. Prostigmin and Tensilon, especially with myasthenic levator involvement
      3. Succinylcholine, subparalytic doses
      4. Thyroid extract
   †B. Fuch phenomenon—healing of injured third nerve, previously ptotic lid has involuntarily spastic raising with movements of eyes
   C. Infant lid retraction—transient because of maternal hyperthyroidism

D. Irritation of cervical sympathetic nerve (Horner syndrome)

†*E. Mechanical suspension of lid such as that due to scar, tumor, surgical attachment to frontalis muscle, or shortening of levator muscle or following glaucoma filtering procedures

†F. Peripheral seventh nerve paresis with loss of orbicularis oculi muscle tone

6. *Lid retraction with myopathic disease:*
   A. Associated with hepatic cirrhosis
   B. Thyroid myopathy (Graves disease, Basedow syndrome):
      1. Dalrymple sign: Widening of palpebral fissure
      2. Stellwag sign: Retraction of upper lid associated with infrequent or incomplete blinking

†7. *Lid retraction following operations on vertical muscles: Recession* of superior rectus muscle or simultaneous recession and restriction of the levator by common fascial check ligament between the two muscles

8. *Paradoxical lid retraction because of paradoxical levator innervation:*
   †A. Defective ocular abduction with abducens palsy
   †B. Lid retraction associated with ptosis of the opposite eyelid (levator denervation supersensitivity)
   †C. Misdirection of third nerve axons (following acquired or congenital lesions): Occurs on attempt to adduct, elevate, or depress eye
   D. Movement of lower jaw:
      1. Contraction of external pterygoid muscle by opening mouth (Marcus Gunn)
      †2. Contraction of internal pterygoid muscle by closing the mouth

†9. *Physiologic*
   A. Act of surprise
   B. Slow onset of blindness, such as that secondary to glaucoma and optic atrophy
   C. Time of attention

---

*Indicates most frequent
†Indicates a general entry and therefore has not been described in detail in the text

🗗 BIBLIOGRAPHY

1. Blaydon SM. (2011). Marcus Gunn jaw-winking syndrome. [online] Available from www.emedicine.com/oph/TOPIC608.HTM. [Accessed September, 2013].
2. Collin JR, Allen L, Castronuovo S. Congenital eyelid retraction. Br J Ophthalmol. 1990;74:542-4.
3. Corenblum B, Adediji OS. (2013). Diffuse toxic goiter. [online] Available from www.emedicine.com/med/TOPIC917.HTM. [Accessed September, 2013].
4. Diaz MM, Foster CS, Walton RC, et al. (2011). Herpes zoster ophthalmicus. [online] Available from www.emedicine.com/oph/TOPIC257.HTM. [Accessed September, 2013].

5. Dixon R. The surgical management of thyroid-related upper eyelid retraction. Ophthalmology. 1982;89:52-7.
6. Eggenberger ER, Clark D. (2013). Progressive supranuclear palsy. [online] Available from www.emedicine.com/neuro/TOPIC328.HTM. [Accessed September, 2013].
7. Ing E. (2012). Thyroid-associated orbitopathy. [online] Available from www.emedicine.com/neuro/TOPIC476.HTM. [Accessed September, 2013].
8. Izquierdo NJ, Townsend W. (2012). Computer vision syndrome. [online] Available from http://www.emedicine.com/oph/TOPIC774.HTM. [Accessed September, 2013].
9. Mercandetti M, Cohen AJ. (2012). Exophthalmos. [online] Available from www.emedicine.com/oph/TOPIC616.HTM. [Accessed September, 2013].
10. Roy FH. Ocular Syndromes and Systemic Diseases, 4th edition. Philadelphia: Lippincott Williams & Wilkins; 2007.
11. Sinha S, Gold JG. (2013). Pediatric hyperthyroidism. [online] Available from www.emedicine.com/ped/TOPIC1099.HTM. [Accessed September, 2013].
12. Walsh FB, Hoyt WF. Clinical Neuro-Ophthalmology, 4th edition. Baltimore: Williams & Wilkins; 1985.
13. Yeung SJ, Habra MA, Chiu AC. (2013). Graves disease. [online] Available from www.emedicine.com/med/TOPIC929.HTM. [Accessed September, 2013].

IGG.2A. PSEUDO-GRAEFE SYNDROME (FUCHS SIGN)

General

Misdirection of regenerating oculomotor nerve (cranial nerve III) fibers to other muscles after injury, aneurysm, tumor, exophthalmic goiter, tabes, anterior poliomyelitis, or vascular lesions of the brainstem.

Ocular

Elevation of the upper lid in downward gaze; lagging in upper lid movement on downward gaze (Graefe sign).

Clinical

None.

Laboratory

Diagnosis is made by clinical findings.

Treatment

See ptosis and lid retraction.

BIBLIOGRAPHY

1. Bender MB. The nerve supply to the orbicularis musxle and the physiology of movements of the upper lid, with particular reference to the pseudo-Graefe phenomenon. Arch Ophthalmol. 1936;15:21.

1GG.2B. BROWN SYNDROME (SUPERIOR OBLIQUE TENDON SHEATH SYNDROME)

General

Etiology unknown; affects both sexes; present from birth; may be congenital or acquired (secondary to trauma, orbital surgery, or injections, or following delivery).

Ocular

Bilateral ptosis with associated backward head tilt; widening of palpebral fissure with attempted upward gaze; ocular movements show failure in the direction of superior oblique action; may be associated with underaction of the inferior oblique; adduction or abduction restricted or completely abolished; choroidal coloboma.

Laboratory

Diagnosis is made by clinical findings.

Treatment

Once systemic disease is excluded, patients' inflammation can be treated with anti-inflammatory medication. Oral ibuprofen is a good first-line choice. Local steroid injections in the area of the trochlea and oral corticosteroids can be used for inflammation. Once the inflammatory disease process is controlled, patients with inflammatory Brown syndrome may show spontaneous resolution. Congenital Brown syndrome is unlikely to improve spontaneously; therefore, surgery is important to consider as an option.

BIBLIOGRAPHY

1. Wright KW, Salvador MG. (2012). Brown syndrome. [online] Available from www.emedicine.com/oph/TOPIC552.HTM. [Accessed September, 2013].
2. Suh DW, Oystreck DT, Hunter DG. Long-term results of an intraoperative adjustable superior oblique tendon suture spacer using nonabsorbable suture for Brown syndrome. Ophthalmology. 2008;115(10):1800-4.

1GG.2C. PARKINSON SYNDROME (PARALYSIS AGITANS; SHAKING PALSY)

General

Late stages of epidemic encephalitis; present with arteriosclerosis and with manganese and carbon monoxide poisoning; widespread destruction of pigmented cells in substantia nigra.

Ocular

Decreased blinking; lid fluttering; blepharospasm; oculogyric crises; ocular hypotony; blepharoplegia; ptosis; nystagmus; paralysis of convergence; paralysis of lateral rectus muscle; absent or sluggish pupillary reactions to light or convergence; mydriasis or anisocoria; optic neuritis; papilledema; abnormal saccades.

Clinical

Slowness of movements; loss of facial expression; "cogwheel" rigidity of the arms; rhythmical tremors; drooling; shuffling gait; stooping; monotonous voice.

Laboratory

Magnetic resonance imaging and CT scan reveal calcium and ceruloplasmin to exclude other conditions.

Treatment

The goal of medical management is to provide control of signs and symptoms for as long as possible while minimizing adverse effects. Medications usually provide good symptomatic control.

BIBLIOGRAPHY

1. Hauser RA, Lyons KE, McClain TA, et al. (2012). Parkinson disease. [online] Available from www.emedicine.com/neuro/TOPIC304.HTM. [Accessed September, 2013].

1GG.2C. STEELE-RICHARDSON-OLSZEWSKI SYNDROME (PROGRESSIVE SUPRANUCLEAR PALSY)

General

Nerve cell degeneration centered in the brainstem; resemblance to Lhermitte pyramidopallidal syndrome and to Jakob disease with dementia and rigidity; onset in the sixth decade of life; prominent in males.

Ocular

Supranuclear ophthalmoplegia affecting chiefly vertical gaze, especially downward.

Clinical

Pseudobulbar palsy; dysarthria; dystonic rigidity of neck and upper trunk; axial rigidity; bradykinesia; pyramidal signs; parkinsonism; frontal lobe-type dementia.

Laboratory

No specific laboratory or imaging findings.

Treatment

No medication is effective and only few patients respond to dopaminergic or anticholineric drugs.

BIBLIOGRAPHY

1. Eggenberger ER, Clark D. (2013). Progressive supranuclear palsy. [online] Available from www.emedicine.com/neuro/TOPIC328.HTM. [Accessed September, 2013].

⊟ 1GG.3A. DUANE SYNDROME (RETRACTION SYNDROME; STILLING SYNDROME; TURK-STILLING SYNDROME)

General

Autosomal dominant; more frequent in females; manifestations in infancy; was thought to be secondary to fibrosis of the LR muscle or abnormal check ligaments; now established to be due to congenital aberrant innervation affecting third and seventh cranial nerves.

Ocular

Narrowing of palpebral fissure on adduction, widening on abduction; primary global retraction; deficiency of medial and lateral recti motility; limitation of abduction in affected eye usually is complete; retraction of the globe with attempted adduction varies from 1 mm to 10 mm; convergence insufficiency; heterochromia irides; left eye is more frequently involved.

Clinical

Associated Klippel-Feil syndrome; malformation of face, ears and teeth.

Laboratory

Diagnosis is made by clinical findings.

Treatment

Indications for surgery include anomalous head position, strabismus in primary gaze, significant upshot or downshoot in adduction and cosmetically significant palpebral fissure. Duane retraction syndrome type 1 (DRS-1) (absent abduction, esotropia in primary position and head turn toward the affected side to fuse) medial recuts recession of the affected eye; DRS with exotropia—recess LR of involved side. Retraction of the globe—recess medial and LR of involved eye. Upshoots and downshoots—recess the LR.

⊟ BIBLIOGRAPHY

1. Verma A. (2011). Duane syndrome. [online] Available from www.emedicine.com/oph/TOPIC326.HTM. [Accessed September, 2013].

⊟ 1GG.4A. POLIOMYELITIS (INFANTILE PARALYSIS)

General

Acute viral infection characterized by varying degrees of neuronal injury, with special localization in the anterior horns and motor nuclei of the brainstem.

Ocular

Diplopia; nystagmus; paralysis of third, fourth, and sixth nerves; paresis of seventh nerve; papilledema; visual agnosia; Homer's syndrome; pupillary paralysis; optic neuritis; ophthalmoparesis; transient visual loss; internuclear ophthalmoplegia; papillary disturbances, spasm of near reflex.

Clinical

Flaccid paralysis of many muscle groups; death from asphyxia and involvement of vital centers in the brainstem.

Laboratory

Obtain specimens from the CSF, stool and throat for viral cultures.

Treatment

No antivirals are effective against polioviruses. The treatment of poliomyelitis is mainly supportive and will involve physical therapist and rehabilitation therapist, pulmonologist, neurologist, immunologist and infectious diseases specialist.

⊟ BIBLIOGRAPHY

1. Estrada B. (2012). Pediatric poliomyelitis. [online] Available from www.emedicine.com/ped/TOPIC1843.HTM. [Accessed September, 2013].

1GG.4B. CHOREA (ACUTE CHOREA; SYDENHAM CHOREA; ST VITUS DANCE; HUNTINGTON HEREDITARY CHOREA)

General

Mendelian dominant trait.

Ocular

Lid retraction; spasmodic closures; apraxia of lid opening; disoriented ocular movements; anisocoria; mydriasis; hippus.

Clinical

Involuntary purposeless movements; emotional ability; muscle weakness.

Laboratory

Diagnosis of the primary choreatic conditions is based on history and clinical findings.

Treatment

The most widely used agents in the treatment of chorea are the neuroleptics. The basis of their mechanism of action is thought to be related to blocking of dopamine receptors.

BIBLIOGRAPHY

1. Vertrees SM, Berman SA. (2012). Chorea in adults. [online] Available from www.emedicine.com/neuro/TOPIC62.HTM. [Accessed September, 2013].

1GG.4E. CRANIOSTENOSIS

General

Skull deformity caused by premature fusion of cranial sutures.

Ocular

Optic atrophy; exophthalmos; strabismus; papilledema; nystagmus; ocular colobomas; swollen optic nerves; dissociated eye movements; ptosis; anisometropia; corneal exposure; amblyopia.

Clinical

Elevated CSF; abnormal development of the skull.

Laboratory

Skull, spine and hand radiography is usually necessary to confirm the diagnosis.

Treatment

Neurosurgical procedure is recommended in cases of intracranial hypertension leading to further optic atrophy.

BIBLIOGRAPHY

1. Chen H. (2013). Genetics of Crouzon syndrome. [online] Available from www.emedicine.com/ped/TOPIC511.HTM. [Accessed September, 2013].

1GG.4F. ENCEPHALITIS, ACUTE

General

In approximately 0.1–0.2% of patients having rubeola (measles), an acute encephalitis is seen within 1 week after the onset of the rash; a case of immunosuppressive encephalitis can present with focal seizures leading to progressive obtundation.

Ocular

Papillitis; optic atrophy; ocular motor palsies; nystagmus; optic neuritis or neuroretinitis.

Clinical

Rise in temperature; drowsiness; irritability; meningismus; vomiting and headache; stupor; convulsions; coma.

Laboratory

Perform head CT, with and without contrast agent, before LP to search for evidence of elevated intracerebral pressure. MRI is useful. Viral serology.

Treatment

Evaluate and treat for shock or hypotension, treat systemic complications, acyclovir.

BIBLIOGRAPHY

1. Howes DS, Lazoff M. (2013). Encephalitis. [online] Available from www.emedicine.com/emerg/TOPIC163.HTM. [Accessed September, 2013].

1GG.4H. HYDROPHOBIA (LYSSA; RABIES)

General

Acute viral zoonosis of the CNS.

Ocular

Lid retraction; widening of palpebral fissure; retinal hemorrhages; mydriasis; paralysis of third, fourth, fifth, or seventh nerve; bilateral optic neuritis; branch retinal artery occlusion; vaccine-induced autoimmune demyelinative optic neuritis.

Clinical

Fever; headache; nausea; numbness; tingling; acute sensitiveness to sound and light; laryngeal and pharyngeal spasms; increased muscle tonus; convulsions; delirium; coma; death.

Laboratory

Saliva can be tested by virus isolation or reverse transcription followed by PCR. Suspected infectious animal should be quarantined for 10 days.

Treatment

Before the onset of symptoms, both passive and active immunizations are effective for preventing progression to full-blown rabies. In exposures to high-risk species, initiate treatment immediately pending laboratory examination of the animal, if it is caught.

BIBLIOGRAPHY

1. Gompf SG. (2011). Rabies. [online] Available from www.emedicine.com/med/TOPIC1374.HTM. [Accessed September, 2013].

1GG.4I. HYSTERIA (MALINGERING; OPHTHALMIC FLAKE SYNDROME)

General

Willful or unwillful exaggeration or simulation of symptoms of an illness without physiologic cause; frequently secondary to a state of anxiety; may be seen more in children; physical or sexual abuse may be a predisposing factor.

Ocular

Anxiety-induced angiospastic or central serous retinopathy; self-induced conjunctivitis; traumatic epithelial erosions; herpetic keratitis; angioneurotic edema; contact dermatitis; ptosis; recurrent herpetic vesicles; anisocoria; peculiar pupillary reflexes; accommodative spasm; amaurosis fugax; anxiety-induced optic neuritis; disturbance of conjugate movement; dyschromatopsia; facial tic; hypersecretion glaucoma; increased or decreased tear secretion; night blindness; nystagmus; photophobia; strabismus; visual loss; psychogenic amaurosis with headaches.

Clinical

Aphonia; deafness; paralysis of limb; hemiplegia; dissociative state; anxiety; insomnia; tachycardia; shortness of breath; fatigue; vertigo, chest pains.

Laboratory

Eye examination to rule out pathology. Visual evoked responses, electro-retinopathy and electro-oculography all should be normal.

Treatment

Psychiatric intervention is required in severe cases.

⊟ BIBLIOGRAPHY

1. Barris MC, Kaufman DI, Barberio D. Visual impairment in hysteria. Doc Ophthalmol. 1992;82:369-82.
2. Catalono RA, Simon JW, Krohel GB, et al. Functional visual loss in children. Ophthalmology. 1986;93:385-90.
3. Kramer KK, La Piana FG, Appleton B. Ocular malingering and hysteria: diagnosis and management. Surv Ophthalmol. 1979;24:89-96.
4. Miller BW. A review of practical tests for ocular malingering and hysteria. Surv Ophthalmol. 1973;17:241-6.
5. Roy FH, Fraunfelder FW, Fraunfelder FT. Roy and Fraunfelder's Current Ocular Therapy, 6th edition. London: Elsevier; 2008.
6. Ziegler DK, Schlemmer RB. Familial psychogenic blindness and headache: a case study. J Clin Psychiatry. 1994;55: 114-7.

⊟ 1GG.4K. MENINGOCOCCEMIA (NEISSERIA MENINGITIDIS; MENINGITIS)

General

Systemic bacterial infection caused by *N. meningitidis*; can be present chronically in patients with immune deficiencies including deficient complement levels.

Ocular

Photophobia; conjunctivitis; chemosis; keratitis; uveitis; panophthalmitis; retinal endophlebitis; macular edema; papillitis; optic neuritis; paresis of sixth or seventh nerve; nystagmus; miosis; hippus; cortical blindness; papilledema (rare); conjunctival petechiae; strabismus.

Clinical

Meningitis; fever; malaise; joint pain; splenic enlargement.

Laboratory

Cultures from blood, spinal fluid, or joint fluid.

Treatment

Treat with antibiotics promptly.

⊟ BIBLIOGRAPHY

1. Javid MH, Ahmed SH. (2013). Meningococcemia. [online] Available from www.emedicine.com/med/TOPIC1445. HTM. [Accessed September, 2013].

⊟ 1GG.4L. DISSEMINATED SCLEROSIS (MULTIPLE SCLEROSIS)

General

Disseminated demyelination affecting white matter of the brain, spinal cord and optic nerves; etiology is unknown.

Ocular

Nystagmus; ptosis; myokymia; optic atrophy; papillitis; optic neuritis; anisocoria; Argyll Robertson pupil; Marcus Gunn pupil; hippus, decreased or absent papillary reaction to light; periphlebitis; visual field defects; gaze palsy; paralysis of third or sixth nerve; uveitis; oscillopsia; Uhthoff symptom (reduction of visual acuity with exercise or ocular hyperthermia); pars planitis; retinal venous sheathing; retinitis; granulomatous uveitis.

Clinical

Incoordination; paresthesia; spasticity; tic douloureux; urinary frequency and infections; progressive disability; paralysis; death.

Laboratory

Magnetic resonance imaging, CSF positive for oligoclonal band, albumin and IgG index; BAER and SEP.

Treatment

Patients with MS may require multiple consultations to rule out other causes for their symptoms. Drugs such as immunomodulators, immunosuppressors, antiparkinson agents, CNS stimulants are all used in the management of the disease.

BIBLIOGRAPHY

1. Luzzio C, Dangond F. (2012). Multiple sclerosis. [online] Available from www.emedicine.com/neuro/topic228.htm. [Accessed September, 2013].

1GG.4M. PARINAUD SYNDROME (DIVERGENCE PARALYSIS; SUBTHALAMIC SYNDROME; PARALYSIS OF VERTICAL MOVEMENTS; PRETECTAL SYNDROME)

General

Various causes, including pineal tumor, supranuclear lesions, vascular lesions, inflammation, hemorrhages, midbrain lesions, lesion of posterior white commissure of pons, red nucleus, or superior cerebellar peduncle; combination of Parinaud and von Monakow syndromes is known as Gruner-Bertolotti syndrome, which consists of paralysis in upward gaze, tremors, hemiplegia and sensory disturbances.

Ocular

Retraction of lids with lesion in mesencephalic gray matter and ptosis with lesions more anteriorly; paralysis of conjugate upward movement of the eye without paralysis of convergence; occasionally paralysis of upward and downward movement; spasm with convergence insufficiency; contralateral hemianopsia occurs when the lateral geniculate body becomes involved in case of infiltrating tumor; wide pupils that fail to react to light but sometimes react during accommodation (Holmes); papilledema (usually severe).

Clinical

Vertigo; contralateral cerebellar ataxia and choreoathetoid movement if lesion involves superior cerebellar peduncle after decussation.

Laboratory

Diagnosis is made by clinical findings, CT and MRI.

Treatment

Papilledema: Underlying cause should be determined and treated. Systemic acetazolamide is the medical therapy of choice.

BIBLIOGRAPHY

1. Zee C, Yao Z, Go JL, et al. (2011). Imaging in pineal germinoma. [online] Available from www.emedicine.com/radio/TOPIC554.HTM. [Accessed September, 2013].

1GG.4N. PARKINSON SYNDROME (PARALYSIS AGITANS; SHAKING PALSY)

General

Late stages of epidemic encephalitis; present with arteriosclerosis and with manganese and carbon monoxide poisoning; widespread destruction of pigmented cells in substantia nigra.

Ocular

Decreased blinking; lid fluttering; blepharospasm; oculogyric crises; ocular hypotony; blepharoplegia; ptosis; nystagmus; paralysis of convergence; paralysis of lateral rectus muscle; absent or sluggish pupillary reactions to light or convergence; mydriasis or anisocoria; optic neuritis; papilledema; abnormal saccades.

Clinical

Slowness of movements; loss of facial expression; "cogwheel" rigidity of the arms; rhythmical tremors; drooling; shuffling gait; stooping; monotonous voice.

Laboratory

Magnetic resonance imaging and CT scan reveal calcium and ceruloplasmin to exclude other conditions.

Treatment

The goal of medical management is to provide control of signs and symptoms as long as possible while minimizing adverse effects. Medications usually provide good symptomatic control.

BIBLIOGRAPHY

1. Hauser RA, Lyons KE, McClain TA, et al. (2012). Parkinson disease. [online] Available from www.emedicine.com/neuro/TOPIC304.HTM. [Accessed September, 2013].
2. Garcia-Martin E, Satue M, Fuertes I, et al. Ability and reproducibility of Fourier-domain optical coherence tomography to detect retinal nerve fiber layer atrophy in Parkinson's disease. Ophthalmology. 2012;119;2161-7.

1GG.4O. RUSSELL SYNDROME (NYSTAGMUS)

General

Onset between 3 months and 2 years; caused by tumors of the anterior portion of the thalamus (usually astrocytoma), optic chiasm, midcerebellar region, and midline ependymoma; erosion under the anterior clinoid processes that causes a characteristic J-shaped sella in lateral skull films.

Ocular

Lid retraction; nystagmus (horizontal, vertical, or rotatory); homonymous hemianopsia; optic nerve atrophy.

Clinical

Extreme emaciation; euphoria; pale skin.

Laboratory

Diagnosis is made by clinical findings.

Treatment

Lid retraction: Identify systemic abnormalities as thyroid treatment—6 months stabilizing before eyelid surgery. Local—ocular lubrication (drops or ointment). Botulism type A may also be useful.

BIBLIOGRAPHY

1. Ciccarelli EC, Huttenlocher PR. Diencephalic tumor: a cause of infantile nystagmus and cachexia. Arch Ophthalmol. 1967;78:350-3.
2. Geeraets WJ. Ocular Syndromes, 3rd edition. Philadelphia: Lea & Febiger; 1976.
3. Russell A. A diencephalic syndrome: emaciation in infancy and childhood. Arch Dis Child. 1951;26:274

1GG.4P. KOERBER-SALUS-ELSCHNIG SYNDROME (SYLVIAN AQUEDUCT SYNDROME; NYSTAGMUS RETRACTORIUS SYNDROME)

General

It is caused by tumor or inflammation in the region of aqueduct of Sylvius, third and fourth ventricle, or corpora quadrigemina.

Ocular

Lid retraction may be associated with midbrain lesions above the posterior commissure; paresis of vertical gaze; tonic spasm of convergence on attempted upward gaze; clonic convergence movements or convergence nystagmus; vertical nystagmus on gaze up or down; nystagmus retractorius with spasmodic retraction of the eyes when an attempt is made to move them in any direction; occasional extraocular muscle paresis.

Clinical

Headaches; dizziness; hypertension; possible hemiparesis; ataxia; hemitremor; Babinski's sign.

Laboratory

Computed tomography and MRI.

Treatment

- *Lid retraction*: Identify systemic abnormalities as thyroid treatment: 6 month stabilizing before eyelid surgery.
- *Local*: Ocular lubrication (drops or ointment). Botulinum toxin type A may also be useful.

BIBLIOGRAPHY

1. Elschnig A. Nystagmus Retractorius, ein Cerebrales Herdsymptom. Med Klin. 1913;9:8.
2. Geeraets WJ. Ocular Syndromes, 3rd edition. Philadelphia, PA: Lea & Febiger; 1976.

1GG.4Q. ACQUIRED LUES (SYPHILIS; ACQUIRED SYPHILIS; LUES VENEREA; MALUM VENEREUM)

General

Causative agent, *T. pallidum*, usually transmitted sexually.

Ocular

Conjunctival chancroid; conjunctivitis; keratitis; blepharitis; ptosis; iris atrophy; hippus; dacryocystitis; optic nerve atrophy; optic neuritis; periostitis; episcleritis; scleritis; nystagmus; uveitis; vitreous hemorrhages; paralysis of sixth nerve; papilledema; retinal hemorrhages; retinitis proliferans; oculogyric crisis; neuroretinitis; papilledema (associated with aseptic meningitis); diffuse or multifocal chorioretinitis; vertical supranuclear gaze palsy; Benedikt syndrome.

Clinical

Primary lesion associated with regional lymphadenopathy; secondary bacteremic stage associated with generalized mucocutaneous lesions; tertiary stage characterized by destructive mucocutaneous, musculoskeletal, or parenchymal lesions, aortitis, or central nervous system disease; syphilis and HIV infection often coexist in the same patient who experiences a higher incidence and greater severity of neurologic and ocular manifestations; a significant percentage of patients infected with HIV-I and *T. pallidum* become seronegative to syphilis testing.

Laboratory

Serologic nontreponemal tests include VDRL and RPR.

Treatment

The goals are to reduce morbidity and to prevent complications. Penicillin is the antibiotic of choice for treating syphilis. Ocular syphilis should be treated the same as patients with neurosyphilis.

BIBLIOGRAPHY

1. Euerle B, Chandrasekar PH, Diaz MM, et al. (2012). Syphilis. [online] Available from www.emedicine.com/med/TOPIC2224.HTM. [Accessed September, 2013].
2. Majmudar PA. (2011). Interstitial keratitis overview of interstitial keratitis. [online] Available from www.emedicine.com/oph/TOPIC453.HTM. [Accessed September, 2013].

1GG.4S. VON ECONOMO SYNDROME (ENCEPHALITIS LETHARGICA; SLEEPING SICKNESS; ICELAND DISEASE) NYSTAGMUS

General

Etiology not known; may be caused by filterable virus; both sexes affected; onset at all ages; epidemic form.

Ocular

Nystagmus; strabismus; diplopia; muscle imbalance; lid retraction; homonymous hemianopsia; cortical blindness.

Clinical

Fever; headache; cramps; lethargy; insomnia; athetoid or choreiform movements; convulsions; depression; unsteady gait; fatigue; Parkinsonism; oculogyric crisis; behavior disorder.

Laboratory

Diagnosis is made by clinical findings.

Treatment

- *Seesaw nystagmus*: Visual field to consider neoplastic or vascular etiologies.
- *Upbeat nystagmus*: May indicate multiple sclerosis, cerbellar degeneration, tumors or infarcts. Treatment is directed toward identification and resolution of underlying cause.
- *Downbeat nystagmus*: Affects the cerebellum or craniocervical junction including Arnold-Chiari malformation, multiple sclerosis, trauma, tumor, infarction and many toxic metabolic entities. MRI may indicate a surgically correctable lesion. Periodic alternating nystagmus is continous horizontal nystagmus from stroke, tumor, multiple sclerosis, trauma, infection, drug intoxication. Can occur from cataract, vitreous hemorrhage or optic atrophy.

BIBLIOGRAPHY

1. Magalini SI, Scrascia E. Dictionary of Medical Syndromes, 2nd edition. Philadelphia: JB Lippincott, 1981.
2. Pruskauer-Apostol B, Popescu-Pretor R, Plăiaşu D, et al. The present status of encephalitis lethargica. Neurol Psychiatr (Bucur). 1977;15:125-8.
3. von Economo C. Encephalitis lethargica. Wien Klin Wochenschr. 1917;30:581.

1GG.5C. BASEDOW SYNDROME (GRAVES DISEASE; HYPERTHYROIDISM; THYROTOXICOSIS; EXOPHTHALMIC GOITER; PARRY DISEASE)

General

Diffuse toxic goiter; inherited as a simple autosomal recessive; penetrance greater in females; however, dominant mode of inheritance and variable penetrance are possible; uncommon in either sex before the age of 15 years.

Ocular

Exophthalmos; swelling of eyelids and discoloration of upper eyelids; lid lag (von Graefe's sign); globe lag (Koeber's sign); lid trembling on gentle closure (Rosenbach's sign); reduced blinking (Stellwag's sign); retraction of upper lid; difficulty in everting upper lid (Gifford's sign); convergence weakness (Möbius's sign); impaired fixation on extreme lateral gaze (Suker's sign); possible external ophthalmoplegia (Ballet's sign); Dalrymple's sign (staring appearance); tearing; photophobia; epiphora; prolapse of lacrimal gland; neuroretinal edema; tortuous vessels; papilledema and papillitis; anisocoria; keratitis; increased IOP on upgaze; decreased visual acuity; enlargement of the extraocular muscles; increased volume of the extraorbital fat; superior rectus muscle enlargement; decreased venous outflow.

Clinical

Tachycardia; anxiety; insomnia; loss of weight; hyperhidrosis; restlessness; myocarditis (toxic); atrial fibrillation.

Laboratory

Visual field testing, forced duction testing for restrictive myopathy, CT, MRI, T_4 and thyroid-stimulating hormone, thyroid-stimulating immunoglobulins.

Treatment

There is no immediate treatment; the disease is self-limited but prolonged course over one or more years. 5% of patients may require surgical intervention which could be orbital decompression, strabismus surgery, lid-lengthening surgery or blepharoplasty.

BIBLIOGRAPHY

1. Ing E. (2012). Thyroid-associated orbitopathy. [online] Available from www.emedicine.com/oph/TOPIC237.HTM. [Accessed September, 2013].
2. Regensburg NI, Wiersinga WM, Berendschot TT, et al. Do subtypes of graves' orbitopathy exist? Ophthalmology. 2011;118:191-6.

🗗 1GG.5D. HORNER SYNDROME (BERNARD-HORNER SYNDROME; CERVICAL SYMPATHETIC PARALYSIS SYNDROME; CLAUDE-BERNARD-HORNER SYNDROME; HORNER OCULOPUPILLARY SYNDROME)

General

Paralysis of cervical sympathetic; hypothalamic lesion with first neuron involved or lesion in the pons or cervical portion of cord; syndrome present in Babinski-Nageotte, Cestan-Chenais, Dejerine-Klumpke, Pancoast, Raeder, and Wallenberg syndromes (*see* Babinski-Nageotte syndrome; Cestan-Chenais syndrome; Dejerine-Klumpke syndrome; Pancoast syndrome; Raeder syndrome; Wallenberg syndrome).

Ocular

Enophthalmos; ptosis or narrowing of palpebral fissure; ocular hypotony; miosis (degree of miosis depends on the site of lesion; most pronounced when roots of cranial nerves VII and VIII, and first thoracic nerve are involved); hypochromic heterochromia (children more than adults); pupil does not dilate with cocaine.

Clinical

Anhidrosis on ipsilateral side of face and neck; transitory rise in facial temperature; hemifacial atrophy; it may result from a variety of conditions, including cluster headache, parasellar neoplasms or aneurysms, internal carotid dissection or occlusion, and Tolosa-Hunt syndrome.

Laboratory

Pharmacologic testing is very helpful in the diagnosis of Horner syndrome; cocaine or apraclonidine (instilled in an eye with intact sympathetic innervation) causes the pupil to dilate. A sympathetically denervated pupil dilates poorly to cocaine, regardless of the level of the sympathetic interruption because of the absence of endogenous norepinephrine in the synapse.

Treatment

Surgical and medical care is dependent upon the particular etiology. Potential surgical care includes neurosurgical care for aneurysm-related Horner syndrome and vascular surgical care for etiologies such as carotid artery dissection/aneurysm.

🗗 BIBLIOGRAPHY

1. Bardorf CM, Stavern GV, Garcia-Valenzuela E. (2012). Horner syndrome. [online] Available from www.emedicine.com/oph/TOPIC336.HTM. [Accessed September, 2013].

🗗 1GG.6A. MOSSE SYNDROME (POLYCYTHEMIA-HEPATIC CIRRHOSIS SYNDROME)

General

Unknown etiology.

Ocular

Scleral icterus; marked retinal venous tortuosity and dilation; retinal artery occlusion (occasionally); papilledema.

Clinical

Thrombosis of portal vein secondary to polycythemia; hepatosplenomegaly; ascites; clinical features of liver cirrhosis.

Laboratory

Diagnosis is made by clinical findings.

Treatment

- *Retinal artery occlusion*: IOP lowering medications, carbogen therapy, hyperbaric oxygen. Vitrectomy may be necessary.
- *Papilledema*: Underlying cause should be determined and treated. Systemic acetazolamide is the medical therapy of choice.

🗗 BIBLIOGRAPHY

1. Barbas AP. Surgical problems associated with polycythemia. Br J Hosp Med. 1980;23:289-90,92,94.
2. Geeraets WJ. Ocular Syndromes, 3rd edition. Philadelphia: Lea & Febiger; 1976.
3. Mosse M. Uber Policythamie mit Urobilinikterus und Milztumor. Dtsch Med Wochenschr. 1907;33:2175.

⊟ 1GG.6B. BASEDOW SYNDROME (GRAVES DISEASE; HYPERTHYROIDISM; THYROTOXICOSIS; EXOPHTHALMIC GOITER; PARRY DISEASE)

General

Diffuse toxic goiter; inherited as a simple autosomal recessive; penetrance greater in females; however, dominant mode of inheritance and variable penetrance are possible; uncommon in either sex before the age of 15 years.

Ocular

Exophthalmos; swelling of eyelids and discoloration of upper eyelids; lid lag (von Graefe's sign); globe lag (Koeber's sign); lid trembling on gentle closure (Rosenbach's sign); reduced blinking (Stellwag's sign); retraction of upper lid; difficulty in everting upper lid (Gifford's sign); convergence weakness (Möbius's sign); impaired fixation on extreme lateral gaze (Suker's sign); possible external ophthalmoplegia (Ballet's sign); Dalrymple's sign (staring appearance); tearing; photophobia; epiphora; prolapse of lacrimal gland; neuroretinal edema; tortuous vessels; papilledema and papillitis; anisocoria; keratitis; increased IOP on upgaze; decreased visual acuity; enlargement of the extraocular muscles; increased volume of the extraorbital fat; superior rectus muscle enlargement; decreased venous outflow.

Clinical

Tachycardia; anxiety; insomnia; loss of weight; hyperhidrosis; restlessness; myocarditis (toxic); atrial fibrillation.

Laboratory

Visual field testing, forced duction testing for restrictive myopathy, CT, MRI, T_4 and thyroid-stimulating hormone, thyroid-stimulating immunoglobulins.

Treatment

There is no immediate treatment; the disease is self-limited but prolonged course over one or more years. 5% of patients may require surgical intervention which could be orbital decompression, strabismus surgery, lid-lengthening surgery or blepharoplasty.

⊟ BIBLIOGRAPHY

1. Ing E. (2012). Thyroid-associated orbitopathy. [online] Available from www.emedicine.com/oph/TOPIC237.HTM. [Accessed September, 2013].
2. Regensburg NI, Wiersinga WM, Berendschot TT, et al. Do subtypes of Graves' orbitopathy exist? Ophthalmology. 2011;118:191-6.

⊟ 1GG.8D1. MARCUS GUNN SYNDROME (JAW-WINKING SYNDROME; CONGENITAL TRIGEMINOOCULOMOTOR SYNKINESIS)

General

Familial occurrence rare, although dominant inheritance has been reported; symptoms are caused by abnormal connections between external pterygoid muscle and levator palpebrae, with supranuclear or supranuclear-nuclear involvement (*See* Marin Amat syndrome).

Ocular

Unilateral congenital ptosis in more than 90% of cases; 10% have spontaneous onset, usually in older persons; lid elevates rapidly when mouth is opened or mandible is moved to one or the other side; left eye seems to be more frequently affected than right eye; high incidences of strabismus (36%); amblyopia (34%); bilateral jaw-winking; decreased abduction.

Clinical

Stimulation of ipsilateral pterygoid with chewing, opening of mouth, sucking or contralateral jaw thrusts.

Laboratory

Diagnosis is made by clinical findings.

Treatment

Treat amblyopia; if mild ptosis and mild jaw-winking, consider Muller's muscle conjunctival resection; severe jaw-winking, release levator and perform a frontalis sling usually bilaterally; unilateral ptosis mild jaw-winking, consider levator release and advance frontalis muscle to the superior tarsus.

BIBLIOGRAPHY

1. Blaydon SM. (2011). Marcus Gunn jaw-winking syndrome. [online] Available from www.emedicine.com/oph/TOP-IC608.HTM. [Accessed September, 2013].
2. Demirci H, Frueh BR, Nelson CC. Marcus Gunn jaw-winking synkinesis. Ophthalmology. 2010;117(7):1447-52.

1HH. TRICHIASIS

General

Acquired condition in which previous normal eyelashes are misdirected toward the globe.

Clinical

Stevens-Johnson syndrome, toxic epidermal necrolysis, and ocular cicatricial pemphigoid.

Ocular

Ocular irritation, chronic eyelid inflammation or infection, foreign body sensation.

Laboratory

Diagnosis is made by clinical findings.

Treatment

Epilation, argon laser ablation, cryosurgery, radiosurgery and full-thickness wedge resection or eyelid margin rotation procedures are all possible therapies.

BIBLIOGRAPHY

1. Graham RH. (2012). Trichiasis. [online] Available from www.emedicine.com/oph/TOPIC609.HTM. [Accessed September, 2013].

1II. XANTHELASMA (XANTHELASMA PALPEBRARUM)

General

Hereditary, isolated disorder associated with aging and hormonal changes. It may occur as a result of hyperlipemia.

Clinical

Hyperlipemia, hypercholesterolemia, obesity, cardiovascular changes.

Ocular

Soft, yellow, plague-like, velvety lesion usually in the medial canthus area.

Laboratory

Lipid profile.

Treatment

Dietary restrictions for obesity and increased triglycerides, dermatologic—trichloroacetic acid, blepharoplasty incision and laser—CO_2 laser.

BIBLIOGRAPHY

1. Roy H. (2011). Xanthelasma. [online] Available from www.emedicine.com/oph/TOPIC610.HTM. [Accessed September, 2013].

⊟ 1JJ. XERODERMA PIGMENTOSUM (SYMBLEPHARON)

General

Rare autosomal recessive disorder characterized by extreme cutaneous photosensitivity; both sexes affected; onset in infancy or early childhood.

Ocular

Conjunctivitis; symblepharon; keratitis; corneal ulcer; blepharitis; uveitis; malignancies of conjunctiva, cornea, eyelids, and iris; ectropion; keratoconus; lid freckles; chronic conjunctival congestion; corneal opacification; bilateral pterygium; epibulbar and palpebral squamous cell corneal carcinoma.

Clinical

Neurologic abnormalities and cutaneous malignancies of ectodermal origin; speech disorders; spastic paralysis; convulsions; mental deficiency; gonadal hypoplasia; stunted growth; carcinoma of tongue.

Laboratory

No consistent laboratory studies.

Treatment

Sunlight protection, treatment of any malignancies, sunscreens, protective clothing, sunglasses and hats.

⊟ BIBLIOGRAPHY

1. Diwan AH. (2011). Xeroderma pigmentosum. [online] Available from www.emedicine.com/derm/TOPIC462. HTM. [Accessed September, 2013].

⊟ 2A. ACQUIRED IMMUNODEFICIENCY SYNDROME (AIDS; ACQUIRED CELLULAR IMMUNODEFICIENCY; ACQUIRED IMMUNODEFICIENCY)

General

Acquired breakdown of the immune system followed by disease that takes advantage of the body's collapsed defenses; acquired by shared drug needles or sexual intercourse; occurs most frequently in homosexually active men (75%), intravenous drug abusers (13%), and Haitian immigrants (6%).

Ocular

Retinal cotton-wool spots; CMV retinitis; retinal periphlebitis; conjunctival Kaposi sarcoma; necrotizing retinitis; retinal hemorrhages; conjunctivitis sicca; orbital Burkitt lymphoma; peripheral retinochoroiditis; vitreitis; fungal corneal ulcer; hypopyon; acute glaucoma; third nerve palsy; anterior uveitis; atypical retinitis; orbital pseudotumor; herpes zoster ophthalmicus; herpes simplex keratitis; bacterial keratitis; molluscum contagiosum; CMV retinitis; toxoplasma retinitis; acute retinal necrosis; HIV retinitis; syphilitic retinitis; *P. carinii* choroiditis; fungal and bacterial endophthalmitis; fungal choroiditis; conjunctival microvasculopathy; keratitis sicca; subconjunctival hemorrhage.

Clinical

Because of lowered immunity, one third develops Kaposi sarcoma; pneumonia caused by *P. carinii*; death.

Laboratory

Enzyme-linked immunosorbent assay (ELISA) test is used for screening other tests are used to evaluate false-positive and false-negative test results.

Treatment

Medical consultations are required for systemic treatment. The treatment of CMV retinitis can include drugs such as ganciclovir, valganciclovir, fomivirsen, foscarnet and cidofovir. All of these drugs have specific adverse effects and complicate the decision to use for treatment.

⊟ BIBLIOGRAPHY

1. Copeland RA, Phillpotts BA. (2011). Ocular manifestations of HIV infection. [online] Available from www.emedicine.com/oph/TOPIC417.HTM. [Accessed September, 2013].
2. Dubin J. (2011). Rapid testing for HIV. [online] Available from www.emedicine.com/emerg/TOPIC253.HTM. [Accessed September, 2013].

⊟ 2B. BLEPHARITIS (SEBORRHEIC BLEPHARITIS, ADULT BLEPHARITIS, MEIBOMIAN GLAND DYSFUNCTION)

General

Common eyelid inflammation. It is seen frequently with seborrheic dermatitis.

Clinical

None.

Ocular

- *Ocular symptoms*: Discharge, foreign body sensation, dryness, uncomfortable sensation, sticky sensation, pain, epiphoria, itching, redness, heavy sensation, glare, excessive blinking, history of chalazion or hordeolum.
- *Lid margin abnormalities*: Irregular lid margin, vascular engorgement, plugged Meibomian gland, anterior or posterior replacement of the mucocutaneous junction. (Meibomian score is graded as 1–3. 1 is less than one-third lid; 2 is one-third to two-thirds lid; 3 is over two-thirds lid.)

Laboratory

Diagnosis is made by clinical findings. Swab of lids usually is *S. aureus*.

Treatment

Oral tetracyclines, omega-3 fatty acids, flax seed oil or fish oil. Ocular therapy includes eyelid scrubs, warm compresses, bacitracin ointment to lid margins, topical cyclosporine A and preservative-free lubricants.

⊟ BIBLIOGRAPHY

1. Ibrahim OM, Matsumoto Y, Dogru M, et al. The efficacy, sensitivity, and specificity of in vivo laser confocal microscopy in the diagnosis of Meibomian gland dysfunction. Ophthalmology. 2010;117(4):665-72.
2. Nemet AY, Vinker S, Kaiserman I. Associated morbidity of blepharitis. Ophthalmology. 2011;118(6):1062-8.
3. Lowery RS. (2011). Adult blepharitis. [online] Available from www.emedicine.com/oph/TOPIC81.HTM. [Accessed September, 2013].

⊟ 2C. CHALAZION

General

Common inflammatory lesion of the eyelid; obstruction of the Meibomian gland with the accumulation of sebaceous material; most frequently seen in individuals between ages of 30 and 50 years.

Clinical

Acne, seborrhea, rosacea.

Ocular

Eyelid swelling; eyelid nodule; injection of the conjunctiva; altered visual acuity; lid tenderness.

Laboratory

Diagnosis is made by clinical findings. Recurrent symptoms may require fine-needle aspiration to exclude malignancy and viral or bacterial cultures.

Treatment

Warm compresses; topical or systemic antibiotics; steroid injections; surgical drainage.

⊟ BIBLIOGRAPHY

1. Fansler JL, Schraga ED, Santen S. (2012). Chalazion in emergency medicine. [online] Available from emedicine.medscape.com/article/797763-overview. [Accessed September, 2013].

2D. TEMPORAL ARTERITIS SYNDROME (CRANIAL ARTERITIS SYNDROME; GIANT CELL ARTERITIS; HUTCHINSON-HORTON-MAGATH-BROWN SYNDROME)

General

Etiology unknown; mainly females; mainly Whites; ages 55–80 years; temporal artery shows inflammatory thickening; arteritis of the vessels supplying the optic nerve.

Ocular

Transient ptosis; partial or complete loss of vision on the affected side; retinal detachment; exudates and hemorrhages; narrowing of retinal vessels; obstruction of the central retinal artery; optic atrophy; ischemic optic neuropathy; acute decreased IOP; corneal hypesthesia; palsies of extraocular muscles; hemorrhagic glaucoma; diplopia; hemorrhages on or around the disk.

Clinical

Throbbing headache; hyperalgesia of the scalp; malaise; anorexia; weakness; weight loss; fever; nodular pulmonary nodules; cough; otitis with deafness.

Laboratory

Elevated ESR greater than 50 mm/hour, positive temporal artery biopsy.

Treatment

Systemic corticosteroids are the therapy of choice.

BIBLIOGRAPHY

1. Allen AW, Biega T, Varma MK. (2012). Temporal arteritis imaging. [online] Available from www.emedicine.com/radio/TOPIC675.HTM. [Accessed September, 2013].
2. Walvick MD, Walvick MP. Giant cell arteritis: laboratory predictors of a positive temporal artery biopsy. Ophthalmology. 2011;118(6):1201-4.

2E. GRANULOMA VENEREUM

General

Donovania granulomatis; infective venereal disease; prevalent in black women; *C. trachomatis* is an intracellular bacterium lacking respiratory enzymes that has an affinity for mucosal epithelium; serotypes A through C have been epidemiologically associated with trachoma; serotypes E through K have been associated with genital infection and keratoconjunctivitis in sexually active adults and neonates; other serotypes have been associated with lymphogranuloma venereum and Reiter syndrome.

Ocular

Lid and orbit granulomas.

Clinical

Painless primary lesions; painful secondarily infected ulcers.

Laboratory

Culturing the organism with best results obtained using aspirates from an involved inguinal lymph node and from bacterial typing of the culture after growth.

Treatment

Recommended treatment is done with doxycycline (100 mg PO BID) or erythromycin (500 mg QID). Continue treatment for 3 weeks, combined with aspiration of the lymph nodes, if needed.

BIBLIOGRAPHY

1. Plaza JA, Prieto VG. (2012). Dermatologic manifestations of lymphogranuloma venereum. [online] Available from www.emedicine.com/derm/TOPIC617.HTM. [Accessed September, 2013].

⊟ 2F. HORDEOLUM (INTERNAL HORDEOLUM, ACUTE MEIBONITIS, EXTERNAL HORDEOLUM, STYE)

General

Acute *Staphylococcal* infection of the sebaceous glands of the eyelids.

Clinical

None.

Ocular

External hordeolum infection (stye) and internal hordeolum is secondary *Staphylococcal* infection of Meibomian gland in the tarsal plate.

Laboratory

Diagnosis is made by clinical findings.

Treatment

Hot moist compresses, topical antibiotic and systemic antibiotics. If the gland does not spontaneously drain, a stab incision of skin or palpebral conjunctiva may be necessary.

⊟ BIBLIOGRAPHY

1. Ehrenhaus MP, Sturridge KA. (2012). Hordeolum. [online] Available from www.emedicine.com/oph/TOPIC606.HTM. [Accessed September, 2013].

⊟ 2G. ORBITAL CELLULITIS AND ABSCESS

General

Potentially life threatening; requires prompt evaluation and treatment.

Clinical

Sinusitis, ear infection, diabetes, dental disease.

Ocular

Orbital pain, proptosis, diplopia, decreased ocular motility, eyelid swelling and erythema, vision loss.

Laboratory

Diagnosis is made by clinical findings.

Treatment

Intravenous and oral antibiotic.

⊟ BIBLIOGRAPHY

1. Harrington JN. (2012). Orbital cellulitis. [online] Available from www.emedicine.com/oph/TOPIC205.HTM. [Accessed September, 2013].

⊟ 2I. STREPTOCOCCUS (SCARLET FEVER)

General

Gram-positive bacteria that can invade any tissue.

Ocular

Conjunctivitis; corneal ulcer; blepharitis; scarlatinal rash of lid; erysipelas dermatitis of lid; gangrene of lid; endophthalmitis; proptosis; dacryocystitis; optic neuritis; orbital cellulitis; uveitis; hypopyon; secondary glaucoma; paralysis of extraocular muscles; infectious crystalline keratopathy; scleritis.

Clinical

Pharyngitis; impetigo; scarlet fever; pneumonia; bacteremia; rheumatic fever; glomerulonephritis.

Laboratory

Gram-positive cocci growing in pairs or chains. Throat culture and sensitivity are useful.

Treatment

Penicillin is the drug of choice.

⊟ BIBLIOGRAPHY

1. Zabawski EJ. (2011). Scarlet fever. [online] Available from www.emedicine.com/emerg/TOPIC518.HTM. [Accessed September, 2013].

⊟ 2J. BASEDOW SYNDROME (GRAVES DISEASE; HYPERTHYROIDISM; THYROTOXICOSIS; EXOPHTHALMIC GOITER; PARRY DISEASE)

General

Diffuse toxic goiter; inherited as a simple autosomal recessive; penetrance greater in females; however, dominant mode of inheritance and variable penetrance are possible; uncommon in either sex before the age of 15 years.

Ocular

Exophthalmos; swelling of eyelids and discoloration of upper eyelids; lid lag (von Graefe's sign); globe lag (Koeber's sign); lid trembling on gentle closure (Rosenbach's sign); reduced blinking (Stellwag's sign); retraction of upper lid; difficulty in everting upper lid (Gifford's sign); convergence weakness (Möbius's sign); impaired fixation on extreme lateral gaze (Suker's sign); possible external ophthalmoplegia (Ballet's sign); Dalrymple's sign (staring appearance); tearing; photophobia; epiphora; prolapse of lacrimal gland; neuroretinal edema; tortuous vessels; papilledema and papillitis; anisocoria; keratitis; increased intraocular pressure on upgaze; decreased visual acuity; enlargement of the extraocular muscles; increased volume of the extraorbital fat; superior rectus muscle enlargement; decreased venous outflow.

Clinical

Tachycardia; anxiety; insomnia; loss of weight; hyperhidrosis; restlessness; myocarditis (toxic); atrial fibrillation.

Laboratory

Visual field testing, forced duction testing for restrictive myopathy, CT, MRI, T_4 and thyroid-stimulating hormone, thyroid-stimulating immunoglobulins.

Treatment

There is no immediate treatment; the disease is self-limited but prolonged course over one or more years. 5% of patients may require surgical intervention which could be orbital decompression, strabismus surgery, lid-lengthening surgery or blepharoplasty.

⊟ BIBLIOGRAPHY

1. Ing E. (2012). Thyroid-associated orbitopathy. [online] Available from www.emedicine.com/oph/TOPIC237.HTM. [Accessed September, 2013].
2. Regensburg NI, Wiersinga WM, Berendschot TT, et al. Do subtypes of Graves' orbitopathy exist? Ophthalmology. 2011;118:191-6.

⊟ 2K. TRACHOMA

General

Most common in rural communities of the Middle East, Africa, Asia, and South and Central America; caused by *C. trachomatis*; associated with poor sanitation and medical care.

Ocular

Chronic keratoconjunctivitis; papillae follicles; keratitis; opacities of cornea; scars of palpebral conjunctiva; ptosis; tearing; entropion.

Clinical

Rhinitis; otitis media; upper respiratory tract infection.

Laboratory

Most endemic areas, laboratory tests are unavailable. Commercial PCR based assay has high sensitivity and specificity.

Treatment

Tetracycline eye ointment for 6 weeks or a single-dose azithromycin systemically.

⊟ BIBLIOGRAPHY

1. Biebesheimer JB, House J, Hong KC, et al. Complete local elimination of infectious trachoma from severely affected communitieis after six biannual mass azithromycin distributions. Ophthalmology. 209;116:2047-50.
2. Solomon AW. (2011). Trachoma. [online] Available from www.emedicine.com/oph/TOPIC118.HTM. [Accessed September, 2013].

2L. WEGENER SYNDROME (WEGENER GRANULOMATOSIS)

General

Etiology unknown; occurs in fourth and fifth decades of life; persistent rhinitis or sinusitis; three characteristic features are: (1) necrotizing granulomatous lesions in the respiratory tract, (2) generalized focal arthritis and (3) necrotizing thrombotic glomerulitis.

Ocular

Exophthalmos; lid and conjunctival chemosis; papillitis; conjunctivitis; corneal ulcer; corneal abscess; optic atrophy; optic neuritis; orbital cellulitis; episcleritis; sclerokeratitis; cataract; peripheral ring corneal ulcers; ptosis; dacryocystitis; retinal periphlebitis; cotton-wool spots; retinal and vitreous hemorrhages; rubeosis iridis; neovascular glaucoma.

Clinical

Severe sinusitis; pulmonary inflammation; arteritis; weakness; fever; weight loss; bony destruction; granulomatous vasculitis of the upper and lower respiratory tracts; glomerulonephritis; diffuse pulmonary infiltrates; lymphadenopathy; diffuse pulmonary hemorrhage; overlap with giant cell arteritis.

Laboratory

Histopathology: Necrotizing, granulomatous vasculitis with infiltrating neutrophils, lymphocytes and giant cells; urine-proteinuria, hematuria and urinary casts.

Treatment

Topical eye lubricants, ophthalmic antibiotic solution or ointments and corticosteroid drops may prove to be beneficial. Orbital decompression is needed when medical treatment is unresponsive to treat optic nerve compression.

BIBLIOGRAPHY

1. Collins JF. Handbook of Clinical Ophthalmology. New York, USA: Year Book Medical Publication; 1982.
2. Flach AJ. Ocular manifestations of Wegener's granulomatosis. JAMA. 1995;274(15):1199-200.
3. Haynes BF, Fishman ML, Fauci AS, et al. The ocular manifestations of Wegener's Wegener's granulomatosis. Fifteen years' experience and review of the literature. Am J Med. 1977;63(1):131-41.
4. Leavitt RY, Fauci AS. Less common manifestations and presentations of Wegener's Wegener's granulomatosis. Curr Opin Rheumatol. 1992;4(1):16-22.
5. Robinson MR, Lee SS, Sneller MC, et al. Tarsal-conjunctival disease associated with Wegener's granulomatosis. Ophthalmology. 2003;110(9): 1770-80.
6. Roy FH, Fraunfelder FW, Fraunfelder FT. Roy and Fraunfelder's Current Ocular Therapy, 6th edition. Philadelphia: WB Saunders; 2008.
7. Straatsma BR. Ocular manifestations of Wegener granulomatosis. Am J Ophthalmol. 1957;44(6):789-99.

2M. YELLOW FEVER

General

Acute infectious disease of short duration and extremely variable severity.

Ocular

Lid edema; orbital pain; subconjunctival, vitreal, and anterior chamber hemorrhages; mydriasis; optic neuritis; partial optic atrophy.

Clinical

Fever; headache; nausea; epistaxis; relative bradycardia; albuminuria; convulsions; tongue shows red margins with white furred center; copious hemorrhages; anuria; delirium; slow pulse; jaundice; "black vomit"; hematemesis; coma; death.

Laboratory

Complete blood count, coagulation studies, urinalysis, chest X-ray, PCR-based assay, monoclonal enzyme immunoassay.

Treatment

No specific treatment.

BIBLIOGRAPHY

1. Busowski MT, Robertson JL, Wallace MR. (2011). Yellow fever. [online] Available from www.emedicine.com/med/TOPIC2432.HTM. [Accessed January, 2013].

⊟ 3A. BASAL CELL CARCINOMA

General

Most common malignant neoplasm of lids; it can occasionally occur as a primary basal cell cancer of the conjunctiva and in the lacrimal canaliculus.

Ocular

Neoplasm most common on lower lid and medial canthus; lacrimation.

Clinical

Tumors of skin and other regions, including sinuses.

Laboratory

Typical histology findings. Imaging studies only for invading or deep tumor in the medial canthus.

Treatment

Surgery involves local excision; advanced and recurrent tumors are best managed by a multidisciplinary approach involving head and neck surgical oncologists. Photodynamic therapy and cryosurgery are also effective.

⊟ BIBLIOGRAPHY

1. Bader RS, Santacroce L, Diomede L, et al. (2012). Basal cell carcinoma. [online] Available from www.emedicine.com/ent/TOPIC722.HTM. [Accessed September, 2013].

⊟ 3B. ACTINIC AND SEBORRHEIC KERATOSIS

General

Actinic keratosis is a precancerous lesion that occurs most commonly on sunlight-exposed areas of the skin. Seborrheic keratosis is a benign epithelial tumor that appears predominantly on the trunk and head.

Clinical

Lupus.

Ocular

Eyebrow and eyelids lesions.

Laboratory

Diagnosis is made by clinical findings.

Treatment

Cryosurgery is the treatment of choice.

⊟ BIBLIOGRAPHY

1. Roy FH, Fraunfelder FW, Fraunfelder FT. Roy and Fraunfelder's Current Ocular Therapy, 6th edition. London, UK: Elsevier; 2008.

⊟ 3C. LYMPHANGIOMA

General

Poorly circumscribed infiltrating lesions consisting of lymphatic/dysplastic blood vessels; occurs predominantly in children and young adults.

Ocular

Conjunctival hemorrhages; cellulitis of lid; ptosis; exophthalmos; amblyopia; astigmatism; extraocular muscle imbalance; optic disk edema; retinal striae.

Clinical

Benign tumors of the lymph system.

Laboratory

Ultrasonography lacks specificity and soft-tissue detail; CT images bone deformity and MRI provides superior soft-tissue details.

Treatment

- *Ptosis*: Most cases require surgical correction if visual acuity is affected and there are several procedures that may be used including levator resection, repair or advancement and Fasanella-Servat procedure.
- *Exophthalmos*: Reversing the problem which is causing the exophthalmos is the treatment of choice and will minimize the ocular complications. Ocular lubricants are beneficial for control of the corneal exposure.

BIBLIOGRAPHY

1. Schwartz RA, Fernandez G. (2012). Lymphangioma. [online] Available from www.emedicine.com/derm/TOPIC866.HTM. [Accessed September, 2013].

3D. MELANOCYTIC LESIONS OF THE EYELIDS (EPHELIS, LENTIGO, NEOVASCULAR NEVUS, DERMAL MELANOCYTOSIS, MALIGNANT MELANOMA)

General

Congenital or acquired eyelid lesions.

Clinical

Benign lesions—frequently from birth to puberity. Sun exposure increases lesion. Large (1 cm or more) from birth may become melanomas and should be removed.

Ocular

Benign lesions and malignant lesions of the eyelid.

Laboratory

Examination with measurement and serial photography to determine if benign or malignant. Histology or biopsy or excisional biopsy.

Treatment

No treatment necessary for benign lesions. Malignant lesions should be dissected.

BIBLIOGRAPHY

1. Bashour M, Bassin R, Benchimol M. (2013). Melanocytic lesions of the eyelid. [online] Availabl;e from www.emedicine.com/oph/TOPIC715.HTM. [Accessed September, 2013].

3E. MALIGNANT MELANOMA OF THE POSTERIOR UVEA (CHOROIDAL MELANOMA, CILIARY BODY MELANOMA, UVEAL MELANOMA, INTRAOCULAR MELANOMA)

General

Most common primary intraocular tumor in adults.

Clinical

Metastatic melanoma can appear in other parts of the body such as skin or liver.

Ocular

Intraocular tumors of the choroid, iris and ciliary body.

Laboratory

Ultrasonography, fluorescein angiography, indocyanine green angiography.

Treatment

Ocular therapy's goal is to eradicate the tumor before metastasis occurs. Diode laser, brachytherapy, stereotactic, local resection, enucleation and exenteration are all used to achieve this. Systemically intravenous therapy; intrahepatic chemoembolization has been used for isolated liver metastases. Proton beam is used to kill the tumor.

BIBLIOGRAPHY

1. Garcia-Valenzuela E, Pons ME, Puklin JE, et al. (2011). Choroidal melanoma. [online] Available from www.emedicine.com/oph/TOPIC403.HTM. [Accessed September, 2013].

🖶 3F. SEBACEOUS GLAND CARCINOMA

General

Ocular adnexa contains various sebaceous glands from which carcinomas may arise; predilection for the upper lids but may involve both lids; usually in older age groups; slight female preponderance.

Ocular

Blepharitis; madarosis; meibomianitis; sebaceous carcinoma of lids or orbit; orbital edema; proptosis; conjunctivitis; superficial keratitis; lacrimal gland tumor.

Clinical

Metastasis to preauricular or cervical lymph nodes, or submandibular area.

Laboratory

Biopsy diagnostic in chronic non-healing chalazia or suspicious unresolved chronic blepharitis.

Treatment

Mohs' technique appears to have the highest success rate.

🖶 BIBLIOGRAPHY

1. Glassman ML, Bashour M. (2012). Sebaceous gland carcinoma. [online] Available from www.emedicine.com/oph/TOPIC716.HTM. [Accessed September, 2013].

CHAPTER
23

Glaucoma

🗗 1A. OPEN ANGLE GLAUCOMA

General

Chronic, bilateral ocular disease characterized by optic nerve damage and visual field defects.

Clinical

Diabetes mellitus, systemic hypertension, migraine headaches.

Ocular

Visual field defects, optic nerve cupping, arcuate scotoma, thin central cornea, high myopia, elevated intraocular pressure (IOP).

Laboratory

Diagnosis is made by clinical findings.

Treatment

Topical anti-glaucoma agents, later trabeculoplasty and surgical interventions—tube-shunt and cyclodestructive procedures.

🗗 BIBLIOGRAPHY

1. Bell JA. (2012). Primary open-angle glaucoma. [online] Available from www.emedicine.com/oph/TOPIC139.HTM. [Accessed October, 2013].

🗗 1A1. NORMAL-TENSION GLAUCOMA (LOW TENSION GLAUCOMA)

General

Normal IOP with progressive optic nerve changes and visual field changes. It is seen more frequently in patients over 50 years of age.

Clinical

None.

Ocular

Normal IOP with cup/disk or visual field changes.

Laboratory

Diagnosis is made by clinical findings.

Treatment

- *Medical*: Glaucoma medications.
- *Surgical*: Argon laser trabeculectomy, selective laser trabeculoplasty, trabeculectomy with or without anti-metabolites, tube shunt surgery and cyclodestructive procedures.

🗗 BIBLIOGRAPHY

1. Roy FH, Fraunfelder FW, Fraunfelder FT. Roy and Fraunfelder's Current Ocular Therapy, 6th edition. London, UK: Elsevier; 2008.

1B1. ANGLE RECESSION GLAUCOMA

General

Manifestation of blunt ocular trauma.

Clinical

None.

Ocular

Angle recession involves rupture of the face of ciliary body, resulting in a tear between the longitudinal and circular fibers of the ciliary muscle, which may cause glaucoma.

Laboratory

Diagnosis is made by clinical findings.

Treatment

- *Topical*: Steroids with cycloplegic agents for inflammation. Anti-glaucoma agents for IOP control.
- *Surgical*: Filtration surgery with the use of antimetabolites appears to be the most effective technique.

BIBLIOGRAPHY

1. Sullivan BR. (2012). Angle recession glaucoma. [online]Available from www.emedicine.com/oph/TOPIC121.HTM. [Accessed October, 2013].

1B3. APHAKIC AND PSEUDOPHAKIC GLAUCOMA

General

Increased IOP following cataract surgery. Pathophysiology may include distortion of chamber angle, retained viscoelastics, inflammation, hemorrhage, ghost cell, vitreous in the anterior chamber, pigment dispersion, aqueous misdirection syndrome and pupillary block.

Clinical

None.

Ocular

Elevated IOP; uveitis; hyphema; retained cortical lens material; shallow anterior chamber; vitreous in anterior chamber.

Laboratory

Imaging studies include ultrasound biomicroscopy; gonioscopy.

Treatment

Mydriasis is the initial treatment to break the block. Iridotomy, trabeculoplasty, cyclophotocoagulation and pars plana vitrectomy may be necessary.

BIBLIOGRAPHY

1. Graham RH. (2012). Aphakic and pseudophakic glaucoma. [online] Available from emedicine.medscape.com/article/1207170-overview. [Accessed October, 2013].

1B4. UGH SYNDROME (UVEITIS-GLAUCOMA-HYPHEMA SYNDROME) GLAUCOMA

General

It is caused by a defective anterior chamber lens; it can be caused by toxic substance incorporated into the plastic of lens during manufacture or warped intraocular lens; syndrome may rarely occur after extracapsular cataract extraction (ECCE) with implantation of a posterior chamber intraocular lens.

Ocular

Uveitis-glaucoma-hyphema (UGH).

Clinical

None.

Laboratory

Diagnosis is made by clinical findings.

Treatment

- *Uveitis*:
  - *Glaucoma*: Glaucoma medication should be the first plan of action. If medication is unsuccessful, a filtering surgical procedure with or without antimetabolites may be beneficial.

- *Hyphema*: Cycloplegia decreased the inflammation and discomfort associated with traumatic iritis.
- Topical beta-adrenergic antagonists are the therapy of choice for elevated IOPs; laser may be used to cauterize the bleeding vessel.

BIBLIOGRAPHY

1. Percival SP, Das SK. UGH syndrome after posterior chamber lens implantation. J Am Intraocul Implant Soc. 1983;9(2):200-1.
2. Masket S. Pseudophakic posterior iris chafing syndrome. J Cataract Refract Surg. 1986;12(3):252-6.

1B5. CORTICOSTEROID-INDUCED GLAUCOMA

General

Oral, inhaled, topical and periocular corticosteroids can cause elevated IOP.

Clinical

None.

Ocular

Open-angle glaucoma is secondary to the use of corticosteroids.

Laboratory

Diagnosis is made by clinical findings.

Treatment

Discontinue the use of steroids if possible; use antiglaucoma agents; filter surgery may be effective.

BIBLIOGRAPHY

1. Rhee DJ, Gedde S. (2012). Drug-induced glaucoma. [online] Available from www.emedicine.com/oph/TOPIC124.HTM. [Accessed October, 2013].

1B6. GLAUCOMA ASSOCIATED WITH ELEVATED VENOUS PRESSURE

General

Systemic disorders that raise the venous pressure to the eye and may cause glaucoma.

Clinical

Elevated episcleral venous pressure as venous obstruction, carotid cavernous fistula and Sturge-Weber syndrome.

Ocular

Prominent veins under the conjunctiva help to diagnose this condition.

Laboratory

Diagnosis is made by clinical findings.

Treatment

Topical—anti-glaucoma agents. Filtering procedure is done if topical treatment is not effective.

BIBLIOGRAPHY

1. Dahl AA, Ebrahim SA. (2012). Intraocular Tumors and Glaucoma. [online] Available from www.emedicine.com/oph/TOPIC143.HTM. [Accessed October, 2013].

🖥 1B7. GHOST CELL GLAUCOMA

General

Usually follows vitreous hemorrhage when the presence of blood debris in the anterior chamber clogs the trabecular meshwork resulting in elevated IOP.

Clinical

Vitreous hemorrhage sometimes is associated with diabetes.

Ocular

Elevated IOP, vitreous hemorrhage, corneal edema, decreased visual acuity, posterior vitreous detachment.

Laboratory

Cytologic examination of the aqueous humor, B-scan ultrasonography.

Treatment

Usually it involves surgical intervention with lavage of the anterior chamber or vitrectomy.

🖥 BIBLIOGRAPHY

1. Campbell DG, Essigmann EM. Hemolytic ghost cell glaucoma. Further studies. Arch Ophthalmol. 1979;97(11): 2141-6.
2. Montenegro MH, Simmons RJ. Ghost cell glaucoma. Int Ophthalmol. 1994;34(1):111-5.
3. Rojas L, Ortiz G, Gutiérrez M, et al. Ghost cell glaucoma related to snake poisoning. Arch Ophthalmol. 2001;119(8): 1212-3.

🖥 1B8. IRIS NEVUS SYNDROME (COGAN-REESE SYNDROME; CHANDLER SYNDROME; IRIDOCORNEAL ENDOTHELIAL SYNDROME; ICE SYNDROME)

General

Usually unilateral but may be bilateral; usually in young adult women; nonfamilial; cause unknown; Chandler, Cogan-Reese, and iridocorneal endothelial (ICE) syndromes have been considered as three separate syndromes but they are now recognized as a single spectrum of diseases.

Ocular

Unilateral glaucoma in eyes with peripheral anterior synechiae; multiple iris nodules; ectopic Descemet's membrane; corneal edema; stromal iris atrophy; iris pigment epithelial atrophy; ectropion uveae; ectopic pupil; keratoconus; herpes simplex virus deoxyribonucleic acid (DNA) has been detected in patients with ICE syndrome from corneal specimens.

Clinical

Glass-like membrane covering the anterior iris surface; corneal endothelial degeneration and accompanying ectopic endothelial membranes are responsible for occlusion of the filtration meshwork and subsequent pressure increase.

Laboratory

Diagnosis is made by clinical findings.

Treatment

This disease does not usually respond to medications and trabeculectomy operations. Glaucoma drainage devices create an alternate aqueous pathway by channeling aqueous from the anterior chamber through a tube to an equatorial plate inserted under the conjunctiva that promotes bleb formation.

🖥 BIBLIOGRAPHY

1. Alvarado JA, Underwood JL, Green WR, et al. Detection of herpes simplex viral DNA in the iridocorneal endothelial syndrome. Arch Ophthalmol. 1994;112(12):1601-9.
2. Buckley RJ. Pathogenesis of the ICE syndrome. Br J Ophthalmol. 1994;78(8):595-6.
3. Chandler PA. Atrophy of the stroma of the iris; endothelial dystrophy, corneal edema, and glaucoma. Am J Ophthalmol. 1956;41(4):607-15.
4. Cogan DG, Reese AB. A syndrome of iris nodules, ectopic Descemet's membrane, and unilateral glaucoma. Doc Ophthalmol. 1969;26:424-33.
5. Radius RL, Herschler J. Histopathology in the irisnevus (Cogan-Reese) syndrome. Am J Ophthalmol. 1980;89(6):780-6.
6. Rodrigues MM, Stulting RD, Waring GO. Clinical, electron microscopic, and immunohistochemical study of the corneal endothelium and Descemet's membrane in the iridocorneal endothelial syndrome. Am J Ophthalmol. 1986;101(1):16-27.

1B9. LENS-INDUCED GLAUCOMA (PHACOLYTIC, LENS PARTICLE AND PHACOANTIGENIC)

General

Open-angle secondary glaucoma can be phacolytic, lens particle and phacoantigenic. Closed-angle secondary lens glaucoma occurs from lens intumescence (phacomorphic glaucoma) or lens dislocation (ectopia lentis).

Clinical

None.

Ocular

Open or closed secondary glaucoma, cataract, retained lens material, uveitis.

Laboratory

Diagnosis is made by clinical findings.

Treatment

- *Mature or hypermature cataract*: Topical steroids, IOP lowering agents, hyperosmotic agents. Removal of cataract will usually restore normal IOP.
- *Lens particle glaucoma*: Topical IOP lowering agents, cycloplegics and steroids. Removal of residual lens material.
- *Phacoantigenic glaucoma*: Topical steroids, IOP lowering agents, and cycloplegics. Pars plana vitrectomy is done to remove all residual lens material and posterior capsule or removal of capsule is done manually with forceps after injection of chymotrypsin beneath the iris.
- *Phacomorphic glaucoma*: Topical IOP lowering agents. Argon laser iridoplasty to open angle, laser iridotomy to bypass papillary black, cataract extraction.
- *Ectopia lentis*: Laser iridotomy is done to bypass papillary block. If lens floats in vitreous, treat conservatively.

BIBLIOGRAPHY

1. Sullivan BR. (2012). Lens-particle glaucoma. [online] Available from www.emedicine.com/oph/TOPIC56.HTM. [Accessed October, 2013].
2. Gill H, Juzych MS, Goyal A. (2012). Phacomorphic glaucoma. [online] Available from www.emedicine.com/oph/TOPIC58.HTM. [Accessed October, 2013].
3. Yi K, Chen TC. (2011). Phacolytic glaucoma. [online] Available from www.emedicine.com/oph/TOPIC57.HTM. [Accessed October, 2013].

1B10. MALIGNANT GLAUCOMA (CILIARY BLOCK GLAUCOMA, AQUEOUS MISDIRECTION, CILOLENTICULAR/CILIOVITREAL BLOCK)

General

Rare; poor response to conventional treatment.

Clinical

None.

Ocular

Shallow angle secondary glaucoma.

Laboratory

Ultrasound biomicroscopy.

Treatment

Argon laser treatment of ciliary processes, yttrium-aluminum-garnet (YAG) laser hyaloidotomy and incisionalsurgery. Pars plana vitrectomy may be necessary sometimes with posterior capsulotomy and lensectomy.

BIBLIOGRAPHY

1. Pons ME, Hughes BA. (2012). Malignant glaucoma. [online] Available from www.emedicine.com/oph/TOPIC134.HTM. [Accessed October, 2013].

⊟ 1B11. GLAUCOMA FOLLOWING PENETRATING KERATOPLASTY

General

Second most common cause for graft failure; etiology varies greatly and include postoperative inflammation, viscoelastic substances in the chamber, hyphema, operative technique, pre-existing glaucoma, misdirected aqueous, epithelial downgrowth and others.

Clinical

None.

Ocular

Elevated IOP; progressive visual field changes; graft edema; graft failure.

Laboratory

Accurate measurement of the IOP with a Mackay-Marg electronic applanation tonometer, the pneumatic applanation tonometer, the Tonon-pen or the dynamic contour tonometer.

Treatment

Treatment is controversial because of the high risk of graft failure. Medical management with topical drops and systemic pills is the treatment of choice; surgical therapy may be necessary and include trabeculoplasty, trabeculectomy, drainage device and cyclodestructive procedures.

⊟ BIBLIOGRAPHY

1. Shetty R, de Resende Moura Filho E, Hasan SA, et al. (2012). Glaucoma and Penetrating Keratoplasty. [online] Available from emedicine.medscape.com/article/1208228-overview. [Accessed October, 2013].

⊟ 1B12. PIGMENTARY DISPERSION SYNDROME AND PIGMENTARY GLAUCOMA

General

Shedding of pigment that is evident as mid-peripheral radial iris transillumination defects. Characterized by pigmentary deposits on the structures of the anterior and posterior chambers.

Clinical

Siderosis, hemosiderosis, diabetes mellitus.

Ocular

Krukenberg's spindles, heterochromia, optic nerve damage, visual field defects, Adie's pupil, chronic open angle glaucoma; concave peripheral iris.

Laboratory

Diagnosis is made by clinical findings.

Treatment

Pilopine HS gel or Ocusert, laser therapy such as trabeculoplasty, iridectomy, iridoplasty and/or filtration surgery are useful.

⊟ BIBLIOGRAPHY

1. Ritch R, Barkana Y. (2012). Pigmentary Glaucoma. [online] Available from www.emedicine.com/oph/TOPIC136.HTM. [Accessed October, 2013].

⊟ 1B13. POSNER-SCHLOSSMAN SYNDROME (GLAUCOMATOCYCLITIC CRISIS)

General

High intraocular tension lasting from hours to several weeks and recurring at varying frequencies; low-grade, intermittent, nongranulomatous inflammation; in one series of patients, human leukocyte antigen (HLA) BW54 was present in 41% of patients.

Ocular

Slight blurring of vision and colored halos during episodes of high intraocular tension; high IOP (unilateral); glaucomatocyclitic crisis (benign and usually unilateral); enlarged pupil; anisocoria; absence of ciliary or conjunctival injection; only trace of aqueous flare; no posterior synechiae; chamber angle open; heterochromia iridis; keratitic precipitates may be present.

Clinical

Allergy; associated with gastrointestinal disease (peptic ulcers).

Laboratory

Diagnosis is made by clinical findings.

Treatment

Ocular hypertension: Timolol and prostaglandin agents; inflammation—topical steroids and cycloplegics.

BIBLIOGRAPHY

1. Oakman JH. (2012). Posner-Schlossman syndrome. [online] Available from www.emedicine.com/oph/TOPIC137.HTM. [Accessed October, 2013].

1B14. PSEUDOEXFOLIATION SYNDROME

General

Prevalent over age of 70 years; rare before age of 40 years; unilateral involvement in 40–50% of cases; asymmetry of severity in bilateral cases; most common in Caucasians, especially from Iceland and Scandinavian countries; pseudoexfoliation fibers were identified in autopsy tissue specimens of skin, heart, lungs, liver and cerebral meninges; consistently associated with connective tissue components, i.e. fibroblasts, collagen and elastic fibers, myocardial tissue and heart muscle cell.

Ocular

Gray or white fluffy material deposited in particles, flakes or sheets on anterior surface of iris, ciliary body, posterior surface of cornea, pupillary margin, lens and trabecular meshwork; increased pigmentation of trabecular meshwork; zonular dialysis; displaced or dislocated lens; anterior chamber depth asymmetry; preoperative phacodonesis; glaucoma; cataract.

Clinical

None.

Laboratory

Diagnosis is made by clinical findings.

Treatment

Annual eye examinations are done for early detection of glaucoma. Glaucoma in pseudoexfoliation is more resistant to medical therapy. If medical therapy is unsuccessful to control the glaucoma, argon laser trabeculoplasty or trabeculectomy may be beneficial.

BIBLIOGRAPHY

1. Pons ME, Eliassi-Rad B. (2011). Pseudoexfoliation glaucoma. [online] Available from www.emedicine.com/oph/TOPIC140.HTM. [Accessed October, 2013].

1B15. PUPILLARY BLOCK GLAUCOMA

General

This condition can occur following cataract surgery with or without an intraocular lens implant. Block is caused by mechanical closure of the pupil by the intraocular lens, by developing synechiae or by lens capsule.

Clinical

Pain in the eye, unilateral headache, nausea, vomiting.

Ocular

Elevated IOP, iris synechiae, anterior pupillary block, posterior pupillary block, postoperative iritis, photophobia, blurred vision, halos around lights.

Laboratory

B-scan to identify retained lens material, lens nucleus, choroidal hemorrhage or aqueous misdirection.

Treatment

Surgically, a peripheral iridectomy to break the block is the treatment of choice. Surgical breaking of the synechiae may be necessary. Vitrectomy may be needed. Filtration surgery may be indicated if the anterior chamber fails to open following the iridectomy. Transciliary filtration can be performed with a Fugo blade to relieve iris bombe.

Medically, analgesics and antiemetics may be beneficial. Dilatation and topical steroids may be useful to relieve inflammation following the episode.

BIBLIOGRAPHY

1. Eezzuduemhoi DR, Wilson D. (2012). Aphakic pupillary block. [online] Available from emedicine.medscape.com/article/1220164-overview. [Accessed October, 2013].

1C1. PRIMARY ANGLE-CLOSURE GLAUCOMA (PRIMARY CLOSED ANGLE GLAUCOMA)

General

Obstruction of aqueous humor outflow forms the anterior chamber which results from closure of the angle by the peripheral root of the iris.

Clinical

Pain, nausea.

Ocular

Flare in the anterior chamber, conjunctival chemosis, hyperemia, corneal epithelial edema, folds in Descemet's membrane, peripheral anterior synechiae, increased IOP, visual field defect.

Laboratory

Diagnosis is made by clinical findings.

Treatment

Systemic hyperosmotic agents, topical pilocarpine every 5 minutes, laser iridotomy and if IOP does not respond, filtering surgery may be necessary.

BIBLIOGRAPHY

1. Noecker RJ, Kahook MY. (2011). Glaucoma, angle closure, acute. [online] Available from www.emedicine.com/oph/TOPIC255.HTM. [Accessed October, 2013].
2. Tham CC, Ritch R. (2012). Glaucoma, angle closure, chronic. [online] Available from www.emedicine.com/oph/TOPIC122.HTM. [Accessed October, 2013].

1C2. CHRONIC ANGLE CLOSURE GLAUCOMA

General

Portion of the anterior chamber angle is closed with peripheral anterior synechiae; five types: (1) chronic angle-closure glaucoma (2) combined mechanism, (3) mixed mechanism, (4) plateau iris and (5) mioticinduced angle-closure glaucoma.

Clinical

Asymptomatic due to the slow onset of the disease.

Ocular

Elevated IOP; peripheral anterior synechiae; deposits of pigment in the angle; plateau iris.

Laboratory

Measurement of IOP; gonioscopy; optic nerve head and retinal nerve fiber layer assessments; visual field testing and slit-lamp examination.

Treatment

Iridotomy is the treatment of choice. Argon laser peripheral iridoplasty and goniosynechialysis may be necessary.

BIBLIOGRAPHY

1. Tham CC, Ritch R. (2012). Glaucoma, angle closure, chronic. [online] Available from emedicine.medscape. com/article/1205154-overview. [Accessed October, 2013].

⊟ 1C4. GLAUCOMA ASSOCIATED WITH INTRAOCULAR TUMORS (TUMOR RELATED GLAUCOMA, MELANOMALYTIC GLAUCOMA, NEOVASCULAR GLAUCOMA, ANGLE CLOSURE GLAUCOMA)

General

Unilateral, closed-angle glaucoma secondary to intraocular tumor.

Clinical

Systemic hamartomatoses, lymphoid tumors, leukemias.

Ocular

Glaucoma in one eye, primarily caused by tumor of eye. Primary tumors of uvea, retina, and pigmented and non-pigmented epithelium.

Laboratory

Ultrasonography, fluorescein angiography or iridocyanine green angiography, magnetic resonance imaging (MRI) and computed tomography (CT) scan of orbit, liver function tests, liver imaging test, general oncologist evaluation.

Treatment

- *Benign tumor*: Treat glaucoma medically.
- *Malignant tumor*: Treat tumor first, antiglaucoma drops and systemic carbonic anhydrase inhibitors are instituted as necessary.
- *Iris and ciliary body tumors*: Observation initially. Uveal metastases and choroidal melanoma treatment consists of serial observation, photocoagulation, transpupillary thermotherapy, radiotherapy, local resection, enucleation and even orbital exenteration. Retinoblastoma may require an enucleation. Irradiation and chemotherapy should be used at the discretion of the oncologist.

⊟ BIBLIOGRAPHY

1. Roy FH, Fraunfelder FW, Fraunfelder FT. Roy and Fraunfelder's Current Ocular Therapy, 6th edition. London, UK: Elsevier; 2008.

⊟ 1C5. IRIDAL ADHESION SYNDROME (IRIS ADHESION SYNDROME, IRIDOCORNEAL ENDOTHELIAL SYNDROME)

General

Surgically related phenomenon following intraocular surgery in which iris pigment epithelium proliferates and adheres to cut edge of anterior capsule, drawing iris posteriorly to posterior and anterior capsules.

Ocular

Posterior synechiae; irregular pupil.

Clinical

None.

Laboratory

Diagnosis is made by clinical findings.

Treatment

Aqueous suppressants can be tried but usually surgery is required.

⊟ BIBLIOGRAPHY

1. Dickerson D. Surgery-related iridal adhesion syndrome. Ophthalmol Times. 1984;9:6.
2. Teekhasaenee C, Ritch R. Iridocorneal endothelial syndrome in Thai patients: clinical variations. Arch Ophthalmol. 2000;118(2):187-92.

⊟ 1C6. MALIGNANT GLAUCOMA (CILIARY BLOCK GLAUCOMA, AQUEOUS MISDIRECTION, CILOLENTICULAR/CILIOVITREAL BLOCK)

General

Rare; poor response to conventional treatment.

Clinical

None.

Ocular

Shallow angle secondary glaucoma.

Laboratory

Ultrasound biomicroscopy.

Treatment

Argon laser treatment of ciliary processes, YAG laser hyaloidotomy and incisional surgery. Pars plana vitrectomy may be necessary sometimes with posterior capsulotomy and lensectomy.

⊟ BIBLIOGRAPHY

1. Pons ME, Hughes BA. (2012). Malignant glaucoma. [online] Available from www.emedicine.com/oph/TOPIC134.HTM. [Accessed October, 2013].

⊟ 1C7. PHACOMORPHIC GLAUCOMA

General

Phacomorphic glaucoma is secondary angle-closure glaucoma due to lens swelling. Pupillary block is caused by the change in size and the position of the anterior lens surface. Causes can include traumatic cataract, intumescent cataract and rapidly developing senile cataract.

Clinical

Nausea; vomiting.

Ocular

Acute pain; blurred vision; rainbow-colored halos; elevated IOP; irregular pupil; corneal edema; shallow central anterior chamber; lens enlargement; weakened zonules.

Laboratory

Optical coherence tomography (OCT) and gonioscopy are useful in visualization of the anterior chamber angle.

Treatment

Beta-blockers and carbonic anhydrase inhibitors are used to initially lower the IOP. Argon iridoplasty can be then used to rapidly reduce the pressure and finally cataract extraction for a definitive treatment.

⊟ BIBLIOGRAPHY

1. Gill H, Juzych MS, Goyal A. (2012). Phacomorphic glaucoma. [online] Available from emedicine.medscape.com/article/1204917-overview. [Accessed October, 2013].

⊟ 1C8. PLATEAU IRIS SYNDROME

General

Rare; occurs in younger age group; presumably due in part to an anterior insertion of the iris; pupillary block is not a significant part of the mechanism leading to angle closure.

Ocular

Spontaneous or mydriasis-induced angle-closure despite a patent iridectomy; anterior chamber is of normal depth axially and the iris plane is flat, but a peripheral roll of iris can close the angle either when the pupil dilates spontaneously or after mydriatic drugs are administered.

Clinical

Nausea; vomiting.

Laboratory

Indentation gonioscopy.

Treatment

Iridotomy.

⊟ BIBLIOGRAPHY

1. Wang JC, Lee PS, Ritch R, et al. (2012). Plateau iris glaucoma. [online] Available from www.emedicine.com/oph/TOPIC574.HTM. [Accessed October, 2013].

🗗 1C9. RUBEOSIS IRIDIS NEOVASCULAR GLAUCOMA

General

Neovascularization of the iris.

Clinical

None.

Ocular

Intractable type of secondary glaucoma, rubeosis iridis, diabetic retinopathy, retinal vein occlusion, carotid occlusive disease, iritis.

Laboratory

Diagnosis is made by clinical findings. Check for diabetes.

Treatment

- Trabeculectomy with the antifibrotic agents, mitomycin-C and 5-fluorouracil (5-FU) is one modality. Trabeculectomy in neovascular glaucoma (NVG) has a significant failure rate. Using standard trabeculectomy (without antifibrosis), an IOP of less than 25 mm Hg on one medication or less has been reported to occur in 67–100% of patients in three studies. Using injections of 5-FU subconjunctivally in the postoperative period, the surgical success has been reported to be 68% over 3 years. Inject 0.1 mL of 5 mg/mL 5-FU subconjunctivally either superiorly above the bleb or inferiorly (just above the lower fornix). Mitomycin-C used intraoperatively has been shown to be more effective than 5-FU in routine trabeculectomies. No significant follow-up studies exist on the use of mitomycin-C with trabeculectomy in NVG.
- Valve implant surgery is another modality, and is indicated when trabeculectomy fails or extensive conjunctival scarring exists, thereby preventing a standard filtering procedure. Molteno, Krupin and Ahmed valve implants commonly are used. One large series using the Krupin valve reported 79% of eyes with NVG had a 67% success rate in controlling IOP (< 24 mm Hg) with mean follow-up of 23 months. Long-term results are mixed. Using the Molteno implant, 60 eyes with NVG achieved a satisfactory IOP (< 21 mm Hg) and maintenance of visual acuity over 5 years of only 10.3%. If combined with the need for vitrectomy, consideration of pars plana tube-shunt insertion may reduce anterior segment complications.
- Avastin injections have shown some promise for the control of iris neovascularization.
- Complications include postoperative hypotony with associated complications, blockage of internal fistula, blockage of external filtration site (fibrosis of the filtering bleb) and corneal endothelial loss.

🗗 BIBLIOGRAPHY

1. Freudenthal J, Khan YA, Ahmed II, et al. (2011). Neovascular glaucoma. [online] Available from www.emedicine.com/oph/TOPIC135.HTM. [Accessed October, 2013].

🗗 2A. ANIRIDIA (CONGENITAL ANIRIDIA, HEREDITARY ANIRIDIA)

General

Hereditary, recessive (two-thirds of cases), can be dominant, sporadic or traumatic; absence of the iris; rare; usually bilateral unless due to trauma.

Ocular

Absence of iris; subluxed lens; iridodialysis; cataract; glaucoma; corneal scarring, vascularization and edema; iris colobomata; round eccentric pupils; keratoconus.

Clinical

Cerebellar ataxia; mental retardation; Wilms' tumor (WT).

Laboratory

Chromosomal deletion, cytogenic analysis, submicroscopic deletions of WT gene with fluorescence in situ hybridization (FISH) technique, polymerase chain reaction (PCR) genotyping halotypes across paired box gene 6 (PAX6)-Wilms' tumor type 1 (WT1) region provides evidence of a chromosomal deletion.

Treatment

Systemic or topical glaucoma therapy.

BIBLIOGRAPHY

1. François J, Coucke D, Coppieters R. Aniridia-Wilms' tumor syndrome. Ophthalmologica. 1977;174(1):35-9.

2. Johns KJ, O'Day DM. Posterior chamber intraocular lenses after extracapsular cataract extraction in patients with aniridia. Ophthalmology. 1991;98(11):1698-702.

3. Kremer I, Rajpal RK, Rapuano CJ, et al. Results of penetrating keratoplasty in aniridia. Am J Ophthalmol. 1993;115(3): 317-20.

4. Magalini SI, Scrascia E. Dictionary of Medical Syndromes, 2nd edition. Philadelphia, PA: Lippincott Williams & Wilkins; 1981.

2B. CONGENITAL CATARACT, MICROCORNEA, ABNORMAL IRIDES, NYSTAGMUS, AND CONGENITAL GLAUCOMA SYNDROME

General

Autosomal dominant.

Ocular

Microphakia; cataract with two concentric disks, with the anterior being swollen; microphthalmos; microcornea; nystagmus; congenital glaucoma; honey-colored iris with absence of pattern; peripheral anterior synechiae; pupillary abnormality; corneal edema; posterior synechiae; vitreous hemorrhage; shallow anterior chamber; vitreous loss; corneal staphyloma; keratoconus.

Clinical

High-arched palate; increased webbing of fingers and toes; deafness.

Laboratory

Diagnosis is made by clinical findings.

Treatment

Cataract surgery if vision decreases.

BIBLIOGRAPHY

1. Cebon L, West RH. A syndrome involving congenital cataracts of unusual morphology, microcornea, abnormal irides, nystagmus and congenital glaucoma, inherited as an autosomal dominant trait. Aust J Ophthalmol. 1982;10(4):237-42.

2. Henkind P, Friedman AH. Iridogoniodysgenesis with cataract. Am J Ophthalmol. 1971;72(5):949-54.

2C. GLAUCOMA, CONGENITAL

General

Autosomal recessive; occurs more frequently in males; can occur isolated or associated with other systemic or ocular malformations (dysgenesis of iris, angle and peripheral cornea).

Ocular

Buphthalmos; corneal haze; glaucoma; epiphora.

Clinical

None.

Laboratory

Tonometry, corneal measurements, gonioscopy, and ophthalmoscopy should be performed in the operating room and carefully documented. IOPs recorded under general anesthesia are usually lower than those obtained in the office due to the effects of the anesthetic agents.

Treatment

Primary congenital glaucoma almost always is managed surgically; both goniotomy and trabeculectomy may be useful. When multiple goniotomies and/or trabeculectomies fail, the surgeon usually resorts to a filtering procedure.

BIBLIOGRAPHY

1. Ben-Zion I, Tomkins O, Moore DB, et al. Surgical results in the management of advanced primary congenital glaucoma in a rural pediatric population. Ophthalmology. 2011;118(2):231-5.e1.

2. Bowman RJ, Dickerson M, Mwende J, et al. Outcomes of goniotomy for primary congenital glaucoma in East Africa. Ophthalmology. 2011;118(2):236-40.

3. Cibis GW, Urban RC, Dahl AA. (2011). Primary congenital glaucoma. [online] Available from www.emedicine.com/oph/TOPIC138.HTM. [Accessed October, 2013].

⊟ 2E. JUVENILE GLAUCOMA

General

Group of glaucomas occurring in later childhood or early adulthood.

Clinical

None.

Ocular

Chronic open-angle glaucoma. Mild cases of infantile glaucoma may have mild corneal enlargement and breaks in Descemet's membrane.

Laboratory

Testing for juvenile rheumatic arthritis, sarcoidosis, ankylosing spondylitis, herpes zoster, syphilis and tuberculosis.

Treatment

Trial topical medical therapy. If IOP is uncontrolled iridectomy, goniotomy, trabeculectomy, filtration surgery or cyclodestructive procedures may be necessary.

⊟ BIBLIOGRAPHY

1. Walton DS. (2011). Juvenile glaucoma. [online] Available from www.emedicine.com/oph/TOPIC333.HTM. [Accessed October, 2013].

⊟ 2F. GLAUCOMA, HEREDITARY JUVENILE

General

Autosomal dominant, present at birth; there has been linkage with chromosome 1q21-q23; age at diagnosis is 5–30 years; positive family history; male-to-female ratio of 2:1.

Ocular

Dysgenesis of the iris and iridocorneal angle; glaucoma; hypoplasia of iris; dark-colored irides; myopia; smooth iris; prominent iris processes; grayish-pale color of trabecular meshwork.

Clinical

None.

Laboratory

Tonometry, corneal measurements, gonioscopy, and ophthalmoscopy should be performed in the operating room and carefully documented. IOPs recorded under general anesthesia are usually lower than those obtained in the office due to the effects of the anesthetic agents.

Treatment

Primary congenital glaucoma almost always is managed surgically, both goniotomy and trabeculectomy may be useful. When multiple goniotomies and/or trabeculectomies fail, the surgeon usually resorts to a filtering procedure.

⊟ BIBLIOGRAPHY

1. Walton DS. (2011). Juvenile glaucoma. [online] Available from www.emedicine.com/oph/TOPIC333.HTM. [Accessed October, 2013].

⊟ 2G. GLAUCOMA, RECESSIVE JUVENILE

General

Autosomal recessive; rare; normal parents and consanguineous marriages; asymptomatic and insidious onset.

Ocular

Buphthalmos; aching of eyes; colored halos around lights; elevated IOP; corneal epithelial edema; severe cupping and atrophy of optic nerve; constriction of visual fields.

Clinical

Headaches.

Laboratory

Tonometry, corneal measurements, gonioscopy, and ophthalmoscopy should be performed in the operating room and carefully documented. IOPs recorded under general anesthesia are usually lower than those obtained in the office due to the effects of the anesthetic agents.

Treatment

Primary congenital glaucoma almost always is managed surgically; both goniotomy and trabeculectomy may be useful. When multiple goniotomies and/or trabeculectomies fail, the surgeon usually resorts to a filtering procedure.

BIBLIOGRAPHY

1. Walton DS. (2011). Juvenile Glaucoma. [online] Available from www.emedicine.com/oph/TOPIC333.HTM. [Accessed October, 2013].

2H. MICROPHTHALMOS, PIGMENTARY RETINOPATHY, GLAUCOMA

General

Autosomal dominant; three disorders are combined.

Ocular

Microphthalmos; pigmentary retinopathy; glaucoma.

Clinical

None.

Laboratory/Glaucoma

Chromosome analysis and genetic counseling.

Treatment/Glaucoma

Beta-blockers, carbonic anhydrase inhibitors and prostaglandin analogs. Surgery may be needed if IOP is uncontrolled.

BIBLIOGRAPHY

1. Hermann P. Syndrome: microphthalmic-retinite pigmentaire-glaucoma. Arch Ophthalmol Rev Gen Ophtalmol. 1958;18(1):17-24.
2. McKusick VA. Mendelian Inheritance in Man; A Catalog of Human Genes and Genetic Disorders, 12th edition. Baltimore, USA: The Johns Hopkins University Press; 1998.
3. Hamosh A, Scott AF, Amberger J, et al. Online Mendelian Inheritance in Man (OMIM), a knowledgebase of human genes and genetic disorders. Nucleic Acids Res. 2002;30(1):52-5.

2I. AXENFELD-RIEGER SYNDROME (POSTERIOR EMBRYOTOXON; AXENFELD SYNDROME)

General

Dominant inheritance; occasionally sporadic; variable in expression.

Ocular

Posterior embryotoxon: ring-like opacity of cornea; long trabecula; prominent Schwalbe line; iris adhesions to Schwalbe line and cornea with large abnormal iris processes or broad sheets of tissues of varying size and location; anterior layer of iris may appear hypoplastic; ectopia of the pupil not uncommon; polycoria occurs; ring-like opacity of the deep corneal layers extending several millimeters from the limbus in continuity with the sclera; keratoconus.

Laboratory

Patients may need workup for associated systemic abnormalities.

Treatment

Patients may need workup for associated systemic abnormalities, so referring to a pediatrician or an internist is important.

BIBLIOGRAPHY

1. Dersu II. (2012). Secondary Congenital Glaucoma. [online] Available from www.emedicine.com/oph/TOPIC141.HTM. [Accessed October, 2013].

2J. RIEGER SYNDROME (AXENFELD-RIEGER SYNDROME; DYSGENESIS MESODERMALIS CORNEAE ET IRIDES; DYSGENESIS MESOSTROMALIS; AXENFELD POSTERIOR EMBRYOTOXON-JUVENILE GLAUCOMA)

General

Autosomal dominant; neural crest abnormality; 50% of patients develop glaucoma.

Ocular

Microphthalmia; congenital glaucoma; iris hypoplasia; deformed and acentric pupil; anterior synechiae; aniridia; microcornea; corneal opacities in Descemet's membrane parallel to the limbus; dislocated lens; optic atrophy; cataract; strabismus; ptosis; hypertelorism; keratoconus; posterior embryotoxon; broad iris processes to embryotoxon; iris stromal hypoplasia; corectopia; polycoria; secondary glaucoma.

Clinical

Face wide; hypodontia; underdeveloped maxilla; teeth deformities; myotonic dystrophy; facial anomalies: maxillary hypoplasia, protrusion of the lower lip, broad, flat nose; dental anomalies include absent teeth, pig-like incisors and decreased crown size; hypospadias.

Laboratory

Diagnosis is made by clinical findings.

Treatment/Ocular

Congenital glaucoma can be treated with beta-blockers, prostaglandin analogs and carbonic anhydrase inhibitors. Surgery such as goniotomy or trabeculectomy can be used if IOP is not controlled.

BIBLIOGRAPHY

1. Eagle RC. Congenital, developmental and degenerative disorders of the iris and ciliary body. In: Albert DM, Jakobiec FA (Eds). Albert & Jakobiec's Principles and Practice of Ophthalmology: Clinical Practice, 3rd edition. Philadelphia, PA: WB Saunders; 1994. pp. 367-87.
2. Montes JG, Montes JC. Syndrome de Rieger, anomalie de axenfeld con glaucoma Juvenil familiar. Arch Soc Ophth Hisp Am. 1967;27:93.
3. Rieger H. Beitrage zur Kenntnis seltener Missbildungen der Iris. Graefes Arch Clin Esp Ophthalmol. 1935;133:602.
4. Wesley RK, Baker JD, Golnick AL. Rieger's syndrome: (oligodontia and primary mesodermal dysgenesis of the iris) clinical features and report of an isolated case. J Pediatr Ophthalmol Strabismus. 1978;15(2):67-70.

2K. RING CHROMOSOME 6 (ANIRIDIA, CONGENITAL GLAUCOMA, AND HYDROCEPHALUS)

General

Rare disorder associated with various congenital anomalies; autosomal dominant with recessive sporadically reported.

Ocular

Microphthalmia; aniridia; congenital uveal ectropion; Rieger anomaly; congenital glaucoma; corneal clouding; prominent Schwalbe's line with attached iris strands; hypopigmented fundi; hypoplasia of iris stroma; strabismus; ptosis; nystagmus; megalocornea; iris coloboma; optic atrophy; hypertelorism; antimongoloid slant of palpebral fissures; ectopic pupils; angle anomalies; posterior embryotoxon; microcornea; colobomatous.

Clinical

Hydrocephalus; agenesis of corpus callosum; congenital heart defects; mental retardation; low-set malformed ears; broad nasal bridge; micrognathia; short neck; hand anomalies; high-arched palate; widely spaced nipples; deformity of feet; respiratory distress syndrome; hyperbilirubinemia; hypocalcemia; anemia; seizure; bulging anterior fontanel.

Laboratory

Diagnosis is made by clinical findings.

Treatment

Ptosis: If visual acuity is affected, most cases require surgical correction and there are several procedures that may be used including levator resection, repair or advancement and Fasanella-Servat procedure.

BIBLIOGRAPHY

1. Bateman JB. Chromosomal anomalies and the eye. In: Wright KW (Ed). Pediatric Ophthalmology and Strabismus. St Louis: Mosby; 1995. p. 595.
2. Chitayat D, Hahm SY, Iqbal MA, et al. Ring chromosome 6: report of a patient and literature review. Am J Med Genet. 1987;26(1):145-51.
3. DeLuise VP, Anderson DR. Primary infantile glaucoma (congenital glaucoma). Surv Ophthalmol. 1983;28(1):1-19.
4. Levin H, Ritch R, Barathur R, et al. Aniridia, congenital glaucoma, and hydrocephalus in a male infant with ring chromosome 6. Am J Med Genet. 1986;25(2):281-7.

3. OCULAR HYPOTONY

General

Low IOP resulting in anatomical or functional abnormalities to the eye.

Clinical

None.

Ocular

Thin corneas, corneal striae, aqueous flare, choroidal folds, effusion, macular folds, low IOP.

Laboratory

Diagnosis is made by clinical findings.

Treatment

Topical corticosteroids and cycloplegic agents are recommended.

BIBLIOGRAPHY

1. Roy FH, Fraunfelder FW, Fraunfelder FT. Roy and Fraunfelder's Current Ocular Therapy, 6th edition. London, UK: Elsevier; 2008.

CHAPTER
24

Globe

⬚ 1. CLINICAL ANOPHTHALMOS (APPARENT ABSENCE OF GLOBE)

1. Anencephaly
2. Gross midline facial defects (median cleft face syndrome)
3. Dyscraniopygophalangea
4. Goldenhar syndrome (oculoauriculovertebral syndrome)
5. Goltz syndrome (focal dermal hypoplasia syndrome)
6. Hallermann-Streiff syndrome (dyscephalic mandibulo-oculofacial syndrome)
7. Hypervitaminosis A
†8. Idiopathic
9. Klinefelter syndrome (gynecomastia-aspermatogenesis)
10. Lanzieri syndrome (craniofacial malformations)
11. Leri syndrome (carpal tunnel syndrome)
12. Meckel syndrome (dysencephalia splanchnocystica syndrome)
13. Oculovertebral dysplasia (Weyers-Thier syndrome)
14. Otocephaly
15. Trisomy 13
†16. Sex-linked or recessive hereditary
17. Waardenburg anophthalmia syndrome* (anophthalmos with limb anomalies)—recessive

⬚ BIBLIOGRAPHY

1. Graham CA, Redmond RM, Nevin NC. X-linked clinical anophthalmos: localization of the gene to Xq27-Xq28. Ophthal Paediatrics Genetics. 1991;12:43-8.
2. Roy FH. Ocular Syndrome and Systemic Diseases, 5th edition. New Delhi: Jaypee Brothers; 2013.

*Indicates most frequent
†Indicates a general entry and therefore has not been described in detail in the text

⬚ 1.1. ANENCEPHALY

General

Congenital neural tube defect that affects the formation of the brain and skull bones. Lethal in all cases.

Ocular

Anophthalmos.

Clinical

Absence of bony covering over the back of the head, cleft palate, heart defects.

Laboratory

Flattened head may be detected by prenatal ultrasound. Alpha-fetoprotein levels are elevated and can be detected in the amniotic fluid. Amniocentesis can be used to determine the chromosomal and genetic disorder.

Treatment

There is no treatment. Grief and genetic counseling should be offered to the parents.

⬚ BIBLIOGRAPHY

1. Best RG, Gregg AR, Lorenzo N. (2011). Anencephaly. [online] Available from emedicine.medscape.com/article/1181570-overview. [Accessed October, 2013].

1.2. FRONTONASAL DYSPLASIA SYNDROME (MEDIAN CLEFT FACE SYNDROME)

General

Congenital disorder without genetic background; condition may present a variety of facial malformations, depending on the stage of embryonic development at which interference occurs.

Ocular

Hypertelorism; anophthalmia or microphthalmia; significant refractive errors; strabismus; nystagmus; eyelid ptosis; optic nerve hypoplasia; optic nerve colobomas; cataract; corneal dermoid; inflammatory retinopathy.

Clinical

Broad nasal root may be associated with median nasal groove and cleft of nose and/or upper lip; cleft of ala nasi (unilateral or bilateral); V-shaped hair prolongation into forehead.

Laboratory

Computed tomography (CT), magnetic resonance imaging (MRI) and physical examination.

Treatment

Reconstruction surgery may be warranted.

BIBLIOGRAPHY

1. Kinsey JA, Streeten BW. Ocular abnormalities in the medial cleft face syndrome. Am J Ophthalmol. 1977;83:261.
2. Roarty JD, Pron GE, Siegel-Bartelt J, et al. Ocular manifestations of frontonasal dysplasia. Plast Reconstr Surg. 1994;93:25-30.
3. Sedano HO, Cohen MM, Jirasek J, et al. Frontonasal dysplasia. J Pediatr. 1970;76:906-13.
4. Weaver D, Bellinger D. Bifid nose associated with midline cleft of the upper lip: case report. Arch Otolaryngol. 1946;44:480.

1.3. ULLRICH SYNDROME (ULLRICH-FEICHTIGER SYNDROME; DYSCRANIOPYLOPHALANGY) CORNEAL ULCER

General

Belongs to trisomy 13–15; unknown etiology; sporadic occurrence.

Ocular

Microphthalmia to anophthalmia; hypertelorism; narrow lid fissures; strabismus; glaucoma; aniridia; cloudy cornea; corneal ulcers; chorioretinal coloboma.

Clinical

Hypoplastic mandible; broad nose; polydactyly; spina bifida; bicornuate uterus or septa vagina; congenital heart disease.

Laboratory/Ocular

Antinuclear antibodies (ANA) test, serum muscle enzyme levels.

Treatment/Ocular/Corneal Ulcer

Topical cycloplegic agents, topical cyclosporin and topical antibiotics.

BIBLIOGRAPHY

1. Geeraets WJ. Ocular Syndromes, 3rd edition. Philadelphia: Lea & Febiger; 1976.

1.4. GOLDENHAR SYNDROME (OCULO-AURICULO-VERTEBRAL DYSPLASIA; GOLDENHAR-GORLIN SYNDROME)

General

Most cases have been sporadic, but cases of autosomal dominant and recessive inheritance have been reported; male preponderance (60%); present at birth.

Ocular

Anophthalmia; colobomata of choroid, iris, and eyelid; antimongolian slant of lid fissure; epibulbar dermoid or lipodermoids of conjunctiva, cornea, and orbit; tilted optic disk; nerve hypoplasia; microphthalmia; macular heterotopia; tortuous retinal vessels.

Clinical

Frontal bulging of the skull; receding chin; malar hypoplasia; micrognathia and macrostomia; auricular appendices (single or multiple); multiple vertebral anomalies; preauricular fistulas; mental retardation.

Laboratory

Clinical.

Treatment

Dermoids: Surgery for function or cosmesis.

🗗 BIBLIOGRAPHY

1. Tewfik TL, Al-Noury KI. (2013). Manifestations of craniofacial syndromes. [online] Available from www.emedicine.com/ent/TOPIC319.HTM. [Accessed October, 2013].

🗗 1.5. GOLTZ SYNDROME (FOCAL DERMAL HYPOPLASIA SYNDROME)

General

X-linked dominant inheritance; lethal in males; skin manifestations present at birth.

Ocular

Microphthalmia; strabismus; coloboma of iris and/or choroid; epiphora; blue sclera; nystagmus; anophthalmos; keratoconus.

Clinical

Skin atrophy and linear pigmentation; telangiectasias of trunk and extremities; superficial, localized fatty skin deposits; multiple papillomas of mucous membranes and periorificial skin (oral, genital, anal); anomalies of extremities with syndactyly, oligodactyly, adactyly; hypohidrosis; paper-thin nails may be present; spina bifida; hypoplasia of right clavicle; umbilical or inguinal hernia.

Laboratory

Radiography may reveal osteopathia striata.

Treatment

Flashlamp-pumped pulse dye laser may ameliorate the pruritic symptoms that sometimes are noted in affected skin and improve the clinical appearance of the telangiectatic and erythematous skin lesions. Papillomas frequently require repeated surgical intervention.

🗗 BIBLIOGRAPHY

1. Goltz RW, Castelo-Soccio L. (2012). Focal dermal hypoplasia syndrome. [online] Available from emedicine.medscape.com/article/1110936-overview. [Accessed October, 2013].

🗗 1.6. HALLERMANN-STREIFF SYNDROME [DYSCEPHALIC-MANDIBULO-OCULO-FACIAL SYNDROME; OCULO-MANDIBULO-DYSCEPHALY; ULLRICH-FREMERY-DOHNA SYNDROME; FRANCOIS DYSCEPHALIC SYNDROME; MANDIBULO-OCULO-FACIAL DYSCEPHALY SYNDROME; FRANCOIS-HALLERMANN-STREIFF SYNDROME; HALLERMANN-STREIFF-FRANCOIS SYNDROME; AUDRY I SYNDROME; DOHNA SYNDROME; FRANCOIS SYNDROME (1); DYSCEPHALY-TEETH ABNORMALITY-DWARFISM; DYSCEPHALIA OCULOMANDIBULARIS-HYPOTRICHOSIS; MANDIBULO-OCULAR DYSCEPHALIA HYPOTRICHOSIS; FREMERY-DOHNA SYNDROME; OCULO-MANDIBULO-FACIAL DYSCEPHALY]

General

Rare; familial occurrence and consanguinity; males and females are equally affected.

Ocular

Microphthalmos (bilateral); proptosis; nystagmus; strabismus; cataracts; bilateral optic atrophy; coloboma of optic disk, choroid, and iris; keratoglobus; microcornea; anti-mongoloid slant; iris atrophy; uveitis; blue sclera; persistent pupillary membrane; secondary glaucoma.

Clinical

Malformations of skull (brachycephaly), facial skeleton and jaws; erupted teeth at birth; diminished hair growth; hyperextensibility of joints; short stature; skin atrophy; mental deficiency; predisposition to upper airway compromise; obstructive sleep apnea.

Laboratory

Diagnosis is made by clinical findings.

Treatment

- *Cataract*: Change in glasses can sometimes improve a patient's visual function temporarily; however the most common treatment is cataract surgery.
- *Strabismus*: Equalized vision with correct refractive error; surgery may be helpful in patients with diplopia.
- *Uveitis*: Topical steroids and cycloplegic medication should be the initial treatment of choice. Oral steroids should be given if not responsive to topical steroids, immunosuppressants if bilateral disease that does not respond to oral steroids, periocular steroids for unilateral or posterior uveitis. Vitrectomy can be used for severe vitreous opacification. Cryotherapy and laser photocoagulation may be used for localized pars plana exudates.
- *Glaucoma*: Glaucoma medication should be the first plan of action. If medication is unsuccessful, a filtering surgical procedure with or without antimetabolites may be beneficial.

BIBLIOGRAPHY

1. François J, Victoria-Troncoso V. François' dyscephalic syndrome and skin manifestations. Ophthalmologica. 1981;183(2):63-7.
2. Roy FH, Fraunfelder FW, Fraunfelder FT. Roy and Fraunfelder's Current Ocular Therapy, 6th edition. Philadelphia, PA: WB Saunders; 2008.
3. Hallermann W. Vogelgesicht und Cataracta Congenita. Klin Monatsbl Augenheilkd. 1948;113:315-8.
4. Ronen S, Rozenmann Y, Isaacson M, et al. The early management of baby with Hallermann-Streiff-Francois syndrome. J Pediatr Ophthalmol Strabismus. 1979;16(2):119-21.
5. Spaepen A, Schrander-Stumpel C, Fryns JP, et al. Hallermann-Streiff syndrome: clinical and psychological findings in children. Nosologic overlap with oculodentodigital dysplasia? Am J Med Genet. 1991;41(4):517-20.
6. Streiff EB. Dysmorphic Mandibulo-faciale (Tete d'Oiseau) et Alterations Oculaires. Ophthalmologica. 1950;120(1-2):79-83.

1.7. HYPERVITAMINOSIS A

General

Excessive vitamin A ingestion.

Ocular

Papilledema; congenital cataract; congenital anophthalmos; night blindness; diplopia; exophthalmos; "hourglass" cornea and iris with reduplicated lens.

Clinical

Elevation of cerebrospinal fluid pressure; migratory polyarthritis; hepatosplenomegaly; skin changes.

Laboratory

Diagnosis is usually based on a high index of suspicion in children who are malnourished or in patients with predisposing factors for its development.

Treatment

Oral administration of vitamin A 200,000 IU at presentation, the following day, and a third dose a week later is recommended. Infants should receive half doses.

BIBLIOGRAPHY

1. Schwartz RA, Centurion SA, Gascon P. (2013). Dermatologic Manifestations of Vitamin A Deficiency. [online] Available from www.emedicine.com/derm/TOPIC794.HTM. [Accessed October, 2013].

🗗 1.9. KLINEFELTER SYNDROME (GYNECOMASTIA-ASPERMATOGENESIS SYNDROME; XXY SYNDROME; XXXY SYNDROME; XXYY SYNDROME; REIFENSTEIN-ALBRIGHT SYNDROME)

General

Occurrence in 1% of retarded males; phenotypically males with positive female sex chromatin; karyotype shows 47 chromosomes, 44 autosomes, and 3 sex chromosomes with the complement XXY.

Ocular

Anophthalmos; coloboma; corneal opacities.

Clinical

Testicular hypoplasia; sterility; gynecomastia; eunuchoid physique; mental retardation; association with progressive systemic sclerosis and systemic lupus erythematosus.

Laboratory

May be diagnosed prenatally based on cytogenetic analysis of a fetus. If not diagnosed prenatally, the 47,XXY karyotype may manifest as various subtle age-related clinical signs that may prompt chromosomal evaluation.

Treatment

Treatment should address three major facets of the disease: (1) hypogonadism, (2) gynecomastia, and (3) psychosocial problems.

🗗 BIBLIOGRAPHY

1. Chen H. (2013). Klinefelter syndrome. [online] Available from www.emedicine.com/ped/TOPIC1252.HTM. [Accessed October, 2013].

🗗 1.10. LANZIERI SYNDROME

General

Developmental anomaly that belongs to group of craniofacial malformations; present from birth.

Ocular

Microphthalmia; anophthalmos; iris coloboma; cataracts; retinal and choroidal coloboma; optic nerve coloboma.

Clinical

Dwarfism; dyscephalia; dental anomalies; hypertrichosis; skin atrophy; absence of fibula, some tarsal and metatarsal bones.

Laboratory

Diagnosis is made by clinical findings.

Treatment

Cataract: Change in glasses can sometimes improve a patient's visual function temporarily; however the most common treatment is cataract surgery.

🗗 BIBLIOGRAPHY

1. Geeraets WJ. Ocular Syndromes, 3rd edition. Philadelphia: Lea & Febiger; 1976.
2. Lanzieri M. On a rare association of craniofacial malformative syndrome and congenital absence of the fibula. Ann Ottal Clin Ocul. 1961;87:667.
3. Magalini SI, Scrascia E. Dictionary of Medical Syndromes, 2nd edition. Philadelphia: JB Lippincott; 1981.

1.11. LERI SYNDROME (PLEONOSTEOSIS SYNDROME; CARPAL TUNNEL SYNDROME)

General

Autosomal dominant type of congenital osseous dystrophy; early epiphyseal bone formation of extremities; Morton metatarsalgia syndrome may result; onset in early infancy.

Ocular

Microphthalmia; anophthalmia; oculomotor paralysis; corneal clouding; cataract.

Clinical

Dwarfism (disproportionate); articular deformities; cutaneous deformities; carpal tunnel syndrome (median nerve compression); deformities of thumbs and great toes; laryngeal stenosis.

Laboratory

Clinical.

Treatment

- *Cataract*: Change in glasses can sometimes improve a patient's visual function temporarily; however the most common treatment is cataract surgery.
- *Corneal clouding*: Check for elevated intraocular pressure. Medical treatment includes the use of hyperosmotic drops, non-steroidal and steroid eye drops. Corneal transplant may be necessary.

BIBLIOGRAPHY

1. Fuller DA. (2012). Orthopedic Surgery for Carpal Tunnel Syndrome. [online] Available from www.emedicine.com/orthoped/TOPIC455.HTM. [Accessed October, 2013].

1.12. MECKEL SYNDROME (DYSENCEPHALIA SPLANCHNOCYSTIC SYNDROME; GRUBER SYNDROME)

General

Autosomal recessive; ocular manifestations are similar to those of trisomy 13–15 syndrome.

Ocular

Cryptophthalmos; clinical anophthalmos; microphthalmos; mongoloid slant of lid fissures; sclerocornea; microcornea; partial aniridia; cataract; retinal dysplasia; posterior staphyloma; optic nerve hypoplasia.

Clinical

Sloping forehead; posterior encephalocele; short neck; polydactyly and syndactyly (hands and feet); polycystic kidneys; cryptorchidism; cleft lip and palate; central nervous system abnormalities, including the Dandy-Walker malformation.

Laboratory

Chromosome analysis, MRI.

Treatment

Cardiac surgery may be warranted.

BIBLIOGRAPHY

1. Jayakar PB, Spiliopoulos M, Jayakar A. (2011). Meckel-Gruber syndrome. [online] Available from www.emedicine.com/ped/TOPIC1390.HTM. [Accessed October, 2013].

1.13. FRANCESCHETTI SYNDROME [FRANCESCHETTI-ZWAHLEN-KLEIN SYNDROME; TREACHER COLLINS SYNDROME; MANDIBULOFACIAL DYSOSTOSIS; MANDIBULOFACIAL SYNDROME; EYELID-MALAR-MANDIBLE SYNDROME; OCULOVERTEBRAL SYNDROME; BERRY SYNDROME; FRANCESCHETTI-ZWAHLEN SYNDROME; ZWAHLEN SYNDROME; BILATERAL FACIAL AGENESIS; BERRY-FRANCESCHETTI-KLEIN SYNDROME; FRANCESCHETTI-KLEIN SYNDROME; FRANCESCHETTI SYNDROME (II); TREACHER COLLINS-FRANCESCHETTI SYNDROME; WEYERS-THIER SYNDROME]

General

Irregular dominant inheritance; Weyers-Thier syndrome has similar features, except it is a unilateral variant; prevalent in Caucasians.

Ocular

Microphthalmia; oblique position of eyes with lateral downward slope of palpebral fissures; temporal lower lid coloboma; lack of cilia on middle third of lower lid; iris coloboma; underdeveloped orbicularis oculi muscle; cataract; optic disk hypoplasia.

Clinical

Fish-like face with sunken cheek bones, receding chin, and large, wide mouth; absent or malformed external ears with auricular appendages; high palate and possible harelip; hypoplastic zygomatic arch with absence of normal malar eminences; prolonged hairline on the cheek; deafness; micrognathia; glossoptosis; cleft palate.

Laboratory

Full craniofacial CT scan (axial and coronal slices from the top of the skull through the cervical spine), brain MRI.

Treatment

Operative repair is based upon the anatomic deformity and timing of correction is done according to physiologic need and development.

BIBLIOGRAPHY

1. Tolarova MM, Wong GB, Varma S. (2012). Mandibulofacial Dysostosis (Treacher Collins Syndrome). [online] Available from www.emedicine.com/ped/TOPIC1364.HTM. [Accessed October, 2013].

1.14. OTOCEPHALY

General

Birth defect; extreme malformation of first brachial arch characterized by almost complete aplasia of its parts.

Ocular

Bilateral anophthalmos.

Clinical

Mouth deformities; absence of lower jaw; joining of ears on the neck.

Laboratory

Diagnosis is made by clinical findings.

Treatment

Expansion of orbit and lid formation.

BIBLIOGRAPHY

1. Duke-Elder S, MacFaul PA. System of Ophthalmology, Volume XIII. St. Louis: CV Mosby; 1974.
2. Glange WD (Ed). The Mosby Medical Encyclopedia. St. Louis: CV Mosby; 1985.

1.15. TRISOMY 13 SYNDROME (TRISOMY D1 SYNDROME, PATAU SYNDROME, REESE SYNDROME) IRIS COLOBOMA

General

Extra chromosome in the D group; fatal in the first few months of life; trisomy 13–15 resembles trisomy D1.

Ocular

Anophthalmia; microphthalmia; iris coloboma; cataracts; retinal dysplasia; optic nerve coloboma; optic atrophy; iris dyplasia; calcified lens; retinal detachment; optic nerve hypoplasia; orbital cysts.

Clinical

Apneic spells; developmental deficiency of the nervous system; seizures (minor motor); deafness; cleft lip and palate; hemangiomata; horizontal palmar creases; hyperconvex fingernails; interventricular septal defects; renal abnormalities; cardiovascular changes; respiratory involvement; gastrointestinal disease; urogenital involvement; cerebral hypoplasia with hydrocephalus; mental retardation.

Laboratory

Immediate conventional cytogenetic test. Ultrasonography for any anomalies. Trisomy 13 is best identified through cytogenetic study of amniotic fluid.

Treatment

Surgical care is usually withheld for the first few months of life.

BIBLIOGRAPHY

1. Best RG, Gregg AR. (2012). Patau syndrome. [online] Available from www.emedicine.com/ped/TOPIC1745.HTM. [Accessed October, 2013].

1.17. WAARDENBURG SYNDROME (VAN DER HOEVE-HALBERSTAM-WAARDEN-BURG SYNDROME; WAARDENBURG-KLEIN SYNDROME; EMBRYONIC FIXATION SYNDROME; INTEROCULO-IRIDODERMATO-AUDITIVE DYSPLASIA; PIEBALDISM) HYPERTELORISM

General

Irregular dominant inheritance; developmental fault in neural crest with absence of the organ of Corti, aplasia of the spiral ganglion, and pigmentary changes; no sex preference; onset at birth.

Ocular

Hyperplasia of the medial portions of the eyebrows; hypertelorism; blepharophimosis; strabismus; heterochromia iridis; aniridia; microcornea; cornea plana; microphakia; abnormal fundus pigmentation; hypoplasia of optic nerve; synophrys; poliosis; hypopigmentation and hypoplasia of retina and choroid; epicanthus; lateral displacement of inferior puncta; lenticonus; underdevelopment of orbital bones; lateral displacement of inner canthi; hypopigmented iris.

Clinical

Congenital deafness; unilateral deafness or deaf-mutism; broad and high nasal root with absent nasofrontal angle; albinotic hair strain (unilateral); faint patches of skin pigmentation; pituitary tumor; nasal atresia; white forelock.

Laboratory

Molecular testing and audiology.

Treatment

Genetic counseling, audiology and otolaryngology management.

BIBLIOGRAPHY

1. Schwartz RA, Bawle EV, Jozwiak S. (2013). Genetics of Waardenburg syndrome. [online] Available from www.emedicine.com/ped/TOPIC2422.HTM. [Accessed October, 2013].

⊟ 2A. BACTERIAL ENDOPHTHALMITIS

General

Rare, intraocular bacteria infection which can follows intraocular surgery or penetrating injury.

Clinical

None.

Ocular

Photophobia, pain, hypoyon, decreased vision.

Laboratory

Vitreous and anterior chamber specimens to determine organism.

Treatment

Systemic steroids, topical, intravitreal and subconjunctival antibiotics and vitrectomy.

⊟ BIBLIOGRAPHY

1. Graham RH, Lawton AW, Law SK, et al. (2013). Bacterial Endophthalmitis. [online] Available from www.emedicine.com/oph/TOPIC393.HTM. [Accessed October, 2013].

⊟ 2B. ESCHERICHIA COLI

General

Gram-negative rod found in the gastrointestinal tract; urinary tract is the usual portal of entry.

Ocular

Uveitis; hyphema; hypopyon; gas bubbles in anterior chamber; purulent conjunctivitis; keratitis; corneal edema; panophthalmitis; endophthalmitis; glaucoma.

Clinical

Diarrhea; gastroenteritis; dehydration.

Laboratory

Anaerobic Gram-negative rod.

Treatment

Antibiotic therapy should start with ampicillin until sensitivity reports return.

⊟ BIBLIOGRAPHY

1. Suh DW. (2011). Ophthalmologic Manifestations of Escherichia Coli. [online] Available from www.emedicine.com/oph/TOPIC496.HTM. [Accessed October, 2013].

⊟ 2C. FUNGAL ENDOPHTHALMITIS

General

Rare, intraocular fungal infection.

Clinical

None.

Ocular

Conjunctival injection; pain; mildly decreased vision; fibrinous membranes in anterior chamber; white fluffy retinal infiltrates.

Laboratory

Fungal tests are done on anterior chamber aspirates and vitreous cavity aspirates.

Treatment

Topical, subconjunctival, intravitreal antifungal agents; pars plana vitrectomy.

⊟ BIBLIOGRAPHY

1. Wu L, Evans T, García RA. (2012). Fungal endophthalmitis. [online] Available from www.emedicine.com/oph/TOPIC706.HTM. [Accessed October, 2013].

2D. METASTATIC BACTERIAL ENDOPHTHALMITIS

General

Causative agents usually of low pathogenicity (e.g. *Staphylococcus albus, Staphylococcus epidermidis*); occasionally organisms of greater pathogenicity (e.g. *Pseudomonas aeruginosa, Diplococcus pneumoniae*); bilateral 45%; organisms originate in the body or are introduced by drug addicts using nonsterile needles.

Ocular

Conjunctival hemorrhages; conjunctivitis; Roth's spots; retinal arterial occlusion; uveitis; hypopyon; chorioretinitis; endophthalmitis; retinal hemorrhages.

Clinical

Manifestations are nonspecific.

Laboratory

Blood, sputum and urine cultures.

Treatment

Aggressive treatment is done with intravitreal and topical antibiotics, steroids and cycloplegics.

BIBLIOGRAPHY

1. Graham RH. (2012). Bacterial endophthalmitis. [online] Available from www.emedicine.com/oph/TOPIC393.HTM. [Accessed October, 2013].

2E. METASTATIC FUNGAL ENDOPHTHALMITIS

General

It usually occurs in immunosuppressed or immunocompromised patients; usually asymmetrical; *Candida albicans* frequent etiologic agent.

Ocular

Anterior uveitis; vitreitis; focal retinitis; Roth's spots; chorioretinitis; *Fusarium solani* also has been isolated from immunocompromised patients with endogenous endophthalmitis.

Clinical

It may be evidence of other monocular foci of metastatic fungal disease.

Laboratory

Blood, sputum and urine cultures. Examination of fungi with Giemsa, Gomori-methenamine-silver (GMS) and periodic-acid Schiff (PAS) stains should be done.

Treatment

Amphotericin B, fluconazole, ketoconazole, miconazole, flucytosine and itraconazole. Amphotericin is the treatment of choice. Vitrectomy may be needed.

BIBLIOGRAPHY

1. Wu L, Evans T, García RA. (2012). Fungal endophthalmitis. [online] Available from www.emedicine.com/oph/TOPIC706.HTM. [Accessed October, 2013].

2F. PHACOANAPHYLACTIC ENDOPHTHALMITIS (ENDOPHTHALMITIS PHACOANAPHYLACTICA, PHACOANAPHYLACTIC UVEITIS, PHACOANTIGENIC UVEITIS)

General

It is an inflammatory disease caused by immunologic sensitization of the individual to lens protein released from the sequestered capsular bag by a lens injury—surgical, traumatic or spontaneous.

Clinical

None.

Ocular

Lid edema, flare and cell of the anterior chamber, hypopyon, corneal edema, mutton-fat precipitates, conjunctival chemosis, anterior and posterior synechiae, papillary membranes, decreased visual acuity, retinal detachment, secondary glaucoma.

Laboratory

Diagnosis is made by clinical findings.

Treatment

Vitrectomy is done to remove lens material; systemic and topical corticosteroids.

BIBLIOGRAPHY

1. Graham RH, Barr CC. (2012). Phacoanaphylaxis. [online] Available from www.emedicine.com/oph/TOPIC600.HTM. [Accessed October, 2013].

3. MIDAS SYNDROME (MICROPHTHALMIA, DERMAL APLASIA AND SCLEROCORNEA)

General

X-linked phenotype; male—lethal trait.

Ocular

Bilateral microphthalmia; sclerocornea; blepharophi-mosis.

Clinical

Dermal aplasia; microcephaly; cardiomyopathy; ventricular fibrillation; congenital heart defect.

Laboratory/Sclerocornea

Diagnosis made by clinical findings.

Treatment/Sclerocornea

Surgical care; penetrating keratoplasty is recommended.

BIBLIOGRAPHY

1. Cape CJ, Zaidman GW, Beck AD, et al. Phenotypic variation in ophthalmic manifestations of MIDAS syndrome (microphthalmia, dermal aplasia, and sclerocornea). Arch Ophthalmol. 2004;122(7):1070-4.
2. Happle R, Daniëls O, Koopman RJ. MIDAS syndrome (microphthalmia, dermal aplasia, and sclerocornea): an X-linked phenotype distinct from Goltz syndrome. Am J Med Genet. 1993;47(5):710-3.

4A. BEHÇET SYNDROME (DERMATO-STOMATO-OPHTHALMIC SYNDROME; OCULOBUCCOGENITAL SYNDROME; GILBERT SYNDROME)

General

Virus infection; occurs in adults; chronic disease; complete remission is rare; etiology is unknown.

Ocular

Muscle palsies (occasional); nystagmus (occasional); conjunctivitis; hypopyon; iritis; recurrent uveitis; keratoconjunctivitis sicca; keratitis; vitreous hemorrhages; thrombophlebitis retinal veins (occasional); retinal hemorrhages; optic neuritis (occasional); macular edema; optic nerve atrophy; retinitis; secondary glaucoma; retinal vasculitis; disk edema; panophthalmitis; optic neuropathy; skin lesions, posterior uveitis and systemic complications have been associated with loss of vision with this disorder; corneal immune ring opacity.

Clinical

Aphthous lesions of mucous membranes of the mouth and genitalia; cerebellar signs; convulsions; paraplegia; skin erythema (multiforme, bullosum); arthritis; urethritis; glossitis; recurrent fever.

Laboratory

Not specific—human leukocyte antigen (HLA) B51 positive may help to support diagnosis.

Treatment

The goals of therapy are to suppress inflammation, to reduce the frequency and severity of recurrences and to minimize involvement of the retina. To be effective, treatment must be started early. Extent of involvement and severity of disease determine the choice of medication. Treatment options include corticosteroids, cytotoxic agents, cyclosporine, and colchicine.

BIBLIOGRAPHY

1. Bashour M. (2012). Ophthalmologic manifestations of Behçet disease. [online] Available from www.emedicine.com/oph/TOPIC425.HTM. [Accessed October, 2013].

4B. FILTERING BLEBS AND ASSOCIATED PROBLEMS

General

Elevation of conjunctiva and Tenon's capsule from anterior chamber fistula caused by antimetabolite/antifibrotic usage, trabeculectomy, bleb leaks or overfiltering blebs.

Clinical

None.

Ocular

Overfiltering blebs, overhanging blebs, bleb dysesthesia. Complications include: hypotony, flat anterior chamber, corneal edema, choroidal effusion, endophthalmitis, dellen, uncontrolled glaucoma, astigmatism, cataract and suprachoroidal hemorrhage.

Laboratory

Diagnosis is made by clinical findings and Seidel test.

Treatment

Conservative treatment includes pressure patching, large diameter bandage contact lens. Cryotherapy, laser thermotherapy and autologous blood injection, cyanoacrylate to dry conjunctiva to close leaking bleb and compression sutures may be used if conservative therapy does not resolve the problem.

BIBLIOGRAPHY

1. Traverso CE. (2012). Filtering bleb complications. [online] Available from www.emedicine.com/oph/TOPIC541.HTM. [Accessed October, 2013].

4C. SCHAUMANN SYNDROME (BESNIER-BOECK-SCHAUMANN SYNDROME; BOECK SARCOID; SARCOIDOSIS)

General

Etiology unknown; theories include tuberculosis, hypersensitivity to pine pollen, virus infection; affects blacks most often; chronic course with spontaneous remissions (*see* Heerfordt's syndrome); hilar or paratracheal nodes with erythema nodosum; onset most often in middle and old age; ocular involvement in 20–25% of all cases.

Ocular

Orbital granulomatous mass; bony defects; cutaneous and subcutaneous nodules; myogenic palsy; lacrimal gland adenopathy; decreased tear formation; secondary glaucoma; granulomatous uveitis with iris nodules, cells and flare; mutton fat keratic precipitates; keratitis sicca; vitreous floaters; band-shaped keratitis; complicated cataract; inflammatory retinal exudates; "candle wax drippings"; optic nerve atrophy; neuritis; eyelid nodules; ocular nerve enlargement (granuloma).

Clinical

Lymphadenopathy; hilar nodes; fatigue; cystic, punched-out or reticulated changes in small bones (mainly, hands and feet); muscle wasting; contractures; weakness in legs and arms.

Laboratory

Chest X-ray, CT scan, and MRI of the brain.

Treatment

Glucocorticoids are the treatment of choice.

BIBLIOGRAPHY

1. Sharma GD. (2011). Pediatric sarcoidosis. [online] Available from www.emedicine.com/ped/TOPIC2043.HTM. [Accessed October, 2013].

4D. SYMPATHETIC OPHTHALMIA

General

Trauma or injury to one eye and later onset of inflammation in the other eye.

Ocular

Iridocyclitis (acute inflammation of iris, ciliary body and anterior chamber); choroiditis; chronic persistent keratitic precipitates; posterior synechiae; phthisis bulbi; it has been reported following laser cyclocoagulation.

Clinical

None.

Laboratory

Diagnosis is made by clinical findings.

Treatment

Aggressive treatment is done with steroids and nonsteroids.

BIBLIOGRAPHY

1. Bechrakis NE, Müller-Stolzenburg NW, Helbig H, et al. Sympathetic ophthalmia following laser cyclocoagulation. Arch Ophthalmol. 1994;112(1):80-4.
2. Boniuk V, Boniuk M. The incidence of phthisis bulbas a complication of cataract surgery in the congenital rubella syndrome. Trans Am Acad Ophthalmol Otolaryngol. 1970;74(2):360-8.
3. Duane TD. Clinical Ophthalmology. Philadelphia, PA: JB Lippincott; 1987.

4E. ACQUIRED LUES (SYPHILIS; ACQUIRED SYPHILIS; LUES VENEREA; MALUM VENEREUM)

General

Causative agent, *Treponema pallidum*, usually transmitted sexually.

Ocular

Conjunctival chancroid; conjunctivitis; keratitis; blepharitis; ptosis; iris atrophy; hippus; dacryocystitis; optic nerve atrophy; optic neuritis; periostitis; episcleritis; scleritis; nystagmus; uveitis; vitreous hemorrhages; paralysis of sixth nerve; papilledema; retinal hemorrhages; retinitis proliferans; oculogyric crisis; neuroretinitis; papilledema (associated with aseptic meningitis); diffuse or multifocal chorioretinitis; vertical supranuclear gaze palsy; Benedikt syndrome.

Clinical

Primary lesion associated with regional lymphadenopathy; secondary bacteremic stage associated with generalized mucocutaneous lesions; tertiary stage characterized by destructive mucocutaneous, musculoskeletal, or parenchymal lesions, aortitis, or central nervous system disease; syphilis and human immunodeficiency virus (HIV) infection often coexist in the same patient who experiences a higher incidence and greater severity of neurologic and ocular manifestations; a significant percentage of patients infected with HIV-I and *T. pallidum* become seronegative to syphilis testing.

Laboratory

Serologic nontreponemal tests include Venereal Disease Research Laboratory (VDRL) and rapid plasma reagin (RPR).

Treatment

The goals are to reduce morbidity and to prevent complications. Penicillin is the antibiotic of choice for treating syphilis. Ocular syphilis should be treated the same as patients with neurosyphilis.

BIBLIOGRAPHY

1. Majmudar PA. (2011). Interstitial Keratitis Overview of Interstitial Keratitis. [online] Available from www.emedicine.com/oph/TOPIC453.HTM. [Accessed October, 2013].

4F. VOGT-KOYANAGI-HARADA DISEASE (HARADA DISEASE; UVEITIS-VITILIGO-ALOPECIA-POLIOSIS SYNDROME)

General

Viral infection; occurs predominantly among Italian and Japanese individuals; young adults; chronic.

Ocular

White lashes; secondary glaucoma; bilateral uveitis; sympathetic ophthalmitis; exudative iridocyclitis; vitreous opacities; bilateral serous retinal detachment and edema with spontaneous reattachment after weeks; depigmentation and patches of scattered pigment later; bilateral acute diffuse exudative choroiditis; papilledema; macular hemorrhage; cataracts; phthisis bulbi; poliosis; scleromalacia; intraocular lymphoma.

Clinical

Poliosis; vitiligo; hearing defect; headache; vomiting; meningeal irritation; reported to occur rarely in children.

Laboratory

Immunohistochemistry specimens demonstrate infiltration of CD4+ T-cells, epithelioid cells and multinucleated giant cells.

Treatment

Systemic therapy involves the use of high-dose corticosteroids. Topical steroids may be needed in conjunction with the use of systemic steroids.

BIBLIOGRAPHY

1. Walton RC, Choczaj-Kukula A, Janniger CK. (2012). Vogt-Koyanagi-Harada Disease. [online] Available from www.emedicine.com/oph/TOPIC459.HTM. [Accessed October, 2013].

5. RETRACTION OF THE GLOBE (ON HORIZONTAL CONJUGATE GAZE)

*1. Duane syndrome (retraction syndrome): Co-contraction of horizontal rectus muscles, lateral rectus, and both vertical muscles, or medial and inferior rectus muscles or fibrotic lateral rectus
   A. Acrorenoocular syndrome
   B. Goldenhar syndrome
   C. Hanhart syndrome
   †D. Isolated
   E. Okihiro syndrome
   F. Wildervanck syndrome (Klippel-Feil anomaly with Duane syndrome)
†2. Fibrosis secondary to strabismus surgery

†3. Medial wall fracture with incarceration of orbit contents: Retraction of globe with attempted abduction
4. Orbital mass
   A. Dermoid cyst
   B. Hemangioma
   C. Lymphangioma
   †D. Osteofibroma
†5. Retraction of convergent non-fixating eye associated with loss of conjugate lateral gaze and occurrence of the near reflex on attempted lateral gaze
†6. Thyroid myopathy

*Indicates most frequent
†Indicates a general entry and therefore has not been described in detail in the text

BIBLIOGRAPHY

1. Yen MT. (2013). Globe Retraction. [online] Available from www.emedicine.com/oph/TOPIC567.HTM. [Accessed October, 2013].

5.1. DUANE SYNDROME (RETRACTION SYNDROME; STILLING SYNDROME; TURK-STILLING SYNDROME)

General

Autosomal dominant; more frequent in females; manifestations in infancy; was thought to be secondary to fibrosis of the LR muscle or abnormal check ligaments; now established to be due to congenital aberrant innervation affecting third and seventh cranial nerves.

Ocular

Narrowing of palpebral fissure on adduction, widening on abduction; primary global retraction; deficiency of medial and lateral recti motility; limitation of abduction in affected eye usually is complete; retraction of the globe with attempted adduction varies from 1 mm to 10 mm; convergence insufficiency; heterochromia irides; left eye is more frequently involved.

Clinical

Associated Klippel-Feil syndrome; malformation of face, ears and teeth.

Laboratory

Diagnosis is made by clinical findings.

Treatment

Indications for surgery include anomalous head position, strabismus in primary gaze, significant upshot or downshoot in adduction and cosmetically significant palpebral fissure. Duane retraction syndrome type 1 (DRS-1) (absent abduction, esotropia in primary position and head turn toward the affected side to fuse) medial rectus recession of the affected eye; DRS with exotropia—recess LR of involved side. Retraction of the globe—recess medial and lateral rectus of involved eye. Upshoots and downshoots—recess the LR.

BIBLIOGRAPHY

1. Verma A. (2011). Duane syndrome. [online] Available from www.emedicine.com/oph/TOPIC326.HTM. [Accessed October, 2013].

5.1A. ACRORENOOCULAR SYNDROME

General

Autosomal dominant; Duane syndrome with radial defects.

Ocular

Complete coloboma; coloboma of optic nerve; ptosis and Duane anomaly.

Clinical

Renal anomalies; hypoplasia of distal part of thumb with lack of motion at phalangeal joint; renal ectopia without fusion; bladder diverticula; malrotation of both kidneys; absence of kidney; clubhand or absence of thumb.

Laboratory

Diagnosis is made by clinical findings.

Treatment

If visual acuity is affected most cases require surgical correction and there are several procedures that may be used including levator resection, repair or advancement and Fasanella-Servat.

BIBLIOGRAPHY

1. Halal F, Homsy M, Perreault G. Acro-renal-ocular syndrome: autosomal dominant thumb hypoplasia; renal ectopia and eye defect. Am J Med Genet. 1984;17:753-62.
2. McKusick VA. Mendelian Inheritance in Man: A Catalog of Human Genes and Genetic Disorders, 12th edition. Baltimore: The Johns Hopkins University Press; 1998.

🗗 5.1B. GOLDENHAR SYNDROME (OCULO-AURICULO-VERTEBRAL DYSPLASIA; GOLDENHAR-GORLIN SYNDROME)

General

Most cases have been sporadic, but cases of autosomal dominant and recessive inheritance have been reported; male preponderance (60%); present at birth.

Ocular

Anophthalmia; colobomata of choroid, iris, and eyelid; antimongolian slant of lid fissure; epibulbar dermoid or lipodermoids of conjunctiva, cornea, and orbit; tilted optic disk; nerve hypoplasia; microphthalmia; macular heterotopia; tortuous retinal vessels.

Clinical

Frontal bulging of the skull; receding chin; malar hypoplasia; micrognathia and macrostomia; auricular appendices (single or multiple); multiple vertebral anomalies; preauricular fistulas; mental retardation.

Laboratory

Clinical.

Treatment

Dermoids: Surgery for function or cosmesis.

🗗 BIBLIOGRAPHY

1. Tewfik TL, Al-Noury KI. (2013). Manifestations of craniofacial syndromes. [online] Available from www.emedicine.com/ent/TOPIC319.HTM. [Accessed October, 2013].

🗗 5.1C. HANHART SYNDROME (RICHNER SYNDROME; RECESSIVE KERATOSIS PALMOPLANTARIS; PSEUDOHERPETIC KERATITIS; RICHNER-HANHART SYNDROME; TYROSINEMIA II; TYROSINOSIS; PSEUDODENDRITIC KERATITIS)

General

Autosomal recessive; consanguinity.

Ocular

Excess tearing; photophobia; dendritic lesions of the cornea with corneal sensitivity not affected; keratitis; papillary hypertrophy of conjunctiva; corneal haze; neovascularization of cornea; cataract; nystagmus.

Clinical

Dyskeratosis palmoplantaris; diffuse keratosis; dystrophy of nails; hypotrichosis; mental retardation (usually pronounced); sensorineural hearing loss.

Laboratory

Serum-plasma tyrosine 16–62 mg/dL; urine-tyrosinuria and tyrosyluria; liver biopsy—decreased cytoplasmic tyrosine aminotransferase (cTAT) activity.

Treatment

Topical keratolytics, topical retinoids, potent topical steroids with or without keratolytics in dermatoses with an inflammatory component.

🗗 BIBLIOGRAPHY

1. Lee RA, Yassaee M, Bowe WP, et al. (2011). Keratosis Palmaris et Plantaris. [online] www.emedicine.com/derm/TOPIC589.HTM. [Accessed October, 2013].

5.1E. OKIHIRO SYNDROME

General

Autosomal recessive syndrome of Duane syndrome (retraction syndrome).

Ocular

Narrowing of palpebral fissures on adduction, widening on abduction; primary global retraction.

Clinical

May be associated with craniofacial abnormalities and various associated syndromes, such as Duane syndrome, cervico-oculo-acoustic syndrome, acrorenoocular syndrome, cat's-eye syndrome; association with cardiac defects, urinary tract anomalies, Duane anomaly associated with mental retardation, thenar hypoplasia, and radial ray abnormalities.

Laboratory

Diagnosis is made by clinical findings.

Treatment

Indications for surgery include anomalous head position, strabismus in primary gaze, significant upshoot or downshoot in adduction and cosmetically significant palpebral fissure. Type 1 DRS (absent abduction, esotropia in primary position and head turn toward the affected side to fuse) medial rectus recession of the affected eye, DRS with exotropia—recess lateral rectus of involved side. Retraction of the globe—recess medial and lateral rectus of involved eye. Upshoots and downshoots—recess the lateral rectus.

BIBLIOGRAPHY

1. Collins A, Baraitser M, Pembrey M. Okihiro syndrome: thenar hypoplasia and Duane anomaly in three generations. Clin Dysmorphol. 1993;2:237-40.
2. McGowan KF, Pagon RA. Okihiro syndrome [Letter]. Am J Med Genet. 1994;51:89.
3. Stoll C, Alembik Y, Dott B. Association of Duane anomaly with mental retardation, cardiac and urinary tract abnormalities: a new autosomal recessive condition? Ann Genet. 1994;37:207-9.

5.1F. WILDERVANCK SYNDROME (CERVICOOCULOACOUSTICUS SYNDROME; FRANCESCHETTI-KLEIN-WILDERVANCK SYNDROME; WILDERVANCK-WAARDENBURG SYNDROME; CERVICOOCULOFACIAL DYSMORPHIA; CERVICOOCULOFACIAL SYNDROME) NYSTAGMUS

General

Etiology unknown; female preponderance; similarities to Klippel-Feil syndrome; onset at birth.

Ocular

Abducens paresis; nystagmus; heterochromia iridis.

Clinical

Deafness or deaf-mutism; torticollis with short, webbed neck; epilepsy; mental retardation; cleft palate; scoliosis; ventricular septal defect; ectopic kidney; hydrocephalus; hypoplastic thumb and growth retardation.

Laboratory

Diagnosis is made by clinical findings.

Treatment

Tape or base-out prism on one eye glass may be useful; botulinum toxin type A into the antagonist medial rectus muscle, if no improvement after 6–12 months—recess/resect of medial and lateral rectus.

BIBLIOGRAPHY

1. Geeraets WJ. Ocular Syndromes, 3rd edition. Philadelphia: Lea & Febiger; 1976.

⊟ 5.4A. DERMOID (DERMOID CHORISTOMA; DERMOID CYST; DERMOLIPOMA; LIPODERMOID)

General

Benign tumors composed of epidermal tissue, dermal adnexal structures, skin appendages, hair follicles, sebaceous gland and sweat glands; slowly growing.

Ocular

Dermoid of conjunctiva, cornea and lids; keratitis; extraocular muscle paralysis; exophthalmos; astigmatism; visual loss; orbital lesions causing diplopia and proptosis; may be connected with the lacrimal canaliculum.

Clinical

Subcutaneous dermoids of the skin; aplasia cutis congenita possibly associated with strabismus has been reported.

Laboratory

Radiographs of the orbit reveal the deeper orbital cysts; CT is commonly used to image orbital cysts; MRI of dermoid cyst is especially valuable in deeper orbital lesions.

Treatment

Surgery for function or cosmesis.

⊟ BIBLIOGRAPHY

1. Schwartz RA, Ruszczak Z. (2012). Dermoid Cyst. [online] Available from www.emedicine.com/derm/TOPIC686. HTM. [Accessed October, 2013].

⊟ 5.4B. HEMANGIOMA

General

It can occur throughout the body, but particularly in the head; primary intraosseous orbital hemangiomas is rare; capillary hemangioma of the orbit and eyelids generally is unilateral.

Ocular

Hemangiomas of lids or orbit; ptosis; strabismus; amblyopia; proptosis; optic atrophy; hypermetropia; cavernous hemangiomas are the most common benign orbital tumors of adults.

Clinical

Ipsilateral hemangiomas of the brain and meninges.

Laboratory

Neuroimaging can be of great assistance in making the diagnosis.

Treatment

Most of these lesions regress on their own; there is no need to intervention. If spontaneous regression does not occur corticosteroids, in various formulations, may be considered. Topical application of timolol has been useful in some cases.

⊟ BIBLIOGRAPHY

1. Karmel M. Topical timolol for capillary hemangioma. Eyenet. 2010.
2. Seiff S, Zwick OM, DeAngelis DD, et al. (2011). Capillary hemangioma. [online] Available from www.emedicine.com/oph/ TOPIC691.HTM. [Accessed October, 2013].

⊟ 5.4C. LYMPHANGIOMA

General

Poorly circumscribed infiltrating lesions consisting of lymphatic/dysplastic blood vessels; occurs predominantly in children and young adults.

Ocular

Conjunctival hemorrhages; cellulitis of lid; ptosis; exophthalmos; amblyopia; astigmatism; extraocular muscle imbalance; optic disk edema; retinal striae.

Clinical

Benign tumors of the lymph system.

Laboratory

Ultrasonography lacks specificity and soft-tissue detail; CT images bone deformity and MRI provides superior soft-tissue details.

Treatment

- *Ptosis*: Most cases require surgical correction if visual acuity is affected and there are several procedures that may be used including levator resection, repair or advancement and Fasanella-Servat procedure.
- *Exophthalmos*: Reversing the problem, which is causing the exophthalmos, is the treatment of choice and will minimize the ocular complications. Ocular lubricants are beneficial for control of the corneal exposure.

BIBLIOGRAPHY

1. Schwartz RA, Fernandez G. (2012). Lymphangioma. [online] Available from www.emedicine.com/derm/TOPIC866.HTM. [Accessed October, 2013].

6. BASEDOW SYNDROME (GRAVES DISEASE; HYPERTHYROIDISM; THYROTOXICOSIS; EXOPHTHALMIC GOITER; PARRY DISEASE)

General

Diffuse toxic goiter; inherited as a simple autosomal recessive; penetrance greater in females; however, dominant mode of inheritance and variable penetrance are possible; uncommon in either sex before the age of 15 years.

Ocular

Exophthalmos; swelling of eyelids and discoloration of upper eyelids; lid lag (von Graefe's sign); globe lag (Koeber's sign); lid trembling on gentle closure (Rosenbach's sign); reduced blinking (Stellwag's sign); retraction of upper lid; difficulty in everting upper lid (Gifford's sign); convergence weakness (Möbius's sign); impaired fixation on extreme lateral gaze (Suker's sign); possible external ophthalmoplegia (Ballet's sign); Dalrymple's sign (staring appearance); tearing; photophobia; epiphora; prolapse of lacrimal gland; neuroretinal edema; tortuous vessels; papilledema and papillitis; anisocoria; keratitis; increased intraocular pressure on upgaze; decreased visual acuity; enlargement of the extraocular muscles; increased volume of the extraorbital fat; superior rectus muscle enlargement; decreased venous outflow.

Clinical

Tachycardia; anxiety; insomnia; loss of weight; hyperhidrosis; restlessness; myocarditis (toxic); atrial fibrillation.

Laboratory

Visual field testing, forced duction testing for restrictive myopathy, CT, MRI, T4 and thyroid-stimulating hormone, thyroid-stimulating immunoglobulins.

Treatment

There is no immediate treatment; the disease is self-limited but prolonged course over 1 or more years. Five percent of patients may require surgical intervention which could be orbital decompression, strabismus surgery, lid-lengthening surgery or blepharoplasty.

BIBLIOGRAPHY

1. Ing E. (2012). Thyroid-associated orbitopathy. [online] Available from www.emedicine.com/oph/TOPIC237.HTM. [Accessed October, 2013].
2. Regensburg NI, Wiersinga WM, Berendschot TT, et al. Do subtypes of Graves' orbitopathy exist? Ophthalmology. 2011;118:191-6.

CHAPTER
25

Headache

⊟ 1. RAEDER SYNDROME (PARATRIGEMINAL PARALYSIS; HORTON HEADACHE; HISTAMINE CEPHALALGIA; CILIARY NEURALGIA; CLUSTER HEADACHE; PERIODIC MIGRAINOUS NEURALGIA)

General

Interruption of sympathetic fibers about the carotid artery and involvement of the fifth nerve; meningioma and aneurysm of the internal carotid artery are the most frequent causes; prominent in males; possible pathogenetic mechanism of this condition is an ischemic injury of the gasserian ganglion.

Ocular

Mild enophthalmos; mild ptosis (unilateral); epiphora; scotoma possible; hypotonia; unilateral miosis; increased tear secretion; periocular pain; Homer syndrome.

Clinical

Facial pain; occasionally weakness of the jaw muscles; headaches (V-region); hypertension; associated inflammatory processes are not infrequent.

Laboratory

Brain scan to rule out meningioma and basilar artery aneurysm.

Treatment

Oxygen inhalation and sumatriptan subcutaneous is useful in acute attacks.

⊟ BIBLIOGRAPHY

1. Bardorf CM, van Stavern G, Garcia-Valenzuela E. (2012). Horner syndrome. [online] Available from www.emedicine.com/oph/TOPIC336.HTM. [Accessed October, 2013].

⊟ 2. TEMPORAL ARTERITIS SYNDROME (CRANIAL ARTERITIS SYNDROME; GIANT CELL ARTERITIS; HUTCHINSON-HORTON-MAGATH-BROWN SYNDROME)

General

Etiology unknown; mainly females; mainly Whites; ages 55–80 years; temporal artery shows inflammatory thickening; arteritis of the vessels supplying the optic nerve.

Ocular

Transient ptosis; partial or complete loss of vision on the affected side; retinal detachment; exudates and hemorrhages; narrowing of retinal vessels; obstruction of the central retinal artery; optic atrophy; ischemic optic neuropathy; acute decreased intraocular pressure (IOP); corneal hypesthesia; palsies of extraocular muscles; hemorrhagic glaucoma; diplopia; hemorrhages on or around the disk.

Clinical

Throbbing headache; hyperalgesia of the scalp; malaise; anorexia; weakness; weight loss; fever; nodular pulmonary nodules; cough; otitis with deafness.

Laboratory

Elevated erythrocyte sedimentation rate (ESR) greater than 50 mm/hour, positive temporal artery biopsy.

Treatment

Systemic corticosteroids are the therapy of choice.

⊟ BIBLIOGRAPHY

1. Allen AW, Biega T, Varma MK. (2012). Temporal arteritis imaging. [online] Available from www.emedicine.com/radio/TOPIC675.HTM. [Accessed October, 2013].
2. Walvick MD, Walvick MP. Giant cell arteritis: laboratory predictors of a positive temporal artery biopsy. Ophthalmology. 2011;118(6):1201-4.

⊟ 3. HYPERTENSION

General

Elevated blood pressure.

Ocular

Retinal arterial narrowing; arteriosclerosis; hemorrhages; retinal edema; cotton-wool spots; fatty exudates; optic disk edema; exudative retinal detachment; optic neuropathy; swollen optic nerve; central retinal vein occlusion; branch retinal vein occlusion; choroidal ischemia.

Clinical

Systemic hypertension; patchy loss of muscle tone in vessel walls; vascular decompensation.

Laboratory

Diagnosis is made from clinical findings; complete blood count, serum electrolytes, serum creatinine, serum glucose, uric acid and urinalysis, lipid profile (total cholesterol, low-density lipoprotein and high-density lipoprotein and triglycerides).

Treatment

Lifestyle modifications: Weight loss, stop smoking, exercise, reduce stress, limit alcohol intake, reduce sodium intake, maintain adequate calcium and potassium intake. Refer to internist for drug therapy.

⊟ BIBLIOGRAPHY

1. Madhur MS, Riaz K, Dreisbach AW, et al. (2012). Hypertension. [online] Available from www.emedicine.com/med/TOPIC1106.HTM. [Accessed October, 2013].

⊟ 4. MIGRAINE (VASCULAR HEADACHE)

General

Recurrent attacks of pain in the head; usually unilateral; often familial.

Ocular

Abnormal visual sensations; scotoma generally restricted to one-half of the visual field; complete blindness; unilateral transient visual loss; photopsia; branch retinal artery occlusions; anisocoria.

Clinical

Nausea; vomiting; anorexia; sensory, motor, and mood disturbances; fluid imbalance; headache.

Laboratory

Investigation studies; rule out comorbid disease, exclude other causes of headaches such as structural and/or metabolic; neurological examination; lumbar puncture followed by computed tomography (CT) scan or magnetic resonance imaging (MRI).

Treatment

Treatment is based on the severity of the case.

BIBLIOGRAPHY

1. Chawla J, Blanda M, Braswell R, et al. (2011). Migraine headache. [online] Available from www.emedicine.com/neuro/TOPIC218.HTM. [Accessed October, 2013].

5. MUSCLE CONTRACTION HEADACHE

General

Chronic recurring; involves both muscular and psychogenic factors; occurs in all ages.

Clinical

Throbbing gradual onset head pain described as a fullness, tightness or squeezing pressure; usual location of the pain is in the frontal-occipital area; it is bilateral and is not aggravated by physical activity. Tenderness of scalp or neck may be present.

Laboratory

Laboratory work is unremarkable. CT or MRI is only necessary if the headache pattern changes.

Treatment

Cold or hot packs, relaxation techniques and regular exercise may be beneficial. Ibuprofen is the usual initial drug of choice though other nonsteroidal anti-inflammatory drugs (NSAIDs) such as indocin, toradol, ketoprofen and naproxen may be beneficial. If NSAIDs are ineffective, barbiturates may be necessary.

BIBLIOGRAPHY

1. Singh MK. (2011). Muscle contraction tension headache. [online] Available from emedicine.medscape.com/article/1142908-overview. [Accessed October, 2013].

6. PSEUDOTUMOR

General

Etiology is unknown; predominantly in obese women of child-bearing age.

Ocular

Papilledema; progressive optic atrophy; blindness; limited abduction of both eyes; diplopia; decreased visual fields.

Clinical

Elevated intracranial pressure; headache, which is nonspecific and occurs in varied locations and frequency.

Laboratory

Blood tests to rule out lupus or other collagen vascular disease may be necessary but typical need; only a routine cerebrospinal fluid investigation is necessary.

Treatment

Carbonic anhydrase inhibitor is useful. Corticosteroids are often used for maximum medical management.

BIBLIOGRAPHY

1. Gans MS. (2012). Idiopathic intracranial hypertension. [online] Available from emedicine.medscape.com/article/1143167-overview. [Accessed October, 2013].

CHAPTER
26

Iris

⊟ 1. ANIRIDIA AND ABSENT PATELLA

General

Autosomal dominant; rare.

Ocular

Absence of iris; cataracts; glaucoma.

Clinical

Absence of knee cap, hypoplastic or aplastic.

Laboratory

Chromosomal deletion is detected by cytogenetic testing with the use of high-resolution banding.

Treatment

The goal is directed toward control of intraocular pressure (IOP), with use of topical drops. Frequently, this goal is not met. Photophobia can be treated with tinted glasses. Strabismus, amblyopia, refractive errors and nystagmus may also require treatment with traditional methods.

⊟ BIBLIOGRAPHY

1. Singh D, Verma A. (2012). Aniridia. [online] Available from www.emedicine.com/oph/TOPIC43.HTM. [Accessed October, 2013].

⊟ 2. ANIRIDIA (ABSENCE OF IRIS, PARTIAL OR COMPLETE)

†1. *AGR triad*: Sporadic (bilateral or unilateral) aniridia, genitourinary abnormalities and mental retardation
†2. Associated ocular findings
  A. Cataracts
  B. Corneal dystrophy
  C. Ectopia lentis
  D. Glaucoma
  E. *Macular aplasia*: Autosomal dominant
  F. Microcornea and subluxated lenses
  G. Nystagmus
  H. Optic nerve hypoplasia
  I. Photophobia
  J. Poor foveal reflex
 *K. Strabismus
†3. Associated with autosomal-recessive inheritance with fully developed macula
†4. Associated with unilateral renal agenesis and psychomotor retardation
†5. Beckwith-Wiedemann syndrome
†6. Deletion of short arm of 11th chromosome

---

*Indicates most frequent
†Indicates a general entry and therefore has not been described in detail in the text

7. Gillespie syndrome (incomplete aniridia, cerebellar ataxia, and oligophrenia)
8. Homocystinuria syndrome
9. Marinesco-Sjögren syndrome (congenital spinocerebellar ataxia)
10. Miller syndrome (Wilms aniridia syndrome)
11. Peters syndrome (oculodental syndrome)
12. Rieger syndrome (dysgenesis mesostromalis)
13. Ring chromosome 6
14. Scaphocephaly syndrome
15. Siemens syndrome (anhidrotic ectodermal dysplasia)
†16. Traumatic
17. Ullrich syndrome (dyscraniopylophalangy)

BIBLIOGRAPHY

1. Bakri S, Simon JW. (2012). Aniridia in the Newborn. [online] Available from http://www.emedicine.com/oph/TOPIC317.HTM. [Accessed October, 2013].
2. Chen H. (2013). Genetics of Crouzon syndrome. [online] Available from www.emedicine.com/ped/TOPIC511.HTM. [Accessed October, 2013].
3. Giri G. (2012). Peters Anomaly. [online] Available fromwww.emedicine.com/oph/TOPIC112.HTM.[Accessed October, 2013].
4. Singh D, Verma A. (2012). Aniridia. [online] Available from www.emedicine.com/oph/TOPIC43.HTM. [Accessed October, 2013].
5. Tekin M, Bodurtha J. (2013). Cornelia De Lange Syndrome. [online] Available from http://www.emedicine.com/ped/TOPIC482.HTM. [Accessed October, 2013].

2.7. ANIRIDIA, CEREBELLAR ATAXIA, AND MENTAL DEFICIENCY (GILLESPIE SYNDROME)

General

Autosomal recessive; onset at birth.

Ocular

Congenital cataracts; incomplete formation of iris; bilateral congenital mydriasis.

Clinical

Cerebellar ataxia; mental deficiency; delayed developmental milestones; persistent hypotonia of muscles; gross incoordination; attention tremor; scanning speech.

Laboratory

Chromosomal deletion is detected by cytogenetic testing with the use of high-resolution banding.

Treatment

The goal is directed toward the control of IOP with use of topical drops. Frequently, this goal is not met. Photophobia can be treated with tinted glasses. Strabismus, amblyopia, refractive errors and nystagmus may also require treatment with traditional methods.

BIBLIOGRAPHY

1. Singh D, Verma A. (2012). Aniridia. [online] Available from www.emedicine.com/oph/TOPIC43.HTM. [Accessed October, 2013].

2.8. HOMOCYSTINURIA SYNDROME

General

Rare disorder of amino acid metabolism; autosomal recessive inheritance; approximately one-third of patients with this disorder have normal intelligence.

Ocular

Dislocated or subluxated lenses; spherophakia; cataract; retinal detachment; optic atrophy; keratitis; ocular hypotony; iris atrophy; uveitis; situs inversus optic disk; central retinal artery occlusion; high myopia; strabismus; pupillary block glaucoma; lens zonular fibers have abnormal glycoprotein with elevated concentration of cystine; ectopia lentis (nearly constant feature).

Clinical

Mental retardation; sparseness of hair; thromboembolism; arachnodactyly; generalized osteoporosis; thrombotic lesions of arteries and veins; abnormal cystathionine synthetase.

Laboratory

Diagnosis is made by clinical findings.

Treatment

Dietary restriction may be partially effective in patients with homocystinuria. Treatment of glaucoma is dependent on the etiologic mechanism. Lens surgery in ectopia lentis is technically challenging.

BIBLIOGRAPHY

1. Cogan D. Dislocated lenses and homocystinuria. Arch Ophthalmol. 1965;74:446.
2. Cross HE, Jensen AD. Ocular manifestations in the Marfan syndrome and homocystinuria. Am J Ophthalmol. 1973;75:405.
3. Roy FH, Fraunfelder FW, Fraunfelder FT. Roy and Fraunfelder's Current Ocular Therapy, 6th edition. Philadelphia: WB Saunders; 2008.
4. McKusick VA. Mendelian Inheritance in Man: A Catalog of Human Genes and Genetic Disorders, 12th edition. Baltimore: The Johns Hopkins University Press; 1998.
5. Streeten BW. The nature of the ocular zonule. Trans Am Ophthalmol Soc. 1982;80:823-54.
6. Ramsey MS, Yanoff M, Fine BS. The ocular histopathology of homocystinuria. A light and electron microscopic study. Am J Ophthalmol. 1972;74:377-85.

2.9. MARINESCO-SJÖGREN SYNDROME (CONGENITAL SPINOCEREBELLAR ATAXIA-CONGENITAL CATARACT-OLIGOPHRENIA SYNDROME)

General

Autosomal recessive trait; onset when child learns to walk; mitochondrial disease.

Ocular

Cataracts; aniridia; rotary and horizontal nystagmus; nystagmus; strabismus; optic atrophy.

Clinical

Cerebellar ataxia; oligophrenia; small stature; scoliosis; genu valgum; restricted extensibility of the knee; defects of fingers and toes; mental retardation; hair sparse; hypersalivation; sensorineural hearing loss.

Laboratory

Diagnosis is made by clinical findings.

Treatment

Cataracts: Change in glasses can sometimes improve a patient's visual function temporarily; however, the most common treatment is cataract surgery.

BIBLIOGRAPHY

1. Dotti MT, Bardelli AM, De Stefano N, et al. Optic atrophy in Marinesco-Sjögren syndrome: an additional ocular feature. Report of three cases in two families. Ophthalmic Genet. 1993;14(1):5-7.
2. Gillespie FD. Aniridia, cerebellar ataxia, and oligophrenia in siblings. Arch Ophthalmol. 1965;73(3):338-41.
3. Lindal S, Lund I, Torbergsen T, et al. Mitochondrial diseases and myopathies: a series of muscle biopsy specimens with ultrastructural changes in the mitochondria. Ultrastruct Pathol. 1992;16:263-75.
4. Marinesco G, Draganesco S, Vasiliu D. Nouvelle Maladie Familiale Caracterisee par une Cataracte Congenitale et un Arret du Developpement Somato-NeuroPsychique. Encephale. 1931;26:97.
5. Sjögren T. Hereditary congenital spinocerebellar ataxia combined with congenital cataracts and oligophrenia. Confinia Neurol. 1950;10:293.

2.10. MILLER SYNDROME (WILMS ANIRIDIA SYNDROME; WAGR SYNDROME; WILMS TUMOR-ANIRIDIA-GENITOURINARY ABNORMALITIES-MENTAL RETARDATION SYNDROME)

General

Etiology is unknown; it manifests an association of aniridia, which is inherited as a dominant autosomal trait and Wilms' tumor (WT); this is one of the best studied continuous gene syndromes as defined by Schmickel.

Ocular

Glaucoma; bilateral aniridia (aniridia often not complete, with remnants of iris root present as rudimentary forms); cataract.

Clinical

Wilms' tumor; mental retardation with microcephaly; genital malformations with cryptorchidism and hypospadias; hemihypertrophy; kidney anomalies (horseshoe kidney).

Laboratory/Glaucoma

Chromosome analysis and genetic counseling.

Treatment/Glaucoma

Beta-blockers, carbonic anhydrase inhibitors and prostaglandin analogs. Surgery may be needed if IOP is uncontrolled.

BIBLIOGRAPHY

1. Fraumeni JF, Glass AG. Wilms' tumor and congenital aniridia. JAMA. 1968;206(4):825-8.
2. Mackintosh TF, Girdwood TG, Parker DJ, et al. Aniridia and Wilms' tumor (nephroblastoma). Br J Ophthalmol. 1968;52(11):846-8.
3. McKusick VA. Mendelian Inheritance in Man: A Catalog of Human Genes and Genetic Disorders, 12th edition. Baltimore, USA: The Johns Hopkins University Press; 1998.
4. Hamosh A, Scott AF, Amberger J, et al. Online Mendelian Inheritance in Man (OMIM), a knowledgebase of human genes and genetic disorders. Nucleic Acids Res. 2002;30(1):52-5.
5. Miller RW, Fraumeni JF, Manning MD. Association of Wilms' tumor with aniridia, hemihypertrophy and other congenital malformations. N Engl J Med. 1964;270:922-7.
6. Schmickel RD. Chromosomal deletions and enzyme deficiencies. J Pediatr. 1986;108(2):244-6.

2.11. OCULODENTAL SYNDROME (PETERS SYNDROME; RUTHERFORD SYNDROME)

General

Similar to Rieger syndrome and Meyer-Schwickerath-Weyer syndrome; Peters syndrome inherited as autosomal recessive with defect of corneogenetic mesoderm characterized by incomplete separation of lens vesicle, causing central opacities of cornea, shallow anterior chamber, synechiae, and remnants of pupillary membrane; anterior pole cataract; Rutherford syndrome inherited as autosomal dominant; exhibits iris and dental anomalies and mental retardation.

Ocular

High myopia; corneoscleral staphyloma; aniridia; macrocornea; opacities of the corneal margin; ectopia lentis with deposits of pigment; macular pigmentation; large excavation of optic nerve with atrophy.

Clinical

Oligodontia; microdontia; hypoplasia of enamel; abnormal tooth positions; hypertrophy of gums; failure of tooth eruption.

Treatment

See oral health specialist.

BIBLIOGRAPHY

1. Houston IB. Rutherford's syndrome. A familial oculodental disorder. A clinical and electrophysiologic study. Acta Paediatr Scand. 1966;55:233-8.
2. McKusick VA. Mendelian Inheritance in Man: A Catalog of Human Genes and Genetic Disorders, 12th edition. Baltimore: The Johns Hopkins University Press; 1998.
3. Online Mendelian Inheritance in Man, OMIM. McKusick-Nathans Institute for Genetic Medicine, Johns Hopkins University and National Center for Biotechnology Information, National Library of Medicine, October 12, 2007. Available from www.ncbi.nlm.nih.gov/omim. [Accessed October, 2013].
4. Peters A. Uber Angeborene Defektbildung der Descemetschen Membran. Klin Monatsbl Augenheilkd. 1906;44:27.
5. Reisner SH, Kott E, Bornstein B, et al. Oculodentodigital dysplasia. Am J Dis Child. 1969;118:600-7.
6. Rutherfurd ME. Three generations of inherited dental defects. Br Med J. 1931;2:9-11.

⊟ 2.12. RIEGER SYNDROME (AXENFELD-RIEGER SYNDROME; DYSGENESIS MESODERMALIS CORNEAE ET IRIDES; DYSGENESIS MESOSTROMALIS; AXENFELD POSTERIOR EMBRYOTOXON-JUVENILE GLAUCOMA)

General

Autosomal dominant; neural crest abnormality; 50% of patients develop glaucoma.

Ocular

Microphthalmia; congenital glaucoma; iris hypoplasia; deformed and acentric pupil; anterior synechiae; aniridia; microcornea; corneal opacities in Descemet's membrane parallel to the limbus; dislocated lens; optic atrophy; cataract; strabismus; ptosis; hypertelorism; keratoconus; posterior embryotoxon; broad iris processes to embryotoxon; iris stromal hypoplasia; corectopia; polycoria; secondary glaucoma.

Clinical

Face wide; hypodontia; underdeveloped maxilla; teeth deformities; myotonic dystrophy; facial anomalies: maxillary hypoplasia, protrusion of the lower lip, broad, flat nose; dental anomalies include absent teeth, pig-like incisors and decreased crown size; hypospadias.

Laboratory

Diagnosis is made by clinical findings.

Treatment/Ocular

Congenital glaucoma can be treated with beta-blockers, prostaglandin analogs and carbonic anhydrase inhibitors. Surgery such as goniotomy or trabeculectomy can be used if IOP is not controlled.

⊟ BIBLIOGRAPHY

1. Eagle RC. Congenital, developmental and degenerative disorders of the iris and ciliary body. In: Albert DM, Jakobiec FA (Eds). Albert & Jakobiec's Principles and Practice of Ophthalmology: Clinical Practice, 3rd edition. Philadelphia, PA: WB Saunders; 1994. pp. 367-87.
2. Montes JG, Montes JC. Syndrome de Rieger, anomalie de axenfeld con glaucoma Juvenil familiar. Arch Soc Ophth Hisp Am. 1967;27:93.
3. Rieger H. Beitrage zur Kenntnis seltener Missbildungen der Iris. Graefes Arch Clin Esp Ophthalmol. 1935;133:602.
4. Wesley RK, Baker JD, Golnick AL. Rieger's syndrome: (oligodontia and primary mesodermal dysgenesis of the iris) clinical features and report of an isolated case. J Pediatr Ophthalmol Strabismus. 1978;15(2):67-70.

⊟ 2.13. RING CHROMOSOME 6 (ANIRIDIA, CONGENITAL GLAUCOMA, AND HYDROCEPHALUS)

General

Rare disorder associated with various congenital anomalies; autosomal dominant with recessive sporadically reported.

Ocular

Microphthalmia; aniridia; congenital uveal ectropion; Rieger anomaly; congenital glaucoma; corneal clouding; prominent Schwalbe's line with attached iris strands; hypopigmented fundi; hypoplasia of iris stroma; strabismus; ptosis; nystagmus; megalocornea; iris coloboma; optic atrophy; hypertelorism; antimongoloid slant of palpebral fissures; ectopic pupils; angle anomalies; posterior embryotoxon; microcornea; colobomatous.

Clinical

Hydrocephalus; agenesis of corpus callosum; congenital heart defects; mental retardation; low-set malformed ears; broad nasal bridge; micrognathia; short neck; hand anomalies; high-arched palate; widely spaced nipples; deformity of feet; respiratory distress syndrome; hyperbilirubinemia; hypocalcemia; anemia; seizure; bulging anterior fontanel.

Laboratory

Diagnosis is made by clinical findings.

Treatment

Ptosis: If visual acuity is affected, most cases require surgical correction and there are several procedures that may be used including levator resection, repair or advancement and Fasanella-Servat procedure.

⊟ BIBLIOGRAPHY

1. Bateman JB. Chromosomal anomalies and the eye. In: Wright KW (Ed). Pediatric Ophthalmology and Strabismus. St Louis: Mosby; 1995. p. 595.
2. Chitayat D, Hahm SY, Iqbal MA, et al. Ring chromosome 6: report of a patient and literature review. Am J Med Genet. 1987;26(1):145-51.
3. deLuise UP, Anderson DR. Primary infantile glaucoma (congenital glaucoma). Surv Ophthalmol. 1983;28(1):1-19.
4. Levin H, Ritch R, Barathur R, et al. Aniridia, congenital glaucoma, and hydrocephalus in a male infant with ring chromosome 6. Am J Med Genet. 1986;25(2):281-7.

⊟ 2.14. SCAPHOCEPHALY SYNDROME (PAPILLEDEMA)

General

Craniofacial dysostoses with failure in the development of the primitive mesoderm; facial features result from premature fusion of the sagittal cranial suture; males more commonly affected (4:1).

Ocular

Shallow orbits; proptosis; nystagmus; exotropia; aniridia; cataract; papilledema; optic atrophy; aniridia; dislocated lens.

Clinical

Long anteroposterior head diameter; short transverse diameter of the head; increased intracranial pressure; flat forehead with absent superciliary arches; prominent nose; mental retardation.

Laboratory

Plain skull radiograph, ultrasound, computed tomography (CT) scan and magnetic resonance imaging (MRI).

Treatment

Molding therapy (helmets) during the 1st year and surgical intervention.

⊟ BIBLIOGRAPHY

1. Podda S, Wolfe SA, Kordestani RK, et al. (2011). Craniosynostosis Management. [online] Available from http://www.emedicine.com/plastic/TOPIC534.HTM. [Accessed October, 2013].

⊟ 2.15. HEREDITARY ECTODERMAL DYSPLASIA SYNDROME (SIEMENS SYNDROME; KERATOSIS FOLLICULARIS SPINULOSA SYNDROME; HYPOHIDROTIC ECTODERMAL DYSPLASIA; CHRIST-SIEMENS-TOURAINE SYNDROME; WEECH SYNDROME; ANHIDROTIC ECTODERMAL DYSPLASIA; ICHTHYOSIS FOLLICULARIS)

General

Autosomal recessive inheritance; strong male preponderance (about 95%); linked to X-chromosome.

Ocular

Complete loss of eyebrows (madarosis); follicular keratosis; blepharitis; entropion or ectropion; reduced tear formation or epiphora; myopia; keratoconjunctivitis; corneal erosions and ulcers (recurrent); corneal dystrophy; cataract; increased periorbital pigmentation; mongoloid lid slant; photophobia; absence of iris; luxation of lens; papillary abnormalities.

Clinical

Mental retardation; dry skin and anhidrosis (reduced number of sweat glands); hypotrichosis; follicular hyperkeratosis (neck, palms, soles); hypohidrosis.

Laboratory

Diagnosis is made by clinical findings.

Treatment

- *Corneal dystrophy*: Mild cases can be observed and soft contact lenses are helpful; penetrating keratoplasty (PK) may be necessary, graft recurrences treated by superficial keratectomy, phototherapeutic keratectomy (PTK) or repeat penetrating keratoplasty.

- *Cataract*: Change in glasses can sometimes improve a patient's visual function temporarily; however, the most common treatment is cataract surgery.

BIBLIOGRAPHY

1. Shah KN. (2012). Ectodermal dysplasia. [online] Available from www.emedicine.com/derm/TOPIC114.HTM. [Accessed October, 2013].

2.17. ULLRICH SYNDROME (ULLRICH-FEICHTIGER SYNDROME; DYSCRANIOPYLOPHALANGY) CORNEAL ULCER

General

Belongs to trisomy 13–15; unknown etiology; sporadic occurrence.

Ocular

Microphthalmia to anophthalmia; hypertelorism; narrow lid fissures; strabismus; glaucoma; aniridia; cloudy cornea; corneal ulcers; chorioretinal coloboma.

Clinical

Hypoplastic mandible; broad nose; polydactyly; spina bifida; bicornuate uterus or septa vagina; congenital heart disease.

Laboratory/Ocular

ANA test, serum muscle enzyme levels.

Treatment/Ocular/Corneal Ulcer

Topical cycloplegic agents, topical cyclosporin and topical antibiotics.

BIBLIOGRAPHY

1. Geeraets WJ. Ocular Syndromes, 3rd edition. Philadelphia: Lea & Febiger; 1976.

3. ANIRIDIA, PARTIAL WITH UNILATERAL RENAL AGENESIS AND PSYCHOMOTOR RETARDATION

General

Autosomal recessive.

Ocular

Congenital glaucoma; telecanthus; absence of iris; hypertelorism.

Clinical

One kidney absent or in failure; motor effects of cerebral or psychic activity retarded or slowed.

Laboratory

Chromosomal deletion is detected by cytogenetic testing with the use of high-resolution banding.

Treatment

The goal is directed toward control of IOP, with use of topical drops. Frequently, this goal is not met. Photophobia can be treated with tinted glasses. Strabismus, amblyopia, refractive errors and nystagmus may also require treatment with traditional methods.

BIBLIOGRAPHY

1. Singh D, Verma A. (2012). Aniridia. [online] Available from www.emedicine.com/oph/TOPIC43.HTM. [Accessed October, 2013].

4A. UVEITIS, ANTERIOR NONGRANULOMATOUS (IRITIS, CHRONIC)

General

Ocular inflammation. Etiology is idiopathic but certain systemic diseases may be the underlying cause.

Clinical

Human leukocyte antigen B27, Behçet disease, herpes zoster, sarcoidosis, syphilis, Lyme disease, JIA, Fuchs heterochromic iridocyclitis, tuberculosis.

Ocular

Photophobia, red eye, dull aching eye pain, perilimbal injection, keratic precipitates, flare and cell of anterior chamber, posterior synechiae, lenticular precipitates.

Laboratory

Diagnosis is made by clinical findings. If nongranulomatous iritis is recurrent, studies are necessary to determine the cause. Human leukocyte antigen B27 typing, serologic testing for syphilis, sarcoidosis rheumatoid factor and Lyme disease may be indicated.

Treatment

Topical corticosteroids are the mainstay of therapy. Subconjunctival corticosteroids may be necessary in non-responding cases. Cycloplegia is useful for controlling pain and photophobia.

BIBLIOGRAPHY

1. Levinson RD. (2012). Uveitis, anterior, nongranulomatous. [online] Available from www.emedicine.com/oph/TOPIC587.HTM. [Accessed October, 2013].

4B. UVEITIS, ANTERIOR GRANULOMATOUS (IRITIS)

General

Ocular inflammation of the iris and ciliary body. Etiology is idiopathic but certain systemic diseases may be the underlying cause.

Clinical

Herpes zoster, sarcoidosis, syphilis, Lyme disease, tuberculosis, multiple sclerosis, leprosy, toxoplasmosis, coccidiodomycosis, Vogt-Koyanagi-Harada disease, brucellosis.

Ocular

Photophobia, red eye, dull aching eye pain, perilimbal injection, keratic precipitates, flare and cell of anterior chamber, posterior synechiae, lenticular precipitates.

Laboratory

Diagnosis is made by clinical findings. If granulomatous iritis is recurrent, studies are necessary to determine the cause. Enzyme-linked immunosorbent assay (ELISA), serologic testing for syphilis, sarcoidosis and Lyme disease may be indicated.

Treatment

Topical corticosteroids are the mainstay of therapy. Subconjunctival corticosteroids may be necessary in non-responding cases. Cycloplegia is useful for control of pain and photophobia.

BIBLIOGRAPHY

1. Levinson RD. (2012). Uveitis, anterior, granulomatous. [online] Available from www.emedicine.com/oph/TOPIC586.HTM. [Accessed October, 2013].

4B1. FUCHS (1) SYNDROME (HETEROCHROMIC CYCLITIS SYNDROME)

General

Etiology is unknown; mild infective cyclitis is the most likely cause; etiology remains unclear, although it is likely to be autoimmune; positive epidemiologic association with ocular toxoplasmosis has been investigated.

Ocular

Secondary glaucoma; unilateral hypochromic heterochromia; painless cyclitis with absence of synechiae and little or no ciliary injection; secondary cataract; vitreous opacities; small white discrete keratic precipitates with fine filaments between the precipitates; corneal epithelium may be slightly edematous; peripheral choroiditis occasionally; keratoconus.

Clinical

Occasional dysraphia of the cervical cord.

Laboratory

Diagnosis is made by clinical findings.

Treatment

Generally no treatment is necessary. Occasionally discomfort and ciliary injection is treated with topical steroids. With cataract surgery, there is a higher rate of vitreous debris and hemorrhage. Glaucoma surgery may be indicated and rubeotic glaucoma may require enucleation.

BIBLIOGRAPHY

1. Arif M, Foster CS, Wong IG. (2011). Fuchs heterochromic uveitis. [online] Available from www.emedicine.com/oph/TOPIC432.HTM. [Accessed October, 2013].

4B2. JUVENILE RHEUMATOID ARTHRITIS (JRA; STILL DISEASE)

General

Onset before age of 16 years; greater occurrence of systemic manifestations, monoarticular and oligoarticular joint involvement and iridocyclitis.

Ocular

Hypopyon; band keratopathy; uveitis; cataract; papillitis; glaucoma; macular edema; ocular pain; vitreous cells; synechiae; scleritis; presumed to have an autoimmune etiology; antiocular antibodies, including iris protein antibodies, have been found in the sera of patients.

Clinical

Salmon pink macular rash; arthritis; hepatosplenomegaly; leukocytosis; chronic pain; joint swelling; low-grade fever; anemia; rheumatoid nodules.

Laboratory

Antinuclear antibody (ANA), rheumatoid factor, HLA-B27, X-ray imaging of joints.

Treatment

Uveitis is treated initially with topical corticosteroids. Systemic immunomodulatory agents may be useful for patients with limited or no response to topical or systemic corticosteroids.

BIBLIOGRAPHY

1. Roque MR, Roque BL, Miserocchi E, et al. (2012). Juvenile idiopathic arthritis uveitis. [online] Available from www.emedicine.com/oph/TOPIC675.HTM. [Accessed October, 2013].
2. Thorne JE, Woreta FA, Dunn JP, et al. Risk of cataract development among children with juvenile idiopathic arthritis-related uveitis treated with topical corticosteroids. Ophthalmology. 2010;117:1436-41.

5. CHARLIN SYNDROME (NASAL NERVE SYNDROME; NASOCILIARIS NERVE SYNDROME; NASOCILIARY SYNDROME)

General

Neuritis of the nasal branch of the trigeminal nerve; three typical spots of pain according to the nerve distribution are: (1) above and outside the nose, (2) above the inner canthus and (3) inferior angle of the medial tarsal ligament (*see* Sluder syndrome).

Ocular

Severe ocular and orbital pain, mainly upper nasal-orbital angle; slight inflammatory swelling of upper lid (occasional); photophobia; ciliary and conjunctival injection; pseudopurulent conjunctivitis; anterior uveitis; iritis; hypopyon; keratitis; corneal ulcers.

Clinical

Rhinorrhea; rhinitis always on same side of the ocular involvement; severe pain of ala nasi.

Laboratory

Diagnosis is made by clinical findings.

Treatment

- *Uveitis*: Topical steroids and cycloplegic medication should be the initial treatment of choice; oral steroids should be given if not responsive to topical steroids, immunosuppressants if bilateral disease that does not respond to oral steroids, periocular steroids for unilateral or posterior uveitis. Vitrectomy can be used for severe vitreous opacification. Cryotherapy and laser photocoagulation may be used for localized pars plana exudates.
- *Corneal ulcer*: Corneal cultures may be taken and treatment is initiated. Treatment includes a broad spectrum of antibiotics and cycloplegic drops.

BIBLIOGRAPHY

1. Charlin C. Le Syndrome du Nerf Nasal. Ann Oculist (Paris). 1931;168:86.
2. Ferrannini G. Charlin's syndrome. Ann Ophthalmol Clin Ocul. 1969;95(10):807-11.
3. Pau H. Differential Diagnosis of Eye Diseases, 2nd edition. New York: Thieme Medical; 1988.

6. CHIKUNGUNYA FEVER

General

Debilitating viral infection spread by the bite of the infected *Aedes albopictus* mosquito and is now thought to have mutated enabling it to be transmitted by *A. albopictus*. The disease was first isolated in Tanzania but no outbreaks have occurred in Africa, Asia, India, Vietnam, Myanmar and Indonesia.

Clinical

Arthritis resulting in a stooped posture, fever, headache, fatigue, nausea, vomiting, renal failure, muscle pain, rash and joint pain.

Ocular

Iridocyclitis, viral retinitis, vitreitis, retinal hemorrhage, conjunctivitis and episcleritis.

Laboratory

Specific diagnosis is based on viral isolation or the demonstration of seroconversion, that is, the presence of specific immunoglobulin M (IgM) antibody or a four-fold increase in the antibody titer.

Treatment

Antiviral therapy may be useful. Acyclovir intravenously (IV) or orally is the drug of choice.

BIBLIOGRAPHY

1. Saemi AM, Anvari EN, Alai NN. (2012). Dermatologic Manifestations of viral hemorrhagic fevers. [online] Available from www.emedicine.com/derm/TOPIC880.HTM. [Accessed October, 2013].

7. COLOBOMA OF IRIS

This condition involves failure of fusions of fetal fissure in optic vesicle, usually inferior or inferonasal.

1. Acrorenoocular syndrome
2. Aicardi syndrome
3. Aniridia
4. Biemond syndrome
5. Cat eye syndrome (partial G-trisomy syndrome)
6. CHARGE association (coloboma, heart anomaly, choanal atresia, retardation, genital, and ear anomalies)
7. Chromosome partial short-arm deletion syndrome
8. Ellis-van Creveld syndrome (chondroectodermal dysplasia)
9. Epidermal nevus syndrome (ichthyosis hystrix)
10. Focal dermal hypoplasia syndrome (Goltz syndrome)
11. Hallermann-Streiff-François syndrome (dyscephalic mandibulooculofacial syndrome)
12. Hemifacial microsoma syndrome (otomandibular dysostosis)
†*13. Hereditary usually dominant may be recessive
14. Hurler syndrome (mucopolysaccharidoses I)
15. Hyperchromic heterochromia
16. Jeune disease (asphyxiating thoracic dystrophy)
17. Joubert syndrome
18. Kartagener syndrome
19. Klinefelter syndrome
20. Klippel-Trenaunay-Weber syndrome (angioosteohypertrophy syndrome)
21. Langer-Giedion syndrome
22. Lanzieri syndrome
23. Laurence-Moon-Bardet-Biedl syndrome (retinitis pigmentosa-polydactyly-adiposogenital syndrome)
*24. Marfan syndrome (dolichostenomelia-arachnodactyly-hyperchondroplasia-dystrophia mesodermalis congenita)

†25. Maternal use of thalidomide
26. Maternal vitamin A deficiency
27. Meckel syndrome
28. Median facial cleft syndrome
29. Microphthalmos syndrome (Meyer-Schwickerath and Weyers syndrome)
30. Nevoid basal cell carcinoma syndrome
31. Nevus sebaceous of Jadassohn (linear sebaceous nevus syndrome of Jadassohn)
32. Obesity-cerebral-ocular-skeletal anomalies syndrome
†33. Oculoauriculovertebral dysplasia syndrome
†34. Organoid nevus syndrome
35. Otomandibular dysostosis (hemifacial microsomia syndrome)
36. Rieger syndrome (dysgenesis mesodermalis corneae et irides)
†37. Retinal dysplasia
38. Rubinstein-Taybi syndrome (broad-thumbs syndrome)
†*39. Sporadic
40. Treacher Collins syndrome (Franceschetti syndrome)
41. Trisomy 13 (D trisomy) (Patau syndrome)
42. Trisomy 18 syndrome (Edwards syndrome)
43. Turner syndrome
44. Warburg syndrome
†45. White sponge nevus
46. Wolf syndrome (monosomy partial syndrome)
47. 11q syndrome
48. 13q syndrome
49. 18q syndrome
50. XYY syndrome

*Indicates most frequent
†Indicates a general entry and therefore has not been described in detail in the text

BIBLIOGRAPHY

1. Isenberg SJ. The Eye in Infancy. Chicago: Year Book Medical; 1989.
2. Roy FH. Ocular Syndromes and Systemic Diseases, 5th edition. New Delhi: Jaypee Brothers Medical Publishers; 2013.

⊟ 7.1. ACRORENOOCULAR SYNDROME

General

Autosomal dominant; Duane syndrome with radial defects.

Ocular

Complete coloboma; coloboma of optic nerve; ptosis and Duane anomaly.

Clinical

Renal anomalies; hypoplasia of distal part of thumb with lack of motion at phalangeal joint; renal ectopia without fusion; bladder diverticula; malrotation of both kidneys; absence of kidney; clubhand or absence of thumb.

Laboratory

Diagnosis is made by clinical findings.

Treatment

If visual acuity is affected most cases require surgical correction and there are several procedures that may be used including levator resection, repair or advancement and Fasanella-Servat.

⊟ BIBLIOGRAPHY

1. Halal F, Homsy M, Perreault G. Acro-renal-ocular syndrome: autosomal dominant thumb hypoplasia; renal ectopia and eye defect. Am J Med Genet. 1984;17:753-62.
2. McKusick VA. Mendelian Inheritance in Man: A Catalog of Human Genes and Genetic Disorders, 12th edition. Baltimore: The Johns Hopkins University Press; 1998.
3. Online Mendelian Inheritance in Man, OMIM. McKusick-Nathans Institute for Genetic Medicine, Johns Hopkins University and National Center for Biotechnology Information, National Library of Medicine, October 12, 2007. Available from www.ncbi.nlm.nih.gov/omim. [Accessed October, 2013].

⊟ 7.2. AICARDI SYNDROME

General

All symptoms present at birth; cause unknown; all findings progress with age; shows X-linked dominant inheritance.

Ocular

Microphthalmia; lid twitching; absent pupillary reflexes; round retinal lacunae up to disk size look like holes with retinal vessels crossing over them; funnel-shaped disk; chorioretinitis.

Clinical

Infantile spasms (tonic seizures in flexion); epileptic seizures; cyanosis; mental anomaly; vertebral anomalies; telangiectasia; hypotonia; head deformities with biparietal bossing, occipital flattening, and plagiocephaly; defects of corpus callosum; cortical heterotopia; characteristic electroencephalogram; dilated intracranial ventricle with leukomalacia.

Laboratory

Generally diagnosis is made by clinical findings. Neuroimaging can delineate the degree of central nervous system (CNS) dysgenesis and help to evaluate other potential etiologies of intractable epilepsy and developmental delay.

Treatment

Consultation with a child neurologist is recommended. Use of traditional epilepsy therapies for seizure manifestations is recommended.

⊟ BIBLIOGRAPHY

1. Davis RG, DiFazio MP. (2012). Aicardi syndrome. [online] Available from www.emedicine.com/ped/TOPIC58.HTM. [Accessed October, 2013].

🗗 7.3. ANIRIDIA (CONGENITAL ANIRIDIA, HEREDITARY ANIRIDIA)

General

Hereditary, recessive (two-thirds of cases), can be dominant, sporadic or traumatic; absence of the iris; rare; usually bilateral unless due to trauma.

Ocular

Absence of iris; subluxed lens; iridodialysis; cataract; glaucoma; corneal scarring, vascularization, and edema; iris colobomata; round eccentric pupils; keratoconus.

Clinical

Cerebellar ataxia; mental retardation; WT.

Laboratory

Chromosomal deletion, cytogenic analysis, submicroscopic deletions of WT gene with fluorescence in situ hybridization (FISH) technique, polymerase chain reaction (PCR) genotyping halotypes across paired box gene 6 (PAX6)-WT1 region provides evidence of a chromosomal deletion.

Treatment

Systemic or topical glaucoma therapy.

🗗 BIBLIOGRAPHY

1. François J, Coucke D, Coppieters R. Aniridia-Wilms' tumor syndrome. Ophthalmologica. 1977;174(1):35-9.
2. Johns KJ, O'Day DM. Posterior chamber intraocular lenses after extracapsular cataract extraction in patients with aniridia. Ophthalmology. 1991;98(11):1698-702.
3. Kremer I, Rajpal RK, Rapuano CJ, et al. Results of penetrating keratoplasty in aniridia. Am J Ophthalmol. 1993;115(3): 317-20.
4. Magalini SI, Scrascia E. Dictionary of Medical Syndromes, 2nd edition. Philadelphia, PA: JB Lippincott; 1981.
5. Mintz-Hittner HA, Ferrell RE, Lyons LA, et al. Criteria to detect minimal expressivity within families with autosomal dominant aniridia. Am J Ophthalmol. 1992;114(6):700-7.
6. Nelson LB, Spaeth GL, Nowinski TS, et al. Aniridia. A review. Surv Ophthalmol. 1984;28(6):621-42.
7. Skeens HM, Brooks BP, Holland EJ. Congenital aniridia variant: minimally abnormal irides with severe limbal stem cell deficiency. Ophthalmology. 2011;118(7):1260-4.

🗗 7.4. BIEMOND SYNDROME

General

Simple recessive; hypophyseal infantilism.

Ocular

Night blindness in the presence of retinal pigment degeneration; iris coloboma (occasionally); retinal pigmentary degeneration.

Clinical

Mental retardation; polydactyly; genital dystrophia (genital organs may have been arrested in their development; absence of secondary sex characteristics); obesity; hypogenitalism; postaxial polydactyly; hydrocephalus; hypospadias.

Laboratory

Clinical.

Treatment

See child endocrinologist.

🗗 BIBLIOGRAPHY

1. Biemond A. Infantilisme Hypophysaire Avec Colobome Irien, Polydactylie et Anomalies Physiques et Sequelettiques. Ned Tijdschr Geneeskd. 1934;78:1801.
2. Duke-Elder S (Ed). System of Ophthalmology, Volume 3. St. Louis: CV Mosby; 1964.
3. McKusick VA. Mendelian Inheritance in Man: A Catalog of Human Genes and Genetic Disorders, 12th edition. Baltimore: The Johns Hopkins University Press; 1998.
4. Online Mendelian Inheritance in Man: OMIM. McKusick-Nathans Institute for Genetic Medicine, Johns Hopkins University and National Center for Biotechnology Information, National Library of Medicine, October 12, 2007. Available from www.ncbi.nlm.nih.gov/omim. [Accessed October, 2013].

⊟ 7.5. CAT'S-EYE SYNDROME (SCHACHENMANN SYNDROME; SCHMID-FRACCARO SYNDROME; PARTIAL TRISOMY G SYNDROME)

General

Causative factor is one extra chromosome, a G chromosome, which may be from a 13–15 or 21–22 chromosome; although the ocular findings of the syndrome are similar to the D 13–15 trisomy group; the systemic manifestations usually are less severe; this syndrome is associated with a supernumerary bisatellited marker chromosome derived from duplicated regions of 22pter'22q11.2; partial cat's-eye syndrome is characterized by the absence of coloboma.

Ocular

Hypertelorism; microphthalmos; antimongoloid slant of palpebral fissures; strabismus; inferior vertical iris coloboma (cat eye); cataract; choroidal coloboma; epicanthal folds.

Clinical

Anal atresia; preauricular fistulae (bilateral); umbilical hernia; heart anomalies.

Laboratory

Chromosome analysis.

Treatment

- *Cataract*: Change in glasses can sometimes improve a patient's visual function temporarily, however the most common treatment is cataract surgery.
- *Strabismus*: Equalized vision with correct refractive error, surgery may be helpful in patient with diplopia.

⊟ BIBLIOGRAPHY

1. Collins JF. Handbook of Clinical Ophthalmology. New York: Masson; 1982.

⊟ 7.6. CHARGE ASSOCIATION (MULTIPLE CONGENITAL ANOMALIES SYNDROME; COLOBOMA, HEART DISEASE, ATRESIA, RETARDED GROWTH, GENITAL HYPOPLASIA, EAR MALFORMATION ASSOCIATION)

General

Syndrome consists of four of six major manifestations of ocular coloboma, heart disease, atresia, retarded growth and development, genital hypoplasia, and ear malformations with or without hearing loss.

Ocular

Blepharoptosis; iris coloboma; optic nerve coloboma; macular hypoplasia; lacrimal canalicular atresia; nasolacrimal duct obstruction.

Clinical

Microcephaly; brachycephaly; malformed ear; bilateral finger contractures; heart disease; genital hypoplasia; heart disease; choanal atresia; retarded growth; hearing loss; facial nerve palsies; mental retardation.

Laboratory

CHD7 mutation analysis is diagnostic in 58–71% of individuals who meet the clinical criteria, head CT and MRI, cranial ultrasound.

Treatment

Secure airway, stabilize the patient, exclude major life-threatening congenital anomalies and transfer the individual with coloboma of the eye, heart defects, atresia of the nasal choanae, retardation of growth and/or development, genital and/or urinary abnormalities, and ear abnormalities and deafness (CHARGE) syndrome to a specialist center with pediatric otolaryngologist and other subspecialty services.

⊟ BIBLIOGRAPHY

1. Tegay DH, Yedowitz JC. (2012). CHARGE syndrome. [online] Available from www.emedicine.com/ped/TOPIC367.HTM. [Accessed October, 2013].

7.7. CHROMOSOME 18 PARTIAL DELETION (SHORT-ARM) SYNDROME [MONOSOMY 18 PARTIAL (SHORT-ARM) SYNDROME]

General

Deletion of the short arm of chromosome 18 (note similarity of clinical features to those of the Cri-du-Chat syndrome or B1 deletion syndrome) (*see* Cri-du-Chat syndrome).

Ocular

Hypertelorism; epicanthal folds; ptosis; mongolian or anti-mongolian slant; strabismus; eccentric pupil; cataract; corneal opacities; concentric visual field defects.

Clinical

Short stature; mental retardation; low-set ears; dysphagia; moon face; oliguria; arhinencephaly; microcephaly; congenital alopecia; flat bridge of nose; pyramidal tract signs; weakness and focal dystonia of the lower extremities.

Laboratory

Clinical.

Treatment

- *Ptosis*: If visual acuity is affected, most cases require surgical correction and there are several procedures that may be used including levator resection, repair or advancement and Fasanella-Servat.
- *Strabismus*: Equalized vision with correct refractive error, surgery may be helpful in patient with diplopia.

BIBLIOGRAPHY

1. Bühler E, Bühler U, Stalder G. Partial monosomy 18 and anomaly of thyroxine synthesis. Lancet. 1964;1:170-1.
2. Levenson JE, Crandall BF, Sparkes RS. Partial deletion syndromes of chromosome 18. Ann Ophthalmol. 1971;3:756-60.
3. Yanoff M, Rorke LB, Niederer BS. Ocular and cerebral abnormalities in chromosome 18 deletion defect. Am J Ophthalmol. 1970;10:391-402.

7.8. ELLIS-VAN CREVELD SYNDROME (CHONDROECTODERMAL DYSPLASIA)

General

Autosomal recessive inheritance; occurs in the Amish; associated with *de novo* chromosomal abnormality: deletion of 12 (p11.21p12.2).

Ocular

Esotropia; iris coloboma; congenital cataract.

Clinical

Bilateral polydactyly; short and plump limbs; genu valgum; talipes (equinovarus, calcaneovalgus); thoracic constriction; fusion of middle part of upper lip to maxillary gingival margin; dental anomalies: number, shape, spacing; congenital heart defect in about 50% of patients; dystrophic fingernails; genital anomalies; mild mental retardation; short stature; hypoplastic hair and skin; oligodontia; small thoracic cage; hypoplastic pelvis; cone-shaped epiphyses of hands.

Laboratory

Clinical.

Treatment

- *Esotropia*: Equalized vision with correct refractive error; surgery may be helpful in patient with diplopia.
- *Retinal detachment*: Scleral buckle, pneumatic retinopexy and vitrectomy may be used to close all the breaks.

BIBLIOGRAPHY

1. Chen H. (2013). Ellis-van Creveld Syndrome. [online] Available from www.emedicine.com/ped/TOPIC660.HTM. [Accessed October, 2013].

⊞ 7.9. EPIDERMAL NEVUS SYNDROME (ICHTHYOSIS HYSTRIX)

General

One or a combination of the following epidermal nevi described as nevus unius lateris, ichthyosis hystrix, linear nevus sebaceous, or congenital acanthosis nigricans; autosomal dominant.

Ocular

Blepharoptosis and fibroma on bulbar conjunctiva; antimongoloid eyelid fissures; eyelid colobomata; horizontal and rotary nystagmus; esotropia; conjunctival tumors; corneal opacities; corectopia and colobomata of the iris.

Clinical

Somatic anomalies involving the skeletal and CNS; anomalies of bone formation; atrophy; ankylosis; vitamin D-resistant rickets; bone cysts; mental retardation; cortical atrophy; hydrocephalus; focal and grand mal epilepsy; cerebrovascular tumors; cortical blindness.

Laboratory

Histologic examination, EEG, MRI.

Treatment

Vitamin D analogs may work by inhibiting epidermal proliferation, promoting keratinocyte differentiation, and/or exerting immunosuppressive effects on lymphoid cells.

⊞ BIBLIOGRAPHY

1. Schwartz RA, Jozwiak S. (2013). Epidermal nevus syndrome. [online] Available from www.emedicine.com/derm/TOPIC732.HTM. [Accessed October, 2013].

⊞ 7.10. GOLTZ SYNDROME (FOCAL DERMAL HYPOPLASIA SYNDROME)

General

X-linked dominant inheritance; lethal in males; skin manifestations present at birth.

Ocular

Microphthalmia; strabismus; coloboma of iris and/or choroid; epiphora; blue sclera; nystagmus; anophthalmos; keratoconus.

Clinical

Skin atrophy and linear pigmentation; telangiectasias of trunk and extremities; superficial, localized fatty skin deposits; multiple papillomas of mucous membranes and periorificial skin (oral, genital, anal); anomalies of extremities with syndactyly, oligodactyly, adactyly; hypohidrosis; paper-thin nails may be present; spina bifida; hypoplasia of right clavicle; umbilical or inguinal hernia.

Laboratory

Radiography may reveal osteopathia striata.

Treatment

Flashlamp-pumped pulse dye laser may ameliorate the pruritic symptoms that sometimes are noted in affected skin and improve the clinical appearance of the telangiectatic and erythematous skin lesions. Papillomas frequently require repeated surgical intervention.

⊞ BIBLIOGRAPHY

1. Goltz RW, Castelo-Soccio L. (2012). Focal dermal hypoplasia syndrome. [online] Available from emedicine.medscape.com/article/1110936-overview. [Accessed October, 2013].

7.11. HALLERMANN-STREIFF SYNDROME (DYSCEPHALIC-MANDIBULO-OCULO-FACIAL SYNDROME; OCULO-MANDIBULO-DYSCEPHALY; ULLRICH-FREMERY-DOHNA SYNDROME; FRANCOIS DYSCEPHALIC SYNDROME; MANDIBULO-OCULO-FACIAL DYSCEPHALY SYNDROME; FRANCOIS-HALLERMANN-STREIFF SYNDROME; HALLERMANN-STREIFF-FRANCOIS SYNDROME; AUDRY I SYNDROME; DOHNA SYNDROME; FRANCOIS SYNDROME (1); DYSCEPHALY-TEETH ABNORMALITY-DWARFISM; DYSCEPHALIA OCULOMANDIBULARIS-HYPOTRICHOSIS; MANDIBULO-OCULAR DYSCEPHALIA HYPOTRICHOSIS; FREMERY-DOHNA SYNDROME; OCULO-MANDIBULO-FACIAL DYSCEPHALY)

General

Rare; familial occurrence and consanguinity; males and females are equally affected.

Ocular

Microphthalmos (bilateral); proptosis; nystagmus; strabismus; cataracts; bilateral optic atrophy; coloboma of optic disk, choroid, and iris; keratoglobus; microcornea; antimongoloid slant; iris atrophy; uveitis; blue sclera; persistent pupillary membrane; secondary glaucoma.

Clinical

Malformations of skull (brachycephaly), facial skeleton and jaws; erupted teeth at birth; diminished hair growth; hyperextensibility of joints; short stature; skin atrophy; mental deficiency; predisposition to upper airway compromise; obstructive sleep apnea.

Laboratory

Diagnosis is made by clinical findings.

Treatment

- *Cataract*: Change in glasses can sometimes improve a patient's visual function temporarily; however, the most common treatment is cataract surgery.
- *Strabismus*: Equalized vision with correct refractive error; surgery may be helpful in patients with diplopia.
- *Uveitis*: Topical steroids and cycloplegic medication should be the initial treatment of choice. Oral steroids should be given if not responsive to topical steroids, immunosuppressants if bilateral disease that does not respond to oral steroids, periocular steroids for unilateral or posterior uveitis. Vitrectomy can be used for severe vitreous opacification. Cryotherapy and laser photocoagulation may be used for localized pars plana exudates.
- *Glaucoma*: Glaucoma medication should be the first plan of action. If medication is unsuccessful, a filtering surgical procedure with or without antimetabolites may be beneficial.

BIBLIOGRAPHY

1. François J, Victoria-Troncoso V. François' dyscephalic syndrome and skin manifestations. Ophthalmologica. 1981;183(2):63-7.
2. Roy FH, Fraunfelder FW, Fraunfelder FT. Roy and Fraunfelder's Current Ocular Therapy, 6th edition. Philadelphia, PA: WB Saunders; 2008.
3. Hallermann W. Vogelgesicht und Cataracta Congenita. Klin Monatsbl Augenheilkd. 1948;113:315-8.
4. Ronen S, Rozenmann Y, Isaacson M, et al. The early management of baby with Hallermann-Streiff-Francois syndrome. J Pediatr Ophthalmol Strabismus. 1979;16(2):119-21.
5. Spaepen A, Schrander-Stumpel C, Fryns JP, et al. Hallermann-Streiff syndrome: clinical and psychological findings in children. Nosologic overlap with oculodentodigital dysplasia? Am J Med Genet. 1991;41(4):517-20.
6. Streiff EB. Dysmorphic Mandibulo-faciale (Tete d'Oiseau) et Alterations Oculaires. Ophthalmologica. 1950;120(1-2):79-83.

⊟ 7.12. HEMIFACIAL MICROSOMIA SYNDROME (UNILATERAL FACIAL AGENESIS; OTOMANDIBULAR DYSOSTOSIS; FRANCOIS-HAUSTRATE SYNDROME)

General

No inheritance pattern; left side of face seems to be more frequently involved; facial asymmetry usually most obvious finding; both sexes affected; alteration of intrauterine environment is possible cause.

Ocular

Microphthalmos; congenital cystic ophthalmia; enophthalmos; strabismus; cataract; colobomata of iris, choroid and retina.

Clinical

Microtia; macrostomia; failure of development of mandibular ramus and condyle; external auditory meatus may be absent; single or numerous ear tags; hypoplasia of facial muscles unilaterally; pulmonary agenesis (ipsilateral side); associated with Goldenhar syndrome.

Laboratory

X-ray, CT and MRI.

Treatment

Silastic implants remain one of the most common materials used for malar and submalar augmentation.

⊟ BIBLIOGRAPHY

1. Francois J, Haustrate L. Anomalies Colobomateuses du Globe Oculaire et Syndrome du Premier arc. Ann Ocul. 1954;187:340-68.
2. Geeraets WJ. Ocular Syndromes, 3rd edition. Philadelphia: Lea & Febiger; 1976.
3. Kobrynski L, Chitayat D, Zahed L, et al. Trisomy 22 and facioauriculovertebral (Goldenhar) sequence. Am J Med Genet. 1993;46:68-71.
4. Magalini SI, Scrascia E. Dictionary of Medical Syndromes, 2nd edition. Philadelphia: JB Lippincott; 1981.

⊟ 7.14. HURLER SYNDROME (PFAUNDLER-HURLER SYNDROME; GARGOYLISM; DYSOSTOSIS MULTIPLEX; MPS IH SYNDROME; SYSTEMIC MUCOPOLYSACCHARIDOSIS TYPE IH; MUCOPOLYSACCHARIDOSIS IH)

General

Autosomal recessive inheritance; in addition to corneal opacities and enlargement of the head at birth, other symptoms become apparent at the end of the 1st year; death occurs usually before 20 years; gross excess of chondroitin sulfate band, heparitin sulfate in the urine (*see* Hunter Syndrome; Sanfilippo-Good Syndrome; Morquio-Brailsford Syndrome; Scheie Syndrome; Maroteaux-Lamy Syndrome). Jensen suggested that the pathogenesis of the various mucopolysaccharidoses is the same but that the variations in the defective enzymes cause the different types; most common mucopolysaccharidosis (MPS), decreased iduronidase.

Ocular

Proptosis; hypertelorism; thick, enlarged lids; esotropia; diffuse haziness of the cornea at birth progressive to milky opacity; retinal pigmentary changes may exist; macular edema and absence of foveal reflex; optic atrophy; megalocornea; bushy eyebrows; coarse eyelashes; mucopolysaccharide deposits of iris, lens, and sclera; enlarged optic foramen; retinal detachment; anisocoria; buphthalmos; nystagmus; secondary open-angle glaucoma; progressive retinopathy with vascular narrowing; hyperpigmentation of the fundus; bone spicule; papilledema.

Clinical

Dorsolumbar kyphosis; head deformities with depressed nose bridge; short cervical spine; short limbs; macroglossia; enlarged liver and spleen; short stature; facial dysmorphism; progressive psychomotor retardation.

Laboratory

Blood smears-abnormal cytoplasmic inclusions in lymphocytes; urine: increased excretion of dermatan sulfate and heparin sulfate.

Treatment

- *Macular edema*: Use of corticosteroids, carbonic anhydrase inhibitors and nonsteroidal anti-inflammatory drugs (NSAIDs) are the mainstay of treatment. If traditional therapy is not effective, intraocular injections of Avastin® may be helpful. In cases that have vitreous strand tugging against the macula, pars plana vitrectomy may be necessary.
- *Retinal detachment*: Scleral buckle, pneumatic retinopexy and vitrectomy may be used to close all the breaks.

- *Glaucoma*: Glaucoma medication should be the first plan of action. If medication is unsuccessful, a filtering surgical procedure with or without antimetabolites may be beneficial.
- *Papilledema*: Underlying cause should be determined and treated. Systemic acetazolamide is the medical therapy of choice.

BIBLIOGRAPHY

1. Banikazemi M. (2012). Genetics of mucopolysaccharidosis type I. [online] Available from www.emedicine.com/ped/TOPIC1031.HTM. [Accessed October, 2013].

7.15. HETEROCHROMIA IRIDIS

General

Autosomal dominant; it can be associated with Horner, Waardenburg and Marfan syndromes; it may occur as an isolated phenomenon.

Ocular

Different pigmentation in the two irides or in the sectors of one iris (heterochromia iridium).

Clinical

None.

Laboratory

Diagnosis is made by clinical findings.

Treatment

None.

BIBLIOGRAPHY

1. Gladstone RM. Development and significance of heterochromia of the iris. Arch Neurol. 1969;21(2):184-91.
2. McKusick VA. Mendelian Inheritance in Man: A Catalog of Human Genes and Genetic Disorders, 12th edition. Baltimore, USA: The Johns Hopkins University Press; 1998.

7.16. JEUNE DISEASE (ASPHYXIATING THORACIC DYSTROPHY; THORACIC-PELVIC-PHALANGEAL DYSTROPHY)

General

Autosomal recessive; similar to Ellis-van Creveld syndrome; positive associations of this disorder with cystinuria has been reported in two sisters.

Ocular

Retinal dysfunction; granular pigmentation of the choroid; nystagmus; small white patches in peripheral fundus; retinal degeneration; coloboma of iris; eyes symmetrically involved; retinal aplasia; photophobia; strabismus; pigmentary retinopathy.

Clinical

Long, narrow thorax; short anteriorly clubbed ribs forming a continuous tube with the abdominal cavity; dwarfing skeletal dysplasia; progressive renal failure; liver abnormalities; severe respiratory insufficiency; long, narrow trunk; dystrophic rib cage with respiratory distress; short limbs; polydactyly.

Laboratory

Newborn and infant radiography show small and bell-shaped thorax with reduced transverse and anterior-posterior diameter. Urinalysis may show hematuria and proteinuria.

Treatment

Chest reconstruction and enlargement of the thoracic cage by sternotomy and fixation with bone grafts or a methyl- methacrylate prosthesis plate provides patients with the time needed for thoracic cage growth may be necessary.

BIBLIOGRAPHY

1. Chen H. (2013). Genetics of Asphyxiating Thoracic Dystrophy (Jeune Syndrome). [online] Available from www.emedicine.com/ped/TOPIC1224.HTM. [Accessed October, 2013].

7.17. JOUBERT SYNDROME (FAMILIAL CEREBELLAR VERMIS AGENESIS)

General

Autosomal recessive; both sexes affected; onset in early infancy.

Ocular

Choroidal coloboma; nystagmus; ocular fibrosis, telecanthus.

Clinical

Episodic hyperpnea; apnea; ataxia; psychomotor retardation; rhythmic protrusion of tongue; mental retardation; micrognathia; complex cardiac malformation; cutaneous dimples over wrists and elbows.

Laboratory

Urine culture, renal ultrasonography, dimercaptosuccinic acid (DMSA) renal scanning.

Treatment

Lifetime follow-up is required whether or not involution has occurred or a nephrectomy.

BIBLIOGRAPHY

1. Swiatecka-Urban A. (2011). Multicystic renal dysplasia. [online] Available from www.emedicine.com/ped/TOPIC1493.HTM. [Accessed October, 2013].

7.18. KARTAGENER SYNDROME (SINUSITIS-BRONCHIECTASIS-SITUS INVERSUS SYNDROME; BRONCHIECTASIS-DEXTROCARDIA-SINUSITIS; KARTAGENER TRIAD)

General

Autosomal recessive; onset in early infancy; occasionally dominant; finding of various structural defects in patients with this condition suggests that there are several genetic determinants.

Ocular

Myopia; glaucoma; conjunctival melanosis; iris coloboma; tortuous and dilated retinal vessels; retinal pigmentary degeneration; pseudopapillitis.

Clinical

Immotile cilia; situs inversus; bronchiectasis; sinusitis; various cardiovascular and renal abnormalities; dyspnea; productive cough; recurrent respiratory infections; palpitation; otitis media; nasal speech; conductive hearing loss; nasal polyps; situs inversus viscerum with hepatic dullness on left side.

Laboratory

High-resolution CT scan of the chest is the most sensitive modality for documenting early and subtle abnormalities within airways and pulmonary parenchyma when compared to routine chest radiographs.

Treatment

Antibiotics, intravenous or oral and continuous or intermittent, are used to treat upper and lower airway infections.

Obstructive lung disease, if present, should be treated with inhaled bronchodilators and aggressive pulmonary toilet. Tympanostomy tubes are required to reduce conductive hearing loss and recurrent infections.

BIBLIOGRAPHY

1. Bent JP, Willis EB. (2013). Kartagener syndrome. [online] Available from www.emedicine.com/med/TOPIC1220.HTM. [Accessed October, 2013].

7.19. KLINEFELTER SYNDROME (GYNECOMASTIA-ASPERMATOGENESIS SYNDROME; XXY SYNDROME; XXXY SYNDROME; XXYY SYNDROME; REIFENSTEIN-ALBRIGHT SYNDROME)

General

Occurrence in 1% of retarded males; phenotypically males with positive female sex chromatin; karyotype shows 47 chromosomes, 44 autosomes, and 3 sex chromosomes with the complement XXY.

Ocular

Anophthalmos; coloboma; corneal opacities.

Clinical

Testicular hypoplasia; sterility; gynecomastia; eunuchoid physique; mental retardation; association with progressive systemic sclerosis and systemic lupus erythematosus.

Laboratory

May be diagnosed prenatally based on cytogenetic analysis of a fetus. If not diagnosed prenatally, the 47,XXY karyotype may manifest as various subtle age-related clinical signs that may prompt chromosomal evaluation.

Treatment

Treatment should address three major facets of the disease: (1) hypogonadism, (2) gynecomastia, and (3) psychosocial problems.

BIBLIOGRAPHY

1. Chen H. (2013). Klinefelter syndrome. [online] Available from www.emedicine.com/ped/TOPIC1252.HTM. [Accessed October, 2013].

7.20. KLIPPEL-TRENAUNAY-WEBER SYNDROME (PARKES-WEBER SYNDROME; ANGIO-OSTEO-HYPERTROPHY SYNDROME)

General

Most frequently inherited as irregular dominant; however, reported to be recessive with parent consanguinity; association of Klippel-Trenaunay-Weber syndrome and Sturge-Weber syndrome has been reported.

Ocular

Enophthalmos; unilateral hydrophthalmos; conjunctival telangiectasia; atypical iris coloboma; cataract; irregular and dilated retinal vessels; choroidal angiomas; exudative outer retinal vascular masses.

Clinical

Vascular nevi; varicose vessels; capillary angiomas; lymphangioma; arteriovenous aneurysm; hypertrophy of soft tissues and bones (local); phlebitis; thrombosis; syndactyly; polydactyly; early eruption of teeth; hemifacial hypertrophy.

Laboratory

Ultrasound, MRI, angiography and X-ray.

Treatment

Compression stockings or pneumatic pumps are usually successful. Surgical intervention (resection or ligation of abnormal blood vessels) is sometimes necessary.

BIBLIOGRAPHY

1. Buehler B. (2012). Genetics of Klippel-Trenaunay-Weber Syndrome. [online] Available from www.emedicine.com/ped/TOPIC1253.HTM. [Accessed October, 2013].

7.21. LANGER-GIEDION SYNDROME (TRICHORHINOPHALANGEAL SYNDROME, TYPE II)

General

Rare congenital condition.

Ocular

Iris colobomata.

Clinical

Mental retardation, bulbous nose, sparse hair, cone-shaped epiphyses, microcephaly, multiple exostoses, redundant skin; less consistently, "floppy infants", hyperextensible joints, recurrent upper respiratory tract infections, delayed speech development and characteristic facies.

Laboratory

Diagnosis is made by clinical findings.

Treatment

None—ocular.

BIBLIOGRAPHY

1. Zeldin AS, Bazzano AT. (2012). Mental Retardation. [online] Available from http://www.emedicine.com/neuro/TOP-IC605.HTM. [Accessed October, 2013].

7.22. LANZIERI SYNDROME

General

Developmental anomaly that belongs to group of craniofacial malformations; present from birth.

Ocular

Microphthalmia; anophthalmos; iris coloboma; cataracts; retinal and choroidal coloboma; optic nerve coloboma.

Clinical

Dwarfism; dyscephalia; dental anomalies; hypertrichosis; skin atrophy; absence of fibula, some tarsal and metatarsal bones.

Laboratory

Diagnosis is made by clinical findings.

Treatment

Cataract: Change in glasses can sometimes improve a patient's visual function temporarily; however, the most common treatment is cataract surgery.

BIBLIOGRAPHY

1. Geeraets WJ. Ocular Syndromes, 3rd edition. Philadelphia: Lea & Febiger; 1976.
2. Lanzieri M. On a rare association of craniofacial malformative syndrome and congenital absence of the fibula. Ann Ottal Clin Ocul. 1961;87:667.
3. Magalini SI, Scrascia E. Dictionary of Medical Syndromes, 2nd edition. Philadelphia: JB Lippincott; 1981.

7.23. LAURENCE-MOON-BARDET-BIEDL SYNDROME (BARDET-BIEDL SYNDROME; RETINITIS PIGMENTOSA-POLYDACTYLY-ADIPOSOGENITAL SYNDROME)

General

Recessive, autosomal dominant, and recessive sex-linked gene; male preponderance; onset in childhood; cases of Laurence-Moon-Bardet-Biedl belong to the group of heredoataxias.

Ocular

Ptosis; epicanthus; nystagmus; strabismus; night blindness; myopia; hypermetropia; iris coloboma; retinitis pigmentosa "bone corpuscles"; macular degeneration; attenuation of retinal vessels; choroidal atrophy; optic nerve atrophy; cataract; microphthalmia; keratoconus.

Clinical

Obesity (Fröhlich type); hypogenitalism; reduced intelligence and mental retardation; turricephaly; shortness of stature; atresia ani; genu valgum; congenital heart disease; polydactyly; body hair scant or absent; pseudogynecomastia.

Laboratory

Chromosomal analysis is recommended to confirm chromosomal sex and to evaluate for associated genetic syndromes.

Treatment

Consultation by pediatric endocrinologist and pediatric urologist is usually necessary.

BIBLIOGRAPHY

1. Telander DG, de Beus A, Small KW. (2012). Retinitis pigmentosa. [online] Available from www.emedicine.com/oph/TOPIC704.HTM. [Accessed October, 2013].

7.24. MARFAN SYNDROME (DOLICHOSTENOMELIA; ARACHNODACTYLY; HYPERCHONDROPLASIA; DYSTROPHIA MESODERMALIS CONGENITA)

General

Hypoplastic form of dystrophia mesodermalis congenita; autosomal dominant; affects both sexes. It has been demonstrated that an abnormality of the gene coding for the connective tissue protein fibrillin is responsible for chronic Marfan syndrome.

Ocular

Exotropia; nystagmus; paralysis of accommodation; myopia (axial or lenticular); iridodonesis; miosis; persistent pupillary membrane; blue sclera; spherophakia; lens dislocation; cataract; megalocornea; retinal detachment (less frequently); pigmentary retinopathy; colobomata of macula, iris, optic nerve, and uveal tract (less frequently); keratoconus; central retinal artery occlusion; rhegmatogenous retinal detachment; syringoma.

Clinical

Arachnodactyly; skeletal anomalies; asymmetric thorax; dolichocephaly and high-arched palate; dissecting aneurysm; mitral valve prolapse; prominent ears; kyphoscoliosis; pectus excavatum; flat feet; hammer toes; pulmonary and kidney defects.

Laboratory

Genetic testing, molecular studies.

Treatment

- *Keratoconus*: Spectacle correction, hard contacts, avoid eye rubbing. If hydrops occur, discontinue contact lens, use sodium chloride (NaCl) drops and ointment, patching, and short course of steroids. As disease advances, PK, deep anterior lamellar keratoplasty intacs with laser grooves or collagen stabilization of cornea.
- *Cataract*: Change in glasses can sometimes improve a patient's visual function temporarily; however, the most common treatment is cataract surgery.
- *Glaucoma*: Glaucoma medication should be the first plan of action. If medication is unsuccessful, a filtering surgical procedure with or without antimetabolites may be beneficial.
- *Strabismus*: Equalized vision with correct refractive error; surgery may be helpful in patient with diplopia.

BIBLIOGRAPHY

1. Chen H. (2011). Genetics of Marfan syndrome. [online] Available from www.emedicine.com/ped/TOPIC1372.HTM. [Accessed October, 2013].

7.26. VITAMIN A DEFICIENCY

General

Worldwide cause of blindness; onset in childhood; dietary vitamin A insufficiency; interference of absorption from the intestinal tract and transport or storage in the liver, as with diarrhea or vomiting; most frequent in young children.

Ocular

Bitot spots; conjunctival xerosis; corneal xerosis; keratomalacia with perforation; photophobia; enlarged tarsal glands; corneal ulcer; nyctalopia; hemeralopia; obstruction of the tear ducts.

Clinical

Diarrhea; malabsorption syndrome; follicular hyperkeratosis; lesions on buttocks, legs, and arms; xerosis of skin; tracheitis; bronchitis; pneumonia; chronic obstruction of pancreatic or biliary ducts; increased infant mortality.

Laboratory

Serum retinol study, serum retinol binding protein (RBP) study, zinc levels, complete blood count (CBC), electrolyte evaluation and liver function studies.

Treatment

Vitamin A rich foods such as beef, chicken, sweet potatoes, mangoes, carrots, eggs, fortified milk and leafy green vegetables.

BIBLIOGRAPHY

1. Ansstas G, Thakore J, Gopalswamy N. (2012). Vitamin A deficiency. [online] Available from www.emedicine.com/med/TOPIC2381.HTM. [Accessed October, 2013].

7.27. MECKEL SYNDROME (DYSENCEPHALIA SPLANCHNOCYSTIC SYNDROME; GRUBER SYNDROME)

General

Autosomal recessive; ocular manifestations are similar to those of trisomy 13–15 syndrome.

Ocular

Cryptophthalmos; clinical anophthalmos; microphthalmos; mongoloid slant of lid fissures; sclerocornea; microcornea; partial aniridia; cataract; retinal dysplasia; posterior staphyloma; optic nerve hypoplasia.

Clinical

Sloping forehead; posterior encephalocele; short neck; polydactyly and syndactyly (hands and feet); polycystic kidneys; cryptorchidism; cleft lip and palate; CNS abnormalities, including the Dandy-Walker malformation.

Laboratory

Chromosome analysis, MRI.

Treatment

Cardiac surgery may be warranted.

BIBLIOGRAPHY

1. Jayakar PB, Spiliopoulos M, Jayakar A. (2011). Meckel-Gruber syndrome. [online] Available from www.emedicine.com/ped/TOPIC1390.HTM. [Accessed October, 2013].

7.28. FRONTONASAL DYSPLASIA SYNDROME (MEDIAN CLEFT FACE SYNDROME)

General

Congenital disorder without genetic background; condition may present a variety of facial malformations, depending on the stage of embryonic development at which interference occurs.

Ocular

Hypertelorism; anophthalmia or microphthalmia; significant refractive errors; strabismus; nystagmus; eyelid ptosis; optic nerve hypoplasia; optic nerve colobomas; cataract; corneal dermoid; inflammatory retinopathy.

Clinical

Broad nasal root may be associated with median nasal groove and cleft of nose and/or upper lip; cleft of ala nasi (unilateral or bilateral); V-shaped hair prolongation into forehead.

Laboratory

CT, MRI and physical examination.

Treatment

Reconstruction surgery may be warranted.

BIBLIOGRAPHY

1. Kinsey JA, Streeten BW. Ocular abnormalities in the medial cleft face syndrome. Am J Ophthalmol. 1977;83:261.
2. Roarty JD, Pron GE, Siegel-Bartelt J, et al. Ocular manifestations of frontonasal dysplasia. Plast Reconstr Surg. 1994;93:25-30.
3. Sedano HO, Cohen MM, Jirasek J, et al. Frontonasal dysplasia. J Pediatr. 1970;76:906-13.
4. Weaver D, Bellinger D. Bifid nose associated with midline cleft of the upper lip: case report. Arch Otolaryngol. 1946;44:480.

7.29. MEYER-SCHWICKERATH-WEYERS SYNDROME (MICROPHTHALMOS SYNDROME; OCULODENTODIGITAL DYSPLASIA)

General

Etiology unknown; two types recognized: (I) dysplasia oculodentodigitalis and (II) dyscraniopygophalangie; type I is characterized by microphthalmia with possible iris pathology and glaucoma, oligodontia and brown pigmentation of teeth, camptodactyly, and possible absence of middle phalanx of second to fifth toes; type II consists of severe microphthalmos to anophthalmos, polydactyly, and developmental anomalies of nose and oral cavity; both sexes affected; present from birth; abnormal cerebral white matter.

Ocular

Microphthalmos; hypotrichosis; glaucoma; iris anomalies (eccentric pupil; changes in normal iris texture; remnants of pupillary membrane along iris margins); microcornea; hypertelorism; myopia; hyperopia; keratoconus.

Clinical

Thin, small nose with anteverted nostrils and hypoplastic alae; syndactyly; camptodactyly (fourth and fifth fingers); anomalies of middle phalanx of fifth finger and toe; hypoplastic teeth; wide mandible; alveolar ridge; sparse hair growth; visceral malformations.

Laboratory

Diagnosis is made by clinical findings.

Treatment

- *Glaucoma*: Glaucoma medication should be the first plan of action. If medication is unsuccessful, a filtering surgical procedure with or without antimetabotites may be beneficial.
- *Keratoconus*: Spectacle correction, hard contacts, avoid eye rubbing. If hydrops occur, discontinue contact lens, use NaCl drops and ointment, patching, and short course of steroids. As disease advances, PK, deep anterior lamellar keratoplasty intacs with laser grooves or collagen stabilization of cornea.

BIBLIOGRAPHY

1. Geeraets WK. Ocular Syndromes, 3rd edition. Philadelphia: Lea & Febiger; 1976.
2. Gutmann DH, Zackai EH, McDonald-McGinn DM, et al. Oculodentodigital dysplasia syndrome associated with abnormal cerebral white matter. Am J Med Genet. 1991;41:18-20.
3. McKusick VA. Mendelian Inheritance in Man: A Catalog of Human Genes and Genetic Disorders, 12th edition. Baltimore: The Johns Hopkins University Press; 1998.

⊟ 7.30. BASAL CELL NEVUS SYNDROME (NEVOID BASAL CELL CARCINOMA SYNDROME; NEVOID BASALIOMA SYNDROME; GORLIN SYNDROME; GORLIN-GOLTZ SYNDROME; MULTIPLE BASAL CELL NEVI SYNDROME)

General

Autosomal dominant; onset of skin lesions in childhood, usually at puberty.

Ocular

Basal cell carcinomas of eyelids; strabismus; hypertelorism; congenital cataracts; choroidal colobomas; glaucoma; medullated nerve fibers; prominence of supraorbital ridges; corneal leukoma; basalioma of the skin; coloboma of the choroid and optic nerve.

Clinical

Basal cell tumors with facial involvement; shallow pits of the skin of the hands and feet; jaw cysts; rib anomalies; kyphoscoliosis and fusion of vertebrae; medulloblastoma; frontal and temporoparietal bossing and broad nasal root.

Laboratory

Computed tomography scanning, ultrasonography, or MRI to evaluate neoplasms. Endoscopy to evaluate for the degree of polyposis and survey for malignant transformation is done.

Treatment

Patients may require medical attention for craniofacial, vertebral, dental and ophthalmologic abnormalities, in addition to diagnosis and treatment of potential neoplasia.

⊟ BIBLIOGRAPHY

1. Hsu EK, Mamula P, Ruchelli ED. (2011). Intestinal Polyposis Syndromes. [online] Available from www.emedicine.com/ped/TOPIC828.HTM. [Accessed October, 2013].

⊟ 7.31. LINEAR NEVUS SEBACEUS OF JADASSOHN (NEVUS SEBACEUS OF JADASSOHN; JADASSOHN-TYPE ANETODERMA; ORGANOID NEVUS SYNDROME; SEBACEUS NEVUS SYNDROME)

General

Skin nevus caused by failure of separation of skin appendages from adjacent epithelium during the third month of gestation.

Ocular

Proptosis; epibulbar lipodermoids; colobomata of eyelids, iris, and choroid; antimongoloid fissures; ocular motor palsies; nystagmus; teratomas of orbit and aberrant lacrimal glands; corneal vascularization; vision defects; conjunctival dermolipomas; choristomas of conjunctiva, sclera; corneal vascularization/opacification; colobomas of uvea, retina, optic disk, and lids; optic nerve hypoplasia; microphthalmia; anophthalmia; hemangioma of the sclera/conjunctiva.

Clinical

Circumscribed lesions of the face and scalp with excessively large sebaceous glands; papillomatous epidermal hyperplasia; seizures; skeletal abnormalities, particularly in skull; failure to thrive; convulsion; mental retardation.

Laboratory

Epidermis shows papillomatous hyperplasia. In the dermis, the numbers of mature sebaceous glands are increased. Ectopic apocrine glands are often found in the deep dermis beneath sebaceous glands.

Treatment

Photodynamic therapy with topical aminolevulinic acid. Full-thickness skin excision is usually required, and topical destruction.

⊟ BIBLIOGRAPHY

1. Al Hammadi A, Lebwohl MG. (2012). Nevus Sebaceus. [online] Available from www.emedicine.com/derm/TOPIC296.HTM. [Accessed October, 2013].

⊟ 7.32. OBESITY-CEREBRAL-OCULAR-SKELETAL ANOMALIES SYNDROME

General

Rare, autosomal recessive disease; similar to Prader-Willi and Laurence-Moon-Bardet-Biedl syndromes.

Ocular

Microphthalmia; antimongoloid slant of lid fissure; asymmetrical size of fissure; strabismus; myopia; iris and chorioretinal colobomata; mottled retina; prominent choroidal vessels.

Clinical

Obesity (mid-childhood onset); hypotonia; mental retardation; craniofacial anomalies with microcephaly; tapering extremities; hyperextensibility at elbows and proximal interphalangeal joints; cubitus valgus; genu valgum; Simian creases; syndactyly.

Laboratory

Diagnosis is made by clinical findings.

Treatment

Strabismus: Equalized vision with correct refractive error; surgery may be helpful in patient with diplopia.

⊟ BIBLIOGRAPHY

1. Cohen MM, Hall BD, Smith DW, et al. A new syndrome with hypotonia, obesity, mental deficiency, and facial, oral, ocular, and limb anomalies. J Pediatr. 1973;83(2):280-4.
2. Hall BD, Smith DW. Prader-Willi syndrome: A resumé of 32 cases including an instance of affected first cousins, one of whom is of normal stature and intelligence. J Pediatr. 1972;81(2):286-93.

⊟ 7.35. HEMIFACIAL MICROSOMIA SYNDROME (UNILATERAL FACIAL AGENESIS; OTOMANDIBULAR DYSOSTOSIS; FRANCOIS-HAUSTRATE SYNDROME)

General

No inheritance pattern; left side of face seems to be more frequently involved; facial asymmetry usually most obvious finding; both sexes affected; alteration of intrauterine environment is possible cause.

Ocular

Microphthalmos; congenital cystic ophthalmia; enophthalmos; strabismus; cataract; colobomata of iris, choroid and retina.

Clinical

Microtia; macrostomia; failure of development of mandibular ramus and condyle; external auditory meatus may be absent; single or numerous ear tags; hypoplasia of facial muscles unilaterally; pulmonary agenesis (ipsilateral side); associated with Goldenhar syndrome.

Laboratory

X-ray, CT and MRI.

Treatment

Silastic implants remain one of the most common materials used for malar and submalar augmentation.

⊟ BIBLIOGRAPHY

1. Francois J, Haustrate L. Anomalies Colobomateuses du Globe Oculaire et Syndrome du Premier arc. Ann Ocul. 1954;187:340.
2. Geeraets WJ. Ocular Syndromes, 3rd edition. Philadelphia: Lea & Febiger; 1976.
3. Kobrynski L, Chitayat D, Zahed L, et al. Trisomy 22 and facioauriculovertebral (Goldenhar) sequence. Am J Med Genet. 1993;46:68-71.
4. Magalini SI, Scrascia E. Dictionary of Medical Syndromes, 2nd edition. Philadelphia: JB Lippincott; 1981.

7.36. RIEGER SYNDROME (AXENFELD-RIEGER SYNDROME; DYSGENESIS MESODERMALIS CORNEAE ET IRIDES;DYSGENESIS MESOSTROMALIS; AXENFELD POSTERIOR EMBRYOTOXON-JUVENILE GLAUCOMA)

General

Autosomal dominant; neural crest abnormality; 50% of patients develop glaucoma.

Ocular

Microphthalmia; congenital glaucoma; iris hypoplasia; deformed and acentric pupil; anterior synechiae; aniridia; microcornea; corneal opacities in Descemet's membrane parallel to the limbus; dislocated lens; optic atrophy; cataract; strabismus; ptosis; hypertelorism; keratoconus; posterior embryotoxon; broad iris processes to embryotoxon; iris stromal hypoplasia; corectopia; polycoria; secondary glaucoma.

Clinical

Face wide; hypodontia; underdeveloped maxilla; teeth deformities; myotonic dystrophy; facial anomalies: maxillary hypoplasia, protrusion of the lower lip, broad, flat nose; dental anomalies include absent teeth, pig-like incisors and decreased crown size; hypospadias.

Laboratory

Diagnosis is made by clinical findings.

Treatment/Ocular

Congenital glaucoma can be treated with beta-blockers, prostaglandin analogs and carbonic anhydrase inhibitors. Surgery such as goniotomy or trabeculectomy can be used if IOP is not controlled.

BIBLIOGRAPHY

1. Eagle RC. Congenital, developmental and degenerative disorders of the iris and ciliary body. In: Albert DM, Jakobiec FA (Eds). Albert & Jakobiec's Principles and Practice of Ophthalmology: Clinical Practice, 3rd edition. Philadelphia, PA: WB Saunders; 1994. pp. 367-87.

7.38. RUBINSTEIN-TAYBI SYNDROME (OPTIC ATROPHY)

General

Inheritance polygenic or multifactorial; rare.

Ocular

Antimongoloid slant of lid fissure; epicanthus; long eyelashes and highly arched brows; strabismus; myopia; hyperopia; iris coloboma; cataract; optic atrophy; ptosis; retinal detachment.

Clinical

Motor and mental retardation; broad thumbs and toes; highly arched palate; allergies; heart murmurs; anomalies of size, shape, and position of ears; dwarfism; cryptorchidism.

Laboratory

CT scan, MRI, chromosomal karyotype analysis, FISH and CBP gene analysis.

Treatment

Physical therapy, speech and feeding therapy. Cardiothoracic intervention may be needed in patients with congenital heart defect.

BIBLIOGRAPHY

1. Mijuskovic ZP, Karadaglic D, Stojanov L. (2013). Dermatologic Manifestations of Rubinstein-Taybi Syndrome. [online] Available from www.emedicine.com/derm/TOPIC711.HTM. [Accessed October, 2013].

7.40. FRANCESCHETTI SYNDROME (FRANCESCHETTI-ZWAHLEN-KLEIN SYNDROME; TREACHER COLLINS SYNDROME; MANDIBULOFACIAL DYSOSTOSIS; MANDIBULOFACIAL SYNDROME; EYELID-MALAR-MANDIBLE SYNDROME; OCULOVERTEBRAL SYNDROME; BERRY SYNDROME; FRANCESCHETTI-ZWAHLEN SYNDROME; ZWAHLEN SYNDROME; BILATERAL FACIAL AGENESIS; BERRY-FRANCESCHETTI-KLEIN SYNDROME; FRANCESCHETTI-KLEIN SYNDROME; FRANCESCHETTI SYNDROME (II); TREACHER COLLINS-FRANCESCHETTI SYNDROME; WEYERS-THIER SYNDROME)

General

Irregular dominant inheritance; Weyers-Thier syndrome has similar features, except it is a unilateral variant; prevalent in Caucasians.

Ocular

Microphthalmia; oblique position of eyes with lateral downward slope of palpebral fissures; temporal lower lid coloboma; lack of cilia on middle third of lower lid; iris coloboma; underdeveloped orbicularis oculi muscle; cataract; optic disk hypoplasia.

Clinical

Fish-like face with sunken cheek bones, receding chin, and large, wide mouth; absent or malformed external ears with auricular appendages; high palate and possible harelip; hypoplastic zygomatic arch with absence of normal malar eminences; prolonged hairline on the cheek; deafness; micrognathia; glossoptosis; cleft palate.

Laboratory

Full craniofacial CT scan (axial and coronal slices from the top of the skull through the cervical spine), brain MRI.

Treatment

Operative repair is based upon the anatomic deformity and timing of correction is done according to physiologic need and development.

BIBLIOGRAPHY

1. Tolarova MM, Wong GB, Varma S. (2012). Mandibulofacial Dysostosis (Treacher Collins Syndrome). [online] Available from www.emedicine.com/ped/TOPIC1364.HTM. [Accessed October, 2013].

7.41. TRISOMY 13 SYNDROME (TRISOMY D1 SYNDROME, PATAU SYNDROME, REESE SYNDROME) IRIS COLOBOMA

General

Extra chromosome in the D group; fatal in the first few months of life; trisomy 13–15 resembles trisomy D1.

Ocular

Anophthalmia; microphthalmia; iris coloboma; cataracts; retinal dysplasia; optic nerve coloboma; optic atrophy; iris dyplasia; calcified lens; retinal detachment; optic nerve hypoplasia; orbital cysts.

Clinical

Apneic spells; developmental deficiency of the nervous system; seizures (minor motor); deafness; cleft lip and palate; hemangiomata; horizontal palmar creases; hyperconvex fingernails; interventricular septal defects; renal abnormalities; cardiovascular changes; respiratory involvement; gastrointestinal disease; urogenital involvement; cerebral hypoplasia with hydrocephalus; mental retardation.

Laboratory

Immediate conventional cytogenetic test. Ultrasonography for any anomalies. Trisomy 13 is best identified through cytogenetic study of amniotic fluid.

Treatment

Surgical care is usually withheld for the first few months of life.

BIBLIOGRAPHY

1. Best RG, Gregg AR. (2012). Patau syndrome. [online] Available from www.emedicine.com/ped/TOPIC1745.HTM. [Accessed October, 2013].

⊟ 7.42. TRISOMY 18 SYNDROME (E SYNDROME; EDWARDS SYNDROME) CONGENITAL GLAUCOMA

General

Chromosome 18 present in triplicate; more common in females (3:1); age of mother over 40 years; onset from fetal life.

Ocular

Unilateral ptosis; epicanthal folds; congenital glaucoma; corneal opacities; lens opacities; optic atrophy.

Clinical

Low-set ears; micrognathia; high-arched palate; prominent occiput; cryptorchidism; failure to thrive; ventricular septal defect; hypertonicity with rigidity in flexion of limbs; mental retardation; umbilical and inguinal hernias.

Laboratory

Cytogenetic test, echocardiography, ultrasonography, and skeletal radiography are used to detect any abnormalities.

Treatment

Treat infections as appropriate. For feeding difficulties nasogastric and gastrostomy supplementation is recommended.

⊟ BIBLIOGRAPHY

1. Chen H. (2013). Trisomy 18. [online] Availble from www.emedicine.com/ped/TOPIC652.HTM. [Accessed October, 2013].

⊟ 7.43. TURNER SYNDROME (TURNER-ALBRIGHT SYNDROME; GONADAL DYSGENESIS; GENITAL DWARFISM SYNDROME; ULLRICH-TURNER SYNDROME; BONNEVIE-ULLRICH SYNDROME; PTERYGOLYMPHANGIECTASIA SYNDROME; ULLRICH-BONNEVIE SYNDROME) CATARACT, POSTERIOR

General

Ovarian or gonadal agenesis; 45 chromosomes with an XO sex-chromosome constitution; females; rare in males; onset in childhood.

Ocular

Exophthalmos; hypertelorism; ptosis; epicanthal folds; blue sclera; corneal nebulae; cataracts; conjunctival lymphedema; keratoconus.

Clinical

Webbed neck (pterygium colli); diminished growth; mandibulofacial disproportion; cubitus valgus; masculine chest and trunk; late appearance of pubic and axillary hair; congenital deafness; mental retardation; coarctation of aorta.

Laboratory

Karyotyping is needed for diagnosis. Y-chromosomal test; luteinizing hormone (LH) and follicle-stimulating hormone (FSH) levels, thyroid function test, fasting glucose levels, echocardiography and MRI.

Treatment

Growth hormone therapy is used to prevent short stature. Estrogen replacement therapy is usually started by the age of 12–15 years.

⊟ BIBLIOGRAPHY

1. Postellon DC, Daniel MS. (2012). Turner syndrome. [online] Available from emedicine.medscape.com/article/949681-overview. [Accessed October, 2013].

🗗 7.44. WALKER-WARBURG SYNDROME (CEREBROOCULAR DYSPLASIA-MUSCULAR DYSTROPHY; WARBURG SYNDROME; COD-MD SYNDROME; FUKUYAMA CONGENITAL MUSCULAR DYSTROPHY; HARD + OR − E SYNDROME) CATARACT

General

Rare; encompassing a triad of brain, eye, and muscle abnormalities; probably autosomal recessive.

Ocular

Microphthalmia; cataract; immature anterior chamber angle; retinal dysplasia; retinal detachment; persistent hyperplastic primary vitreous; optic nerve hypoplasia; iris coloboma; opaque cornea; myopia; orbicularis weakness; irregular gray subretinal mottling; optic atrophy.

Clinical

Cerebral and cerebellar agyria-micropolygyria; cortical disorganization; glial mesodermal proliferation; neuronal heterotopias; hypoplasia of nerve tracts; hydrocephalus; encephalocele; muscular dystrophy; seizures; mental retardation; hypotonia; abnormal facies.

Laboratory

MRI, creatine kinases levels, electromyography and nerve conduction study.

Treatment

No specific treatment is available.

🗗 BIBLIOGRAPHY

1. Lopate G. (2013). Congenital Muscular Dystrophy. [online] Available from www.emedicine.com/neuro/TOPIC549.HTM. [Accessed October, 2013].

🗗 7.46. WOLF SYNDROME (MONOSOMY 4 PARTIAL SYNDROME; CHROMOSOME 4 PARTIAL DELETION SYNDROME; HIRSCHHORN-COOPER SYNDROME) PTOSIS

General

Partial deletion of chromosome 4 of the B group; short life expectancy; present from birth (*see* Cri-Du-Chat syndrome).

Ocular

Hypertelorism; antimongoloid slanting of palpebral fissures; ptosis; nystagmus; strabismus; iris coloboma; retinal coloboma.

Clinical

Microcephaly; mental retardation; seizures; ear malformations; hypospadias; beaked nose; broad nasal root; cleft lip and palate; hypotonia.

Laboratory

High-resolution cytogenetic studies, conventional cytogenetic, FISH.

Treatment

No known treatment exist for the underlying disorder.

🗗 BIBLIOGRAPHY

1. Chen H. (2013). Wolf-Hirschhorn syndrome. [online] Available from www.emedicine.com/ped/TOPIC2446.HTM. [Accessed October, 2013].

🗗 7.47. 11Q- SYNDROME

General

Chromosome II deletion syndrome.

Ocular

Telecanthus/hypertelorism; rarely, congenital glaucoma, cyclopia.

Clinical

Psychomotor retardation, trigonocephaly, broad depressed nasal bridge, micrognathia, low-set abnormal ears, cardiac anomalies, hand and foot anomalies, renal agenesis, anal atresia, supratentorial white matter abnormality on CT or MRI; microphallus; holoprosencephaly; female preponderance.

Laboratory

Clinical.

Treatment

See congenital glaucoma.

🗗 BIBLIOGRAPHY

1. Helmuth RA, Weaver DD, Wills ER. Holoprosencephaly, ear abnormalities, congenital heart defect, and microphallus in a patient with 11q- mosaicism. Am J Med Genet. 1989;32:178-81.
2. Ishida Y, Watanabe N, Ishihara Y, et al. The 11q- syndrome with mosaic partial deletion of 11q. Acta Paediatr Jpn. 1992;34:592-6.
3. Leegte B, Kerstjens-Frederikse WS, Deelstra K, et al. 11q-syndrome: three cases and a review of the literature. Genet Couns. 1999;10:305-13.

🗗 7.48. CHROMOSOME 13Q PARTIAL DELETION (LONG-ARM SYNDROME; 13Q SYNDROME)

General

No hereditary factor.

Ocular

Microphthalmos; antimongoloid slant of lid fissures; bilateral epicanthus; esotropia; cataract; choroidal coloboma; ptosis; retinoblastoma.

Clinical

Genital malformations; meningocele; short neck; small mouth; mental and physical retardation; small head; short stature; broad nasal bridge; simian crease; microcephaly; high nasal bridge; thumb hypoplasia.

Laboratory

The red blood cells are usually normochromic normocytic. An elevated white blood cell count (> 12,000/μL) occurs in approximately 60% of patients.

Treatment

Phlebotomy is the mainstay of therapy for this disease. The object is to remove excess cellular elements, mainly red blood cells, to improve the circulation of blood by lowering the blood viscosity.

🗗 BIBLIOGRAPHY

1. Besa EC, Woermann UJ. (2012). Polycythemia Vera. [online] Available from www.emedicine.com/med/TOPIC1864.HTM. [Accessed October, 2013].

🗗 7.49. 18Q- SYNDROME (18Q DELETION SYNDROME)

General

Chromosome 18q deletion syndrome.

Ocular

Macular "fibrosis"; optic disk abnormalities with tractional retinal detachment, retinal degeneration, and tilting of the optic disk.

Clinical

Microcephaly; short stature; hypotonia; hypothyroidism; diabetes mellitus; short neck; sensorineural hearing loss; sensorimotor axonal neuropathy; mild-to-moderate mental retardation; chronic arthritis; seizures.

Laboratory

Clinical.

Treatment

Retinal detachment: Scleral buckle, pneumatic retinopexy and vitrectomy may be used to close all the breaks.

BIBLIOGRAPHY

1. Gordon MF, Bressman S, Brin MF, et al. Dystonia in a patient with deletion of 18q. Mov Disord. 1995;10:496-9.
2. Hansen US, Herline T. Chronic arthritis in a boy with 18q-syndrome. J Rheumatol. 1994;21:1958-9.
3. Smith A, Caradus V, Henry JG. Translocation 46X6 t(17;18) (q25;q21) in a mentally retarded boy with progressive eye abnormalities. Clin Genet. 1979;16:156162.

7.50. XYY SYNDROME

General

Y chromosome polysomy syndrome.

Ocular

Colobomata.

Clinical

Mild mental retardation; autism; impulsiveness; aggressive behavior; developmental motor and language delays; excessive height for age; frequent antisocial behavior.

Laboratory

Chromosome studies.

Treatment

None.

BIBLIOGRAPHY

1. Onwochei BC, Simon JW, Bateman JB, et al. Ocular colobomata: major review. Surv Ophthalmol. 2000;45:175-94.
2. Von Gontard A, Hillig U. Ein Kind mit XYY-Syndrom im Erleben seiner Mutter. Ein Bericht nach Tagebuchaufzeichnungen. A child with XYY syndrome as experienced by his mother. A report of daily journal recordings. Z Kinder Jugendpsychiatr. 1992;20:46-53.

8. CONCAVE PERIPHERAL IRIS

1. Increased accommodation
2. Myopia
3. Pigment dispersion syndrome
4. Pseudoexfoliation syndrome
5. Retinal detachment
6. Younger age

BIBLIOGRAPHY

1. Laemmer R, Mardin CY, Juenemann AG, et al. Visualization of changes of the iris configuration after peripheral laser iridotomy in primary melamin dispersion syndrome using optical coherence tomography. J Glaucoma. 2008;17:569-70.
2. Liu L, Ong EL, Crowston J. The concave iris in pigment dispersion syndrome. Ophthalmology. 2011;118:66-70.

8.3. PIGMENTARY DISPERSION SYNDROME AND PIGMENTARY GLAUCOMA

General

Shedding of pigment that is evident as mid-peripheral radial iris transillumination defects. Characterized by pigmentary deposits on the structures of the anterior and posterior chambers.

Clinical

Siderosis, hemosiderosis, diabetes mellitus.

Ocular

Krukenberg's spindles, heterochromia, optic nerve damage, visual field defects, Adie's pupil, chronic open angle glaucoma; concave peripheral iris.

Laboratory

Diagnosis is made by clinical findings.

Treatment

Pilopine HS gel or Ocusert, laser therapy such as trabeculoplasty, iridectomy, iridoplasty and/or filtration surgery are useful.

⊟ BIBLIOGRAPHY

1. Ritch R, Barkana Y. (2012). Pigmentary Glaucoma. [online] Available from www.emedicine.com/oph/TOPIC136.HTM. [Accessed October, 2013].

⊟ 8.4. PSEUDOEXFOLIATION SYNDROME

General

Prevalent over age of 70 years; rare before age of 40 years; unilateral involvement in 40–50% of cases; asymmetry of severity in bilateral cases; most common in Caucasians, especially from Iceland and Scandinavian countries; pseudoexfoliation fibers were identified in autopsy tissue specimens of skin, heart, lungs, liver and cerebral meninges; consistently associated with connective tissue components, i.e. fibroblasts, collagen and elastic fibers, myocardial tissue and heart muscle cell.

Ocular

Gray or white fluffy material deposited in particles, flakes or sheets on anterior surface of iris, ciliary body, posterior surface of cornea, pupillary margin, lens and trabecular meshwork; increased pigmentation of trabecular meshwork; zonular dialysis; displaced or dislocated lens; anterior chamber depth asymmetry; preoperative phacodonesis; glaucoma; cataract.

Clinical

None.

Laboratory

Diagnosis is made by clinical findings.

Treatment

Annual eye examinations are done for early detection of glaucoma. Glaucoma in pseudoexfoliation is more resistant to medical therapy. If medical therapy is unsuccessful to control the glaucoma, argon laser trabeculoplasty or trabeculectomy may be beneficial.

⊟ BIBLIOGRAPHY

1. Pons ME, Eliassi-Rad B. (2011). Pseudoexfoliation glaucoma. [online] Available from www.emedicine.com/oph/TOPIC140.HTM. [Accessed October, 2013].

⊟ 9. FLOPPY IRIS SYNDROME

General

Flomax (tamsulosin) is the causative agent during cataract. It is commonly prescribed for benign prostate hypertrophy.

Ocular

Floppy iris.

Clinical

Benign prostate hypertrophy; noted during cataract surgery.

Laboratory

Diagnosis is made by clinical findings.

Treatment

Stop tamsulosin at least 3 days before cataract surgery.

⊟ BIBLIOGRAPHY

1. Chang DF, Campbell JR. Intraoperative floppy iris syndrome associated with tamsulosin. J Cataract Refract Surg. 2005;31(4):664-73.
2. Gurbaxani A, Packard R. Intracameral phenylephrine to prevent floppy iris syndrome during cataract surgery in patients on tamsulosin. Eye (Lond). 2007;21(3):331-2.
3. Schlötzer-Schrehardt U, Stojkovic M, Hofmann-Rummelt C, et al. The pathogenesis of floppy eyelid syndrome: involvement of matrix metalloproteinases in elastic fiber degradation. Ophthalmology. 2005;112(4):694-704.
4. Lorente R, de Rajas V, Vázquez de Parga P, et al. Intracameral phenylephrine 1.5% for prophylaxis against intraoperative floppy iris syndrome: prospective, randomized fellow eye study. Ophthalmology. 2012;119(10):2053-8.

🗗 10. FUCHS (1) SYNDROME (HETEROCHROMIC CYCLITIS SYNDROME)

General

Etiology is unknown; mild infective cyclitis is the most likely cause; etiology remains unclear, although it is likely to be autoimmune; positive epidemiologic association with ocular toxoplasmosis has been investigated.

Ocular

Secondary glaucoma; unilateral hypochromic heterochromia; painless cyclitis with absence of synechiae and little or no ciliary injection; secondary cataract; vitreous opacities; small white discrete keratic precipitates with fine filaments between the precipitates; corneal epithelium may be slightly edematous; peripheral choroiditis occasionally; keratoconus.

Clinical

Occasional dysraphia of the cervical cord.

Laboratory

Diagnosis is made by clinical findings.

Treatment

Generally no treatment is necessary. Occasionally discomfort and ciliary injection is treated with topical steroids. With cataract surgery, there is a higher rate of vitreous debris and hemorrhage. Glaucoma surgery may be indicated and rubeotic glaucoma may require enucleation.

🗗 BIBLIOGRAPHY

1. Arif M, Foster CS, Wong IG. (2011). Fuchs heterochromic uveitis. [online] Available from www.emedicine.com/oph/TOPIC432.HTM. [Accessed October, 2013].

🗗 11. GRAY IRIS SYNDROME

General

Excessive trauma of iris at the time of lens implantation with loss of posterior iris pigment; originally had blue irides.

Ocular

Pigmentary glaucoma; gray iris; massive pigment deposits in chamber angle; nonfixated intraocular lens (IOL).

Clinical

None.

Laboratory

Diagnosis is made by clinical findings.

Treatment

If glaucoma occurs, topical glaucoma drops can be used; laser trabeculoplasty, laser iridectomy and filtering surgery may be necessary.

🗗 BIBLIOGRAPHY

1. Ritch R, Barkana Y. (2012). Pigmentary glaucoma. [online] Available from www.emedicine.com/oph/TOPIC136.HTM. [Accessed October, 2013].

🗗 12. HETEROCHROMIA IRIDIS

General

Autosomal dominant; it can be associated with Horner, Waardenburg and Marfan syndromes; it may occur as an isolated phenomenon.

Ocular

Different pigmentation in the two irides or in the sectors of one iris (heterochromia iridium).

Clinical

None.

Laboratory

Diagnosis is made by clinical findings.

Treatment

None.

BIBLIOGRAPHY

1. Gladstone RM. Development and significance of heterochromia of the iris. Arch Neurol. 1969;21(2):184-91.

2. McKusick VA. Mendelian Inheritance in Man: A Catalog of Human Genes and Genetic Disorders, 12th edition. Baltimore, USA: The Johns Hopkins University Press; 1998.

13. IRIDAL ADHESION SYNDROME (IRIS ADHESION SYNDROME, IRIDOCORNEAL ENDOTHELIAL SYNDROME)

General

It is surgically related phenomenon following intraocular surgery in which iris pigment epithelium proliferates and adheres to cut edge of anterior capsule, drawing iris posteriorly to posterior and anterior capsules.

Ocular

Posterior synechiae; irregular pupil.

Clinical

None.

Laboratory

Diagnosis is made by clinical findings.

Treatment

Aqueous suppressants can be tried but usually surgery is required.

BIBLIOGRAPHY

1. Dickerson D. Surgery-related iridal adhesion syndrome. Ophthalmol Times. 1984;9:6.
2. Teekhasaenee C, Ritch R. Iridocorneal endothelial syndrome in Thai patients: clinical variations. Arch Ophthalmol. 2000;118(2):187-92.

14. IRIS BOMBE

General

Peripheral iris bowed forward while the central iris remains deep. Most commonly, it is seen as primary pupillary block.

Clinical

Pain, nausea.

Ocular

Bowing forward of the peripheral iris, corneal edema, ciliary body, pain, elevated IOP.

Laboratory

Diagnosis is made by clinical findings.

Treatment

Systemic IV mannitol, IV or oral acetazolamide, topical antiglaucoma agents, yttrium-aluminum-garnet (YAG) laser peripheral iridotomy.

BIBLIOGRAPHY

1. Roy FH, Fraunfelder FW, Fraunfelder FT. Roy and Fraunfelder's Current Ocular Therapy, 6th edition. London, UK: Elsevier; 2008.

15. IRIS CYSTS

General

Intraepithelial cyst originating between the epithelial layers and stromal cysts that are congenital or caused by surgery or trauma.

Clinical

None.

Ocular

Keratopathy, iridocyclitis, glaucoma, iris cysts.

Laboratory

Diagnosis is made by clinical findings.

Treatment

Chemical cauterization, laser photocoagulation, diathermy, cryocoagulation and block excision with cornea sclera transplant.

📄 BIBLIOGRAPHY

1. Roy FH, Fraunfelder FW, Fraunfelder FT. Roy and Fraunfelder's Current Ocular Therapy, 6th edition. London, UK: Elsevier; 2008.

📄 16. IRIS DYSPLASIA HYPERTELORISM-PSYCHOMOTOR RETARDATION SYNDROME

General

Autosomal dominant inheritance; some features in common with Rieger syndrome.

Ocular

Hypertelorism; telecanthus; hypoplasia of the iris stroma; abnormally prominent Schwalbe's line; synechiae between iris and cornea; pear-shaped pupils.

Clinical

Bilateral or unilateral hip dislocation; facial anomalies; psychomotor retardation; hypotonia and hyperlaxity of joints.

Laboratory

Diagnosis is made by clinical findings.

Treatment

No ocular treatment.

📄 BIBLIOGRAPHY

1. De Hauwere RC, Leroy JG, Adriaenssens K, et al. Iris dysplasia, orbital hypertelorism, and psychomotor retardation: a dominantly inherited developmental syndrome. J Pediatr. 1973;82(4):679-81.
2. Rieger H. Beitrage zur Kenntnis seltener Missbildungen der Iris. Graefes Arch Ophthalmol. 1935;133:602.
3. McKusick VA. Mendelian Inheritance in Man: A Catalog of Human Genes and Genetic Disorders, 12th edition. Baltimore, USA: The Johns Hopkins University Press; 1998.
4. Hamosh A, Scott AF, Amberger J, et al. Online Mendelian Inheritance in Man (OMIM), a knowledgebase of human genes and genetic disorders. Nucleic Acids Res. 2002;30(1):52-5.
5. von Noorden GK, Baller RS. The chamber angle in split-pupil. Arch Ophthalmol. 1963;70:598-602.

📄 17. IRIS MELANOMA

General

Malignant neoplasm.

Clinical

None.

Ocular

Iris melanoma, ectropion uvea, sector cataract, sentinel vessels, heterochromia, hyphema, chronic uveitis, glaucoma.

Laboratory

Diagnosis is made by clinical findings.

Treatment

Resection with iridectomy/iridocyclectomy or radiotherapy and enucleation.

📄 BIBLIOGRAPHY

1. Waheed NK, Foster CS. (2012). Iris melanoma. [online] Available from www.emedicine.com/oph/TOPIC405.HTM. [Accessed October, 2013].

⊟ 18. IRIS PIGMENT LAYER CLEAVAGE

General

Autosomal dominant; cleavage of pigment of iris and ciliary body.

Ocular

Cataracts; reduced sagittal and spherical lens diameters; glaucoma; retinal detachment; microphakia; spherophakia.

Clinical

None.

Laboratory

Diagnosis is made by clinical findings.

Treatment

See cataract, glaucoma and retinal detachment.

⊟ BIBLIOGRAPHY

1. Käfer O. Dominant Vererbte Spaltung des Pigmentblattes van Iris und Ciliarkoeper mit Consekutiver Microphakie, Ectopia Lentis and Cataract. Albrecht Von Graefes Arch Klin Exp Ophthalmol. 1977;202(2):133-41.
2. McKusick VA. Mendelian Inheritance in Man: A Catalog of Human Genes and Genetic Disorders, 12th edition. Baltimore, USA: The Johns Hopkins University Press; 1998.
3. Hamosh A, Scott AF, Amberger J, et al. Online Mendelian Inheritance in Man (OMIM), a knowledgebase of human genes and genetic disorders. Nucleic Acids Res. 2002;30(1):52-5.

⊟ 19. IRIS PROLAPSE

General

Uncommon intraoperative or postoperative complications of intraocular surgery or a penetrating injury.

Clinical

None.

Ocular

Floppy iris, papillary block, retro-orbital or expulsive hemorrhage, poor wound healing.

Laboratory

Diagnosis is made by clinical findings.

Treatment

Reduce wound leak, decrease the wound size by placing sutures, excision of prolapsed iris.

⊟ BIBLIOGRAPHY

1. Giri G. (2011). Iris prolapse. [online] Available from www.emedicine.com/oph/TOPIC584.HTM. [Accessed October, 2013].

⊟ 20. IRIS RETRACTION SYNDROME (POSTERIOR SYNECHIAE AND IRIS RETRACTION SYNDROME)

General

Rhegmatogenous retinal detachment, hypotony, and retrodisplacement of the iris with seclusion of the pupil, often associated with ciliochoroidal detachment, inflammation, and posterior vitreous retraction; caused by lowering of pressure behind iris partially due to posterior removal of fluid from subretinal space.

Ocular

Retinal detachment; hypotony; iris retraction; angle closure glaucoma; iris bombe; cataract; vitreous retraction; seclusion of the pupil; following intraocular surgery.

Clinical

None.

Laboratory

Diagnosis is made by clinical findings.

Treatment

The surgical goals are to identify and close all the breaks with minimum iatrogenic damage. Scleral buckles, scleral implant, vitrectomy and pneumatic retinopexy may be useful.

🖻 BIBLIOGRAPHY

1. Wu L, Evans T. (2011). Rhegmatogenous retinal detachment. [online] Available from www.emedicine.com/oph/ TOPIC410.HTM. [Accessed October, 2013].

🖻 21. JABS SYNDROME (SYNOVITIS, GRANULOMATOUS UVEITIS, AND CRANIAL NEUROPATHIES)

General

Autosomal dominant.

Ocular

Granulomatous uveitis; iritis; sixth nerve palsy.

Clinical

Granulomatous synovitis; corticosteroid responsive hearing loss; boggy polysynovitis; boutonneuse deformities; granulomatous arthritis; skin involvement; fever; hypertension; large-vessel vasculitis.

Laboratory

Diagnosis is made by clinical findings.

Treatment

Cycloplegics; corticosteroids; aqueous suppressant should be prescribed if the IOP is elevated.

🖻 BIBLIOGRAPHY

1. Levinson RD. (2012). Uveitis, anterior, granulomatous. [online] Available from www.emedicine.com/oph/TOPIC586.HTM. [Accessed October, 2013].

🖻 22. JUVENILE XANTHOGRANULOMA (JXG; NEVOXANTHOENDOTHELIOMA)

General

Childhood disease; unknown etiology.

Ocular

Uveal tract tumor presenting as spontaneous hyphema; secondary glaucoma; uveitis; corneal, lid and epibulbar tumors; proptosis; retinal and choroidal lesions (rare).

Clinical

Multiple benign tumors, primarily of the skin; usually appear in the first 3 years of life; lesions appear as yellow-to-brown papules or nodules.

Laboratory

Diagnostic techniques include biomicroscopy, high frequency ultrasound and cytologic examination of anterior chamber parencentesis material.

Treatment

Topical, subconjunctival, intralesional and systemic corticosteroids are useful. Low-dose radiation may be the treatment of choice for diffuse uveal lesions. Glaucoma medications should be used in the setting of hyphema and increased IOP.

🖻 BIBLIOGRAPHY

1. Curtis T, Wheeler DT. (2012). Juvenile xanthogranuloma. [online] Available from www.emedicine.com/oph/TOPIC588.HTM. [Accessed October, 2013].

23. IRIS LACERATION AND IRIS HOLES, AND IRIDODIALYSIS

General

Partial or full thickness iris defects that are most often caused by trauma. Iridodialysis is a separation of the thin, weak iris root from its attachment to the ciliary body and sclera spur.

Clinical

None.

Ocular

Transillumination defects, corneal edema, traumatic cataract, hyphema, retinal tears, vitreous hemorrhage, retinal detachment, choroidal rupture and traumatic optic neuropathy.

Laboratory

Diagnosis is made by clinical findings.

Treatment

Cycloplegics and steroid drops for traumatic iritis.

BIBLIOGRAPHY

1. Roy FH, Fraunfelder FW, Fraunfelder FT. Roy and Fraunfelder's Current Ocular Therapy, 6th edition. London, UK: Elsevier; 2008.

24. LENS-IRIS DIAPHRAM RETROPULSION SYNDROME

General

It is associated with small incision phacoemulsification.

Ocular

Infusion of fluid into the anterior chamber; posterior displacement of the lens-iris diaphragm; posterior iris bowing; pupil dilatation; ocular discomfort.

Clinical

Deep anterior chamber with small incision phacoemulsification.

Laboratory

Diagnosis is made by clinical findings.

Treatment

Consider YAG iridotomy.

BIBLIOGRAPHY

1. Ocampo VV, Foster CS. (2013). Senile cataract. [online] Available from www.emedicine.com/oph/TOPIC49.HTM. [Accessed October, 2013].

25. IRIS MELANOMA

General

Malignant neoplasm.

Clinical

None.

Ocular

Iris melanoma, ectropion uvea, sector cataract, sentinel vessels, heterochromia, hyphema, chronic uveitis, glaucoma.

Laboratory

Diagnosis is made by clinical findings.

Treatment

Resection with iridectomy/iridocyclectomy or radiotherapy and enucleation.

BIBLIOGRAPHY

1. Waheed NK, Foster CS. (2012). Iris melanoma. [online] Available from www.emedicine.com/oph/TOPIC405.HTM. [Accessed October, 2013].

26. MILLER SYNDROME (WILMS' ANIRIDIA SYNDROME; WAGR SYNDROME; WILMS' TUMOR-ANIRIDIA-GENITOURINARY ABNORMALITIES-MENTAL RETARDATION SYNDROME)

General

Etiology is unknown; it manifests an association of aniridia, which is inherited as a dominant autosomal trait and WT; this is one of the best studied continuous gene syndromes as defined by Schmickel.

Ocular

Glaucoma; bilateral aniridia (aniridia often not complete, with remnants of iris root present as rudimentary forms); cataract.

Clinical

Wilms' tumor; mental retardation with microcephaly; genital malformations with cryptorchidism and hypospadias; hemihypertrophy; kidney anomalies (horseshoe kidney).

Laboratory/Glaucoma

Chromosome analysis and genetic counseling.

Treatment/Glaucoma

Beta-blockers, carbonic anhydrase inhibitors and prostaglandin analogs. Surgery may be needed if IOP is uncontrolled.

BIBLIOGRAPHY

1. Fraumeni JF, Glass AG. Wilms' tumor and congenital aniridia. JAMA. 1968;206(4):825-8.
2. Mackintosh TF, Girdwood TG, Parker DJ, et al. Aniridia and Wilms' tumor (nephroblastoma). Br J Ophthalmol. 1968;52(11):846-8.
3. McKusick VA. Mendelian Inheritance in Man: A Catalog of Human Genes and Genetic Disorders, 12th edition. Baltimore, USA: The Johns Hopkins University Press; 1998.
4. Hamosh A, Scott AF, Amberger J, et al. Online Mendelian Inheritance in Man (OMIM), a knowledgebase of human genes and genetic disorders. Nucleic Acids Res. 2002;30(1):52-5.
5. Miller RW, Fraumeni JF, Manning MD. Association of Wilms' tumor with aniridia, hemihypertrophy and other congenital malformations. N Engl J Med. 1964;270:922-7.
6. Schmickel RD. Chromosomal deletions and enzyme deficiencies. J Pediatr. 1986;108(2):244-6.

27. IRIS NEOVASCULARIZATION WITH PSEUDOEXFOLIATION SYNDROME

General

Anoxia secondary to iris vessel obstruction; electron microscopic studies reveal endothelial thickening with decreased lumen size and fenestration of vessel walls.

Ocular

Materials found on posterior and anterior iris surface, anterior lens surface, ciliary processes, zonules and anterior hyaloid membranes; neovascularization of iris stroma; increased permeability of iris vessels.

Clinical

None.

Laboratory

Diagnosis is made by clinical findings.

Treatment

Patients with pseudoexfoliation syndrome should have annual eye examinations for early detection of glaucoma.

BIBLIOGRAPHY

1. Pons ME, Eliassi-Rad B. (2011). Pseudoexfoliation glaucoma. [online] Available from www.emedicine.com/oph/TOPIC140.HTM. [Accessed October, 2013].

⊟ 28. ALBINISM (BROWN OCULOCUTANEOUS ALBINISM; NETTLESHIP FALLS SYNDROME)

General

Congenital hypopigmentation.

- *Complete*
  - *Ocular*: Iris thin, pale blue; prominent choroidal vessels with poorly defined fovea; nystagmus; head nodding; frequently myopic astigmatism and strabismus; marked photophobia; eyelashes and eyebrows are white; optic atrophy; cataract; abnormal decussation of retinogeniculate axons at the chiasm.
  - *Clinical*: White hair, eyebrows and skin; autosomal recessive.
- *Modified complete*
  - *Ocular*: Marked deficiency of pigment in iris and choroid; nystagmus and myopic astigmatism; iris of female carrier frequently is translucent; macular hypoplasia; photophobia; pigmentation of retinal pigment epithelium.
  - *Clinical*: Normal pigmentation elsewhere; autosomal recessive.
- *Amish*
  - *Ocular*: At birth, complete albinism with blue translucent irides and albinotic fundal reflex; nystagmus; photophobia; increasing pigmentation with age; abnormal decussation of retinogeniculate axons at the chiasm.
  - *Clinical*: White hair and skin at birth; increasing pigmentation with yellow hair and normal skin that tans; autosomal recessive.

Laboratory

The most definitive test in determining the albinism type is genetic sequence analysis. This test is useful only for families with individuals who have albinism. The test cannot be used as a screening tool.

Treatment

Currently, there is no therapy for albinism. Sunglasses to reduce photophobia, low-vision aids and treatment for strabismus might be useful.

⊟ BIBLIOGRAPHY

1. Bashour M, Hasanee K, Ahmed II. (2012). Albinism. [online] Available from www.emedicine.com/oph/TOPIC315.HTM. [Accessed October, 2013].

⊟ 29. IRIS PIGMENT LAYER CLEAVAGE

General

Autosomal dominant; cleavage of pigment of iris and ciliary body.

Ocular

Cataracts; reduced sagittal and spherical lens diameters; glaucoma; retinal detachment; microphakia; spherophakia.

Clinical

None.

Laboratory

Diagnosis is made by clinical findings.

Treatment

See cataract, glaucoma and retinal detachment.

⊟ BIBLIOGRAPHY

1. Käfer O. Dominant Vererbte Spaltung des Pigmentblattes van Iris und Ciliarkoeper mit Consekutiver Microphakie, Ectopia Lentis und Cataract. Albrecht Von Graefes Arch Klin Exp Ophthalmol. 1977;202(2):133-41.
2. McKusick VA. Mendelian Inheritance in Man: A Catalog of Human Genes and Genetic Disorders, 12th edition. Baltimore, USA: The Johns Hopkins University Press; 1998.
3. Hamosh A, Scott AF, Amberger J, et al. Online Mendelian Inheritance in Man (OMIM), a knowledgebase of human genes and genetic disorders. Nucleic Acids Res. 2002;30(1):52-5.

30. PLATEAU IRIS SYNDROME

General

Rare; occurs in younger age group; presumably due in part to an anterior insertion of the iris; pupillary block is not a significant part of the mechanism leading to angle closure.

Ocular

Spontaneous or mydriasis-induced angle closure despite a patent iridectomy; anterior chamber is of normal depth axially and the iris plane is flat, but a peripheral roll of iris can close the angle either when the pupil dilates spontaneously or after mydriatic drugs are administered.

Clinical

Nausea; vomiting.

Laboratory

Indentation gonioscopy.

Treatment

Iridotomy.

BIBLIOGRAPHY

1. Wang JC, Lee PS, Ritch R, et al. (2012). Plateau iris glaucoma. [online] Available from www.emedicine.com/oph/TOPIC574.HTM. [Accessed October, 2013].

31. POSTERIOR IRIS CHAFING SYNDROME

General

Complication following IOL implantation attributed to sulcus-fixed posterior chamber lenses, decentration of the lens, traumatic insertion, movement of the lens during dilation and constriction of the pupil, or difficulty with positioning of the lens.

Ocular

Iris transillumination defects; recurrent microhyphemas; pigment dispersion glaucoma; pigment deposition in trabecular meshwork; iris pigment atrophy.

Clinical

None.

Laboratory

Diagnosis is made by clinical findings.

Treatment

Glaucoma therapy, repositioning of IOL, suturing of the IOL.

BIBLIOGRAPHY

1. Jaffe NS. Current concepts in posterior chamber lens technology. J Am Intraocul Implant Soc. 1985;11(5):456-60.
2. Johnson SH, Kratz RP, Olson PF. Iris transillumination defect and microhyphema syndrome. J Am Intraocul Implant Soc. 1984;10(4):425-8.
3. Smiddy WE, Ibanez GV, Alfonso E, et al. Surgical management of dislocated intraocular lenses. J Cataract Refract Surg. 1995;21(1):64-9.
4. Smith SG, Lindstrom RL. Malpositioned posterior chamber lenses: etiology, prevention, and management. J Am Intraocul Implant Soc. 1985;11(6):584-91.
5. Woodhams JT, Lester JC. Pigmentary dispersion glaucoma secondary to posterior chamber intraocular lenses. Ann Ophthalmol. 1984;16(9):852-5.

32. RING CHROMOSOME 6 (ANIRIDIA, CONGENITAL GLAUCOMA, AND HYDROCEPHALUS)

General

Rare disorder associated with various congenital anomalies; autosomal dominant with recessive sporadically reported.

Ocular

Microphthalmia; aniridia; congenital uveal ectropion; Rieger anomaly; congenital glaucoma; corneal clouding;

prominent Schwalbe's line with attached iris strands; hypopigmented fundi; hypoplasia of iris stroma; strabismus; ptosis; nystagmus; megalocornea; iris coloboma; optic atrophy; hypertelorism; antimongoloid slant of palpebral fissures; ectopic pupils; angle anomalies; posterior embryotoxon; microcornea; colobomatous.

Clinical

Hydrocephalus; agenesis of corpus callosum; congenital heart defects; mental retardation; low-set malformed ears; broad nasal bridge; micrognathia; short neck; hand anomalies; high-arched palate; widely spaced nipples; deformity of feet; respiratory distress syndrome; hyperbilirubinemia; hypocalcemia; anemia; seizure; bulging anterior fontanel.

Laboratory

Diagnosis is made by clinical findings.

Treatment

Ptosis: If visual acuity is affected, most cases require surgical correction and there are several procedures that may be used including levator resection, repair or advancement and Fasanella-Servat procedure.

BIBLIOGRAPHY

1. Bateman JB. Chromosomal anomalies and the eye. In: Wright KW (Ed). Pediatric Ophthalmology and Strabismus. St Louis: Mosby; 1995. p. 595.
2. Chitayat D, Hahm SY, Iqbal MA, et al. Ring chromosome 6: report of a patient and literature review. Am J Med Genet. 1987;26(1):145-51.
3. deLuise UP, Anderson DR. Primary infantile glaucoma (congenital glaucoma). Surv Ophthalmol. 1983;28(1):1-19.
4. Levin H, Ritch R, Barathur R, et al. Aniridia, congenital glaucoma, and hydrocephalus in a male infant with ring chromosome 6. Am J Med Genet. 1986;25(2):281-7.

33. RUBEOSIS IRIDIS [NEOVACULARIZATION (NEWLY FORMED BLOOD VESSELS) ON THE IRIS]

1. *Proximal vascular disease*
   A. Aortic arch syndrome (pulseless disease; Takayasu syndrome)
   B. Carotid-cavernous fistula (carotid artery syndrome)
   †C. Carotid ligation
   †D. Carotid occlusive disease
   E. Cranial arteritis syndrome (giant cell arteritis)
2. *Ocular vascular disease*
   *A. Central retinal artery thrombosis
   †*B. Central retinal vein thrombosis
   †C. Long posterior ciliary artery occlusion
   †D. Reversed flow through the ophthalmic artery
3. *Retinal diseases*
   †A. Coats disease (retinal telangiectasia)
   *B. Diabetes mellitus
   C. Eales disease (periphlebitis)
   D. Glaucoma, chronic
   †E. Melanoma of choroid
   F. Norrie disease (oligophrenia-microphthalmos syndrome)
   G. Persistent hyperplastic primary vitreous
   H. Retinal detachment
   I. Retinal hemangioma
   J. Retinoblastoma
   K. Retrolental fibroplasia
   L. Sickle cell disease (Herrick syndrome)
4. *Iris tumors*
   A. Hemangioma
   †B. Melanoma
   †C. Metastatic carcinoma
5. *Postinflammatory*
   †A. Argon laser coreoplasty
   B. Exfoliation syndrome
   C. Fibrinoid syndrome
   D. Fungal endophthalmitis
   E. Iris neovascularization with pseudoexfoliation
   †F. Radiation
   G. Surgery for retinal detachment
   H. Uveitis, chronic
6. *Vascular tufts at the pupillary margin*
   A. Cataract
   B. Diabetes mellitus
   C. Myotonic dystrophy syndrome (myotonia atrophica syndrome)
   D. Ocular hypotony
   †E. Respiratory failure

*Indicates most frequent
†Indicates a general entry and therefore has not been described in detail in the text

Treatment

- Trabeculectomy with the antifibrotic agents mitomycin-C and 5-fluorouracil (5-FU) is one modality. Trabeculectomy in neovascular glaucoma (NVG) has a significant failure rate. Using standard trabeculectomy (without antifibrosis), an IOP of less than 25 mm Hg on one medication or less has been reported to occur in 67–100% of patients in three studies. Using injections of 5-FU subconjunctivally in the postoperative period, the surgical success has been reported to be 68% over 3 years. Inject 0.1 mL of 5 mg/mL 5-FU subconjunctivally either superiorly above the bleb or inferiorly (just above the lower fornix). Mitomycin-C used intraoperatively has been shown to be more effective than 5-FU in routine trabeculectomies. No significant follow-up studies exist on the use of mitomycin-C with trabeculectomy in NVG.
- Valve implant surgery is another modality and is indicated when trabeculectomy fails or extensive conjunctival scarring exists, thereby preventing a standard filtering procedure. Molteno, Krupin and Ahmed valve implants commonly are used. One large series using the Krupin valve reported 79% of eyes with NVG had a 67% success rate in controlling IOP (< 24 mm Hg) with mean follow-up of 23 months. Long-term results are mixed. Using the Molteno implant, 60 eyes with NVG achieved a satisfactory IOP (< 21 mm Hg) and maintenance of visual acuity over 5 years of only 10.3%. If combined with the need for vitrectomy, consideration of pars plana tube-shunt insertion may reduce anterior segment complications.
- Complications include postoperative hypotony with associated complications, blockage of internal fistula, blockage of external filtration site (fibrosis of the filtering bleb), and corneal endothelial loss.

BIBLIOGRAPHY

1. Freudenthal J, Khan YA, Ahmed II, et al. (2011). Neovascular glaucoma. [online] Available from www.emedicine.com/oph/TOPIC135.HTM. [Accessed October, 2013].

33.1A. TAKAYASU SYNDROME (MARTORELL SYNDROME; AORTIC ARCH SYNDROME; PULSELESS DISEASE; REVERSED COARCTATION SYNDROME)

General

Two types are: (1) occlusive inflammatory lesion (seen in young Japanese women) and (2) occlusive vascular disease without inflammation, associated with atherosclerosis and syphilis; onset in between 5th and 6th decades; both sexes affected; can involve the aorta and its major branches as well as the coronary, hepatic, mesenteric, pulmonary and renal arteries.

Ocular

Iris atrophy; cataracts; retinal microaneurysms; sausage-shaped venous dilations; reduced central retinal artery pressure; optic atrophy; cotton-wool spots; anterior segment ischemia; retinal arteriovenous shunts.

Clinical

Diminished or absent pulsation of arteries (head, neck, upper limbs); orthostatic syncope; facial atrophy; epileptiform seizures; intermittent claudication.

Laboratory

Arteriography, magnetic resonance angiography, MRI, CT scan, Gallium-67 radionuclide scan, or chest radiography.

Treatment

Corticosteroids, methotrexate or intravenous cyclophosphamide can be used in patients with glucocorticoid-resistant Takayasu arteritis (TA).

BIBLIOGRAPHY

1. Hom C. (2013). Pediatric Takayasu Arteritis. [online] Available from www.emedicine.com/ped/TOPIC1956.HTM. [Accessed October, 2013].

🗗 33.1B. CAROTID ARTERY SYNDROME (CAVERNOUS SINUS FISTULA SYNDROME; RED-EYED SHUNT SYNDROME)

General

Seventy-five percent of cases caused by trauma; others occur spontaneously or are congenital; fistula from carotid artery to cavernous sinus.

Ocular

Progressive, pulsating exophthalmos; distended pulsating superior orbital vein; venous congestion of lids; variable ophthalmoplegia, depending on involvement of cranial nerves III to VI; secondary glaucoma; congestion of conjunctiva with chemosis; corneal ulcerations; eversion of the lower lid; loss of corneal sensation; retinal edema; engorgement of retinal veins; papilledema; optic atrophy; ocular bruit that may be subjective and/or objective; diplopia; visual decrease; choroidal folds; dilated superior ophthalmic vein.

Clinical

Severe unilateral headache; buzzing noise.

Laboratory

Orbital ultrasonography, CT, six-vessel cranial digital subtraction angiography—characterization of the arterial supply and venous drainage of fistula.

Treatment

Use of intraocular lowering agent and topical lubrication is the ocular treatment of choice.

🗗 BIBLIOGRAPHY

1. Dailey EJ, Holloway JA, Murto RE, et al. Evaluation of ocular signs and symptoms in cerebral aneurysms. Arch Ophthalmol. 1964;71:463-74.
2. Duane TD. Clinical Ophthalmology. Philadelphia: JB Lippincott; 1987.
3. Flaharty PM, Lieb WE, Sergott RC, et al. Color Doppler imaging. A new noninvasive technique to diagnose and monitor carotid cavernous sinus fistulas. Arch Ophthalmol. 1991;109:522-6.
4. Gonshor LG, Kline LB. Choroidal folds and dural cavernous sinus fistula. Arch Ophthalmol. 1991;109:1065-6.
5. Phelps CD, Thompson HS, Ossoinig KC. The diagnosis and prognosis of atypical carotid cavernous fistula. Am J Ophthalmol. 1982;93:423-36.
6. Roy FH, Fraunfelder FW, Fraunfelder FT. Roy and Fraunfelder's Current Ocular Therapy, 6th edition. Philadelphia: WB Saunders; 2008.
7. Travers B. A case of aneurysm by anastomosis in the orbit, cured by ligation of common carotid artery. Med Chir Trans. 1917;2:1-420.

🗗 33.1E. TEMPORAL ARTERITIS SYNDROME (CRANIAL ARTERITIS SYNDROME; GIANT CELL ARTERITIS; HUTCHINSON-HORTON-MAGATH-BROWN SYNDROME)

General

Etiology unknown; mainly females; mainly Whites; ages 55–80 years; temporal artery shows inflammatory thickening; arteritis of the vessels supplying the optic nerve.

Ocular

Transient ptosis; partial or complete loss of vision on the affected side; retinal detachment; exudates and hemorrhages; narrowing of retinal vessels; obstruction of the central retinal artery; optic atrophy; ischemic optic neuropathy; acute decreased IOP; corneal hypesthesia; palsies of extraocular muscles; hemorrhagic glaucoma; diplopia; hemorrhages on or around the disk.

Clinical

Throbbing headache; hyperalgesia of the scalp; malaise; anorexia; weakness; weight loss; fever; nodular pulmonary nodules; cough; otitis with deafness.

Laboratory

Elevated erythrocyte sedimentation rate (ESR) greater than 50 mm/hour, positive temporal artery biopsy.

Treatment

Systemic corticosteroids are the therapy of choice.

BIBLIOGRAPHY

1. Allen AW, Biega T, Varma MK. (2012). Temporal arteritis imaging. [online] Available from www.emedicine.com/radio/TOPIC675.HTM. [Accessed October, 2013].

2. Walvick MD, Walvick MP. Giant cell arteritis: laboratory predictors of a positive temporal artery biopsy. Ophthalmology. 2011;118(6):1201-4.

33.2A. CENTRAL OR BRANCH RETINAL ARTERY OCCLUSION

General

Present with profound monocular vision loss. In branch occlusion, the visual loss is partial with a scotoma or visual field loss.

Clinical

None.

Ocular

Vision loss, macular edema, macular ischemia, vitreous hemorrhage, traction detachment, rubeosis irides.

Laboratory

Complete blood count, ESR, fasting blood sugar, cholesterol, triglyceride and lipid panels, coagulopathy screen and blood cultures, carotid Doppler ultrasound, ERG, electrocardiogram (ECG) and echocardiogram to identify the cause; optical coherence tomography (OCT) to identify area of occlusion.

Treatment

Acetazolamide intravenously, distal ocular massage, hyperbaric oxygen, grid laser photocoagulation for macular edema, vitrectomy without sheathotomy.

BIBLIOGRAPHY

1. Campochiaro PA, Heier JS, Feiner L, et al. Ranibizumab for macular edema following branch retinal vein occlusion: six-month primary end point results of a phase III study. Ophthalmology. 2010;117(6):1102-12.e1.
2. Rogers SL, McIntosh RL, Lim L, et al. Natural history of branch retinal vein occlusion: an evidence-based systematic review. Ophthalmology. 2010;117(6):1094-101.e5.

33.3B. DIABETES MELLITUS

General

Complex disorder of carbohydrate, lipid and protein metabolism characterized by hyperglycemia and a relative or total lack of insulin. Development is influenced by both genetic and environmental factors. Most commonly occurs in middle or late life (type II) and is seen most commonly in the obese. Diabetes can occur in the 1st or 2nd decade of life (type I) and usually involves the lack of insulin production by the pancreas and the need for insulin therapy.

Clinical

Atherosclerosis; nephropathy; neuropathy; polyuria; polydipsia; polyphagia; obesity; elevated plasma glucose and elevated glycated hemoglobin (A1C).

Ocular

Diabetic retinopathy; vitreous hemorrhage; macular edema; cataract; glaucoma; asteroid hyalosis; extraocular muscle paralysis; rubeosis iridis; corneal hypesthesia; optic nerve atrophy; papillopathy.

Laboratory

Diagnosis made by fasting plasma glucose of greater than 126 mg/dL and 2 hours post glucose load (75 g) plasma glucose of greater than 200 mg/dL and confirmed by repeat test.

Treatment

Goals include elimination of symptoms, by reduction of blood sugar and blood pressure. Smoking cessation, aspirin therapy, weight loss, exercise, diabetic diet as well as oral medication and/or insulin are all used in the treatment of diabetes. Diabetic retinopathy is most successfully treated with retinal photocoagulation. Pars plana vitrectomy is sometimes necessary to remove vitreous hemorrhage. Other ocular problems caused by diabetes such as cataracts and glaucoma are treated in traditional methods.

BIBLIOGRAPHY

1. Khardori R. (2012). Type 2 diabetes mellitus. [online] Available from emedicine.medscape.com/article/117853-overview. [Accessed October, 2013].

⊟ 33.3C. EALES DISEASE (PERIPHLEBITIS)

General

Common; young adults.

Ocular

Sheathing of peripheral veins; hemorrhage in new vessels and later retinal detachment; retinal vascular tortuosity; microaneurysms of retina; postneovascularization of vitreous; internuclear ophthalmoplegia.

Clinical

Epilepsy and hemiplegia have been reported; chronic encephalitis; ulcerative colitis; central nervous infarction.

Laboratory

Fluorescein angiography and tuberculosis screening test.

Treatment

Thyroid extract, osteogenic hormones, androgenic hormones and systemic steroids are recommended. The antioxidant vitamins A, C and E have been suggested as a possible therapy because antioxidizing enzymes are deficient in the vitreous samples.

⊟ BIBLIOGRAPHY

1. Roth DB, Fine HF. (2012). Eales disease. [online] Available from emedicine.medscape.com/article/1225636-overview. [Accessed October, 2013].

⊟ 33.3F. ANDERSEN-WARBURG SYNDROME (WHITNALL-NORMAN SYNDROME; OLIGOPHRENIA MICROPHTHALMOS SYNDROME; NORRIE DISEASE; ATROPHIA OCULI CONGENITAL FETAL IRITIS SYNDROME; CONGENITAL PROGRESSIVE OCULO-ACOUSTICO-CEREBRAL DYSPLASIA)

General

Sex-linked inheritance; gross deformation of both eyes; only males affected; onset at birth; putative gene for Norrie disease has been isolated and mapped to Xp11.3.

Ocular

Bilateral microphthalmos with extensive destruction of all ocular structures often resembling a pseudotumor; blindness at birth; iris atrophy; iritis; corneal opacification and lenticular destruction with a mass visible behind the lens as long as the lens is still clear; malformed retina and choroid with retinal pseudotumors; retinal detachment; retrolental vascular mass.

Clinical

Mental retardation ranging from imbecility to idiocy (may begin at any age) in about two-thirds of the cases; deafness of differing severity with onset between ages 9 and 45 years.

Laboratory

Diagnosis is made by clinical findings.

Treatment

Topical treatment for iritis; retinal detachment surgery and vitrectomy may be necessary. Immediate laser treatment is recommended following birth.

⊟ BIBLIOGRAPHY

1. Andersen SR, Warburg M. Norrie's disease: congenital bilateral pseudotumor of the retina with recessive X-chromosomal inheritance; Preliminary Report. Arch Ophthalmol. 1961;66(5):614-8.
2. Black G, Redmond RM. The molecular biology of Norrie's disease. Eye (Lond). 1994;8(5):491-6.
3. Chow CC, Kiernam DF, Chau FY, et al. Laser photocoagulation at birth prevents blindness in Norrie's disease diagnosed using amniocentesis. Ophthalmology. 2010;117(12):2402-6.
4. Enyedi LB, de Juan E, Gaitan A. Ultrastructural study of Norrie's disease. Am J Ophthalmol. l991;111(4):439-45.
5. Liberfarb RM, Eavey RD, De Long GR, et al. Norrie's disease: a study of two families. Ophthalmology. 1985;92(10):1445-51.
6. Norrie G. Causes of blindness in children; Twenty-five years' experience of Danish institutes for the blind. Acta Ophthalmologica. 1927;5(1-3):357-86.
7. Warburg M. Norrie's disease: differential diagnosis and treatment. Acta Ophthalmologica. 1975;53(2):217-36.
8. Wong F, Goldberg MF, Hao Y. Identification of a nonsense mutation at codon 128 of the Norrie's disease gene in a male infant. Arch Ophthalmol. 1993;111(11):1553-7.

⊟ 33.3G. PERSISTENT HYPERPLASTIC PRIMARY VITREOUS (PHPV, PERSISTENT FETAL VASCULATURE)

General

Congenital ocular disorder with the potential to affect the eye's anterior and posterior anatomy. Usually only affects one eye.

Clinical

Systemic abnormalities may include polydactyly, microcephaly, and cleft palate and lip as well as CNS abnormalities.

Ocular

Anterior persistent hyperplastic primary vitreous (PHPV) includes engorged radial iris vessels, microcornea, Mittendorf' dot, elongated ciliary processes, microophthalmia, cataract.

Laboratory

Diagnosis is made by clinical findings.

Treatment

Monocular congenital cataract surgery and amblyopia therapy. Posterior transciliary for pars plana vitrectomy and removal of tissue.

⊟ BIBLIOGRAPHY

1. Roy FH, Fraunfelder FW, Fraunfelder FT. Roy and Fraunfelder's Current Ocular Therapy, 6th edition. London: WB Saunders; 2008.

⊟ 33.3H. RETINAL DETACHMENT, RHEGMATOGENOUS

General

Subretinal fluid accumulation in the space between the neurosensory retina and the underlying RPE. Most common type of retinal detachment and occurs with a retinal tear that allows liquefied vitreous to seep under the tear leading to the detachment.

Clinical

None.

Ocular

Vitreous traction, cut in visual field; vitreous floaters; decreased visual acuity; scleritis.

Laboratory

Diagnosis is generally made by clinical observation. Ultrasound may be necessary if the media is hazy.

Treatment

Scleral buckle, pneumatic retinopexy and vitrectomy are used for this type of detachment and the goal is to close all the breaks.

⊟ BIBLIOGRAPHY

1. Wu L, Evans T. (2011). Rhegmatogenous retinal detachment treatment and management. [online] Available from emedicine.medscape.com/article/1224737-treatment. [Accessed October, 2013].

⊟ 33.3I. HEMANGIOMA

General

It can occur throughout the body, but particularly in the head; primary intraosseous orbital hemangiomas is rare; capillary hemangioma of the orbit and eyelids generally is unilateral.

Ocular

Hemangiomas of lids or orbit; ptosis; strabismus; amblyopia; proptosis; optic atrophy; hypermetropia; cavernous hemangiomas are the most common benign orbital tumors of adults.

Clinical

Ipsilateral hemangiomas of the brain and meninges.

Laboratory

Neuroimaging can be of great assistance in making the diagnosis.

Treatment

Most of these lesions regress on their own; there is no need to intervention. If spontaneous regression does not occur

corticosteroids, in various formulations, may be considered. Topical application of timolol has been useful in some cases.

BIBLIOGRAPHY

1. Karmel M. Topical timolol for capillary hemangioma. Eyenet. 2010.
2. Seiff S, Zwick OM, DeAngelis DD, et al. (2011). Capillary hemangioma. [online] Available from www.emedicine.com/oph/TOPIC691.HTM. [Accessed October, 2013].

33.3J. RETINOBLASTOMA

General

Retinoblastoma is a malignant tumor arising in one or both retinas of young children, usually under the age of 2 years; usually unilateral; autosomal dominant; this is the most common intraocular malignancy of childhood; incidence is 1 in 20,000 live births; origin is questionably neuroectodermal cells capable of multipotentiality; one-third of patients have heritable (bilateral or have a positive family history) autosomal dominant and two-thirds are sporadic; genetic transmission obeys two-mutation hypothesis of Knudson; trilateral retinoblastoma is bilateral retinoblastoma plus midline CNS tumor (most commonly pinealoma); most common second tumor is an osteogenic sarcoma (begins in 2nd decade).

Ocular

Hyphema; hypopyon; corneal tumor; lid edema; endophthalmitis; exophthalmos; intraocular calcification of globe; heterochromia; neovascularization of iris or retina; papilledema; panophthalmitis; retinoblastoma extension into orbit and choroid; cat's-eye reflex; leukocoria; mydriasis; vitreous hemorrhage tumor seeding; esotropia; exotropia; glaucoma; visual loss.

Clinical

Metastasis into the lymph system, bone marrow, and subarachnoid space; basal meningitis; death.

Laboratory

Computed tomography—calcification of lesion hallmark of disease; ultrasound demonstrates calcification and MRI demonstrates presence and extent of extraocular disease.

Treatment

External beam radiation therapy is recommended on patients with significant vitreous seeding. Radioactive isotope plaques and chemotherapy are also an option. Removal of the tumor is the standard management for retinoblastoma.

BIBLIOGRAPHY

1. Isidro MA, Roque MR, Aaberg TM, et al. (2012). Retinoblastoma. [online] Available from www.emedicine.com/oph/TOPIC346.HTM. [Accessed October, 2013].

33.3K. RETROLENTAL FIBROPLASIA (RLF; RETINOPATHY OF PREMATURITY)

General

Bilateral disease seen primarily in premature infants with immature retinal vessels; excessive use of oxygen is responsible for the majority of cases, but disease is seen despite oxygen restrictions or even when no oxygen supplementation is used; known factors that correlate with degrees of retinopathy of prematurity are low birth weight, short

gestational age, length of time with supplemental oxygen, length of time on a mechanical ventilator; role of excessive light in newborn nurseries also has been proposed.

Ocular

Anterior or posterior synechiae; neovascularization of iris; pallor of optic disk; dragged disk; attenuated vessels;

retinal detachment; dilation of veins; retinal folds; retinal hemorrhage; retrolental mass; vascular tortuosity; vasoconstriction of retina; retinal pigmentary changes; vitreous haze; vitreous traction; vitreous hemorrhages; cataract; glaucoma; leukocoria; myopia; shallow anterior chamber; opaque retrolental membrane; ciliary body drawn anteriorly; ciliary process around dilated pupil; absent pupillary reflexes; keratoconus; associated strabismus; amblyopia.

Clinical

Low birth weight; prematurity.

Laboratory

Diagnosis is made by clinical findings.

Treatment

Cryotherapy and laser surgery can be effective. Vitrectomy may be necessary.

⊟ BIBLIOGRAPHY

1. Bashour M, Menassa J, Gerontis CC. (2013). Retinopathy of prematurity. [online] Available from www.emedicine.com/oph/TOPIC413.HTM. [Accessed October, 2013].

⊟ 33.3L. HERRICK SYNDROME (DRESBACH SYNDROME; SICKLE CELL DISEASE; DREPANOCYTIC ANEMIA)

General

It usually occurs in members of the black race; poor prognosis.

Ocular

Secondary glaucoma; telangiectasis of conjunctival vessels; scleral icterus; vitreous hemorrhages; cataract; retinal hemorrhages, exudates, and neovascularization; retinitis proliferans; microaneurysms; thrombosis of retinal venules; retinal vascular sheathing; central vein occlusion; angioid streaks; retinopathy with "black sunburst sign" in patients with SS hemoglobin; "sea fan sign" in patients with SC hemoglobin; comma signs of conjunctiva; fan-shaped neovascularization of iris; sector ischemic atrophy of iris; optic atrophy; white cotton mass of vitreous; retinal holes; color vision defects; central retinal artery obstruction; branch retinal artery obstruction; white without pressure; venous tortuosity; sickling maculopathy.

Clinical

Severe anemia with hemolytic crises; bone and joint aches; hemarthrosis; jaundice; hepatosplenomegaly.

Laboratory

Blood-sickling of red blood cells, newborn screening for hemoglobin disorders.

Treatment

Transfusion is required in an aplastic crisis, erythrocytapheresis is an automated red-cell exchange and bone marrow transplantation may be useful. Pain is the hallmark of SC disease. While frequency and severity vary greatly, most patients have interval symptoms. Once pain has begun, no therapy reverses the process. Analgesics may provide a reasonable degree of comfort. While certain dosing guidelines are available, the amount of drug given should be titrated to the degree of pain experienced. Vitrectomy may be necessary.

⊟ BIBLIOGRAPHY

1. Maakaron JE, Taher AT. (2013). Sickle cell anemia. [online] Available from www.emedicine.com/ped/TOPIC2096.HTM. [Accessed October, 2013].

⊟ 33.4A. HEMANGIOMA

General

It can occur throughout the body, but particularly in the head; primary intraosseous orbital hemangiomas is rare; capillary hemangioma of the orbit and eyelids generally is unilateral.

Ocular

Hemangiomas of lids or orbit; ptosis; strabismus; amblyopia; proptosis; optic atrophy; hypermetropia; cavernous hemangiomas are the most common benign orbital tumors of adults.

Clinical

Ipsilateral hemangiomas of the brain and meninges.

Laboratory

Neuroimaging can be of great assistance in making the diagnosis.

Treatment

Most of these lesions regress on their own; there is no need to intervention. If spontaneous regression does not occur corticosteroids, in various formulations, may be considered. Topical application of timolol has been useful in some cases.

BIBLIOGRAPHY

1. Karmel M. Topical timolol for capillary hemangioma. Eyenet. 2010.
2. Seiff S, Zwick OM, DeAngelis DD, et al. (2011). Capillary hemangioma. [online] Available from www.emedicine.com/oph/TOPIC691.HTM. [Accessed October, 2013].

33.5B. EXFOLIATION SYNDROME (CAPSULAR EXFOLIATION SYNDROME)

General

Only in men older than 60 years.

Ocular

Iridodonesis; rubeosis iridis; cataract; phacodonesis; dislocated lens; corneal dystrophy; choroidal sclerosis; primary optic atrophy; lens capsule exfoliation; lower endothelial cell density.

Clinical

None.

Laboratory

Diagnosis is made by clinical findings.

Treatment

Aggressive open angle glaucoma therapy with topical agents is the initial treatment. Laser trabeculectomy and filtering surgery may be necessary.

BIBLIOGRAPHY

1. Pons ME, Eliassi-Rad B. (2013). Pseudoexfoliation Glaucoma. [online] Available from www.emedicine.com/oph/TOPIC140.HTM. [Accessed October, 2013].

33.5C. FIBRINOID SYNDROME

General

From 2 days to 14 days postvitrectomy, white-gray crisscross layers of fibrin appear on the surface of the retina and immediately behind the plane of the iris; occurs only in patients with diabetes mellitus and usually in those requiring insulin; seen more frequently in people who have been diabetic for 15 years or more.

Ocular

Fibrin material interlaced on the surface of the retina and behind the iris; retinal detachment; neovascular glaucoma; rubeosis irides.

Clinical

Diabetes mellitus.

Laboratory

Diagnosis is made by clinical findings.

Treatment

Although prognosis is poor, lensectomy (in phakic eyes), excision of the posterior hyaloid face and vitreous base dissection, extensive pan-retinal photocoagulation (to induce regression of or prevent anterior hyaloidal fibrovascular proliferation) and silicone oil infusion can be useful.

BIBLIOGRAPHY

1. Ho T, Smiddy WE, Flynn HW. Vitrectomy in the management of diabetic eye disease. Surv Ophthalmol. 1992;37:190-202.
2. Schepens CL. Clinical and research aspects of subtotal open-sky vitrectomy: 439VII Edward Jackson Memorial Lecture. Am J Ophthalmol. 1981;92:143-71.
3. Sebestzen JG. Fibrinoid syndrome: a severe complication of vitrectomy surgery in diabetes. Ann Ophthalmol. 1982;14:853-6.

⊟ 33.5D. FUNGAL ENOPHTHALMITIS

General

Rare, intraocular fungal infection.

Clinical

None.

Ocular

Conjunctival injection; pain; mildly decreased vision; fibrinous membranes in anterior chamber; white fluffy retinal infiltrates.

Laboratory

Fungal tests are done on anterior chamber aspirates and vitreous cavity aspirates.

Treatment

Topical, subconjunctival, intravitreal antifungal agents; pars plana vitrectomy.

⊟ BIBLIOGRAPHY

1. Wu L, Evans T, García RA. (2012). Fungal endophthalmitis. [online] Available from www.emedicine.com/oph/TOP-IC706.HTM. [Accessed October, 2013].

⊟ 33.5E. IRIS NEOVASCULARIZATION WITH PSEUDOEXFOLIATION SYNDROME

General

Anoxia secondary to iris vessel obstruction; electron microscopic studies reveal endothelial thickening with decreased lumen size and fenestration of vessel walls.

Ocular

Materials found on posterior and anterior iris surface, anterior lens surface, ciliary processes, zonules and anterior hyaloid membranes; neovascularization of iris stroma; increased permeability of iris vessels.

Clinical

None.

Laboratory

Diagnosis is made by clinical findings.

Treatment

Patients with pseudoexfoliation syndrome should have annual eye examinations for early detection of glaucoma.

⊟ BIBLIOGRAPHY

1. Pons ME, Eliassi-Rad B. (2011). Pseudoexfoliation glaucoma. [online] Available from www.emedicine.com/oph/TOPIC140.HTM. [Accessed October, 2013].

⊟ 33.5H. UVEITIS, ANTERIOR GRANULOMATOUS (IRITIS)

General

Ocular inflammation of the iris and ciliary body. Etiology is idiopathic but certain systemic diseases may be the underlying cause.

Clinical

Herpes zoster, sarcoidosis, syphilis, Lyme disease, tuberculosis, multiple sclerosis, leprosy, toxoplasmosis, coccidiodomycosis, Vogt-Koyanagi-Harada disease, brucellosis.

Ocular

Photophobia, red eye, dull aching eye pain, perilimbal injection, keratic precipitates, flare and cell of anterior chamber, posterior synechiae, lenticular precipitates.

Laboratory

Diagnosis is made by clinical findings. If granulomatous iritis is recurrent, studies are necessary to determine the cause. ELISA, serologic testing for syphilis, sarcoidosis and Lyme disease may be indicated.

Treatment

Topical corticosteroids are the mainstay of therapy. Subconjunctival corticosteroids may be necessary in non-responding cases. Cycloplegia is useful for control of pain and photophobia.

BIBLIOGRAPHY

1. Levinson RD. (2012). Uveitis, anterior, granulomatous. [online] Available from www.emedicine.com/oph/TOPIC586.HTM. [Accessed October, 2013].

33.6A. ADULT CATARACTS

General

Cataract is a disorder in which the crystalline lens becomes opacified.

Clinical

None.

Ocular

Glare, monocular diplopia, changes in refractive error, decreased visual acuity.

Laboratory

Diagnosis is made by clinical findings.

Treatment

Change in glasses can sometimes improve a patient's visual function temporarily; however, the most common treatment is cataract surgery.

BIBLIOGRAPHY

1. Roy FH, Fraunfelder FW, Fraunfelder FT. Roy and Fraunfelder's Current Ocular Therapy, 6th edition. London, UK: Elsevier; 2008.

33.6B. DIABETES MELLITUS

General

Complex disorder of carbohydrate, lipid and protein metabolism characterized by hyperglycemia and a relative or total lack of insulin. Development is influenced by both genetic and environmental factors. Most commonly occurs in middle or late life (type II) and is seen most commonly in the obese. Diabetes can occur in the first or second decade of life (type I) and usually involves the lack of insulin production by the pancreas and the need for insulin therapy.

Clinical

Atherosclerosis; nephropathy; neuropathy; polyuria; polydipsia; polyphagia; obesity; elevated plasma glucose and elevated glycated hemoglobin (A1C).

Ocular

Diabetic retinopathy; vitreous hemorrhage; macular edema; cataract; glaucoma; asteroid hyalosis; extraocular muscle paralysis; rubeosis iridis; corneal hypesthesia; optic nerve atrophy; papillopathy.

Laboratory

Diagnosis made by fasting plasma glucose of greater than 126 mg/dL and 2 hours post glucose load (75 g) plasma glucose of greater than 200 mg/dL and confirmed by repeat test.

Treatment

Goals include elimination of symptoms, by reduction of blood sugar and blood pressure. Smoking cessation, aspirin therapy, weight loss, exercise, diabetic diet as well as oral medication and/or insulin are all used in the treatment of diabetes. Diabetic retinopathy is most successfully treated with retinal photocoagulation. Pars plana vitrectomy is sometimes necessary to remove vitreous hemorrhage. Other ocular problems caused by diabetes such as cataracts and glaucoma are treated in traditional methods.

BIBLIOGRAPHY

1. Khardori R. (2012). Type 2 diabetes mellitus. [online] Available from emedicine.medscape.com/article/117853-overview. [Accessed October, 2013].
2. Ostri C, Lund-Andersen H, Sander B, et al. Bilateral diabetic papillopathy and metabolic control. Ophthalmology. 2010;117:2214-7.
3. Richter GM, Torres M, Choudhury F, et al. Risk Factors for Cortical, Nuclear, Posterior Subcapsular, and Mixed Lens Opacities: The Los Angeles Latino Eye Study. Ophthalmology. 2012;119:547-54.

🗗 33.6C. MYOTONIC DYSTROPHY SYNDROME (MYOTONIA ATROPHICA SYNDROME; DYSTROPHIA MYOTONICA; CURSCHMANN-STEINERT SYNDROME)

General

Rare autosomal dominant disease; onset at the age of 20 years; condition is worsened by administration of neostigmine (Prostigmin); associated with an unstable deoxyribonucleic acid (DNA) sequence composed of varying numbers of CTG triplet repeats (which allows a specific molecular test for this disorder).

Ocular

Mild ptosis (occasionally); myotonic cataract with small, dot-like subcapsular cortical opacities during early stage, with polychromatic properties on biomicroscopic examination; corneal epithelial dystrophy; loss of corneal sensitivity; tapetoretinal degeneration; macular red spot; macular degeneration; chorioretinitis; pilomatrixomas; ocular hypotony; pattern pigmentary changes; abnormal saccades.

Clinical

Progressive muscular atrophy with selection of certain muscles (mainly sternocleidomastoid, temporalis, dorsiflexor muscles of the ankle, anterior oblique); myotonia; bland facial expression; speech disturbance due to involvement of vocal cords and palatal muscles; dysphagia; endocrine disturbances.

Laboratory

Diagnosis is made by clinical findings.

Treatment

- *Ptosis*: If visual acuity is affected, most cases require surgical correction and there are several procedures that may be used including levator resection, repair or advancement and Fasanella-Servat procedure.
- *Cataract*: Change in glasses can sometimes improve a patient's visual function temporarily; however, the most common treatment is cataract surgery.
- *Corneal dystrophy*: Mild cases—can be observed and soft contact lenses are helpful; PK may be necessary; graft recurrences are treated by superficial keratectomy, PTK or repeat PK.
- *Macular degeneration*: No treatment is available for non-neovascular age-related macular degeneration (AMD). Preventative therapy includes no smoking, control of hypertension, cholesterol, and blood sugar, exercise and vitamins. Neovascular AMD treatment consists of laser, avastin and lucentis.

🗗 BIBLIOGRAPHY

1. Brooke NM, Cwik VE. Myotonic dystrophy. In: Bradley WG (Ed). Neurology in Clinical Practice: Principles of Diagnosis and Management, 2nd edition. Boston, USA: Butterworth-Heinemann; 1995. pp. 2020-2.
2. Gjertsen IK, Sandvig KU, Eide N, et al. Recurrence of secondary opacification and development of a dense posterior vitreous membrane in patients with myotonic dystrophy. J Cataract Refract Surg. 2003;29(1):213-6.
3. Kimizuka Y, Kiyosawa M, Tamai M, et al. Retinal changes in myotonic dystrophy. Clinical and follow-up evaluation. Retina. 1993;13(2):129-35.
4. Koca MR, Horn F, Korth M. Alterations of saccadic eye movements in myotonic dystrophy. Graefes Arch Clin Exp Ophthalmol. 1992;230(5):437-41.
5. Kuwabara T, Lessell S. Electron microscopic study of extraocular muscles in myotonic dystrophy. Am J Ophthalmol. 1976;82(2):303-9.
6. Mausolf FA, Burns CA, Burian HM. Morphologic and functional retinal changes in myotonic dystrophy unrelated to quinine therapy. Am J Ophthalmol. 1972;74(6):1141-3.
7. Meyer E, Navon D, Auslender L, et al. Myotonic dystrophy: pathological study of the eyes. Ophthalmologica. 1980;181(3-4):215-20.
8. Reardon W, MacMillan JC, Myring J, et al. Cataract and myotonic dystrophy: the role of molecular diagnosis. Br J Ophthalmol. 1993;77(9):579-83.
9. Rosa N, Lanza M, Borrelli M, et al. Low intraocular pressure resulting from ciliary body detachment in patients with myotonic dystrophy. Ophthalmology. 2011;118(2):260-4.

33.6D. OCULAR HYPOTONY

General

Low IOP resulting in anatomical or functional abnormalities to the eye.

Clinical

None.

Ocular

Thin corneas, corneal striae, aqueous flare, choroidal folds, effusion, macular folds, low IOP.

Laboratory

Diagnosis is made by clinical findings.

Treatment

Topical corticosteroids and cycloplegic agents are recommended.

BIBLIOGRAPHY

1. Roy FH, Fraunfelder FW, Fraunfelder FT. Roy and Fraunfelder's Current Ocular Therapy, 6th edition. London, UK: Elsevier; 2008.

34. UVEITIS, ANTERIOR GRANULOMATOUS (IRITIS)

General

Ocular inflammation of the iris and ciliary body. Etiology is idiopathic but certain systemic diseases may be the underlying cause.

Clinical

Herpes zoster, sarcoidosis, syphilis, Lyme disease, tuberculosis, multiple sclerosis, leprosy, toxoplasmosis, coccidiodomycosis, Vogt-Koyanagi-Harada disease, brucellosis.

Ocular

Photophobia, red eye, dull aching eye pain, perilimbal injection, keratic precipitates, flare and cell of anterior chamber, posterior synechiae, lenticular precipitates.

Laboratory

Diagnosis is made by clinical findings. If granulomatous iritis is recurrent studies are necessary to determine the cause. ELISA, serologic testing for syphilis, sarcoidosis and Lyme may be indicated.

Treatment

Topical corticosteroids are the mainstay of therapy. Subconjunctival corticosteroids may be necessary in nonresponding cases. Cycloplegia is useful for control of pain and photophobia.

BIBLIOGRAPHY

1. Levinson RD. (2012). Uveitis, Anterior, Granulomatous. [online] Available from www.emedicine.com/oph/TOPIC586.HTM. [Accessed October, 2013].

34A. UVEITIS, ANTERIOR NONGRANULOMATOUS (IRITIS, CHRONIC)

General

Ocular inflammation. Etiology is idiopathic but certain systemic diseases may be the underlying cause.

Clinical

Human leukocyte antigen B27, Behçet disease, herpes zoster, sarcoidosis, syphilis, Lyme disease, juvenile idiopathic arthritis, Fuchs heterochromic iridocyclitis, tuberculosis.

Ocular

Photophobia, red eye, dull aching eye pain, perilimbal injection, keratic precipitates, flare and cell of anterior chamber, posterior synechiae, lenticular precipitates.

Laboratory

Diagnosis is made by clinical findings. If nongranulomatous iritis is recurrent, studies are necessary to determine the cause. Human leukocyte antigen B27 typing, serologic testing for syphilis, sarcoidosis rheumatoid factor and Lyme disease may be indicated.

Treatment

Topical corticosteroids are the mainstay of therapy. Subconjunctival corticosteroids may be necessary in non-responding cases. Cycloplegia is useful for controlling pain and photophobia.

🗗 BIBLIOGRAPHY

1. Levinson RD. (2012). Uveitis, anterior, nongranulomatous. [online] Available from www.emedicine.com/oph/TOP-IC587.HTM. [Accessed October, 2013].

🗗 34B. UVEITIS (IRITIS, IRIDOCYSTITIS, INTERMEDIATE AND POSTERIOR UVEITIS, NONINFECTIOUS CHORIORETINITIS)

General

Mostly idiopathic or post-traumatic but other causes include infections, malignancies, autoimmune diseases and pharmaceutical.

Clinical

None.

Ocular

Photophobia, ciliary flush, decreased vision.

Laboratory

Chest X-ray—sarcoid; purified protein derivative (PPD), fluorescent treponemal antibody-absorption (FTA-ABS)—syphilis; Lyme C6 peptide—Lyme disease.

Treatment

Oral steroids should be given if not responsive to topical steroids; immunosuppressants if bilateral disease that does not respond to oral steroids; periocular steroids for unilateral or posterior uveitis. Vitrectomy can be used for severe vitreous opacification. Cryotherapy and laser photocoagulation may be used for localized pars plana exudates. Fluocinolone acetonide intravitreal implants may also be useful.

🗗 BIBLIOGRAPHY

1. Levinson RD. (2012). Uveitis, anterior, nongranulomatous. [online] Available from www.emedicine.com/oph/TOP-IC587.HTM. [Accessed October, 2013].
2. Levinson RD. (2012). Uveitis, anterior, granulomatous. [online] Available from www.emedicine.com/oph/TOP-IC586.HTM. [Accessed October, 2013].

🗗 35. UVEITIS MASQUERADE SYNDROME(S) (VMS) UVEITIS 1286

General

Uveitis masquerade syndrome is a group of disorders that mimic uveitis; cells seen may be of non-inflammatory origin or are inflammatory and secondary to another disorder.

Ocular

Uveitis; panuveitis; pars planitis; vitreitis; papillitis; anterior segment cells; hypopyon; vitreal infiltrates.

Clinical

Causes may be malignant such as lymphoma, leukemia, retinoblastoma, melanoma and lung cancer metastasis, or nonmalignant such as ocular toxoplasmosis, diabetic retinopathy, hypertension and radiation retinopathy.

Laboratory/Ocular

Diagnosis is made by clinical findings.

Treatment/Ocular

Uveitis: Topical steroids and cycloplegic medication should be the initial treatment of choice. Oral steroids should be given if not responsive to topical steroids, immunosuppressants if bilateral disease that does not respond to oral steroids, periocular steroids for unilateral or posterior uveitis. Vitrectomy can be used for severe vitreous opacification. Cryotherapy and laser photocoagulation may be used for localized pars plana exudates.

🗗 BIBLIOGRAPHY

1. Nussenblatt RB, Whitcup SM. Uveitis: Fundamentals and Clinical Practice, 2nd edition. St Louis: Mosby; 1996. pp. 385-95.
2. To KW, Rankin GA, Jakobiec FA, et al. Intraocular lymphoproliferations simulating uveitis. In: Albert DM, Jakobiec FA (Eds). Albert & Jakobiec's Principles and Practice of Ophthalmology. Philadelphia, PA: WB Saunders; 1994. pp. 524-48.

⊟ 36. UGH SYNDROME (UVEITIS-GLAUCOMA-HYPHEMA SYNDROME) GLAUCOMA

General

Uveitis-glaucoma-hyphema (UGH) syndrome is caused by a defective anterior chamber lens; it can be caused by toxic substance incorporated into the plastic of lens during manufacture or warped IOL; syndrome may rarely occur after extracapsular cataract extraction with implantation of a posterior chamber IOL.

Ocular

Uveitis-glaucoma-hyphema.

Clinical

None.

Laboratory

Diagnosis is made by clinical findings.

Treatment

- *Uveitis*:
  - *Glaucoma*: Glaucoma medication should be the first plan of action. If medication is unsuccessful, a filtering surgical procedure with or without antimetabolites may be beneficial.
  - *Hyphema*: Cycloplegia decreased the inflammation and discomfort associated with traumatic iritis. Topical beta-adrenergic antagonists are the therapy of choice for elevated IOPs; laser may be used to cauterize the bleeding vessel.

⊟ BIBLIOGRAPHY

1. Percival SP, Das SK. UGH syndrome after posterior chamber lens implantation. J Am Intraocul Implant Soc. 1983;9(2):200-1.
2. Masket S. Pseudophakic posterior iris chafing syndrome. J Cataract Refract Surg. 1986;12(3):252-6.

CHAPTER
27

Lacrimal System

🔲 1A. ALACRIMA

General

Autosomal recessive; wide spectrum of lacrimal secretory disorders that are mostly congenital in origin. Symptoms of these disorders can range from a complete absence of tears to hyposecretion of tears; symptoms of rarer disorders include a selective absence of tearing in response to emotional stimulation but a normal secretory response to mechanical stimulation. It may be associated with syndromes such as Riley-Day, anhidrotic ectodermal dysplasia, Sjögren and Allgrove.

Clinical

Decreased salivation and sweating; osteoporosis; short stature; adrenocortical insufficiency.

Ocular

Foreign body sensation; photophobia, decreased visual acuity; absence of tears; chronic blepharoconjunctivitis; hyperemia; thick mucoid discharge; keratinization; pannus; corneal ulcers or perforation; tonic pupils; optic atrophy.

Laboratory

Computed tomography (CT) scan of orbits to determine aplastic lacrimal glands; Schirmer testing; conjunctival and lacrimal gland biopsy.

Treatment

Artificial tears, gels and ointments are used as the primary treatment. Permanent or temporary punctal occlusion can be effective. Tarsorrhaphy may be necessary if the corneal health has been compromised.

🔲 BIBLIOGRAPHY

1. DeAngelis DD, Hurwitz J. (2012). Alacrima. [online] Available from emedicine.medscape.com/article/1210539-overview. [Accessed October, 2013].

🔲 1B. BRANCHIAL CLEFTS WITH CHARACTERISTIC FACIES, GROWTH RETARDATION, IMPERFORATE NASOLACRIMAL DUCT, AND PREMATURE AGING

General

Autosomal dominant.

Ocular

Strabismus; obstructed nasolacrimal ducts.

Clinical

Low birth weight; retarded growth; bilateral bronchial cleft sinuses; broad nasal bridge; protruding upper lip; carp mouth; premature aging; malformed ears; linear skin lesions behind the ears.

Laboratory

Diagnosis is made by clinical findings.

Treatment

- *Strabismus*: Equalized vision with correct refractive error; surgery may be helpful in patients with diplopia.
- *Obstructed nasolacrimal ducts*: It may spontaneously resolve during the 1st year of life with massage if not probing and irrigation of the nasolacrimal duct can be done.

BIBLIOGRAPHY

1. Tewfik TL, Al-Noury KI. (2011). Manifestations of craniofacial syndromes. [online] Available from www.emedicine.com/ent/TOPIC319.HTM. [Accessed October, 2013].

1C. CONGENITAL ANOMALIES OF THE LACRIMAL SYSTEM (CONGENITAL NASOLACRIMAL DUCT OBSTRUCTION, DACRYOCYSTITIS, DACRYOCYSTOCELE, ACCESSORY PUNCTUM, PUNCTAL STENOSIS, CANALICULAR STENOSIS)

General

It is the common congenital abnormality of lacrimal drainage system.

Clinical

None.

Ocular

Tearing, recurrent mucopurulent discharge, reflux of tears and mucopurulent material from the punctum with pressure in the nasolacrimal sac.

Laboratory

Diagnosis is made by clinical findings.

Treatment

Spontaneously resolves during the 1st year of life if not probing and irrigation of the nasolacrimal duct can be done in an office setting.

BIBLIOGRAPHY

1. Bashour M. (2012). Congenital anomalies of the nasolacrimal duct. [online] Available from www.emedicine.com/oph/TOPIC592.HTM. [Accessed October, 2013].

1D. DACRYOADENITIS

General

Acute or chronic inflammatory enlargement of lacrimal gland generally caused by a virus, however immunoglobulin G4 (IgG4) systemic disease has also been linked as a cause.

Clinical

Sarcoid, Sjögren's syndrome, Graves' disease, lupus, Wegener's granulomatosis, benign lymphoepithelial lesions.

Ocular

Orbital pain, edema of upper lid, S-shaped upper lid.

Laboratory

CT scan of enlarged gland.

Treatment

Determine the cause and treat; systemic steroids or antibiotics, lavage the conjunctival sac if discharge is present, ocular therapy with tear substitutes, incision of lacrimal palpebral lobe if involved.

BIBLIOGRAPHY

1. Singh GJ, Ahuja R. (2011). Dacryoadenitis. [online] Available from www.emedicine.com/oph/TOPIC594.HTM. [Accessed October, 2013].

🗗 1E. AUTOIMMUNOLOGICALLY MEDIATED SYNDROME (LYMPHOCYTIC HYPOPHYSITIS ASSOCIATED WITH DACRYOADENITIS SYNDROME)

General

Lymphocytes infiltrate the hypophysis.

Ocular

Dacryoadenitis.

Clinical

Lymphocytic infiltration of the hypophysis by CD3 cells, T cells, and CD20+ B cells is an autoimmune process that may rarely cause lacrimal gland swelling.

Laboratory

CT scan of the orbits with contrast can be helpful. The affected lacrimal gland shows diffuse enlargement, oblong shape, and marked enhancement with contrast.

Treatment

Warm compresses, oral nonsteroidal anti-inflammatories are useful. Treat the underlying systemic condition. If the enlargement does not subside after 2 weeks, consider lacrimal gland biopsy.

🗗 BIBLIOGRAPHY

1. Singh GJ, Ahuja R. (2013). Dacryoadenitis. [online] Available from http://www.emedicine.com/oph/TOPIC594.HTM. [Accessed October, 2013].

🗗 1F. DRY EYE SYNDROME

General

Multifactorial disease of the tears and the ocular surface that results in symptoms of discomfort, visual disturbance, and tear film instability with potential damage to the ocular surface, increased osmolarity of the tear film and inflammation of the ocular surface. The most common cause is aqueous tear deficiency. Keratoconjunctivitis sicca, which is an ocular surface disorder, may also be a cause. It is associated with connective tissue disease such as rheumatoid arthritis and systemic sclerosis; postmenopausal women; pregnant women; and individuals taking oral contraceptives and hormone replacement therapy.

Clinical

Rheumatoid arthritis; systemic sclerosis; menopause; pregnancy, prostate disease.

Ocular

Foreign body sensation; burning; itching; photophobic; blurred vision; excessive tearing; irregular corneal surface; decreased tear breakup time; punctate epithelial keratopathy; debris in the tear film; corneal ulcer.

Laboratory

Diagnosis is generally made by clinical observation; careful history; tear breakup test; Schirmer's test and the use of Rose Bengal and fluorescein to check for staining is useful. Additional testing can be used to determine the tear components. These include conjunctival biopsy, tear function index, tear ferning test, impression cytology and meibometry.

Treatment

Environmental and dietary modifications; elimination of systemic medications if possible; artificial tears, gels and ointments; anti-inflammatory agents such as topical corticosteroids, cyclosporine A and omega-3 fatty acids; and tetracyclines for meibomianitis. Punctal plugs; moisture chamber spectacles and autologous serum tears may be necessary if the symptoms persist. Sometimes systemic anti-inflammatory agents, tarsorrhaphy, mucous membrane grafting; amniotic membrane transplantation and salivary gland duct transposition may be necessary in the worst cases.

🗗 BIBLIOGRAPHY

1. Foster CS, Yuksel E, Anzaar F, et al. (2012). Dry eye syndrome. [online] Available from emedicine.medscape.com/article/1210417-overview. [Accessed October, 2013].
2. Liang L, Sheha H, Fu Y, et al. Ocular surface morbidity in eyes with senile sunken upper eyelids. Ophthalmology. 2011;118:2487-92.

⊟ 1G. EPIPHORIA

General

Hypersecretion or failure of the lacrimal excretory system to function.

Clinical

Nasal pathology.

Ocular

Epiphoria, corneal foreign body, trichiasis, corneal ulcer, entropion, ectropion or lid retraction.

Laboratory

Diagnosis is made by clinical findings.

Treatment

Treat the underlying cause, massage the tear sac and antibiotics, conjunctival dacryocystorhinostomy (DCR) with Jones tube.

⊟ BIBLIOGRAPHY

1. Roy FH, Fraunfelder FW, Fraunfelder FT. Roy and Fraunfelder's Current Ocular Therapy, 6th edition. London, UK: Elsevier; 2008.

⊟ 1H. HEERFORDT SYNDROME (UVEOPAROTID FEVER; UVEOPAROTITIS; UVEOPAROTITIC PARALYSIS)

General

It occurs in young adults, more frequently in females than in males; usual cause is sarcoidosis.

Ocular

Band keratopathy; keratoconjunctivitis sicca; uveitis; optic atrophy; papilledema; episcleritis; snowball opacity of vitreous; retinal vasculitis; proptosis; cataract; paralysis of seventh nerve; sarcoid nodules of eyelid, iris, ciliary body, choroid, and sclera; dacryoadenitis.

Clinical

Parotid gland swelling; facial paralysis; lymphadenopathy; splenomegaly; cutaneous nodules; facial nerve palsy.

Laboratory

Biopsy of liver, skin, lymph nodes or conjunctiva show noncaseating epithelioid cell follicles; X-ray shows lung changes; low tuberculin sensitivity; elevated angiotensin-converting enzyme level.

Treatment

Systemic corticosteroids are the treatment of choice.

⊟ BIBLIOGRAPHY

1. Dahl AA. (2011). Ophthalmologic manifestations of sarcoidosis. [online] Available from www.emedicine.com/oph/TOPIC451.HTM. [Accessed October, 2013].

⊟ 1I. LACRIMAL DUCT DEFECT

General

Autosomal dominant.

Ocular

Imperforate nasolacrimal ducts with or without absence of puncta and canaliculi.

Clinical

None.

Laboratory

Diagnosis is made by clinical findings.

Treatment

Most congenital nasolacrimal duct obstructions sponta-neously resolve, probing, nasolacrimal intubation, bal-loon catheter dilatation of the nasolacrimal system, DCR.

⊟ BIBLIOGRAPHY

1. Bashour M. (2012). Congenital anomalies of the nasolac-rimal duct. [online] Available from www.emedicine.com/oph/TOPIC592.HTM. [Accessed October, 2013].

⊟ 1J. LACRIMAL GLAND TUMORS

General

Swelling of lateral superior orbit, tumors can be benign or malignant.

Clinical

None.

Ocular

Tumor of the lacrimal gland, globe may be pushed down and medial from the tumor, diplopia, proptosis, ptosis and pain.

Laboratory

CT scan of orbit.

Treatment

Biopsy, excise of tumor with the capsule for benign tumor, malignant tumors may require large excision or orbital exenteration, chemotherapy or radiation.

⊟ BIBLIOGRAPHY

1. DeAngelis DD, Pang NK, Hurwitz J. (2011). Lacrimal gland tumors. [online] Available from www.emedicine.com/oph/TOPIC694.HTM. [Accessed October, 2013].
2. McNab AA, Satchi K. Recurrent lacrimal gland pleomor-phic adenoma: clinical and computed tomography fea-tures. Ophthalmology. 2011;118(10):2088-92.

⊟ 1K. LACRIMAL HYPERSECRETION

General

Excessive secretion of tears from the main or accessory lacrimal glands.

Clinical

None.

Ocular

Excess tears.

Laboratory

Diagnosis is made by clinical findings.

Treatment

Botulinum toxin injected into the lacrimal gland is effec-tive for excess tears.

⊟ BIBLIOGRAPHY

1. Roy FH, Fraunfelder FW, Fraunfelder FT. Roy and Fraun-felder's Current Ocular Therapy, 6th edition. London, UK: Elsevier, 2008.

⊟ 1L. LACRIMAL SYSTEM CONTUSIONS AND LACERATIONS

General

Sharp and blunt trauma.

Clinical

None.

Ocular

Laceration of upper or lower eyelid medially.

Laboratory

Diagnosis is made by clinical findings.

Treatment

Repair canaliculus.

BIBLIOGRAPHY

1. Mawn LA. (2012). Canalicular laceration. [online] Available from www.emedicine.com/oph/TOPIC218.HTM. [Accessed October, 2013].

1M. PARINAUD OCULOGLANDULAR SYNDROME (PARINAUD CONJUNCTIVA-ADENITIS SYNDROME; CATSCRATCH OCULOGLANDULAR SYNDROME; CATSCRATCH DISEASE; BARTONELLA HENSELAE)

General

It is most frequently seen in children; incubation time is 7–10 days; caused by small pleomorphic Gram-negative bacillus; good prognosis; affects both sexes; about 90% of patients with this condition have serologic evidence of infection by *Rochalimaea henselae*.

Ocular

Conjunctivitis; retrotarsal conjunctival granulations; formation of granulomata in anterior segment about 3 mm high and 2–6 mm in diameter; inferior fornix is usually affected; ulceration common; neuroretinitis; optic neuritis.

Clinical

Tender, red papule at the site of a cat scratch; regional preauricular and cervical lymphadenitis (often only one gland is involved); irregular fever for 4–5 days and malaise; fever; parotid gland swelling.

Laboratory

Histopathology of biopsied lymph node of Warthin-Starry's silver stain.

Treatment

Symptomatic treatment includes warm compresses, analgesics and antipyretics; aspiration of lymph node if distention causes pain. Antibiotics may be necessary in severe cases.

BIBLIOGRAPHY

1. Chi SL, Stinnett S, Eggenberger E, et al. Clinical characteristics in 53 patients with cat scratch optic neuropathy. Ophthalmology. 2012;119:183-7.
2. Nervi SJ, Ressner RA, Drayton JR, et al. (2011). Catscratch disease. [online] Available from www.emedicine.com/med/TOPIC304.HTM. [Accessed October, 2013].

1N. PAROTID APLASIA OR HYPOPLASIA (SALIVARY GLAND ABSENCE; LACRIMAL PUNCTA ABSENCE)

General

Autosomal dominant.

Ocular

Lacrimal gland aplasia; absence or severe dysfunction of lacrimal glands.

Clinical

Aplasia of parotid salivary glands; hemifacial microsomia; mandibulofacial dysostoses; xerostomia; rampant caries; edentulous, salivary gland dysfunction; parotid agenesis or hypoplasia; impalpable parotid gland; absence of the orifice of Stensen's duct; bilateral parotid gland aplasia.

Laboratory

Diagnosis is made by clinical findings.

Treatment

Ocular lubrication with topical drops and ointments. Bandage contact lens may sometimes be necessary.

BIBLIOGRAPHY

1. DeAngelis DD, Hurwitz J. (2012). Alacrima. [online] Available from www.emedicine.com/oph/TOPIC693.HTM. [Accessed October, 2013].

⬚ 1O. RILEY-DAY SYNDROME (CONGENITAL FAMILIAL DYSAUTONOMIA)

General

It is autosomal recessive; it occurs in Ashkenazi Jewish population; impaired catechol metabolism; manifested in first few days of life; it is characterized by developmental loss of neurons from the sensory and autonomic nervous systems.

Ocular

Congenital failure of tear production; corneal anesthesia; neuroparalytic keratitis; keratitis sicca; corneal ulcers; optic atrophy.

Clinical

Excessive salivation; failure to thrive; recurrent respiratory infections; diarrhea; insensitivity to pain; spontaneous fractures; pandysautonomia; orthostatic hypotension; gastrointestinal paresis; decreased fungiform papillae on the tongue.

Laboratory

Deoxyribonucleic acid (DNA) test is used to confirm the diagnosis.

Treatment

Artificial drops and/or gels are useful in any dry eye condition. Tarsorrhaphy is an effective treatment of the decompensated neurotrophic cornea.

⬚ BIBLIOGRAPHY

1. D'Amico RA, Axelrod FB. (2011). Familial dysautonomia. [online] Available from www.emedicine.com/oph/TOPIC678.HTM. [Accessed October, 2013].

⬚ 1P. KERATOCONJUNCTIVITIS SICCA AND SJÖGREN'S SYNDROME

General

Autoimmune disease, seen more frequently in females.

Clinical

Xerostomia (dry mouth), dry nasal and genital mucosa.

Ocular

Severe dry eyes, corneal ulceration, corneal perforation, corneal scarring and vascularization.

Laboratory

Biopsy of lip and lachrymal gland positive, anti-nuclear antibody rheumatoid factor (RF) and anti-ro (Sjögren's specific A) and anti-La (Sjögren's specific B). Elevated IgG level positive—predication for positive biopsy.

Treatment

Severe cases—immunosuppressive agents as cyclosporin A and corticosteroids. Frequent application of tear substitutes, steroids, punctal plugs, bandage contacts and partial tarsorrhaphy.

⬚ BIBLIOGRAPHY

1. Foster CS, Yuksel E, Anzaar F, et al. (2013). Dry eye syndrome. [online] Available from www.emedicine.com/oph/TOPIC597.HTM. [Accessed October, 2013].

⬚ 1Q. WERNER SYNDROME (PROGERIA OF ADULTS) BLUE SCLERA

General

Etiology unknown; recessive inheritance; consanguinity; between 2nd decade and 3rd decade; possible mechanisms have been proposed to explain mutation of a gene causing inhibition of DNA synthesis and early cellular senescence.

Ocular

Absence of eyelashes and scanty eyebrows; blue sclera; juvenile cataracts; bullous keratitis; trophic corneal defects; paramacular retinal degeneration; proptosis; telangiectasia of lid; astigmatism; nystagmus; presbyopia; uveitis.

Clinical

Leanness; short stature (160 cm maximum); thin limbs; short, deformed fingers; small mouth; early baldness; stretched, atrophic skin (scleropoikiloderma); telangiectasia and trophic indolent ulcers on toes, heels, and ankles; arteriosclerosis with secondary heart failure.

Laboratory

Fasting blood glucose test, oral glucose tolerance test, tri-iodothyronine levothyroxide and thyrotropin test.

Treatment

No specific treatment exists.

BIBLIOGRAPHY

1. Janniger CK, Wozniacka A. (2013). Werner Syndrome. [online] Available from www.emedicine.com/derm/TOPIC697.HTM. [Accessed October, 2013].

2A. CONGENITAL ANOMALIES OF THE LACRIMAL SYSTEM (CONGENITAL NASOLACRIMAL DUCT OBSTRUCTION, DACRYOCYSTITIS, DACRYOCYSTOCELE, ACCESSORY PUNCTUM, PUNCTAL STENOSIS, CANALICULAR STENOSIS)

General

Common congenital anomalies of lacrimal drainage system.

Clinical

None.

Ocular

Tearing, recurrent mucopurulent discharge, reflux of tears and mucopurulent material from the punctum with pressure in the nasolacrimal sac.

Laboratory

Diagnosis is made by clinical findings.

Treatment

Spontaneously resolves during the 1st year of life if not probing and irrigation of the nasolacrimal duct can be done in an office setting.

BIBLIOGRAPHY

1. Bashour M. (2012). Congenital Anomalies of the Nasolacrimal Duct. [online] Available from www.emedicine.com/oph/TOPIC592.HTM. [Accessed October, 2013].

2B. STASIS

General

Inflammation in the lacrimal sac resulting from stasis of tears in lacrimal drainage system and secondary infection by bacteria or fungus. Dacryolith is concretion of material in canaliculi or lacrimal sac.

Clinical

None.

Ocular

Redness and tenderness of medial area.

Laboratory

Diagnosis is made by clinical findings.

Treatment

Warm compresses and topical antibiotics, pressure over the sac to express material into conjunctiva, topical nystatin, external DCR.

BIBLIOGRAPHY

1. Gilliland GD. (2012). Dacryocystitis. [online] Available from www.emedicine.com/oph/TOPIC708.HTM. [Accessed October, 2013].

2C. EPIPHORIA

General

Hypersecretion or failure of the lacrimal excretory system to function.

Clinical

Nasal pathology.

Ocular

Epiphoria, corneal foreign body, trichiasis, corneal ulcer, entropion, ectropion or lid retraction.

Laboratory

Diagnosis is made by clinical findings.

Treatment

Treat the underlying cause, massage the tear sac and antibiotics, conjunctival dacryocystorhinostomy (DCR) with Jones tube.

BIBLIOGRAPHY

1. Roy FH, Fraunfelder FW, Fraunfelder FT. Roy and Fraunfelder's Current Ocular Therapy, 6th edition. London, UK: Elsevier; 2008.

2D1. BRANCHIAL CLEFTS WITH CHARACTERISTIC FACIES, GROWTH RETARDATION, IMPERFORATE NASOLACRIMAL DUCT, AND PREMATURE AGING

General

Autosomal dominant.

Ocular

Strabismus; obstructed nasolacrimal ducts.

Clinical

Low-birth weight; retarded growth; bilateral bronchial cleft sinuses; broad nasal bridge; protruding upper lip; carp mouth; premature aging; malformed ears; linear skin lesions behind the ears.

Laboratory

Diagnosis is made by clinical findings.

Treatment

- *Strabismus*: Equalized vision with correct refractive error; surgery may be helpful in patients with diplopia.
- *Obstructed nasolacrimal ducts*: It may spontaneously resolve during the 1st year of life with massage if not probing and irrigation of the nasolacrimal duct can be done.

BIBLIOGRAPHY

1. Tewfik TL, Al-Noury KI. (2011). Manifestations of craniofacial syndromes. [online] Available from www.emedicine.com/ent/TOPIC319.HTM. [Accessed October, 2013].

2D2. WALKER-CLODIUS SYNDROME (LOBSTER CLAW DEFORMITY WITH NASOLACRIMAL OBSTRUCTION; EEC; ECTRODACTYLY, ECTODERMAL DYSPLASIA, AND CLEFT LIP/PALATE)

General

Autosomal dominant; both sexes are affected; onset from birth; association with chromosome 7 abnormalities.

Ocular

Hypertelorism; nasolacrimal obstruction with constant epiphora; mucopurulent conjunctival discharge; keratitis; nanocanalization of the lacrimal duct.

Clinical

Deformities of hands and feet (lobster claw); absence of both index and middle fingers and second metacarpals with rudimentary third metacarpals; syndactylism; cleft palate and lips; deafness; ear malformation; renal anomalies.

Laboratory

Chromosomal evaluation.

Treatment

See a specialist for general body problems.

⊟ BIBLIOGRAPHY

1. Fukushima Y, Ohashi H, Hasegawa T. The breakpoints of the EEC syndrome (ectrodactyly, ectodermal dysplasia and cleft lip/palate) confirmed to 7q11.21 and 9p12 by fluorescence in situ hybridization. Clin Genet. 1993;44(1):50.
2. Walker JC, Clodius L. The syndromes of cleft lip, cleft palate and lobster-claw deformities of hands and feet. Plast Reconstr Surg. 1963;32:627-36.
3. Wiegmann OA, Walker FA. The syndrome of lobster claw deformity and nasolacrimal obstruction. J Pediatr Ophthalmol. 1970;7:79.

CHAPTER

28

Lens

🗗 1. ADULT CATARACTS

General

Cataract is a disorder in which the crystalline lens becomes opacified.

Clinical

None.

Ocular

Glare, monocular diplopia, changes in refractive error, decreased visual acuity.

Laboratory

Diagnosis is made by clinical findings.

Treatment

Change in glasses can sometimes improve a patient's visual function temporarily; however the most common treatment is cataract surgery.

🗗 BIBLIOGRAPHY

1. Roy FH, Fraunfelder FW, Fraunfelder FT. Roy and Fraunfelder's Current Ocular Therapy, 6th edition. London, UK: Elsevier; 2008.

🗗 2. AFTER CATARACTS

General

"After cataract" is a term originally used to describe lens epithelial cell proliferation following cataract surgery.

Clinical

None.

Ocular

Posterior capsule opacification, delayed endophthalmitis.

Laboratory

Diagnosis is made by clinical findings.

Treatment

Laser posterior capsulotomy.

🗗 BIBLIOGRAPHY

1. Roy FH, Fraunfelder FW, Fraunfelder FT. Roy and Fraunfelder's Current Ocular Therapy, 6th edition. London, UK: Elsevier; 2008.

⊟ 3. ALSTRÖM DISEASE (CATARACT AND RETINITIS PIGMENTOSA)

General

Retinal lesion associated with deafness; severe visual loss in the 1st decade.

Ocular

Cataract; retinitis pigmentosa; optic atrophy; salt and pepper pigment epithelial abnormalities. Electroretinogram pathognomonic findings include initially normal rod component, which can become undetectable as early as 5 years of age; undetectable cone activity at 18 months.

Clinical

Nerve deafness; diabetes mellitus in childhood; obesity; renal disease; baldness; hyperuricemia; hypogenitalism; acanthosis nigricans; skeletal anomalies; diabetes mellitus; deafness.

Laboratory

Diagnosis is made by clinical findings.

Treatment

- *Cataract*: Change in glasses can sometimes improve a patient's visual function temporarily; however the most common treatment is cataract surgery.
- *Retinitis pigmentosa*: Vitamin A 15,000 IU/day is thought to slow the decline of retinal function; dark sunglasses for outdoor use; surgery for cataract; genetic counseling.

⊟ BIBLIOGRAPHY

1. Geeraets WJ. Ocular Syndromes, 3rd edition. Philadelphia, PA: Lea & Febiger; 1976.
2. Konigsmark BW, Knox DL, Hussels IE, et al. Dominant congenital deafness and progressive optic nerve atrophy. Occurrence in four generations of a family. Arch Ophthalmol. 1974;91(2):99-103.
3. Millay RH, Weleber RG, Heckenlively JR. Ophthalmologic and systemic manifestations of Alström's disease. Am J Ophthalmol. 1986;102(4):482-90.
4. Nelson LB, Harley RD (Eds). Harley's Pediatric Ophthalmology, 4th edition. Philadelphia, PA: WB Saunders; 1998.
5. Tremblay F, LaRoche RG, Shea SE, et al. Longitudinal study of the early electroretinographic changes in Alström's syndrome. Am J Ophthalmol. 1993;115(5):657-65.

⊟ 4. ANDOGSKY SYNDROME (ATOPIC CATARACT SYNDROME; DERMATOGENOUS CATARACT)

General

Inherited abnormality involving the skin and lens with an altered reactivity to antigen.

Ocular

Atopic keratoconjunctivitis; keratoconus; uveitis; dense subcapsular cataract developing to a complete dense opacification.

Clinical

Atopic dermatitis as erythematous thickening of the skin with papular hyperpigmented and scaly changes; most frequently found in regions of the wrist, popliteal fossa, neck and sometimes forehead.

Laboratory

Diagnosis is made by clinical findings.

Treatment

Uveitis treatment includes topical steroids and cycloplegic medication should be the initial treatment of choice. Oral steroids should be given if not responsive to topical steroids, immunosuppressants if bilateral disease that does not respond to oral steroids, periocular steroids for unilateral or posterior uveitis. Vitrectomy can be used for severe vitreous opacification. Cryotherapy and laser photocoagulation may be used for localized pars plana exudates. Cataract can be treated by change in glasses which can sometimes improve a patient's visual function temporarily; however the most common treatment is cataract surgery.

⊟ BIBLIOGRAPHY

1. Andogsky N. Cataracts Dermatogenes. Ein Beitrag zur Aetiologieder Linsentrubung. Klin Monatsbl Augenheilk. 1914;52:824.
2. Coles RS, Laval J. Retinal detachments occurring in cataract associated with neurodermatitis. AMA Arch Ophthalmol. 1952;48(1):30-9.
3. Geeraets WJ. Ocular Syndromes, 3rd edition. Philadelphia, PA: Lea & Febiger; 1976.
4. Magalini SI, Scrascia E. Dictionary of Medical Syndromes, 2nd edition. Philadelphia, PA: JB Lippincott; 1981.

🖻 5. CATARACT, ANTERIOR POLAR

General

Autosomal dominant; imperfect separation of lens from the surface of ectoderm during 5th week of embryologic development; abnormal mass in the region of anterior pole and incomplete resorption of blood vessels and mesoderm at anterior pole of embryonic lens; they can be associated with chromosomal abnormalities including 3;18 chromosomal translocation.

Ocular

Small opacities on anterior surface of lens; microphthalmia; cataracts usually do not interfere with vision; corneal astigmatism.

Clinical

None.

Laboratory

Diagnosis is made by clinical findings.

Treatment

Cataract surgery if vision decreases.

🖻 BIBLIOGRAPHY

1. Bouzas AG. Anterior polar congenital cataract and corneal astigmatism. J Pediatr Ophthalmol Strabismus. 1992;29(4): 210-2.
2. McKusick VA. Mendelian Inheritance in Man: A Catalog of Human Genes and Genetic Disorders, 12th edition. Baltimore, USA: The Johns Hopkins University Press; 1998.
3. Moross T, Vaithilingam SS, Styles S, et al. Autosomal dominant anterior polar cataracts associated with a familial 2;14 translocation. J Med Genet. 1984;21(1):52-3.
4. Online Mendelian Inheritance in Man, OMIM. (2007). McKusick-Nathans Institute for Genetic Medicine, Johns Hopkins University and National Center for Biotechnology Information, National Library of Medicine, February 12, 2007. [online] Available from www.ncbi.nlm.nih.gov/omim. [Accessed October, 2013].
5. Rubin SE, Nelson LB, Pletcher BA. Anterior polar cataract in two sisters with an unbalanced 3;18 chromosomal translocation. Am J Ophthalmol. 1994;117(4):512-5.

🖻 6. CATARACT AND CONGENITAL ICHTHYOSIS

General

Autosomal recessive; rare.

Ocular

Cortical cataract.

Clinical

Ichthyosis.

Laboratory

Diagnosis is made by clinical findings.

Treatment

Cataract: Change in glasses can sometimes improve a patient's visual function temporarily; however the most common treatment is cataract surgery.

🖻 BIBLIOGRAPHY

1. McKusick VA. Mendelian Inheritance in Man: A Catalog of Human Genes and Genetic Disorders, 12th edition. Baltimore, USA: The Johns Hopkins University Press; 1998.
2. Online Mendelian Inheritance in Man, OMIM. (2007). McKusick-Nathans Institute for Genetic Medicine, Johns Hopkins University and National Center for Biotechnology Information, National Library of Medicine, February 12, 2007. [online] Available from www.ncbi.nlm.nih.gov/omim. [Accessed October, 2013].
3. Pinkerton OD. Cataract associated with congenital ichthyosis. AMA Arch Ophthalmol. 1958;60(3):393-6.

7. CATARACT, CONGENITAL OR JUVENILE (CATARACT, JUVENILE, HUTTERITE TYPE)

General

Autosomal recessive; seen most frequently in the people of Japanese origin; autosomal dominant inheritance also has been reported.

Ocular

Retinitis pigmentosa; Usher syndrome (retinitis pigmentosa and congenital deafness); congenital cataract of the "i" phenotype; microphthalmos; keratoconus.

Clinical

Congenital deafness; galactokinase deficiency; epimerase deficiency.

Laboratory

Diagnosis is made by clinical findings.

Treatment

- *Cataract*: Change in glasses can sometimes improve a patient's visual function temporarily; however the most common treatment is cataract surgery.
- *Retinitis pigmentosa*: Vitamin A 15,000 IU/day is thought to slow the decline of retinal function; dark sunglasses for outdoor use; surgery for cataract; genetic counseling.

BIBLIOGRAPHY

1. McKusick VA. Mendelian Inheritance in Man: A Catalog of Human Genes and Genetic Disorders, 12th edition. Baltimore, USA: The Johns Hopkins University Press; 1998.
2. Online Mendelian Inheritance in Man, OMIM. (2007). McKusick-Nathans Institute for Genetic Medicine, Johns Hopkins University and National Center for Biotechnology Information, National Library of Medicine, February 12, 2007. [online] Available from www.ncbi.nlm.nih.gov/omim. [Accessed October, 2013].

8. CATARACT, CONGENITAL TOTAL WITH POSTERIOR SUTURAL OPACITIES

General

Sex-linked; initial lens changes occur in both men and women with continuation of process in men; women show progression at much later age; it has been suggested that several X-linked cataract syndromes are due to deletions of different sizes in the X chromosome.

Ocular

Y-shaped sutural cataracts; congenital cataracts; nuclear cataract; cortical cataract; posterior subcapsular cataract; asymptomatic posterior Y-sutural cataracts; severe visual impairment; bilateral pendular nystagmus; bilateral microcornea; exotropia; keratoconus.

Clinical

Mental retardation.

Laboratory

Diagnosis is made by clinical findings.

Treatment

Cataract surgery.

BIBLIOGRAPHY

1. Crews SJ, Bundey SE. Is there an X-linked form of congenital cataracts? Clin Genet. 1982;21(5):351-3.
2. McKusick VA. Mendelian Inheritance in Man: A Catalog of Human Genes and Genetic Disorders, 12th edition. Baltimore, USA: The Johns Hopkins University Press; 1998.
3. Online Mendelian Inheritance in Man, OMIM. (2007). McKusick-Nathans Institute for Genetic Medicine, Johns Hopkins University and National Center for Biotechnology Information, National Library of Medicine, February 12, 2007. [online] Available from www.ncbi.nlm.nih.gov/omim/. [Accessed October, 2013].
4. Warburg M. X-linked cataract and X-linked microphthalmos: how many deletion families? Am J Med Genet. 1989;34(3):451-3.

9. CATARACT, CRYSTALLINE ACULEIFORM OR FROSTED

General

Autosomal dominant.

Ocular

Small crystal-like opacities of lens.

Clinical

None.

Laboratory

Diagnosis is made by clinical findings.

Treatment

Cataract surgery if vision decreases.

BIBLIOGRAPHY

1. Gifford SR, Puntenney I. Coralliform cataract and a new form of congenital cataract with crystals in the lens. Arch Ophthalmol. 1937;17(5):885-92.
2. McKusick VA. Mendelian Inheritance in Man: A Catalog of Human Genes and Genetic Disorders, 12th edition. Baltimore, USA: The Johns Hopkins University Press; 1998.
3. Online Mendelian Inheritance in Man, OMIM. (2007). McKusick-Nathans Institute for Genetic Medicine, Johns Hopkins University and National Center for Biotechnology Information, National Library of Medicine, February 12, 2007. [online] Available from www.ncbi.nlm.nih.gov/omim. [Accessed October, 2013].

10. CATARACT, CRYSTALLINE CORALLIFORM

General

Autosomal dominant.

Ocular

Cataracts characterized by fine crystals in the axial region of the lens.

Clinical

None.

Laboratory

Diagnosis is made by clinical findings.

Treatment

Cataract surgery if vision decreases.

BIBLIOGRAPHY

1. Bey MR. Congenital familial cataract with cholesterin deposits. Br J Ophthalmol. 1938;22(12):745-9.
2. McKusick VA. Mendelian Inheritance in Man: A Catalog of Human Genes and Genetic Disorders, 12th edition. Baltimore, USA: The Johns Hopkins University Press; 1998.
3. Online Mendelian Inheritance in Man, OMIM. (2007). McKusick-Nathans Institute for Genetic Medicine, Johns Hopkins University and National Center for Biotechnology Information, National Library of Medicine, February 12, 2007. [online] Available from www.ncbi.nlm.nih.gov/omim. [Accessed October, 2013].

11. CATARACT, FLORIFORM

General

Autosomal dominant; rare.

Ocular

Lens opacity takes the form of annular elements, arranged either independently or grouped together like petals of a flower; lenticonus; aniridia.

Clinical

None.

Laboratory

Diagnosis is made by clinical findings.

Treatment

Cataract surgery if vision decreases.

BIBLIOGRAPHY

1. Doggart JH. Congenital cataract. Trans Opthal Soc UK. 1957;77:31-7.
2. McKusick VA. Mendelian Inheritance in Man: A Catalog of Human Genes and Genetic Disorders, 12th edition. Baltimore, USA: The Johns Hopkins University Press; 1998.
3. Online Mendelian Inheritance in Man, OMIM. (2007). McKusick-Nathans Institute for Genetic Medicine, Johns Hopkins University and National Center for Biotechnology Information, National Library of Medicine, February 12, 2007. [online] Available from www.ncbi.nlm.nih.gov/omim. [Accessed October, 2013].

⊟ 12. CATARACT, MEMBRANOUS

General

Autosomal dominant.

Ocular

Total cataract that has undergone regression or resorption.

Clinical

None.

Laboratory

Diagnosis is made by clinical findings.

Treatment

Cataract surgery if vision decreases.

⊟ BIBLIOGRAPHY

1. Gruber M. Ueber Primaere Familaere Linsendysplasie. Ophthalmologica. 1945;110:60-72.
2. McKusick VA. Mendelian Inheritance in Man: A Catalog of Human Genes and Genetic Disorders, 12th edition. Baltimore, USA: The Johns Hopkins University Press; 1998.
3. Online Mendelian Inheritance in Man, OMIM. (2007). McKusick-Nathans Institute for Genetic Medicine, Johns Hopkins University and National Center for Biotechnology Information, National Library of Medicine, February 12, 2007. [online] Available from www.ncbi.nlm.nih.gov/omim. [Accessed October, 2013].

⊟ 13. CATARACT, MICROCORNEA SYNDROME

General

Autosomal dominant; prominent in Sicilian families.

Ocular

Cataracts; microcornea; myopia.

Clinical

None.

Laboratory

Diagnosis is made by clinical findings.

Treatment

Cataract surgery if vision decreases.

⊟ BIBLIOGRAPHY

1. McKusick VA. Mendelian Inheritance in Man: A Catalog of Human Genes and Genetic Disorders, 12th edition. Baltimore, USA: The Johns Hopkins University Press; 1998.
2. Mollica F, Li Volti S, Tomarchio S, et al. Autosomal dominant cataract and microcornea associated with myopia in a Sicilian family. Clin Genet. 1985;28(1):42-6.
3. Online Mendelian Inheritance in Man, OMIM. (2007). McKusick-Nathans Institute for Genetic Medicine, Johns Hopkins University and National Center for Biotechnology Information, National Library of Medicine, February 12, 2007. [online] Available from www.ncbi.nlm.nih.gov/omim. [Accessed October, 2013].
4. Polomeno RC, Cummings C. Autosomal dominant cataracts and microcornea. Can J Ophthalmol. 1979;14(4):227-9.
5. Salmon JF, Wallis CE, Murray AD. Variable expressivity of autosomal dominant microcornea with cataract. Arch Ophthalmol. 1988;106(4):505-10.

⊟ 14. CATARACT, MICROPHTHALMIA AND NYSTAGMUS

General

Autosomal recessive.

Ocular

Miosis; cataract; nystagmus; microphthalmia.

Clinical

None.

Laboratory

Diagnosis is made by clinical findings.

Treatment

Cataract surgery if vision decreases.

BIBLIOGRAPHY

1. McKusick VA. Mendelian Inheritance in Man: A Catalog of Human Genes and Genetic Disorders, 12th edition. Baltimore, USA: The Johns Hopkins University Press; 1998.
2. Online Mendelian Inheritance in Man, OMIM. (2007). McKusick-Nathans Institute for Genetic Medicine, Johns Hopkins University and National Center for Biotechnology Information, National Library of Medicine, February 12, 2007. [online] Available from www.ncbi.nlm.nih.gov/omim. [Accessed October, 2013].
3. Temtamy SA, Shalash BA. Genetic heterogeneity of the syndrome: microphthalmos with congenital cataract. Birth Defects Orig Artic Ser. 1974;10(4):292-3.
4. Zeiter HJ. Congenital microphthalmos. A pedigree of four affected siblings and an additional report of forty-four sporadic cases. Am J Ophthalmol. 1963;55:910-22.

15. CATARACT, NUCLEAR (COPPOCK CATARACT; CATARACT, DISCOID)

General

Autosomal dominant; epidemiologic evidence suggests that a single major gene can account for the correlation among siblings of nuclear sclerosis.

Ocular

Congenital zonular cataract; total nuclear cataract; fetal nucleus with scattered fine diffuse cortical opacities and incomplete cortical riders.

Clinical

None.

Laboratory

Diagnosis is made by clinical findings.

Treatment

Cataract surgery.

BIBLIOGRAPHY

1. Harman NB. Congenital cataract: a pedigree of five generations. Trans Opthal Soc UK. 1909;29:101-8.
2. Heiba IM, Elston RC, Klein BE, et al. Genetic etiology of nuclear cataract: evidence for a major gene. Am J Med Genet. 1993;47(8):1208-14.
3. Lee JB, Benedict WL. Hereditary nuclear cataract. AMA Arch Ophthalmol. 1950;44(5):643-50.
4. McKusick VA. Mendelian Inheritance in Man: A Catalog of Human Genes and Genetic Disorders, 12th edition. Baltimore, USA: The Johns Hopkins University Press; 1998.
5. Merin S. Inherited cataracts. In: Merin S (Ed). Inherited Eye Diseases. New York, USA: Marcel Dekker; 1991. pp. 86-120.
6. Online Mendelian Inheritance in Man, OMIM. (2007). McKusick-Nathans Institute for Genetic Medicine, Johns Hopkins University and National Center for Biotechnology Information, National Library of Medicine, February 12, 2007. [online] Available from www.ncbi.nlm.nih.gov/omim. [Accessed October, 2013].

16. CATARACT, NUCLEAR DIFFUSE NONPROGRESSIVE

General

Autosomal dominant; nonprogressive.

Ocular

Opacity of fetal nucleus resembles senile nuclear sclerosis.

Clinical

None.

Laboratory

Diagnosis is made by clinical findings.

Treatment

Cataract surgery if vision decreases.

BIBLIOGRAPHY

1. McKusick VA. Mendelian Inheritance in Man: A Catalog of Human Genes and Genetic Disorders, 12th edition. Baltimore, USA: The Johns Hopkins University Press; 1998.
2. Online Mendelian Inheritance in Man, OMIM. (2007). McKusick-Nathans Institute for Genetic Medicine, Johns Hopkins University and National Center for Biotechnology Information, National Library of Medicine, February 12, 2007. [online] Available from www.ncbi.nlm.nih.gov/omim. [Accessed October, 2013].

⊟ 17. CATARACT, POSTERIOR POLAR

General

Autosomal dominant; onset in childhood; progressive.

Ocular

Congenital posterior polar opacity; scattered cortical opacities; choroideremia; myopia.

Clinical

None.

Laboratory

Diagnosis is made by clinical findings.

Treatment

Cataract surgery if vision decreases.

⊟ BIBLIOGRAPHY

1. Binkhorst PG, Valk LE. A case of familial dwarfism, with choroideremia, myopia, posterior polar cataract, and zonular cataract. Ophthalmologica. 1956;132(5):299.
2. McKusick VA. Mendelian Inheritance in Man: A Catalog of Human Genes and Genetic Disorders, 12th edition. Baltimore, USA: The Johns Hopkins University Press; 1998.
3. Online Mendelian Inheritance in Man, OMIM. (2007). McKusick-Nathans Institute for Genetic Medicine, Johns Hopkins University and National Center for Biotechnology Information, National Library of Medicine, February 12, 2007. [online] Available from www.ncbi.nlm.nih.gov/omim. [Accessed October, 2013].

⊟ 18. CEREBELLAR ATAXIA, CATARACT, DEAFNESS, AND DEMENTIA OR PSYCHOSIS (HEREDOPATHIA OPHTHALMO-OTO-ENCEPHALICA)

General

Autosomal dominant.

Ocular

Posterior polar cataracts.

Clinical

Tremor, paranoid psychosis; dementia; deafness.

Laboratory

None.

Treatment

Cataract surgery if vision decreases.

⊟ BIBLIOGRAPHY

1. McKusick VA. Mendelian Inheritance in Man: A Catalog of Human Genes and Genetic Disorders, 12th edition. Baltimore, USA: The Johns Hopkins University Press; 1998.
2. Online Mendelian Inheritance in Man, OMIM. (2007). McKusick-Nathans Institute for Genetic Medicine, Johns Hopkins University and National Center for Biotechnology Information, National Library of Medicine, February 12, 2007. [online] Available from www.ncbi.nlm.nih.gov/omim. [Accessed October, 2013].
3. Stromgren E. Heredopathia Ophthalmo-oto-encephalica. Neurogenetic Directory. Handbook Clin Neurol. 1981;42: 150-2.

⊟ 19. CEREBELLAR ATAXIA, INFANTILE, WITH PROGRESSIVE EXTERNAL OPHTHALMOPLEGIA

General

Autosomal recessive; neurologic lesion.

Ocular

Paralysis of all extraocular muscles; ptosis; retinal degeneration; blindness.

Clinical

Spinocerebellar degeneration; ataxia.

Laboratory

None.

Treatment

None.

BIBLIOGRAPHY

1. Jampel RS, Okazaki H, Bernstein H. Ophthalmoplegia and retinal degeneration associated with spinocerebellar ataxia. Arch Ophthalmol. 1961;66:247-59.
2. McKusick VA. Mendelian Inheritance in Man: A Catalog of Human Genes and Genetic Disorders, 12th edition. Baltimore, USA: The Johns Hopkins University Press; 1998.
3. Online Mendelian Inheritance in Man, OMIM. (2007). McKusick-Nathans Institute for Genetic Medicine, Johns Hopkins University and National Center for Biotechnology Information, National Library of Medicine, February 12, 2007. [online] Available from www.ncbi.nlm.nih.gov/omim. [Accessed October, 2013].

20. CONGENITAL CATARACTS FACIAL DYSMORPHISM NEUROPATHY SYNDROME

General

Autosomal recessive; motor and sensory neuropathy.

Ocular

Congenital cataracts, microcorneas, strabismus, pendular nystagmus, bilateral blepharoptosis.

Clinical

Patients are recognized in infancy by the presence of congenital cataracts and microcorneas; initially, a predominantly motor neuropathy begins in the lower limbs followed by upper limb involvement; severe disability occurs by the 3rd decade; short stature, moderate nonprogressive cognitive deficits, pyramidal signs and mild chorea are characteristic.

Laboratory

Diagnosis is made by clinical findings.

Treatment

Change in glasses can sometimes improve a patient's visual function temporarily; however the most common treatment is cataract surgery.

BIBLIOGRAPHY

1. Müllner-Eidenböck A, Moser E, Klebermass N, et al. Ocular features of the congenital cataracts facial dysmorphism neuropathy syndrome. Ophthalmology. 2004;111(7):1415-23.
2. Tournev I, Kalaydjieva L, Youl B, et al. Congenital cataracts facial dysmorphism neuropathy syndrome, a novel complex genetic disease in Balkan Gypsies: clinical and electrophysiological observations. Ann Neurol. 1999;45(6):742-50.

21. CONGENITAL CATARACT, MICROCORNEA, ABNORMAL IRIDES, NYSTAGMUS AND CONGENITAL GLAUCOMA SYNDROME

General

Autosomal dominant.

Ocular

Microphakia; cataract with two concentric disks, with the anterior being swollen; microphthalmos; microcornea; nystagmus; congenital glaucoma; honey-colored iris with absence of pattern; peripheral anterior synechiae; pupillary abnormality; corneal edema; posterior synechiae; vitreous hemorrhage; shallow anterior chamber; vitreous loss; corneal staphyloma; keratoconus.

Clinical

High-arched palate; increased webbing of fingers and toes; deafness.

Laboratory

Diagnosis is made by clinical findings.

Treatment

Cataract surgery if vision decreases.

BIBLIOGRAPHY

1. Cebon L, West RH. A syndrome involving congenital cataracts of unusual morphology, microcornea, abnormal irides, nystagmus, and congenital glaucoma, inherited as an autosomal dominant trait. Aust J Ophthalmol. 1982;10(4):237-42.
2. Henkind P, Friedman AH. Iridogoniodysgenesis with cataract. Am J Ophthalmol. 1971;72(5):949-54.

22. CONGENITAL CATARACT WITH OXYCEPHALY (TOWER SKULL SYNDROME)

General

Autosomal dominant; craniostenosis.

Ocular

Congenital cataracts; keratoconus.

Clinical

Large fontanels; deformed skull; dwarfing; osteopetrosis.

Laboratory

Diagnosis is made by clinical findings.

Treatment

Cataract surgery if vision decreases.

BIBLIOGRAPHY

1. McKusick VA. Mendelian Inheritance in Man: A Catalog of Human Genes and Genetic Disorders, 12th edition. Baltimore, USA: The Johns Hopkins University Press; 1998.
2. Online Mendelian Inheritance in Man, OMIM. (2007). McKusick-Nathans Institute for Genetic Medicine, Johns Hopkins University and National Center for Biotechnology Information, National Library of Medicine, February 12, 2007. [online] Available from www.ncbi.nlm.nih.gov/omim. [Accessed October, 2013].
3. Roy FH. Ocular Differential Diagnosis, 9th edition. New Delhi, India: Jaypee Brothers Medical Publishers (P) Ltd; 2012.

23. DESERT LUNG AND CATARACT SYNDROME

General

Non-occupational pneumoconiosis; common in desert areas; excessive exposure to atmospheric dust; inhalant of fine, sandy dust.

Ocular

Cataracts (posterior subcapsular most prevalent); corneal opacities.

Clinical

Miliary infiltrates; thickening of bronchial walls; mild restrictive changes with pulmonary function.

Laboratory

Chest X-ray, ultrasound, computed tomography (CT) and bronchoscopy.

Treatment

Maintenance of airways and clearance of secretions with tracheal suctioning; oxygen supplementation; antibiotics.

BIBLIOGRAPHY

1. Ocampo VV, Foster CS. (2013). Senile cataract. [online] Available from www.emedicine.com/oph/TOPIC49.HTM. [Accessed October, 2013].

24. DISLOCATION OF INTRAOCULAR LENS

General

Following cataract surgery or yttrium aluminum garnet (YAG) posterior capsulotomy. Intraocular lens (IOL) malpositions range from decentration to luxation into the posterior segment. Subluxated IOLs involve such extreme decentration that the IOL optic covers only a small fraction of the pupillary space. Luxation involves total dislocation of the IOL into the posterior segment. Causes include improper fixation, trauma, internal forces such as scarring, anterior synechiae and capsular contraction with pseudoexfoliation syndrome.

Clinical

Facial trauma.

Ocular

Pseudoexfoliation; decreased vision, edge glare, diplopia streaks of light; haloes; photophobia; ghost images; aphakia; retinal detachment; cystoid macular edema; vitreous hemorrhage; irregular pupil; corneal decompensation; torn zonules.

Laboratory

Generally diagnosis is made by clinical observation. If vitreous hemorrhage or severe corneal edema is present, B-scan ultrasonic imaging may be necessary to determine the position of the IOL.

Treatment

In the absence of symptoms, observation is the necessary treatment. Intraocular lens repositioning with or without a McConnell's suture; IOL exchange and IOL explantation are all surgical procedures used in the more severe, symptomatic cases.

BIBLIOGRAPHY

1. Wu L, Evans T, García RA, et al. (2011). Intraocular lens dislocation. [online] Available from emedicine.medscape.com/article/1211310-overview. [Accessed October, 2013].

25. DISLOCATION OF THE LENS

General

Ectopia lentis, occurs when the lens is not in its normal position.

Clinical

Marfan syndrome, Weill-Marchesani syndrome, sulfite-oxidase deficiency.

Laboratory

Diagnosis is made by clinical findings.

Treatment

Careful phacoemulsification; topical steroids should be given to control ocular inflammation.

BIBLIOGRAPHY

1. Eifrig CW. (2011). Ectopia lentis. [online] Available from www.emedicine.com/oph/TOPIC55.HTM. [Accessed October, 2013].

26. FOVEAL HYPOPLASIA AND PRESENILE CATARACT SYNDROME (O'DONNELL-PAPPAS SYNDROME)

General

Autosomal dominant.

Ocular

Foveal hypoplasia; nystagmus; presenile cataract; peripheral corneal pannus.

Clinical

None.

Laboratory

Diagnosis is made by clinical findings.

Treatment

Cataract: Change in glasses can sometimes improve a patient's visual function temporarily; however the most common treatment is cataract surgery.

BIBLIOGRAPHY

1. Roy FH. Ocular Syndromes and Systemic Diseases, 5th edition. New Delhi: Jaypee Brothers Medical Publishers; 2013.

27. HYPOGONADISM-CATARACT SYNDROME

General

Autosomal recessive.

Ocular

Cataracts.

Clinical

Elevated follicle-stimulating hormone levels; myotonic dystrophy; infertility.

Laboratory

Diagnosis is made by clinical findings.

Treatment

Cataract surgery is the therapy of choice if there is visual limitation.

BIBLIOGRAPHY

1. Lubinsky MS. Cataracts and testicular failure in three brothers. Am J Med Genet. 1983;16(2):149-52.
2. McKusick VA. Mendelian Inheritance in Man: A Catalog of Human Genes and Genetic Disorders, 12th edition. Baltimore, USA: The Johns Hopkins University Press; 1998.

28.1. IRIDESCENT CRYSTALLINE DEPOSITS IN LENS

1. Idiopathic
2. Hypothyroid (cretinism)
3. Hypocalcemia
   A. Postoperative: Removal of thyroid and accidental parathyroid removal
   B. Idiopathic hypoparathyroidism
   C. Pseudohypoparathyroidism or with hyperphosphatemia
4. Myotonic dystrophy (Curschmann-Steinert syndrome)
5. Drugs, including the following:
   - Acetophenazine
   - Amiodarone
   - Auranofin
   - Aurothioglucose
   - Aurothioglycanide
   - Butaperazine
   - Carphenazine
   - Chlorpromazine
   - Chlorprothixene
   - Colloidal silver
   - Diazepam (?)
   - Diethazine
   - Ethopropazine
   - Fluphenazine
   - Gold (Au) 198
   - Gold sodium thiomalate
   - Gold sodium thiosulfate
   - Mercuric oxide
   - Mesoridazine
   - Methdilazine
   - Methotrimeprazine
   - Mild silver protein
   - Perazine
   - Pericyazine
   - Perphenazine
   - Phenylmercuric acetate
   - Phenylmercuric nitrate
   - Piperacetazine
   - Prochlorperazine
   - Promazine
   - Promethazine
   - Propiomazine
   - Silver nitrate
   - Silver protein
   - Thiethylperazine
   - Thiopropazate
   - Thioridazine
   - Thiothixene
   - Trifluoperazine
   - Triflupromazine
   - Trimeprazine
6. Cataract (coralliform and aculeiform) usually autosomal dominant; sometimes recessive.

BIBLIOGRAPHY

1. Fraunfelder FT, Fraunfelder FW. Drug-induced ocular side effects. Woburn, MA: Butterworth-Heinemann; 2001.

⌸ 28.2. CRETINISM (HYPOTHYROID GOITER; HYPOTHYROIDISM; JUVENILE HYPOTHYROIDISM; MYXEDEMA)

General

Deficient thyroid function.

Ocular

Blepharitis; ptosis; enophthalmos; temporal madarosis; decreased tear secretion; glaucoma; proptosis; optic atrophy; optic neuritis; blue dot cataract; conjunctivitis; scleritis; optic disk hemorrhage and arcuate scotoma associated with glaucoma.

Clinical

Myxedema; larynx and tongue swollen; hoarse speech; dry, yellowish skin; slow pulse; mental retardation; infertility; pericardial effusion; cardiac enlargement; physical development retarded.

Laboratory

Clinical.

Treatment

- *Blepharitis*: Oral tetracyclines, omega-3 fatty acids, flax seed oil or fish oil. Ocular therapy include eyelid scrubs, warm compresses, bacitricin ointment to lid margins, topical cyclosporine A and preservative free lubricants.
- *Ptosis*: If visual acuity is affected, most cases require surgical correction and there are several procedures that may be used including levator resection, repair or advancement and Fasanella-Servat.
- *Glaucoma*: Glaucoma medication should be the first plan of action. If medication is unsuccessful, a filtering surgical procedure with or without antimetabotites may be beneficial.
- *Cataract*: Change in glasses can sometimes improve a patient's visual function temporarily; however the most common treatment is cataract surgery.

⌸ BIBLIOGRAPHY

1. Daniel MS, Postellon DC. (2013). Congenital hypothyroidism. [online] Available from www.emedicine.com/ped/TOPIC501.HTM. [Accessed October, 2013].

⌸ 28.3. HYPOCALCEMIA

General

Serum calcium level depressed; secondary hypocalcemia can result following foscarnet treatment for cytomegalovirus retinitis in patients with acquired immunodeficiency syndrome.

Ocular

Conjunctivitis; blepharitis; blepharospasm; madarosis; ptosis; cataract; papilledema; strabismus.

Clinical

Chronic renal failure; hypoparathyroidism; hypoproteinemia; hypomagnesemia; malabsorption; acute pancreatitis; osteoblastic metastases; rickets; osteomalacia; medullary carcinoma of the thyroid; neuromuscular abnormalities.

Laboratory

Serum calcium, magnesium level, serum electrolyte and glucose levels, phosphorus levels and parathyroid hormone (PTH) levels.

Treatment

Intravenous treatment is usually indicated in patients having seizures, those who are critically ill, and those who are planning to have surgery. Oral calcium therapy is used in asymptomatic patients and as follow-up to intravenous calcium therapy.

⌸ BIBLIOGRAPHY

1. Sinha S, Singhal A, Campbell DE. (2012). Pediatric Hypocalcemia. [online] Available from www.emedicine.com/ped/TOPIC1111.HTM. [Accessed October, 2013].

28.3A. CRETINISM (HYPOTHYROID GOITER; HYPOTHYROIDISM; JUVENILE HYPOTHYROIDISM; MYXEDEMA)

General

Deficient thyroid function.

Ocular

Blepharitis; ptosis; enophthalmos; temporal madarosis; decreased tear secretion; glaucoma; proptosis; optic atrophy; optic neuritis; blue dot cataract; conjunctivitis; scleritis; optic disk hemorrhage and arcuate scotoma associated with glaucoma.

Clinical

Myxedema; larynx and tongue swollen; hoarse speech; dry, yellowish skin; slow pulse; mental retardation; infertility; pericardial effusion; cardiac enlargement; physical development retarded.

Laboratory

Clinical.

Treatment

- *Blepharitis*: Oral tetracyclines, omega-3 fatty acids, flax seed oil or fish oil. Ocular therapy include eyelid scrubs, warm compresses, bacitracin ointment to lid margins, topical cyclosporine A and preservative free lubricants.
- *Ptosis*: If visual acuity is affected, most cases require surgical correction and there are several procedures that may be used including levator resection, repair or advancement and Fasanella-Servat.
- *Glaucoma*: Glaucoma medication should be the first plan of action. If medication is unsuccessful, a filtering surgical procedure with or without antimetabolites may be beneficial.
- *Cataract*: Change in glasses can sometimes improve a patient's visual function temporarily; however the most common treatment is cataract surgery.

BIBLIOGRAPHY

1. Daniel MS, Postellon DC. (2013). Congenital hypothyroidism. [online] Available from www.emedicine.com/ped/TOPIC501.HTM. [Accessed October, 2013].

28.3B. HYPOPARATHYROIDISM

General

Deficient secretion of PTH.

Ocular

Keratitis; blepharospasm; ptosis; cataract; madarosis; optic neuritis; papilledema; conjunctivitis; myopia; ocular colobomata.

Clinical

Decreased blood calcium; increased serum phosphate; tetany; muscle cramps; stridor; carpopedal spasms; convulsions; lethargy; personality changes; mental retardation; intracranial calcification; choreoathetosis; hemiballismus; renal agenesis.

Laboratory

Diagnosis made rests on the functional capacity of the adrenal cortex to synthesize cortisol. This is accomplished primarily by use of the rapid adrenocorticotropic hormone (ACTH) stimulation test (Cortrosyn, Cosyntropin, or Synacthen).

Treatment

Endocrinologist should be consulted for the acute care and chronic care.

BIBLIOGRAPHY

1. Gonzalez-Campoy JM. (2012). Hypoparathyroidism. [online] Available from www.emedicine.com/med/TOPIC1131.HTM. [Accessed October, 2013].

28.3C. PSEUDOHYPOPARATHYROIDISM SYNDROME (CHRONIC RENAL TUBULAR INSUFFICIENCY SYNDROME; SEABRIGHT-BANTAM SYNDROME; ALBRIGHT HEREDITARY OSTEODYSTROPHY)

General

Etiology unknown; autosomal dominant; more common in females (2:1); present from birth; kidney and skeleton fail to respond to PTH; if patients receive parathyroid extract, their kidneys fail to respond with phosphate diuresis; genetic form of hypoparathyroidism resulting from end-organ resistance to PTH; resulting hypocalcemia is responsible for many of the clinical features of this syndrome.

Ocular

Strabismus; blue sclera; punctate cataracts (white opacities and polychromatic cortex); papilledema; hypertelorism; keratitis; scleral and choroidal calcifications; blepharospasm; cataracts.

Clinical

Short stature; short metacarpals; short limbs; round face with short neck; decalcification of teeth; obesity; fat, stubby hands; tetany with positive Chvostek and Trousseau signs; atypical seizure disorder.

Laboratory

Hypocalcemia, hyperphosphatemia, and low PTH levels in the absence of renal failure or intestinal malabsorption.

Treatment

See papilledema and cataracts.

BIBLIOGRAPHY

1. Gliwa A, Wallace DJ. (2012). Hypoparathyroidism in Emergency Medicine. [online] Available from www.emedicine.com/emerg/TOPIC276.HTM. [Accessed October, 2013].

28.4. MYOTONIC DYSTROPHY SYNDROME (MYOTONIA ATROPHICA SYNDROME; DYSTROPHIA MYOTONICA; CURSCHMANN-STEINERT SYNDROME)

General

Rare autosomal dominant disease; onset at the age of 20 years; condition is worsened by administration of neostigmine (Prostigmin); associated with an unstable DNA sequence composed of varying numbers of CTG triplet repeats (which allows a specific molecular test for this disorder).

Ocular

Mild ptosis (occasionally); myotonic cataract with small, dot-like subcapsular cortical opacities during early stage, with polychromatic properties on biomicroscopic examination; corneal epithelial dystrophy; loss of corneal sensitivity; tapetoretinal degeneration; macular red spot; macular degeneration; chorioretinitis; pilomatrixomas; ocular hypotony; pattern pigmentary changes; abnormal saccades.

Clinical

Progressive muscular atrophy with selection of certain muscles (mainly sternocleidomastoid, temporalis, dorsiflexor muscles of the ankle, anterior oblique); myotonia; bland facial expression; speech disturbance due to involvement of vocal cords and palatal muscles; dysphagia; endocrine disturbances.

Laboratory

Diagnosis is made by clinical findings.

Treatment

- *Ptosis*: If visual acuity is affected, most cases require surgical correction and there are several procedures that may be used including levator resection, repair or advancement and Fasanella-Servat procedure.
- *Cataract*: Change in glasses can sometimes improve a patient's visual function temporarily; however, the most common treatment is cataract surgery.
- *Corneal dystrophy*: Mild cases can be observed and soft contact lenses are helpful; penetrating keratoplasty (PK) may be necessary; graft recurrences are treated by superficial keratectomy, phototherapeutic keratectomy (PTK) or repeat PK.

- *Macular degeneration*: No treatment is available for non-neovascular age-related macular degeneration (AMD). Preventative therapy includes no smoking, control of hypertension, cholesterol, and blood sugar, exercise and vitamins. Neovascular AMD treatment consists of laser, avastin and lucentis.

BIBLIOGRAPHY

1. Brooke NM, Cwik VE. Myotonic dystrophy. In: Bradley WG (Ed). Neurology in Clinical Practice: Principles of Diagnosis and Management, 2nd edition. Boston, USA: Butterworth-Heinemann; 1995. pp. 2020-2.
2. Gjertsen IK, Sandvig KU, Eide N, et al. Recurrence of secondary opacification and development of a dense posterior vitreous membrane in patients with myotonic dystrophy. J Cataract Refract Surg. 2003;29(1):213-6.
3. Kimizuka Y, Kiyosawa M, Tamai M, et al. Retinal changes in myotonic dystrophy. Clinical and follow-up evaluation. Retina. 1993;13(2):129-35.
4. Koca MR, Horn F, Korth M. Alterations of saccadic eye movements in myotonic dystrophy. Graefes Arch Clin Exp Ophthalmol. 1992;230(5):437-41.
5. Kuwabara T, Lessell S. Electron microscopic study of extraocular muscles in myotonic dystrophy. Am J Ophthalmol. 1976;82(2):303-9.
6. Mausolf FA, Burns CA, Burian HM. Morphologic and functional retinal changes in myotonic dystrophy unrelated to quinine therapy. Am J Ophthalmol. 1972;74(6):1141-3.
7. Meyer E, Navon D, Auslender L, et al. Myotonic dystrophy: pathological study of the eyes. Ophthalmologica. 1980; 181(3-4):215-20.
8. Reardon W, MacMillan JC, Myring J, et al. Cataract and myotonic dystrophy: the role of molecular diagnosis. Br J Ophthalmol. 1993;77(9):579-83.
9. Rosa N, Lanza M, Borrelli M, et al. Low intraocular pressure resulting from ciliary body detachment in patients with myotonic dystrophy. Ophthalmology. 2011;118(2):260-4.

28.5. CATARACT, CRYSTALLINE CORALLIFORM

General

Autosomal dominant.

Ocular

Cataracts characterized by fine crystals in the axial region of the lens.

Clinical

None.

Laboratory

Diagnosis is made by clinical findings.

Treatment

Cataract surgery if vision decreases.

BIBLIOGRAPHY

1. Bey MR. Congenital familial cataract with cholesterin deposits. Br J Ophthalmol. 1938;22(12):745-9.
2. McKusick VA. Mendelian Inheritance in Man: A Catalog of Human Genes and Genetic Disorders, 12th edition. Baltimore, USA: The Johns Hopkins University Press; 1998.
3. Online Mendelian Inheritance in Man, OMIM. (2007). McKusick-Nathans Institute for Genetic Medicine, Johns Hopkins University and National Center for Biotechnology Information, National Library of Medicine, February 12, 2007. [online] Available from www.ncbi.nlm.nih.gov/omim. [Accessed October, 2013].

28.6. CATARACT, CRYSTALLINE ACULEIFORM OR FROSTED

General

Autosomal dominant.

Ocular

Small crystal-like opacities of lens.

Clinical

None.

Laboratory

Diagnosis is made by clinical findings.

Treatment

Cataract surgery if vision decreases.

🗗 BIBLIOGRAPHY

1. Gifford SR, Puntenney I. Coralliform cataract and a new form of congenital cataract with crystals in the lens. Arch Ophthalmol. 1937;17(5):885-92.

2. McKusick VA. Mendelian Inheritance in Man: A Catalog of Human Genes and Genetic Disorders, 12th edition. Baltimore, USA: The Johns Hopkins University Press; 1998.

3. Online Mendelian Inheritance in Man, OMIM. (2007). McKusick-Nathans Institute for Genetic Medicine, Johns Hopkins University and National Center for Biotechnology Information, National Library of Medicine, February 12, 2007. [online] Available from www.ncbi.nlm.nih.gov/omim. [Accessed October, 2013].

🗗 29. KOBY SYNDROME (FLORIFORM CATARACT)

General

Autosomal dominant; both sexes are affected.

Ocular

Multiple opacities of different shapes (annular, floriform and polychromatic); found especially around embryonic nucleus.

Clinical

None.

Laboratory

Diagnosis is made by clinical findings.

Treatment

Cataract surgery should be considered if visual acuity is decreased.

🗗 BIBLIOGRAPHY

1. Bashour M, Menassa J, Gerontis CC. (2012). Congenital cataract. [online] Available from www.emedicine.com/oph/TOPIC45.HTM. [Accessed October, 2013].

🗗 30. LENS INDUCED GLAUCOMA (PHACOLYTIC, LENS PARTICLE AND PHACOANTIGENIC)

General

Open angle secondary glaucoma can be phacolytic, lens particle and phacoantigenic. Closed angle secondary lens glaucoma occurs from lens intumescence (phacomorphic glaucoma) or lens dislocation (ectopia lentis).

Clinical

None.

Ocular

Open or closed secondary glaucoma, cataract, retained lens material, uveitis.

Laboratory

Diagnosis is made by clinical findings.

Treatment

- *Mature or hypermature cataract*: Topical steroids, IOP lowering agents, hyperosmotic agents. Removal of cataract will usually restore normal IOP.
- *Lens particle glaucoma*: Topical IOP lowering agents, cycloplegics and steroids. Removal of residual lens material.
- *Phacoantigenic glaucoma*: Topical steroids, IOP lowering agents and cycloplegics. Pars plana vitrectomy is done to remove all residual lens material and posterior capsule or removal of capsule manually with forceps after injection of chymotrypsin beneath the iris.
- *Phacomorphic glaucoma*: Topical IOP lowering agents. Argon laser iridoplasty for open angle, laser iridotomy for bypass papillary block, cataract extraction.
- *Ectopia lentis*: Laser iridotomy for bypass papillary block. If lens floats in vitreous, treat conservatively.

🗗 BIBLIOGRAPHY

1. Sullivan BR. (2012). Lens-particle glaucoma. [online] Available from www.emedicine.com/oph/TOPIC56.HTM. [Accessed October, 2013].

2. Gill H, Juzychc MS, Goyal A. (2012). Phacomorphic glaucoma. [online] Available from www.emedicine.com/oph/TOPIC58.HTM. [Accessed October, 2013].

3. Yi K, Chen TC. (2011). Phacolytic glaucoma. [online] Available from www.emedicine.com/oph/TOPIC57.HTM. [Accessed October, 2013].

31. LENS-IRIS DIAPHRAGM RETROPULSION SYNDROME

General

It is associated with small incision phacoemulsification.

Ocular

Infusion of fluid into the anterior chamber; posterior displacement of the lens-iris diaphragm; posterior iris bowing; pupil dilatation; ocular discomfort.

Clinical

Deep anterior chamber with small incision phacoemulsification.

Laboratory

Diagnosis is made by clinical findings.

Treatment

Consider YAG iridotomy.

BIBLIOGRAPHY

1. Ocampo VV, Foster CS. (2013). Senile cataract. [online] Available from www.emedicine.com/oph/TOPIC49.HTM. [Accessed October, 2013].

32. LENTICONUS AND LENTIGLOBUS

General

Lenticonus is a circumscribed conical bulge of the anterior or more commonly, posterior lens capsule and cortex. In lentiglobus, the entire posterior capsule has a globular shape.

Clinical

Alport's syndrome, Waardenburg's syndrome.

Ocular

Oil droplet appearance, amblyopia, strabismus.

Laboratory

Diagnosis is made by clinical findings.

Treatment

Lens extraction with irrigation-aspiration.

BIBLIOGRAPHY

1. Roy FH, Fraunfelder FW, Fraunfelder FT. Roy and Fraunfelder's Current Ocular Therapy, 6th edition. London, UK: Elsevier; 2008.

33. LOST LENS SYNDROME

General

It occurs when IOL is completely dislocated into the vitreous cavity; it is caused by luxation of the implant through a zonular disinsertion or an unrecognized opening in the posterior capsule or trauma.

Ocular

Decreased visual acuity; retinal detachment; cystoid macular edema.

Clinical

None.

Laboratory

Diagnosis is made by clinical findings.

Treatment

If IOL is mobile, options include removal, exchange or repositioning of the IOL. Repositioning of the IOL into the ciliary sulcus or over capsular remnants with less than a total of 6 hours of inferior capsular support is not a stable situation, as many of those repositioned IOLs will end up dislocating again. Trans-scleral suturing or IOL exchange [removal of the dislocated IOL and placement of a flexible open loop anterior chamber intraocular lens (ACIOL)] is recommended in these cases.

BIBLIOGRAPHY

1. Wu L, Evans T, García RA, et al. (2011). Intraocular lens dislocation. [online] Available from www.emedicine.com/oph/TOPIC392.HTM. [Accessed October, 2013].

34. MALIGNANT HYPERPYREXIA SYNDROME (POSTCATARACT HYPERPYREXIA SYNDROME; POSTINDUCTION HYPERPYREXIA SYNDROME)

General

Etiology is uncertain, but is believed to be a secondary response to suxamethonium and halothane used with general anesthesia; high mortality rate of about 70%.

Ocular

Malignant hyperpyrexia following congenital cataract or strabismus surgery under general anesthesia.

Clinical

Rapid elevation of body temperature and vastly enhanced metabolic activity; hyperapnea; tachycardia.

Laboratory

Diagnosis is made by clinical findings.

Treatment

Early detection, if occurs, reduce temperature.

BIBLIOGRAPHY

1. Geeraets WJ. Ocular Syndromes, 3rd edition. Philadelphia, PA: Lea & Febiger; 1976.
2. Petersdorf RG. Malignant hyperthermia. In: Isselbacher KJ (Ed). Harrison's Principles of Internal Medicine, 13th edition. New York, USA: McGraw-Hill; 1994. p. 2476.
3. Rosenberg H, Fletcher JE. An update on the malignant hyperthermia syndrome. Ann Acad Med Singapore. 1994;23(6):84-97.
4. Snow JC, Kerman TJ. Malignant hyperpyrexia. Eye Ear Nose Throat Mon. 1970;49(9):427-30.

35. MARINESCO-SJÖGREN SYNDROME (CONGENITAL SPINOCEREBELLAR ATAXIA-CONGENITAL CATARACT-OLIGOPHRENIA SYNDROME)

General

Autosomal recessive trait; onset when child learns to walk; mitochondrial disease.

Ocular

Cataracts; aniridia; rotary and horizontal nystagmus; nystagmus; strabismus; optic atrophy.

Clinical

Cerebellar ataxia; oligophrenia; small stature; scoliosis; genu valgum; restricted extensibility of the knee; defects of fingers and toes; mental retardation; hair sparse; hypersalivation; sensorineural hearing loss.

Laboratory

Diagnosis is made by clinical findings.

Treatment

Cataracts: Change in glasses can sometimes improve a patient's visual function temporarily; however the most common treatment is cataract surgery.

BIBLIOGRAPHY

1. Dotti MT, Bardelli AM, De Stefano N, et al. Optic atrophy in Marinesco-Sjögren syndrome: an additional ocular feature. Report of three cases in two families. Ophthalmic Paediatr Genet. 1993;14(1):5-7.
2. Gillespie FD. Aniridia, cerebellar ataxia, and oligophrenia in siblings. Arch Ophthalmol. 1965;73:338-41.
3. Lindal S, Lund I, Torbergsen T, et al. Mitochondrial diseases and myopathies: a series of muscle biopsy specimens with ultrastructural changes in the mitochondria. Ultrastruct Pathol. 1992;16(3):263-75.
4. Marinesco G, Draganesco S, Vasiliu D. Nouvelle maladie familiale caracterisee par une cataracte congenitale et un arret du developpement somato-neuro-psychique. Encephale. 1931;26:97-109.
5. Sjögren T. Hereditary congenital spinocerebellar ataxia accompanied by congenital cataracts and oligophrenia; a genetic and clinical investigation. Confin Neurol. 1950;10(5):293-308.

36. MICROCEPHALY, MICROPHTHALMIA, CATARACTS, AND JOINT CONTRACTURES

General

Autosomal dominant; ocular features like Hagberg-Santavuori syndrome.

Ocular

Microphthalmia; cataracts; hypopigmented retinal degeneration.

Clinical

Microcephaly; shortening or wasting of muscle fibers, causing excess scar tissue over joints.

Laboratory

Diagnosis is made by clinical findings.

Treatment

Cataracts: Change in glasses can sometimes improve a patient's visual function temporarily; however the most common treatment is cataract surgery.

BIBLIOGRAPHY

1. Bateman JB, Philippart M. Ocular features of Hagberg-Santavuori syndrome. Am J Ophthalmol. 1986;102(2):262-71.
2. McKusick VA. Mendelian Inheritance in Man: A Catalog of Human Genes and Genetic Disorders, 12th edition. Baltimore, USA: The Johns Hopkins University Press; 1998.
3. Online Mendelian Inheritance in Man, OMIM. (2007). McKusick-Nathans Institute for Genetic Medicine, Johns Hopkins University and National Center for Biotechnology Information, National Library of Medicine, February 12, 2007. [online] Available from www.ncbi.nlm.nih.gov/omim. [Accessed October, 2013].

37. MICROSPHEROPHAKIA

General

Small and spherical lens, larger in the anteroposterior diameter and the equatorial diameter is smaller than normal.

Clinical

Weill-Marchesani syndrome.

Ocular

Secondary glaucoma, peripheral anterior synechiae, myopia, lens dislocation.

Laboratory

Diagnosis is made by clinical findings.

Treatment

Glaucoma control is of primary concern; mydriatics are used to control pupillary block; laser iridectomy.

BIBLIOGRAPHY

1. Roy FH, Fraunfelder FW, Fraunfelder FT. Roy and Fraunfelder's Current Ocular Therapy, 6th edition. London, UK: Elsevier; 2008.

38. MICROSPHEROPHAKIA WITH HERNIA

General

Autosomal dominant.

Ocular

Microspherophakia; glaucoma.

Clinical

Inguinal hernia.

Laboratory/Glaucoma

Chromosome analysis and genetic counseling.

Treatment/Glaucoma

Beta-blockers, carbonic-anhydrase inhibitors and prostaglandin analogs. Surgery may be needed if IOP is uncontrolled.

BIBLIOGRAPHY

1. Johnson VP, Grayson M, Christian JC. Dominant microspherophakia. Arch Ophthalmol. 1971;85(5):534-7.
2. McKusick VA. Mendelian Inheritance in Man: A Catalog of Human Genes and Genetic Disorders, 12th edition. Baltimore, USA: The Johns Hopkins University Press; 1998.
3. Online Mendelian Inheritance in Man, OMIM. (2007). McKusick-Nathans Institute for Genetic Medicine, Johns Hopkins University and National Center for Biotechnology Information, National Library of Medicine, February 12, 2007. [online] Available from www.ncbi.nlm.nih.gov/omim. [Accessed October, 2013].

39. MYOPATHY, MITOCHONDRIAL, WITH CATARACT

General

Autosomal dominant.

Ocular

Early-onset bilateral cataracts; severe ophthalmoplegia; mitochondrial abnormalities in the inferior oblique muscle.

Clinical

Facial weakness; myocardial and skeletal myopathy of the mitochondrial type.

Laboratory

Diagnosis is made by clinical findings.

Treatment

Cataracts: Change in glasses can sometimes improve a patient's visual function temporarily; however the most common treatment is cataract surgery.

BIBLIOGRAPHY

1. McKusick VA. Mendelian Inheritance in Man: A Catalog of Human Genes and Genetic Disorders, 12th edition. Baltimore, USA: The Johns Hopkins University Press; 1998.
2. Online Mendelian Inheritance in Man, OMIM. (2007). McKusick-Nathans Institute for Genetic Medicine, Johns Hopkins University and National Center for Biotechnology Information, National Library of Medicine, February 12, 2007. [online] Available from www.ncbi.nlm.nih.gov/omim. [Accessed October, 2013].
3. Pepin B, Mikol J, Goldstein B, et al. Familial mitochondrial myopathy with cataract. J Neurol Sci. 1980;45(2-3):191-203.

40. NIEDEN SYNDROME (TELANGIECTASIA-CATARACT SYNDROME)

General

Etiology is unknown; familial occurrence; onset from birth.

Ocular

Sparse eyebrows; glaucoma; dyscoria; defects of iris mesenchyme; bilateral cataract (cortical or mature).

Clinical

Telangiectasia of face and upper extremities; pigmentary changes of the neck; thick, atrophic skin; heart enlargement; congenital valvular defect.

Laboratory

Diagnosis is made by clinical findings.

Treatment

Glaucoma: Glaucoma medication should be the first plan of action. If medication is unsuccessful, a filtering surgical procedure with or without antimetabolites may be beneficial.

BIBLIOGRAPHY

1. Geeraets WJ. Ocular Syndromes, 3rd edition. Philadelphia, PA: Lea & Febiger; 1976.
2. Nieden A. Cataractbildung bei Teleangiectatischer Ausdehnung der Capillaren der Ganzen Gesichtshaut. Zentbl Parkt Augenheilkd. 1887;11:353.
3. Petersen HP. Telangiectasis and cataract. Acta Ophthalmol (Copenh). 1954;32(5):565-71.

🗗 41. OSTEOGENESIS IMPERFECTA CONGENITA, MICROCEPHALY AND CATARACTS

General

Autosomal recessive.

Ocular

Cataracts; blue sclera; keratoconus.

Clinical

Brain abnormally small; multiple prenatal bone fractures; calvaria soft; shortening and bowing of lower limbs.

Laboratory

Diagnosis is made by clinical findings.

Treatment

Spectacle correction, hard contacts, avoid eye rubbing. If hydrops occur, discontinue contact lens, use sodium chloride (NaCl) drops and ointment, patching and short course of steroids. As disease advances, penetrating keratoplasty, deep anterior lamellar keratoplasty intacs with laser grooves or collagen stabilization of cornea.
Cataract: Change in glasses can sometimes improve a patient's visual function temporarily; however the most common treatment is cataract surgery.

🗗 BIBLIOGRAPHY

1. Plotkin H. (2012). Genetics of osteogenesis imperfecta. [online] Available from www.emedicine.com/ped/TOPIC1674.HTM. [Accessed October, 2013].

🗗 42. PSEUDOEXFOLIATION SYNDROME

General

Prevalent over age of 70 years; rare before age of 40 years; unilateral involvement in 40–50% of cases; asymmetry of severity in bilateral cases; most common in Caucasians, especially from Iceland and Scandinavian countries; pseudoexfoliation fibers were identified in autopsy tissue specimens of skin, heart, lungs, liver and cerebral meninges; consistently associated with connective tissue components, i.e. fibroblasts, collagen and elastic fibers, myocardial tissue and heart muscle cell.

Ocular

Gray or white fluffy material deposited in particles, flakes or sheets on anterior surface of iris, ciliary body, posterior surface of cornea, pupillary margin, lens and trabecular meshwork; increased pigmentation of trabecular meshwork; zonular dialysis; displaced or dislocated lens; anterior chamber depth asymmetry; preoperative phacodonesis; glaucoma; cataract.

Clinical

None.

Laboratory

Diagnosis is made by clinical findings.

Treatment

Annual eye examinations for early detection of glaucoma. Glaucoma in pseudoexfoliation is more resistant to medical therapy, which is unsuccessful to control the glaucoma. Argon laser trabeculoplasty or trabeculectomy may be beneficial.

🗗 BIBLIOGRAPHY

1. Pons ME, Eliassi-Rad B. (2011). Pseudoexfoliation glaucoma. [online] Available from www.emedicine.com/oph/TOPIC140.HTM. [Accessed October, 2013].

43. RUBELLA SYNDROME (CONGENITAL RUBELLA SYNDROME; GERMAN MEASLES; GREGG SYNDROME)

General

Rubella infection of the mother during 1st trimester of pregnancy; ocular disease is the most commonly found abnormality in patients with congenital rubella syndrome (75%), multiorgan disease is common (> 75%); no significant association has been found between gestational age and time of maternal infection and incidence of individual ocular conditions.

Ocular

Nystagmus; glaucoma; corneal haziness; cataracts; retinal pigmentary changes; appearance and central distribution of lesions are quite distinguishable from retinitis pigmentosa; retinopathy is not progressive and has little, if any, effect on vision; waxy atrophy of optic disk; conjunctivitis; megalocornea or microcornea; buphthalmos; microphthalmos; uveitis; iris atrophy; spherophakia; strabismus.

Clinical

Low birth weight; diarrhea; pneumonia; urinary infection; hearing loss; heart disease; hepatosplenomegaly; mental retardation; inguinal hernias; ataxia; cardiac abnormalities.

Laboratory

Diagnosis is made by clinical findings; if in doubt a rising titer of immunoglobulin M will indicate a recent infection.

Treatment

Treatment for rubella of the eye centers on glaucoma and cataract.

BIBLIOGRAPHY

1. Lombardo PC. (2011). Dermatologic manifestations of rubella. [online] Available from www.emedicine.com/derm/TOPIC380.HTM. [Accessed October, 2013].

44. TOXIC LENS SYNDROME (TOXIC ANTERIOR SEGMENT SYNDROME; TASS)

General

Syndrome occurs within a few days to several weeks of implantation of an IOL; with therapy, vision is restored in the majority of cases; increased incidence of disease caused by usc of ethylene oxide sterilization (dry pack IOLs); toxic lens syndrome may be prevented by treating the lens with sodium hydroxide and by using modem lathe-cut or compression-molded lenses with polypropylene loops; risk factors include uveitis in history, pseudoexfoliation syndrome, inadequate mydriasis at the start of surgery, problems with IOL implantation and pigment effusion during surgery.

Ocular

Pigment precipitation on the surface of IOL; hypopyon; vitreous opacification; chronic uveitis; secondary glaucoma.

Clinical

None.

Laboratory

Anterior chamber aspiration, vitreous tap and/or vitreous biopsy for Gram stain and microbiologic cultures.

Treatment

Topical steroids and nonsteroidal anti-inflammatory drugs (NSAIDs); patients should be evaluated the same or the next day to rule out infectious endophthalmitis, in which case, steroids would worsen the condition.

BIBLIOGRAPHY

1. Al-Ghoul AR, Charukamnoetkanok P, Dhaliwal DK. (2012). Toxic anterior segment syndrome. [online] Available from www.emedicine.com/oph/TOPIC779.HTM. [Accessed October, 2013].
2. Rishi E, Rishi P, Sengupta S, et al. Acute postoperative bacillus cereus endophthamitis mimicking Toxic Anterior Segment Syndrome. Ophthalmology. 2013:120:181-5.

🗗 45. TRAUMATIC CATARACT

General

Injury resulting in lens opacification which can be diagnosed at the time of the trauma or years later.

Clinical

None.

Ocular

Visual loss, amblyopia, trauma to cornea, loose iris zonules.

Laboratory

Diagnosis is made by clinical findings.

Treatment

Extracapsular cataract extraction or phacoemulsification is the procedure of choice.

🗗 BIBLIOGRAPHY

1. Graham RH, Mulrooney BC. (2012). Traumatic cataract. [online] Available from www.emedicine.com/oph/TOPIC52.HTM. [Accessed October, 2013].

🗗 46. Z SYNDROME

General

Occurs with hinged accommodating IOL such as the Crystalens, the capsule contracts and causes long-axis compression resulting in the asymmetric folding; Z syndrome—so named because the shape of the distorted IOL resembles a stretched-out "Z".

Ocular

Increased myopia and astigmatism; coma aberration; tilting of the IOL optic; striae/fibrosis of posterior capsule.

Laboratory

Diagnosis is made by clinical observation.

Treatment

YAG capsulotomy is the treatment of choice and works well unless there is a gap between the posterior capsule and any part of the IOL. If there is a gap, a surgical procedure is used to reposition the IOL or in severe cases removal of the IOL may be necessary.

🗗 BIBLIOGRAPHY

1. Yuen L, Trattler W, Boxer Wachler BS. Two cases of Z syndrome with the Crystalens after uneventful cataract surgery. J Cataract Refract Surg. 2008;34(11):1986-9.

CHAPTER
29

Macula

1. AGE-RELATED MACULAR DEGENERATION

General

Pathologic changes of this chronic degenerative condition occur primarily in the retinal pigment epithelium (RPE), Bruch's membrane and the choriocapillaris of the macular region.

Clinical

Hypertension, high cholesterol level.

Ocular

Vision loss, choroidal neovascularization.

Laboratory

Diagnosis is made by clinical findings.

Treatment

No treatment is available for non-neovascular age-related macular degeneration (AMD). Preventative therapy includes no smoking, control of hypertension, cholesterol, and blood sugar, exercise and vitamins. Neovascular AMD treatment consists of laser, avastin and lucentis.

BIBLIOGRAPHY

1. Lima LH, Schubert C, Ferrara DC, et al. Three major loci involved in age-related macular degeneration are also associated with polypoidal choroidal vasculopathy. Ophthalmology. 2010;117(8):1567-70.
2. Maturi RK. (2012). Nonexudative ARMD. [online] Available from www.emedicine.com/oph/TOPIC383.HTM. [Accessed October, 2013].
3. Prall FR, Ciulla T, Criswell MH, et al. (2012). Exudative ARMD. [online] Available from www.emedicine.com/oph/TOPIC653.HTM. [Accessed October, 2013].
4. Singer MA, Awh CC, Sadda S, et al. HORIZON: An open-label extension trial of ranibizumab for choroidal neovascularization secondary to age-related macular degeneration. Ophthalmology. 2012;119(6):1175-83.

2. BATTEN-MAYOU SYNDROME (SPIELMEYER-VOGT SYNDROME; MAYOU-BATTEN DISEASE; STOCK-SPIELMEYER-VOGT SYNDROME; CEREBRORETINAL DEGENERATION; PIGMENTARY RETINAL LIPOID NEURONAL HEREDODEGENERATION; VOGT-SPIELMEYER SYNDROME; JUVENILE GANGLIOSIDE LIPIDOSIS; NEURONAL CEROID LIPOFUSCINOSIS; MYOCLONIC VARIANT OF CEREBRAL LIPIDOSIS; BATTEN DISEASE; CEREBROMACULAR DYSTROPHY; JUVENILE AMAUROTIC FAMILY IDIOCY; SPIELMEYER-SJÖGREN SYNDROME)

General

Autosomal recessive; some cases of autosomal dominant; possible disturbance in lipid metabolism; most common in Jewish families; onset between ages 5 years and 8 years; mean age at death is 17 years; poor prognosis (*see* Tay-Sachs disease; Dollinger-Bielschowsky syndrome). The lipopigment storage diseases are divided into four types based on the clinical and electron microscopic features: (1) infantile (Hagberg-Santavuori syndrome), (2) late infantile (Jansky-Bielschowsky disease), (3) juvenile (Spielmeyer-Vogt disease) and (4) adult (Kufs disease).

Ocular

Vision initially reduced, progressing to total blindness; fat deposition in the retina with gradual development of pigment disturbances resembling retinitis pigmentosa; progressive primary optic atrophy; granular pigmentary change of macula; there is clinical evidence supporting the idea that the primary lesion of the retina is in the inner layers.

Clinical

Mental disturbances; convulsions (later); apathy; irritability; ataxia; upper and lower motor neuron palsies; rigidity; complete paralysis and dementia in terminal stage; hypertonus; death from intercurrent infection.

Laboratory

Palmitoyl protein thioesterase (PPT) and tripeptidyl peptidase 1 (TTP1) levels can be measured in leukocytes, cultured fibroblasts, dried blood spots and saliva. Fibroblast TTP1 activity is approximately 17,000 µM of amino acids produced per hour per mg of protein. The TTP1 activity in CLN2 is less than 4% of normal.

Treatment

No specific treatment is available for these diseases.

BIBLIOGRAPHY

1. Chang CH. (2009). Neuronal ceroid lipofuscinoses. [online] Available from www.emedicine.com/neuro/TOPIC498.HTM. [Accessed October, 2013].

3. CENTRAL SEROUS CHORIORETINOPATHY

General

Disorder of the central macula.

Clinical

None.

Ocular

Decreased visual acuity, metamorphopsia, micropsia, central color vision deficiency, central scotoma.

Laboratory

Fluorescein angiopathy for "expansile dot" pattern, a "smokestack" pattern or diffuse hyperfluorescence.

Treatment

Observation in most cases; thermal or photodynamic therapy is necessary in some cases.

BIBLIOGRAPHY

1. Oh KT. (2011). Central serous chorioretinopathy. [online] Available from www.emedicine.com/oph/TOPIC689.HTM. [Accessed October, 2013].

🗗 4. CHOROIDORETINAL DEGENERATION WITH RETINAL REFLEX IN HETEROZYGOUS WOMEN

General

Sex-linked; choroidoretinal degeneration is differentiated by presence in heterozygous women of a tapetal-like retinal reflex; there is probably more than one X-linked locus leading to a retinitis pigmentosa type of picture.

Ocular

Retinitis pigmentosa; golden-hued, patchy appearance around macula.

Clinical

None.

Laboratory

Diagnosis is made by clinical findings.

Treatment

Retinitis pigmentosa: Vitamin A 15,000 IU/day is thought to slow the decline of retinal function, dark sunglasses for outdoor use; surgery for cataract; genetic counseling.

🗗 BIBLIOGRAPHY

1. Hamosh A, Scott AF, Amberger J, et al. Online Mendelian Inheritance in Man (OMIM), a knowledgebase of human genes and genetic disorders. Nucleic Acids Res. 2002;30(1):52-5.
2. McKusick VA. Mendelian Inheritance in Man: A Catalog of Human Genes and Genetic Disorders, 12th edition. Baltimore, USA: The Johns Hopkins University Press; 1998.
3. Musarella MA, Anson-Cartwright L, Leal SM, et al. Multipoint linkage analysis and heterogeneity testing in 20 X-linked retinitis pigmentosa families. Genomics. 1990;8(2):286-96.
4. Nussbaum RL, Lewis RA, Lesko JG, et al. Mapping X-linked ophthalmic diseases: II. Linkage relationship of X-linked retinitis pigmentosa to X chromosomal short arm markers. Hum Genet. 1985;70(1):45-50.

🗗 5. COLOBOMA OF MACULA (AGENESIS OF MACULA)

General

Autosomal dominant; can be caused by intrauterine inflammation, birth hemorrhage; infantile inflammation.

Ocular

Defect in central area of fundus; coloboma can be pigmented, nonpigmented or have abnormal vessels associated or completely absent; visual defect; absolute central scotoma; nystagmus; myopia; destruction of pigment epithelium; microphthalmos; coloboma of optic nerve (rare); keratoconus; paravenous retinochoroidal atrophy.

Clinical

Microencephaly.

Laboratory

Diagnosis is made by clinical findings.

Treatment

Keratoconus: Spectacle correction, hard contacts, avoid eye rubbing. If hydrops occur, discontinue contact lens, use sodium chloride (NaCl) drops and ointment, patching and short course of steroids. As disease advances, penetrating keratoplasty, deep anterior lamellar keratoplasty intacs with laser grooves or collagen stabilization of cornea.

🗗 BIBLIOGRAPHY

1. Chen MS, Yang CH, Huang JS. Bilateral macular coloboma and pigmented paravenous retinochoroidal atrophy. Br J Ophthalmol. 1992;76(4):250-1.
2. Duane TD. Clinical Ophthalmology. Philadelphia, PA: JB Lippincott; 1987.
3. McKusick VA. Mendelian Inheritance in Man: A Catalog of Human Genes and Genetic Disorders, 12th edition. Baltimore, USA: The Johns Hopkins University Press; 1998.
4. Online Mendelian Inheritance in Man, OMIM. McKusick-Nathans Institute for Genetic Medicine, Johns Hopkins University and National Center for Biotechnology Information, National Library of Medicine, February 12, 2007. Available from www.ncbi.nlm.nih.gov/omim. [Accessed October, 2013].
5. Ranchod TM, Quiram PA, Hathaway N, et al. Microcornea, posterior megalolenticonus, persistent fetal vasculature, and coloboma: a new syndrome. Ophthalmology. 2010;117(9):1843-7.

6. COLOBOMA OF MACULA WITH TYPE B BRACHYDACTYLY (APICAL DYSTROPHY)

General

Autosomal dominant; bilateral pigmented macular coloboma and brachydactyly.

Ocular

Myopia; retinal detachment; coloboma of retina, choroid, sclera and macula.

Clinical

Cleft palate; flexion deformity of distal interphalangeal joints of little fingers of hand; retarded growth; delayed sexual maturity; recurrent dislocation of left patella; short feet; coxa valga; genu valgum.

Laboratory

Diagnosis is made by clinical findings.

Treatment

See myopia and retinal detachment.

BIBLIOGRAPHY

1. Hamosh A, Scott AF, Amberger J, et al. Online Mendelian Inheritance in Man (OMIM), a knowledgebase of human genes and genetic disorders. Nucleic Acids Res. 2002;30(1):52-5.
2. McKusick VA. Mendelian Inheritance in Man: A Catalog of Human Genes and Genetic Disorders, 12th edition. Baltimore, USA: The Johns Hopkins University Press; 1998.
3. Smith RD, Fineman RM, Sillence DO, et al. Congenital macular colobomas and short-limb skeletal dysplasia. Am J Med Genet. 1980;5(4):365-71.
4. Sorsby A. Congenital coloboma of the macula: together with an account of the familial occurrence of bilateral macular coloboma in association with apical dystrophy of hands and feet. Br J Ophthalmol. 1935;19(2):65-90.

7. DIABETIC MACULAR EDEMA

General

Diabetes is a major medical problem that is growing in numbers. It is seen most commonly in Western countries in individuals that consume more calories than they use each day. It is caused by the pancreas not making enough insulin.

Clinical

Renal, neuropathic and cardiovascular disease, polyuria, polydipsia, polyphagia and weight loss.

Ocular

Cataracts, glaucoma, corneal abnormalities, iris neovascularization, macular edema, microaneurysms, retinal hemorrhage, cotton-wool spots and changes in refractive error.

Laboratory

Fasting glucose and hemoglobin A1c, fluorescein angiography and optical coherence tomography (OCT), color stereo fundus photographs.

Treatment

Glucose can be controlled with diet, exercise and medication, lowering blood pressure and lipid levels, laser photocoagulation, intravitreal triamcinolone acetonide and anti-vascular endothelial growth factor (VEGF) agents. Ranibizumab injection may be useful. Pars plana vitrectomy may also be necessary.

BIBLIOGRAPHY

1. Campochiaro PA, Brown DM, Pearson A, et al. Sustained delivery fluocinolone acetonide vitreous inserts provide benefit for at least 3 years in patients with diabetic macular edema. Ophthalmology. 2012;119(10):2125-32.
2. Kozak I, Oster SF, Cortex MA, et al. Clinical evaluation and treatment accuracy in diabetic macular edema using navigated laser photocoagulator NAVILAS. Ophthalmology. 2011;118(6):1119-24.
3. Murakami T, Nishijima K, Sakamoto A, et al. Foveal cystoid spaces are associated with enlarged foveal avascular zone and microaneurysms in diabetic macular edema. Ophthalmology. 2011;118(2):359-67.
4. Nguyen QD, Brown DM, Marcus DM, et al. Ranibizumab for diabetic macular edema: results from 2 phase III randomized trials: RISE and RIDE. Ophthalmology. 2012;119(4):789-801.
5. Sultan, MB, Zhou D, Loftus J, et al. A phase 2/3, multicenter, randomized, double-masked, 2-year trial of pegaptanib sodium for the treatment of diabetic macular edema. Ophthalmology. 2011;118(6):1107-18.

⊟ 8. DIALINAS-AMALRIC SYNDROME (AMALRIC-DIALINAS SYNDROME; DEAF MUTISM-RETINAL DEGENERATION SYNDROME)

General

Retinal pigmentary disturbances and deafness as outstanding findings but without severe general systemic disorders as seen in the syndromes of Hallgren, Cockayne, Alport, Laurence-Moon-Bardet-Biedl (*see* Hallgren syndrome; Cockayne syndrome; Alport syndrome; Laurence-Moon-Bardet-Biedl syndrome).

Ocular

No night blindness but heterochromia iridis; atypical retinitis pigmentosa with small, scattered, fine-pigmented deposits in the macular region with some accumulations and accompanied by small white and yellow spots.

Clinical

Deaf mutism.

Laboratory

None—ocular.

Treatment

Retinitis pigmentosa: Vitamin A 15,000 IU/day is thought to slow the decline of retinal function, dark sunglasses for outdoor use; surgery for cataract; genetic counseling.

⊟ BIBLIOGRAPHY

1. Amalric P. Nouveau Type de Degenerescence Tapeto-Retinienne au Cours de la Surdumutite. Bull Soc Ophthalmol Fr. 1960;196:211.
2. Charamis J, Tsamparlakis J, Palimeris G, et al. Deaf-mutism and ophthalmic lesions. J Pediatr Ophthalmol. 1968;5:230-7.
3. Dialinas NP. Les Alterations Oculaires chez les Sourds-Muets. Genet Hum. 1959;8:225.
4. Geeraets WJ. Ocular Syndromes, 3rd edition. Philadelphia, PA: Lea & Febiger; 1976.

⊟ 9. EPIMACULAR PROLIFERATION (MACULAR PUCKER)

General

It is a condition in which the macular region is destroyed by the contraction of a fibrocellular epiretinal membrane that has grown across the inner retinal surface.

Clinical

None.

Laboratory

Optical coherence tomography demonstrates the extent of epiretinal membrane; fluorescein angiography.

Treatment

Three port pars plana vitrectomy.

⊟ BIBLIOGRAPHY

1. Oh KT, Hughes BM, Drouilhet JH. (2012). Epimacular membrane. [online] Available from www.emedicine.com/oph/TOPIC396.HTM. [Accessed October, 2013].

⊟ 10. FRANCESCHETTI DISEASE (FUNDUS FLAVIMACULATUS)

General

It affects both sexes; onset between ages 10 years and 25 years; autosomal recessive; genetic linkage analysis has assigned the disease locus to chromosome 1p21-p13.

Ocular

Irregular yellowish deposit in and around the macula lutea forming a garland; impaired central vision with intact peripheral retinal function; bilateral retinal dystrophy;

progressive subretinal fibrosis; chorioretinal punched-out spots in the posterior pole and midperiphery of the retina.

Clinical

None.

Laboratory

Diagnosis is made by clinical findings.

Treatment

Ocular—ocular.

BIBLIOGRAPHY

1. Magalini SI, Scrascia E. Dictionary of Medical Syndromes, 2nd edition. Philadelphia, PA: JB Lippincott; 1981.
2. Parodi MB. Progressive subretinal fibrosis in fundus flavi-maculatus. Acta Ophthalmol (Copenh). 1994;72(2):260-4.

11. GROUPED PIGMENTATION OF THE MACULA

General

Autosomal recessive.

Ocular

Grouped pigmentation limited to foveal area; metamorphopsia; pigmented spots around a clear hole in the foveal area.

Clinical

None.

Laboratory

Diagnosis is made by clinical findings.

Treatment

None—ocular.

BIBLIOGRAPHY

1. Forsius H, Eriksson A, Nuutila A, et al. A genetic study of three rare retinal disorders: dystrophia retinae dysacusis syndrome, x-chromosomal retinoschisis and grouped pigments of the retina. Birth Defects Orig Artic Ser. 1971;7(3):83-98.
2. McKusick VA. Mendelian Inheritance in Man: A Catalog of Human Genes and Genetic Disorders, 12th edition. Baltimore, USA: The Johns Hopkins University press; 1998.

12. HISTOPLASMOSIS (HISTOPLASMOSIS CHOROIDITIS; HISTOPLASMOSIS MACULOPATHY; PRESUMED OCULAR HISTOPLASMOSIS SYNDROME)

General

It is a fungal infection caused by *Histoplasma capsulatum*.

Ocular

Circumpapillary atrophy; maculopathy; scattered yellow "histo" spots; optic disk edema; disseminated choroiditis (immunocompromised patients); vitreous hemorrhage; punched-out chorioretinal lesions; choroidal neovascular membrane; exogenous endophthalmitis (isolated report).

Clinical

Pulmonary infection; fever; malaise.

Laboratory

Sixty percent of the adult populations come from the Ohio and Mississippi river valleys have a positive histoplasmin skin test, therefore clinic course is most helpful.

Treatment

Although the diagnosis is clinical, certain ancillary tests help in confirming it; fluorescein angiography; human leukocyte antigen (HLA) types B7 and DRw2 may be indicated.

BIBLIOGRAPHY

1. Wu L, Evans T. (2012). Presumed ocular histoplasmosis syndrome. [online] Available from www.emedicine.com/oph/TOPIC406.HTM. [Accessed October, 2013].

13. JENSEN DISEASE (JUXTAPAPILLARY RETINOPATHY)

General

Etiology is unknown.

Ocular

Circumscribed inflammatory changes of the choroid; field defect.

Clinical

None.

Laboratory

Diagnosis is made by clinical findings.

Treatment

None—ocular.

BIBLIOGRAPHY

1. Harley RD, Nelson LB, Olitsky SE (Eds). Harley's Pediatric Ophthalmology, 5th illustrated edition. Philadelphia, PA: Lippincott Williams & Wilkins; 2005.
2. Magalini SI, Scrascia E. Dictionary of Medical Syndromes, 2nd edition. Philadelphia, PA: JB Lippincott; 1981.

14. JUNIUS-KUHNT SYNDROME [KUHNT-JUNIUS DISEASE; MACULAR SENILE DISCIFORM DEGENERATION (1); MACULA LUTEA JUVENILE DEGENERATION (2)]

General

Onset in advanced age or in juvenile period; etiology is unknown; possible autosomal dominant or recessive inheritance.

Ocular

Impairment of central vision; central scotoma; atrophic macular degeneration surrounded by retinal hemorrhages, resulting in mount-like lesion; exudative and atrophic reaction with deposit in and about macula.

Clinical

None.

Laboratory

Diagnosis is made by clinical findings.

Treatment

Macular degeneration: No treatment is available for non-neovascular AMD. Preventative therapy includes no smoking, control of hypertension, cholesterol and blood sugar, exercise and vitamins. Neovascular AMD treatment consists of laser, avastin and lucentis.

BIBLIOGRAPHY

1. Deutman AF. Hereditary dystrophies of the central retina and choroid. In: Winkelman JE, Crone RA (Eds). Perspectives in Ophthalmology. Amsterdam: Excerpta Medica; 1970.
2. Deutman AF. Macular dystrophies. In: Ryan SJ (Ed). Retina, 2nd edition. St. Louis: Mosby; 1994.
3. Kimura SJ, Caygill WM (Eds). Retinal Diseases. Philadelphia, PA: Lea & Febiger; 1966.
4. Magalini SJ, Scrascia E. Dictionary of Medical Syndromes, 2nd edition. Philadelphia, PA: JB Lippincott; 1981. p. 440.

🗗 15. MACULAR EDEMA, PSEUDOPHAKIC (IRVINE-GASS)

General

Painless loss of vision due to swelling or thickening of the macula. Frequently associated with cataract surgery (Irvine-Gass), AMD, uveitis, injury, diabetes and retinal vein occlusion.

Clinical

Diabetes; renal failure, following cataract surgery.

Ocular

Decreased visual acuity; uveitis; retinal vein occlusion; macular degeneration; macular pucker.

Laboratory

Fluorescein angiography and OCT are helpful in determining the disease.

Treatment

Use of corticosteroids, carbonic anhydrase inhibitors and nonsteroidal anti-inflammatory drugs (NSAIDs) are the mainstay of treatment. If traditional therapy is not effective, intraocular injections of avastin may be helpful. In cases that have vitreous strand tugging against the macula, pars plana vitrectomy may be necessary.

🗗 BIBLIOGRAPHY

1. Telander DG, Cessna CT. (2012). Pseudophakic (Irvine-Gass) macular edema. [online] Available from emedicine.medscape.com/article/1224224-overview. [Accessed October, 2013].

🗗 16. MACULAR HOLE

Macular hole must be differentiated from macular cyst with Hruby lens or contact lens and slit lamp)

†1. Idiopathic (most common, may be bilateral)
2. From the following:
   A. Edema
      †1. Inflammatory
      †2. Toxic
      †3. Vascular
      4. Following papilledema
   †B. High myopia
   C. Ischemic, such as with retinal detachment or choroidal tumor—the macula is separated from choriocapillaris
   †D. Degenerative conditions of the retina and retinal dystrophy
   †E. Trauma
   †F. Radiation injury
   G. Glaucoma
   H. Posterior senile retinoschisis (RS)
   I. High tension electric shock
   J. Central serous chorioretinopathy
   K. Optic disk coloboma
   †L. Posterior retinal detachment associated with optic pits
   †M. Industrial laser bums
   †N. Lightening-induced
   †O. Posterior microphthalmos
   †P. Septic embolization
   †Q. Subhyaloid hemorrhage
   †R. Topical pilocarpine use
   †S. Yttrium-aluminum-garnet (YAG) laser
3. Dawson disease (subacute sclerosing panencephalitis)
†4. Foveomacular retinitis-usually young males
†5. Pseudohole due to epiretinal membrane (may differentiated from true hole by fluorescein angiography)
6. Sickle cell disease

🗗 BIBLIOGRAPHY

1. Oh KT, Hughes BM, Atebara NH, et al. (2012). Macular hole. [online] Available from www.emedicine.com/oph/TOPIC401.HTM. [Accessed October, 2013].

---

†Indicates a general entry and therefore has not been described in detail in the text

🖶 16.2A4. PAPILLEDEMA

General

Papilledema is the swelling of the optic disk due to increased intracranial pressure.

Clinical

Holocranial headaches, neck and back pain, pulsatile tinnitus, nausea and vomiting.

Ocular

Visual loss, nerve fiber loss, intermittent or constant diplopia.

Laboratory

Lumbar puncture to determine if intracranial pressure is elevated.

Treatment

Underlying cause should be determined and treated. Systemic acetazolamide is the medical therapy of choice.

🖶 BIBLIOGRAPHY

1. Gossman MV, Giovannini J. (2012). Papilledema. [online] Available from www.emedicine.com/oph/TOPIC187.HTM. [Accessed October, 2013].

🖶 16.2C. RETINAL DETACHMENT, RHEGMATOGENOUS

General

Subretinal fluid accumulation in the space between the neurosensory retina and the underlying RPE. Most common type of retinal detachment and occurs with a retinal tear that allows liquefied vitreous to seep under the tear leading to the detachment.

Clinical

None.

Ocular

Vitreous traction, cut in visual field; vitreous floaters; decreased visual acuity; scleritis.

Laboratory

Diagnosis is generally made by clinical observation. Ultrasound may be necessary if the media is hazy.

Treatment

Scleral buckle, pneumatic retinopexy and vitrectomy are used for this type of detachment and the goal is to close all the breaks.

🖶 BIBLIOGRAPHY

1. Wu L, Evans T. (2011). Rhegmatogenous retinal detachment treatment and management. [online] Available from emedicine.medscape.com/article/1224737-treatment. [Accessed October, 2013].

🖶 16.2H. RETINOSCHISIS

General

Sex-linked; may not manifest until middle life.

Ocular

Intraretinal splitting due to degeneration or detachment of retina; retinal atrophy with sclerosis of the choroid; cystic maculopathy.

Clinical

None.

Laboratory

Optical coherence tomography provides high resolution of the macula region. Fluorescein angiography, indocyanine green angiography (ICGA) and electroretinography (ERG) are helpful tools in finding a diagnosis.

Treatment

No treatment is available.

🖶 BIBLIOGRAPHY

1. Small KW, McLellan CM, Song MK. (2012). Juvenile retinoschisis. [online] Available from www.emedicine.com/oph/TOPIC639.HTM. [Accessed October, 2013].

🗗 16.2I. ELECTRICAL INJURY

General

Electric current passes through the body; voltage ranging from 100 million volts to 200 million volts may cause electrical burns.

Ocular

Choroidal atrophy; corneal perforation; necrosis of cornea or lids; blepharospasm; anterior or posterior subcapsular cataracts and vacuoles; optic neuritis; optic nerve atrophy; retinal edema; retinal hemorrhage; pigmentary degeneration; retinal holes; anterior uveitis; hyphema; hypotony; glaucoma; night blindness; nystagmus; paralysis of extraocular muscles; visual field defects; dilation of retinal veins.

Clinical

Skin burns; injury to cardiovascular, central nervous and musculoskeletal systems; tissue necrosis; vascular injury.

Laboratory

Diagnosis is made by clinical findings.

Treatment

Basics of supportive care and appropriate advanced cardiac life support measures should be administered. Limb-saving measures, such as escharotomy and fasciotomy, may be needed to restore tissue perfusion.

🗗 BIBLIOGRAPHY

1. Cushing TA, Wright RK. (2010). Electrical Injuries in Emergency Medicine. [online] Available from www.emedicine.com/derm/TOPIC859.HTM. [Accessed October, 2013].

🗗 16.2J. CENTRAL SEROUS CHORIORETINOPATHY

General

Disorder of the central macula.

Clinical

None.

Ocular

Decreased visual acuity, metamorphopsia, micropsia, central color vision deficiency, central scotoma.

Laboratory

Fluorescein angiopathy for "expansile dot" pattern, a "smokestack" pattern or diffuse hyperfluorescence.

Treatment

Observation in most cases. Thermal or photodynamic therapy is necessary in some cases.

🗗 BIBLIOGRAPHY

1. Oh KT. (2011). Central Serous Chorioretinopathy. [online] Available from www.emedicine.com/oph/TOPIC689.HTM. [Accessed October, 2013].

🗗 16.2K. COLOBOMA OF MACULA (AGENESIS OF MACULA)

General

Autosomal dominant; can be caused by intrauterine inflammation, birth hemorrhage; infantile inflammation.

Ocular

Defect in central area of fundus; coloboma can be pigmented, nonpigmented or have abnormal vessels associated or completely absent; visual defect; absolute central scotoma; nystagmus; myopia; destruction of pigment epithelium; microphthalmos; coloboma of optic nerve (rare); keratoconus; paravenous retinochoroidal atrophy.

Clinical

Microencephaly.

Laboratory

Diagnosis is made by clinical findings.

Treatment

Keratoconus: Spectacle correction, hard contacts, avoid eye rubbing. If hydrops occur, discontinue contact lens, use NaCl drops and ointment, patching and short course of steroids. As disease advances, penetrating keratoplasty, deep anterior lamellar keratoplasty intacs with laser grooves or collagen stabilization of cornea.

⊟ BIBLIOGRAPHY

1. Chen MS, Yang CH, Huang JS. Bilateral macular coloboma and pigmented paravenous retinochoroidal atrophy. Br J Ophthalmol. 1992;76(4):250-1.
2. Duane TD. Clinical Ophthalmology. Philadelphia, PA: JB Lippincott; 1987.
3. Hamosh A, Scott AF, Amberger J, et al. Online Mendelian Inheritance in Man (OMIM), a knowledgebase of human genes and genetic disorders. Nucleic Acids Res. 2002;30(1):52-5.
4. McKusick VA. Mendelian Inheritance in Man: A Catalog of Human Genes and Genetic Disorders, 12th edition. Baltimore, USA: The Johns Hopkins University Press; 1998.
5. Ranchod TM, Quiram PA, Hathaway N, et al. Microcornea, posterior megalolenticonus, persistent fetal vasculature, and coloboma: a new syndrome. Ophthalmology. 2010;117(9): 1843-7.

⊟ 16.3. DAWSON DISEASE (DAWSON ENCEPHALITIS; SUBACUTE SCLEROSING PANENCEPHALITIS; INCLUSION-BODY)

General

Sclerosing panencephalitis classified as a degenerative, progressive neurologic disorder caused by a measles virus infection of the central nervous system.

Ocular

Nystagmus; ptosis; papilledema; optic neuritis; macular pigmentation and degeneration; focal retinitis; ocular motor palsies; optic atrophy; preretinal vitreous membrane; exophthalmos; visual agnosia; chorioretinitis; retinal vasculitis; macular chorioretinitis.

Clinical

Chronic inflammation of brain with neuronal degeneration; gliosis; eosinophilic inclusion bodies in brain tissue; decline in intellect; behavioral changes; slurred speech; drooling; motor abnormalities; disorientation; seizures; death.

Laboratory

Refer to neurologist.

Treatment

- *Ptosis*: If visual acuity is affected most cases require surgical correction and there are several procedures that may be used including levator resection, repair or advancement and Fasanella-Servat.
- *Optic neuritis*: Intravenous steroids may be used with optic neuritis or ischemic neuropathy. Stem cell treatment may be the future treatment of choice.

⊟ BIBLIOGRAPHY

1. Fenichel GM. Subacute sclerosing panencephalitis. In: Fenichel GM (Ed). Clinical Pediatric Neurology, 2nd edition. Philadelphia: WB Saunders; 1993. p. 137.
2. Gravina RF, Nakanishi AS, Faden A. Subacute sclerosing panencephalitis. Am J Ophthalmol. 1978;86:106-9.
3. Johnston HM, Wise GA, Henry JG. Visual deterioration as presentation of subacute sclerosing panencephalitis. Arch Dis Child. 1980;55:899-90l.
4. Kovacs B, Vastag O. Fluoroangiographic picture of the acute stage of the retinal lesion in subacute sclerosing panencephalitis. Ophthalmologica. 1978;177:264-9.
5. Meyer E, Majlin M, Zonis S. Subacute sclerosing panencephalitis: clinicopathological study of the eyes. J Pediatr Ophthalmol Strabismus. 1978;15:19-23.
6. Miller JR, Jubelt B. Viral infections. In: Rowland LP (Ed). Merritt's Textbook of Neurology, 9th edition. Baltimore: Williams & Wilkins; 1995. pp. 164-5.
7. Miller NR. SSPE. In: Miller NR (Ed). Walsh and Hoyt's Clinical Neuro-Ophthalmology, 4th edition. Baltimore: Williams & Wilkins; 1995. pp. 4048-58.
8. Salmon JF, Pan EL, Murray AD. Visual loss with dancing extremities and mental disturbances. Surv Ophthalmol. 1991;35:299-306.
9. Takayama S, Iwasaki Y, Yamanouchi H, et al. Characteristic Clinical features in a case of fulminant subacute sclerosing panencephalitis. Brain Dev. 1994;16:132-5.
10. Vignaendra V, Lim CL, Chen ST, et al. Subacute sclerosing panencephalitis with unusual ocular movements: polygraphic studies. Neurology. 1978;28:1052-6.
11. Zagami AS, Lethlean AK. Chorioretinitis as a possible very early manifestation of subacute sclerosing panencephalitis. Aust N Z J Med. 1991;21:350-2.

🗗 16.6. HERRICK SYNDROME (DRESBACH SYNDROME; SICKLE CELL DISEASE; DREPANOCYTIC ANEMIA)

General

Usually occurs in members of the black race; poor prognosis.

Ocular

Secondary glaucoma; telangiectasia of conjunctival vessels; scleral icterus; vitreous hemorrhages; cataract; retinal hemorrhages; exudates, and neovascularization; retinitis proliferans; microaneurysms; thrombosis of retinal venules; retinal vascular sheathing; central vein occlusion; angioid streaks; retinopathy with "black sunburst sign" in patients with SS hemoglobin; "sea-fan sign" in patients with sickle cell (SC) hemoglobin; comma signs of conjunctiva; fan-shaped neovascularization of iris; sector ischemic atrophy of iris; optic atrophy; white cotton mass of vitreous; retinal holes; color vision defects; central retinal artery obstruction; branch retinal artery obstruction; white without pressure; venous tortuosity; sickling maculopathy.

Clinical

Severe anemia with hemolytic crises; bone and joint aches; hemarthrosis; jaundice; hepatosplenomegaly.

Laboratory

Blood-sickling of red blood cells, newborn screening for hemoglobin disorders.

Treatment

Transfusion is required in an aplastic crisis; erythrocytapheresis is an automated red-cell exchange and bone marrow transplantation may be useful. Pain is the hallmark of SC disease. While frequency and severity vary greatly, most patients have interval symptoms. Once pain has begun, no therapy reverses the process. Analgesics may provide a reasonable degree of comfort. While certain dosing guidelines are available, the amount of drug given should be titrated to the degree of pain experienced. Vitrectomy may be necessary.

🗗 BIBLIOGRAPHY

1. Maakaron JE, Taher A, Woermann UJ. (2012). Sickle cell anemia. [online] Available from www.emedicine.com/ped/TOPIC2096.HTM. [Accessed October, 2013].

🗗 17. MARSEILLES FEVER (BOUTONNEUSE FEVER)

General

It is caused by *Rickettsia conorii* and transmitted by ticks.

Ocular

Conjunctivitis; central serous retinopathy; retinal detachment; perivasculitis; uveitis; papillitis; keratitis.

Clinical

Fever; lymph node enlargement; papular rash.

Laboratory

Serology is usually a confirmatory method; however, these tests are useful only after an acute infection. Culture of the organism may be used for diagnosis early in the course of the disease.

Treatment

Tetracyclines with chloramphenicol and quinolones may be considered as the first-line antibiotics. Patients with the benign form are usually treated with antibiotics for 7 days. Patients with the malignant form are usually treated with antibiotics for 2 weeks.

🗗 BIBLIOGRAPHY

1. Zalewska A, Schwartz RA. (2011). Boutonneuse fever. [online] Available from www.emedicine.com/derm/TOPIC759.HTM. [Accessed October, 2013].

18. PROGRESSIVE FOVEAL DYSTROPHY (CENTRAL RETINAL PIGMENT EPITHELIAL DYSTROPHY)

General

Autosomal dominant; onset late in the first decade of life.

Ocular

Progressive foveal dystrophy; pigmentary changes and drusen of the macula; normal electroretinogram; subnormal electro-oculogram.

Clinical

Generalized aminoaciduria; increased glycine levels.

Laboratory

Fluorescein angiogram, electro-oculogram.

Treatment

No treatment exists. Secondary choroidal neovascularization can be managed with direct laser treatment.

BIBLIOGRAPHY

1. McKusick VA. Mendelian Inheritance in Man: A Catalog of Human Genes and Genetic Disorders, 12th edition. Baltimore, USA: The Johns Hopkins University Press; 1998.
2. Sohn EH, Mullins RF, Stone EM. Macular dystrophies. In: Ryan SJ, Schachat AP, Wilkinson CP, Hinton DR, Sadda S, Wiedemann P (Eds). Retina, 5th edition. Philadelphia, USA: Elsevier Saunders; 2013. pp. 852-90.

19. SOLAR RETINOPATHY

General

Photochemical injury to the retina.

Clinical

None.

Ocular

Central scotoma, micron lamellar defect.

Laboratory

Optical coherence tomography can be normal or tiny hyperreflective spots.

Treatment

No effective treatment is available.

BIBLIOGRAPHY

1. Roy FH, Fraunfelder FW, Fraunfelder FT. Roy and Fraunfelder's Current Ocular Therapy, 6th edition. London, UK: Elsevier; 2008.

20. SORSBY I SYNDROME (HEREDITARY MACULAR COLOBOMA SYNDROME)

General

Autosomal dominant; related to Laurence-Moon-Bardet-Biedl and Biemond syndromes; apical dystrophy of the extremities and bilateral macular colobomata; both sexes are affected; onset from birth.

Ocular

Hypermetropia; nystagmus; bilateral macular colobomata with various degrees of pigmentation but sharply lined borders.

Clinical

Distal dystrophy of the hands and feet; rudimentary or absent index fingernails; absence of big toe; cleft palate.

Laboratory

Diagnosis is made by clinical findings.

Treatment

None.

BIBLIOGRAPHY

1. François J. Heredity in Ophthalmology. St. Louis: Mosby; 1961. p. 694.
2. Magalini SI, Scrascia E. Dictionary of Medical Syndromes, 2nd edition. Philadelphia, PA: JB Lippincott; 1981.
3. Sorsby A. Congenital coloboma of the macula: together with an account of the familial occurrence of bilateral macular coloboma in association with apical dystrophy of hands and feet. Br J Ophthalmol. 1935;19(2):65-90.

21. STARGARDT DISEASE (JUVENILE MACULAR DEGENERATION)

General

Onset between ages 8 years and 14 years; variable appearance in different families.

Ocular

Heredomacular dystrophy; bilateral lesions showing some degree of symmetry; chorioretinal heredodegeneration; abnormal color vision.

Clinical

Possible association with neurologic deficits, including spastic tetraparesis and cerebellar involvement.

Laboratory

Diagnosis is made by clinical findings.

Treatment

No effective treatment. Ultraviolet sunglasses may be beneficial.

BIBLIOGRAPHY

1. Cibis GW, Morey M, Harris DJ. Dominantly inherited macular dystrophy with flecks (Stargardt). Arch Ophthalmol. 1980;98(10):1785-9.
2. Hadden OB, Gass JD. Fundus flavimaculatus and Stargardt's disease. Am J Ophthalmol. 1976;82(4):527-39.
3. Kalfakis N, Grivas I, Panayiotidou E, et al. Stargardt's disease with neurological involvement: case report. Funct Neurol. 1994;9(2):97-100.
4. Mäntyjärvi M, Tuppurainen K. Color vision in Stargardt's disease. Int Ophthalmol. 1992;16(6):423-8.
5. Moloney JB, Mooney DJ, O'Connor MA. Retinal function in Stargardt's disease and fundus flavimaculatus. Am J Ophthalmol. 1983;96(1):57-65.
6. Noble KG, Carr RE. Stargardt's disease and fundus flavimaculatus. Arch Ophthalmol. 1979;97(7):1281-5.

CHAPTER 30

Optic Nerve

1. CROWDED DISK SYNDROME (BILATERAL CHOROIDAL FOLDS AND OPTIC NEUROPATHY)

Ocular

Bilateral choroidal folds; optic disk congestion; optic atrophy; hyperopia; shortened axial length.

Clinical

Elevated intracranial pressure is ruled out.

Laboratory

Fluorescein angiogram, computed tomography (CT) or magnetic resonance imaging (MRI) when orbital tumor or inflammation is suspected; ultrasonography when posterior scleritis is suspected.

Treatment

Reversal of underlying cause is the therapy of choice.

BIBLIOGRAPHY

1. Kim JW, Lee DK, Cooper T. (2011). Compressive optic neuropathy. [online] Available from www.emedicine.com/oph/TOPIC167.HTM. [Accessed January, 2013].
2. Younge BR. (2012). Anterior ischemic optic neuropathy. [online] Available from www.emedicine.com/oph/TOPIC161.HTM. [Accessed January, 2013].

2. MENINGIOMA, OPTIC NERVE SHEATH

General

Primary meningioma arises from the cap cells of the arachnoid surrounding the intraorbital, or less frequently, the intracanalicular optic nerve. Secondary meningioma is extensions of intracranial meningioma into the orbit. Secondary meningioma is much more common than primary meningioma, but the unqualified term "optic nerve sheath meningioma" ordinarily refers to primary meningioma. It may be caused by radiation; head trauma, hormonal factors and infectious agents.

Clinical

Headache, head trauma.

Ocular

Compressive optic neuropathy; transient visual obscurations; visual loss; proptosis; exophthalmos; ptosis; diplopia.

Laboratory

Computed tomography and MRI are the best imaging techniques.

Treatment

Radiotherapy is followed with surgical removal. Chemotherapy is reserved for unresectable or recurrent meningiomas.

BIBLIOGRAPHY

1. Gossman MV, Zachariah SB, Khoromi S. (2012). Optic nerve sheath meningioma. [online] Available from emedicine.medscape.com/article/1217466-overview. [Accessed January, 2013].

3. NASAL RETINAL NERVE FIBER LAYER ATTENUATION

General

It is associated with the use of the antiepileptic drug vigabatrin.

Clinical

Epilepsy, seizures.

Ocular

Visual field loss—severe bilateral and symmetric, "concentric" constriction of sudden/rapid but variable onset; p deep and steeply bordered bilateral nasal annulus with a relative sparing of the temporal field.

Laboratory

Visual field testing, optical coherence tomography (OCT) testing.

Treatment

Visual field and OCT testing should be done routinely. 3.4 retinal nerve fiber layer (RNFL) thickness can be used as a biomarker of vigabatrin toxicity and when that is noted, vigabatrin should be stopped.

BIBLIOGRAPHY

1. Hardus P, Verduin W, Berendschot T, et al. Vigabatrin: longterm follow-up of electrophysiology and visual field examinations. Acta Ophthalmol Scand. 2003;81(5):459-65.
2. Lawthom C, Smith PE, Wild JM. Nasal retinal nerve fiber layer attenuation: a biomarker for vigabatrin toxicity. Ophthalmology. 2009;116(3):565-71.

4. OPTIC ATROPHY

[†]A. Demyelinating and degenerative disease
[†]B. Dermatologic disorders
[†]C. Drugs, poisons and vaccines
 D. GAPO syndrome
[†]E. Infections
 F. Leber hereditary optic neuropathy
 G. Marquardt-Loriaux syndrome
 H. Optic atrophy, nerve deafness
 I. Optic atrophy, non-Leber-type with early onset
 J. Spastic paraplegia optic atrophy, dementia
 K. Toxic /Nutritional optic neuropathy
[†]L. Trauma
[†]M. Vascular
 N. X-Chromosomal deletion
 O. Yellow fever

[†]Indicates a general entry and therefore has not been described in detail in the text

General

Axon degeneration in the retinogeniculate pathway; causes vary from hereditary, circulatory, metabolic, postinflammatory, traumatic and consecutive.

Clinical

Multiple sclerosis; orbit tumors.

Ocular

Axial myopia; myelinated nerve fibers; optic nerve pit; tilted disk; optic nerve hypoplasia; scleral crescent areas; optic disk drusen; papilledema.

Laboratory

Magnetic resonance imaging to look for solid lesions; B-scan to look for sheath dilatation; CT if associated with trauma; contrast sensitivity, color vision and pupillary evaluation are also useful.

Treatment

Intravenous steroids may be used with optic neuritis or ischemic neuropathy. Stem cell treatment may be the future treatment of choice.

BIBLIOGRAPHY

1. Gandhi R, Amula GM. (2012). Optic atrophy treatment and management. [online] Available from emedicine.medscape.com/article/1217760-treatment. [Accessed January, 2013].

4D. GAPO SYNDROME (GROWTH RETARDATION, ALOPECIA, PSEUDOANODONTIA, OPTIC ATROPHY SYNDROME)

General

Autosomal recessive.

Ocular

Progressive optic atrophy; glaucoma; keratoconus.

Clinical

Growth retardation; alopecia; pseudoanodontia; frontal bossing; high forehead; midfacial hypoplasia; wide-open anterior fontanel; retarded bone age; premature aged appearance; hypogonadism; hepatomegaly; muscular body build.

Laboratory

Erythrocyte sedimentation rate (ESR).

Treatment

Initial dose is 40–60 mg/day of prednisone, depending on the size of the patient and the severity of the disease.

BIBLIOGRAPHY

1. Gagliardi AR, González CH, Pratesi R. GAPO syndrome: report of three affected brothers. Am J Med Genet. 1984;19(2):217-23.
2. McKusick VA. Mendelian Inheritance in Man: A Catalog of Human Genes and Genetic Disorders, 12th edition. Baltimore, USA: The Johns Hopkins University Press; 1998.

4F. LEBER HEREDITARY OPTIC NEUROPATHY (OPTIC ATROPHY AMAUROSIS; PITUITARY SYNDROME; LEBER SYNDROME)

General

Male preponderance; in acute phase of neuropathy, there are three characteristic fundus changes: (1) circumpapillary microangiopathy, (2) pseudoedema around the disk and (3) absence of staining on fluorescein angiography; possibly a toxic metabolic disorder, an abnormality of cyanide metabolism, or an effect of smoking; maternally inherited disease affecting young males presenting with unilateral or bilateral visual loss; second eye becomes involved within weeks to months later; positive association with an inherited mutation in mitochondrial deoxyribonucleic acid (DNA).

Ocular

Sudden severe loss of vision, which usually reaches its maximum after 1 or 2 months; complete blindness rare; central vision remains seriously impaired; occasional considerable visual improvement; sheathing of retinal vessels; circumpapillary telangiectatic microangiopathy; initial low-grade optic neuritis, then bilateral optic atrophy (partial or complete); possible swelling of the disk with hemorrhages and exudates, but usually transitory; nystagmus; macular colobomas; optic disk edema; cataracts; keratoconus; hyperemia of the disk; swelling of peripapillary nerve fiber layer.

Clinical

Headaches and vertigo; Uhthoff's sign.

Laboratory

Diagnosis is made by clinical findings.

Treatment

• Intravenous steroids may be used with optic neuritis or ischemic neuropathy. Stem cell treatment may be the future treatment of choice.

- *Cataract*: Change in glasses can sometimes improve a patient's visual function temporarily; however the most common treatment is cataract surgery.
- *Keratoconus*: Spectacle correction, hard contacts, avoid eye rubbing. If hydrops occur, discontinue contact lens, use sodium chloride (NaCl) drops and ointment, patching and short course of steroids. As disease advances penetrating keratoplasty, deep anterior lamellar keratoplasty intacs with laser grooves or collagen stabilization of cornea.

BIBLIOGRAPHY

1. Younge BR. (2012). Anterior ischemic optic neuropathy. [online] Available from www.emedicine.com/oph/TOPIC161.HTM. [Accessed January, 2013].

4G. MARQUARDT-LORIAUX SYNDROME (WOLFRAM SYNDROME; DIABETES INSIPIDUS-DIABETES MELLITUS-OPTIC ATROPHY-DEAFNESS SYNDROME; DIDMOAD SYNDROME)

General

Autosomal recessive; present from childhood; age of onset varies.

Ocular

Optic nerve atrophy; color blindness; visual field defects; anisocoria; diabetic retinopathy; nystagmus; cataract; pigmentation of retina.

Clinical

Juvenile diabetes mellitus; diabetes insipidus; neurosensory hearing loss; hypertension; cerebellar dysfunction; vertigo; atony of urinary tract; anosmia; peripheral neuropathy; mitochondrial abnormalities; moderate hearing loss.

Laboratory

Diagnosis is made by clinical findings.

Treatment

Optic nerve atrophy: Intravenous steroids may be used with optic neuritis or ischemic neuropathy. Stem cell treatment may be the future treatment of choice.

BIBLIOGRAPHY

1. Bundey S, Poulton K, Whitwell H, et al. Mitochondrial abnormalities in the DIDMOAD syndrome. J Inherit Metab Dis. 1992;15(3):315-9.
2. Higashi K. Otologic findings of DIDMOAD syndrome. Am J Otol. 1991;12(1):57-60.
3. Mtanda AT, Cruysberg JR, Pinckers AJ. Optic atrophy in Wolfram syndrome. Ophthalmic Paediatr Genet. 1986;7(3):159-65.
4. Niemeyer G, Marquardt JL. Retinal function in an unique syndrome of optic atrophy, juvenile diabetes mellitus, diabetes insipidus, neurosensory hearing loss, autonomic dysfunction, and hyperalanineuria. Invest Ophthalmol. 1972;11(7):617-24.
5. Wolfram DJ. Diabetes mellitus and simple optic atrophy among siblings: report of four cases. Mayo Clin Proc. 1938;13:715.

4H. OPTIC ATROPHY, NERVE DEAFNESS

General

Autosomal recessive.

Ocular

Degeneration of optic nerves.

Clinical

Degeneration of the acoustic nerves; progressive polyneuropathy, distally.

Laboratory

Study depends on the disease process.

Treatment

No treatment is available.

BIBLIOGRAPHY

1. Gandhi R, Amula GM. (2012). Optic atrophy. [online] Available from www.emedicine.com/oph/TOPIC777.HTM. [Accessed January, 2013].

4I. OPTIC ATROPHY, NON-LEBER-TYPE, WITH EARLY ONSET

General

Sex-linked; onset early in life.

Ocular

Optic atrophy.

Clinical

Mental retardation; hyperactive knee jerks; absent ankle jerks, extensor plantar reflexes; dysarthria; tremor; dysdiadochokinesia; difficulty with tandem gait.

Laboratory

Study depends on the disease process.

Treatment

No treatment is available.

BIBLIOGRAPHY

1. Gandhi R, Amula GM. (2012). Optic atrophy. [online] Available from www.emedicine.com/oph/TOPIC777.HTM. [Accessed January, 2013].

4J. SPASTIC PARAPLEGIA, OPTIC ATROPHY, DEMENTIA

General

Autosomal dominant.

Ocular

Pallor of optic disk; constricted visual fields; optic atrophy; visible deficit in retinal fiber layer; deficit in color vision; slight decrease in visual acuity; pupillary reflex sluggishness to light.

Clinical

Dementia; spastic paraparesis; stiff gait; increased deep tendon reflexes; bilateral extensor plantar responses; euphoria; pseudobulbar speech; incontinence.

Laboratory

Erythrocyte sedimentation rate, C-reactive protein (CRP).

Treatment

Control of blood pressure and diabetes. In giant cell arteritis, systemic steroids are used.

BIBLIOGRAPHY

1. Younge BR. (2012). Anterior ischemic optic neuropathy. [online] Available from www.emedicine.com/oph/TOPIC161.HTM. [Accessed January, 2013].

4K. TOXIC/NUTRITIONAL OPTIC NEUROPATHY

General

It is caused by deficit nutrition or abuse of ethanol and tobacco; is seen more frequently in underdeveloped countries but is seen in United States undernourished tobacco and alcohol abusers. It can also be associated with ingestion of toxic substances, workplace exposure or systemic medications.

Clinical

Alcoholism; drug and tobacco abuse.

Ocular

Papillomacular bundle damage; central scotoma; decreased color vision; bilateral vision loss; hyperemic disk; optic atrophy; temporal disk pallor; flame-shaped hemorrhages.

Laboratory

Clinical observation is used to make the diagnosis. Blood work for serum vitamin B_{12} and red cell folate levels should be obtained. Urinalysis and other blood work may be needed to identify the possible toxin.

Treatment

Correction of the underlying etiology includes improving nutrition and eliminating the toxin is critical.

BIBLIOGRAPHY

1. Zafar A. (2011). Toxic/nutritional optic neuropathy. [online] Available from emedicine.medscape.com/article/1217661-overview. [Accessed January, 2013].

⊟ 4N. X-CHROMOSOMAL DELETION (OPTIC ATROPHY)

General

Deletion of proximal part of long arm of the X chromosome; deletion covers part of region Xq21.1-Xq21.31, the locus for choroideremia; congenital deafness; probable mental retardation.

Ocular

Choroideremia, translucent pigment epithelium; peripheral hyperpigmentation; diffuse choriocapillary layer and retinal pigment epithelium; decreased night vision; optic atrophy; excessive myopia; nystagmus.

Clinical

Congenital deafness; mental retardation; corpus callosum agenesia; cleft lip and palate; anhidrotic ectodermal dysplasia; agammaglobulinemia.

Laboratory

Chromosome studies.

Treatment

None.

⊟ BIBLIOGRAPHY

1. Bleeker-Wagemakers LM, Friedrich U, Gal A, et al. Close linkage between Norrie disease, a cloned DNA sequence from the proximal short arm, and the centromere of the X chromosome. Hum Genet. 1985;71(3):211-4.
2. Rosenberg T, Niebuhr E, Yang HM, et al. Choroideremia, congenital deafness and mental retardation in a family with an X chromosomal deletion. Ophthalmic Paediatr Genet. 1987;8(3):139-43.

⊟ 4O. YELLOW FEVER

General

Acute infectious disease of short duration and extremely variable severity.

Ocular

Lid edema; orbital pain; subconjunctival, vitreal and anterior chamber hemorrhages; mydriasis; optic neuritis; partial optic atrophy.

Clinical

Fever; headache; nausea; epistaxis; relative bradycardia; albuminuria; convulsions; tongue shows red margins with white furred center; copious hemorrhages; anuria; delirium; slow pulse; jaundice; "black vomit"; hematemesis; coma; death.

Laboratory

Complete blood count, coagulation studies, urinalysis, chest X-ray, polymerase chain reaction (PCR) assay, monoclonal enzyme immunoassay.

Treatment

No specific treatment.

⊟ BIBLIOGRAPHY

1. Busowski MT, Robertson JL, Wallace MR. (2012). Yellow fever. [online] Available from www.emedicine.com/med/TOPIC2432.HTM. [Accessed January, 2013].

⊟ 5. OPTIC NEURITIS

†A. Drugs, poisons, vaccines
 B. Optic neuropathy, anterior ischemic
 C. Botulism
 D. Optic neuritis, childhood
 E. Optic neuropathy, compressive
 F. Optic nerve decompression for traumatic neuropathy
 G. Lyme disease
 H. Rocky Mountain Spotted fever

†Indicates a general entry and therefore has not been described in detail in the text

General

Inflammatory demyelinating condition of the optic nerve that usually presents a subacute painful unilateral impairment of vision, although bilateral visual loss can occur.

Clinical

Multiple sclerosis.

Ocular

Retro-ocular pain, visual loss, decreased color vision, central scotoma.

Laboratory

Orbital MRI, cerebrospinal fluid examination is done to rule out infectious or other inflammatory optic neuropathy.

Treatment

Systemic corticosteroids.

⎙ BIBLIOGRAPHY

1. Ergene E, Machens NA. (2012). Adult optic neuritis. [online] Available from www.emedicine.com/oph/TOPIC186.HTM. [Accessed January, 2013].
2. Schatz MP, Carter JE. (2011). Childhood optic neuritis. [online] Available from www.emedicine.com/oph/TOPIC343.HTM. [Accessed January, 2013].

⎙ 5B. OPTIC NEUROPATHY, ANTERIOR ISCHEMIC

General

Ischemic process affecting the posterior circulation of the globe. It may be arteritic or nonarteritic; usually occurs in individuals over age of 50 years.

Clinical

Hypertension; myocardial infarction; atherosclerosis; giant cell arteritis; malaise; headache; scalp tenderness; jaw pain; diabetes mellitus; migraine; Takayasu's disease; polycythemia vera; sickle cell disease; hypotension; syphilis; lupus; Buerger's disease; postimmunization; radiation necrosis; sleep apnea.

Ocular

Visual loss; ocular palsies; temporal pain.

Laboratory

Erythrocyte sedimentation rate is the most important test to determine if it is elevated; temporal artery biopsy is used to diagnose giant cell arteritis.

Treatment

Comanagement with an internist is recommended; large dose of systemic prednisone on a tapered scale is the usual treatment.

⎙ BIBLIOGRAPHY

1. Younge BR. (2012). Anterior ischemic optic neuropathy. [online] Available from emedicine.medscape.com/article/1216891-overview. [Accessed January, 2013].

⎙ 5C. BOTULISM

General

It is caused by a toxin-producing strain of *Clostridium botulinum*; it occurs primarily after the ingestion of contaminated food; the organism can produce a neurotoxin, the effect of which can be life threatening.

Ocular

Absent optokinetic nystagmus, absent vertical gaze; marked limitation of horizontal gaze; ptosis; diplopia; decreased tear secretion; mydriasis; paralysis of accommodation; nystagmus; optic atrophy; optic neuritis; extraocular muscle paresis.

Clinical

Dizziness; severe respiratory impairment; gastrointestinal disturbances; dysphagia; dysarthria; postural hypotension.

Laboratory

Toxin assay for early diagnosis, whereas later cases are more likely to yield a positive specimen culture.

Treatment

Antitoxin appears to be the only effective medication. Supportive care such as ventilation and parenteral nutrition are necessary for the duration of the paralytic illness.

⎙ BIBLIOGRAPHY

1. Patel B, Taylor SF. (2012). Ophthalmologic manifestations of botulism. [online] Available from www.emedicine.com/oph/TOPIC493.HTM. [Accessed January, 2013].

⎘ 5D. OPTIC NEURITIS, CHILDHOOD

General

Inflammatory process of the optic nerve. In children, most cases of optic neuritis are due to a viral or other infection or with immunization.

Clinical

Multiple sclerosis; acute disseminated encephalomyelitis; neuromyelitis; injections of sinuses or orbital structures; Lyme disease; syphilis; leukemia; wasp stings; cat scratch disease; toxoplasmosis; toxocariasis; helminths.

Ocular

Visual loss; change in color perception; loss of visual field change in brightness sense; afferent pupil defect; disk edema.

Laboratory

Magnetic resonance imaging and lumbar puncture help to determine the cause.

Treatment

Some propose no treatment. Some give intravenous steroids for initial therapy. Plasma exchange and intravenous immunoglobulin have also been used.

⎘ BIBLIOGRAPHY

1. Schatz MP, Carter JE. (2011). Childhood optic neuritis. [online] Available from emedicine.medscape.com/article/1217290-overview. [Accessed January, 2013].

⎘ 5E. OPTIC NEUROPATHY, COMPRESSIVE

General

Injury to the optic nerve anywhere along this pathway by an extrinsic lesion by compressive force. Typically, it is caused by optic nerve glioma or rhabdomyosarcoma.

Clinical

Endocrine dysfunction; cranial nerve palsies; stroke; tumors within the orbit; facial numbness; pituitary dysfunction; glioma; rhabdomyosarcoma.

Ocular

Slow progressive vision loss; dyschromatopsia; relative afferent pupillary defect; visual field defect; optic atrophy; papilledema; proptosis; strabismus; eyelid malposition.

Laboratory

Magnetic resonance imaging is generally the test of choice; ultrasonography and CT can also be useful.

Treatment

Corticosteroids are useful for inflammatory and thyroid issues; radiation therapy and surgical excision may be necessary with malignant lesions.

⎘ BIBLIOGRAPHY

1. Kim JW, Lee DK, Cooper T. (2011). Compressive optic neuropathy. [online] Available from emedicine.medscape.com/article/1217005-overview. [Accessed January, 2013].

⎘ 5F. OPTIC NERVE DECOMPRESSION FOR TRAUMATIC NEUROPATHY

General

It is a complication of closed head injury. It can be temporary or permanent.

Clinical

Closed head injury.

Ocular

Afferent pupillary defect; decreased visual function; subnormal color vision; visual field loss; optic nerve sheath hematoma; optic nerve impingement.

Laboratory

Thin slice CT provides the best imaging of orbital soft tissue.

Treatment

Contemporary treatments for traumatic optic neuropathy have included observation, steroids and surgical decompression.

⊟ BIBLIOGRAPHY

1. O'Brien EK, Leopold D, Gigantelli JW, et al. (2012). Optic nerve decompression for traumatic optic neuropathy. [online] Available from emedicine.medscape.com/article/868252-overview. [Accessed January, 2013].

⊟ 5G. LYME DISEASE

General

Lyme disease is caused by tick bite; symptoms resolve after treatment.

Ocular

Keratitis may occur up to 5 years of age after the first episode; diplopia; photophobia; ischemic optic neuropathy; iritis; panophthalmitis; conjunctivitis; exudative retinal detachment; choroiditis; vitreitis; multiple cranial nerve palsies; association with acute, posterior, multifocal, placoid, pigment epitheliopathy; branch retinal artery occlusion.

Clinical

Arthritis; increased intracranial pressure; effusion of knees; swelling of wrists.

Laboratory

Immunofluorescent assay and enzyme-linked immunosorbent assay.

Treatment

Oral antibiotics for 2–3 weeks: tetracycline 500 mg four times a day, doxycycline 100 mg two times a day, phenoxymethyl penicillin 500 mg four times a day or amoxicillin 500 mg three to four times a day.

⊟ BIBLIOGRAPHY

1. Zaidman GW. (2011). Ophthalmic aspects of Lyme disease overview of Lyme disease. [online] Available from www.emedicine.com/oph/TOPIC262.HTM. [Accessed January, 2013].

⊟ 5H. ROCKY MOUNTAIN SPOTTED FEVER

General

An acute systemic disease caused by *Rickettsia rickettsii* and transmitted by a wood tick or dog tick.

Ocular

Conjunctivitis; optic atrophy; cotton-wool spots; scotoma; uveitis; optic neuritis; paralysis of accommodation; paralysis of extraocular muscles; retinal vascular occlusion; vitreal opacity; hypopyon; anterior uveitis with fibrin clots.

Clinical

Fever; chills; headache; muscle aches; rash.

Laboratory

Early diagnosis depends on clinical and epidemiologic grounds. PCR has high sensitivity and specificity.

Treatment

Intravenous tetracycline and chloramphenicol should be started as soon as possible. Oral doxycycline, tetracycline and chloramphenicol may be considered but only if patient is not acutely ill.

⊟ BIBLIOGRAPHY

1. Cunha BA, O'Brien MS. (2012). Rocky mountain spotted fever. [online] Available from www.emedicine.com/oph/TOPIC503.HTM. [Accessed January, 2013].

6. PSEUDOPAPILLEDEMA (OPTIC NERVE HEAD DRUSEN)

General

Autosomal dominant; incidence in males and females is approximately the same; two-thirds of the cases are bilateral; visual acuity is usually unaffected; it may cause slowly progressive visual field defect.

Ocular

Elevation of optic disk; drusen; injected conjunctiva; associated with retinitis pigmentosa, subretinal pigment epithelium hemorrhages (rare).

Clinical

None.

Laboratory

B-scan ultrasonography, fluorescein angiography.

Treatment

No treatment is needed for most causes of pseudopapilledema because they represent normal physiologic variants.

BIBLIOGRAPHY

1. Gossman MV, Giovannini J. (2011). Pseudopapilledema. [online] Available from www.emedicine.com/oph/TOPIC615.HTM. [Accessed January, 2013].

7. OPTIC NERVE HYPOPLASIA, FAMILIAL (BILATERAL, UNILATERAL)

General

Autosomal dominant; congenital defect of optic nerve and retina that occurs in both unilateral and bilateral forms; onset at birth; majority of cases are sporadic, although there are reports of familial cases; association of this condition with maternal ingestion of various substances including quinine, lysergic acid diethylamide and anticonvulsants.

Ocular

Optic nerve hypoplasia; diameter of optic disk is one-third of normal size; nystagmus; peripapillary halos; situs inversus of disk; strabismus; choroidal atrophy; microphthalmos; coloboma of choroid and/or optic disk; blepharophimosis; ptosis; aniridia; ocular motor nerve palsy.

Clinical

Central nervous system defects; chromosomal abnormalities; cerebral malformations; vascular hypertension.

Laboratory

Diagnosis is made by clinical findings.

Treatment

None.

BIBLIOGRAPHY

1. Hackenbruch Y, Meerhoff E, Besio R, et al. Familial bilateral optic nerve hypoplasia. Am J Ophthalmol. 1975;79(2): 314-20.

8. OPTIC PIT SYNDROME

General

Congenital.

Ocular

Serous detachment of macula; situs inversus; peripapillary chorioretinal changes; cilioretinal vessels; large optic disk; tortuous retinal vessels; retinoschisis.

Clinical

None.

Laboratory

Diagnosis is made by clinical findings.

Treatment

Retinal detachment: Scleral buckle, pneumatic retinopexy and vitrectomy may be used to close all the breaks.

⊟ BIBLIOGRAPHY

1. Gass JD. Serous detachment of the macula. Secondary to congenital pit of the optic nervehead. Am J Ophthalmol. 1969;67(6):821-41.

2. Giuffrè G. Optic pit syndrome. Doc Ophthalmol. 1986;64(2): 187-99.
3. Lineoff H, Lopez R, Kreissig I, et al. Retinoschisis associated with optic nerve pits. Arch Ophthalmol. 1988;106(1): 61-7.

⊟ 9. PAPILLEDEMA

General

Papilledema is the swelling of the optic disk due to increased intracranial pressure.

Clinical

Holocranial headaches, neck and back pain, pulsatile tinnitus, nausea and vomiting.

Ocular

Visual loss, nerve fiber loss, intermittent or constant diplopia.

Laboratory

Lumbar puncture to determine if intracranial pressure is elevated.

Treatment

Underlying cause should be determined and treated. Systemic acetazolamide is the medical therapy of choice.

⊟ BIBLIOGRAPHY

1. Gossman MV, Giovannini J. (2012). Papilledema. [online] Available from www.emedicine.com/oph/TOPIC187.HTM. [Accessed January, 2013].

⊟ 10. SYMONDS SYNDROME (OTITIC HYDROCEPHALUS SYNDROME; SEROUS MENINGITIS SYNDROME; BENIGN INTRACRANIAL HYPERTENSION; PSEUDOTUMOR CEREBRI)

General

Children and adolescents; protracted course; increased cerebrospinal fluid, but without increase in protein or cells.

Ocular

Sixth nerve palsy, ipsilateral side with otitis media; retinal hemorrhages and exudates; moderate-to-marked papilledema followed by secondary optic atrophy; unilateral or bilateral swelling of the optic nerve head has been reported; cranial nerve third and fourth involvement; bilateral retinal vein occlusion.

Clinical

Greatly increased pressure of spinal fluid, often greater than 300 mm, without increased cells or protein; intermittent headaches; otitis media; chronic renal failure; chronic myeloid leukemia.

Laboratory

Imaging studies such as MRI are done to rule out tumors of brain and spinal cord, and lumbar puncture.

Treatment

Carbonic anhydrase inhibitors such as acetazolamide and furosemide are useful.

⊟ BIBLIOGRAPHY

1. Chang D, Nagamoto G, Smith WE. Benign intracranial hypertension and chronic renal failure. Cleve Clin J Med. 1992;59(4):419-22.
2. Chari C, Rao NS. Benign intracranial hypertension–its unusual manifestations. Headache. 1991;31(9):599-600.
3. Chern S, Magargal LE, Brav SS. Bilateral central retinal vein occlusion as an initial manifestation of pseudotumor cerebri. Ann Ophthalmol. 1991;23(2):54-7.
4. Roy FH, Fraunfelder FW, Fraunfelder FT. Roy and Fraunfelder's Current Ocular Therapy, 6th edition. Philadelphia, PA: WB Saunders; 2008.
5. Venable HP. Pseudo-tumor cerebri. J Natl Med Assoc. 1970;62(6):435-40.
6. Venable HP. Pseudo-tumor cerebri: further studies. J Natl Med Assoc. 1973;65(3):194-7.

CHAPTER 31

Orbit

⊟ 1A. ACUTE ORBITAL COMPARTMENT SYNDROME

General

Increased pressure within the confined orbital space generally secondary to facial trauma or surgery; blindness can occur without prompt treatment.

Clinical

Facial trauma; head trauma.

Ocular

Decreased visual acuity; ischemic optic neuropathy; retrobulbar hematoma; diplopia; proptosis; eye pain; reduction of ocular motility; papilledema; cherry-red macula; ecchymosis of lids; chemosis; increased intraocular pressure; afferent pupillary defect; ophthalmoplegia.

Laboratory

Computed tomography (CT) or magnetic resonance imaging (MRI) may be useful to identify the etiology of compression.

Treatment

Immediate osmotic agents and carbonic anhydrase inhibitors should be used; lateral orbital canthotomy should be used as soon as diagnosis is made and life-threatening injuries are stabilized to prevent permanent visual loss.

⊟ BIBLIOGRAPHY

1. Peak DA, Green TE. (2011). Acute orbital compartment syndrome. [online] Available from emedicine.medscape.com/article/799528-overview. [Accessed October, 2013].

⊟ 1B. FORAMEN LACERUM SYNDROME
(ANEURYSM OF INTERNAL CAROTID ARTERY SYNDROME)

General

Most commonly caused by congenital aneurysm involving the intradural portion of the carotid artery.

Ocular

Periorbital pain; ptosis; oculomotor paralysis with ptosis, diplopia and internal ophthalmoplegia; cranial nerves IV and VI may be involved; homonymous hemianopia (occasionally); loss of pupillary reflexes for light and accommodation; papilledema; optic atrophy.

Clinical

Meningism; mental disturbances; unilateral frontal or orbital headache; migraine attacks.

Laboratory

Computed tomography, MRI, angiography, magnetic resonance angiography (MRA).

Treatment

Endovascular balloon occlusion.

🗗 BIBLIOGRAPHY

1. Dailey EJ, Holloway JA, Murto RE, et al. Evaluation of ocular signs and symptoms in cerebral aneurysms. Arch Ophthalmol. 1964;71:463-74.
2. Geeraets WJ. Ocular Syndromes, 3rd edition. Philadelphia, PA: Lea & Febiger; 1976.
3. Misra M, Mohanty AB, Rath S. Giant aneurysm of internal carotid artery presenting features of retrobulbar neuritis. Indian J Ophthalmol. 1991;39(1):28-9.

🗗 1C. BLATT SYNDROME (CRANIO-ORBITO-OCULAR DYSRAPHIA)

General

Autosomal dominant; characterized by distichiasis and anisometropia; both sexes are affected; present from birth.

Ocular

Hypertelorism; microphthalmos; distichiasis with the meibomian glands usually absent; anisometropia.

Clinical

Meningocele or meningoencephalocele; cranial deformities; malformations of facial bones.

Laboratory

Diagnosis is made by clinical findings.

Treatment

- *Distichiasis*:
  - Symptomatic: Therapeutic contact lenses as well as lubricating drops and ointments. Epilation with electrolysis cryosurgery; double freeze-thaw down to –20°C; lid splitting procedure.

🗗 BIBLIOGRAPHY

1. Blatt N. [Cranio-orbito-ocular dysraphia and meningocele]. Rev Otoneuroophtalmol. 1961;33:185-232.
2. Duke-Elder S (Ed). System of Ophthalmology. St Louis: CV Mosby; 1976.
3. Magalini SI, Scrascia E. Dictionary of Medical Syndromes, 2nd edition. Philadelphia, PA: Lippincott Williams and Wilkins; 1981.

🗗 1D. CAROTID ARTERY SYNDROME (CAVERNOUS SINUS FISTULA SYNDROME; RED-EYED SHUNT SYNDROME)

General

Seventy-five percent of cases are caused by trauma; others occur spontaneously or are congenital; fistula from carotid artery to cavernous sinus.

Ocular

Progressive, pulsating exophthalmos; distended pulsating superior orbital vein; venous congestion of lids; variable ophthalmoplegia, depending on involvement of cranial nerves III to VI; secondary glaucoma; congestion of conjunctiva with chemosis; corneal ulcerations; eversion of the lower lid; loss of corneal sensation; retinal edema; engorgement of retinal veins; papilledema; optic atrophy; ocular bruit that may be subjective and/or objective; diplopia; decreased vision; choroidal folds; dilated superior ophthalmic vein.

Clinical

Severe unilateral headache; buzzing noise.

Laboratory

Orbital ultrasonography, CT, six-vessel cranial digital subtraction angiography—characterization of the arterial supply and venous drainage of fistula.

Treatment

Use of intraocular lowering agent and topical lubrication is the ocular treatment of choice.

BIBLIOGRAPHY

1. Dailey EJ, Holloway JA, Murto RE, et al. Evaluation of ocular signs and symptoms in cerebral aneurysms. Arch Ophthalmol. 1964;71:463-74.
2. Duane TD. Clinical Ophthalmology. Philadelphia, PA: JB Lippincott; 1987.
3. Flaharty PM, Lieb WE, Sergott RC, et al. Color Doppler imaging. A new noninvasive technique to diagnose and monitor carotid cavernous sinus fistulas. Arch Ophthalmol. 1991;109(4):522-6.
4. Roy FH, Fraunfelder FW, Fraunfelder FT. Roy and Fraunfelder's Current Ocular Therapy, 6th edition. Philadelphia, PA: WB Saunders; 2008.
5. Gonshor LG, Kline LB. Choroidal folds and dural cavernous sinus fistula. Arch Ophthalmol. 1991;109(8):1065-6.
6. Phelps CD, Thompson HS, Ossoinig KC. The diagnosis and prognosis of atypical carotid-cavernous fistula (red-eyed shunt syndrome). Am J Ophthalmol. 1982;93(4):423-36.
7. Travers B. A case of Aneurysm by Anastomosis in the Orbit, cured by the Ligature of the common Carotid Artery. Med Chir Trans. 1811;2:1-420.1.

1E. FOIX SYNDROME (CAVERNOUS SINUS SYNDROME; HYPOPHYSEAL-SPHENOIDAL SYNDROME; CAVERNOUS SINUS NEURALGIA SYNDROME; GODTFREDSEN SYNDROME; CAVERNOUS SINUS-NASOPHARYNGEAL TUMOR SYNDROME; CAVERNOUS SINUS THROMBOSIS)

General

Causes include tumor of lateral sinus wall or sphenoid bone, intracranial aneurysm, cavernous and lateral sinus thrombosis, or lesions; multiple myeloma; may result from infarctions or cancer or be idiopathic.

Ocular

Proptosis; severe ocular and periorbital pain; lid edema; paresis or paralysis of cranial nerves III, IV, V and VI; corneal anesthesia; optic atrophy.

Clinical

Postauricular edema; trigeminal neuralgia; deviation of the tongue toward paralyzed side; patients usually have prominent manifestations of sepsis and paranasal sinus; local skin infections are the most common cause.

Laboratory

Computed tomography and MRI.

Treatment

Radiotherapy, anticoagulation, high-dose antibiotic therapy.

BIBLIOGRAPHY

1. Kattah JC, Pula JH. (2012). Cavernous sinus syndromes. [online] Available from www.emedicine.com/neuro/TOPIC572.HTM. [Accessed October, 2013].

1F. ORBITAL CELLULITIS AND ABSCESS

General

Potentially life threatening, requires prompt evaluation and treatment.

Clinical

Sinusitis, ear infection, diabetes, dental disease.

Ocular

Orbital pain, proptosis, diplopia, decreased ocular motility, eyelid swelling and erythema, vision loss.

Laboratory

Diagnosis is made by clinical findings.

Treatment

Intravenous and oral antibiotic.

BIBLIOGRAPHY

1. Harrington JN. (2012). Orbital cellulitis. [online] Available from www.emedicine.com/oph/TOPIC205.HTM. [Accessed October, 2013].

1G. EXOPHTHALMOS (PROPTOSIS)

General

Abnormal protrusion of the eyeball. Etiology is varied and can include inflammatory, vascular or infections. Thyroid disease is the most frequent cause for both unilateral and bilateral exophthalmos.

Clinical

Thyroid disease, lymphoma, cavernous hemangiomas, leukemia, sinus disease.

Ocular

Proptosis, orbital cellulitis, orbital emphysema, lid retraction, punctate keratopathy, corneal ulcer, corneal perforation, diplopia.

Laboratory

Thyroid function studies, CT, MRI, ocular ultrasonography can all be used to determine the cause.

Treatment

Reversing the problem, which is causing the exophthalmos, is the treatment of choice and will minimize the ocular complications. Ocular lubricants are beneficial for controlling the corneal exposure.

BIBLIOGRAPHY

1. Mercandetti M, Cohen AJ. (2012). Exophthalmos. [online] Available from www.emedicine.com/oph/TOPIC616.HTM. [Accessed October, 2013].

1H. GENERAL FIBROSIS SYNDROME [CONGENITAL ENOPHTHALMOS WITH OCULAR MUSCLE FIBROSIS AND PTOSIS; CONGENITAL FIBROSIS OF THE INFERIOR RECTUS WITH PTOSIS; STRABISMUS FIXUS; VERTICAL RETRACTION SYNDROME (CONGENITAL FIBROSIS SYNDROME)]

General

Present from birth; familial history; apparent autosomal dominant transmission; sex-linked recessive transmission is also reported.

Ocular

Ptosis; enophthalmos; disk hypoplasia; astigmatism; esotropia; exotropia; hypotropia; nystagmus; visual loss; positive forced duction test; may be associated with Marcus Gunn jaw-winking and synergistic divergence in attempted right gaze.

Clinical

None.

Laboratory

Neuroimaging is the most essential laboratory study.

Treatment

Surgically approximating normal orbital bone positions before addressing soft tissue volume loss.

BIBLIOGRAPHY

1. Soparkar CN. (2012). Enophthalmos. [online] Available from www.emedicine.com/oph/TOPIC617.HTM. [Accessed October, 2013].

⊟ 1I. ORBITAL INFARCTION SYNDROME

General

Rare disorder secondary to ischemia of the intraorbital tissue due to occlusion of the ophthalmic artery and its branches.

Clinical

Occlusion of carotid artery; giant-cell arteritis; mucormycosis; systemic vasculitis; acute perfusion failure; sickle cell disease.

Ocular

Proptosis; ophthalmoplegia; lid edema; restricted motility; compressive optic neuropathy; reduced visual acuity; pain.

Laboratory

Magnetic resonance imaging is more specific than CT or nuclear scintigraphy in the evaluation of orbital changes.

Treatment

Orbital decompression.

⊟ BIBLIOGRAPHY

1. Maier P, Feltgen N, Lagrèze WA. Bilateral orbital infarction syndrome after bifrontal craniotomy. Arch Ophthalmol. 2007;125(3):422-3.

⊟ 1J. SPHENOCAVERNOUS SYNDROME

General

Lesion in the cavernous sinus; similar to the superior orbital fissure syndrome (Rochon-Duvigneaud syndrome) and orbital apex syndrome (Rochon-Duvigneaud syndrome).

Ocular

Proptosis; edema; paresis of cranial nerves III, IV and VI (paralysis of the abducens nerve precedes paralysis of the oculomotor nerve, because the abducens is situated between the internal carotid artery and the cavernous sinus wall); conjunctival edema.

Laboratory

Computed tomography and MRI.

Clinical

Paresis of the first (sometimes second and third) division of cranial nerve V; sinusitis.

Treatment

- *Proptosis*: Ocular lubricants are beneficial for controlling the corneal exposure.
- *Paresis of cranial nerve III*: Prism therapy, surgical—muscle surgery on the affected muscle, occlusion of the involved eye to relieve diplopia.

⊟ BIBLIOGRAPHY

1. Geeraets WJ. Ocular Syndromes, 3rd edition. Philadelphia, PA: Lea & Febiger; 1976.
2. Jefferson G. Concerning injuries, aneurysms and tumours involving the cavernous sinus. Trans Ophthalmol Soc UK. 1953;73:117.
3. Sekhar LN, Linskey ME, Sen CN, et al. Surgical management of lesions within the cavernous sinus. Clin Neurosurg. 1991;37:440-89.
4. Watson NJ, Dick AD, Hutchinson CH. A case of sinusitis presenting with spheno-cavernous syndrome: discussion of the differential diagnosis. Scott Med J. 1991;36(6): 179-80.

🗗 1K. YELLOW FEVER

General

Acute infectious disease of short duration and extremely variable severity.

Ocular

Lid edema; orbital pain; subconjunctival, vitreal and anterior chamber hemorrhages; mydriasis; optic neuritis; partial optic atrophy.

Clinical

Fever; headache; nausea; epistaxis; relative bradycardia; albuminuria; convulsions; tongue shows red margins with white furred center; copious hemorrhages; anuria; delirium; slow pulse; jaundice; "black vomit"; hematemesis; coma; death.

Laboratory

Complete blood count (CBC), coagulation studies, urinalysis, chest X-ray, polymerase chain reaction (PCR) assay, monoclonal enzyme immunoassay.

Treatment

No specific treatment.

🗗 BIBLIOGRAPHY

1. Busowski MT, Robertson JL, Wallace MR. (2011). Yellow fever. [online] Available from www.emedicine.com/med/TOPIC2432.HTM. [Accessed October, 2013].

🗗 2A. CAROTID ARTERY SYNDROME (CAVERNOUS SINUS FISTULA SYNDROME; RED-EYED SHUNT SYNDROME)

General

Seventy-five percent of cases caused by trauma; others occur spontaneously or are congenital; fistula from carotid artery to cavernous sinus.

Ocular

Progressive, pulsating exophthalmos; distended pulsating superior orbital vein; venous congestion of lids; variable ophthalmoplegia, depending on involvement of cranial nerves III to VI; secondary glaucoma; congestion of conjunctiva with chemosis; corneal ulcerations; eversion of the lower lid; loss of corneal sensation; retinal edema; engorgement of retinal veins; papilledema; optic atrophy; ocular bruit that may be subjective and/or objective; diplopia; visual decrease; choroidal folds; dilated superior ophthalmic vein.

Clinical

Severe unilateral headache; buzzing noise.

Laboratory

Orbital ultrasonography, CT, six-vessel cranial digital subtraction angiography—characterization of the arterial supply and venous drainage of fistula.

Treatment

Use of intraocular lowering agent and topical lubrication is the ocular treatment of choice.

🗗 BIBLIOGRAPHY

1. Dailey EJ, Holloway JA, Murto RE, et al. Evaluation of ocular signs and symptoms in cerebral aneurysms. Arch Ophthalmol. 1964;71:463-74.
2. Duane TD. Clinical Ophthalmology. Philadelphia: JB Lippincott; 1987.
3. Flaharty PM, Lieb WE, Sergott RC, et al. Color Doppler imaging. A new noninvasive technique to diagnose and monitor carotid cavernous sinus fistulas. Arch Ophthalmol. 1991;109:522-6.
4. Gonshor LG, Kline LB. Choroidal folds and dural cavernous sinus fistula. Arch Ophthalmol. 1991;109:1065-6.
5. Phelps CD, Thompson HS, Ossoinig KC. The diagnosis and prognosis of atypical carotid cavernous fistula. Am J Ophthalmol. 1982;93:423-36.
6. Roy FH, Fraunfelder FW, Fraunfelder FT. Roy and Fraunfelder's Current Ocular Therapy, 6th edition. Philadelphia: WB Saunders; 2008.

⊟ 2B. FOIX SYNDROME (CAVERNOUS SINUS SYNDROME; HYPOPHYSEAL-SPHENOIDAL SYNDROME; CAVERNOUS SINUS NEURALGIA SYNDROME; GODTFREDSEN SYNDROME; CAVERNOUS SINUS-NASOPHARYNGEAL TUMOR SYNDROME; CAVERNOUS SINUS THROMBOSIS)

General

Causes include tumor of lateral sinus wall or sphenoid bone, intracranial aneurysm, cavernous and lateral sinus thrombosis, or lesions; multiple myeloma; may result from infarctions or cancer or be idiopathic.

Ocular

Proptosis; severe ocular and periorbital pain; lid edema; paresis or paralysis of cranial nerves III, IV, V and VI; corneal anesthesia; optic atrophy.

Clinical

Postauricular edema; trigeminal neuralgia; deviation of the tongue toward paralyzed side; patients usually have prominent manifestations of sepsis and paranasal sinus; local skin infections are the most common cause.

Laboratory

Computed tomography and MRI.

Treatment

Radiotherapy, anticoagulation, high-dose antibiotic therapy.

⊟ BIBLIOGRAPHY

1. Kattah JC, Pula JH. (2012). Cavernous sinus syndromes. [online] Available from www.emedicine.com/neuro/TOPIC572.HTM. [Accessed October, 2013].

⊟ 2C. EXTERNAL ORBITAL FRACTURES

General

External fracture of the orbit results in direct disjunction of any portion of the orbital rim usually with bony orbital wall involvement.

Clinical

Tripod fractures of the zygoma, naso-orbito-ethmoid fractures.

Laboratory

Computed tomography and ultrasound.

Treatment

Surgery is indicated when bone displacement causes cosmetic or functional defects.

⊟ BIBLIOGRAPHY

1. Seiff S, Torres J, DeAngelis DD, et al. (2012). Zygomatic Orbital Fracture. [online] Available from www.emedicine.com/oph/TOPIC231.HTM. [Accessed October, 2013].

⊟ 2D. INTERNAL ORBITAL FRACTURES (BLOWOUT FRACTURE)

General

Trauma that involves the walls of the orbit leaving the bony rim intact.

Clinical

Tripod fracture of the zygoma.

Ocular

Proptosis, enophthalmos, diplopia.

Laboratory

Computed tomography.

Treatment

The transconjunctival approach with lateral canthotomy and cantholysis is preferred to expose the orbital floor, nasal approach to further expose the medial wall.

🗗 BIBLIOGRAPHY

1. Cohen AJ, Mercandetti M. (2012). Orbital floor fractures (blowout). [online] Available from www.emedicine.com/plastic/TOPIC485.HTM. [Accessed October, 2013].

🗗 2E. ORBITAL FRACTURE, APEX

General

Apex orbital fracture affects the most posterior portion of the pyramidal-shaped orbit, positioned at the craniofacial junction. Usually, it is associated with blunt or penetrating trauma to the face or skull.

Clinical

Intracranial or facial trauma.

Ocular

Visual loss; optic neuropathy; optic nerve sheath hematoma; optic nerve impingement; optic nerve compression; retrobulbar hemorrhage; extraocular muscle nerve palsy; diplopia; afferent pupil defect; periocular ecchymosis; proptosis.

Laboratory

Computed tomography scan is the most appropriate method to make diagnosis.

Treatment

In cases that involve decreased vision and optic nerve injury, medical or surgical nerve decompression should be considered. Corticosteroids should be the initial treatment and if it is not effective, surgical intervention is necessary.

🗗 BIBLIOGRAPHY

1. Patel B, Taylor SF. (2012). Apex orbital fracture. [online] Available from emedicine.medscape.com/article/1218196-overview. [Accessed October, 2013].

🗗 2F. OPTIC FORAMEN FRACTURES

General

It is caused by non-penetrating blow to the head with subsequent transfer of force to the optic canal and its contents or with basilar skull fractures.

Clinical

Loss of consciousness, cerebrospinal fluid (CSF) leak.

Ocular

Traumatic optic neuropathy hematoma, ischemic necrosis.

Laboratory

Computed tomography is done to identify bony anomaly.

Treatment

Intravenous steroids are recommended alone or in conjunction with optic canal decompression.

🗗 BIBLIOGRAPHY

1. Patel B, Taylor SF. (2012). Apex orbital fracture. [online] Available from www.emedicine.com/oph/TOPIC228.HTM. [Accessed October, 2013].

⊡ 2G. ORBITAL HEMORRHAGES

General

Orbital hemorrhage occurs acutely; substantial hemorrhage behind the orbit septum will raise intraorbital and intraocular pressure.

Clinical

None.

Ocular

Elevated intraocular pressure, orbital pain, diplopia, vision loss, ptosis, lid retraction, immobile globe, cloudy cornea, hemorrhagic conjunctiva, disk pallor, hyperemia of the disk, disk edema, choroidal folds.

Laboratory

Diagnosis is made by clinical findings.

Treatment

Topical medication is recommended to lower intraocular pressure, lateral canthotomy and inferior cantholysis.

⊡ BIBLIOGRAPHY

1. Roy FH, Fraunfelder FW, Fraunfelder FT. Roy and Fraunfelder's Current Ocular Therapy, 6th edition. London, UK: Elsevier; 2008.

⊡ 3A. DERMOID, ORBITAL

General

Choristomas, tumors that originate from aberrant primordial tissue; may displace structures in the orbit, especially the globe. If the displacement is great, interference with vision by compression of the optic nerve.

Ocular

Mass in the orbital area; decreased visual acuity, color vision and brightness perception; afferent pupillary defect; optic nerve compression.

Laboratory

Radiography, CT, MRI and ultrasound can be used for diagnosis.

Treatment

No treatment is generally required unless there is optic nerve compression or for cosmetic problems. If surgery is required, the location of the cyst helps to determine the appropriate type of orbitotomy.

⊡ BIBLIOGRAPHY

1. Cooper T, Nugent AK. (2012). Orbital dermoid. [online] Available from emedicine.medscape.com/article/1218740-overview. [Accessed October, 2013].

⊡ 3B. BASEDOW SYNDROME (GRAVES DISEASE; HYPERTHYROIDISM; THYROTOXICOSIS; EXOPHTHALMIC GOITER; PARRY DISEASE)

General

Diffuse toxic goiter; inherited as a simple autosomal recessive; penetrance greater in females; however, dominant mode of inheritance and variable penetrance are possible; uncommon in either sex before the age of 15 years.

Ocular

Exophthalmos; swelling of eyelids and discoloration of upper eyelids; lid lag (von Graefe's sign); globe lag (Koeber's sign); lid trembling on gentle closure (Rosenbach's sign); reduced blinking (Stellwag's sign); retraction of upper lid; difficulty in everting upper lid (Gifford's sign); convergence weakness (Möbius's sign); impaired fixation on extreme lateral gaze (Suker's sign); possible external ophthalmoplegia (Ballet's sign); Dalrymple's sign (staring appearance); tearing; photophobia; epiphora; prolapse of lacrimal gland; neuroretinal edema; tortuous vessels; papilledema and papillitis; anisocoria; keratitis; increased intraocular pressure on upgaze; decreased visual acuity; enlargement of the extraocular muscles; increased volume of the extraorbital fat; superior rectus muscle enlargement; decreased venous outflow.

Clinical

Tachycardia; anxiety; insomnia; loss of weight; hyperhidrosis; restlessness; myocarditis (toxic); atrial fibrillation.

Laboratory

Visual field testing, forced duction testing for restrictive myopathy, CT, MRI, thyroxine (T4) and thyroid-stimulating hormone, thyroid-stimulating immunoglobulins.

Treatment

There is no immediate treatment; the disease is self-limited but prolonged course over 1 or more years. Five percent of patients may require surgical intervention which could be orbital decompression, strabismus surgery, lid-lengthening surgery or blepharoplasty.

BIBLIOGRAPHY

1. Ing E. (2012). Thyroid-associated orbitopathy. [online] Available from www.emedicine.com/oph/TOPIC237.HTM. [Accessed September, 2013].
2. Regensburg NI, Wiersinga WM, Berendschot TT, et al. Do subtypes of Graves' orbitopathy exist? Ophthalmology. 2011;118:191-6.

3C. HEMANGIOMA

General

Hemangioma can occur throughout the body, but particularly in the head; primary intraosseous orbital hemangiomas are rare; capillary hemangioma of the orbit and eyelids generally is unilateral.

Ocular

Hemangiomas of lids or orbit; ptosis; strabismus; amblyopia; proptosis; optic atrophy; hypermetropia; cavernous hemangiomas are the most common benign orbital tumors of adults.

Clinical

Ipsilateral hemangiomas of the brain and meninges.

Laboratory

Neuroimaging can be of great assistance in making the diagnosis.

Treatment

Most of these lesions regress on their own; there is no need to intervention. If spontaneous regression does not occur corticosteroids, in various formulations, may be considered. Topical application of timolol has been useful in some cases.

BIBLIOGRAPHY

1. Karmel M. Topical timolol for capillary hemangioma. Eyenet. 2010.
2. Seiff S, Zwick OM, DeAngelis DD, et al. (2011). Capillary hemangioma. [online] Available from www.emedicine.com/oph/TOPIC691.HTM. [Accessed October, 2013].

3D. HEMANGIOMA, CAPILLARY

General

Benign orbital tumors of infancy, rapid growth; thought to be of placental origin due to a unique microvascular phenotype shared by juvenile hemangiomas and human placenta.

Clinical

Kasabach-Merritt syndrome; congestive heart failure; nasopharyngeal obstruction; thrombocytopenia; hemolytic anemia.

Ocular

Red, thickened spot in the periorbital area, lid or brow; amblyopia; anisometropia.

Laboratory

Neuroimaging studies are useful to establish the diagnosis; CT, MRI and ultrasound may be beneficial.

Treatment

Corticosteroids topically, systemically and injection are the first line of treatment. Interferon may also be used in resistant cases. Laser and incisional surgical techniques have had variable success.

BIBLIOGRAPHY

1. Al Dhaybi R, Superstein R, Milet A, et al. Treatment of periocular infantile hemangiomas with propranolol: case series of 18 children. Ophthalmology. 2011;118(6):1184-8.
2. Seiff S, Zwick OM, DeAngelis DD, et al. (2011). Capillary hemangioma. [online] Available from emedicine.medscape.com/article/1218805-overview. [Accessed October, 2013].

3E. HEMANGIOMA, CAVERNOUS

General

They are the most common intraorbital tumors found in adults; benign, vascular lesions; slow growing; usually unilateral; first symptoms include bulging of the globe and eyelid fullness; usually found in the intracorneal space between the optic nerve and extraocular muscles.

Clinical

Neurosurgical or otolaryngologic issues may be present of the hemangioma extends to the facial structure outside of the orbit.

Ocular

Decreased visual acuity and visual field; diplopia; proptosis; extraocular and pupillary dysfunction; lagophthalmos; exposure keratopathy; keratitis; corneal perforation.

Laboratory

Computed tomography, MRI scan, ultrasound studies are commonly used to make the diagnosis.

Treatment

Most require no intervention; some cases do require surgical treatment.

BIBLIOGRAPHY

1. Cohen AJ, Mercandetti M, Weinberg DA. (2011). Cavernous hemangioma. [online] Available from emedicine.medscape.com/article/1218120-overview. [Accessed October, 2013].

3F. LACRIMAL GLAND TUMORS

General

Swelling of lateral superior orbit, tumors can be benign or malignant.

Clinical

None.

Ocular

Tumor of the lacrimal gland, globe may be pushed down and medial from the tumor, diplopia, proptosis, ptosis, pain.

Laboratory

Computed tomography scan of orbit.

Treatment

Biopsy, excise of tumor with the capsule for benign tumor, malignant tumors may require large excision or orbital exenteration, chemotherapy or radiation.

BIBLIOGRAPHY

1. DeAngelis DD, Pang NK, Hurwitz J. (2011). Lacrimal gland tumors. [online] Available from www.emedicine.com/oph/TOPIC694.HTM. [Accessed October, 2013].

🗗 3G. LEUKEMIA

General

Acute or chronic blood disorder.

Ocular

Engorgement of conjunctival vessels; papillary hypertrophy; aggregations of tumor cells in conjunctiva, choroid and orbit; secondary glaucoma; retinal venous engorgement and tortuosity with pronounced constrictions; retinal hemorrhages; retinal detachment; cotton-wool spots; macular edema; papilledema; optic atrophy; optic neuritis; paralysis of extraocular muscles; hypopyon; vitreous opacities; retinal sea fans; perilimbal subconjunctival infiltrates; corneal leukemic infiltration (rare); shallow serous retinal detachments; hyphema; iris neovascularization; central retinal vein occlusion; vitreous infiltrates.

Clinical

Frequent involvement of central nervous system; intracranial hemorrhage; thrombocytopenia; rising white cell count.

Laboratory

Complete blood count and differential, bone marrow aspiration, immunophenotyping, chromosomal analysis.

Treatment

Chemotherapy with or without radiotherapy.

🗗 BIBLIOGRAPHY

1. Wu L, Evans T, Martinez J. (2012). Leukemias. [online] Available from www.emedicine.com/oph/TOPIC489.HTM. [Accessed October, 2013].

🗗 3H. LYMPHOID HYPERPLASIA (REACTIVE LYMPHOID HYPERPLASIA; LYMPHOID TUMORS; MALIGNANT LYMPHOMA; PSEUDOLYMPHOMA; PSEUDOTUMOR; BURKITT LYMPHOMA; NEOPLASTIC ANGIOENDOTHELIOMATOSIS)

General

It occurs in tropical Africa; young children; idiopathic orbital inflammation; systemic disease is rarely associated but occasionally occurs with either vasculitis or lymphomas; etiology of Burkitt's lymphoma currently includes three factors: (1) Epstein-Barr virus, (2) malaria and (3) chromosomal translocations activating the *c-Myc* oncogene, which induces uncontrolled B-cell proliferation.

Ocular

Proptosis; extraocular motility disturbances; lesions of orbit, lacrimal gland, conjunctiva and uvea; cortical blindness; retinal artery occlusion; retinal vascular and pigment epithelial alterations; vitreitis.

Clinical

Maxillary tumor; Epstein-Barr virus; cranial neuropathy.

Laboratory

Generally, it is diagnosed with a lymph node biopsy.

Treatment

Chemotherapy, monoclonal antibody therapy and bone marrow or stem cell infusions may be chosen as therapy.

🗗 BIBLIOGRAPHY

1. Brooks HL, Downing J, McClure JA, et al. Orbital Burkitt's lymphoma in a homosexual man with acquired immune deficiency. Arch Ophthalmol. 1984;102(10):1533-7.
2. Cheung MK, Martin DF, Chan CC, et al. Diagnosis of reactive lymphoid hyperplasia by chorioretinal biopsy. Am J Ophthalmol. 1994;118(4):457-62.

3I. MENINGIOMA, OPTIC NERVE SHEATH

General

Primary meningioma arises from the cap cells of the arachnoid surrounding the intraorbital or less frequently, the intracanalicular optic nerve. Secondary meningioma is the extensions of intracranial meningioma into the orbit. Secondary meningioma is much more common than primary, but the unqualified term "optic nerve sheath meningioma" ordinarily refers to primary meningioma. They may be caused by radiation; head trauma, hormonal factors and infectious agents.

Clinical

Headache, head trauma.

Ocular

Compressive optic neuropathy; transient visual obscurations; visual loss; proptosis; exophthalmos; ptosis; diplopia.

Laboratory

Computed tomography and MRI are the best imaging techniques.

Treatment

Radiotherapy is performed following the surgical removal. Chemotherapy is reserved for unresectable or recurrent meningiomas.

BIBLIOGRAPHY

1. Gossman MV, Zachariah SB, Khoromi S. (2012). Optic nerve sheath meningioma. [online] Available from emedicine.medscape.com/article/1217466-overview. [Accessed October, 2013].

3J. MENINGIOMA, SPHENOID WING

General

It arises from arachnoid cap cells which are attached to the dura at any location where meninges exist; it may be associated with hyperostosis of the sphenoid ridge and be very invasive; it may expand into the wall for the cavernous sinus and anteriorly into the orbit.

Clinical

Diffuse tumor infiltration; transient ischemic attack; anosmia; mental changes; increased intracranial pressure.

Ocular

Unilateral exophthalmos; proptosis; oculomotor palsy; painful ophthalmoplegia; blindness; papilledema.

Laboratory

Endocrine testing; CT and MRI allow definitive diagnosis.

Treatment

Tumor resection without injury to the optic nerve if the bone has not been invaded; if resection is not complete, radiation therapy will be necessary; antihormonal agents may be useful in a typical and malignant meningiomas as an adjunct to surgery.

BIBLIOGRAPHY

1. Zachariah SB, Khoromi S. (2012). Sphenoid wing meningioma. [online] Available from emedicine.medscape.com/article/1215752-overview. [Accessed October, 2013].

⊟ 3K. NEUROBLASTOMA

General

Highly malignant solid tumor arising from undifferentiated sympathetic neuroblasts of the adrenal medulla, sympathetic ganglia, ectopic adrenal, and theoretically the ciliary ganglion; autosomal dominant.

Ocular

Ptosis; exophthalmos; optic atrophy; optic neuritis; papilledema; metastatic tumor of orbit; retinal hemorrhage; convergent strabismus; paralysis of VIth or VIIth nerve; nonreactive pupil; primary differentiated neuroblastoma of the orbit also has been reported; tonic pupils; microphthalmia; choroidal metastases (rare); iris metastases (rare).

Clinical

Skeletal metastasis to the cranium.

Laboratory

Serum lactate dehydrogenase (LDH), ferritin, CBC count, serum creatine, liver function test, CT and MRI test, echocardiogram.

Treatment

Treatment is provided by a multidisciplinary team.

⊟ BIBLIOGRAPHY

1. Lacayo NJ, Davis KL. (2012). Pediatric neuroblastoma. [online] Available from www.emedicine.com/ped/TOPIC1570.HTM. [Accessed October, 2013].

⊟ 3L. VON RECKLINGHAUSEN SYNDROME (NEUROFIBROMATOSIS TYPE I; NEURINOMATOSIS)

General

Dominant inheritance activated at puberty, during pregnancy and at menopause; strong evidence supports the existence of neurofibromatosis type 1 (NF-l) as a tumor suppressor gene.

Ocular

Proptosis; displacement of the globe; pulsation of the globe; ptosis; elephantiasis of the lids; pigment spots on lids; hydrophthalmos; nodular swelling of corneal nerves; cataracts; optic atrophy; choroidal melanoma; neurofibroma of the choroid, iris, eyelid and ciliary body; enlarged optic foramen; underdevelopment of orbital bones; café-au-lait spots on fundus; hamartoma of retina; congenital glaucoma; focal iris nodules; choroidal nevi; optic nerve gliomas; orbital neurofibroma; keratoconus.

Clinical

Café-au-lait skin pigmentations; fibroma molluscum; lipomas and sebaceous adenomas; schwannomas; growth abnormalities; spontaneous fractures; facial hemihypertrophy.

Laboratory

T2-weighted MRI images demonstrate multiple bright lesions in the basal ganglia, cerebellum, and brain in 80% optic nerve gliomas often develop perineural arachnoidal hyperplasia which appears as an expanded CSF space around the nerve.

Treatment

Oral ketotifen may reduce the pain, tenderness and itchiness associated with neurofibromas.

⊟ BIBLIOGRAPHY

1. Dahl AA. (2011). Ophthalmologic manifestations of neurofibromatosis type 1. [online] Available from www.emedicine.com/oph/TOPIC338.HTM. [Accessed October, 2013].

⊟ 3M. ORBITAL LYMPHOMA

General

Orbital lymphoma is localized form of systemic lymphoma affecting the orbit, lacrimal gland, lid and conjunctiva.

Clinical

Systemic lymphoma.

Ocular

Diplopia; exophthalmos; ocular pain; salmon-colored mass of the conjunctiva or eyelid.

Laboratory

Open biopsy and MRI or CT scan of the orbit.

Treatment

Radiation is the most frequently used treatment. Chemotherapy may be indicated for large diffuse B-cell lymphoma or with systemic treatment; excision of localized lesions; cryotherapy may be beneficial.

⊟ BIBLIOGRAPHY

1. EyeWikiTM. (2010). Orbital lymphoma. [online] Available from eyewiki.aao.org/Orbital_Lymphoma. [Accessed October, 2013].

⊟ 3N. RHABDOMYOSARCOMA (CORNEAL EDEMA)

General

Most common malignant orbital neoplasm of childhood; usually occurs before age of 10 years; more commonly seen in males; rarely may develop in adults; shows evidence of striated muscle differentiation; has been divided into three histopathologic types: (1) embryonal, (2) alveolar and (3) pleomorphic.

Ocular

Choroidal folds; corneal edema; exposure keratitis; rhabdomyosarcoma (RMS) of orbit or extraocular muscles; decreased motility; proptosis; papilledema; orbital edema; enlarged optic foramen; erosion of bony walls of orbit; pupil irregularity; epiphora; glaucoma; visual loss; nasolacrimal duct obstruction; conjunctival mass.

Clinical

Metastasis to the lymph system, bone marrow and lungs; headaches.

Laboratory

Live, renal and cytogenetic testing; CT and bone scanning; MRI, ultrasonography and echocardiography.

Treatment

Chemotherapy radiation and surgically removing the tumor are used to treat patients with RMS.

⊟ BIBLIOGRAPHY

1. Cripe TP. (2011). Pediatric rhabdomyosarcoma. [online] Available from www.emedicine.com/ped/TOPIC2005. HTM. [Accessed October, 2013].

1. HORNER SYNDROME (BERNARD-HORNER SYNDROME; CERVICAL SYMPATHETIC PARALYSIS SYNDROME; CLAUDE-BERNARD-HORNER SYNDROME; HORNER OCULOPUPILLARY SYNDROME)

General

Paralysis of cervical sympathetic; hypothalamic lesion with first neuron involved or lesion in the pons or cervical portion of cord; syndrome present in Babinski-Nageotte, Cestan-Chenais, Dejerine-Klumpke, Pancoast, Raeder, and Wallenberg syndromes (Babinski-Nageotte syndrome; Cestan-Chenais syndrome; Dejerine-Klumpke syndrome; Pancoast syndrome; Raeder syndrome; Wallenberg syndrome).

Ocular

Enophthalmos; ptosis or narrowing of palpebral fissure; ocular hypotony; miosis (degree of miosis depends on the site of lesion; most pronounced when roots of cranial nerves VII and VIII, and first thoracic nerve are involved); hypochromic heterochromia (children more than adults); pupil does not dilate with cocaine.

Clinical

Anhidrosis on ipsilateral side of face and neck; transitory rise in facial temperature; hemifacial atrophy; it may result from a variety of conditions, including cluster headache, parasellar neoplasms or aneurysms, internal carotid dissection or occlusion and Tolosa-Hunt syndrome.

Laboratory

Pharmacologic testing is very helpful in the diagnosis of Horner syndrome; cocaine or apraclonidine (instilled in an eye with intact sympathetic innervation) causes the pupil to dilate. A sympathetically denervated pupil dilates poorly to cocaine, regardless of the level of the sympathetic interruption because of the absence of endogenous norepinephrine in the synapse.

Treatment

Surgical and medical care is dependent upon the particular etiology. Potential surgical care includes neurosurgical care for aneurysm-related Horner syndrome and vascular surgical care for etiologies such as carotid artery dissection/aneurysm.

BIBLIOGRAPHY

1. Bardorf CM, Stavern GV, Garcia-Valenzuela E. (2012). Horner syndrome. [online] Available from www.emedicine.com/oph/TOPIC336.HTM. [Accessed October, 2013].

2. PUPILLARY MEMBRANE, PERSISTENT

General

Autosomal dominant.

Ocular

Remnants of pupillary membrane persist as strands and other irregular tissue in pupil; congenital cataract; corneal edema; Rieger syndrome; keratoconus.

Clinical

None.

Laboratory

Diagnosis is made by clinical findings.

Treatment

Cataract surgery may be necessary if vision is affected; steroids and Muro 128 may be used for corneal edema; keratoconus may be treated with spectacle correction, hard contacts, avoid eye rubbing. If hydrops occur, discontinue contact lens, use sodium chloride (NaCl) drops and ointment, patching and short course of steroids. As disease advances, penetrating keratoplasty, deep anterior lamellar keratoplasty intacs with laser grooves or collagen stabilization of cornea.

BIBLIOGRAPHY

1. Duane TD. Clinical Ophthalmology. Philadelphia, PA: JB Lippincott; 1987.
2. McKusick VA. Mendelian Inheritance in Man: A Catalog of Human Genes and Genetic Disorders, 12th edition. Baltimore, USA: The Johns Hopkins University Press; 1998.

CHAPTER
33

Retina

⊟ 1A. ACUTE POSTERIOR MULTIFOCAL PLACOID PIGMENT EPITHELIOPATHY (WHITE DOT SYNDROME)

General

Inflammatory chorioretinopathy; etiology unknown but can be associated with systemic conditions such as viral disease, thyroiditis, Lyme disease, tuberculosis and nephritis.

Clinical

Thyroiditis, erythema nodosum, Wegener's granulomatosis, polyarteritis nodosa, nephritis, sarcoidosis, central nervous system (CNS) vasculitis.

Ocular

Blurred vision, central and paracentral scotomas.

Laboratory

Clinical observation is made by funduscopic examination and fluorescein angiography.

Treatment

There is no current consensus on treatment and most resolve without treatment. Systemic and intravitreal steroids may be beneficial to shorten the duration and for those cases involving the fovea.

⊟ BIBLIOGRAPHY

1. Mansour SE, Cook GR. (2012). Multifocal choroidopathy syndromes. [online] Available from emedicine.medscape.com/article/1190935-overview. [Accessed October, 2013].

⊟ 1B. ACUTE RETINAL NECROSIS SYNDROME (ARN SYNDROME; BILATERAL ACUTE RETINAL NECROSIS; BARN SYNDROME)

General

Evidence of association with herpes-type deoxyribonucleic acid (DNA) virus; occurs both unilaterally and bilaterally; includes varicella-zoster virus and herpes simplex virus type 1.

Ocular

Uveitis; vasculitis; vitreitis; retinal detachment; vitreous opacification; retinal periarteritis; exudates of peripheral retina; retinal necrosis; optic nerve enlargement; papillitis; arcuate neuroretinitis; arteritis and phlebitis (affecting the retinal vasculature); necrotizing retinitis; moderate-to-severe vitreitis; anterior segment inflammation; optic neuritis; late retinal detachment.

Clinical

None.

Laboratory

Diagnosis is made by clinical findings.

Treatment

Antiviral therapy, anti-inflammatory therapy, antithrombotic therapy and retinal detachment prophylaxis. Vitrectomy may be necessary.

🗗 BIBLIOGRAPHY

1. Tibbetts MD, Shah CP, Young LH, et al. Treatment of acute retinal necrosis. Ophthalmology. 2010;117(4):818-24.
2. Wong R, Pavesio CE, Laidlaw AH, et al. Acute retinal necrosis: the effects of intravitreal foscarnet and virus type on outcome. Ophthalmology. 2010;117(3):556-60.

🗗 1C. ALBINISM (BROWN OCULOCUTANEOUS ALBINISM; NETTLESHIP FALLS SYNDROME)

General

Congenital hypopigmentation.
- *Complete*
  - *Ocular*: Iris thin, pale blue; prominent choroidal vessels with poorly defined fovea; nystagmus; head nodding; frequently myopic astigmatism and strabismus; marked photophobia; eyelashes and eyebrows are white; optic atrophy; cataract; abnormal decussation of retinogeniculate axons at the chiasm.
  - *Clinical*: White hair, eyebrows and skin; autosomal recessive.
- *Modified complete*
  - *Ocular*: Marked deficiency of pigment in the iris and choroid; nystagmus and myopic astigmatism; iris of female carrier frequently is translucent; macular hypoplasia; photophobia; pigmentation of retinal pigment epithelium (RPE).
  - *Clinical*: Normal pigmentation elsewhere; autosomal recessive.
- *Amish*
  - *Ocular*: At birth, complete albinism with blue translucent irides and albinotic fundal reflex; nystagmus; photophobia; increasing pigmentation with age; abnormal decussation of retinogeniculate axons at the chiasm.
  - *Clinical*: White hair and skin at birth; increasing pigmentation with yellow hair and normal skin that tans; autosomal recessive.

Laboratory

The most definitive test in determining the albinism type is genetic sequence analysis. This test is useful only for families with individuals who have albinism. The test cannot be used as a screening tool.

Treatment

Currently, there is no therapy for albinism. Sunglasses to reduce photophobia, low-vision aids and treatment for strabismus might be useful.

🗗 BIBLIOGRAPHY

1. Bashour M, Hasanee K, Ahmed II. (2012). Albinism. [online] Available from www.emedicine.com/oph/TOPIC315.HTM. [Accessed October, 2013].

🗗 1D. BEST DISEASE (BEST MACULAR DEGENERATION; VITELLIRUPTIVE MACULAR DYSTROPHY; POLYMORPHIC MACULAR DEGENERATION OF BRALEY; VITELLIFORM DYSTROPHY)

General

Up to 7 years of age; a type of heredomacular dystrophy; autosomal dominant with variable expressivity.

Ocular

Egg yolk lesion at macula, later absorbed to leave atrophic scar; hemorrhagic or serous exudates beneath pigment epithelium; hyperopia; esotropia; strabismic amblyopia; unusual associations with full-thickness macular hole and extramacular multifocal vitelliform disease have been reported.

Laboratory

Fluorescein angiogram reveals blockage of choroidal fluorescence by the vitelliform lesion.

Treatment

No treatment exists. Secondary choroidal neovascularization can be managed with direct laser treatment.

⊟ BIBLIOGRAPHY

1. Meunier I, Sénéchal A, Dhaenens CM, et al. Systematic screening of BEST1 and PRPH2 in juvenile and adult vitelliform macular dystrophies: a rational for molecular analysis. Ophthalmology. 2011:118(6):1130-6.
2. Altaweel M. (2012). Best disease. [online] Available from www.emedicine.com/oph/TOPIC700.HTM. [Accessed October, 2013].

⊟ 1E. BIRDSHOT RETINOPATHY (VITILIGINOUS CHORIORETINITIS)

General

Uncommon; may relate to an inherited immune dysregulation but exact cause is unknown; average presenting age is 50 years; spots in the retina resemble the pattern seen with birdshot scatter from the shotgun.

Clinical

None.

Ocular

Gradual painless loss of vision; vitreous floaters; photopsia; vitritis; multiple ovoid spots that are orange to cream in color and hypopigmented in the posterior pole and midperiphery of the retina.

Laboratory

Human leukocyte antigen (HLA) A29 blood testing; fluorescein angiography; indocyanine green angiography (ICGA); optical coherence tomography (OCT); and electrophysiologic testing.

Treatment

Topical, systemic and regional steroids may be useful. Cyclosporine, ketoconazole and other immunomodulatory therapies may also be necessary.

⊟ BIBLIOGRAPHY

1. Samson CM, Mohamoud Ali AM, Foster CS. (2011). Birdshot retinopathy. [online] Available from emedicine.medscape.com/article/1223257-overview. [Accessed October, 2013].

⊟ 1F. BLACKWATER FEVER

General

Blackwater fever usually occurs in association with malaria, *Plasmodium falciparum* infection; mortality 20–30%; recurrent hemolytic episodes with subsequent malarial infections.

Ocular

Scleral icterus; cotton-wool spots; retinal edema; optic disk edema; conjunctival calcium deposits; band keratopathy; cortical blindness; epibulbar hemorrhage of conjunctiva and episclera; retinal hemorrhages.

Clinical

Fever; hemolysis; icterus; hemoglobinuria; malaria; uremia; nausea; vomiting; vertigo; convulsions; coma; acute renal failure; hypertension, azotemia; hypervolemia; metabolic disturbances; hyponatremia; hypercalcemia.

Laboratory

Complete blood count (CBC), electrolyte panel, renal function tests, pregnancy test, urinalysis, free serum haptoglobin, urine and blood cultures, and thick and thin blood smears are useful.

Treatment

If the patient is experiencing life-threatening complications (coma, respiratory failure, coagulopathy, fulminant kidney failure), then investigate exchange transfusion as a treatment option.

⊟ BIBLIOGRAPHY

1. Fernandez MC. (2012). Emergent management of malaria. [online] Available from www.emedicine.com/emerg/TOPIC305.HTM. [Accessed October, 2013].

⌸ 1G. CAR SYNDROME (CANCER-ASSOCIATED RETINOPATHY SYNDROME)

General

Rare; antiretinal antibodies in blood of cancer patients experiencing concomitant loss of vision; vision loss may be noted before cancer is diagnosed; mechanisms involved in the vision loss experienced by patients is not understood, but serologic studies indicate that they may include a series of autoimmune reactions directed at specific components of the retina.

Ocular

Vision loss usually progressive; retinal degeneration; retinal hole; abnormal visual fields; loss of color vision; retinal detachment; optic atrophy; ring-like scotoma; night blindness; retinal phlebitis.

Clinical

Carcinoma with or without metastasis to any part of the body.

Laboratory

Diagnosis is made by clinical findings.

Treatment

Treat the antiretinal antibodies.

⌸ BIBLIOGRAPHY

1. Keltner JL, Roth AM, Chang RS. Photoreceptor degeneration. Possible autoimmune disorder. Arch Ophthalmol. 1983;101(4):564-9.
2. Ohnishi Y, Ohara S, Sakamoto T, et al. Cancer-associated retinopathy with retinal phlebitis. Br J Ophthalmol. 1993;77(12):795-8.
3. Thirkill CE, Roth AM, Keltner JL. Cancer-associated retinopathy. Arch Ophthalmol. 1987;105(3):372-5.
5. Thirkill CE, Tait RC, Tyler NK, et al. The cancer-associated retinopathy antigen is a recovering-like protein. Invest Ophthalmol Vis Sci. 1992;33(10):2768-72.

⌸ 1H. CEROID LIPOFUSCINOSIS

General

Ceroid lipofuscinoses are disorders characterized by the accumulation of fluorescent lipopigments in a number of body tissues; included in this group are several diseases that were once considered variants of Tay-Sachs disease but are now classified separately; it may be divided into infantile, late infantile (Bielschowsky-Jansky), juvenile (Spielmeyer-Vogt), adult (Kufs) and atypical forms (Dollinger-Bielschowsky syndrome; Kufs disease; infantile neuronal ceroid lipofuscinosis; Batten-Mayou syndrome).

Ocular

Tapetoretinal degeneration; pigmentary macular changes.

Clinical

Seizures; ataxia; dementia; cerebellar and extrapyramidal signs; "release" hallucinations.

Laboratory

Enzyme levels, magnetic resonance imaging (MRI), positron-emission tomography.

Treatment

No specific treatment is available for these diseases.

⌸ BIBLIOGRAPHY

1. Chang CH. (2009). Neuronal ceroid lipofuscinoses. [online] Available from www.emedicine.com/neuro/TOPIC498. HTM. [Accessed October, 2013].

1I. CHLOROQUINE/HYDROXYCHLOROQUINE TOXICITY (BULL'S EYE MACULOPATHY)

General

Toxicity caused by using chloroquine or hydroxychloroquine incidence increased with both dose and duration of treatment.

Clinical

Malaria; lupus; rheumatoid arthritis; nausea; rash; sensitivity to ultraviolet light; vertigo; muscle weakness; cranial nerve palsies.

Ocular

Corneal deposits; white flake-like lens opacity; scotoma; stippling of macular pigmentation; concentric zone of hypopigmentation of the retina; generalized hypopigmentation; bone spicule formation; vascular attenuation; optic disk pallor.

Laboratory

Fluorescein angiography; Amsler grid; perimetry; retinal examination and photography; color vision; photostress testing; and electrophysiologic studies are useful. A yearly visual field examination is useful to detect charges from hydroxychloroquine. A small case series study revealed the evidence of retinal toxicity that included difficulty with reading, variation in fundus findings from normal to bull's eye maculopathy, electroretinogram (ERG) findings of reduced rod and cone function and abnormal visual fields. Cessation of the study drug did not result in sustained improved visual function. Chloroquine and hydroxychloroquine are associated with substantial retinal toxicities that require diligent monitoring and management.

Treatment

Withdrawal of the medication; ammonium chloride systemically made be necessary if severe toxic symptoms occur.

BIBLIOGRAPHY

1. Michaelides M, Stover NB, Francis PJ, et al. Retinal toxicity associated with hydroxychloroquine and chloroquine. Arch Ophthalmol. 2011;129(1);30-9.
2. Roque MR, Roque BL, Foster CS. (2011). Chloroquine/hydroxychloroquine toxicity. [online] Available from emedicine.medscape.com/article/1229016-overview. [Accessed October, 2013].

1J. CHOROIDORETINAL DYSTROPHY

General

Sex-linked; similar to retinitis pigmentosa (RP) with absence of annular scotoma and little vascular change.

Ocular

Early poor central vision; RP; night blindness.

Clinical

None.

Laboratory

Diagnosis is made by clinical findings.

Treatment

Retinitis pigmentosa: Vitamin A 15,000 IU/day is thought to slow the decline of retinal function; dark sunglasses for outdoor use; surgery for cataract; genetic counseling.

BIBLIOGRAPHY

1. Hoare GW. Choroido-retinal dystrophy. Br J Ophthalmol. 1965;49(9):449-59.
2. McKusick VA. Mendelian Inheritance in Man: A Catalog of Human Genes and Genetic Disorders, 12th edition. Baltimore, USA: The Johns Hopkins University Press; 1998.

1K. COATS DISEASE (LEBER MILIARY ANEURYSM; RETINAL TELANGIECTASIA)

General

Exudative retinitis; rare; more common in males than females; 95% unilateral.

Ocular

Leukocoria; telangiectatic retinal vessels; solid gray-yellow retinal detachment; optic atrophy; vitreous hemorrhage; anterior uveitis; glaucoma; intraocular calcification (rare); fibro-osseous retinal nodules (atypical); hemorrhagic retinal macrocysts; cystoid macular edema.

Clinical

None.

Laboratory

Fluorescein angiography demonstrates large aneurismal (light bulb) dilatation of the retinal vessels.

Treatment

Cryotherapy and vitrectomy can be used to obliterate the vascular abnormalities.

BIBLIOGRAPHY

1. Cameron JD, Yanoff M, Frayer WC. Coats' disease and Turner's syndrome. Am J Ophthalmol. 1974;78(5):852-4.
2. Senft SH, Hidayat AA, Cavender JC. Atypical presentation of Coats disease. Retina. 1994;14(1):36-8.

1L. CONGENITAL HEREDITARY RETINOSCHISIS (CHRS; JUVENILE X-LINKED RETINOSCHISIS)

General

X-linked recessive; bilateral; develops early in life but often stabilized toward the end of the second decade; severity varies widely.

Ocular

Bilateral vitreoretinal dystrophy; retinoschisis (RS); vitreous veil; vitreous detachment; vitreous hemorrhage; decreased visual fields; maculopathy; cataract; neovascular glaucoma; vitreoretinopathy; proliferative retinal detachment; Mizuo's phenomenon.

Laboratory

Optical coherence tomography provides high-resolution cross-sectional images of the macular region ICGA performed on patients with X-linked juvenile retinoschisis (XJR) shows a distinct hyperfluorescence in the macular region that is associated with radial lines of hypofluorescence centered on the foveola in the early phase.

Treatment

No treatment is available to halt the natural progression of schisis formation.

BIBLIOGRAPHY

1. Small KW, McLellan CM, Song MK. (2012). Juvenile retinoschisis. [online] Available from emedicine.medscape.com/article/1225857-overview. [Accessed October, 2013].

1M. CENTRAL SEROUS CHORIORETINOPATHY

General

Central serous chorioretinopathy is a disorder of the central macula.

Clinical

None.

Ocular

Decreased visual acuity, metamorphopsia, micropsia, central color vision deficiency, central scotoma.

Laboratory

Fluorescein angiopathy for "expansile dot" pattern, a "smokestack" pattern or diffuse hyperfluorescence.

Treatment

Observation in most cases. Thermal or photodynamic therapy is necessary in some cases.

BIBLIOGRAPHY

1. Oh KT. (2011). Central serous chorioretinopathy. [online] Available from www.emedicine.com/oph/TOPIC689.HTM. [Accessed October, 2013].

1N. CYTOMEGALOVIRUS RETINITIS

General

Cytomegalovirus (CMV) is a ubiquitous DNA virus that infects the majority of adults and generally, only an issue in immunocompromised individuals such as with acquired immunodeficiency syndrome (AIDS), transplant and those immunosuppressive medication.

Clinical

Acquired immunodeficiency syndrome, transplantation patients; myalgia, cervical lymphadenopathy; hepatitis.

Ocular

Decrease visual acuity; blindness; retinitis; retinal detachment; retinal breaks; necrotic retina.

Laboratory

Laboratory testing is performed to determine the cause; ultrasound is done to evaluate for retinal detachment; dilated fundus examination.

Treatment

Intravitreal ganciclovir implant or injection may be used; retinal detachment surgery may be necessary.

BIBLIOGRAPHY

1. Altaweel M, Youssef PN, Reed MD. (2012). CMV retinitis. [online] Available from emedicine.medscape.com/article/1227228-overview. [Accessed October, 2013].

1O. DIFFUSE UNILATERAL SUBACUTE NEURORETINITIS SYNDROME (DUSN; UNILATERAL WIPEOUT SYNDROME; WIPEOUT SYNDROME)

General

It is caused by a nematode that is not *Toxocara canis*, i.e. at least two nematodes of different sizes; usually occurs in children or young adults; nematode may remain viable in the eye for 3 years or longer.

Ocular

Vitreitis; papillitis; gray-white lesions of retina; optic atrophy; retinal vessel narrowing; diffuse pigment epithelial degeneration; endophthalmitis; nematode in fundus; the pathognomonic finding in diffuse unilateral subacute neuroretinities (DUSN) syndrome is the presence of a motile intraocular nematode.

Clinical

Weight loss; lack of appetite; cough; fever; pulmonary infiltration; hepatomegaly; leukocytosis; persistent eosinophilia.

Laboratory

Electroretinopathy, enzyme-linked immunosorbent assays for individual nematode species.

Treatment

Direct laser photocoagulation of the nematode is the treatment of choice for DUSN; surgical transvitreal removal of the nematode may be indicated in selected cases.

BIBLIOGRAPHY

1. Kooragayala LM. (2011). Diffuse unilateral subacute neuroretinitis. [online] Available from emedicine.medscape.com/article/1226931-overview. [Accessed October, 2013].

1P. EALES DISEASE (PERIPHLEBITIS)

General

Common; young adults.

Ocular

Sheathing of peripheral veins; hemorrhage in new vessels and later retinal detachment; retinal vascular tortuosity; microaneurysms of retina; postneovascularization of vitreous; internuclear ophthalmoplegia.

Clinical

Epilepsy and hemiplegia have been reported; chronic encephalitis; ulcerative colitis; central nervous infarction.

Laboratory

Fluorescein angiography and tuberculosis screening test.

Treatment

Thyroid extract, osteogenic hormones, androgenic hormones and systemic steroids are recommended. The antioxidant vitamins A, C and E have been suggested as a possible therapy because antioxidizing enzymes are deficient in the vitreous samples.

BIBLIOGRAPHY

1. Roth DB, Fine HF. (2012). Eales disease. [online] Available from emedicine.medscape.com/article/1225636-overview. [Accessed October, 2013].

1Q. FLECK RETINA OF KANDORI SYNDROME (KANDORI SYNDROME)

General

Possibly hereditary; onset at young age; focal disturbance of the RPE; affects both sexes; toxic causes are also considered.

Ocular

Relatively large, irregular, yellowish flecks, sharply borderlined without pigmentation underneath retinal vessels and usually in the midperiphery; poor dark adaptation; normal photopic electroretinographic response; delay in generation of the scotopic response.

Clinical

None.

Laboratory

Diagnosis is made by clinical findings.

Treatment

None—ocular.

BIBLIOGRAPHY

1. Bullock JD, Albert DM. Flecked retina. Appearance secondary to oxalate crystals from methoxyflurane anesthesia. Arch Ophthalmol. 1975;93(1):26-31.
2. Carr RE. Abnormalities of cone and rod function. In: Ryan SJ (Ed). Retina, 2nd edition. St Louis: Mosby; 1994. pp. 512-3.
3. Kandori F. Very rare cases of congenital non-progressive night blindness with fleck retina. Jpn J Ophthal. 1959;13:384-6.

1R. GIANT RETINAL TEARS

General

Giant retinal tears are seen most commonly in the highly myopic; tear extends across at least 25% of the retina; tear commonly folds over itself.

Clinical

None.

Ocular

Lesions of the retina; loss of vision.

Laboratory

Diagnosis is made by clinical findings.

Treatment

Perfluoron can be used to unravel the retina and then laser is applied to reattach the retina.

BIBLIOGRAPHY

1. Retina San Antonio and MedNet Technologies, Inc. (2010). Giant retinal tear treatment. [online] Available from www.retinasanantonio.com/services/giant-retinal-tear-treatment. [Accessed October, 2013].

🗗 1S. GYRATE ATROPHY (ORNITHINE KETOACID AMINOTRANSFERASE DEFICIENCY)

General

Deficiency of the enzyme ornithine aminotransferase; autosomal recessive; chronic, progressive dystrophy; responsible human gene has been localized to chromosome 10.

Ocular

Chorioretinal atrophy; crystalline deposits associated with brown pigment in fundus; myopia; cataract; keratoconus; night blindness; constricted visual fields; axial hypermetropia; cobblestone-like peripheral lesions; blunting of ciliary processes; iris atrophy.

Clinical

Absence of enzyme ornithine ketoacid transaminase; elevated levels of amino acid ornithine in the body fluids; seizures; abnormal electroencephalography; eosinophilic sub-sarcolemmal deposits are seen on muscle biopsy; massive cystinuria and lysinuria; diabetes.

Laboratory

Visual field test, ERG and electrooculogram (EOG).

Treatment

- *Cataract*: Change in glasses can sometimes improve a patient's visual function temporarily; however the most common treatment is cataract surgery.
- *Keratoconus*: Spectacle correction, hard contacts, avoid eye rubbing. If hydrops occur, discontinue contact lens, use sodium chloride (NaCl) drops and ointment, patching and short course of steroids. As disease advances, penetrating keratoplasty, deep anterior lamellar keratoplasty intacs with laser grooves or collagen stabilization of cornea.

🗗 BIBLIOGRAPHY

1. Weissman BA, Yeung KK. (2011). Keratoconus. [online] Available from www.emedicine.com/oph/TOPIC104.HTM. [Accessed October, 2013].

🗗 1T. JENSEN DISEASE (JUXTAPAPILLARY RETINOPATHY)

General

Etiology is unknown.

Ocular

Circumscribed inflammatory changes of the choroid; field defect.

Clinical

None.

Laboratory

Diagnosis is made by clinical findings.

Treatment

None—ocular.

🗗 BIBLIOGRAPHY

1. Harley RD (Ed). Pediatric Ophthalmology, 4th edition. Philadelphia, PA: WB Saunders; 1998.
2. Magalini SI, Scrascia E. Dictionary of Medical Syndromes, 2nd edition. Philadelphia, PA: JB Lippincott; 1981.

🗗 1V. LATTICE DEGENERATION AND RETINAL DETACHMENT

General

Autosomal dominant; progressive; lattice degeneration precedes retinal detachment by about 20 years of age; familial occurrence of lattice degeneration in nonmyopes has been reported.

Ocular

Myopia; RS; peripheral retinal degeneration; lattice degeneration.

Clinical

None.

Laboratory

Diagnosis is made by clinical findings.

Treatment

Laser photocoagulation, cryotherapy, scleral buckling procedure and/or pars plana vitrectomy and gas administration.

⊟ BIBLIOGRAPHY

1. Sarraf D, Yuan A, Saulny SM. (2012). Lattice degeneration. [online] Available from www.emedicine.com/oph/TOPIC397.HTM. [Accessed October, 2013].

⊟ 1W. METAPHYSEAL CHONDRODYSPLASIA WITH RETINITIS PIGMENTOSA

General

Autosomal recessive.

Ocular

Retinitis pigmentosa.

Clinical

Defective cartilage and growth of long bones, particularly the metacarpals and phalanges.

Laboratory/Ocular

Diagnosis is made by clinical findings.

Treatment/Ocular

Low-vision clinic, vitamin A/beta-carotene.

⊟ BIBLIOGRAPHY

1. Telander DG, de Beus A, Small KW. (2012). Retinitis pigmentosa. [online] Available from www.emedicine.com/oph/TOPIC704.HTM. [Accessed October, 2013].

⊟ 1X. MICROCEPHALY WITH CHORIORETINOPATHY

General

Autosomal dominant; congenital infection; exposure to irradiation, chemical agents, mother's infection or injury.

Ocular

Chorioretinopathy is usually inactive.

Clinical

Microcephaly; slow growth of brain; mild mental retardation.

Laboratory

None.

Treatment

Laser photocoagulation, photodynamic therapy.

⊟ BIBLIOGRAPHY

1. Oh KT, Phillpotts BA, Law SK, et al. (2011). Central serous chorioretinopathy. [online] Available from www.emedicine.com/oph/TOPIC689.HTM. [Accessed October, 2013].

⊟ 1Y. PERIPHERAL RETINAL BREAKS AND DEGENERATION

General

Causes are related to the development of rhegmatogenous retinal detachment.

Clinical

None.

Ocular

Lattice lesions of the retina, tractional horseshoe breaks in the retina.

Laboratory

Diagnosis is made by clinical findings.

Treatment

Cryotherapy and laser use prophylactically.

🖿 BIBLIOGRAPHY

1. Sarraf D, Yuan A, Saulny SM. (2012). Lattice degeneration. [online] Available from www.emedicine.com/oph/TOPIC397.HTM. [Accessed October, 2013].
2. Small KW, McLellan CM, Song MK. (2012). Juvenile retinoschisis. [online] Available from www.emedicine.com/oph/TOPIC639.HTM. [Accessed October, 2013].

🖿 1Z. PROLIFERATIVE VITREORETINOPATHY (PVR)

General

Repair process with full or partial thickness retinal breaks, retinopexy or other types of retinal damage.

Ocular

Multiple starfolds and fixed retinal folds.

Clinical

None.

Laboratory

Diagnosis is made by clinical findings.

Treatment

Encircling buckle, gas injection, vitreous surgery and peeling epiretinal membrane.

🖿 BIBLIOGRAPHY

1. Roy FH, Fraunfelder FW, Fraunfelder FT. Roy and Fraunfelder's Current Ocular Therapy, 6th edition. London, UK: Elsevier; 2008.

🖿 1BB. REFSUM SYNDROME (HEREDOPATHIA ATACTICA POLYNEURITIFORMIS SYNDROME; PHYTANIC ACID OXIDASE DEFICIENCY; PHYTANIC ACID STORAGE DISEASE; REFSUM-THIEBAUT SYNDROME)

General

Autosomal recessive; disorder of lipid metabolism; interstitial hypertrophic polyneuropathy; delamination of myelin sheaths; onset usually between ages 4 and 7 years; caused by deficiency of phytanic acid hydroxylase.

Ocular

Progressive external ophthalmoplegia; night blindness; visual field constriction; pupillary abnormalities; corneal opacities; retinal degeneration beginning in macula; atypical RP; cataracts.

Clinical

Spinocerebellar ataxia; deafness (progressive); polyneuritis-like effect on limbs; CNS degeneration; ichthyosis; sensory changes; wasting of extremities; complete heart block; relapses and remissions in adolescence; normal intelligence.

Laboratory

Check phytanic acid in serum.

Treatment

Dietary restriction of phytanic acid, plasma exchange.

🖿 BIBLIOGRAPHY

1. Zalewska A, Schwartz RA. (2011). Refsum disease. [online] Available from www.emedicine.com/derm/TOPIC705.HTM. [Accessed October, 2013].

🗗 1CC. RETINAL CAPILLARITIS

General

Rare; frequently associated with uveitis.

Clinical

Tubulointerstitial nephritis; inflammatory bowel disease.

Ocular

Decreased visual acuity; dilation and leakage of capillary.

Laboratory

Fluorescein angiography; OCT/scanning laser ophthalmoscopy (SLO); ICGA; fundus autofluorescence (FAF).

Treatment

Traditional treatment for uveitis with topical steroids.

🗗 BIBLIOGRAPHY

1. Ozmert E, Batioglu F. An unusual case of acute unilateral uveitis with retinal capillaritis. Ann Ophthalmol (Skokie). 2009;41(3-4):184-8.

🗗 1DD. RETINOBLASTOMA

General

Retinoblastoma is a malignant tumor arising in one or both retinas of young children, usually under the age of 2 years; usually unilateral; autosomal dominant; this is the most common intraocular malignancy of childhood; incidence is 1 in 20,000 live births; origin is questionably neuroectodermal cells capable of multipotentiality; one-third of patients have heritable (bilateral or have a positive family history) autosomal dominant and two-thirds are sporadic; genetic transmission obeys two-mutation hypothesis of Knudson; trilateral retinoblastoma is bilateral retinoblastoma plus midline CNS tumor (most commonly pinealoma); most common second tumor is an osteogenic sarcoma (begins in second decade).

Ocular

Hyphema; hypopyon; corneal tumor; lid edema; endophthalmitis; exophthalmos; intraocular calcification of globe; heterochromia; neovascularization of iris or retina; papilledema; panophthalmitis; retinoblastoma extension into orbit and choroid; cat's-eye reflex; leukocoria; mydriasis; vitreous hemorrhage tumor seeding; esotropia; exotropia; glaucoma; visual loss.

Clinical

Metastasis into the lymph system, bone marrow, and subarachnoid space; basal meningitis; death.

Laboratory

Computed tomography (CT)—calcification of lesion hallmark of disease; ultrasound demonstrates calcification and MRI demonstrates presence and extent of extraocular disease.

Treatment

External beam radiation therapy is recommended on patients with significant vitreous seeding. Radioactive isotope plaques and chemotherapy are also an option. Removal of the tumor is the standard management for retinoblastoma.

🗗 BIBLIOGRAPHY

1. Isidro MA, Roque MR, Aaberg TM, et al. (2012). Retinoblastoma. [online] Available from www.emedicine.com/oph/TOPIC346.HTM. [Accessed October, 2013].

🗗 1EE. RETROLENTAL FIBROPLASIA (RLF; RETINOPATHY OF PREMATURITY)

General

Bilateral disease seen primarily in premature infants with immature retinal vessels; excessive use of oxygen is responsible for the majority of cases, but disease is seen despite oxygen restrictions or even when no oxygen supplementation is used; known factors that correlate with degrees of retinopathy of prematurity are low birth weight, short gestational age, length of time with supplemental oxygen, length of time on a mechanical ventilator; role of excessive light in newborn nurseries also has been proposed.

Ocular

Anterior or posterior synechiae; neovascularization of iris; pallor of optic disk; dragged disk; attenuated vessels; retinal detachment; dilation of veins; retinal folds; retinal hemorrhage; retrolental mass; vascular tortuosity; vasoconstriction of retina; retinal pigmentary changes; vitreous haze; vitreous traction; vitreous hemorrhages; cataract; glaucoma; leukocoria; myopia; shallow anterior chamber; opaque retrolental membrane; ciliary body drawn anteriorly; ciliary process around dilated pupil; absent pupillary reflexes; keratoconus; associated strabismus; amblyopia.

Clinical

Low birth weight; prematurity.

Laboratory

Diagnosis is made by clinical findings.

Treatment

Cryotherapy and laser surgery can be effective. Vitrectomy may be necessary.

🗗 BIBLIOGRAPHY

1. Bashour M, Menassa J, Gerontis CC. (2013). Retinopathy of prematurity. [online] Available from www.emedicine.com/oph/TOPIC413.HTM. [Accessed October, 2013].

🗗 1FF1. DIVERTICULOSIS OF BOWEL, HERNIA, RETINAL DETACHMENT

General

Autosomal recessive.

Ocular

Severe myopia; esotropia; retinal detachment.

Clinical

Femoral or inguinal hernias; diverticula of bowel or bladder.

Laboratory

Diagnosis is made by clinical findings.

Treatment

- *Esotropia*: Equalized vision with correct refractive error; surgery may be helpful in patient with diplopia.
- *Retinal detachment*: Scleral buckle, pneumatic retinopexy and vitrectomy may be used to close all the breaks.

🗗 BIBLIOGRAPHY

1. Clunie GJ, Mason JM. Visceral diverticula and the Marfan syndrome. Br J Surg. 1962;50:51-2.
2. McKusick VA. Mendelian Inheritance in Man; A Catalog of Human Genes and Genetic Disorders, 12th edition. Baltimore, USA: The Johns Hopkins University Press; 1998.
3. Online Mendelian Inheritance in Man, OMIM. McKusick-Nathans Institute for Genetic Medicine, Johns Hopkins University and National Center for Biotechnology Information, National Library of Medicine, February 12, 2007. Available from www.ncbi.nlm.nih.gov/omim. [Accessed October, 2013].

⊟ 1FF2. RETINAL DETACHMENT, EXUDATIVE

General

Subretinal fluid accumulation in the space between the neurosensory retina and the underlying RPE.

Clinical

Rheumatoid arthritis; pre-eclampsia; Coats disease; Vogt-Koyanagi-Harada syndrome; sarcoidosis; syphilis; toxoplasmosis; CMV; Lyme disease; lupus; rean; disease.

Ocular

Bullous retinal detachment, cut in visual field; vitreous floaters; decreased visual acuity; scleritis.

Laboratory

Diagnosis is generally made by clinical observation. Ultrasound may be necessary if the media is hazy.

Treatment

Medical and surgical treatment of exudative retinal detachment is tailored to the underlying condition and may include laser, cryotherapy and vitrectomy.

⊟ BIBLIOGRAPHY

1. Wu L, Evans T. (2012). Exudative retinal detachment. [online] Available from emedicine.medscape.com/article/1224509-overview. [Accessed October, 2013].

⊟ 1FF3. RETINAL DETACHMENT, PROLIFERATIVE

General

Subretinal fluid accumulation in the space between the neurosensory retina and the underlying RPE. Proliferative vitreoretinopathy (PVR) is the most common cause of failure in retinal detachment surgery.

Clinical

Diabetes; injury; following pneumatic retinopexy, cryotherapy, laser retinopexy, scleral buckling or vitrectomy.

Ocular

Vitreous traction, cut in visual field; vitreous floaters; decreased visual acuity; scleritis; retinal breaks.

Laboratory

Diagnosis is generally made by clinical observation. Ultrasound may be necessary if the media is hazy.

Treatment

Corticosteroids (topical, subconjunctival or retrobulbar) are beneficial at the time of surgery. Scleral buckle and vitrectomy are the treatments of choice for this type of detachment.

⊟ BIBLIOGRAPHY

1. Charles S. (2012). Proliferative retinal detachment. [online] Available from emedicine.medscape.com/article/1226426-overview. [Accessed October, 2013].

⊟ 1FF4. RETINAL DETACHMENT, RHEGMATOGENOUS

General

Subretinal fluid accumulation in the space between the neurosensory retina and the underlying RPE. Most common type of retinal detachment and occurs with a retinal tear that allows liquefied vitreous to seep under the tear leading to the detachment.

Clinical

None.

Ocular

Vitreous traction, cut in visual field; vitreous floaters; decreased visual acuity; scleritis.

Laboratory

Diagnosis is generally made by clinical observation. Ultrasound may be necessary if the media is hazy.

Treatment

Scleral buckle, pneumatic retinopexy and vitrectomy are used for this type of detachment and the goal is to close all the breaks.

BIBLIOGRAPHY

1. Wu L, Evans T. (2011). Rhegmatogenous retinal detachment treatment and management. [online] Available from emedicine.medscape.com/article/1224737-treatment. [Accessed October, 2013].

1FF5. SCHWARTZ SYNDROME (RETINAL DETACHMENT)

General

Glaucoma associated with retinal detachment; caused by inflammation of trabecula or pigment granules obstructing outflow; photoreceptor outer segments identified in the aqueous humor of patients with this syndrome are thought to play a role in the elevation of intraocular pressure.

Ocular

Secondary open-angle glaucoma; retinal detachment; uveitis; myopia; blepharophimosis; long eyelashes; microcornea.

Clinical

Small stature; myotonia; expressionless facies; joint limitation in hips; dystrophy of epiphyseal cartilage, vertical shortness of vertebrae, short neck; low hairline.

Laboratory

Blood test, muscle biopsy, electromyography (EMG) and nerve conduction studies.

Treatment

Botulinum toxin type A is used to treat problems such as blepharospasm, blepharophimosis and ptosis; surgery may also be necessary.

BIBLIOGRAPHY

1. Ault J, Berman SA, Dinnerstein E. (2012). Schwartz-Jampel syndrome. [online] Available from www.emedicine.com/neuro/TOPIC337.HTM. [Accessed October, 2013].

1FF6. RETINAL DETACHMENT, TRACTIONAL

General

Subretinal fluid accumulation in the space between the neurosensory retina and the underlying RPE; caused by traction on the retina secondary to injury, subretinal membranes; retinopathy of prematurity and PVR.

Clinical

Diabetes; injury.

Ocular

Vitreous traction, cut in visual field; vitreous floaters; decreased visual acuity; scleritis; retinal breaks.

Laboratory

Diagnosis is generally made by clinical observation. Ultrasound may be necessary if the media is hazy.

Treatment

Scleral buckle and vitrectomy are used to relieve vitreoretinal traction.

BIBLIOGRAPHY

1. Wu L, Evans T. (2012). Tractional retinal detachment. [online] Available from emedicine.medscape.com/article/1224891-overview. [Accessed October, 2013].

⊟ 1GG1. ALSTROM DISEASE (CATARACT AND RETINITIS PIGMENTOSA)

General

Retinal lesion associated with deafness; severe visual loss in the first decade.

Ocular

Cataract; RP; optic atrophy; salt and pepper pigment epithelial abnormalities. ERG pathognomonic findings include initially normal rod component, which can become undetectable as early as 5 years of age; undetectable cone activity at 18 months.

Clinical

Nerve deafness; diabetes mellitus in childhood; obesity; renal disease; baldness; hyperuricemia; hypogenitalism; acanthosis nigricans; skeletal anomalies; diabetes mellitus; deafness.

Laboratory

Diagnosis is made by clinical findings.

Treatment

- *Cataract*: Change in glasses can sometimes improve a patient's visual function temporarily; however the most common treatment is cataract surgery.
- *Retinitis pigmentosa*: Vitamin A 15,000 IU/day is thought to slow the decline of retinal function; dark sunglasses for outdoor use; surgery for cataract; genetic counseling.

⊟ BIBLIOGRAPHY

1. Geeraets WJ. Ocular Syndromes, 3rd edition. Philadelphia, PA: Lea & Febiger; 1976.
2. Harley RD (Ed). Pediatric Ophthalmology, 4th edition. Philadelphia, PA: WB Saunders; 1998.
3. Konigsmark BW, Knox DL, Hussels IE, et al. Dominant congenital deafness and progressive optic nerve atrophy. Occurrence in four generations of a family. Arch Ophthalmol. 1974;91(2):99-103.
4. Millay RH, Weleber RG, Heckenlively JR. Ophthalmologic and systemic manifestations of Alström's disease. Am J Ophthalmol. 1986;102(4):482-90.
5. Tremblay F, LaRoche RG, Shea SE, et al. Longitudinal study of the early electroretinographic changes in Alström's syndrome. Am J Ophthalmol. 1993;115(5):657-65.

⊟ 1GG2. LAURENCE-MOON-BARDET-BIEDL SYNDROME (BARDET-BIEDL SYNDROME; RETINITIS PIGMENTOSA-POLYDACTYLY-ADIPOSOGENITAL SYNDROME)

General

Recessive, autosomal dominant and recessive sex-linked gene; male preponderance; onset in childhood; cases of Laurence-Moon belong to the group of heredoataxias.

Ocular

Ptosis; epicanthus; nystagmus; strabismus; night blindness; myopia; hypermetropia; iris coloboma; RP "bone corpuscles"; macular degeneration; attenuation of retinal vessels; choroidal atrophy; optic nerve atrophy; cataract; microphthalmia; keratoconus.

Clinical

Obesity (Fröhlich type); hypogenitalism; reduced intelligence and mental retardation; turricephaly; shortness of stature; atresia ani; genu valgum; congenital heart disease; polydactyly; body hair scant or absent; pseudogynecomastia.

Laboratory

Chromosomal analysis is recommended to confirm chromosomal sex and to evaluate for associated genetic syndromes.

Treatment

Consultation by pediatric endocrinologist and pediatric urologist is usually necessary.

⊟ BIBLIOGRAPHY

1. Telander DG, de Beus A, Small KW. (2012). Retinitis pigmentosa. [online] Available from www.emedicine.com/oph/TOPIC704.HTM. [Accessed October, 2013].

1GG3. USHER SYNDROME (HEREDITARY RETINITIS PIGMENTOSA-DEAFNESS SYNDROME) RETINITIS PIGMENTOSA

General

Retinitis pigmentosa associated with deaf-mutism; dominantly inherited; anatomic and metabolic condition; onset unknown (Hallgren syndrome).

Ocular

Concentric contraction of visual fields; RP with dotted, fine pigmentation in midperiphery; bone-corpuscle configured pigment deposits mainly along the vessels toward the periphery; yellow-white dots in outer retina and choroid; poor night vision.

Clinical

Deaf-mutism; however, deafness is not always complete; multiple sclerosis.

Laboratory

Diagnosis is made by clinical findings.

Treatment

Retinitis pigmentosa may be treated with vitamin A 15,000 IU/day, which is thought to slow the decline of retinal function; dark sunglasses for outdoor use; surgery for cataract; genetic counseling.

BIBLIOGRAPHY

1. Berson EL, Adamian M. Ultrastructural findings in an autopsy eye from a patient with Usher's syndrome type II. Am J Ophthalmol. 1992;114(6):748-57.
2. Holland MG, Cambie E, Kloepfer W. An evaluation of genetic carriers of Usher's syndrome. Am J Ophthalmol. 1972;74(5):940-7.
3. Lynch SG, Digre K, Rose JW. Usher's syndrome and multiple sclerosis. Review of an individual with Usher's syndrome with a multiple sclerosis-like illness. J Neuroophthalmol. 1994;14(1):34-7.
4. Müftüoglu AU, Akman N, Savaş I. Polycythemia vera associated with Usher's syndrome. Am J Ophthalmol. 1975;80(1): 93-5.
5. Usher CH. On the Inheritance of Retinitis Pigmentosa, with Notes of Cases. R Lond Ophthalmol Hosp Rep. 1913;19:130.

1GG4. HALLGREN SYNDROME (RETINITIS PIGMENTOSA-DEAFNESS-ATAXIA SYNDROME; USHER SYNDROME TYPE I)

General

Autosomal recessive inheritance.

Ocular

Horizontal nystagmus (10%); cataract; RP; retinal atrophy; narrow retinal vessels; optic atrophy; keratoconus.

Clinical

Congenital deafness (complete or at least severe auditory impairment); mental deficiency (25%); vestibulocerebellar ataxia (90%); schizophrenia-like symptoms (25%).

Laboratory

Diagnosis is made by clinical findings.

Treatment

Low-vision evaluation, vitamin A/beta-carotene may be helpful.

BIBLIOGRAPHY

1. Telander DG, de Beus A, Small KW. (2012). Retinitis pigmentosa. [online] Available from www.emedicine.com/oph/TOPIC704.HTM. [Accessed October, 2013].

1GG5. RETINOPATHY, PIGMENTARY, AND MENTAL RETARDATION (MIRHOSSEINI-HOLMES-WALTON SYNDROME)

General

Autosomal recessive; this disorder may be the same as (or allele) to Cohen syndrome.

Ocular

Pigmentary retinal degeneration; cataract; keratoconus.

Clinical

Microcephaly; severe mental retardation; hyperextensible joints; scoliosis; arachnodactyly; hypogonadism.

Laboratory

Diagnosis is made by clinical findings.

Treatment

Vitamin A 15,000 IU/day is thought to slow the decline of retinal function; dark sunglasses for outdoor use; surgery for cataract, genetic counseling.

BIBLIOGRAPHY

1. McKusick VA. Mendelian Inheritance in Man: A Catalog of Human Genes and Genetic Disorders, 12th edition. Baltimore, USA: The Johns Hopkins University Press; 1998.
2. Hamosh A, Scott AF, Amberger J, et al. Online Mendelian Inheritance in Man (OMIM), a knowledgebase of human genes and genetic disorders. Nucleic Acids Res. 2002;30(1):52-5.
3. Mendez HM, Paskulin GA, Vallandro C. The syndrome of retinal pigmentary degeneration, microcephaly, and severe mental retardation (Mirhosseini-Holmes-Walton syndrome): report of two patients. Am J Med Genet. 1985;22(2):223-8.
4. Steinlein O, Tariverdian G, Boll HU, et al. Tapetoretinal degeneration in brothers with apparent Cohen syndrome: nosology with Mirhosseini-Holmes-Walton syndrome. Am J Med Genet. 1991;41(2):196-200.

1GG6. PALLIDAL DEGENERATION, PROGRESSIVE, WITH RETINITIS PIGMENTOSA (HYPOPREBETALIPOPROTEINEMIA, ACANTHOCYTOSIS, RETINITIS PIGMENTOSA, AND PALLIDAL DEGENERATION; HARP SYNDROME)

General

Autosomal recessive; destruction of global pallida and reticular portions of substantia nigra; also may be associated with hypoprebetalipoproteinemia and acanthocytosis; various combinations of components of hypoprebetalipoproteinemia, acanthocytosis, retinitis pigmentosa, and pallidal degeneration (HARP) syndrome may be caused by several distinct genetic diseases or may represent variable manifestations of a contiguous gene defect.

Ocular

Retinitis pigmentosa.

Clinical

Progressive extrapyramidal rigidity; dysarthria.

Laboratory

Diagnosis is made by clinical findings and visual fields.

Treatment

Maximize with the refraction and low-vision evaluation; vitamin A/beta-carotene antioxidants may be useful.

BIBLIOGRAPHY

1. Telander DG, de Beus A, Small KW. (2012). Retinitis pigmentosa. [online] Available from www.emedicine.com/oph/TOPIC704.HTM. [Accessed October, 2013].

1GG7. SPASTIC QUADRIPLEGIA, RETINITIS PIGMENTOSA, MENTAL RETARDATION

General

Autosomal recessive; consanguineous parents.

Ocular

Granular pigmented retina; pale optic disk; retinal degeneration; exotropia; miotic pupils; ptosis; nystagmus; small optic disk; RP.

Clinical

Expressionless face; drooling; spastic contractures; scissoring; spastic gait; mental retardation; brachydactyly; hypoplasia; tremors; hearing impairment.

Laboratory

Fluorescent treponemal antibody absorption test, inherited/syndromic disease laboratory test, neoplasm-related laboratory test and OCT can be helpful.

Treatment/Ocular

Antioxidants may be useful; very high daily doses of vitamin A palmitate slow the progress of RP; beta-carotene has been recommended.

BIBLIOGRAPHY

1. Telander DG, de Beus A, Small KW. (2012). Retinitis pigmentosa. [online] Available from www.emedicine.com/oph/TOPIC704.HTM. [Accessed October, 2013].

1HH1. RETINOSCHISIS, ACQUIRED [ACQUIRED RETINOSCHISIS (RS)]

General

Present in 4–22% of normal population over the age of 40 years; splitting in the outer plexiform layer; occasionally in the inner nuclear layer; generally asymptomatic.

Ocular

Slowly progressive; may cause retinal detachment when there are breaks in both outer and inner layers of RS.

Clinical

None.

Laboratory

Visual field—absolute scotoma versus relative scotoma in retinal detachment; ultrasonography including B-scan and ultrasonic biomicroscopy; OCT to differentiate between schisis and detachment.

Treatment

Photocoagulation and/or cryotherapy can be used if RS is extending into the posterior pole.

BIBLIOGRAPHY

1. Phillpotts BA, Gounder R. (2012). Senile retinoschisis. [online] Available from www.emedicine.com/oph/TOPIC640.HTM. [Accessed October, 2013].

1HH2. RETINOSCHISIS, AUTOSOMAL DOMINANT

General

Autosomal dominant; degenerative abnormal splitting of retinal sensory layers.

Ocular

Loss of retinal function; retinal degeneration; macular degeneration.

Clinical

None.

Laboratory

Diagnosis is made by clinical findings.

Treatment

Photocoagulation and/or cryotherapy.

BIBLIOGRAPHY

1. http://www.emedicine.com/oph/TOPIC1083.HTM.

1HH3. RETINOSCHISIS, CONGENITAL

General

X-linked recessive; nearly always found in males.

Ocular

Retinal splitting usually occurs in the nerve fiber layer; slow progression; frequently affects the macula; associated with vitreous hemorrhage; strabismus; nystagmus; retinal folds radiating from the fovea; macular pigmentary mottling; retinal detachment (rare complication).

Clinical

None.

Laboratory

Diagnosis is made by clinical findings.

Treatment

Photocoagulation and/or cryotherapy.

BIBLIOGRAPHY

1. Condon GP, Brownstein S, Wang NS, et al. Congenital hereditary (juvenile X-linked) retinoschisis. Histopathologic and ultrastructural findings in three eyes. Arch Ophthalmol. 1986;104(4):576-83.
2. Hirose T. Retinoschisis. In: Albert DM, Jakobiec FA (Eds). Albert & Jakobiec's Principles and Practice of Ophthalmology: Clinical Practice, 5th edition. Philadelphia, PA: WB Saunders; 1994. pp. 1071-84.
3. Regillo CD, Tasman WS, Brown GC. Surgical management of complications associated with X-linked retinoschisis. Arch Ophthalmol. 1993;111(8):1080-6.

1HH4. RETINOSCHISIS OF FOVEA

General

Autosomal recessive.

Ocular

Foveal dystrophy; rod-cone dystrophy; nyctalopia; hyperopia; paramacular tapetal sheen reflex.

Clinical

None.

Laboratory

Diagnosis is made by clinical findings.

Treatment

Photocoagulation and/or cryotherapy.

BIBLIOGRAPHY

1. McKusick VA. Mendelian Inheritance in Man: A Catalog of Human Genes and Genetic Disorders, 12th edition. Baltimore, USA: The Johns Hopkins University Press; 1998.
2. Hamosh A, Scott AF, Amberger J, et al. Online Mendelian Inheritance in Man (OMIM), a knowledgebase of human genes and genetic disorders. Nucleic Acids Res. 2002;30(1):52-5.
3. Noble KG, Carr RE, Siegel IM. Familial foveal retinoschisis associated with a rod-cone dystrophy. Am J Ophthalmol. 1978;85(4):551-7.

1II. TERSON SYNDROME (SUBARACHNOID HEMORRHAGE SYNDROME)

General

Spontaneous rupture of aneurysm or traumatic intracerebral hemorrhage; onset at all ages.

Ocular

Weakness of extraocular muscles; disarranged and uncoordinated gaze; severe intraocular hemorrhage; preretinal hemorrhages; peripapillary hemorrhages; papilledema secondary to optic nerve sheath hemorrhages; pigmentary changes in macula and retina; preretinal membrane formation; vitreous detachment; amblyopia; anisocoria; bilateral retinal detachments have been associated with this disorder; epiretinal membranes (sequelae).

Clinical

Sudden unconsciousness; elevated cerebrospinal fluid pressure.

Laboratory

Sickle cell (SC) preparation, CT scan, MRI and angiography.

Treatment

Vitrectomy is required if vitreous hemorrhage does not clear by itself.

🖶 BIBLIOGRAPHY

1. Ou RJ, Yoshizumi MO. (2012). Terson syndrome. [online] Available from www.emedicine.com/oph/TOPIC753.HTM. [Accessed October, 2013].
2. Ko F, Knox DL. The ocular pathology of Terson's syndrome. Ophthalmology. 2010;117(7):1423-9.e2.

🖶 1JJ. ABDOMINAL TYPHUS (ENTERIC FEVER; TYPHOID FEVER)

General

Causative agent, *Salmonella typhi*.

Ocular

Conjunctivitis; chemosis; corneal ulcer; tenonitis; paralysis of extraocular muscles; endophthalmitis; panophthalmitis; optic neuritis; retinal detachment; central scotoma; central retinal artery emboli; iritis with or without hypopyon; choroiditis; retinal hemorrhages; bilateral optic neuritis; abnormal ocular motility (likely secondary to thrombotic infarcts affecting the ocular motor nerve nuclei, fascicles, brainstem, or cerebral hemispheres).

Clinical

Fever; headache; bradycardia; splenomegaly; maculopapular rash; leukopenia; encephalitis. Salmonella may produce an illness characterized by fever and bacteremia without any other manifestations of enterocolitis or enteric fever, which is particularly common in patients with AIDS.

Laboratory

Gram-negative bacillus isolation from blood culture (50–70% of cases). Positive stool culture is less frequent.

Treatment

Early detection, antibiotic therapy and adequate fluids, electrolytes, and nutrition reduce the rate of complications and reduce the case-fatality rate.

🖶 BIBLIOGRAPHY

1. Brusch JL. (2011). Typhoid fever. [online] Available from www.emedicine.com/med/TOPIC2331.HTM. [Accessed October, 2013].

🖶 1KK. OCULAR TOXOPLASMOSIS (TOXOPLASMIC RETINOCHOROIDITIS; TOXOPLASMOSIS)

General

Parasite infestation caused by *Toxoplasma gondii*; cell-mediated immunity is believed to be the major defence mechanism against *Toxoplasma* infection; ocular toxoplasmosis occurs in approximately 1% of patients with AIDS; AIDS-related toxoplasma retinochoroiditis may have several atypical clinical manifestations.

Ocular

Keratitis; uveitis; optic atrophy; papillitis; anisocoria; persistent pupillary membrane; focal retinochoroiditis; scleritis; cataract; microphthalmos; myopia; nystagmus; esotropia.

Clinical

Cysts are seen in many organs, including brain and muscle; hydrocephalus; intracerebral calcification; various CNS complaints.

Laboratory

Serologic tests for anti-*T. gondii*. Antibodies are common.

Treatment

Triple drug therapy pyrimethamine, sulfadiazine and prednisone. Pyrimethamine should be combined with folinic acid. Surgical care includes photocoagulation, cryotherapy or vitrectomy.

BIBLIOGRAPHY

1. Lasave AF, Llopis MD, Muccioli C, et al. Intravitreal clindamycin and dexamethasone for zone 1 toxoplasmic retinochoroiditis at twenty-four months. Ophthalmology. 2010;1831-8.
2. Soheilian M, Ramezani A, Azimzadeh A, et al. Randomized trial of intravitreal clindamycin and dexamethasone versus pyrimethamine, sulfadiazine and prednisolone in treatment of ocular toxoplasmosis. Ophthalmology. 2011;118:134-41.
3. Wuh L. (2011). Ophthalmologic Manifestations of Toxoplasmosis. [online] Available from www.emedicine.com/oph/TOPIC707.HTM. [Accessed October, 2013].

1LL. OLIVER-MCFARLANE SYNDROME (TRICHOMEGALY SYNDROME)

General

Rare syndrome.

Ocular

Trichomegaly; pigmentary retinal degeneration.

Clinical

Prenatal onset growth failure; anterior pituitary deficiencies; peripheral neuropathy; mental retardation, sparse scalp hair, endocrinologic deficiencies and koilonychias may be found.

Laboratory

Diagnosis is made by clinical findings.

Treatment

None—ocular.

BIBLIOGRAPHY

1. Sampson JR, Tolmie JL, Cant JS. Oliver McFarlane syndrome: a 25 year follow-up. Am J Med Genet. 1989;34(2):199-201.
2. Shaker AG, Fleming R, Jamieson ME, et al. Ovarian stimulation in an infertile patient with growth hormone-deficient Oliver-McFarlane syndrome. Hum Reprod. 1994;9(11):1997-8.
3. Zaun H, Stenger D, Zabransky S, et al. [The long-eyelash syndrome (trichomegaly syndrome, Oliver-McFarlane)]. Hautarzt. 1984;35(3):162-5.

1MM. USHER SYNDROME (HEREDITARY RETINITIS PIGMENTOSA-DEAFNESS SYNDROME) RETINITIS PIGMENTOSA

General

Retinitis pigmentosa associated with deaf-mutism; dominantly inherited; anatomic and metabolic condition; onset unknown (Hallgren syndrome).

Ocular

Concentric contraction of visual fields; RP with dotted, fine pigmentation in midperiphery; bone-corpuscle configured pigment deposits mainly along the vessels toward the periphery; yellow-white dots in outer retina and choroid; poor night vision.

Clinical

Deaf-mutism; however, deafness is not always complete; multiple sclerosis.

Laboratory

Diagnosis is made by clinical findings.

Treatment

Retinitis pigmentosa may be treated with vitamin A 15,000 IU/day, which is thought to slow the decline of retinal function; dark sunglasses for outdoor use; surgery for cataract; genetic counseling.

BIBLIOGRAPHY

1. Berson EL, Adamian M. Ultrastructural findings in an autopsy eye from a patient with Usher's syndrome type II. Am J Ophthalmol. 1992;114(6):748-57.
2. Holland MG, Cambie E, Kloepfer W. An evaluation of genetic carriers of Usher's syndrome. Am J Ophthalmol. 1972;74(5):940-7.
3. Lynch SG, Digre K, Rose JW. Usher's syndrome and multiple sclerosis. Review of an individual with Usher's syndrome with a multiple sclerosis-like illness. J Neuroophthalmol. 1994;14(1):34-7.
4. Müftüoglu AU, Akman N, Savaş I. Polycythemia vera associated with Usher's syndrome. Am J Ophthalmol. 1975;80(1):93-5.
5. Usher CH. On the Inheritance of Retinitis Pigmentosa, with Notes of Cases. R Lond Ophthalmol Hosp Rep. 1913;19:130.

🗗 1NN. VON HIPPEL-LINDAU SYNDROME (RETINOCEREBRAL ANGIOMATOSIS; ANGIOMATOSIS RETINAE; CEREBELLORETINAL HEMANGIOBLASTOMATOSIS; LINDAU SYNDROME; RETINAL CAPILLARY HAMARTOMA) GLAUCOMA

General

Dominant inheritance; angiomata in the cerebellum and the walls of the fourth ventricle; young adults.

Ocular

Secondary glaucoma; angiomatosis of the iris; vitreous hemorrhages; tortuosity of dilated retinal artery and vein (feeder vessels); retinal exudates and hemorrhages; retinitis proliferans; angiomata of optic nerve and retina; papilledema; retinal detachment; lipid accumulation in macula; keratoconus; bilateral macular holes; choroid plexus papilloma; bilateral optic nerve hemangioblastomas.

Clinical

Cerebellar angiomatosis; epilepsy; psychic disturbances to dementia.

Laboratory

Diagnosis is made by clinical findings.

Treatment

Smaller tumors can be treated with argon laser photocoagulation. Cryotherapy is used to treat larger posterior angiomas. Vitreoretinal surgery is effective for the treatment of severe von Hippel-Lindau (VHL) retinal hemangiomas.

🗗 BIBLIOGRAPHY

1. Khan AN, Turnbull I, Al-Okaili R. (2011). Imaging in Von Hippel-Lindau syndrome. [online] Available from www.emedicine.com/radio/TOPIC742.HTM. [Accessed October, 2013].
2. Gaudric A, Krivosic V, Duguid G, et al. Vitreoretinal surgery for severe retinal capillary hemangiomas in von Hippel-Lindau disease. Ophthalmology. 2011;118(1):142-9.

🗗 100. WAGNER SYNDROME (HYALOIDEORETINAL DEGENERATION; HEREDITARY HYALOIDEORETINAL DEGENERATION AND PALATOSCHISIS; CLEFTING SYNDROME; GOLDMANN-FAVRE SYNDROME; FAVRE HYALOIDEORETINAL DEGENERATION; RETINOSCHISIS WITH EARLY HEMERALOPIA) NYSTAGMUS

General

Irregular dominant inheritance; both sexes are affected.

Ocular

Epicanthus; nystagmus; myopia; iris atrophy; vitreous opacities with dense streaks and folds in posterior hyaloid membrane; corneal degeneration, including band-shaped keratopathy; cataracts; hyaloideoretinal degeneration (usually apparent after 15 years of age); narrowing of retinal vessels; pigmentary changes; type of retinal degeneration varies from case to case; retinal detachment and avascular preretinal membranes; marked choroidal sclerosis; pale optic disk; Bergmeister's papilla.

Clinical

Palatoschisis; genua valga; facial anomalies; hypoplastic maxilla; saddle nose; hyperextensible fingers, elbows and knees; tapering fingers.

Laboratory

Diagnosis is made by clinical findings.

Treatment

- *Seesaw nystagmus*: Visual field to consider neoplastic or vascular etiologies.
- *Upbeat nystagmus*: It may indicate multiple sclerosis, cerebellar degeneration, tumors or infarcts. Treatment is directed toward identification and resolution of underlying cause.
- *Downbeat nystagmus*: It affects the cerebellum or craniocervical junction including Arnold-Chiari malformation, multiple sclerosis, trauma, tumor, infarction and many toxic metabolic entities. MRI may indicate a surgically correctable lesion. Periodic alternating nystagmus is continuous horizontal nystagmus from stroke, tumor, multiple sclerosis, trauma, infection, drug intoxication. It can occur from cataract, vitreous hemorrhage or optic atrophy.

- *Corneal opacity*: Medical treatment includes the use of hyperosmotic drops, nonsteroidal and steroid eye drops. Corneal transplant may be necessary.
- *Cataract*: Change in glasses can sometimes improve a patient's visual function temporarily; however, the most common treatment is cataract surgery.

BIBLIOGRAPHY

1. Black GC, Perveen R, Wiszniewski W, et al. A novel hereditary developmental vitreoretinopathy with multiple ocular abnormalities localizing to a 5-cM region of chromosome 5q13-q14. Ophthalmology. 1999;106(11):2074-81.
2. Frandsen E. Hereditary hyaloideoretinal degeneration (Wagner) in a Danish family. Arch Ophthalmol (Kbh). 1966;74:223.
3. Hirose T, Lee KY, Schepens CL. Wagner's hereditary vitreoretinal degeneration and retinal detachment. Arch Ophthalmol. 1973;89(3):176-85.
4. Kaiser-Kupfer M. Ectrodactyly, ectodermal dysplasia, and clefting syndrome. Am J Ophthalmol. 1973;76(6):992-8.
5. Wagner H. Ein Bisher Unbekanntes Erbleiden des Auges (Degeneratio Hyaloideo Hereditaria), Beobachtet im Kanton Zurich. Klin Monatsbl Augenheilkd. 1938;100:840.

2A. CENTRAL OR BRANCH RETINAL ARTERY OCCLUSION

General

Present with profound monocular vision loss. In branch occlusion, the visual loss is partial with a scotoma or visual field loss.

Clinical

None.

Ocular

Vision loss, macular edema, macular ischemia, vitreous hemorrhage, traction detachment, rubeosis irides.

Laboratory

Complete blood count, erythrocyte sedimentation rate (ESR), fasting blood sugar, cholesterol, triglyceride and lipid panels, coagulopathy screen and blood cultures, carotid Doppler ultrasound, ERG, electrocardiogram (ECG) and echocardiogram to identify the cause; OCT to identify area of occlusion.

Treatment

Acetazolamide intravenously, distal ocular massage, hyperbaric oxygen, grid laser photocoagulation for macular edema, vitrectomy without sheathotomy.

BIBLIOGRAPHY

1. Campochiaro PA, Heier JS, Feiner L, et al. Ranibizumab for macular edema following branch retinal vein occlusion: six-month primary end point results of a phase III study. Ophthalmology. 2010;117(6):1102-12.e1.
2. Rogers SL, McIntosh RL, Lim L, et al. Natural history of branch retinal vein occlusion: an evidence-based systematic review. Ophthalmology. 2010;117(6):1094-101.e5.

2B. CAROTID ARTERY SYNDROME (CAROTID VASCULAR INSUFFICIENCY SYNDROME; OCULAR ISCHEMIC SYNDROME)

General

Causes include microemboli, atherosclerotic plaques, arteritis, arterial compression by cicatricial tissue surrounding the vessel and tumors; male preponderance; onset between ages of 50 years and 70 years.

Ocular

Lacrimation; homolateral transient, painless visual loss; photopsia; hemianopsia; retinal infarcts; cholesterol plaques may be seen in retinal arteries on funduscopic examination; optic atrophy; hypoxic retinopathy; low-tension glaucoma; anterior uveitis; cataract; visual acuity 20/400 or less; iris neovascularization; angle neovascularization; optic disk pale; retinal hemorrhages; Homer syndrome; amaurosis fugax; retinal artery occlusion; ophthalmoparesis; proptosis; chemosis; conjunctival hyperemia; acute orbital infarction.

Clinical

Transient cerebral ischemia with contralateral weakness of arm and leg; hemisensory disturbances; mental confusion and dysphasia; headache; dizziness; epileptiform seizures; carotid dissection.

Laboratory

Erythrocyte sedimentation rate and C-reactive protein levels in patients with suspected giant cell arteritis (GCA); fluorescein angiography.

Treatment

Panretinal photocoagulation is used to treat neovascularization of the iris, optic nerve or retina. It was reported to cause regression of neovascularization. Antiplatelet therapy may be useful. Carotid endarterectomy has shown to benefit symptomatic patients.

BIBLIOGRAPHY

1. Leibovitch I, Calonje D, El-Harazi SM. (2011). Ocular ischemic syndrome. [online] Available from www.emedicine.com/oph/TOPIC487.HTM. [Accessed October, 2013].

2C. DIABETES MELLITUS

General

Complex disorder of carbohydrate, lipid and protein metabolism characterized by hyperglycemia and a relative or total lack of insulin. Development is influenced by both genetic and environmental factors. Most commonly occurs in middle or late life (type II) and is seen most commonly in the obese. Diabetes can occur in the first or second decade of life (type I) and usually involves the lack of insulin production by the pancreas and the need for insulin therapy.

Clinical

Atherosclerosis; nephropathy; neuropathy; polyuria; polydipsia; polyphagia; obesity; elevated plasma glucose and elevated glycated hemoglobin (HbA_{1c}).

Ocular

Diabetic retinopathy; vitreous hemorrhage; macular edema; cataract; glaucoma; asteroid hyalosis; extraocular muscle paralysis; rubeosis iridis; corneal hypesthesia; optic nerve atrophy; papillopathy.

Laboratory

Diagnosis is made by fasting plasma glucose of greater than 126 mg/dL and 2 hours post-glucose load (75 g) plasma glucose of greater than 200 mg/dL and confirmed by repeat test.

Treatment

Goals include elimination of symptoms, by reduction of blood sugar and blood pressure. Smoking cessation, aspirin therapy, weight loss, exercise, diabetic diet as well as oral medication and/or insulin are all used in the treatment of diabetes. Diabetic retinopathy is most successfully treated with retinal photocoagulation. Pars plana vitrectomy is sometimes necessary to remove vitreous hemorrhage. Other ocular problems caused by diabetes such as cataracts and glaucoma are treated in traditional methods.

BIBLIOGRAPHY

1. Khardori R. (2012). Type 2 diabetes mellitus. [online] Available from emedicine.medscape.com/article/117853-overview. [Accessed October, 2013].

2C1. DIABETIC RETINOPATHY, BACKGROUND

General

Diabetes is a major medical problem that is growing in numbers. It is seen most commonly in Western countries in individuals that consume more calories than they use each day. It is caused by the pancreas not making enough insulin.

Clinical

Renal, neuropathic and cardiovascular disease, polyuria, polydipsia, polyphagia and weight loss.

Ocular

Cataracts, glaucoma, corneal abnormalities, iris neovascularization, macular edema, microaneurysms, retinal hemorrhage, cotton-wool spots, changes in refractive error.

Laboratory

Fasting glucose and HbA_{1c}, fluorescein angiography and OCT.

Treatment

Glucose control with diet, exercise and medication, daily dose of aspirin (650 mg), laser photocoagulation, Avastin and Lucentis is also being used off label.

⊟ BIBLIOGRAPHY

1. Bhavsar AR, Atebara NH, Drouilhet JH. (2012). Diabetic retinopathy. [online] Available from emedicine.medscape.com/article/1225122-overview. [Accessed October, 2013].

⊟ 2C2. DIABETIC RETINOPATHY, PROLIFERATIVE

General

Diabetes is a major medical problem that is growing in numbers. It is seen most commonly in Western countries in individuals that consume more calories than they use each day. It is caused by the pancreas not making or not making enough insulin.

Clinical

Renal, neuropathic and cardiovascular disease, polyuria, polydipsia, polyphagia and weight loss.

Ocular

Cataracts, glaucoma, corneal abnormalities, iris neovascularization, macular edema, microaneurysms, retinal hemorrhage, cotton-wool spots changes in refractive error.

Laboratory

Fasting glucose and HbA_{1c}, fluorescein angiography and OCT; B-scan may be necessary to evaluate the retina if vitreous hemorrhage is present.

Treatment

Glucose control with diet, exercise and medication, daily dose of aspirin (650 mg), laser photocoagulation, intravitreal injections of triamcinolone, Avastin and Lucentis can be used. The use of avastin and lucentis is off label. Vitrectomy and cryotherapy may also be necessary.

Treatment

Goals include elimination of symptoms, by reduction of blood sugar and blood pressure. Smoking cessation, aspirin therapy, weight loss, exercise, diabetic diet as well as oral medication and/or insulin are all used in the treatment of diabetes. Diabetic retinopathy is most successfully treated with retinal photocoagulation. Pars plana vitrectomy is sometimes necessary to remove vitreous hemorrhage. Other ocular problems caused by diabetes such as cataracts and glaucoma are treated in traditional methods.

⊟ BIBLIOGRAPHY

1. http://emedicine.medscape.com/article/117853-overview
2. Ostri C, Lund-Andersen H, Sander B, et.al.: Bilateral diabetic papillopathy and metabolic control. Ophthalmology 2010; 117: 2214-7.
3. Richter GM, Torres M, Choudhury F, et al: Risk Factors for Cortical, Nuclear, Posterior Subcapsular, and Mixed Lens Opacities: The Los Angeles Latino Eye Study. Ophthalmology 2012; 119: 547-54.

⊟ 2D. HYPERTENSION

General

Elevated blood pressure.

Ocular

Retinal arterial narrowing; arteriosclerosis; hemorrhages; retinal edema; cotton-wool spots; fatty exudates; optic disk edema; exudative retinal detachment; optic neuropathy; swollen optic nerve; central retinal vein occlusion; branch retinal vein occlusion; choroidal ischemia.

Clinical

Systemic hypertension; patchy loss of muscle tone in vessel walls; vascular decompensation.

Laboratory

Diagnosis is made from clinical findings, CBC count, serum electrolytes, serum creatinine, serum glucose, uric acid and urinalysis, lipid profile [total cholesterol, low-density lipoprotein (LDL) and high-density lipoprotein (HDL), and triglycerides].

Treatment

Lifestyle modifications: Weight loss, stop smoking, exercise, reduce stress, limit alcohol intake, reduce sodium intake, maintain adequate calcium and potassium intake. Refer to internist for drug therapy.

BIBLIOGRAPHY

1. Madhur MS, Riaz K, Dreisbach AW, et al. (2013). Hypertension. [online] Available from www.emedicine.com/med/TOPIC1106.HTM. [Accessed October, 2013].

2E. JENSEN DISEASE (JUXTAPAPILLARY RETINOPATHY)

General

Etiology is unknown.

Ocular

Circumscribed inflammatory changes of the choroid; field defect.

Clinical

None.

Laboratory

Diagnosis is made by clinical findings.

Treatment

None—ocular.

BIBLIOGRAPHY

1. Harley RD (Ed). Pediatric Ophthalmology, 4th edition. Philadelphia, PA: WB Saunders; 1998.
2. Magalini SI, Scrascia E. Dictionary of Medical Syndromes, 2nd edition. Philadelphia, PA: JB Lippincott; 1981.

2F. MACROANEURYSM

General

Dilation of the large arterioles of the retina; associated with systemic hypertension and atherosclerotic disease; most commonly seen between sixth decade and seventh decade.

Clinical

Hypertension; elevated cholesterol; atherosclerosis disease.

Ocular

Retinal edema; sudden painless vision loss; retinal hemorrhage; retinal exudate.

Laboratory

Fluorescein angiography is most helpful in diagnosis.

Treatment

Control hypertension and serum lipids. Many cases resolve without treatment. Laser photocoagulation may be necessary if the disease is persistent or progressive.

BIBLIOGRAPHY

1. Chaum E. (2012). Macroaneurysm. [online] Available from emedicine.medscape.com/article/1224043-overview. [Accessed October, 2013].

⊟ 2G. HERRICK SYNDROME (DRESBACH SYNDROME; SICKLE CELL DISEASE; DREPANOCYTIC ANEMIA)

General

It usually occurs in members of the black race; poor prognosis.

Ocular

Secondary glaucoma; telangiectasis of conjunctival vessels; scleral icterus; vitreous hemorrhages; cataract; retinal hemorrhages, exudates, and neovascularization; retinitis proliferans; microaneurysms; thrombosis of retinal venules; retinal vascular sheathing; central vein occlusion; angioid streaks; retinopathy with "black sunburst sign" in patients with SS hemoglobin; "sea fan sign" in patients with SC hemoglobin; comma signs of conjunctiva; fan-shaped neovascularization of iris; sector ischemic atrophy of iris; optic atrophy; white cotton mass of vitreous; retinal holes; color vision defects; central retinal artery obstruction; branch retinal artery obstruction; white without pressure; venous tortuosity; sickling maculopathy.

Clinical

Severe anemia with hemolytic crises; bone and joint aches; hemarthrosis; jaundice; hepatosplenomegaly.

Laboratory

Blood-sickling of red blood cells, newborn screening for hemoglobin disorders.

Treatment

Transfusion is required in an aplastic crisis, erythrocytapheresis is an automated red-cell exchange and bone marrow transplantation may be useful. Pain is the hallmark of SC disease. While frequency and severity vary greatly, most patients have interval symptoms. Once pain has begun, no therapy reverses the process. Analgesics may provide a reasonable degree of comfort. While certain dosing guidelines are available, the amount of drug given should be titrated to the degree of pain experienced. Vitrectomy may be necessary.

⊟ BIBLIOGRAPHY

1. Maakaron JE, Taher AT. (2013). Sickle cell anemia. [online] Available from www.emedicine.com/ped/TOPIC2096.HTM. [Accessed October, 2013].

⊟ 2H. RENDU-OSLER SYNDROME [RENDU-OSLER-WEBER SYNDROME; HEREDITARY HEMORRHAGIC TELANGIECTASIS; BABINGTON DISEASE; GOLDSTEIN HEMATEMESIS; OSLER SYNDROME (2)]

General

Etiology unknown; autosomal dominant in Jews; repeated epistaxis begins in childhood; gastrointestinal hemorrhages with melena and hematemesis manifest in middle and later life.

Ocular

Star-shaped angiomas of the palpebral conjunctiva; intermittent filamentary keratitis; small retinal angiomas and occasionally retinal hemorrhages; subconjunctival hemorrhages; small retinal arteriovenous malformations; bloody tears; conjunctival telangiectasias.

Clinical

Epistaxis; hematuria; melena; angiomata of the pharynx and oral and nasal mucosa; angiomas on lips, face and upper extremities; cyanosis; polycythemia.

Laboratory

Anemia usually present; hematuria and stool evaluation. CT and/or MRI to evaluate internal arteriovenous malformations.

Treatment

In mild cases of hereditary hemorrhagic telangiectasia (HHT), no treatment is necessary. In severe cases, estrogen therapy may be useful.

⊟ BIBLIOGRAPHY

1. Klaus-Dieter L, Lanza J, Soriano PA, et al. (2013). Osler-Weber-Rendu Disease. [online] Available from www.emedicine.com/derm/TOPIC782.HTM. [Accessed October, 2013].

21. RETINAL VENOUS OBSTRUCTION

General

Occlusion at the level of either the branch or central retinal venous system, causing a reduction in venous return.

Clinical

None.

Ocular

Painless visual loss, ischemic central retinal vein occlusion, branch retinal vein occlusion.

Laboratory

Fluorescein angiography, OCT for assessment of macular edema.

Treatment

Anticoagulation, surgical adventitial shealthotomy, radial optic neurotomy, intravitreal injection of triamcinolone acetonide for macular edema. Vitrectomy may be necessary.

BIBLIOGRAPHY

1. Campochiaro PA, Hafiz G, Channa R, et al. Antagonism of vascular endothelial growth factor for macular edema caused by retinal vein occlusions: two-year outcomes. Ophthalmology. 2010;117:2387-94.
2. Kooragayala LM. (2012). Central retinal vein occlusion. [online] Available from www.emedicine.com/oph/TOPIC388.HTM. [Accessed October, 2013].
3. Scott IU, Van Velhuisen PC, Oden NL, et al. Baseline predictors of visual acuity and retinal thickness outcomes in patients with retinal vein occlusion: standard care versus corticosteroid for retinal vein occlusion study report 10. Ophthalmology. 2011;118:345-52.

CHAPTER
34

Sclera

1. EPISCLERITIS

General

Benign, recurrent, self-limiting inflammation of the highly vascularized episclera which is closely attached to the underlying sclera and the mobile Tenon's capsule.

Clinical

Episcleritis may be the first sign of a systemic connective tissue disorder.

Ocular

Pain, redness and swelling around the eyes.

Laboratory

Diagnosis is made by clinical findings.

Treatment

Topical prednisolone, artificial tears and cold compresses.

BIBLIOGRAPHY

1. Roy H. (2012). Episcleritis. [online] Available from www.emedicine.com/oph/TOPIC641.HTM. [Accessed October, 2013].
2. de la Maza MS. (2012). Scleritis. [online] Available from www.emedicine.com/oph/TOPIC642.HTM. [Accessed October, 2013].

2. BLUE SCLERA

Blue sclera is characterized by localized or generalized blue coloration of sclera because of thinness and loss of water content, which allow underlying dark choroid to be seen.

A1. Folling syndrome (phenylketonuria)
A2. Hypophosphatasia (phosphoethanolaminuria)
A3. Lowe syndrome (oculocerebrorenal syndrome; chondroitin-4-sulfate-uria)
B1. de Lange syndrome
B2. Brittle cornea syndrome (blue sclera syndrome)-recessive
B3. Crouzon disease (craniofacial dysostosis)
B4. Hallermann-Streiff syndrome (dyscephalia mandibulooculofacial syndrome)
B5. Marfan syndrome (dystrophia mesodermalis congenita)
B6. Marshall-Smith syndrome
B7. Mucopolysaccharidosis VI (Maroteaux-Lamy syndrome)
B8. Osteogenesis imperfecta (van der Hoeve syndrome)
B9. Paget syndrome (osteitis deformans)
B10. Pierre Robin syndrome (micrognathia-glossoptosis syndrome)
B11. Robert Pseudothalidomide syndrome
B12. Werner syndrome (progeria of adults)
C. Turner syndrome
D. Scleral staphyloma

E1. Ehlers-Danlos syndrome (fibrodysplasia elastica generalisata)

E2. Goltz syndrome (focal dermal hypoplasia syndrome)

E3. Incontinentia pigmenti (Bloch-Sulzberger syndrome)

E4. Ota syndrome

E5. Pseudoxanthoma elasticum (Grönblad-Strandberg syndrome)

E6. Relapsing polychondritis

3. Infection- Systemic

    A. Aspergillosis

    B. Candidiasis

    C. Cytomegalovirus retinitis

    D. Diffuse unilateral subacute neuroretinitis syndrome (DUSN, Unilateral wipeout syndrome)

    E. Histoplasmosis

    F. Propionibacterium acnes

    G. Ocular toxoplasmosis

4. Viral infection and metabolic abnormality

    A. Behcet syndrome

    B. Blackwater fever

    C. Familial Mediterranean fever

D. Kussmaul Disease

E. Porphyria cutanea tarda

F. Relapsing polychondritis

G. Rheumatoid arthritis

H. Schaumann syndrome

I. Disseminated lupus erythematosus

J. Takayasu syndrome

K. Temporal arteritis syndrome (Giant cell arteritis)

L. Wegener syndrome

BIBLIOGRAPHY

1. Cameron JA, Cotter JB, Risco JM, et al. Epikeratoplasty for keratoglobus associated with blue sclera. Ophthalmology 1991; 98:446-52.
2. Fraunfelder FT, Randall JA. Minocycline-induced sclera pigmentation. Ophthalmology 1997;104(6):936-8.
3. Khan AO. Blue sclera with or without corneal fragility (Brittle cornea syndrome) in a cansanguineous family harboring ZNF469 mutation Arch Ophthal. 2010; 128: 1376-79.
4. Roy FH. Ocular Syndromes and Systemic Diseases, 5th edition. New Delhi: Jaypee Brothers Medical Publishers (P) Ltd; 2013.

2A1. FOLLING SYNDROME (PHENYLKETONURIA; PHENYLPYRUVIC OLIGOPHRENIA; IKIOTIA PHENYLKETONURIA SYNDROME)

General

Rare; autosomal recessive; phenylalanine cannot be converted to tyrosine; poor prognosis without early diet therapy; both sexes affected.

Ocular

Blue sclera; severe photophobia; corneal opacities; cataracts (controversial); partial ocular albinism; macular atrophy.

Clinical

Phenylketonuria (PKU); oligophrenia; partial albinism; muscle hypertonicity; hyper-reflexia of tendons; epilepsy; microcephaly; mousy odor of habitus; fair skin.

Laboratory

Newborn screening, low-grade elevations of phenylalanine may require repeat screening. More significant elevations may require definitive testing and/or referral to a metabolic treatment facility experienced with PKU.

Treatment

Most patients are treated in a specialty metabolic clinic, usually under the auspices of a genetics or pediatric endocrinology clinic. Treatment consists of dietary restriction of phenylalanine with tyrosine supplementation.

BIBLIOGRAPHY

1. Georgianne L Arnold, Robert D Steiner. (2013). Phenylketonuria. [online] Available from www.emedicine.com/ped/TOPIC1787.HTM. [Accessed October, 2013].

⊟ 2A2. HYPOPHOSPHATASIA (PHOSPHOETHANOLAMINURIA)

General

Inborn error of metabolism that entails increased urinary excretion of phosphoethanolamine (PEA) and associated low alkaline phosphatase and hypercalcemia, prevalent in females, may result from absence or abnormal circulating factor regulating expression of alkaline phosphatase.

Ocular

Papilledema; optic atrophy; exophthalmos; blue sclera; conjunctival calcification; lid retraction; cataract; corneal subepithelial calcifications.

Clinical

Defect in true bone formation associated with widespread skeletal abnormalities; low serum alkaline phosphatase activity; hypercalcemia; nausea; vomiting; bowing of legs; convulsions; premature loss of teeth.

Laboratory

Assess the alkaline phosphatase levels. The levels are low in all types of hypophosphatasia. Fasting laboratory evaluations should include levels of calcium, phosphorus, magnesium, alkaline phosphatase, creatinine, parathyroid hormone (PTH), 25-hydroxy (OH) vitamin D, and 1,25(OH)2 vitamin D. Levels of pyridoxal-5'-phosphate (PLP), inorganic pyrophosphate (PPi), and PEA in serum and urine determine the diagnosis.

Treatment

No medical therapy is available. Supportive care is necessary to decrease the morbidity associated with hypophosphatasia. Regularly examine infants and children to check for evidence of increased intracranial pressure. Observe fractures closely. Adult pseudofractures may require orthopedic care to heal properly. A dentist should closely monitor all individuals with hypophosphatasia.

⊟ BIBLIOGRAPHY

1. Plotkin H, Anadiotis GA. (2012). Hypophosphatasia. [online] Available from www.emedicine.com/ped/TOPIC1126.HTM. [Accessed October, 2013].

⊟ 2A3. LOWE SYNDROME (OCULO-CEREBRO-RENAL SYNDROME)

General

Essential enzyme or protein abnormality is unknown; sex-linked recessive trait (male incidence only); onset in early infancy.

Ocular

Nystagmus; congenital glaucoma; miotic pupils; no pupillary reaction; ectropion uveae; malformation of the anterior chamber angle and of the iris; Schlemm canal may be absent with imperfect angle cleavage; blue sclera; cloudy cornea; cataracts; megalocornea; corneal dystrophy; buphthalmos; microphthalmos; microphakia; mydriasis; strabismus; lens punctate cortical opacities.

Clinical

Mental, psychomotor and growth retardation; aminoaciduria; albuminuria; glycosuria; renal tubular acidosis; rickets; osteomalacia; muscular hypotony; hyporeflexia; hyperactivity with bizarre choreoathetoid movements and screaming.

Laboratory

Urine-aminoaciduria, proteinuria, calciuria, phosphaturia; serum-elevated acid phosphate; imaging studies—brain magnetic resonance imaging (MRI), mild ventriculomegaly (1/3 cases); ocular ultrasound—if dense cataract rule out mass or retinal detachment posterior.

Treatment

Monitor and treat for glaucoma. If glaucoma develops, intraocular pressure (IOP) lowering agents must be used. Often, these patients require surgical intervention with goniotomy, trabeculotomy, or a drainage filtration device. Congenital cataracts should be removed, ideally in the first 6 weeks of life, to optimize the visual potential.

⊟ BIBLIOGRAPHY

1. Alcorn DM. (2012). Oculocerebrorenal syndrome. [online] Available from www.emedicine.com/oph/TOPIC516.HTM. [Accessed October, 2013].

2B1. DE LANGE SYNDROME (I) (CONGENITAL MUSCULAR HYPERTROPHY CEREBRAL SYNDROME; BRACHMANN-DE LANGE SYNDROME)

General

Etiology not known; autosomal recessive inheritance.

Ocular

Antimongoloid slant of palpebral fissures; mild exophthalmos; hypertrichosis of eyebrows; long eyelashes; telecanthus; ptosis; blepharophimosis; nystagmus on lateral gaze; constant coarse nystagmus; strabismus; alternating exotropia; high myopia; anisocoria; chronic conjunctivitis; blue sclera; pallor of optic disk.

Clinical

Mental retardation; growth retardation; extrapyramidal motor disturbances; multiple skeletal abnormalities with congenital muscular hypertrophy; long philtrum; thin lips; crescent-shaped mouth.

Laboratory

Molecular diagnosis with screening of the *NIPBL* gene, X-ray, ultrasonography and echocardiography.

Treatment

Early intervention for feeding problems, hearing and visual impairment, congenital heart disease, urinary system abnormalities and psychomotor delay.

BIBLIOGRAPHY

1. Tekin M, Bodurtha J. (2013). Cornelia De Lange syndrome. [online] Available from www.emedicine.com/ped/TOPIC482.HTM. [Accessed October, 2013].

2B2. BRITTLE CORNEA SYNDROME (BRITTLE CORNEA, BLUE SCLERA AND RED HAIR SYNDROME; BLUE SCLERA SYNDROME)

General

Autosomal recessive; rare.

Ocular

Spontaneous perforation of cornea (brittle cornea); blue sclera; acute hydrops; microcornea; sclerocornea; cornea plana; keratoconus; keratoglobus.

Clinical

Red hair; associated with Ehlers-Danlos syndrome, osteogenesis imperfecta and Marfan syndrome.

Laboratory

Diagnosis is made by clinical findings.

Treatment

Surgical correction of deformities, physiotherapy, and the use of orthotic support and devices to assist mobility were the primary means of treatment for osteogenesis imperfecta. With the more recent understanding of the molecular mechanisms of the disease, medical treatment to increase bone mass and strength are gaining popularity.

BIBLIOGRAPHY

1. Ramachandran M, Achan P, Jones DH, et al. (2012). Osteogenesis imperfecta. [online] Available from www.emedicine.com/orthoped/TOPIC530.HTM. [Accessed October, 2013].

⊟ 2B3. CROUZON SYNDROME (DYSOSTOSIS CRANIOFACIALIS; OXYCEPHALY; CRANIOFACIAL DYSOSTOSIS; PARROT-HEAD SYNDROME; MÖBIUS-CROUZON SYNDROME; HEREDITARY CRANIOFACIAL DYSOSTOSIS)

General

Autosomal dominant; manifestations present at birth.

Ocular

Bilateral exophthalmos; hypertelorism (wide interpupillary distance); obliquity of palpebral fissures with outer canthus slanting downward; nystagmus; exotropia; upper field defects due to pressure upon the optic nerve on its lower part; bluish sclera; exposure keratitis in extreme exophthalmos; cataract; papilledema; secondary optic atrophy; corneal dystrophy; ptosis; strabismus; keratoconus.

Clinical

Prognathism; maxillary hypoplasia with short upper lip; synostosis of coronal and lambda sutures; parrot-beaked nose (psittachosrhina); widening temporal fossae; headaches.

Laboratory

Skull, spine and hand radiography is usually necessary to confirm the diagnosis.

Treatment

Neurosurgical procedure is recommended in cases of intracranial hypertension leading to further optic atrophy.

⊟ BIBLIOGRAPHY

1. Chen H. (2013). Genetics of Crouzon syndrome. [online] Available from www.emedicine.com/ped/TOPIC511.HTM. [Accessed October, 2013].

⊟ 2B4. HALLERMANN-STREIFF SYNDROME [DYSCEPHALIC-MANDIBULO-OCULO-FACIAL SYNDROME; OCULO-MANDIBULO-DYSCEPHALY; ULLRICH-FREMERY-DOHNA SYNDROME; FRANCOIS DYSCEPHALIC SYNDROME; MANDIBULO-OCULO-FACIAL DYSCEPHALY SYNDROME; FRANCOIS-HALLERMANN-STREIFF SYNDROME; HALLERMANN-STREIFF-FRANCOIS SYNDROME; AUDREY I SYNDROME; DOHNA SYNDROME; FRANCOIS SYNDROME (1); DYSCEPHALY- TEETH ABNORMALITY-DWARFISM; DYSCEPHALIA OCULOMANDIBULARIS-HYPOTRICHOSIS; MANDIBULO-OCULAR DYSCEPHALIA HYPOTRICHOSIS; FREMERY-DOHNA SYNDROME; OCULO-MANDIBULO-FACIAL DYSCEPHALY]

General

Rare; familial occurrence and consanguinity; males and females equally affected.

Ocular

Microphthalmos (bilateral); proptosis; nystagmus; strabismus; cataracts; bilateral optic atrophy; coloboma of optic disk, choroid and iris; keratoglobus; microcornea; antimongoloid slant; iris atrophy; uveitis; blue sclera; persistent pupillary membrane; secondary glaucoma.

Clinical

Malformations of skull (brachycephaly), facial skeleton, and jaws; erupted teeth at birth; diminished hair growth; hyperextensibility of joints; short stature; skin atrophy; mental deficiency; predisposition to upper airway compromise; obstructive sleep apnea.

Laboratory

Clinical.

Treatment

- *Cataract*: Change in glasses can sometimes improve a patient's visual function temporarily; however the most common treatment is cataract surgery.
- *Strabismus*: Equalized vision with correct refractive error, surgery may be helpful in patient with diplopia.
- *Uveitis*: Topical steroids and cycloplegic medication should be the initial treatment choice. Oral steroids if not responsive to topical steroids, immunosuppressants if bilateral disease that does not respond to oral steroids, periocular steroids for unilateral or posterior uveitis. Vitrectomy can be used for severe vitreous opacification. Cryotherapy and laser photocoagulation may be used for localized pars plana exudates.
- *Glaucoma*: Glaucoma medication should be the first plan of action. If medication is unsuccessful, a filtering surgical procedure with or without antimetabolites may be beneficial.

⊟ BIBLIOGRAPHY

1. François J, Victoria-Troncoso V. François' dyscephalic syndrome and skin manifestations. Ophthalmologica. 1981;183(2):63-7.
2. Roy FH, Fraunfelder FW, Fraunfelder FT. Roy and Fraunfelder's Current Ocular Therapy, 6th edition. Philadelphia: WB Saunders; 2008.
3. Hallermann W. Vogelgesicht und Cataracta Congenita. Klin Monatsbl Augenheilkd. 1948;113:315.
4. Ronen S, Rozenmann Y, Isaacson M, et al. The early management of baby with Hallermann-Streiff-Francois syndrome. J Pediatr Ophthalmol Strabismus. 1979;16(2): 119-21.
5. Spaepen A, Schrander-Stumpel C, Fryns JP, et al. Hallermann-Streiff syndrome: clinical and psychological findings in children. Nosologic overlap with oculodentodigital dysplasia? Am J Med Genet. 1991;41(4):517-20.
6. Streiff EB. [Mandibulofacial dysmorphia with ocular abnormalities]. Ophthalmologica. 1950;120(1-2):79-83.

⊟ 2B5. MARFAN SYNDROME (DOLICHOSTENOMELIA; ARACHNODACTYLY; HYPERCHONDROPLASIA; DYSTROPHIA MESODERMALIS CONGENITA)

General

Hypoplastic form of dystrophia mesodermalis congenita, autosomal dominant, affects both sexes, has been demonstrated that an abnormality of the gene coding for the connective tissue protein fibrillin is responsible for chronic Marfan syndrome.

Ocular

Exotropia; nystagmus; paralysis of accommodation; myopia (axial or lenticular); iridodonesis; miosis; persistent pupillary membrane; blue sclera; spherophakia; lens dislocation; cataract; megalocornea; retinal detachment (less frequently); pigmentary retinopathy; colobomata of macula, iris, optic nerve and uveal tract (less frequently); keratoconus; central retinal artery occlusion; rhegmatogenous retinal detachment; syringoma.

Clinical

Arachnodactyly; skeletal anomalies; asymmetric thorax; dolichocephaly and high-arched palate; dissecting aneurysm; mitral valve prolapse; prominent ears; kyphoscoliosis; pectus excavatum; flat feet; hammer toes; pulmonary and kidney defects.

Laboratory

Genetic testing, molecular studies.

Treatment

Keratoconus—spectacle correction, hard contacts, avoid eye rubbing. If hydrops occur—discontinue contact lens, use sodium chloride (NaCl) drops and ointment, patching and short course of steroids. As disease advances penetrating keratoplasty, deep anterior lamellar keratoplasty intacs with laser grooves or collagen stabilization of cornea. Cataract—change in glasses can sometimes improve a patient's visual function temporarily; however the most common treatment is cataract surgery. Glaucoma—glaucoma medication should be the first plan of action. If medication is unsuccessful, a filtering surgical procedure with or without antimetabolites may be beneficial. Strabismus—equalized vision with correct refractive error, surgery may be helpful in patient with diplopia.

⊟ BIBLIOGRAPHY

1. Chen H. (2013). Genetics of Marfan syndrome. [online] Available from www.emedicine.com/ped/TOPIC1372. HTM. [Accessed October, 2013].

⊟ 2B6. MARSHALL-SMITH SYNDROME

General

Rare congenital condition with advanced bone age, facial anomalies and relative failure to thrive.

Ocular

Hypertelorism, protuberant eyes with shallow orbits.

Clinical

Feeding and respiratory difficulties; developmental delay; advanced bone age; characteristic facies.

Laboratory

Diagnosis is made by clinical findings.

Treatment

Ocular lubricants.

⊟ BIBLIOGRAPHY

1. Summers DA, Cooper HA, Butler MG. Marshall-Smith syndrome: case report of a newborn male and review of the literature. Clin Dysmorphol. 1999;8(3):207-10.
2. Williams DK, Carlton DR, Green SH, et al. Marshall-Smith syndrome: the expanding phenotype. J Med Genet. 1997;34(10):842-5.
3. Yoder CC, Wiswell T, Cornish JD, et al. Marshall-Smith syndrome: further delineation. South Med J. 1988;81(10): 1297-300.

⊟ 2B7. MAROTEAUX-LAMY SYNDROME (SYSTEMIC MUCOPOLYSACCHARIDOSIS TYPE VI; MPS VI SYNDROME; MUCOPOLYSACCHARIDOSIS VI)

General

Onset in infancy; etiology unknown; autosomal recessive; excessive urinary excretion of chondroitin sulfate B; lysosomal storage disease; deficiency of the enzyme aryl-sulfatase B; multiple clinical phenotypes.

Ocular

Corneal haziness and opacities; pupillary membrane remnants.

Clinical

Skeleton deformities; restriction of articular movements; dyspnea; heart murmur; hearing impairment.

Laboratory

Urine-excessive glycosaminoglycan dermatan sulfate or chondroitin sulfate B.

Treatment

Enzyme replacement, bone marrow transplant and stem cell therapy is in the experimental.

⊟ BIBLIOGRAPHY

1. Kenyon KR, Topping TM, Green WR, et al. Ocular pathology of the Maroteaux-Lamy syndrome. (systemic mucopolysaccharidosis type VI). Histologic and ultrastructural report of two cases. Am J Ophthalmol. 1972;73(5):718-41.
2. Matalon R, Arbogast B, Dorfman A, et al. Deficiency of chondroitin sulfate N-acetylgalactosamine 4-sulfate sulfatase in Maroteaux-Lamy syndrome. Biochem Biophys Res Commun. 1974;61(4):1450-7.
3. Quigley HA, Kenyon KR. Ultrastructural and histochemical studies of a newly recognized form of systemic mucopolysaccharidosis. (Maroteaux-Lamy syndrome, mild phenotype). Am J Ophthalmol. 1974;77(6):809-18.
4. Roy FH, Fraunfelder FW, Fraunfelder FT. Roy and Fraunfelder's Current Ocular Therapy, 6th edition. Philadelphia: WB Saunders; 2008.
5. Voskoboeva E, Isbrandt D, von Figura K, et al. Four novel mutant alleles of the arylsulfatase B gene in two patients with intermediate form of mucopolysaccharidosis VI (Maroteaux-Lamy syndrome). Hum Genet. 1994;93(3):259-64.

⊟ 2B8. OSTEOGENESIS IMPERFECTA CONGENITA, MICROCEPHALY AND CATARACTS

General

Autosomal recessive.

Ocular

Cataracts; blue sclera; keratoconus.

Clinical

Brain abnormally small; multiple prenatal bone fractures; calvaria soft; shortening and bowing of lower limbs.

Laboratory

Diagnosis is made by clinical findings.

Treatment

Spectacle correction, hard contacts and avoid eye rubbing. If hydrops occur—discontinue contact lens, use NaCl drops and ointment, patching and short course of steroids. As disease advances penetrating keratoplasty, deep anterior lamellar keratoplasty intacs with laser grooves or collagen stabilization of cornea. Cataract—Change in glasses can sometimes improve a patient's visual function temporarily; however the most common treatment is cataract surgery.

⊟ BIBLIOGRAPHY

1. Plotkin H. (2012). Genetics of osteogenesis imperfecta. [online] Available from www.emedicine.com/ped/TOPIC1674.HTM. [Accessed October, 2013].

⊟ 2B9. PAGET DISEASE (OSTEITIS DEFORMANS; CONGENITAL HYPERPHOSPHATEMIA; HYPEROSTOSIS CORTICALIS DEFORMANS; POZZI SYNDROME; CHRONIC CONGENITAL IDIOPATHIC HYPERPHOSPHATEMIA; OSTEOCHALASIS DESMALIS FAMILIARIS; FAMILIAL OSTEOECTASIA)

General

Autosomal dominant; more frequent in men, but more severe in women; onset after age 40 years; characterized by diffuse cortical thickening of involved bones with osteoporosis, bowing deformities and shortening of stature; osteogenic sarcoma not infrequent.

Ocular

Shallow orbits with progressive unilateral or bilateral proptosis palsy of extraocular muscles; corneal ring opacities; cataract; retinal hemorrhages; pigmentary retinopathy; macular changes resembling Kuhnt-Junius degeneration; angioid streaks; papilledema; optic nerve atrophy; blue sclera; exophthalmos.

Clinical

Skull deformities; kyphoscoliosis; hypertension and arteriosclerosis; muscle weakness; waddling gait; hearing impairment; osteoarthritis.

Laboratory

Bone-specific alkaline phosphatase (BSAP) levels, radiographs may demonstrate both osteolysis and excessive bone formation. Bone biopsies may be necessary for diagnostic purposes in rare cases.

Treatment

Medical therapy for Paget disease should include bisphosphonate treatment with serial monitoring of bone markers. Nonsteroidal anti-inflammatory drugs (NSAIDs) and acetaminophen may be effective for pain management. Chemotherapy, radiation, or both may be used to treat neoplasms arising from pagetic bone.

⊟ BIBLIOGRAPHY

1. Alikhan MA, Driver K. (2013). Paget disease. [online] Available from www.emedicine.com/med/TOPIC2998.HTM. [Accessed October, 2013].

2B10. PIERRE-ROBIN SYNDROME (ROBIN SYNDROME; MICROGNATHIA-GLOSSOPTOSIS SYNDROME)

General

Etiology unknown; manifestations at birth; pathogenesis based on arrested fetal development; history of intrauterine disturbance in early pregnancy (25% of cases); also increased incidence in offspring of mothers age 35 years or older; pathogenesis is thought to be incomplete development of the first brachial arch, which forms the maxilla and mandible.

Ocular

Microphthalmos; proptosis; ptosis; high myopia; glaucoma; cataract (rare); retinal disinsertion; megalocornea; iris atrophy; blue sclera; esotropia; conjunctivitis; distichiasis; vitreoretinal degeneration; retinal detachments.

Clinical

Micrognathia; cleft palate; glossoptosis; cyanosis; facial expression birdlike with flat base of nose and high-arched deformed palate with or without cleft; difficulty in breathing.

Laboratory

Diagnosis is made by clinical findings.

Treatment

Multidisciplinary approach is required to manage the complex features involved in the care of these children and their families.

BIBLIOGRAPHY

1. Tewfik TL, Trinh N, Teebi AS. (2012). Pierre Robin syndrome. [online] Available from www.emedicine.com/ent/TOPIC150.HTM. [Accessed October, 2013].

2B11. ROBERTS PSEUDOTHALIDOMIDE SYNDROME (GLAUCOMA)

General

Rare autosomal recessive disorder characterized by prenatal and postnatal growth retardation, limb defects and craniofacial anomalies.

Ocular

Cataracts; glaucoma; microcornea; corneal clouding.

Clinical

Patients usually do not survive past 1 month; patients often are mentally retarded.

Laboratory

Diagnosis is made by clinical findings.

Treatment

Cataract—change in glasses can sometimes improve a patient's visual function temporarily; however the most common treatment is cataract surgery. Glaucoma—glaucoma medication should be the first plan of action. If medication is unsuccessful, a filtering surgical procedure with or without antimetabolites may be beneficial.

BIBLIOGRAPHY

1. Holden KR, Jabs EW, Sponseller PD. Roberts/pseudothalidomide syndrome and normal intelligence: approaches to diagnosis and management. Dev Med Child Neurol. 1992;34(6):534-9.
2. Otano L, Matayoshi T, Gadow EC. Roberts syndrome: first-trimester prenatal diagnosis. Prenat Diagn. 1996;16(8):770-1.

🖶 2B12. WERNER SYNDROME (PROGERIA OF ADULTS) BLUE SCLERA

General

Etiology unknown; recessive inheritance; consanguinity; second and third decades; possible mechanisms have been proposed to explain mutation of a gene causing inhibition of deoxyribonucleic acid (DNA) synthesis and early cellular senescence.

Ocular

Absence of eyelashes and scanty eyebrows; blue sclera; juvenile cataracts; bullous keratitis; trophic corneal defects; paramacular retinal degeneration; proptosis; telangiectasia of lid; astigmatism; nystagmus; presbyopia; uveitis.

Clinical

Leanness; short stature (160 cm maximum); thin limbs; short, deformed fingers; small mouth; early baldness; stretched, atrophic skin (scleropoikiloderma); telangiectasia and trophic indolent ulcers on toes, heels and ankles; arteriosclerosis with secondary heart failure.

Laboratory

Fasting blood glucose test, oral glucose tolerance test, triiodothyronine, levothyroxide and throtropin test.

Treatment

No specific treatment exists.

🖶 BIBLIOGRAPHY

1. Janniger CK, Wozniacka A. (2013). Werner syndrome. [online] Available from www.emedicine.com/derm/TOPIC697.HTM. [Accessed October, 2013].

🖶 2C. TURNER SYNDROME (TURNER-ALBRIGHT SYNDROME; GONADAL DYSGENESIS; GENITAL DWARFISM SYNDROME; ULLRICH-TURNER SYNDROME; BONNEVIE-ULLRICH SYNDROME; PTERYGOLYMPHANGIECTASIA SYNDROME; ULLRICH-BONNEVIE SYNDROME) CATARACT, POSTERIOR

General

Ovarian or gonadal agenesis; 45 chromosomes with an XO sex chromosome constitution; females; rare in males; onset in childhood.

Ocular

Exophthalmos; hypertelorism; ptosis; epicanthal folds; blue sclera; corneal nebulae; cataracts; conjunctival lymphedema; keratoconus.

Clinical

Webbed neck (pterygium colli); diminished growth; mandibulofacial disproportion; cubitus valgus; masculine chest and trunk; late appearance of pubic and axillary hair; congenital deafness; mental retardation; coarctation of aorta.

Laboratory

Karyotyping is needed for diagnosis. Y chromosomal test. Luteinizing hormone (LH) and follicle-stimulating hormonc (FSH) levels, thyroid function test, fasting glucose levels, echocardiography and MRI.

Treatment

Growth hormone therapy is used to prevent short stature. Estrogen replacement therapy is usually started by the age of 12–15 years old.

🖶 BIBLIOGRAPHY

1. Daniel MS, Postellon DC. (2013). Turner syndrome. [online] Available from www.emedicine.com/ped/TOPIC2330.HTM. [Accessed October, 2013].

⊟ 2D. SCLERAL STAPHYLOMAS AND DEHISCENCES

General

Staphylomas may be congenital or acquired. They are anterior or posterior.

Clinical

None

Ocular

Posterior staphylomas are associated with myopia greater than 8 diopters as well as Ehler-Danlos and Marfan syndromes, elevated IOP.

Laboratory

Diagnosis is made by clinical findings.

Treatment

Lower IOP with topical agents if elevated, consider pars plana vitrectomy internal drainage with endophotocoagulation and air-gas exchange.

⊟ BIBLIOGRAPHY

1. Roy FH, Fraunfelder FW, Fraunfelder FT. Roy and Fraunfelder's Current Ocular Therapy, 6th edition. Philadelphia: WB Saunders; 2008.

⊟ 2E1. EHLERS-DANLOS SYNDROME (FIBRODYSPLASIA ELASTICA GENERALISATA; CUTIS HYPERELASTICA; MEEKEREN-EHLERS-DANLOS SYNDROME; INDIAN RUBBER MAN SYNDROME; CUTIS LAXA)

General

Present at birth; autosomal dominant; two groups: cutaneous and articular; syndrome is one of three primary disorders of elastic tissue [other two are pseudoxanthoma elasticum (Grönblad-Strandberg syndrome) and senile elastosis]; inherited disorder of collagen biosynthesis.

Ocular

Hyperelasticity of palpebral skin; easy eversion of upper lid; ptosis; epicanthal folds; hypotony of extraocular muscles; strabismus; microcornea; thinning of cornea with keratoconus; thinning of sclera (blue sclera); subluxation of lens; angioid streaks; chorioretinal hemorrhages; retinitis proliferans with secondary detachment; macular degeneration; myopia; ruptured globe after minor trauma; limbus-to-limbus corneal thinning; acute hydrops; cornea plana; keratoglobus.

Clinical

Cutaneous manifestations include thin, atrophic, fragile skin, cutaneous hyperelasticity and pseudomolluscoid tumors; articular manifestations include excessive articular laxity and luxations; hypermobile joints.

Laboratory

Biochemical studies can detect alterations in collagen molecules in cultured skin fibroblasts. Molecular (DNA-based) testing is available. Diagnosis may by urinary analyte assay and clinical examination is the most common.

Treatment

Ascorbic acid therapy, in the event of skin lacerations seriously consider alternatives to sutures, including adhesive strips and wound glues, monitor for cardiac conditions and scolosis.

⊟ BIBLIOGRAPHY

1. Defendi GL. (2013). Genetics of Ehlers-Danlos Syndrome. [online] Available from www.emedicine.com/ped/TOPIC654.HTM. [Accessed October, 2013].

⧉ 2E2. GOLTZ SYNDROME (FOCAL DERMAL HYPOPLASIA SYNDROME)

General

X-linked dominant inheritance; lethal in males; skin manifestations present at birth.

Ocular

Microphthalmia; strabismus; coloboma of iris and/or choroid; epiphora; blue sclera; nystagmus; anophthalmos; keratoconus.

Clinical

Skin atrophy and linear pigmentation; telangiectasias of trunk and extremities; superficial, localized fatty skin deposits; multiple papillomas of mucous membranes and periorificial skin (oral, genital and anal); anomalies of extremities with syndactyly, oligodactyly, adactyly; hypo-hidrosis; paper-thin nails may be present; spina bifida; hypoplasia of right clavicle; umbilical or inguinal hernia.

Laboratory

Radiography may reveal osteopathia striata.

Treatment

Flashlamp-pumped pulsed dye laser may ameliorate the pruritic symptoms that sometimes are noted in affected skin and improve the clinical appearance of the telangiectatic and erythematous skin lesions. Papillomas frequently require repeated surgical intervention.

⧉ BIBLIOGRAPHY

1. Goltz RW, Castelo-Soccio L. (2012). Focal dermal hypoplasia syndrome. [online] Available from www.emedicine.com/derm/TOPIC155.HTM. [Accessed October, 2013].

⧉ 2E3. BLOCH-SULZBERGER SYNDROME (INCONTINENTIA PIGMENTI; SIEMENS-BLOCH-SULZBERGER SYNDROME)

General

Familial disorder affecting ectoderm; manifestations at birth; female predominance; X-linked dominant phenotype; disturbance of skin pigmentation.

Ocular

Orbital mass; retrolental fibroplasia; pseudoglioma; strabismus; blue sclera; cataract; optic nerve atrophy; papillitis; nystagmus; chorioretinitis; anomalies of chamber angle; neovascularization of retina; retinal hemorrhages and edema; microphthalmia; tractional retinal detachment.

Clinical

Dental and skeletal anomalies common; neurologic abnormalities; recurrent inflammatory lesions; skin melanin pigmentation on the trunk: (Marble cake); occipital lobe infarct; neonatal infarction of the macula.

Laboratory

Computed tomography (CT) scan or MRI of brain should be performed.

Treatment

No specific treatment. Lesions should be left intact and kept clean and meticulous dental care is very important.

⧉ BIBLIOGRAPHY

1. Chang CH. (2012). Neurologic manifestations of incontinentia pigmenti. [online] Available from www.emedicine.com/neuro/TOPIC169.HTM. [Accessed October, 2013].

2E4. OTA SYNDROME (NEVUS OF OTA; OCULODERMAL MELANOCYTOSIS; NEVUS FUSCOCERULEUS OPHTHALMOMAXILLARIS SYNDROME)

General

Affects mainly black and Japanese populations; female preponderance (4:1); mode of transmission unknown; most frequently unilateral; pigmentary changes frequently spread during puberty, but no malignant transformation occurs; malignant transformation to melanoma in the uvea and orbit has been reported.

Ocular

Congenital benign periorbital pigmentation of brown, slate to bluish-black coloration, involving area of first and second (rarely third) division of trigeminal nerve; unilateral hyperchromic heterochromia iridis; possible scleral and conjunctival pigmentation; trabeculae heavily pigmented; slate-gray hyperpigmentation of fundus; optic disk pigmentation (occasionally).

Clinical

Pigmentation of temples, nose, forehead and malar region; "Mongolian spot" in sacral area (present at birth but usually disappears after puberty).

Laboratory

Diagnosis is made by clinical findings.

Treatment

Observation.

BIBLIOGRAPHY

1. Lui H, Zhou Y, Zandi S. (2013). Nevi of Ota and Ito. [online] Available from www.emedicine.com/derm/TOPIC290.HTM. [Accessed October, 2013].

2E5. GRÖNBLAD-STRANDBERG SYNDROME (SYSTEMIC ELASTODYSTROPHY; PSEUDOXANTHOMA ELASTICUM; ELASTORRHEXIS; DARIER-GRÖNBLAD-STRANDBERG SYNDROME)

General

Autosomal recessive; female-to-male ratio of 2:1; inheritance is usually autosomal recessive, but it also has reported as autosomal dominant.

Ocular

"Angioid streaks" of the retina; macular hemorrhages and transudates not infrequent; choroidal sclerosis; retinal detachment; keratoconus; cataract; paralysis of extraocular muscles [secondary to vascular lesions of central nervous system (CNS)]; subluxation of lens; exophthalmos; optic atrophy; vitreous hemorrhages; Salmon spot multiple atrophic peripheral retinal pigment epithelium (RPE) lesions; reticular pigment dystrophy of the macula; optic disk drusen; multiple small crystalline bodies associated with atrophic RPE changes.

Clinical

Pseudoxanthoma elasticum with thickening, softening and relaxation of the skin; skin changes are symmetrical in skin folds near large joints (axilla, elbow, inguinal region, lower abdomen and neck); flattening of the pulse curve and peripheral vascular disturbances; gastrointestinal hemorrhages.

Laboratory

Characteristic skin and retinal findings. Fluorescein angiography to detect angioid streaks and choroidal neovascular membranes.

Treatment

Dietary calcium and phosphorus restriction to minimum daily requirement levels has shown arrest in progression of the disease.

BIBLIOGRAPHY

1. Dahl AA, Calonje D, El-Harazi SM. (2012). Ophthalmologic manifestations of pseudoxanthoma elasticum. [online] Available from www.emedicine.com/oph/TOPIC475.HTM. [Accessed October, 2013].

🗗 2E6. RELAPSING POLYCHONDRITIS (JAKSCH-WARTENHOST SYNDROME; MEYEN-BURG-ALTHERZ-VEHLINGER SYNDROME; VON MEYENBERG II SYNDROME)

General

Episodic, yet generally progressive; onset usually in middle life; possibly caused by lysosomal labilizing factor of endogenous or exogenous toxic nature or immunologic reactions; possible association with Reiter syndrome.

Ocular

Conjunctivitis; corneal ulcer; exophthalmos; panophthalmitis; phthisis bulbi; proptosis; optic neuritis; papilledema; retinal detachment; blue sclera; episcleritis; scleromalacia; vitreous opacity; cataracts; nystagmus; retinal artery thrombosis; keratoconjunctivitis sicca; secondary glaucoma; scotoma; uveitis; paresis of third or sixth nerve; conjunctival mass (salmon patch); chorioretinitis.

Clinical

Destruction of cartilage and eventual replacement with connective tissue; polyarthritis; chondritis; tracheal collapse; bronchial collapse; anemia; liver dysfunction; death; malaise; fever; dyspnea; changes in pitch of voice; hearing impairment; vertigo; deformed ears; aortic valve insufficiency.

Laboratory

No specific serologic markers.

Treatment

No therapy.

🗗 BIBLIOGRAPHY

1. Compton N, Buckner JH, Harp KI. (2012). Polychondritis. [online] Available from emedicine.medscape.com/article/331475-overview. [Accessed October, 2013].

🗗 3A. ASPERGILLOSIS

General

Systemic infection common in poultry farmers, feeders or breeders of pigeons, and persons who work with grains; should be considered in immunocompromised patients.

Ocular

Corneal ulcer; blepharitis; keratitis; scleritis; endophthalmitis; exophthalmos; retinal hemorrhages; retinal detachment; vitreitis; cataract; conjunctivitis; orbital cellulitis; paresis of extraocular muscles; secondary glaucoma; scleromalacia perforans; endogenous endophthalmitis; anterior chamber mass; invasion of choroid and anterior optic nerve.

Clinical

Pulmonary infections; invasive fungal disease.

Laboratory

Culture from superficial scrapings from bed of infection.

Treatment

Voriconazole is the drug of choice. Although disease outcomes substantially improve with antifungal treatment, patient survival and infection resolution depend on improved immunosuppression.

🗗 BIBLIOGRAPHY

1. Batra V, Asmar B, Ang JY. (2013). Pediatric aspergillosis. [online] Available from www.emedicine.com/ped/TOPIC148.HTM. [Accessed October, 2013].

3B. CANDIDIASIS

General

Yeastlike opportunistic fungal infection caused by *Candida albicans*.

Ocular

Uveitis; hypopyon; conjunctivitis; keratitis; corneal ulcer; blepharitis; endophthalmitis; dacryocystitis; papillitis; retinal atrophy; Roth spot; vitreous abscess; retrobulbar abscess; retinal detachment; panophthalmitis; chorioretinitis; infectious crystalline keratopathy.

Clinical

C. albicans normally is present as an intestinal saprophyte in 35–75% of the human population; in situations of internal environmental change, however, *Candida* can become pathogenic (obesity, diabetes mellitus, malignancy, and other debilitating conditions).

Laboratory

Common yeast from up to 50% of healthy individuals isolate directly from the eye should be attempted to confirm the presence of organism. Blood agar and Sabouraud's dextrose agar may be used. Polymerase chain reaction (PCR) for species identification.

Treatment

Mucocutaneous infection typically responds to topical therapy. Antifungal therapy should be started immediately after necessary cultures have been obtained from all suspected sites of infection. Infectious disease specialists are typically involved in cases of invasive candidiasis.

BIBLIOGRAPHY

1. Hedayati T, Shafiei G. (2012). Candidiasis in emergency medicine. [online] Available from www.emedicine.com/emerg/TOPIC76.HTM. [Accessed October, 2013].

3C. CYTOMEGALOVIRUS RETINITIS

General

Ubiquitous DNA virus that infects the majority of adults and generally only an issue in immunocompromised individuals such as with acquired immunodeficiency syndrome (AIDS), transplant and those immunosuppressive medications.

Clinical

Acquired immunodeficiency syndrome, transplantation patients; myalgia, cervical lymphadenopathy; hepatitis.

Ocular

Decrease visual acuity; blindness; retinitis; retinal detachment; retinal breaks; necrotic retina.

Laboratory

Laboratory testing to determine the cause; ultrasound to evaluate for retinal detachment; dilated fundus examination.

Treatment

Intravitreal ganciclovir implant or injection may be used; retinal detachment surgery may be necessary.

BIBLIOGRAPHY

1. Altaweel M, Youssef PN, Reed MD. (2012). CMV retinitis. [online] Available from emedicine.medscape.com/article/1227228-overview. [Accessed October, 2013].

3D. DIFFUSE UNILATERAL SUBACUTE NEURORETINITIS SYNDROME (DUSN; UNILATERAL WIPEOUT SYNDROME; WIPEOUT SYNDROME)

General

It is caused by a nematode that is not *Toxocara canis*, i.e. at least two nematodes of different sizes; usually occurs in children or young adults; nematode may remain viable in eye for 3 years or longer.

Ocular

Vitreitis; papillitis; gray-white lesions of retina; optic atrophy; retinal vessel narrowing; diffuse pigment epithelial degeneration; endophthalmitis; nematode in fundus; the pathognomonic finding in diffuse unilateral subacute neuroretinitis (DUSN) syndrome is the presence of a motile intraocular nematode.

Clinical

Weight loss; lack of appetite; cough; fever; pulmonary infiltration; hepatomegaly; leukocytosis; persistent eosinophilia.

Laboratory

Electroretinopathy, enzyme-linked immunosorbent assays for individual nematode species.

Treatment

Direct laser photocoagulation of the nematode is the treatment of choice for DUSN, surgical transvitreal removal of the nematode may be indicated in selected cases.

BIBLIOGRAPHY

1. Kooragayala LM. (2013). Diffuse unilateral subacute neuroretinitis. [online] Available from www.emedicine.com/oph/TOPIC684.HTM. [Accessed October, 2013].

3E. HISTOPLASMOSIS (HISTOPLASMOSIS CHOROIDITIS; HISTOPLASMOSIS MACULOPATHY; PRESUMED OCULAR HISTOPLASMOSIS SYNDROME)

General

Fungal infection caused by *Histoplasma capsulatum*.

Ocular

Circumpapillary atrophy; maculopathy; scattered yellow "histo" spots; optic disk edema; disseminated choroiditis (immunocompromised patients); vitreous hemorrhage; punched-out chorioretinal lesions; choroidal neovascular membrane; exogenous endophthalmitis (isolated report).

Clinical

Pulmonary infection; fever; malaise.

Laboratory

Sixty percent of the adult population from the Ohio and Mississippi river valleys has a positive histoplasmin skin test, therefore clinic course is most helpful.

Treatment

Although the diagnosis is clinical, certain ancillary tests help in confirming it, fluorescein angiography, human leukocyte antigen (HLA) typing B7 and DRw2 may be indicated.

BIBLIOGRAPHY

1. Wu L, Evans T. (2012). Presumed ocular histoplasmosis syndrome. [online] Available from www.emedicine.com/oph/TOPIC406.HTM. [Accessed October, 2013].

3F. PROPIONIBACTERIUM ACNES

General

Gram-positive, pleomorphic, non-spore forming bacillus that is considered part of the normal eyelid and conjunctival anaerobic flora. Pathogenic if introduced intraocular.

Clinical

None.

Ocular

Chronic keratitis, endophthalmitis and vitritis.

Laboratory

Aerobic and anaerobic cultures must be incubated for 14 days. Capsular biopsy may demonstrate Gram-positive, pleomorphic, non-spore forming bacillus or Gram stain.

Treatment

Vancomycin intravitreal or systemic initiate.

BIBLIOGRAPHY

1. Roy FH, Fraunfelder FW, Fraunfelder FT. Roy and Fraunfelder's Current Ocular Therapy, 6th edition. Philadelphia: WB Saunders; 2008.

3G. OCULAR TOXOPLASMOSIS (TOXOPLASMIC RETINOCHOROIDITIS; TOXOPLASMOSIS)

General

Parasite infestation caused by *Toxoplasma gondii*; cell-mediated immunity is believed to be the major defense mechanism against *Toxoplasma* infection; ocular toxoplasmosis occurs in approximately 1% of patients with AIDS; AIDS-related toxoplasma retinochoroiditis may have several atypical clinical manifestations.

Ocular

Keratitis; uveitis; optic atrophy; papillitis; anisocoria; persistent pupillary membrane; focal retinochoroiditis; scleritis; cataract; microphthalmos; myopia; nystagmus; esotropia.

Clinical

Cysts are seen in many organs, including brain and muscle; hydrocephalus; intracerebral calcification; various CNS complaints.

Laboratory

Serologic tests for anti *T. gondii*. Antibodies are common.

Treatment

Triple drug therapy pyrimethamine, sulfadiazine and prednisone. Pyrimethamine should be combined with folinic acid, surgical care including photocoagulation, cryotherapy or vitrectomy.

BIBLIOGRAPHY

1. Wu L, Evans T, GarcÃa RA. (2013). Ophthalmologic manifestations of toxoplasmosis. [online] Available from www.emedicine.com/oph/TOPIC707.HTM. [Accessed October, 2013].
2. Lasave AF, Díaz-Llopis M, Muccioli C, et al. Intravitreal clindamycin and dexamethasone for zone 1 toxoplasmic retinochoroiditis at twenty-four months. Ophthalmology. 2010;117(9):1831-8.

4A. BEHÇET SYNDROME (DERMATO-STOMATO-OPHTHALMIC SYNDROME; OCULOBUCCOGENITAL SYNDROME; GILBERT SYNDROME)

General

Virus infection; occurs in adults; chronic disease; complete remission is rare; etiology is unknown.

Ocular

Muscle palsies (occasional); nystagmus (occasional); conjunctivitis; hypopyon; iritis; recurrent uveitis; keratoconjunctivitis sicca; keratitis; vitreous hemorrhages; thrombophlebitis retinal veins (occasional); retinal hemorrhages; optic neuritis (occasional); macular edema; optic nerve atrophy; retinitis; secondary glaucoma; retinal vasculitis; disk edema; panophthalmitis; optic neuropathy; skin lesions, posterior uveitis and systemic complications have been associated with loss of vision with this disorder; corneal immune ring opacity.

Clinical

Aphthous lesions of mucous membranes of the mouth and genitalia; cerebellar signs; convulsions; paraplegia; skin erythema (multiforme, bullosum); arthritis; urethritis; glossitis; recurrent fever.

Laboratory

None. Specific HLA-B51 positive may help to support diagnosis.

Treatment

The goals of therapy are to suppress inflammation, to reduce the frequency and severity of recurrences, and to minimize involvement of the retina. To be effective, treatment must be started early. Extent of involvement and severity of disease determine the choice of medication. Treatment options include corticosteroids, cytotoxic agents, cyclosporine and colchicine.

BIBLIOGRAPHY

1. Bashour M. (2012). Ophthalmologic manifestations of Behcet disease. [online] Available from www.emedicine.com/oph/TOPIC425.HTM. [Accessed October, 2013].

4B. BLACKWATER FEVER

General

Usually occurs in association with malaria, *Plasmodium falciparum* infection; mortality 20–30%; recurrent hemolytic episodes with subsequent malarial infections.

Ocular

Scleral icterus; cotton-wool spots; retinal edema; optic disk edema; conjunctival calcium deposits; band keratopathy; cortical blindness; epibulbar hemorrhage of conjunctiva, and episclera; retinal hemorrhages.

Clinical

Fever; hemolysis; icterus; hemoglobinuria; malaria; uremia; nausea; vomiting; vertigo; convulsions; coma; acute renal failure; hypertension, azotemia; hypervolemia; metabolic disturbances; hyponatremia; hypercalcemia.

Laboratory

Complete blood count, electrolyte panel, renal function tests, pregnancy test, urinalysis, free serum haptoglobin, urine and blood cultures; thick and thin blood smears are useful.

Treatment

If the patient is experiencing life-threatening complications (coma, respiratory failure, coagulopathy and fulminant kidney failure), then investigate exchange transfusion as a treatment option.

BIBLIOGRAPHY

1. Fernandez MC. (2012). Emergent management of malaria. [online] Available from www.emedicine.com/emerg/TOPIC305.HTM. [Accessed October, 2013].

4C. FAMILIAL MEDITERRANEAN FEVER

General

Recessive inherited polyserositis; progressive, fatal complications are renal failure and amyloidosis.

Ocular

Episcleritis; uveitis; colloid bodies; optic neuritis.

Clinical

Peritonitis; pleuritis; arthritis; fever; skin rash; renal failure; amyloidosis; recurrent attacks of fever and polyserositis of unknown origin.

Laboratory

Synovial fluid is inflammatory, with cell counts high.

Treatment

Colchicine therapy daily is the treatment of choice.

BIBLIOGRAPHY

1. Meyerhoff JO. (2012). Familial mediterranean fever. [online] Available from www.emedicine.com/med/TOPIC1410.HTM. [Accessed October, 2013].

4D. KUSSMAUL DISEASE (KUSSMAUL-MAIER DISEASE; NECROTIZING ANGIITIS; PAN; POLYARTERITIS NODOSA)

General

Progressive process of vascular inflammation and necrosis, manifested by numerous nodules along the course of small-sized and medium-sized arteries; lesions are segmental in distribution, have a predilection for bifurcation and involve all but the pulmonary arteries; arteries in gastrointestinal tract, kidneys and muscles are particularly affected; affects primarily males between ages 20 years and 50 years.

Ocular

Retinal detachment; cotton-wool patches; polyarteritis nodosa (PAN) lesion of arteries; pseudoretinitis pigmentosa; conjunctivitis; corneal ulcer; tenonitis; ptosis; exophthalmos; uveitis; optic atrophy; cataract; scleritis; paralysis of extraocular muscles; neuroretinitis; macular star; peripheral ulcerative keratitis; retinal vasculitis; pseudotumor of the orbit; central retinal artery occlusion.

Clinical

Fever; myalgia; hypertension; gastrointestinal disorders; neuropathy; respiratory infection; weight loss; anginal pain; hemiplegia; convulsion; acute brain syndrome; skin lesions; diffuse erythema; purpura; urticaria; gangrene; tachycardia; pericarditis; aortitis; painful facial swelling; diplopia.

Laboratory

Diagnosis is made by clinical findings.

Treatment

Retinal detachment—scleral buckle, pneumatic retinopexy and vitrectomy may be used to close all the breaks. Corneal ulcer—corneal cultures may be taken and treatment initiated. Treatment includes a broad spectrum of antibiotics and cycloplegic drops. Uveitis—topical steroids and cycloplegic medication should be the initial treatment choice. Oral steroids if not responsive to topical steroids, immunosuppressants if bilateral disease that does not respond to oral steroids, periocular steroids for unilateral or posterior uveitis. Vitrectomy can be used for severe vitreous opacification. Cryotherapy and laser photocoagulation may be used for localized pars plana exudates.

BIBLIOGRAPHY

1. Akova YA, Jabbur NS, Foster CS. Ocular presentation of polyarteritis nodosa. Clinical course and management with steroid and cytotoxic therapy. Ophthalmology. 1993;100:1775-81.
2. Kussmaul A, Maier R. Ueber Eine Bisher Nicht Beschriebene Eigenthumliche Artenener Krankung (Periarteritis Nodosa), die Mit Morbus Brightii und Rapid Fortschreitender Allgemeiner Muskellahumung Einhergeht. Dtsch Arch Klin Med. 1866;1:484-518.
3. Matsuda A, Chin S, Ohashi T. A case of neuroretinitis associated with long-standing polyarteritis nodosa. Ophthalmologica. 1994;208(3):168-71.
4. Roy FH, Fraunfelder FW, Fraunfelder FT. Roy and Fraunfelder's Current Ocular Therapy, 6th edition. Philadelphia: WB Saunders; 2008.
5. Solomon SM. Solomon JH. Bilateral central retinal artery occlusions in polyarteritis nodosa. Ann Ophthalmol. 1978;10:567-69.

4E. PORPHYRIA CUTANEA TARDA

General

Disorder of porphyria metabolism; highest incidence in Bantu population; both sexes affected; onset between ages 40 years and 60 years; insidious onset; autosomal dominant; light-sensitive dermatitis in later adult life; associated with excretion of large amounts of uroporphyrin in urine.

Ocular

Synophrys; keratitis; palsies of third and seventh cranial nerves; scleromalacia perforans; optic atrophy; retinal hemorrhages and cotton-wool spots; macular edema; pinguecula; pterygium; brownish pigmentation in conjunctiva and lid margin.

Clinical

Cutaneous manifestations are solar hypersensitivity, vesiculobullous lesions, ulcerations, severe scarring and hypertrichosis; erythrodontia.

Laboratory

Urinary porphyrin levels are abnormally high, with several hundred to several thousand micrograms excreted in a 24-hour period. Direct immunofluorescence examination can help to differentiate porphyria cutanea tarda (PCT) from immunobullous diseases with dermoepidermal junction cleavage (epidermolysis bullosa acquisita, lupus erythematosus) in which the perivascular immunoglobulin deposition found in PCT is not observed.

Treatment

Sunlight avoidance, therapeutic phlebotomy to reduce iron stores, chelation with desferrioxamine, iron-rich foods should be consumed in moderation.

BIBLIOGRAPHY

1. Poh-Fitzpatrick MB. (2012). Porphyria cutanea tarda. [online] Available from www.emedicine.com/derm/TOPIC344.HTM. [Accessed October, 2013].

4F. RELAPSING POLYCHONDRITIS (JAKSCH WARTENHOST SYNDROME; MEYENBURG-ALTHERZ-VEHLINGER SYNDROME; VON MEYENBERG II SYNDROME)

General

Episodic, yet generally progressive; onset usually in middle life; possibly caused by lysosomal labilizing factor of endogenous or exogenous toxic nature or immunologic reactions; possible association with Reiter syndrome.

Ocular

Conjunctivitis; corneal ulcer; exophthalmos; panophthalmitis; phthisis bulbi; proptosis; optic neuritis; papilledema; retinal detachment; blue sclera; episcleritis; scleromalacia; vitreous opacity; cataracts; nystagmus; retinal artery thrombosis; keratoconjunctivitis sicca; secondary glaucoma; scotoma; uveitis; paresis of third or sixth nerve; conjunctival mass (salmon patch); chorioretinitis.

Clinical

Destruction of cartilage and eventual replacement with connective tissue; polyarthritis; chondritis; tracheal collapse; bronchial collapse; anemia; liver dysfunction; death; malaise; fever; dyspnea; changes in pitch of voice; hearing impairment; vertigo; deformed ears; aortic valve insufficiency.

Laboratory

No specific serologic markers.

Treatment

No therapy.

BIBLIOGRAPHY

1. Compton N, Buckner JH, Harp KI. (2012). Polychondritis. [online] Available from emedicine.medscape.com/article/331475-overview. [Accessed October, 2013].

🗗 4G. RHEUMATOID ARTHRITIS (ADULT)

General

Systemic disease of unknown cause; more common in women (3:1); thought to have a strong autoimmune pathogenesis with positive immunoglobulins M, G and A directed against the fragment, crystallizable (Fc) portion of immunoglobulin G.

Ocular

Sjögren syndrome; episcleritis; scleritis; keratitis; corneal ulcers; corneal perforation; uveitis; motility disorders; dry eyes; posterior scleritis (rare).

Clinical

Synovitis; stiffness; swelling; cartilaginous hypertrophy; joint pain; fibrous ankylosis; malaise; weight loss; vasomotor disturbance.

Laboratory

About 80% are positive for rheumatoid factor but is also found in systemic lupus erythematosus (SLE), Sjögren syndrome, sarcoidosis, hepatitis B and tuberculosis.

Treatment

Nonsteroidal anti-inflammatory drugs, disease-modifying anti-rheumatologic drugs (DMARD's), corticosteroids and immunosuppressant can be used.

🗗 BIBLIOGRAPHY

1. Temprano KK, Smith HR. (2013). Rheumatoid arthritis. [online] Available from www.emedicine.com/emerg/TOPIC48.HTM. [Accessed October, 2013].

🗗 4H. SCHAUMANN SYNDROME (BESNIER-BOECK-SCHAUMANN SYNDROME; BOECK SARCOID; SARCOIDOSIS)

General

Etiology unknown; theories include tuberculosis, hypersensitivity to pine pollen, virus infection; affects blacks most often; chronic course with spontaneous remissions (Heerfordt Syndrome); hilar or paratracheal nodes with erythema nodosum; onset most often in middle and old age; ocular involvement in 20–25% of all cases.

Ocular

Orbital granulomatous mass; bony defects; cutaneous and subcutaneous nodules; myogenic palsy; lacrimal gland adenopathy; decreased tear formation; secondary glaucoma; granulomatous uveitis with iris nodules, cells and flare; mutton fat keratitic precipitates; keratitis sicca; vitreous floaters; band-shaped keratitis; complicated cataract; inflammatory retinal exudates; "candle wax drippings"; optic nerve atrophy; neuritis; eyelid nodules; ocular nerve enlargement (granuloma).

Clinical

Lymphadenopathy; hilar nodes; fatigue; cystic, punched-out or reticulated changes in small bones (mainly hands and feet); muscle wasting; contractures; weakness in legs and arms.

Laboratory

Chest X-ray, CT scan and MRI of the brain.

Treatment

Glucocorticoids is the treatment of choice.

🗗 BIBLIOGRAPHY

1. Sharma GD. (2012). Pediatric sarcoidosis. [online] Available from www.emedicine.com/ped/TOPIC2043.HTM. [Accessed October, 2013].

🔲 4I. DISSEMINATED LUPUS ERYTHEMATOSUS (SYSTEMIC LUPUS ERYTHEMATOSUS; LUPUS ERYTHEMATOSUS; KAPOSI-LIBMAN-SACK SYNDROME, SLE)

General

Possible etiology includes viral infections and genetic predisposition; immunologic abnormalities.

Ocular

Keratitis; keratoconjunctivitis sicca; corneal ulcer; optic nerve atrophy; optic neuritis; papilledema; arteritis; central retinal vein occlusion; retinal detachment; microaneurysm; scleritis; uveitis; ptosis; conjunctivitis; paralysis of third nerve; homonymous hemianopsia; multifocal microinfarcts; mydriasis; nystagmus; proptosis; orbital myositis; pseudoretinitis pigmentosa; photophobia.

Clinical

Polyarthritis; morning stiffness; fever; malaise; fatigue; polyserositis; renal disease; CNS disease; anemia; leukopenia; maculopapular rash in a "butterfly" distribution over malar region; alopecia.

Laboratory

Antibodies to double-stranded DNA or the SM antigen or a false-positive serology test for syphilis; positive antinuclear antibody test that is caused by a medication.

Treatment

Fever, rash, musculoskeletal and serositis manifestations respond to hydroxychloroquine and NSAIDs. Low-to-moderate–dose steroids are necessary for acute flares. CNS involvement and renal disease constitute more serious disease and often require high-dose steroids and other immunosuppression agents. Diffuse proliferative lupus nephritis has been treated with cyclophosphamide induction therapy.

🔲 BIBLIOGRAPHY

1. Bartels CM, Muller D. (2013). Systemic lupus erythematosus (SLE). [online] Available from www.emedicine.com/med/TOPIC2228.HTM. [Accessed October, 2013].

🔲 4J. TAKAYASU SYNDROME (MARTORELL SYNDROME; AORTIC ARCH SYNDROME; PULSELESS DISEASE; REVERSED COARCTATION SYNDROME)

General

Two types are occlusive inflammatory lesion (seen in young Japanese women) and occlusive vascular disease without inflammation, associated with atherosclerosis and syphilis; onset in fifth and sixth decades; both sexes affected; can involve the aorta and its major branches as well as the coronary, hepatic, mesenteric, pulmonary and renal arteries.

Ocular

Iris atrophy; cataracts; retinal microaneurysms; sausage-shaped venous dilations; reduced central retinal artery pressure; optic atrophy; cotton-wool spots; anterior segment ischemia; retinal arteriovenous shunts.

Clinical

Diminished or absent pulsation of arteries (head, neck and upper limbs); orthostatic syncope; facial atrophy; epileptiform seizures; intermittent claudication.

Laboratory

Arteriography, magnetic resonance angiography (MRA), MRI, CT scan, Gallium-67 radionuclide scan or chest radiography.

Treatment

Corticosteroids, methotrexate or intravenous cyclophosphamide can be used in patients with glucocorticoid resistant triamcinolone acetonide (TA).

🔲 BIBLIOGRAPHY

1. Hom C. (2013). Pediatric takayasu arteritis. [online] Available from www.emedicine.com/ped/TOPIC1956.HTM. [Accessed October, 2013].

🗗 4K. TEMPORAL ARTERITIS SYNDROME (CRANIAL ARTERITIS SYNDROME; GIANT CELL ARTERITIS; HUTCHINSON-HORTON-MAGATH-BROWN SYNDROME)

General

Etiology unknown; mainly females; mainly whites; ages 55–80 years; temporal artery shows inflammatory thickening; arteritis of the vessels supplying the optic nerve.

Ocular

Transient ptosis; partial or complete loss of vision on the affected side; retinal detachment; exudates and hemorrhages; narrowing of retinal vessels; obstruction of the central retinal artery; optic atrophy; ischemic optic neuropathy; acute decreased IOP; corneal hypesthesia; palsies of extraocular muscles; hemorrhagic glaucoma; diplopia; hemorrhages on or around the disk.

Clinical

Throbbing headache; hyperalgesia of the scalp; malaise; anorexia; weakness; weight loss; fever; nodular pulmonary nodules; cough; otitis with deafness.

Laboratory

Elevated erythrocyte sedimentation rate (ESR) greater than 50 mm/hr, positive temporal artery biopsy.

Treatment

Systemic corticosteroid is the therapy of choice.

🗗 BIBLIOGRAPHY

1. Walvick MD, Walvick MP. Giant cell arteritis: laboratory predictors of a positive temporal artery biopsy. Ophthalmology. 2011;118(6):1201-4.
2. Allen AW, Biega T, Varma MK. (2012). Temporal arteritis imaging. [online] Available from www.emedicine.com/radio/TOPIC675.HTM. [Accessed October, 2013].

🗗 4L. WEGENER SYNDROME (WEGENER GRANULOMATOSIS)

General

Etiology unknown; occurs in the fourth and fifth decades of life; persistent rhinitis or sinusitis; three characteristic features are: (1) necrotizing granulomatous lesions in the respiratory tract, (2) generalized focal arthritis and (3) necrotizing thrombotic glomerulitis.

Ocular

Exophthalmos; lid and conjunctival chemosis; papillitis; conjunctivitis; corneal ulcer; corneal abscess; optic atrophy; optic neuritis; orbital cellulitis; episcleritis; sclerokeratitis; cataract; peripheral ring corneal ulcers; ptosis; dacryocystitis; retinal periphlebitis; cotton-wool spots; retinal and vitreous hemorrhages; rubeosis iridis; neovascular glaucoma.

Clinical

Severe sinusitis; pulmonary inflammation; arteritis; weakness; fever; weight loss; bony destruction; granulomatous vasculitis of the upper and lower respiratory tracts; glomer-ulonephritis; diffuse pulmonary infiltrates; lymphadenopathy; diffuse pulmonary hemorrhage; overlap with giant cell arteritis.

Laboratory

Histopathology: Necrotizing, granulomatous vasculitis with infiltrating neutrophils, lymphocytes and giant cells; urine-proteinuria, hematuria and urinary casts.

Treatment

Topical eye lubricants, ophthalmic antibiotic solution or ointment and corticosteroid drops may prove to be beneficial. Orbital decompression needed when medical treatment is unresponsive to treat optic nerve compression.

🗗 BIBLIOGRAPHY

1. Collins JF. Handbook of Clinical Ophthalmology. New York: Masson; 1982.
2. Flach AJ. Ocular manifestations of Wegener's granulomatosis. JAMA. 1995;274(15):1199-200.

CHAPTER
35

Vitreous

🗗 1. ANTERIOR VITREOUS DETACHMENT

General

Vitreous cortex is separated from the posterior lens or zonular fibers; usually caused by vitreous shrinkage.

Ocular

Vitreous floaters, peripheral flashes of light.

Laboratory

Diagnosis is made by clinical findings.

Treatment

No treatment is necessary unless the detachment causes a retinal detachment or macular hole. It is important to be followed by an ophthalmologist so that if complications occur they can be treated promptly.

🗗 BIBLIOGRAPHY

1. Tolentino FI, Schepens CL, Freeman HM. Vitreoretinal Disorders: Diagnosis and Management. Philadelphia, USA: WB Saunders; 1976.

🗗 2. FAMILIAL EXUDATIVE VITREORETINOPATHY

General

Hereditary abnormality characterized by abnormal vascularization of the peripheral retina, which may appear similar to retinopathy of prematurity.

Clinical

Norrie disease gene mutation.

Laboratory

Fluorescein angiography, especially temporal periphery.

Treatment

Ablation of the peripheral avascular zone, sclera buckling, vitrectomy or both.

🗗 BIBLIOGRAPHY

1. Roy FH, Fraunfelder FW, Fraunfelder FT. Roy and Fraunfelder's Current Ocular Therapy, 6th edition. Philadelphia, USA: WB Saunders; 2008.

3. VITREOUS HEMORRHAGE

General

Hemorrhage into vitreous.

Clinical

Reduced vision secondary to bleeding in vitreous.

Ocular

Retinal vascular with proliferation or nonproliferation of retinal vessels, traction on retinal vessel, trauma, uveal tract.

Laboratory

Identify the cause with complete blood count (CBC), sickle cell prep, fasting blood sugar (FBS), clotting time, B-scan ultrasonography.

Treatment

- *Prophylaxis*: Treat the underlying pathology
- *Vitreous surgery*: Vitrectomy for nonclearing

BIBLIOGRAPHY

1. Phillpotts BA, Blair NP, Gieser JP. (2013). Vitreous hemorrhage. [online] Available from www.emedicine.com/oph/TOPIC421.HTM. [Accessed October, 2013].

4. HYDATID CYST (ECHINOCOCCOSIS)

General

It is caused by *Echinococcus granulosus* acquired by contact with a dog host.

Ocular

Conjunctivitis; keratitis; exophthalmos; phthisis bulbi; optic atrophy; optic neuritis; papilledema; abscesses of orbit and cornea; retinal detachment; retinal hemorrhages; cataract; hypopyon; secondary glaucoma; hydatid cysts of the conjunctiva, eyelid, orbit and lacrimal system; acute visual loss; vitreous mass.

Clinical

Pruritus; urticaria; pulmonary cysts; brain cysts; anaphylactic shock; death.

Laboratory

Plain orbital radiographs may show enlarged orbital diameters and increased soft-tissue density. Ultrasonography demonstrates a cystic lesion without internal reflectivity computed tomography (CT) discloses a well-defined cystic mass.

Treatment

Echinococcosis is rare and can be severe. Refer patients to reference centers to confirm their diagnosis and to obtain advice on therapeutic strategy.

BIBLIOGRAPHY

1. Vuitton DA. (2011). Echinococcosis. [online] Available from www.emedicine.com/med/TOPIC326.HTM. [Accessed October, 2013].

5. INTRAOCULAR FOREIGN BODY: COPPER

General

Injury with copper foreign body; ocular response results from the chemistry of the copper ion and the eye.

Clinical

None.

Ocular

Endophthalmitis, recurrent nongranulomatous inflammation, fibrous encapsulation.

Laboratory

Computed tomography to localize the foreign body, B-scan ultrasonography, radiographic spectrometry to define the presence of intraocular copper ions.

Treatment

Antibiotics to prevent endophthalmitis; oral prednisone to reduce intraocular inflammation; repair of laceration; vitrectomy may be needed.

⊟ BIBLIOGRAPHY

1. Kuhn F, Wong DT, Giavedoni L. (2013). Intraocular foreign body. [online] Available from www.emedicine.com/oph/ TOPIC648.HTM. [Accessed October, 2013].

⊟ 6. INTRAOCULAR FOREIGN BODY: NONMAGNETIC CHEMICALLY INERT

General

Intraocular foreign bodies that are nonmagnetic and chemically inert.

Clinical

None.

Ocular

Endophthalmitis, ocular laceration.

Laboratory

Computed tomography to localize foreign body and B-scan ultrasonography.

Treatment

Topical antibiotics are recommended. Topical steroid may be useful with traumatic uveitis. Repair of ocular laceration; vitrectomy may be needed.

⊟ BIBLIOGRAPHY

1. Ferenc Kuhn, Wong DT, Giavedoni L. (2013). Intraocular foreign body. [online] Available from www.emedicine. com/oph/TOPIC648.HTM. [Accessed October, 2013].

⊟ 7. INTRAOCULAR FOREIGN BODY: STEEL OR IRON

General

Intraocular foreign body of either steel or iron; foreign bodies are the major cause of ocular trauma legal blindness.

Clinical

None.

Ocular

Subconjunctival hemorrhage or edema, iris defect, lens disruption, retinal hemorrhage, inflammation or edema, endophthalmitis.

Laboratory

Computed tomography to define and localize the foreign body and B-scan ultrasonography; magnetic resonance imaging (MRI) is contraindicated because it may shift the position of the foreign body.

Treatment

Antibiotics via intravenous (IV) are recommended to prevent endophthalmitis, intravitreal antibiotics, repair of laceration and other ocular injury. Vitrectomy may be needed.

⊟ BIBLIOGRAPHY

1. Ferenc Kuhn, Wong DT, Giavedoni L. (2013). Intraocular foreign body. [online] Available from www.emedicine. com/oph/TOPIC648.HTM. [Accessed October, 2013].

8. PERSISTENT FETAL VASCULATURE

General

Spectrum of conditions caused by failure of apoptosis of the primary hyaloidal vasculature system, incomplete ocular neurovascular development.

Ocular

Amblyopia, persistent hyaloid stalk; persistent hyperplastic primary vitreous (PHPV); cataract; progressive retinal detachment; vitreous hemorrhage; ciliary body detachment; decreased visual acuity.

Laboratory

Diagnosis is based on clinical findings.

Treatment

Surgical procedure may be necessary to eliminate media opacities and relieve tractional forces.

BIBLIOGRAPHY

1. Sisk RA, Berrocal AM, Feuer WJ, et al. Visual and anatomic outcomes with or without surgery in persistent fetal vasculature. Ophthalmology. 2010;117(11):2178-83.e1-2.

9. PERSISTENT HYPERPLASTIC PRIMARY VITREOUS (PHPV, PERSISTENT FETAL VASCULATURE)

General

Congenital ocular disorder with the potential to affect the eye's anterior and posterior anatomy. Usually, it only affects one eye.

Clinical

Systemic abnormalities may include polydactyly, microcephaly and cleft palate and lip as well as central nervous system abnormalities.

Ocular

Anterior PHPV includes engorged radial iris vessels, microcornea, Mittendorf's dot, elongated ciliary processes, microphthalmia and cataract.

Laboratory

Diagnosis is made by clinical findings.

Treatment

Monocular congenital cataract surgery and amblyopia therapy; posterior transciliary for pars plana vitrectomy and removal of tissue.

BIBLIOGRAPHY

1. Roy FH, Fraunfelder FW, Fraunfelder FT. Roy and Fraunfelder's Current Ocular Therapy, 6th edition. Philadelphia, USA: WB Saunders; 2008.

10. PROLIFERATIVE VITREORETINOPATHY (PVR)

General

Repair process with full or partial thickness retinal breaks, retinopexy or other types of retinal damage.

Ocular

Multiple starfolds and fixed retinal folds.

Clinical

None.

Laboratory

Diagnosis is made by clinical findings.

Treatment

Encircling buckle, gas injection, vitreous surgery and peeling epiretinal membrane.

BIBLIOGRAPHY

1. Roy FH, Fraunfelder FT, Fraunfelder FW. Roy and Fraunfelder's Current Ocular Therapy, 6th edition. Philadelphia, USA: WB Saunders; 2008.

🖻 11. RETINAL VASCULAR HYPOPLASIA WITH PERSISTENCE OF PRIMARY VITREOUS

General

Bilateral congenital retinopathy is characterized by retinal vascular hypoplasia and persistence of primary vitreous; etiology is unknown.

Ocular

Buphthalmos; microphthalmia; fixed and dilated pupils; neovascularization of iris; glaucoma; cataract; white opaque fibrovascular retrolental membrane; retinal detachment; vitreous hemorrhage; retinal vascular hypoplasia.

Clinical

None.

Laboratory

Diagnosis is made by clinical findings.

Treatment

- *Cataract*: Change in glasses can sometimes improve a patient's visual function temporarily; however, the most common treatment is cataract surgery.
- *Retinal detachment*: Scleral buckle, pneumatic retinopexy and vitrectomy may be used to close all the breaks.

🖻 BIBLIOGRAPHY

1. Ryan SJ, Ogden TE (Eds). Retina, 2nd edition. St Louis, USA: Mosby, 1994.
2. Pollard JF. Treatment of persistent hypoplastic primary vitreous. J Pediatr Ophthalmol Strabismus. 1985;22(5):180-3.

🖻 12. VITREOUS WICK SYNDROME

General

Vitreous incarcerated in corneal or corneoscleral wound.

Clinical

None.

Ocular

Anterior chamber cells and flare, hypopyon, strands of vitreous in anterior chamber, distorted pupil, cystoid macular edema, retinal tears, retinal detachment.

Laboratory

Fluorescein angiography.

Treatment

Topical steroids for 2 weeks, followed by nonsteroid drops, if no improvement sub-Tenon's injection of steroids; surgical sponge vitrectomy at time of initial surgery.

🖻 BIBLIOGRAPHY

1. Roque MR, Roque BL, Foster CS. (2013). Vitreous wick syndrome. [online] Available from http://www.emedicine.com/oph/TOPIC649.HTM. [Accessed October, 2013].

Index

11Q syndrome 473, 781, 1018
13Q
    deletion syndrome 782
    syndrome 677, 782, 1018
18Q
    deletion syndrome 474, 681, 782, 1018
    syndrome 474, 681, 782, 1018
21Q deletion syndrome 799
4Q
    deletion syndrome 683
    syndrome 683, 781

A

Aarskog
    syndrome 423
    Scott syndrome 739
Abdominal typhus 27, 141, 576, 831
Abducens
    facial hemiplegia alternans 501, 525, 702
    palsy 497
Aberfeld syndrome 436, 638, 681
Abetalipoproteinemia 194, 601, 672, 743
Abnormal irides 960, 1063
Absent-digits-cranial-defects
        syndrome 402, 741
Acanthamoeba 29, 141, 149
Acanthocytosis 194, 601, 672, 743, 1138
Accessory punctum 1046, 1052
Accommodative
    esotropia 525
    spasm 267
Achondroplastic dwarfism 653, 691
Acid burns 114
    of eye 333, 362
Acinetobacter 342, 345
    iwoffi 342
ACL syndrome 467
Acne
    erythematosa 55, 305, 480, 898
    rosacea 55, 305, 480, 898
Acoustic neuroma syndrome 80, 505, 586
Acquired
    cellular immunodeficiency 11, 141, 234,
        248, 580, 629, 940
    exotropia 557
    immunodeficiency 1, 141, 234, 248, 580,
        629, 940

syndrome 1, 141, 234, 248, 580, 629,
        940
Lues 25, 232, 241, 253, 275, 315, 512, 547,
        592, 598, 619, 707, 713, 715, 740,
        836, 837, 861, 908, 935, 977
    nonaccommodative esotropia 526
    retinoschisis 1139
    syphilis 25, 232, 241, 253, 275, 315, 512,
        547, 592, 598, 619, 704, 707, 713,
        715, 836, 837, 861, 908, 935, 977
Acrocephalopolysyndactyly 437, 674
Acrocephalosyndactylism syndrome 402,
        741
Acrocraniodysphalangia 402, 741
Acrodermatitis enteropathica 663
Acrodysplasia 402, 741
Acropachyderma 813
Acroreno-ocular syndrome 739, 979, 998
Actinic
    keratosis 93
    seborrheic keratosis 295, 946
Actinomycosis 150, 336, 372, 456, 879, 915
Acute
    chorea 930
    Epstein-Barr virus 12, 238, 807
    febrile polyneuritis 579, 611, 657, 701,
        833
    follicular conjunctivitis 18, 278, 882
    hemorrhagic conjunctivitis 2, 278
    histiocytosis X 160, 484
    idiopathic polyneuritis 579, 611, 657,
        701, 833
    infectious neuritis 579, 611, 657, 701, 833
    meibonitis 943
    mucopurulent conjunctivitis 279
    onset of extraocular muscle palsy 567
    ophthalmoplegia 567
    orbital compartment syndrome 1104
    polyradiculitis 579, 611, 657, 701, 833
    posterior multifocal placoid pigment
        epitheliopathy 1121
    retinal necrosis syndrome 1121
Addison pernicious anemia syndrome 225,
        610
Adenoviral conjunctivitis 18, 278, 882
Adrenal cortex neuroblastoma 102
Adult
    blepharitis 941
    cataracts 1040, 1055

Agenesis of macula 1081, 1088
Age-related macular degeneration 1079
Aicardi syndrome 204, 771, 998
Alacrima 325, 740, 1045
Alagille
    syndrome 379, 401
    Watson syndrome 379, 401
Aland disease 791
Albers-Schonberg disease 553, 740, 866
Albinism 1028
Albright hereditary osteodystrophy 1069
Alcoholism 544
Alkaline injury of eye 114, 143, 305, 334, 362,
        898
Allergic
    conjunctivitis 285, 377, 491
    rhinoconjunctivitis 285
Alopecia 1095
Alport syndrome 379
Alström
    disease 1056, 1136
    Olsen syndrome 409
Alternating oculomotor paralysis 92, 535,
        557, 700, 848
Alveolar capillary block syndrome 60
Amalric-Dialinas syndrome 1083
Amaurosis congenital 409
Amblyopia 71, 100, 454
Amebiasis 150, 536, 849
Amebic dysentery 150, 536, 849
Amendola syndrome 658, 669
Amino diabetes 39, 794
Aminopterin-induced syndrome 671
Amish oculocerebral syndrome 85, 793
Amniogenic band syndrome 641, 786
Amyloidosis 57, 600, 741, 822, 924
    of gingiva and conjunctiva 58, 286
Anaphylactoid purpura 135, 180
Andersen-Warburg syndrome 72, 172, 188,
        271, 790, 1034
Andogsky syndrome 1056
Anemia 187
Aneurysm of internal carotid artery
        syndrome 49, 504, 551, 601, 864, 1104
Angelucci syndrome 286, 888
Angiohyalitis 231, 259
Angioid streaks 193

Bietti
    disease 393
    marginal crystalline dystrophy 393
Bilateral
    acute retinal necrosis 1121
    choroidal folds 256, 1093
    complete ophthalmoplegia 586
    facial agenesis 645, 649, 779, 971, 1015
    palsy of ocular muscles 586
Birdshot retinopathy 235, 1123
Bitot spots 288
Blackwater fever 1123, 1167
Blastomycosis 4, 659
Blatt syndrome 795, 1105
Blepharitis 941
Blepharochalasis 639, 822, 871
Blepharoconjunctivitis 291, 304, 897
Blepharophimosis 692
    syndrome 639, 655, 673, 744
Blepharoptosis 640
Blepharospasm-oromandibular dystonia 653, 811
Bloch-Sulzberger syndrome 95, 208, 270, 772, 1161
Blocked nystagmus syndrome 561
Blowout fracture 570, 593, 1110
Blue
    diaper syndrome 386, 680
    nevus 199, 316
    sclera 419, 1051, 1150, 1153, 1159
        syndrome 419, 1153
Boeck sarcoid 63, 232, 240, 244, 275, 302, 384, 524, 556, 582, 870, 895, 976, 1170
Bonnet-Dechaume-Blanc syndrome 75, 744
Bonnevie-Ullrich syndrome 217, 673, 694, 745, 1016, 1159
Botulism 539, 582, 699, 823, 850, 870, 1099
Bourneville
    Pringle syndrome 202, 210, 376, 391, 780
    syndrome 202, 210, 376, 381, 391, 780
Boutonneuse fever 14, 1090
Bowen disease 376
Brachmann-De Lange syndrome 80, 752, 1153
Brachymorphy with spherophakia 67
Brailsford-Morquio dystrophy 43, 461, 760, 809
Branch retinal artery occlusion 1033, 1144
Branched-chain ketoaciduria 759
Branchial clefts 1053
Brandt syndrome 663
Bremer status dysraphicus 514, 555, 596, 702, 715, 816, 837, 869, 937
Brittle
    bone disease 404, 428
    cornea 419, 1153
        syndrome 419, 1153

Broad-thumbs syndrome 215
Bronchiectasis-dextrocardia-sinusitis 208, 774, 1006
Brown
    Marie
        ataxic syndrome 595
        syndrome 595
    oculocutaneous albinism 1028, 1122
    syndrome 559, 745, 823, 927
Brucellosis 4, 513
Brugsch syndrome 813
Bruns syndrome 533, 846
Bull's eye maculopathy 1125
Bullous
    ichthyosiform erythroderma 52, 310, 312, 388, 657, 903, 905
    keratopathy 482, 492
Buphthalmos 650
Burkitt lymphoma 106, 179, 294, 297, 387, 1115
Burnett syndrome 387

C

Calcinosis universalis 675, 792
Camurati-Engelmann disease 521, 753
Canalicular stenosis 1046, 1052
Cancer-associated retinopathy syndrome 1124
Candidiasis 5, 142, 152, 236, 283, 360, 372, 875, 915, 1164
Canine tooth syndrome 559
Capillary angioma 197
    thrombocytopenia 104, 226
Caprolalia generalized tic 418
Capsular exfoliation syndrome 1038
CAR syndrome 1124
Carbamyl phosphate synthetase deficiency 766
Carcinoma in situ 376
Carotid
    artery syndrome 48, 49, 170, 548, 549, 863, 1032, 1105, 1109, 1144
    vascular insufficiency syndrome 49, 1144
Carpal Tunnel syndrome 796, 970
Carpenter syndrome 437, 674, 746
Cat's-eye syndrome 205, 674, 786
Cataract 76, 217, 419, 420, 437, 468, 562, 673, 694, 745, 777, 1016, 1017, 1056-1062, 1070, 1075, 1136, 1159
    congenital ichthyosis 1057
    syndrome 1064
Cat-cry syndrome 96, 679, 750
Catscratch
    disease 5, 236, 347, 532, 590, 885, 1050
    oculoglandular syndrome 5, 236, 347, 532, 590, 885, 1050

Cavernous sinus 517, 841
    fistula syndrome 48, 107, 548, 549, 863, 1032, 1105, 1109
    nasopharyngeal tumor syndrome 627, 720, 862, 865, 1106, 1110
    neuralgia syndrome 517, 627, 720, 841, 862, 865, 1106, 1110
    syndrome 517, 627, 720, 841, 862, 865, 1106, 1110
    thrombosis 517, 627, 720, 841, 862, 865, 1106, 1110
Central
    cloudy dystrophy 397
    retinal pigment epithelial dystrophy 1091
    serous chorioretinopathy 203, 1080, 1088, 1126
    sterile corneal ulceration 457
Cerebellar
    ataxia 71, 75, 76, 593, 988, 1062
        syndrome 847
    degeneration with slow movements 76
    peduncle syndrome 92, 535, 557, 700, 848
Cerebellomedullary malformation
    syndrome 72, 502, 617, 712, 835
Cerebellopontine angle syndrome 80, 505, 586
Cerebelloretinal hemangioblastomatosis 69, 1143
Cerebral
    autosomal dominant arteriopathy 76
    cholesterolosis 77
    gigantism 88
    palsy 77, 746
Cerebrohepatorenal syndrome 675, 815
    of Zellweger 780
Cerebromacular dystrophy 73, 1080
Cerebro-ocular dysplasia-muscular
    dystrophy 217, 777, 1017
Cerebro-oculo-facio-skeletal syndrome 464, 650, 792
Cerebroretinal
    arteriovenous aneurysm syndrome 75, 744
    degeneration 73, 1080
Cerebroside lipidosis 499
Cerebrotendinous xanthomatosis 77
Ceroid lipofuscinosis 1124
Cervical sympathetic paralysis syndrome 819, 826, 834, 937, 1119
Cervicooculoacousticus syndrome 981
Cervicooculofacial
    dysmorphia 981
    syndrome 981
Cestan
    Chenais syndrome 824
    syndrome 515

Chalazion 941
Chandler syndrome 405, 952
Charlin syndrome 996
Chauffard-Still syndrome 59, 390
Chickenpox 28, 243, 505, 537, 574, 807, 843, 850
Chikungunya fever 996
Child abuse syndrome 122, 177
Chlamydia 12, 306, 328, 485, 883, 887, 899
Chloroquine 1125
Cholestasis with peripheral pulmonary stenosis 379
Cholesterolosis of anterior chamber 126
Chondrodysplasia punctata 675, 792
Chondrodystrophia
    foetalis hypoplastica 675, 792
    tarda 43, 461, 760, 809
Chondrodystrophicus congenita 500, 508
Chondroectodermal dysplasia 773, 1001
Chondro-osteodystrophy 43, 461, 760, 809
Chorea 930
Chorioretinitis 448, 804
Choroid 193
    coloboma 203
Choroidal
    atrophy 266
    detachment 200, 218, 222
    folds 218
    hemorrhage 223
    melanoma 171, 219, 258, 273, 277, 293, 920, 947
    ruptures 229
    sclerosis 229
Choroideremia 229
Choroiditis 230, 243
Choroidoretinal
    degeneration 255, 1081
    dystrophy 255, 1125
Christ-Siemens-Touraine syndrome 656, 666, 992
Chromosome
    11 long-arm deletion syndrome 747
    13Q partial deletion syndrome 1018
    18 partial deletion syndrome 437, 676, 747, 748, 1001
    4 partial deletion syndrome 677, 1017
Chronic
    angle closure glaucoma 269, 956
    cicatricial conjunctivitis 288, 303, 312, 318, 894, 899, 906
    congenital idiopathic hyperphos-phatemia 195, 200, 227, 387, 1157
    cyclitis 231, 259
    follicular conjunctivits 295
    hereditary
        edema 653, 811
        lymphedema 653, 811
        trophedema 653, 811

mucopurulent conjunctivitis 297
ophthalmoplegia 594
progressive external ophthalmoplegia 78, 598, 602
renal tubular insufficiency syndrome 1069
serpiginous ulcer of cornea 478
trophedema 653, 811
uveitis 126
Cicatricial
    conjunctivitis 299
    pemphigoid 288, 299, 303, 312, 318, 894, 899, 906
Ciliary
    block glaucoma 953, 958
    body 267
        concussions and lacerations 115, 267
        detachment 268
        melanoma 171, 219, 258, 273, 277, 293, 920, 947
    neuralgia 88, 520, 719, 720, 828, 842, 984
Ciliochoroidal detachment 200, 218
Circumscribed scleroderma 62
Cirsoid aneurysm 263, 549, 819, 863
Claude
    Bernard-Horner syndrome 826, 834, 819, 937, 1119
    syndrome 78, 533, 847
Cleft lip/palate 1053
Clefting syndrome 392, 1143
Clinical anophthalmos 965
Clostridium perfringens 130, 345
Cloudy central corneal dystrophy 397
Cloverleaf skull syndrome 500, 508
Cluster headache 88, 520, 719, 720, 828, 842, 984
Coats disease 97, 171, 1126
Coccidioidomycosis 6, 152, 238, 265, 506
Cockayne syndrome 458, 755
Cod-MD syndrome 217, 777, 1017
Coenurosis 30, 153
COFS syndrome 464, 650, 792
Cogan
    Guerry syndrome 395
    Reese syndrome 405, 952
    syndrome 59, 479, 491, 527
Cole-Rauschkolb-Toomey syndrome 663
Collodion baby 52, 310, 312, 388, 659, 903, 905
Coloboma 206, 640, 703, 787, 1000
    of iris 997
    of macula 1081, 1082, 1088
Colobomatous, microphthalmia and microcornea syndrome 420, 434
Combined dystrophy of Fuchs' 399, 408, 483
Compound nevus 199, 316
Comprehensive ptosis classification 727

Concave peripheral iris 1019
Congenital
    amaurosis 409
    and infantile cataracts 424
    aniridia 268, 402, 432, 959, 999
    anomalies of
        heart and peripheral vasculature 648
        lacrimal system 1046, 1052
    blepharophimosis 436, 638, 681
    calcifying chondrodystrophy 675, 792
    cataract 446, 776, 960, 1063, 1064
    clouding of cornea 421
    cytomegalic inclusion disease 237, 247, 256
    dyslexia syndrome 79
    encephalo-ophthalmic dysplasia 759, 802, 827
    enophthalmos 636, 748, 757
        with ocular muscle fibrosis and ptosis 667, 1107
    epiblepharon inferior oblique insuffi-ciency syndrome 560
    esotropia 527
    eyelid tetrad 686, 767
    facial diplegia 510, 678, 699, 809
    familial dysautonomia 326, 821, 1051
    fibrosis
        of inferior rectus with ptosis 636, 667, 748, 757, 1107
        syndrome 636, 667, 748, 757, 1107
    generalized lipodystrophy 419, 466
    glaucoma 216, 447, 691, 694, 785, 963, 991, 1016, 1029
        syndrome 960, 1063
    hemolytic jaundice 197, 806
    hereditary retinoschisis 1126
    hyperphosphatemia 195, 200, 227, 387, 1157
    ichthyosis 52, 310, 312, 388, 659, 903, 905
    idiopathic nystagmus 565
    Lues 25, 306, 900
    melanocytosis 199, 316
    muscular hypertrophy cerebral syndrome 80, 752, 1153
    nasolacrimal duct obstruction 1046, 1052
    nystagmus 566
    oculofacial paralysis 510, 678, 699, 809
    paralysis of sixth and seventh nerves 510, 678, 699, 809
    poikiloderma 296
        with juvenile cataract 891
    progressive oculo-acoustico-cerebral dysplasia 72, 172, 188, 271, 790, 1034
    rubella syndrome 22, 252, 281, 430, 448, 459, 469, 802, 873, 1077

spherocytic anemia 197, 806
spinocerebellar ataxia-congenital
cataract-oligophrenia syndrome
83, 775, 989, 1073
syphilis 306, 900
trigeminooculomotor synkinesis 528,
724, 820, 938
trophedema 653, 811
varicella syndrome 722
vertical retraction syndrome 635, 847
word blindness 79
of Hermann 79
Conical cornea 400
Conjunctiva 278
Conjunctival
juncional nevus 199, 316
lacerations 115, 332
malignant melanoma 199, 316
melanoma 199, 316
melanotic lesions 199, 316
nevus 199, 316
xerosis 317
Conjunctivitis 327, 328, 884
giant papillary 295
Conjunctivochalasis 329
Conjunctivourethro-synovial syndrome
251, 282, 313, 359, 874, 907
Connective tissue disorders 57
Conradi
Hünermann syndrome 675, 792
syndrome 675, 792
Contact dermatitis 53, 310, 904
Cooley anemia 51, 194, 693
Coppock cataract 1061
Cornea 378
plana 422
Corneal
abrasions 491, 925
and conjunctival calcifications 328
cerebellar syndrome 421
contact lens 162, 405, 481, 495
dermoids 95
dystrophy 395, 398, 470
of Bowman's layer 396
with spinocerebellar degeneration
421
edema 113, 482, 492, 572, 920, 1118
foreign body 115, 493
graft rejection 493
involvement 455, 476
leukoma syndrome 467
mucous plaques 495
opacity 455, 457, 467, 805
snowflake dystrophy 290, 400
ulcer 373, 457, 787, 916, 966, 993
Cortical degeneration syndrome 79
Corticosteroid-induced glaucoma 951

Corticostriatospinal degeneration 79
Coxiella burnetii 21
Cranial
arteritis syndrome 65, 170, 260, 547, 585,
588, 620, 631, 861, 942, 984, 1032,
1172
neuropathies 1025
Craniocarpo-tarsal dysplasia 676, 682, 749,
756
Craniocervical syndrome 620, 824
Craniofacial dysostosis 206, 406, 429, 751,
778, 1154
Cranio-orbito-ocular dysraphia 795, 1105
Craniopharyngioma 99, 503, 537, 851
Craniostenosis 930
Craniosynostosis
mental retardation-clefting syndrome
424
radial aplasia 678
Cretinism 520, 750, 825, 1067, 1068
Creutzfeldt-Jakob syndrome 79
Cri-du-chat syndrome 96, 679, 750
Critical allergic conjunctivitis syndrome
286, 888
Crohn disease 34, 320
Cross syndrome 85, 793
Crouzon syndrome 206, 406, 429, 751, 778,
1154
Crowded disk syndrome 256, 1093
Crying cat syndrome 96, 679, 750
Cryoinjury 117
Cryptococcosis 237, 581, 622
Cryptogenic polycythemia 51
Cryptophthalmia syndrome 642, 755
Cryptophthalmos syndactyly syndrome 642,
755
Crystalline
aculeiform 1070
coralliform 1059, 1070
Curschmann-Steinert syndrome 452, 607,
797, 810, 1041, 1067
Cushing syndrome 80, 505, 585
Cutis
hyperelastica 195, 227, 406, 438, 665, 680,
753, 1160
laxa 195, 227, 406, 434, 665, 680, 753,
1160
verticis gyrate 467
Cyclic oculomotor paralysis 526, 533, 742,
846
Cyclitis peripheral uveitis 231, 259
Cystic fibrosis syndrome 319
Cysticercosis 153
Cystine storage-aminoaciduria-dwarfism
syndrome 388, 458
Cystinosis syndrome 387, 458
Cytomegalic inclusion disease 237, 247, 256

Cytomegalovirus 237, 247, 256
retinitis 807, 1127, 1164

D

Dacryoadenitis 1046
Dacryocystitis 1046, 1052
Dacryocystocele 1046, 1052
Dacryosialoadenopathy 709
Danbolt-Closs syndrome 663
Dandy-Walker syndrome 506, 751
Darier
Grönblad-Strandberg syndrome 60, 201,
408, 1162
White syndrome 290
Dawson
disease 252, 1089
encephalitis 252, 1089
De Grouchy syndrome 437, 676, 747
De Lange syndrome 80, 752, 1153
De Toni-Fanconi syndrome 39, 794
Deaf mutism-retinal degeneration
syndrome 1083
Deafness 76, 599, 646, 1062
Debarsy syndrome 382
Debré-Lamy-Lyell syndrome 284, 311, 904
Deerfly
fever 6, 482
tularemia 6, 482
Degeneration 378
Dejean syndrome 825
Dejerine-Klumpke syndrome 717, 826, 839
Dementia 76, 1062, 1097
Demodicosis 30
Dengue fever 6, 538, 851
Dental-ocular-cutaneous syndrome 666
Dentoirideal dysplasia 455, 805
Dermal melanocytosis 922, 947
Dermatitis
contusiformis 54
herpetiformis 307, 482, 900
venenata 53, 310, 904
Dermatochalasis 646
Dermatogenous cataract 1056
Dermatophytosis 7
Dermatostomatitis 53, 162, 309, 360, 374,
902
Dermato-stomato-ophthalmic syndrome
58, 148, 151, 159, 184, 235, 246, 624,
975, 1167
Dermoid 99, 100, 982, 1112
choristoma 99, 293, 982
cyst 99, 293, 982
Dermolipoma 99, 293, 982
Descemet membrane folds 493
Desert lung 1064
Developmental dyslexia of critchley 79

Devergie disease 324
Devic syndrome 538, 852
Diabetes
    insipidus-diabetes mellitus-optic
        atrophy-deafness syndrome 41,
        1096
    mellitus 38, 184, 226, 510, 583, 602, 1033,
        1040, 1145
        hypertension-nephrosis syndrome
           41, 123
        nephrosis syndrome 41, 123
Diabetic
    glomerulosclerosis 41, 123
    macular edema 1082
    retinopathy 1145, 1146
Dialinas-Amalric syndrome 1083
Diamond Blackfan syndrome 793
Diaphyseal dysplasia 521, 753
Didmoad syndrome 41, 1096
Diencephalic
    epilepsy syndrome 835
    syndrome 835
Diffuse
    angiokeratosis 46, 617, 762
    lamellar keratitis 474
    pulmonary fibrosis syndrome 60
    unilateral subacute neuroretinitis
        syndrome 247, 1127, 1165
Diktyoma 106
Dimmer syndrome 477
Diphtheria 7, 301, 334, 340, 352, 506, 539,
    581, 603, 852, 894
Diplopia 501, 525, 702
Disassociation of lateral gaze syndrome 515
Dislocation of
    intraocular lens 1064
    lens 269, 433, 1065
Disorders of
    carbohydrate metabolism 38
    lipid metabolism 46
    protein metabolism 36
Disseminated
    encephalopathy 79
    lupus erythematosus 54, 64, 241, 260,
        263, 383, 522, 554, 867, 1171
    sclerosis 81, 239, 274, 512, 541, 589, 597,
        618, 623, 714, 856, 932
Distichiasis 648
Divergence paralysis 845, 892, 933
Diverticulosis of bowel, hernia, retinal
    detachment 1133
Dohna syndrome 196, 207, 439, 801, 967,
    1003, 1154
Dolichostenomelia 61, 411, 425, 443, 778,
    1009, 1155
Dominant
    epidermolysis bullosa dystrophiea
        albopapuloidea 308, 902

optic atrophy 599, 646
    syndrome 599, 646
    Orbruch membrane drusen 256
Dorsolateral medullary syndrome 714, 830,
    836
Down syndrome 68, 412, 422, 424, 651, 679
Doyne honeycomb choroiditis 223, 256
Drepanocytic anemia 50, 136, 175, 201,
    1037, 1090, 1148
Dresbach syndrome 50, 136, 175, 201, 1036,
    1090, 1148
Drummond syndrome 386, 680
Dry eye 924
    syndrome 329, 1047
Dryness of conjunctiva 317
Duane
    retinopathy 228
    syndrome 96, 521, 636, 756, 929, 979
Dubowitz syndrome 679, 752
Duck-bill lips and ptosis 647, 752
Duhring-Brocq disease 307, 482, 900
Dwarf-cardiopathy syndrome 692
Dwarfism
    eczema-peculiar facies 679, 752
    hepatomegaly-obesity-juvenile diabetes
        syndrome 40
    with retinal atrophy and deafness 458,
        755
Dyscephalia oculomandibularis-hypotri-
    chosis 196, 207, 439, 801, 967, 1003,
    1154
Dyscephalic-mandibulo-oculo-facial
    syndrome 196, 207, 439, 801, 967,
    1003, 1154
Dyscephaly-teeth abnormality-dwarfism
    439, 801, 967, 1003
Dyscraniopylophalangy 966
Dysembryogenesis 166
Dysencephalia splanchnocystic syndrome
    214, 435, 444, 776, 970, 1010
Dysgenesis
    iridodentalis 455, 805
    mesodermalis corneae et irides 289, 418,
        430, 446, 472, 805, 798, 963, 991,
        1014
        with digodontia 455
    mesostromalis 289, 418, 430, 446, 472,
        798, 962, 991, 1014
    neuroepithelialis retinae 409
Dyskeratosis 376
    congenita with pigmentation 663
    follicularis syndrome 290
Dyslexia syndrome 79
Dysmorphic sialidosis 36
Dysostosis
    craniofacialis 206, 406, 429, 751, 778,
        1154

enchondralis meta-epiphysaria 43, 461,
    760, 809
    multiplex 40, 460, 684, 765, 1004
Dysphagia 726
Dysplasia
    epiphysealis congenita 675, 792
    linguofacialis 813
Dystaxia 599, 646
Dystrophia 61
    mesodermalis congenita 411, 425, 443,
        778, 1009, 1155
        hyperplastica 67, 425, 442
    myotonica 452, 607, 797, 810, 1041, 1069
Dystrophy 395

E

E syndrome 216, 217, 694, 777, 785, 1016,
    1017
Eales disease 127, 171, 1028, 1034
Eccentro-osteochondrodysplasia 43, 461,
    760, 809
Echinococcosis 31, 154, 1174
Eclampsia 524
Ectodermal syndrome 296, 891
Ectopia lentis 640
    et pupillae 816
    with ectopia of pupil 816
Ectrodactyly, ectodermal dysplasia 1053
Ectropion 299, 647, 654, 658, 663
Edwards syndrome 216, 404, 428, 694, 785,
    1016
Ehlers-Danlos syndrome 195, 227, 406, 438,
    665, 680, 753, 1160
Ekman syndrome 404, 428
Elastorrhexis 60, 201, 4081162
Electrical injury 116, 1088
Elephantiasis
    arabum congenita 653, 811
    congenita hereditaria 653, 811
Ellis-Van Creveld syndrome 773, 1001
Elschnig syndrome 330, 664
Embryonic fixation syndrome 451, 473, 695,
    818, 972
Encephalitis 539, 587, 853, 930
    hemorrhagica superioris 615, 504, 583,
        592, 621, 703
    lethargica 935
Encephalofacial angiomatosis 70, 202, 224,
    431
Encephalo-ophthalmic syndrome 759, 802,
    827
Encephalotrigeminal syndrome 70, 202,
    224, 431
Endophthalmitis phacoanaphylactica 974
Endothelial dystrophy of cornea 399, 408,
    483

Engelmann syndrome 521, 753
Enophthalmus 391, 814
Entamoeba histolytica 150, 536, 849
Enteric fever 27, 576, 831, 1141
Enterobiasis 368
Entropion 665
Eosinophilic granuloma 160, 484
Ephelis 922, 947
Epicanthus 670
Epidemic
    hemorrhagic keratoconjunctivitis 2, 278
    keratoconjunctivitis 8, 307, 330, 338, 358,
        879, 882, 901
Epidermal nevus syndrome 641, 762, 1002
Epidermolysis
    acuta toxica 308, 361, 875, 901
    bullosa 308, 902
Epidermolytic hyperkeratosis 52, 310, 312,
        388, 659, 903, 905
Epidermomycosis 7
Epiloia 202, 210, 376, 391, 780
Epimacular proliferation 1083
Epiphoria 1048, 1053
Epiphyseal dysplasia 562
Episcleritis 1150
Episkopi blindness 381
Epithelial
    downgrowth 129
    dystrophy of Fuchs' 408, 399, 483
    edema 482, 492
    erosion syndrome 477
    ingrowth 129
Epstein-Barr virus 12, 238, 807
Erb
    Goldflam syndrome 523, 531, 554, 571,
        606, 618, 623, 655, 725, 832, 844,
        868
    II syndrome 523, 531, 554, 571, 606, 618,
        623, 655, 698, 725, 832, 868
Erosion syndrome 393
Erysipelas 8
Erythema
    multiforme exudativum 51, 53, 162, 309,
        360, 374, 902
    nodosum 54
Erythrocytosis megalosplenica 51
Escherichia coli 9, 131, 143, 342, 356, 368,
        911, 973
Esotropia 528, 818
    syndrome 526
Essential shrinkage of conjunctiva 288, 303,
        312, 318, 894, 899, 906
Ewing
    sarcoma 101
    syndrome 101

Exfoliation syndrome 1038
Exophthalmic goiter 220, 324, 597, 605, 831,
        936, 938, 944, 983, 1112
Exophthalmos 182, 220, 318, 1107
Exotropia 783
    syndrome 558
Expulsive choroidal hemorrhage 257
Extending aroundentire limbus 479
External
    hordeolum 943
    ophthalmoplegia 599
    orbital fractures 1110
Extraocular muscle 497
    lacerations 116
Extreme hydrocephalus syndrome 500, 508
Eyelid 638
    coloboma 288, 649
    contusions, lacerations and avulsions
        117, 646
    malar-mandible syndrome 645, 649, 779,
        971, 1015

F

Fabry
    Anderson syndrome 46, 617, 762
    disease 46, 617, 762
Facial
    digital-genital syndrome 423
    dysmorphism neuropathy syndrome
        1063
    hemiatrophy 391, 612, 761, 814
    palsy 696
Faciogenital dysplasia 739
Facio-skeleto-genital dysplasia 692, 815
Falciform detachment 270
Familial
    cerebellar vermis agenesis 83, 212, 774,
        1006
    exudative vitreoretinopathy 1173
    hemolytic icterus 439, 683, 795
    hereditary edema 653, 811
    hypolipoproteinemia 194, 601, 672, 743
    mediterranean fever 1168
    myloid polyneuropathy 398, 404
    nephritis 379
    osseous dystrophy 43, 461, 760, 809
    osteoectasia 195, 200, 227, 387, 1157
    progressive cerebral sclerosis 463
    thyrocerebral-retinal syndrome 90
Fanconi
    Lignac syndrome 387, 458
    syndrome 39, 794
Fat embolism syndrome 228
Favre hyaloideoretinal degeneration 392,
        1143
Felty syndrome 59, 390

Fetal alcohol syndrome 468, 682, 808
Fibrinoid syndrome 1038
Fibrocystic disease of pancreas 319
Fibrodysplasia elastica generalisata 195,
        227, 406, 438, 665, 680, 753, 1160
Fibrosarcoma 101
Fiessinger-Leroy syndrome 251, 282, 313,
        359, 874, 907
Filamentary keratitis 474
Filtering blebs 976
Fisher syndrome 573, 587, 611, 616
Fleck retina of Kandori syndrome 1128
Floppy
    eyelid syndrome 407, 709, 889, 917
    iris syndrome 1020
Floriform 1059
    cataract 1071
Focal dermal hypoplasia syndrome 211,
        407, 772, 967, 1002, 1161
Foix syndrome 517, 627, 720, 841, 862, 865,
        1106, 1110
Fold of skin over inner canthus of eye 670
Folling syndrome 808, 1151
Foramen lacerum syndrome 49, 504, 551,
        601, 791, 864, 1104
Fourth nerve palsy 561
Foveal hypoplasia 1065
Foville
    peduncular syndrome 499, 701
    syndrome 499, 701
Fowlpox 16
Franceschetti
    disease 1083
    dystrophy 477
    Klein
        syndrome 645, 649, 779, 971, 1015
        Wildervanck syndrome 981
    syndrome 645, 649, 779, 971, 1015
    Zwahlen
        Klein syndrome 645, 649, 779, 971,
            1015
        syndrome 645, 649, 779, 971, 1015
Francis disease 6, 482
Francois
    dyscephalic syndrome 196, 207, 439, 801,
        967, 1003, 1154
    dystrophy 397, 422
    Evens syndrome 422
    Hallermann-Streiff syndrome 196, 207,
        439, 801, 967, 1003, 1154
    Haustrate syndrome 440, 758, 789, 1004,
        1013
    Neetens syndrome 397
    syndrome 196, 207, 439, 801, 967, 1003,
        1154
Fraser syndrome 642, 755
Freeman-Sheldon syndrome 676, 682, 749,
        756

Fremery-Dohna syndrome 196, 207, 439, 801, 967, 1003, 1154
Frenkel syndrome 130
Friedreich ataxia 81, 595, 604
Friedrich-Erb-Arnold syndrome 813
Frontonasal dysplasia syndrome 214, 642, 788, 966, 1011
Frostbite 117
Fuchs'
    corneal dystrophy 399, 408, 483
    endothelial dystrophy of cornea 399, 408, 483
        Lyell syndrome 284, 311, 904
        Salzmann-Terrien syndrome 394
        sign 927
        syndrome 53, 132, 162, 309, 360, 374, 902, 995, 1021
Fukuyama congenital muscular dystrophy 217, 777, 1017
Functional amblyopia 71
Fundus
    albipunctatus 325
    flavimaculatus 1083
Fungal
    endophthalmitis 168, 973, 1039
    keratitis 475
Fusobacterium 144, 154

G

Galactokinase deficiency 45
Galactosemia 45
Galactosemic syndrome 45
Gansslen syndrome 439, 683, 795
Gapo syndrome 1095
Garcin syndrome 604
Gargoylism 40, 460, 684, 765, 1004
Gaucher syndrome 499
Gayet-Wernicke syndrome 504, 583, 592, 615, 621, 703
Genee-Wiedemann syndrome 643, 652
General fibrosis syndrome 636, 667, 748, 757, 1107
Generalized
    gangliosidosis 459
    myopathy syndrome 436, 638, 681
Geniculate neuralgia 630
Genital
    dwarfism syndrome 217, 673, 694, 745, 1016, 1159
    hypoplasia 206, 640, 703, 787, 1000
German measles 22, 252, 281, 430, 448, 459, 469, 805, 873, 1077
Ghost cell glaucoma 164, 952
Giant
    cell arteritis 65, 170, 260, 547, 585, 588, 620, 631, 861, 942, 984, 1032, 1172

edema 56
    papillary conjunctivitis 285, 377, 491
        syndrome 332, 890
    retinal tears 128, 1128
Gibraltar fever 4, 513
Gilbert syndrome 58, 148, 151, 159, 184, 235, 246, 624, 975, 1167
Gilles De La Tourette syndrome 418
Gillespie syndrome 71, 988
Gillum-Anderson syndrome 763
Glander syndrome 880
Glandular fever 12, 238, 807
Glaucoma 131, 139, 404, 425, 428, 434, 443, 447, 695, 949, 950, 960-962, 990, 1027, 1044, 1074, 1075, 1143, 1158
    associated with intraocular tumors 957
Glaucomatocyclitic crisis 954
Glucocerebroside storage disease 499
Glucosyl ceramide lipidosis 46, 499
Glycosphingolipid lipidosis 617, 762
Glycosphingolipidosis 46, 617, 762
Godtfredsen syndrome 517, 627, 720, 841, 862, 865, 1106, 1110
Goldberg disease 467
Goldenhar
    Gorlin syndrome 98, 211, 643, 788, 966, 9080
    syndrome 98, 211, 643, 788, 966, 980
Goldmann-Favre syndrome 392, 1143
Goldscheider syndrome 308, 902
Goldstein hematemesis 1148
Goltz syndrome 211, 407, 772, 967, 1002, 1161
Gonadal dysgenesis 217, 673, 694, 745, 1016, 1159
Gonorrhea 9, 133, 146, 185, 343, 353, 370, 913
Gorlin
    Chaudhry-Moss syndrome 800
    Goltz syndrome 94, 204, 672, 922, 1012
    syndrome 94, 204, 672, 813, 922, 1012
Gougerot-Sjögren syndrome 285, 314, 327, 877
Gout 383
Gradenigo syndrome 507, 552, 865
Granular corneal dystrophy 396, 397
Granuloma
    faciale 710
    venereum 942
Granulomatous
    ileocolitis 34, 320
    uveitis 1025
Graves disease 220, 324, 597, 605, 831, 936, 938, 944, 983, 1112
Gray iris syndrome 1021
Greenfield disease 463
Gregg syndrome 22, 252, 281, 430, 448, 459, 469, 507, 683, 757, 805, 873, 1077

Grob linguofacial dysplasia 813
Groenouw type II corneal dystrophy 398
Grönblad-Strandberg syndrome 60, 201, 408, 1162
Grouped pigmentation of macula 1084
Growth retardation 1053, 1095
Gruber syndrome 214, 435, 444, 776, 970, 1010
Guillain-Barré syndrome 579, 611, 657, 701, 833
Guinon myospasia impulsiva 418
Gutter dystrophy 394, 486
Gynecomastia 969
    aspermatogenesis syndrome 212, 685, 1007
Gyrate atrophy 1129

H

H disease 82
Haemophilus
    aegyptius 10, 280, 355, 363, 872
    influenzae 10, 342, 355, 369, 483, 911
Half-base syndrome 604
Hallermann-Streiff
    Francois syndrome 207, 439, 196, 801, 967, 1003, 1154
    syndrome 196, 207, 439, 801, 967, 1003, 1154
Hallgren syndrome 1137
Hamman-Rich syndrome 60
Hand-Schuller-Christian syndrome 160, 484
Hanhart syndrome 37, 472, 488, 980
Hansen disease 10, 660, 668, 707
Harada disease 124, 234, 245, 265, 978
Hare syndrome 717, 828, 840
Harlequin syndrome 659
Harp syndrome 1138
Hartnup syndrome 82, 651
Hay
    bacillus 356
    fever 403
        conjunctivitis 285
Headache 984
Hearing impairment 624
Heart disease 206, 640, 703, 7871000
Hebra disease 324
Heerfordt syndrome 385, 708, 1048
Hehlinger syndrome 813
Heidenhain syndrome 79
Hemangioma 101, 167, 173, 197, 292, 503, 763, 918, 982, 1035, 1037, 1113, 1114
    thrombocytopenia 104, 226
Hematologic
    and cardiovascular disorders 48
    metabolic bone disorder 439, 683, 795
Hemeralopia 325

Hemifacial microsomia syndrome 440, 758, 789, 1004, 1013
Hemochromatosis 197
Hemophilia 135, 178
Hemorrhagic polioencephalitis superior syndrome 504, 583, 592, 615, 621, 703
Hennebert syndrome 563
Henoch-Schönlein purpura 135, 180
Heparitinuria 42
Hepatic
  cirrhosis syndrome 322
  ductular hypoplasia 379, 401
  failure 853
Hereditary
  aniridia 268, 402, 432, 959, 999
  ataxia syndrome 595
  craniofacial dysostosis 206, 406, 429, 751, 778, 1154
  ectodermal dysplasia syndrome 656, 666, 992
  edema 653, 811
  familial congenital hemorrhagic nephritis 379
  hemorrhagic telangiectasis 1148
  hyaloideoretinal degeneration 392 and palatoschisis 1143
  macular coloboma syndrome 1091
  multiple diaphyseal sclerosis 521, 753
  nephritis 379
  osteochondrodystrophy 43, 461, 760, 809
  osteo-onycho-dysplasia 411, 442, 769
  polytopic enchondral dysostosis 43, 461, 760, 809
  progressive arthro-ophthalmopathy 210, 779
  retinitis pigmentosa-deafness syndrome 1137, 1142
  spherocytosis 197, 806
Heredopathia
  atactica polyneuritiformis syndrome 612, 1131
  ophthalmo-oto-encephalica 76, 1062
Herpes
  simplex 11, 144, 186, 230, 248, 331, 338, 344, 358, 494, 881
    masquerade syndrome 11
  zoster 133, 144, 185, 231, 331, 358, 511, 544, 576, 706, 721, 842, 858, 883, 885
    auricularis 630
Herrick syndrome 50, 136, 175, 201, 1037, 1090, 1148
Heterochromia iridis 1005, 1021
Heterochromic cyclitis syndrome 132, 995, 1021
Hirschhorn-Cooper syndrome 677, 1017
Histamine cephalalgia 88, 520, 719, 720, 828, 842, 984

Histiocytosis X 484
Histoplasmosis 239, 257, 1084, 1165
  choroiditis 19, 239, 257, 1084, 1165
  maculopathy 19, 239, 257, 1084, 1165
  syndrome 19
Hodgkin disease 102, 553, 718, 840, 867
Holthouse-Batten superficial choroiditis 223, 256
Homocystinuria syndrome 988
Hood syndrome 769
Hoof and mouth disease 363
Hookworm disease 322
Hoppe-Goldflam disease 523, 531, 554, 606, 618, 623, 655, 698, 725, 832, 844, 868
Hordeolum 943
Horizontal conjugate gaze 978
Horner
  oculopupillary syndrome 819, 826, 834, 937, 1119
  syndrome 710, 819, 826, 834, 937, 1119
Horton headache 88, 719, 720, 828, 842, 984
Hunt syndrome 630
Hunter syndrome 39, 764
Huntington hereditary chorea 930
Hurler syndrome 40, 460, 684, 765, 1004
Hutchinson
  Gilford syndrome 441, 802
  Horton-Magath-Brown syndrome 65, 170, 260, 547, 585, 588, 620, 631, 861, 942, 984, 1032, 1172
  syndrome 102
  Tays central guttate choroiditis 223, 256
Hyalinosis cutis et mucosae 364, 924
Hyaloideoretinal degeneration 392, 1143
Hydatid cyst 31, 154, 1174
Hydroa vacciniforme 311, 905
Hydrocephalus 447, 500, 508, 691, 963, 991, 1029
Hydrophobia 21, 508, 545, 573, 859, 931
Hydroxychloroquine toxicity 1125
Hyper-alpha-alaninemia 768
Hyperammonemia 766
  hyperornithinemia-homocitrullinuria syndrome 766
Hypercalcemia supravalvular aortic stenosis 384
Hypercalcemic face 384
Hypercholester 400
Hyperchondroplasia 61, 411, 425, 443, 778, 1009, 1155
Hyperlipoproteinemia 47
Hyperopia 221, 434
Hyperostosis
  corticalis deformans 195, 200, 227, 387, 1157
  frontalis interna syndrome 445
Hyperparathyroidism 385

Hyperpyruvicemia 768
Hypersplenism 390, 507, 972
Hypertelorism 473, 683, 696, 757, 784
  ocularis 507, 683, 757
Hypertension 181, 706, 985, 1146
Hyperthyroidism 220, 324, 597, 605, 831, 936, 938, 944, 983, 1112
Hyperuricemia 383
Hypervitaminosis A 968
Hyphema 131, 132, 139
Hypoacusis 590, 626
Hypocalcemia 1067
Hypochloremic-glycosuric osteonephropathy syndrome 39, 794
Hypogonadism-cataract syndrome 1066
Hypohidrotic ectodermal dysplasia 66, 656, 992
Hypomelanosis of Ito syndrome 722, 796
Hypoparathyroidism 485, 1068
Hypophosphatasia 386, 1152
Hypophyseal-sphenoidal syndrome 517, 627, 720, 841, 862, 865, 1106, 1110
Hypopigmentation 85, 793
Hypoplasia 1050
Hypoprebetalipoproteinemia 1138
Hypopyon 139
Hypothermal injury 117
Hypothyroid goiter 520, 750, 825, 1067, 1068
Hypothyroidism 520, 750, 825, 1067, 1068
Hypotonia 590, 626
Hypovitaminosis A 35
Hysteria 82, 931

I

Ice syndrome 405
Iceland disease 935
Ichthyosiform erythroderma 455, 476
Ichthyosis 52, 310, 312, 388, 659, 903, 905
  follicularis 656, 666, 992
  hystrix 641, 762, 1002
  vulgaris 52, 310, 312, 388, 659, 903, 905
Idiopathic
  amyloidosis 57, 600, 741, 822, 924
  blennorrheal arthritis syndrome 251, 282, 313, 359, 874, 907
  facial paralysis 74, 638, 656, 705
  hereditary lymphedema 653, 811
  hypercalcemia 386, 680
Ikiotia phenylketonuria syndrome 808, 1151
Imperforate nasolacrimal duct 1053
Impetigo 311, 905
Inclusion
  body encephalitis 252
  conjunctivitis 12, 306, 328, 485
Incontinentia pigmenti 95, 208, 270, 772, 1161
  achromians 722, 796

Indian Rubber Man syndrome 195, 227, 406, 438, 665, 680, 733, 1160
Infantile
    esotropia 527
    hereditary chondrodysplasia 43, 461, 760, 809
    metachromatic leukodystrophy 463
    paralysis 511, 543, 716, 838, 858, 929,
    progressive cerebral sclerosis 463
    subacute necrotizing encephalomyelo-
        pathy 768
Infectious
    diseases 1
    mononucleosis 12, 238, 807
Infective conjunctivitis 287
Inferior nucleus ruber syndrome 78, 533, 847
Inflammatory
    bowel disease 35, 276, 321
    polyradiculoneuropathy 579, 611, 657, 701, 833
Influenza 13, 155, 539, 575, 853, 874, 884
Intercapillary glomerulosclerosis 41, 123
Intermediate and posterior uveitis 249, 1043
Internal
    hordeolum 943
    ophthalmoplegia 624
    orbital fractures 570, 593, 1110
Internuclear ophthalmoplegia 74, 585, 616, 622
Interoculo-iridodermato-auditive dysplasia 451, 473, 695, 818, 972
Interstitial keratitis 390, 476
Intestinal lipodystrophy 456, 593
Intracorneal rings 495
Intracranial exostosis 445
Intraepithelial epithelioma 376
Intranuclear ophthalmoplegia 502, 534
Intraocular
    epithelial cysts 165
    foreign body 117, 118, 1174, 1175
    melanoma 171, 219, 258, 273, 277, 293, 920, 947
Inversion of lid margin 665
Inverted
    Marcus Gunn phenomenon 724, 820
    Marfan syndrome 67, 425, 442
Iridal adhesion syndrome 957, 1022
Iridocorneal endothelial syndrome 405, 952, 957, 1022
Iridocystitis 249, 1043
Iridodental dysplasia 455, 805
Iridodialysis 1026
Iris 987
    adhesion syndrome 957, 1022
    bombe 1022
    coloboma 215, 216, 272, 450, 783, 784, 972, 1015

cysts 269, 1022
dysplasia hypertelorism-psychomotor retardation syndrome 1023
laceration 1026
melanoma 167, 713, 1023, 1026
neovascularization 1027
    with pseudoexfoliation syndrome 137, 1039
nevus syndrome 405, 952
pigment layer cleavage 1024, 1028
prolapse 1024
retraction syndrome 1024
Iritis 169, 222, 249, 264, 994, 1042, 1043
Ivic syndrome 624

J

Jabs syndrome 1025
Jacobs syndrome 685
Jadassohn
    Lewandowsky syndrome 464
    type anetoderma 98, 213, 608, 644, 789, 1012
Jaksch Wartenhost syndrome 62, 284, 516, 546, 860, 876, 1163, 1169
Japanese river fever 578
Jaw-Winking syndrome 724, 528, 820, 938
Jensen disease 246, 1005, 1085, 1129, 1147
Joubert syndrome 83, 212, 774, 1006
Jugular foramen syndrome 830
Junius-Kuhnt syndrome 219, 1085
Juvenile
    amaurotic family idiocy 73, 1080
    cataract 296
    diabetes-dwarfism-obesity syndrome 40
    ganglioside lipidosis 73, 1080
    glaucoma 961
    hypothyroidism 520, 750, 825, 1067, 1068
    idiopathic arthritis 65
    macular degeneration 1092
    muscular atrophy 700, 767
    Paget disease 521, 753
    rheumatoid arthritis 61, 134, 160, 186, 250, 389, 995
    xanthogranuloma 103, 137, 182, 188, 919, 1025
    X-linked retinoschisis 1126
Juxtapapillary retinopathy 246, 1085, 1129, 1147

K

Kabuki makeup syndrome 660
Kahler disease 103, 324, 522
Kandori syndrome 1128
Kaposi
    disease 664

hemorrhagic sarcoma 103, 664
Libman-Sack syndrome 54, 64, 241, 260, 263, 383, 522, 554, 867, 1171
sarcoma 103, 664
varicelliform eruption 103, 664
Karsch-Neugebauer syndrome 563
Kartagener
    syndrome 208, 774, 1006
    triad 208, 774, 1006
Kasabach-Merritt syndrome 104, 197, 226
Kaufman syndrome 477
Kearns
    disease 606, 625
    Sayre syndrome 606, 625
    Shy syndrome 606, 625
Keratitis 316, 359, 372, 455, 456, 476, 909, 914
    fugax hereditaria 476
    ichthyosis-deafness syndrome 455, 476
    nummularis 477
    superficialis punctata 396
Keratoacanthoma 104, 376
Keratoconjunctivitis sicca 326, 486, 907, 1051
Keratoconus 400, 416, 804, 891
    posticus circumscriptus 469
Keratodermia palmaris et plantaris 661
Keratosis
    follicularis 290
        spinulosa syndrome 656, 666, 992
    palmoplantaris 661
Keratosulfaturia 43, 461, 760, 809
Kid syndrome 455, 476
Kiloh-Nevin syndrome 588, 766
Kimmelstiel-Wilson syndrome 41, 123
Klebsiella rhinoscleromatis 369, 912
Kleeblattschädel syndrome 500, 508
Klinefelter syndrome 212, 685, 969, 1007
Klippel-Trenaunay-Weber syndrome 758, 1007
Klumpke
    paralysis 717, 826, 839
    syndrome 717, 826, 839
Koby syndrome 934
Koch-Weeks bacillus 10, 280, 355, 363, 872
Koerber-Salus-elschnig syndrome 532, 564, 934
Kohn-Romano syndrome 685, 767
Komoto syndrome 686, 767
Krause syndrome 759, 802, 827
Kugelberg-Welander syndrome 700, 767
Kuhnt-Junius disease 219, 1085
Kuru syndrome 410
Kussmaul
    disease 261, 543, 857, 1168
    Maier disease 261, 543, 857, 1168

L

Lacerations 925
Lacrimal
    duct defect 1048
    gland tumors 1049, 1114
    hypersecretion 1049
    puncta absence 1050
    system 1045
        contusions and lacerations 118, 1049
Lagophthalmos 657, 723
Lamellar ichthyosis 52, 310, 312, 388, 659,
        903, 905
Landry
    Guillain-Barré-Strohl syndrome 579,
        611, 657, 701, 833
    paralysis 579, 611, 657, 701, 833
Langer-Giedion syndrome 1008
Lannois-Gradenigo syndrome 507, 552, 865
Lanzieri syndrome 969, 1008
Lateral bulbar syndrome 714, 830, 836
Lattice
    corneal dystrophy 398, 404
    degeneration 1129
    dystrophy 398, 404
Laughing death 410
Laurence-Moon-Bardet-Biedl syndrome
        209, 410, 441, 686, 768, 775, 834, 1008,
        1136
Lazy eye 71
Lead poisoning 198
Leber
    hereditary optic neuropathy 1095
    miliary aneurysm 97, 171, 1126
    syndrome 1095
    tapetoretinal dystrophy syndrome 409
Leigh syndrome 768
Leiomyoma 105, 664
Leishmaniasis 486
Lejeune syndrome 96, 679, 750
Lenoble-Aubineau syndrome 564
Lens 1055
    induced glaucoma 953, 1071
    iris diaphragm retropulsion syndrome
        1026, 1072
Lenticonus and lentiglobus 415, 1072
Lentigo 922, 947
Lenz microphthalmia syndrome 213, 442,
        773
Leopard syndrome 687
Leprosy 10, 660, 668, 707
Leptospirosis 13, 163
Leri syndrome 796, 970
Leroy syndrome 687
Lesions of caruncle 292
Letterer-Siwe syndrome 160, 484
Leukemia 135, 161, 179, 187, 225, 500, 584,
        718, 841, 1115

Leukodystrophia cerebri progressiva
        metachromatica diffusa 463
Lichen
    planus 303, 313, 896, 906
    ruber 324
        acuminatus 324
    simplex chronicus 413
Lid
    coloboma 641
    myokymia 723
    retraction 925
Lignac-Fanconi syndrome 387, 458
Ligneous conjunctivitis 333, 335, 364
Lindau syndrome 69, 1143
Linear
    IgA disease 304, 897
    nevus sebaceus of Jadassohn 98, 213,
        608, 644, 789, 1012
Linguofacial dysplasia of grob 813
Lipodermoid 99, 982
Lipoid
    granuloma 160, 484
    proteinosis 364, 924
Lipomucopolysaccharidosis 36
Lipoproteinosis 364, 924
Liposarcoma 105
Listerellosis 155, 346, 910
Listeriosis 155, 346, 910
Little syndrome 411, 442, 688, 769
Lobstein syndrome 404, 428
Lobster claw deformity with nasolacrimal
        obstruction 1053
Localized scleroderma 62
Lockjaw 156, 540, 582, 854
Long-arm syndrome 677
Loss of lashes 723
Lost lens syndrome 1072
Low tension glaucoma 949
Lowe syndrome 36, 427, 652, 689, 791, 1152
Lower
    facial neuralgia syndrome 518
    lid ptosis 925
    radicular syndrome 717, 826, 839
Lubarsch-Pick syndrome 57, 600, 741, 822,
        924
Lues venerea 25, 232, 241, 253, 275, 315, 512,
        547, 592, 598, 619, 704, 707, 713, 715,
        836, 837, 861, 908, 935, 977
Luetic-otitic-nystagmus syndrome 563
Lupus erythematosus 54, 64, 241, 260, 263,
        383, 522, 554, 867, 1171
Lyell syndrome 308, 361, 875, 901
Lyme disease 14, 238, 614, 1101
Lymphangioma 105, 919, 946, 982
Lymphedema 668
Lymphocytic hypophysitis associated with
        dacryoadenitis syndrome 1047

Lymphogranuloma
    inguinale 411
    venereum 411
Lymphoid
    follicles cobblestoning of conjunctiva
        295
    hyperplasia 106, 179, 294, 297, 1115
    tumors 106, 179, 294, 297, 1115
Lyssa 508, 859

M

Macroaneurysm 1147
Macrocytic anemia 225, 610
Macula 1079
    lutea juvenile degeneration 219, 1085
Macular
    edema 1086
    hole 1086
    pucker 1083
    senile disciform degeneration 219, 1085
Madarosis 723
Malaria 322, 509, 540, 579, 855
Malattia-Leventinese syndrome 223, 256
Male Turner syndrome 414, 689, 812
Malignant
    cutaneous reticulosis syndrome 662
    glaucoma 958
    hyperpyrexia syndrome 1073
    lymphoma 106, 179, 294, 297, 1115
    melanoma 199, 316, 922, 947
        of posterior uvea 171, 219, 258, 273,
        277, 293, 920, 947
Malta fever 4, 513
Malum venereum 25, 232, 241, 253, 275, 315,
        512, 547, 592, 598, 619, 704, 707, 713,
        715, 836, 837, 861, 908, 935, 977
Mandibulofacial
    dysostosis 645, 649, 779, 971, 1015
    syndrome 645, 649, 779, 971, 1015
Mandibulo-ocular dyscephalia hypotri-
        chosis 196, 207, 439, 801, 967, 1003,
        1154
Mandibulo-oculo-facial dyscephaly syn-
        drome 196, 207, 439, 801, 967, 1003,
        1154
Map-dot fingerprint dystrophy 395
Maple syrup urine disease 759
Marble bone disease 553, 740, 866
Marchesani syndrome 67, 425, 442
Marcus gunn syndrome 528, 724, 820, 938
Marfan syndrome 61, 411, 425, 443, 778,
        1009, 1155
Marie
    hereditary ataxia 595
    Strumpell spondylitis 66, 134, 161, 244,
        764

Marin Amat syndrome 724, 820

Marinesco-Sjögren syndrome 83, 775, 989, 1073

Maroteaux-Lamy syndrome 41, 44, 461, 1096, 1156

Marseilles fever 14, 1090

Marshall-Smith syndrome 1156

Martorell syndrome 169, 1031, 1171

Mast cell leukemia 55

Mastocytosis 55

Mauriac syndrome 40

Mayou-Batten disease 73, 1080

Measles 23, 145, 281, 336, 412, 509, 541, 574, 855, 873

Mechanical and non-mechanical injuries 114

Meckel syndrome 214, 435, 444, 776, 970, 1010

Median cleft face syndrome 214, 642, 788, 966, 1011

Mediterranean fever 4, 513

Medulloepithelioma 106

Meekeren-Ehlers-Danlos syndrome 195, 227, 406, 438, 665, 680, 753, 1160

Meesmann epithelial 395
  dystrophy of cornea 395, 470

Megalocornea 423, 426, 427, 452

Meibomian
  conjunctivitis 330, 664
  gland dysfunction 941

Meige
  disease 653, 811
  Milroy syndrome 653, 811

Melanocytic lesions of eyelids 922, 947

Melanomalytic glaucoma 957

Melanosis oculi 199, 316

Melkersson
  idiopathic fibroedema 708, 725
  Rosenthal syndrome 708, 725

Membrane pemphigus 288, 303, 312, 318, 894, 899, 906

Membranous conjunctivitis 333

Meningioma 107, 108, 1093, 1116

Meningitis 338, 343, 353, 370, 509, 541, 716, 838, 855, 880, 913, 932

Meningococcemia 338, 343, 353, 370, 509, 541, 716, 838, 855, 880, 913, 932

Meningocutaneous syndrome 70, 202, 224, 431

Mental
  deficiency 71, 988
  motor retardation 426, 427, 452
  retardation 58, 286, 1139

Mercury poisoning 382

Meretoja's syndrome 398, 404

Merrf syndrome 769

Mesodermal dysgenesis 166

Mesodermalis congenita 61

Mesomelic dwarfism 653, 691

Metabolic craniopathy 445

Metachromatic leukodystrophy 463

Metaherpetic keratitis 477

Metaphyseal chondrodysplasia 1130

Metastatic
  bacterial endophthalmitis 156, 974
  fungal endophthalmitis 974

Meyenburg-Altherz-Vehlinger syndrome 62, 284, 516, 546, 860, 876, 1163, 1169

Meyer-Schwickerath-Weyers syndrome 444, 690, 803, 1011

Michel syndrome 688

Mickey mouse syndrome 458, 755

Micro syndrome 446, 776

Microcephaly
  microphthalmia, cataracts, and joint contractures 128, 1074
  with chorioretinopathy 1130

Microcornea 960, 1063
  syndrome 419, 437, 468, 770, 1060

Microcystic corneal dystrophy 395

Micrognathia-glossoptosis syndrome 209, 429, 727, 803, 1158

Microphthalmia 562, 770, 1060
  dermal aplasia and sclerocornea 451, 975

Microphthalmos 962
  syndrome 444, 690, 803, 1011

Microspherophakia 1074
  with hernia 1074

Microsporidial infection 14

Midas syndrome 451, 975

Miescher cheilitis granulomatosis 708, 725

Migraine 535, 721, 843, 848, 985

Mikulicz
  Radecki syndrome 709
  Sjögren syndrome 709
  syndrome 709

Milk
  alkali syndrome 387
  drinker syndrome 387

Millard-Gubler syndrome 501, 525, 702

Miller
  Fisher syndrome 573, 587, 611, 616
  syndrome 643, 652, 989, 1027

Milroy disease 653, 811

Mima polymorpha 1, 342

Minamata syndrome 382

Minimal brain dysfunction syndrome 79

Mirhosseini-Holmes-Walton syndrome 1138

Misdirected third nerve syndrome 821

Mite-borne typhus 578

MMMM syndrome 426, 452

Möbius
  Crouzon syndrome 206, 406, 429, 751, 778, 1154
  II syndrome 510, 678, 699, 809

Moderate hyperemia 297

Mohr-Claussen syndrome 688

Molluscum contagiosum 15, 892, 917

Mongolism 68

Mongoloid idiocy 68, 422, 424, 651, 679

Mononucleosis 12, 238, 807

Monosomy
  18 partial syndrome 437, 676, 747, 748, 1001
  4 partial syndrome 677, 1017

Mooren's ulcer 478

Morax-Axenfeld bacillus 287, 298, 877, 891

Moraxella lacunata 15, 145, 156, 182, 346, 370, 886, 912

Morbilli 145, 281, 336, 412, 509, 541, 574, 855

Morgagni syndrome 445

Morphea 62

Morquio
  Brailsford syndrome 43, 461, 760, 809
  syndrome 43, 461, 760, 809
  Ullrich syndrome 43, 461, 760, 809

Mosse syndrome 322, 937

Mucocele 108, 923

Mucocutaneous ocular syndrome 53, 162, 309, 360, 374, 902

Mucopolysaccharidosis 39, 42-44, 50, 426, 461, 465, 760, 765, 809, 1156

Mucopurulent
  conjunctivitis 287
  discharge 297

Mucormycosis 16, 157, 589, 628

Mucosal-respiratory syndrome 53, 162, 309, 360, 374, 902

Mucous membrane pemphigoid 339, 496

Multiple
  basal cell nevi syndrome 94, 204, 672, 922, 1012
  congenital anomalies syndrome 206, 640, 703, 1000
  endocrine adenomatosis partial syndrome 207
  endocrine neoplasia 453
  epiphyseal dysplasia congenita 675, 792
  idiopathic hemorrhagic sarcoma 103, 664
  lentigines syndrome 687
  myeloma 522
  sclerosis 81, 239, 274, 512, 541, 589, 597, 618, 623, 714, 856, 932

Multiplex infantilis 521, 753

Mulvihill-Smith syndrome 413

Mumps 16, 282, 545, 575, 606, 859, 874

Muscle contraction headache 986

Muscular dystrophy of external ocular muscles 588, 766
Myasthenia gravis 523, 531, 554, 571, 606, 618, 623, 655, 698, 725, 832, 844, 868
Mycosis fungoides syndrome 662
Myelomatosis 522
Myelopathic polycythemia 51
Myoclonic variant of cerebral lipidosis 73, 1080
Myopathy 599, 646, 1075
Myopia 495, 640
    ophthalmoplegia syndrome 625
Myotonia atrophica syndrome 452, 607, 797, 810, 1041, 1069
Myotonic dystrophy syndrome 452, 607, 797, 810, 1041, 1069
Mystagmus 1063
Myxedema 520, 750, 825, 1067, 1068

N

Naffziger syndrome 827
Nager
    acrofacial dyostosis 644
    syndrome 644
Nail-patella syndrome 411, 442, 688, 769
Nasal
    nerve syndrome 996
    retinal nerve fiber layer attenuation 1094
Nasociliaris nerve syndrome 996
Nasociliary syndrome 996
Nasopalpebral lipoma-coloboma 645, 726
Nasopharyngeal tumor syndrome 517, 841
Necrotizing angiitis 261, 543, 857, 1168
Negri-Jacod syndrome 605
Neisseria meningitides 338, 343, 353, 370, 509, 541, 716, 835, 855, 880, 913, 932
Nematode ophthalmia syndrome 31, 242, 250
Neonatal conjunctivitis 888
Neoplasms 93
Neoplastic angioendotheliomatosis 106, 179, 294, 297, 1115
Neovacularization 1030
Neovascular
    glaucoma 957
    nevus 922, 947
Neovascularization 405, 481, 495
    of anterior chamber angle 166
Nephropathic cystinosis 388, 458
Nerve deafness 1096
Nettleship falls syndrome 1028, 1122
Neuhauser syndrome 426, 427, 452
Neurilemmoma 108
Neurinoma 108
Neurinomatosis 69, 198, 414, 760, 811, 1117
Neuroblastoma 109, 1117

Neurocutaneous syndrome 97, 892
Neurodermatitis 413
Neurofibromatosis 414, 760, 1117
Neurologic disorders 71
Neuromyelitis optica 538, 852
Neuronal
    ceroid lipofuscinosis 1080
    ceroid lipofuscinosis 73
Neuro-oculocutaneous angiomatosis 70, 202, 224, 431
Neuroparalytic keratitis 84, 478
Neuroretinoangiomatosis syndrome 744, 75
Neurotropic keratitis 84
Nevoid
    basal cell carcinoma syndrome 94, 204, 672, 922, 1012
    basalioma syndrome 94, 204, 672, 922, 1012
Nevoxanthoendothelioma 103, 137, 182, 188, 919, 1025
Nevus
    fuscoceruleus ophthalmomaxillaris syndrome 1162
    of Ota 1162
    sebaceus of Jadassohn 98, 213, 608, 644, 789, 1012
Newcastle disease 16, 884
Niacin deficiency 82, 651
Nicolas-Favre disease 411
Nieden syndrome 1075
Night blindness 325
Niikawa-Kuroki syndrome 660
Nocardiosis 17, 373, 916
Nonbullous ichthyosiform erythroderma 52, 310, 312, 388, 659, 903, 905
Non-Hodgkin lymphoma 112, 165, 251, 854
Noninfectious chorioretinitis 249, 1043
Nonne-Milroy
    Meige disease 653, 811
    syndrome 653, 811
Nonsyphilitic interstitial keratitis 479, 491
Nonvenereal treponematosis 887
Noonan syndrome 414, 689, 812
Normal tension glaucoma 949
Norman-Landing syndrome 459
Norrie disease 72, 172, 188, 271, 790, 1034
Nothnagel syndrome 84, 534, 608, 626, 847
Nutritional disorders 34
Nystagmus 45, 91, 289, 561, 562, 565, 566, 934, 935, 960, 981, 1060, 1143
    blockage syndrome 561
    compensation syndrome 561, 565
    myoclonia syndrome 564
    retractorius syndrome 532, 564, 934
    split hand syndrome 563

O

O'Donnell-Pappas syndrome 1065
Obesity-cerebral-ocular-skeletal anomalies syndrome 84, 794, 1013
Ocular
    and facial abnormalities syndrome 436
    contusion syndrome 130
    hypertelorism syndrome 507, 683, 757
    hypertension 415
    hypotony 221, 964, 1042
    ischemic syndrome 49, 1144
    larva migrans 29
    metastatic tumors 111
    muscle fibrosis and ptosis 636, 748, 757
    myopathy 588, 766
    pemphigoid 288, 303, 312, 318, 894, 899
    rosacea 55, 305, 480, 898
    toxoplasmosis 32, 233, 242, 258, 254, 276, 806, 1141, 1166
Ocularpemphigoid 906
Oculo-auriculo-vertebral dysplasia 98, 211, 643, 788, 966, 980
Oculobuccogenital syndrome 58, 148, 151, 159, 184, 235, 246, 624, 975, 1167
Oculocerebellar tegmental syndrome 85, 619
Oculocerebral syndrome 85, 793
Oculo-cerebro-renal syndrome 36, 427, 652, 689, 791, 1152
Oculodental syndrome 428, 465, 990
Oculodentodigital dysplasia 444, 690, 803, 1011
Oculodermal melanocytosis 1162
Oculo-mandibulo-dyscephaly 196, 207, 439, 801, 967, 1003, 1154
Oculo-mandibulo-facial dyscephaly 196, 207, 439, 801, 967, 1003, 1154
Oculomotor
    apraxia syndrome 59, 527
    nerve 528
    paralysis 843, 849
Oculopalatocerebral dwarfism 86
Oculopharyngeal
    muscular dystrophy 609, 726, 812
    syndrome 609, 726, 812
Oculorenocerebellar syndrome 86
Oculovertebral syndrome 645, 649, 779, 971, 1015
OFD syndrome 813
Ohaha syndrome 590, 626
Okihiro syndrome 981
Olemia and genu valgum 400
Oligophrenia
    ichthyosis spastic diplegia syndrome 654, 770, 777
    microphthalmos syndrome 72, 172, 188, 271, 790, 1034

Oliver-McFarlane syndrome 1142
Olivopontocerebellar atrophy 87, 609
Open angle glaucoma 949
Ophthalmia neonatorum 339, 888
Ophthalmic flake syndrome 82, 931
Ophthalmoencephalomyelopathy 538, 852
Ophthalmomandibulomelic dysplasia 471
Ophthalmoplegia 567, 590, 594, 599, 626,
        627, 632, 633, 646, 749, 847
    ataxia areflexia syndrome 573, 587, 611,
        616
    cerebellar ataxia syndrome 84, 534, 608,
        626
    plus 78, 598, 602
    plus syndrome 606, 625
Ophthalmoplegic migraine syndrome 513,
        542, 571, 628, 856
Optic
    atrophy 66, 134, 161, 207, 244, 519, 550,
        552, 591, 631, 692, 764, 790, 799,
            817, 866, 1014, 1094, 1096,
            1097, 1098
        amaurosis 1095
        syndrome 1095
        with demyelinating disease of CNS 87
    disk 798
    foramen fractures 1111
    gliomas 109
    myelitis 538, 852
    nerve 1093
        decompression for traumatic neuro-
            pathy 1100
        head drusen 199, 1102
        hypoplasia 1102
        sheath 107, 1093, 1116
    neuritis 591, 629, 1098, 1100
    neuropathy 256, 1093, 1099, 1100
    pit syndrome 1102
Opticochleodentate degeneration 463
Oral-facial-digital syndrome 688
Orbit 1104
Orbital
    apex-sphenoidal syndrome 591, 629
    cellulitis and abscess 119, 570, 943, 1106
    compartment syndrome 119
    floor syndrome 825
    fracture 120, 517, 661, 1111
    hemorrhages 120, 1112
    implant extrusion 120
    infarction syndrome 121, 1108
    lymphoma 110, 1118
    metastasis 102
    rhabdomyosarcoma 110
Organoid nevus syndrome 98, 213, 608, 644,
        789, 1012

Ornithine
    ketoacid aminotransferase deficiency
        1129
    transcarbamylase deficiency 766
Oro-digital-facial
    dysostosis 813
    syndrome 813
Orofaciodigital syndrome 688
Oromandibular dystonia 653, 811
Orthostatic hypotension syndrome 613
Osler syndrome 1148
Osteitis deformans 195, 200, 227, 387, 1157
Osteochalasis desmalis familiaris 195, 200,
        227, 387, 1157
Osteochondrodystrophia deformans 43,
        461, 760, 809
Osteogenesis imperfecta 404, 428
    congenita, microcephaly and cataracts
        1076, 1157
Osteopathia hyperostotica 521, 753
Osteopetrosis 553, 740, 866
Osteopoikilosis 553, 740, 866
Osteopsathyrosis 404, 428
Osteosclerosis
    congenita diffusa 553, 740, 866
    fragilis generalisata 553, 740, 866
Ota syndrome 1162
Otitic hydrocephalus syndrome 90, 515,
        1103
Otocephaly 971
Otomandibular dysostosis 440, 758, 789,
        1004, 1013
Oxycephaly 368, 778, 1154

P

Pachydermoperiostosis 813
Pachyonychia congenita 464
Paget disease 195, 200, 227, 387, 1157
Painful ophthalmoplegia 91, 519, 550, 627,
        632, 635, 864
Palatoschisis 392
Pallidal degeneration 1138
Palmoplantar keratodermia 661
Palpebral coloboma-lipoma syndrome 645,
        726
Palsy of ocular muscles with pain 627
Pancoast syndrome 717, 828, 840
Pancreatitis 321
Pannus 479
Papilledema 221, 456, 593, 992, 1087, 1103
Papilloma 110, 294, 921
Papillon-Leage-Psaume syndrome 813
Papillorenal syndrome 123
Pappataci fever 17
Paralysis
    agitans 87, 928, 933

of ocular muscles 599
of sixth nerve 497
of third nerve 528
of vertical movements 845, 892, 933
Parasitic diseases 29
Paratrachoma 12, 328, 485
Paratrigeminal paralysis 88, 520, 719, 720,
        828, 842, 984
Parinaud
    conjunctiva-adenitis syndrome 5, 236,
        347, 532, 590, 885, 1050
    oculoglandular syndrome 5, 236, 347,
        532, 590, 885, 1050
    syndrome 845, 892, 933
Parkes-Weber syndrome 758, 1007
Parkinson syndrome 87, 928, 933
Parotid aplasia 1050
Parrot-head syndrome 206, 406, 429, 751,
        778, 1154
Parry
    disease 220, 324, 597, 605, 831, 936, 938,
        944, 983, 1112
    Romberg syndrome 391, 612, 761, 814
Pars planitis 231, 259, 761
Partial trisomy G syndrome 205, 674, 786,
        1000
Passow syndrome 514, 555, 596, 702, 715,
        761, 816, 837, 869, 921
Patau syndrome 216, 272, 450, 784, 972, 1015
Pediatric congenital glaucoma 650
Pediculosis 32, 298, 878
Pellagra 481
    cerebellar ataxia-renal aminoaciduria
        syndrome 82, 651
Pellucid marginal degeneration 415
Pemphigus vulgaris 361
Penfield syndrome 835
Penta X syndrome 696
Pepper syndrome 102
Perforations 925
Periocular
    merkel cell carcinoma 111
    metastatic tumors 111
Periodic migrainous neuralgia 88, 520, 719,
        720, 828, 842, 984
Peripheral
    furrow keratitis 394, 486
    pulmonary stenosis 401
    retinal breaks and degeneration 1130
    ulcerative keratitis 487, 490
    uveitis 273
    uveoretinitis vitritis 231, 259
Periphlebitis 127, 171, 1034, 1128
Pernicious anemia syndrome 225, 610
Persistence of primary vitreous 1177

Persistent
  fetal vasculature 189, 272, 1035, 1176
  hyperplastic primary vitreous 189, 272,
    1035, 1176
Pertussis 577
Peters
  anomaly 176, 470
  plus syndrome 125, 471
  syndrome 428, 465, 990
Petrosphenoidal space syndrome 605
Petzetakis-Takos syndrome 347
Pfaundler-Hurler syndrome 40, 460, 684,
    765, 1004
Phacoanaphylactic
  endophthalmitis 974
  uveitis 974
Phacoantigenic uveitis 974
Phacomorphic glaucoma 958
Phakomatoses 69
Pharyngoconjunctival fever 18, 278, 882
Phenylketonuria 808, 1151
Phenylpyruvic oligophrenia 808, 1151
Phlebotomus fever 17
Phlyctenular keratoconjunctivitis 347
Phosphoethanolaminuria 386, 1152
Phthiriasis 32, 298, 878
Phthisis bulbi 128, 389
Phycomycosis 16, 157, 589, 628
Phytanic acid
  oxidase deficiency 612, 1131
  storage disease 612, 1131
Piebaldism 972
Pierre-Marie syndrome 66, 134, 161, 244,
    764
Pierre-Robin syndrome 209, 429, 727, 803,
    1158
Pig breeder disease 4, 513
Pigmentary
  dispersion syndrome 954, 1019
  glaucoma 954, 1019
  retinal lipoid neuronal heredodege-
    neration 73, 1080
  retinitis 409
  retinopathy 962
Pigmented ciliary body lesions 277
Pillay syndrome 471
Pinworm 368
Pituitary syndrome 1095
Pityriasis
  pilaris 324
  rubra pilaris 324
Plateau iris syndrome 270, 958, 1029
Platybasia syndrome 72, 502, 617, 712, 835
Pleonosteosis syndrome 796, 970
Pneumococcal infections 18, 279, 335, 341,
    353, 367, 501, 578, 871, 910
Poliomyelitis 511, 543, 716, 838, 858, 929

Polyarteritis
  nodosa 261, 857, 1168
  enterica 251, 282, 313, 359, 874, 907
Polycythemia 322
  hepatic cirrhosis syndrome 937
  rubra 51
  vera 51
Polyglandular adenomatosis syndrome 207
Polymorphic macular degeneration of
    Braley 1122
Pontine syndrome 515
Pontocerebellar angle tumor syndrome 80,
    505, 586
Porphyria cutanea tarda 555, 584, 869, 1169
Posner-Schlossman syndrome 954
Postaxial acrofacial dysostosis 643, 652
Postcataract hyperpyrexia syndrome 1073
Postconcussion syndrome 91
Posterior
  embryotoxon 433, 962
  iris chafing syndrome 1029
  polymorphous dystrophy 399, 416
  retroparotid space syndrome 829
  synechiae 1024
  uveitis 230, 243
Postinduction hyperpyrexia syndrome 1073
Postinfectious polyneuritis 579, 611, 657,
    701, 833
Post-traumatic
  general cerebral syndrome 91
  keratitis 477
Postural change syndrome 533, 846
Pozzi syndrome 195, 200, 227, 387, 690, 1157
Preeclampsia 524
Presenile
  cataract syndrome 1065
  dementia 79
Pressure induced intralamellar stromal
    keratitis 487
Presumed ocular histoplasmosis 19
  syndrome 239, 257, 1084, 1165
Pretectal syndrome 845, 892, 933
Primary
  acquired melanosis 199, 316
  amyloidosis 57, 600, 741, 822, 924
  angle-closure glaucoma 164, 435, 956
  closed angle glaucoma 164, 435, 956
  dyslexia 79
  embryonic hypertelorism 507, 683, 757
  infantile glaucoma 650
  splenic neutropenia 390
    with arthritis 59
  systemic amyloidosis 58, 286
Progeria 441
  of adults 1051, 1159
Progressive
  external ophthalmoplegia 75, 593, 1062
    and scoliosis 610, 634

facial hemiatrophy 391, 612, 761, 814
foveal dystrophy 1091
hemifacial atrophy 391, 612, 761, 814
muscular dystrophy 609, 726
  with ptosis and dysphagia 812
supranuclear palsy 596, 928
systemic sclerosis 64, 302, 315, 613, 716,
    839, 896, 909
Proliferative vitreoretinopathy 1131, 1176
Propionibacterium acnes 19, 346, 1166
Proptosis 182, 220, 318, 1107
Proteinosis lipoidosis 924
Proteus
  infections 19, 146, 344, 371
  syndrome 20, 913
Proximal and distal click syndrome of
    superior oblique tendon 560
Pseudoanodontia 1095
Pseudodendritic keratitis 37, 472, 488, 980
Pseudoedematous hypodermal hypertrophy
    653, 811
Pseudoelephantiasis neuroarthritica 653,
    811
Pseudoexfoliation syndrome 955, 1020,
    1027, 1076
Pseudo-Graefe syndrome 927
Pseudoherpetic keratitis 37, 472, 488, 980
Pseudo-Hurler
  lipoidosis 459
  polydystrophy 462
Pseudohypoparathyroidism syndrome 1069
Pseudolymphoma 106, 179, 294, 297, 1115
Pseudomembranous conjunctivitis 348
Pseudomonas aeruginosa 147, 337, 344, 356,
    371, 914
  infections 20, 157, 881
Pseudo-ophthalmoplegia syndrome 634
Pseudopapilledema 199, 1102
Pseudoparalytic syndrome 523, 531, 554,
    571, 606, 618, 623, 655, 698, 725, 832,
    844, 868
Pseudotumor 106, 179, 294, 297, 986, 1115
  cerebri 90, 515, 1103
Pseudoxanthoma elasticum 60, 201, 408,
    1162
Psoriasis 56, 661
  vulgaris 56, 661
Psoriatic arthritis 249
Psorospermosis 290
Psychosis 76, 1062
Pterygium of conjunctiva and cornea 366,
    394
Pterygolymphangiectasia syndrome 217,
    673, 694, 745, 1016, 1159
Ptosis 92, 504, 535, 557, 583, 586, 592, 599,
    615, 621, 646, 677, 700, 703, 714, 726,
    822, 830, 836, 848, 1017

Pulseless disease 169, 1031, 1171
Punch-drunk syndrome 91
Punctal stenosis 1046, 1052
Pupil 1119
Pupillary
    block glaucoma 955
    membrane 138, 1120
Purtscher syndrome 228
Purulent conjunctivitis 366
Pyocele 108, 923

Q

Q fever 21
Quincke disease 56

R

Rabbit fever 6, 482
Rabies 21, 508, 859
Racemose hemangioma 263, 549, 819, 863
Racial melanosis 199, 316
Radial ray defects 624
Raeder syndrome 88, 520, 719, 720, 828,
    842, 984
Ramsay-Hunt syndrome 630
Raymond
    Cestan syndrome 515
    syndrome 515
Reactive lymphoid hyperplasia 106, 179,
    294, 297, 1115
Recessive keratosis palmoplantaris 37, 472,
    488, 980
Recurrent
    fever 158, 488
    hyphema 177
Red hair syndrome 419, 1153
Red-eyed shunt syndrome 48, 170, 548, 549,
    863, 1032, 1105, 1109
Reese
    Ellsworth syndrome 125, 471
    syndrome 216, 272, 450, 784, 972, 1015
Refsum
    syndrome 612, 1131
    Thiebaut syndrome 612, 1131
Regional enteritis 35, 276, 321
Reifenstein-Albright syndrome 212, 685,
    969, 1007
Reis-Bucklers corneal dystrophy 396
Reiter syndrome 251, 282, 313, 359, 874, 902
Relapsing
    fever 158, 488
    polychondritis 62, 284, 512, 546, 860, 876,
        1163, 1169
Renal
    agenesis syndrome 690

coloboma syndrome 123
glomerulohyalinosis-diabetic syndrome
    41, 123
rickets 388, 458
Rendu-Osler
    syndrome 1148
    Weber syndrome 1148
Renofacial syndrome 690
Retarded growth 206, 640, 703, 787, 1000
Reticuloendotheliosis syndrome 160, 484
Reticulum cell sarcoma 112, 165, 251, 854
Retina 1121
Retinal
    abiotrophy 409
    aplasia 409
    artery occlusion 173, 572
    capillaritis 1132
    capillary hamartoma 69, 1143
    detachment 128, 168, 172, 222, 449, 1035,
        1087, 1129, 1134, 1135
    disinsertion syndrome 416, 804
    telangiectasia 97, 171, 1126
    vascular hypoplasia 1177
    venous obstruction 168, 1149
Retinitis pigmentosa 416, 742, 771, 1056,
    1130, 1136-1139, 1142
    deafness-ataxia syndrome 1137
    polydactyly-adiposogenital syndrome
        209, 410, 441, 686, 768, 775, 834,
            1008, 1136
Retinoblastoma 112, 138, 174, 189, 214,
    1036, 1132
Retinocerebral angiomatosis 69, 1143
Retinopathy of prematurity 174, 181, 190,
    272, 417, 1036, 1133
Retinoschisis 180, 190, 392, 1087, 1139, 1140
    of fovea 1140
    with early hemeralopia 1143
Retraction
    of globe 978
    syndrome 521, 636, 756, 929, 979
Retrolental fibroplasia 174, 181, 190, 272,
    417, 1036, 1133
Retroparotid space syndrome 829
Reversed coarctation syndrome 169, 1031,
    1171
Rhabdomyosarcoma 113, 572, 920, 1118
Rhegmatogenous 168, 172
Rheumatoid
    arthritis 59, 63, 262, 274, 389, 390, 1170
    lung syndrome 60
    spondylitis 66, 134, 161, 244, 764
Rhinoscleroma 369, 912
Rhinosporidiosis 22
Richner
    Hanhart syndrome 37, 472, 488, 980
    syndrome 37, 472, 488, 980

Rieger syndrome 289, 418, 430, 446, 472,
    798, 963, 991, 1014
Riley-Day syndrome 326, 821, 1051
Ring
    chromosome 447, 691, 963, 991, 1029
    constriction 641, 786
    dermoid syndrome 99, 100, 454
Ritter disease 308, 361, 875, 901
Roberts pseudothalidomide syndrome 447,
    1158
Robin syndrome 209, 429, 727, 803, 1158
Robinow
    dwarfism 653, 691
    Silverman-Smith syndrome 653, 691
Rochon-Duvigneaud syndrome 519, 550,
    552, 591, 631, 866
Rocky mountain spotted fever 22, 489, 615,
    1101
Rollet syndrome 591, 629
Romberg syndrome 391, 612, 761, 814
Rossle-Urbach-Wiethe syndrome 364, 924
Roth-Bielschowsky syndrome 634
Rothmund
    syndrome 296, 891
    Thomson syndrome 296, 891
Rubella syndrome 22, 252, 281, 430, 448, 459,
    469, 805, 873, 1077
Rubeola 23, 145, 281, 336, 412, 509, 541, 574,
    855
Rubeosis iridis 183, 1030
    neovascular glaucoma 959
Rubinstein-Taybi syndrome 215, 692, 790,
    1014
Rubrophytia 7
Rubrospinal-cerebellar-peduncle syndrome
    78, 533, 847
Rural typhus 578
Russell syndrome 934
Rutherford syndrome 428, 465, 990

S

Sabin-Feldman syndrome 448, 804
Salivary gland absence 1050
San Joaquin fever 6, 152, 238, 265, 506
Sandfly fever 17
Sands of Sahara syndrome 474
Sandwich infectious keratitis syndrome 489
Sanfilippo-good syndrome 42
Sanger brown syndrome 595
Sarcoidosis 63, 232, 240, 244, 275, 302, 384,
    524, 556, 582, 870, 895, 976, 1170
Scalded skin syndrome 308, 361, 875, 901
Scalenus anticus syndrome 827
Scaphocephaly syndrome 992
Scarlet fever 24, 148, 159, 283, 301, 336, 341,
    354, 368, 577, 895, 943

Scarring of conjunctiva 299

Schachenmann syndrome 205, 674, 786, 1000

Schaumann syndrome 63, 232, 240, 244, 275, 302, 384, 524, 556, 582, 870, 895, 976, 1170

Scheie syndrome 43, 50, 426, 465

Schmid-Fraccaro syndrome 205, 674, 786, 1000

Schmincke tumor-unilateral cranial paralysis 604

Schnyder's crystalline corneal dystrophy 380, 400

Scholz
   Bielschowsky-Henneberg syndrome 463
   syndrome 463

Schonenberg syndrome 692

Schuller-Christian-Hand syndrome 160, 484

Schwannoma 108

Schwartz
   Jampel syndrome 436, 638, 681
   syndrome 449, 1135

Sclera 1150

Scleral
   ruptures and lacerations 121
   staphylomas and dehiscences 1160

Sclerocornea 436, 451, 454, 466, 975

Scleroderma 64, 302, 315, 521, 613, 716, 839, 896, 909

Scleroticans 753

Scrub typhus 578

Scurvy 136, 180

Seabright-Bantam syndrome 1069

Seatworm 368

Sebaceous
   gland carcinoma 113, 923, 948
   nevus syndrome 98, 213, 608, 644, 789, 1012

Seborrheic
   blepharitis 941
   keratosis 93

Secretoinhibitor syndrome 285, 314, 327, 877

Segment of cornea 479

Senile marginal atrophy 394, 486

Senter syndrome 455, 476

Serous meningitis syndrome 90, 515, 1103

Serpiginous choroidopathy 240, 259

Sézary syndrome 662

Shaken baby syndrome 122, 177

Shaking palsy 87, 928, 933

Shigellosis 357

Short-arm syndrome 748

Shy-Drager syndrome 613

Shy-Gonatas syndrome 614, 814

Shy-Megee-Drager syndrome 613

Sicca syndrome 285, 314, 327, 877

Sickle cell disease 50, 136, 175, 201, 1037, 1090, 1148

Siemens
   Bloch-Sulzberger syndrome 95, 208, 270, 772, 1161
   syndrome 656, 666, 992

Silent sinus syndrome 829

Silverman syndrome 122, 177

Simosa syndrome 639, 655, 673, 744

Simulated superior oblique tendon syndrome 560

Sinusitis-bronchiectasis-situs inversus syndrome 208, 774, 1006

Sjögren
   Larsson syndrome 654, 770, 777
   syndrome 285, 314, 326, 327, 486, 877, 907, 1051

Skeletal disorders 68

Sleeping sickness 935

Slow onset of extraocular muscle palsy 594

Sluder syndrome 518

Smallpox 147, 337, 546, 574, 670, 860, 881

Smith
   Lemli-Opitz syndrome 675, 815
   Magenis syndrome 449
   syndrome 692, 815

Snail tracks of cornea 455

Solar retinopathy 1091

Sorsby I syndrome 1091

Sotos syndrome 88

Spastic
   paralysis 79
   paraplegia 1097
   pseudosclerosis 79
   quadriplegia 1139

Speckled corneal dystrophy 422

Sphenoacrocranio-syndactyly 402, 741

Sphenocavernous syndrome 518, 551, 1108

Sphenoid wing 108, 1116

Sphenopalatine ganglion neuralgia syndrome 518

Spielmeyer
   Sjögren syndrome 73, 1080
   Vogt syndrome 73, 1080

Spinocerebellar
   ataxia 81, 595, 604
   atrophy with pupillary paralysis 89
   degeneration and corneal dystrophy 421

Splenomegalic polycythemia 51

Spondyloepiphyseal dysplasia 43, 461, 760, 809

Spontaneous hyphema 178, 186

Sporotrichosis 23

Spranger syndrome 36, 404, 428

Squamous cell carcinoma 94, 295
   of eyelid 95, 918

St Vitus dance 930

Stannus cerebellar syndrome 89

Staphylococcal scalded skin syndrome 308, 361, 875, 901

Staphylococcus 872, 878, 908, 911

Stargardt disease 1092

Stasis 1052

Status dysraphicus syndrome 514, 555, 596, 702, 715, 761, 816, 837, 869, 921

Steele-Richardson-Olszewski syndrome 596, 928

Stevens-Johnson syndrome 53, 162, 309, 360, 374, 902

Stickler syndrome 210, 779

Still
   Chauffard syndrome 59, 390
   disease 61, 134, 160, 186, 250, 389, 995

Stilling syndrome 521, 636, 756, 929, 979

Stippled epiphyses syndrome 675, 792

Stock-Spielmeyer-Vogt syndrome 73, 1080

Strabismus fixus 636, 667, 748, 757, 1107

Streeter dysplasia 641, 786

Streptococcus pneumoniae infections 18, 279, 335, 341, 353, 367, 501, 578, 871, 910

Stromal edema 482, 492

Sturge-Weber syndrome 70, 202, 224, 431

Subacute
   necrotizing encephalomyelopathy 768
   sclerosing panencephalitis 252, 1089

Subarachnoid hemorrhage syndrome 1140

Sub-epithelial
   melanocytosis 199, 316
   nevus 199, 316

Subluxation, dislocation of lens 127

Subthalamic syndrome 845, 892, 933

Sulfatide lipoidosis syndrome 463

Super female syndrome 685

Superficial
   variant of granular dystrophy 396
   vascular invasion 479

Superior
   hemorrhagic polioencephalopathic syndrome 504, 583, 592, 615, 621, 703
   limbic keratoconjunctivitis 365, 374, 489
   oblique
     myokymia 561
     tendon sheath syndrome 559, 745, 823, 927
   orbital fissure syndrome 519, 550, 552, 591, 631, 866
   pulmonary sulcus syndrome 717, 828, 840

Supravalvular aortic stenosis 384

Sydenham chorea 930

Sylvian aqueduct syndrome 532, 564, 934

Symblepharon 361, 875, 901, 940

Symonds syndrome 90, 515, 1103

Sympathetic
  heterochromia 822
  ophthalmia 245, 259, 264, 977
Syndroma mucocutaneo-oculare 53, 162,
  309, 360, 374, 902
Synechiae 175
Synovitis 1025
Syphilis 25, 232, 241, 253, 275, 315, 512, 547,
  592, 598, 619, 707, 713, 715, 836, 836,
  837, 861, 908, 935, 977
Syringobulbia 514, 555, 596, 702, 715, 761,
  816, 837, 869, 921
Syringomyelia 514, 555, 596, 702, 715, 761,
  816, 837, 869, 921
Systematized achromic nevus 722, 796
Systemic
  elastodystrophy 60, 201, 408, 1162
  lupus erythematosus 54, 64, 241, 260,
    263, 384, 522, 554, 867, 1171
  mucopolysaccharidosis 39, 40, 44, 460,
    461, 765, 1004, 1156
  scleroderma 64, 302, 315, 613, 716, 839,
    896, 909

T

Takayasu syndrome 169, 1031, 1171
Tapetochoroidal dystrophy 229
Tapeworm 30, 153
Tar syndrome 693
Tarral-Besnier disease 324
Tegmental syndrome 531, 844
Telangiectasia
  cataract syndrome 1075
  pigmentation-cataract syndrome 296,
    891
Temporal
  arteritis syndrome 65, 170, 260, 547, 585,
    588, 620, 631, 861, 942, 984, 1032,
    1172
  syndrome 507, 552, 865
Terrien
  disease 394, 486
  marginal degeneration 394, 486
Terson syndrome 1140
Tetanus 26, 156, 540, 854
Tetra X syndrome 696
Thalassemia 51, 194, 693
  major 51, 194, 693
  minor 51, 693
Theodores superior limbic keratoconjuncti-
  vitis 365, 374, 489
Thermal burns 122
Thiamine deficiency 504, 583, 592, 615, 621,
  703
Thoracic-pelvic-phalangeal dystrophy 1005
Thrombocytopenia 197, 624
  absent radius syndrome 693

purpura 197
  hemangioma 104, 226
Thrombocytopenic purpura 135, 178
Thygeson syndrome 396
Thyrocerebroretinal syndrome 90
Thyrotoxicosis 220, 324, 597, 605, 831, 936,
  938, 944, 983, 1112
Tic douloureux 632
Tinea 7
Tolosa-Hunt syndrome 91, 519, 550, 632,
  635, 864
Toni-Fanconi syndrome 39, 794
Torulosis 237, 581, 622
Touraine-Solente-Gole syndrome 813
Tourette syndrome 418
Tower skull syndrome 1064
Toxemia of pregnancy 524
Toxic
  anterior segment syndrome 149, 191,
    1077
  epidermal necrolysis 284, 308, 311, 361,
    875, 901, 904
    of Lyell 308, 361, 875, 901
  lens syndrome 149, 177, 191, 1077
Toxocariasis 31, 242, 250
Toxoplasmic retinochoroiditis 32, 233, 242,
  254, 256, 276, 806, 1141, 1166
Toxoplasmosis 32, 233, 242, 254, 258, 276,
  806, 1141, 1166
Trachoma 26, 304, 669, 886, 893, 897, 944
Trauma 491
Traumatic
  cataract 129, 1078
  encephalopathy syndrome 91
  hyphema 139
  liporrhagia 228
  retinal angiopathy 228
Treacher Collins
  Franceschetti syndrome 645, 649, 779,
    971, 1015
  syndrome 645, 649, 779, 971, 1015
Treft syndrome 817
Trichiasis 939
Trichinellosis 33, 516
Trichinosis 33, 516
Trichomegaly syndrome 1142
Trichophytosis 7
Trichorhinophalangeal syndrome 1008
Trigeminal
  neuralgia 632
  neuropathic keratopathy 84, 478
Triple X syndrome 685
Triploidy syndrome 215, 450, 783
Trisomy
  10Q syndrome 798
  13 syndrome 216, 272, 450, 784, 972, 1015
  18 syndrome 216, 694, 785, 1016
  21 syndrome 68, 422, 651, 679
  21Q- syndrome 799
  8 mosaicism syndrome 783

9Q syndrome 784
D1 syndrome 216, 272, 450, 784, 972,
  1015
G 68, 422, 424, 651, 679
Trochlear nerve palsy 561
Tropholymphedema 653, 811
Trophoneurosis 653, 811
Tropical
  bubo LGV 411
  pancreatic diabetes 45
  typhus 578
Tsutsugamushi disease 578
Tuberculosis 27, 163, 233, 254, 323, 357, 548,
  580, 704, 862, 919
Tuberous sclerosis 202, 210, 376, 391, 780
Tularemia 6, 482
Tumor
  of conjunctiva 375
  related glaucoma 957
Tunbridge-Paley disease 817
Turk-Stilling syndrome 521, 636, 756, 929,
  979
Turner
  Albright syndrome 217, 673, 694, 745,
    1016
  syndrome 217, 673, 694, 745, 1016, 1159
Typhoid fever 27, 576, 1141, 831
Typhus 578
Tyrosinosis 37, 472

U

Ugh syndrome 139, 950, 1044
Ulcerative colitis 35, 276, 321
Ullrich
  Bonnevie syndrome 217, 673, 694, 745,
    1016, 1159
  Feichtiger syndrome 787, 966, 993
  Fremery-Dohna syndrome 196, 207, 439,
    801, 967, 1003, 1154
  syndrome 787, 766, 993
  Turner syndrome 217, 673, 694, 745,
    1016, 1159
Ultraviolet keratitis 490, 496
Undulant fever 4, 513
Unilateral
  facial agenesis 440, 758, 789, 1004, 1013
  subacute neuroretinitis 29
  wipeout syndrome 247, 1127, 1165
Urbach-Wiethe syndrome 364, 924
Urticaria 55
Usher syndrome 1137, 1142
Uveal
  effusion 263
  melanoma 171, 219, 258, 273, 277, 293,
    920, 947